Microbiology

Medical Microbiology

FOURTH EDITION

Patrick R. Murray, PhD

Director, Clinical Microbiology Laboratory
Professor, Department of Pathology
University of Maryland School of Medicine
Baltimore, Maryland

Ken S. Rosenthal, PhD

Professor
Department of Microbiology and Immunology
Northeastern Ohio Universities College of Medicine
Rootstown, Ohio

George S. Kobayashi, PhD

Professor, Departments of Medicine and Molecular Microbiology
Washington University School of Medicine
Associate Director, Clinical Microbiology Laboratory
Barnes-Jewish Hospital
St. Louis, Missouri

Michael A. Pfaller, MD

Professor
Department of Pathology
University of Iowa College of Medicine
Iowa City, Iowa

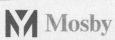

Mosby

A Harcourt Health Sciences Company

St. Louis   London   Philadelphia   Sydney   Toronto

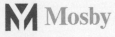

An Affiliate of Elsevier Science

Acquisitions Editor: William Schmitt
Manuscript Editor: Linda Lewis Grigg
Production Manager: Peter Faber
Designer: Gene Harris
Illustration Specialist: Lisa Lambert

FOURTH EDITION
Copyright © 2002 by Mosby, Inc.

Previous editions copyrighted 1998, 1994, 1990

NOTICE

Microbiology is an ever-changing field. Standard safety precautions must be followed, but as new research and clinical experience broaden our knowledge, changes in treatment and drug therapy may become necessary or appropriate. Readers are advised to check the product information currently provided by the manufacturer of each drug to be administered to verify the recommended dose, the method and duration of administration, and the contraindications. It is the responsibility of the treating physician, relying on experience and knowledge of the patient, to determine dosages and the best treatment for each individual patient. Neither the publisher nor the editor assumes any liability for an injury and/or damage to persons or property arising from this publication.

THE PUBLISHER

Permissions may be sought directly from Elsevier's Health Sciences Rights Department in Philadelphia, USA: phone: (+1)215-238-7869, fax: (+1)215-238-2239, email: healthpermissions@elsevier.com. You may also complete your request on-line via the Elsevier Science homepage (http://www.elsevier.com), by selecting 'Customer Support' and then 'Obtaining Permissions'.

Mosby, Inc.
An Affiliate of Elsevier Science
11830 Westline Industrial Drive
St. Louis, Missouri 63146

Printed in Chile

Library of Congress Cataloging-in-Publication Data

Medical microbiology / Patrick R. Murray ... [et al.].—4th ed.
    p. ; cm.
  Includes bibliographical references and index.
  ISBN 0-323-01213-2
  1. Medical microbiology. I. Murray, Patrick R.
  [DNLM: 1. Microbiology. 2. Microbiological Techniques. 3. Parasitology. QW 4
M4862 2002]
   QR46 .M4683 2002
   616'.01—dc211
                                                      2001042766

03 04 / 9 8 7 6 5 4

To all who use
this textbook,
that they may benefit
from its use
as much as we did
in the preparation.

Preface

Medical microbiology can be a bewildering field to the novice. The student is faced with many questions when learning microbiology. How do I learn all the names? Which infectious agents cause which diseases? Why? When? Who is at risk? Is there a treatment? However, all these concerns can be reduced to one essential question: What information do I need to know which will help me understand how to diagnose and treat an infected patient?

Certainly, there are a number of theories about what a student needs to know and how to teach it, which supposedly validates the plethora of microbiology textbooks that have flooded the bookstores in recent years. Although we do not claim to have the one right approach to teaching medical microbiology (there is truly no one perfect approach to medical education), we have founded the revisions of this textbook on our experience gained through years of teaching medical students, residents, and infectious disease fellows as well as on the work devoted to the three previous editions. We have tried to present the basic concepts of medical microbiology clearly and succinctly in a manner that addresses different types of learners. The text is written in a straightforward manner with, it is hoped, uncomplicated explanations of difficult concepts. Details are summarized in tabular format rather than in lengthy text, and there are colorful illustrations for the visual learner. Important points are emphasized in boxes to aid the student, especially in their review; and the study questions address relevant aspects of each chapter, including clinical cases.

The material included in this text—and maybe more important, the material excluded—can be a subject for debate, but we have used our perception of the practical needs of the student as our guide. We are faced with the dilemma that new and exciting discoveries add not only to our foundation of knowledge but can also add to the length of the book. We used our experience as authors and teachers to choose the most important information and explanations for inclusion in this textbook. Each chapter has been carefully updated and expanded to include new, medically relevant discoveries. In each of these chapters, we have attempted to present the material that we feel will help the student gain a clear understanding of the significance of the individual microbes and their diseases.

To the Student

How can the student digest what appear to be innumerable facts? On first impression, success in medical microbiology would seem to depend on memorization. Although memorization is an important part of any medical discipline, understanding the basic principles and developing a system for storing this information plays an important role in mastering this science. We suggest that the student concentrate on learning what is important by **thinking like a physician.** Continue to ask seven basic questions as you approach this material: Who? Where? When? Why? Which? What? and How? For example: Who is at risk for disease? Where does this organism cause infections (both body site and geographic area)? When is isolation of this organism important? Why is this organism able to cause disease? Which species and genera are medically important? What diagnostic tests should be performed? How is this infection managed? Each organism that is encountered can be systematically examined. Know the specifics about how the organism grows, the virulence properties of the organism, and the diseases it causes; understand the epidemiology of infections; know what specimens should be collected and the basic identification tests that should be performed; and be familiar with preventive and therapeutic strategies. Learn three to five words or phrases that are associated with the microbe—words that will stimulate your memory **(trigger words)** and organize the diverse facts into a logical picture. Develop **alternative associations.** For example, this textbook presents organisms in the systematic taxonomic structure (frequently called a "bug parade," but which the authors think is the easiest way to introduce the organisms). Take a given virulence property (e.g., toxin production) or type of disease (e.g., meningitis) and list the organisms that share this property. Pretend that an imaginary patient is infected with a specific agent and create the case history. In other words, do not simply attempt to memorize page after page of facts; rather, use techniques that stimulate your mind and challenge your understanding of the facts presented throughout the text.

No textbook of this magnitude would be successful without the contributions of numerous individuals. We are grateful for the valuable professional help and support provided by the staff at Harcourt Health Sciences, particularly William Schmitt, Antony Galbraith, Linda Grigg, and Peter Faber. We also want to thank the many students and professional colleagues who have offered their advice and constructive criticism throughout the development of this fourth edition of *Medical Microbiology*.

Patrick R. Murray
Ken S. Rosenthal
George S. Kobayashi
Michael A. Pfaller

Contents

CHAPTER 1

Introduction to Medical Microbiology

Since the last edition of this textbook, wondrous discoveries in outer space have been made—new planets, galaxies, black holes, and unimaginable details of our sun and the neighboring planets. On our planet Earth, we have seen the escalation of wars, the discovery of peace, and the human struggles to understand our neighbors' needs. We have also discovered new pathogens and their diseases, old pathogens causing new diseases, and the increased threat of biologic terrorism. Diseases such as smallpox, anthrax, and brucellosis have taken on renewed interest. Finally, the antibiotics that were so effective in the past are now impotent against some very common and important pathogens because these drugs have been freely prescribed to humans and farm animals alike. Thus, we find that the science of microbiology is in dynamic flux—an intellectually satisfying but socially alarming development.

The Microbial World

Imagine the excitement felt by the Dutch biologist Anton van Leeuwenhoek in 1674 as he peered through his carefully ground microscopic lenses at a drop of water and discovered a world of millions of tiny "animalcules." Almost 100 years later the Danish biologist Otto Müller extended van Leeuwenhoek's studies and organized bacteria into genera and species according to the classification methods of Linnaeus. This was the beginning of the taxonomic classification of microbes. In 1840, the German pathologist Friedrich Henle proposed criteria for proving that microorganisms were responsible for causing human disease (the "germ theory" of disease). Koch and Pasteur confirmed this theory in the 1870s and 1880s with a series of elegant experiments proving that microorganisms were responsible for causing anthrax, rabies, plague, cholera, and tuberculosis. Other brilliant scientists went on to prove that a diverse collection of microbes was responsible for causing human disease. The era of chemotherapy was begun in 1910 when the German chemist Paul Ehrlich discovered the first antibacterial agent, a compound effective against the spirochete that causes syphilis. This was followed by Alexander Fleming's discovery of penicillin in 1928, Gerhard Domagk's discovery of sulfanilamide in 1935, and Selman Waksman's discovery of streptomycin in 1943. In 1946, the American microbiologist John Enders was the first to cultivate viruses in cell cultures, leading the way to the large-scale production of virus cultures for vaccine development. Thousands of scientists have followed these pioneers, each building on the foundation established by his or her predecessors, and each adding an observation that expanded our understanding of microbes and their role in disease.

The world that van Leeuwenhoek discovered was complex, consisting of protozoa and bacteria of all shapes and sizes. However, the complexity of medical microbiology we know today rivals the limits of the imagination. We now know that there are thousands of different types of microbes that live in, on, and around us—and hundreds that cause serious human diseases. To understand this information and organize it in a useful manner, it is important to understand some of the basic aspects of medical microbiology. To start, the microbes can be subdivided into four groups: viruses, bacteria, fungi, and parasites, each having its own level of complexity.

Viruses

Viruses are the smallest infectious particles, ranging in diameter from 18 to almost 300 nm (particles less than 200 nm cannot be seen with a light microscope). More than 40 genera of viruses have been implicated in human disease, and, certainly, more will be discovered each year. Viruses consist of either DNA or RNA (but not both) and proteins required for replication and pathogenesis. These components are then enclosed in a protein coat with or without a lipid membrane coat. These organisms are true parasites, requiring host cells for replication. The cells they infect and the outcome of the infection dictate the nature of the clinical manifestation. Infection can lead either to rapid replication of the organisms and destruction of the cell or to a long-term latent relationship with possible integration of the viral genetic information into the host genome. The factors that determine which of these takes place are only partially understood. For example, infection with the human immunodeficiency virus, the etiologic agent of the acquired immunodeficiency syndrome (AIDS), can result in the latent infection of CD4 lymphocytes or the active replication and destruction of these immunologically important cells. Likewise, infection can spread to other susceptible cells, such as the microglial cells of the brain, resulting in the neurologic manifestations of AIDS. Thus, the diseases caused by viruses can range from the common cold to gastroenteritis to fatal catastrophes such as rabies, smallpox, and AIDS.

Bacteria

Bacteria are relatively simple in structure. They are **prokaryotic** organisms—a simple unicellular organism with no nuclear membrane, mitochondria, Golgi bodies, or endoplasmic reticulum that reproduces by asexual division. Although the cell wall encircling bacteria is itself complex, there are two basic forms: a gram-positive cell wall with a thick peptidoglycan layer and a gram-negative cell wall with a thin peptidoglycan layer and an overlying outer membrane (additional information about this structure is presented in Chapter 3). Some bacteria lack this cell wall structure and compensate by surviving only inside host cells or in a hypertonic environment. The size (1 to 20 μm or longer), shape (spheres, rods, spirals), and spatial arrangement (single cells, chains, clusters) of the cells are used for the preliminary classification of bacteria, and the phenotypic and genotypic properties of the bacteria form the basis for the definitive classification. The human body is inhabited by thousands of different bacterial species—some living transiently, others in a permanent parasitic relationship. Likewise, the environment that surrounds us, including the air we breathe, water we drink, and food we eat, is inhabited by bacteria, many of which are relatively avirulent and some of which are capable of producing life-threatening disease.

Fungi

In contrast to bacteria, the cellular structure of fungi is more complex. These are **eukaryotic** organisms that contain a well-defined nucleus, mitochondria, Golgi bodies, and endoplasmic reticulum. Fungi can exist either in a unicellular form (**yeast**) that can replicate asexually or in a filamentous form (**mold**) that can replicate asexually and sexually. Most fungi exist as either yeasts or molds; some can assume either morphology, however. These are known as **dimorphic** fungi and consist of such organisms as *Histoplasma*, *Blastomyces*, and *Coccidioides*.

Parasites

Parasites are the most complex microbes. Although all parasites are classified as eukaryotic, some are unicellular and others are multicellular. They range in size from tiny protozoa as small as 1 to 2 μm in diameter (the size of many bacteria) to arthropods and tapeworms that can measure up to 10 m in length. Indeed, considering the size of some of these parasites, it is hard to imagine how these organisms came to be classified as microbes. Their life cycles are equally complex, with some parasites establishing a permanent relationship with humans and others going through a series of developmental stages in a progression of animal hosts. One of the difficulties confronting students is not only an understanding of the spectrum of diseases caused by parasites, but also an appreciation of the epidemiology of these infections, which is vital for an understanding of the control and prevention of these infections.

Microbial Disease

One of the most important reasons for studying microbes is to understand the diseases they cause and the ways to control them. Unfortunately, the relationship between many organisms and their diseases is not simple. Specifically, organisms rarely cause a single well-defined disease, although there are certainly ones that do (e.g., *Treponema pallidum*, syphilis; poliovirus, polio; *Plasmodium* species, malaria). Instead, it is more common for a particular organism to produce many manifestations of disease (e.g., *Staphylococcus aureus*—endocarditis, pneumonia, wound infections, food poisoning) or for many organisms to produce the same disease (e.g., meningitis caused by viruses, bacteria, fungi, and parasites). In addition, relatively few organisms can be classified as always pathogenic, though some do belong in this category (e.g., rabies virus, *Brucella* species, *Sporothrix schenckii*, *Plasmodium* species). Instead, most are able to establish disease only under well-defined circumstances (e.g., the introduction of an organism with a potential for causing disease into a normally sterile site, such as the brain, lungs, and peritoneal cavity). Some diseases arise when a person is exposed to organisms from external sources. These are known as **exogenous infections**, and examples include diseases caused by influenza virus, *Neisseria gonorrhoeae*, *Coccidioides immitis*, and *Entamoeba histolytica*. Most human diseases, however, are produced by organisms in the person's own microbial flora that spread to body sites where disease can ensue (**endogenous infections**).

The interaction between an organism and the human host is complex. The interaction can result in transient colonization, a long-term symbiotic relationship, or disease. The outcome of this interaction is determined by the virulence of the organism, the site of exposure, and the host's ability to respond to the organism. Thus, the manifestations of disease can range from mild symptoms to organ failure and death. The role of microbial virulence and the host's immunologic response is discussed in depth in subsequent chapters.

Although the human body is remarkably adapted to controlling exposure to pathogenic microbes, the physical barriers that prevent invasion by the organism and the immunologic response to infection are frequently inadequate. To improve the human body's ability to prevent infection, the immune system can be augmented either through the passive transfer of antibodies present in immune globulin preparations or through active immunization with microbial antigens. Infections can also be controlled with a variety of chemotherapeutic agents. Unfortunately, microbes can alter their antigenic complexion (**antigenic variation**) or develop resistance to even the most potent antibiotics. Thus, the battle for control between microbe and host continues, with neither side yet able to claim victory (although the microbes have demonstrated remarkable ingenuity).

Diagnostic Microbiology

The clinical microbiology laboratory plays an important role in the diagnosis and control of infectious diseases. However, the ability of the laboratory to perform these functions is limited by the quality of the specimen collected from the patient, the means by which it is transported from the patient to the laboratory, and the techniques used to demonstrate the microbe in the sample. Because most diagnostic tests are based on the ability of the organism to grow, transport conditions must ensure the viability of the pathogen.

In addition, the most sophisticated testing protocols are of little value if the collected specimen is not representative of the site of infection. This seems obvious, but many specimens sent to laboratories for analysis are contaminated during collection with the organisms that colonize the mucosal surfaces. Because most infections are caused by endogenous organisms, it is virtually impossible to interpret the testing results with contaminated specimens.

The laboratory is also able to determine the antimicrobial activity of selected chemotherapeutic agents, although the value of these tests is limited. The laboratory must test only organisms capable of producing disease and only medically relevant antimicrobials. To test all isolated organisms or an indiscriminate selection of drugs can yield misleading results, with potentially dangerous consequences. Not only can a patient be treated inappropriately with unnecessary antibiotics, but the true pathogenic organism may not be recognized among the plethora of organisms isolated and tested. Finally, the in vitro determination of an organism's susceptibility to a variety of antibiotics is only one aspect of a complex picture. The virulence of the organism, site of infection, and patient's ability to respond to the infection influence the host-parasite interaction and must also be considered when planning treatment.

Summary

It is important to realize that, as was stated in the introduction of this chapter, our knowledge of the microbial world is evolving continually. Just as the early microbiologists built their discoveries on the foundations established by their predecessors, so, too, will we and future generations continue to discover new microbes, new diseases, and new therapies. The following chapters are intended as a foundation of knowledge that can be used to enrich your understanding of microbes and their diseases.

Basic Principles of Medical Microbiology

CHAPTER 2

Bacterial Classification

Understanding the relevance and complex nomenclature of literally hundreds of "important" bacteria can be challenging. The mastery of this exercise depends on the systematic organization of the bewildering array of different organisms into logical relationships (i.e., the taxonomic classification of the organisms).

Phenotypic Classification

The **microscopic** and **macroscopic morphologies** of bacteria were the first characteristics used to identify bacteria and form the cornerstones for most identification algorithms used today (Box 2–1). For example, bacteria can be classified by their ability to retain the Gram stain (gram-positive or gram-negative) and by the shape of the individual organisms (cocci, bacilli, curved, or spiral). The macroscopic appearance of colonies of bacteria can also be used to identify bacteria (e.g., hemolytic properties on agar containing blood, pigmentation of the colonies, size and shape of the colonies). Thus, *Streptococcus pyogenes* is a gram-positive bacterium that forms long chains of cocci and appears as small, white, hemolytic colonies on blood agar plates. Because many organisms can appear very similar on microscopic and macroscopic examination, morphologic characteristics are used to provide a tentative identification of the organism and to select more discriminating classification methods.

The most common methods that are still used to identify bacteria consist of measuring the presence or absence of specific biochemical markers (e.g., ability to ferment specific carbohydrates or use different compounds as a source of carbon for growth; presence of specific proteases, lipases, or nucleases; presence of various aminopeptidases). With the use of carefully selected biochemical tests, most clinically significant isolates can be identified with a high degree of precision. These methods have also been used for subdividing groups of organisms beyond the species level, primarily for epidemiologic purposes (e.g., to determine whether a group of organisms from the same genus and species is from a common source or from distinct sources). These techniques are referred to as **biotyping**.

Many bacteria possess antigens that are unique, and antibodies used to detect these antigens are powerful tools for their identification (**serotyping**). These serologic tests can be used to identify organisms that are inert in biochemical testing (e.g., *Francisella*, the organism that causes tularemia), difficult or impossible to grow (e.g., *Treponema pallidum*, the organism responsible for syphilis), associated with specific disease syndromes (e.g., *Escherichia coli* serotype O157, responsible for hemorrhagic colitis), or need to be identified rapidly (e.g., *S. pyogenes*, responsible for streptococcal pharyngitis). Serotyping is also used to subdivide bacteria below the species level for epidemiologic purposes.

Other examples of phenotypic methods used to classify bacteria include analysis of **antibiogram patterns** (patterns of susceptibility to different antibiotics) and **phage typing** (susceptibility to viruses that infect bacteria—bacteriophages). Assessment of antibiotic susceptibility patterns is commonly performed but has limited discriminatory power. Phage typing is technically cumbersome and has now been replaced by more sensitive genetic techniques.

Analytic Classification

Analysis of the analytic characteristics of bacteria has also been used to classify bacteria at the genus, species, or subspecies level (Box 2–2). The chromatographic

---

BOX 2–1. Phenotypic Classification of Bacteria

Microscopic morphology
Macroscopic morphology
Biotyping
Serotyping
Antibiogram patterns
Phage typing

BOX 2-2. Analytic Classification of Bacteria

Cell wall fatty acid analysis
Whole cell lipid analysis
Whole cell protein analysis
Multifocus locus enzyme electrophoresis

BOX 2-3. Genotypic Classification of Bacteria

Guanine plus cytosine ratio
DNA hybridization
Nucleic acid sequence analysis
Plasmid analysis
Ribotyping
Chromosomal DNA fragment

pattern of cell wall mycolic acids is unique for many of the individual species of mycobacteria and has been used for more than 25 years to identify the most commonly isolated species. Analysis of the lipids in the entire cell has also proved to be a useful method for characterizing many bacterial species, as well as yeasts. Analyses of the whole cell proteins and cellular enzymes **(multilocus enzyme electrophoresis)** are also techniques that have been used to characterize bacteria, most typically at the subspecies level for epidemiologic investigations. Although these analytic methods are accurate and reproducible, they are labor intensive, and the instrumentation is expensive. For these reasons the analyses are used primarily in reference laboratories.

Genotypic Classification

The most precise method for classifying bacteria is by analysis of their genetic material (Box 2-3). Organisms were initially classified by the **ratio of guanine to cytosine;** this procedure has largely been forsaken for more discriminating methods, however. **DNA hybridization** was used initially to determine the relationship among bacterial isolates (e.g., to determine whether two isolates were in the same genus or species). More recently, this technique has been exploited for the rapid identification of organisms by use of molecular probes. That is, DNA from an organism to be identified is extracted and exposed to species-specific molecular probes. If the probe binds to the DNA, then the organism's identity is confirmed. This technique has also been used to detect organisms directly in clinical specimens, thus avoiding the need to grow the organisms. DNA hybridization has proved to be a valuable tool for the rapid detection and identification of slow-growing organisms such as mycobacteria and fungi.

An extension of the hybridization method is **nucleic acid sequence analysis.** Probes are used to localize specific nucleic acid sequences that are unique to a genus, species, or subspecies. These sequences are amplified so that millions of copies are produced, and then the amplified genetic material is sequenced to define the precise identity of the isolate. This method primarily analyzes sequences of ribosomal DNA (because highly conserved [family- or genus-specific] sequences and highly variable [species- or subspecies-spe-

cific] sequences are present). It has also been used to define the evolutionary relationship among organisms and to identify organisms that are difficult or impossible to grow. Most of the recent changes in taxonomic nomenclature were determined by nucleic acid sequence analysis. An extension of this work is the complete sequencing of a bacterium's entire genome, a technique that has now become technically feasible.

Various other methods have been used, primarily to classify organisms at the subspecies level for epidemiologic investigations: **plasmid analysis, ribotyping,** and **analysis of chromosomal DNA fragments.** In recent years, the technical aspects of these methods have been simplified to the point that most clinical laboratories use variations of these methods in their day-to-day practice.

Boxes 2-4 through 2-8 provide a useful classification scheme for organizing the many bacteria that are discussed in subsequent chapters. It should be noted that the list of organisms is not exhaustive. Many genera that are recovered in clinical specimens are omitted for the sake of simplifying this presentation. The organisms that are included in these summary boxes are only those that are discussed in subsequent chapters. In addition, the precise arrangement of bacteria in families, genera, and species continues to change. In Section IV,

BOX 2-4. Aerobic, Gram-Positive Cocci

Catalase-Positive Cocci

Micrococcus
Staphylococcus
Stomatococcus

Catalase-Negative Cocci

Aerococcus
Alloiococcus
Enterococcus
Lactococcus
Leuconostoc
Pediococcus
Streptococcus

BOX 2–5. Aerobic, Gram-Positive Bacilli

Actinomycetes with Cell Wall Mycolic Acids

Corynebacteriaceae
  Corynebacterium
Nocardiaceae
  Gordona
  Nocardia
  Rhodococcus
  Tsukamurella
Mycobacteriaceae
  Mycobacterium

Actinomycetes with No Cell Wall Mycolic Acids

Actinomadura
Dermatophilus
Nocardiopsis
Oerskovia

Rothia
Streptomyces
Thermophilic actinomycetes
  Saccharomonospora
  Saccharopolyspora
  Thermoactinomyces
Tropheryma

Miscellaneous Gram-Positive Bacilli

Arcanobacterium
Bacillus
Brevibacterium
Erysipelothrix
Gardnerella
Listeria
Turicella

BOX 2–6. Aerobic, Gram-Negative Cocci, Coccobacilli, and Bacilli

Cocci and Coccobacilli

Branhamella
Moraxella
Neisseria

Bacilli

Enterobacteriaceae
  Citrobacter
  Enterobacter
  Escherichia
  Klebsiella
  Morganella
  Proteus
  Salmonella
  Serratia
  Shigella
  Yersinia

Vibrionaceae
  Vibrio
Aeromonadaceae
  Aeromonas
Plesiomonadaceae
  Plesiomonas
Campylobacteriaceae
  Arcobacter
  Campylobacter
Helicobacteriaceae
  Helicobacter
Pseudomonadaceae
  Pseudomonas
Pasteurellaceae
  Actinobacillus
  Haemophilus
  Pasteurella

Miscellaneous genera
  Acinetobacter
  Bartonella
  Bordetella
  Brucella
  Burkholderia
  Capnocytophaga
  Cardiobacterium
  Eikenella
  Francisella
  Kingella
  Legionella
  Spirillum
  Stenotrophomonas
  Streptobacillus

BOX 2–7. Anaerobic Gram-Positive and Gram-Negative Bacteria

Gram-Positive Cocci

Peptostreptococcus

Gram-Negative Cocci

Veillonella

Gram-Positive Bacilli

Actinomyces
Bifidobacterium
Clostridium

Eubacterium
Lactobacillus
Mobiluncus
Propionibacterium

Gram-Negative Bacilli

Bacteroides
Fusobacterium
Porphyromonas
Prevotella

BOX 2–8. Miscellaneous, Medically Important Bacteria

Mycoplasmataceae
  Mycoplasma
  Ureaplasma
Spirochaetaceae
  Borrelia
  Treponema
Leptospiraceae
  Leptospira

Chlamydiaceae
  Chlamydia
  Chlamydophila
Other bacteria
  Coxiella
  Ehrlichia
  Orientia
  Rickettsia

Bacteriology, we identify newly defined relationships among bacteria and predict where reorganization of the bacteria will occur.

QUESTIONS

1. Name three examples each of phenotypic, analytic, and genotypic characteristics used to classify bacteria.

2. Describe the microscopic morphology (e.g., Gram-stain characteristic, shape of organism) of the following bacteria: *Staphylococcus, Escherichia, Neisseria, Clostridium, Enterococcus,* and *Pseudomonas.*

3. Which of the following organisms have mycolic acids in their cell walls: *Staphylococcus, Nocardia, Mycobacterium,* and *Klebsiella?*

BIBLIOGRAPHY

Balows A et al, editors: *The prokaryotes,* ed 2, New York, 1992, Springer-Verlag.

Borriello P, Murray P, editors: *Systematic bacteriology,* vol 2 in Topley and Wilson's *Microbiology and microbial infections,* ed 9, London, 1999, Arnold.

Borriello P, Murray P, editors: *Bacterial infections,* vol 3 in Topley and Wilson's *Microbiology and microbial infections,* ed 9, London, 1999, Arnold.

Murray PR: *Pocket guide to clinical microbiology,* ed 2, Washington, DC, 1998, American Society for Microbiology.

Murray PR et al, editors: *Manual of clinical microbiology,* ed 7, Washington, DC, 1999, American Society for Microbiology.

CHAPTER 3

Bacterial Morphology and Cell Wall Structure and Synthesis

Cells are the fundamental units of living things, from the smallest bacterium to the largest of the plants and animals. Bacteria, the smallest cells, are visible only with the aid of a microscope. The smallest bacteria (*Chlamydia* and *Rickettsia*) are only 0.1 to 0.2 μm in diameter, whereas larger bacteria may be many microns in length. A newly described species is hundreds of times larger than the average bacterial cell and is visible to the naked eye. Most species, however, are approximately 1 μm in diameter and are therefore visible using the light microscope, which has a resolution of 0.2 μm. In comparison, animal and plant cells are much larger, ranging from 7 μm (the diameter of a red blood cell) to several feet (the length of certain nerve cells).

Each cell contains the genetic basis for reproduction in its DNA genome, the biochemical machinery for transcribing genetic information into messenger RNA (mRNA) and translating the mRNA into proteins, and the machinery for energy production and biosynthesis, which is all packaged by a membrane. In addition, each cell replicates by cell division. The mechanisms and machinery for accomplishing these functions are basically similar, but the specifics may be different for bacteria and for the higher-order organisms. These differences are influenced by the structure of the cell, the environment in which the cell lives, the source and means of the cell's energy production, and the nature of and requirement for cell interaction (or lack thereof).

Differences Between Eukaryotes and Prokaryotes

Cells from animals, plants, and fungi are **eukaryotes** (Greek for "true nucleus"), whereas bacteria and the blue-green algae belong to the **prokaryotes** (Greek for "primitive nucleus"). In addition to lacking a nucleus and other organelles, prokaryotes use a smaller ribosome, the 70S ribosome, and in most bacteria, a mesh-like peptidoglycan cell wall surrounds the membranes to protect it against the environment. Bacteria can survive and, in some cases, grow in hostile environments in which the osmotic pressure outside the cell is so low that most eukaryotic cells would lyse, at temperature extremes (both hot and cold), with dryness, and with very dilute and diverse energy sources. Bacteria have evolved the structures and functions to adapt to these conditions. These and other distinguishing features are depicted in Figure 3–1 and outlined in Table 3–1. Several of these distinctions provide the basis for antimicrobial action.

Differences Among Prokaryotes

Bacteria can be distinguished from one another by their morphology (size, shape, and staining characteristics) and metabolic, antigenic, and genetic characteristics. Although bacteria are difficult to differentiate by size, they do have different shapes. A spherical bacterium, such as *Staphylococcus*, is a **coccus**; a rod-shaped bacterium, such as *Escherichia coli*, is a **bacillus**; and the snakelike treponeme is a **spirillum**. In addition, *Nocardia* and *Actinomyces* species have **branched filamentous** appearances similar to those of fungi. Some bacteria form aggregates such as the grapelike clusters of *Staphylococcus aureus* or the **diplococcus** (two cells together) observed in *Streptococcus* or *Neisseria* species.

Gram stain is a powerful, easy test that allows clinicians to distinguish between the two major classes of bacteria and to initiate therapy (Fig. 3–2). Bacteria that are heat-fixed or otherwise dried onto a slide are stained with **crystal violet** (Fig. 3–3); this stain is precipitated with **Gram iodine**, and then the unbound and excess stain is removed by washing with the acetone-based decolorizer. A counterstain, **safranin**, is added to stain any decolorized cells red. This process takes less than 10 minutes.

For **gram-positive bacteria**, which turn **purple**, the stain gets trapped in a thick, cross-linked, meshlike

Prokaryote

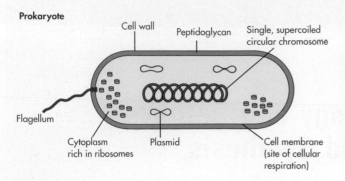

Eukaryote

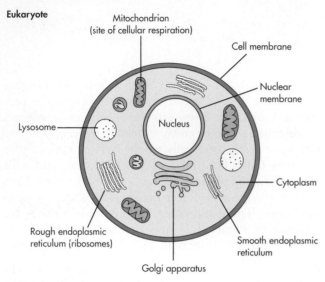

FIGURE 3–1. Major features of prokaryotes and eukaryotes.

structure, the peptidoglycan layer, which surrounds the cell. **Gram-negative bacteria** have a thin peptidoglycan layer that does not retain crystal violet stain, so the cells must be counterstained with safranin and turned red (Fig. 3–4). A mnemonic device that may help is **"P-Purple-Positive."** Gram stain is not a dependable test for bacteria that are starved (e.g., old or stationary phase cultures).

Bacteria that cannot be classified by Gram stain include mycobacteria, which have a waxy outer shell and are distinguished with the acid-fast stain, and mycoplasmas, which have no peptidoglycan.

Bacterial Ultrastructure

Cytoplasmic Structures

Gram-positive and gram-negative bacteria have similar internal but very different external structures. The cytoplasm of the bacterial cell contains the DNA chromosome, the mRNA, ribosomes, proteins, and metabolites (see Fig. 3–4). Unlike eukaryotes, the **bacterial chromosome** is a single, double-stranded circle that is contained not in a nucleus but in a discrete area known as the **nucleoid.** Histones are not required to maintain the conformation of the DNA, and the DNA does not form nucleosomes. **Plasmids**, which are smaller, circular, extrachromosomal DNAs, may also be present. Plasmids are most commonly found in gram-negative bacteria, and although not usually essential for cellular survival, they often provide a selective advantage: many confer resistance to one or more antibiotics.

TABLE 3–1. Major Characteristics of Eukaryotes and Prokaryotes

Characteristic	Eukaryote	Prokaryote
Major groups	Algae, fungi, protozoa, plants, animals	Bacteria
Size (approximate)	>5 μm	0.5 to 3 μm
Nuclear structures		
Nucleus	Classic membrane	No nuclear membrane
Chromosomes	Strands of DNA	Single, circular DNA
	Diploid genome	Haploid genome
Cytoplasmic structures		
Mitochondria	Present	Absent
Golgi bodies	Present	Absent
Endoplasmic reticulum	Present	Absent
Ribosomes (sedimentation coefficient)	80S (60S + 40S)	70S (50S + 30S)
Cytoplasmic membrane	Contains sterols	Does not contain sterols
Cell wall	Is absent or is composed of chitin	Is a complex structure containing protein, lipids, and peptidoglycans
Reproduction	Sexual and asexual	Asexual (binary fission)
Movement	Complex flagellum, if present	Simple flagellum, if present
Respiration	Via mitochondria	Via cytoplasmic membrane

From Holt S: In Slots J, Taubman M, editors: *Contemporary oral microbiology and immunology*, St Louis, 1992, Mosby.

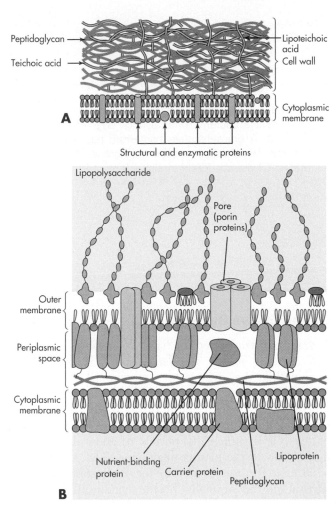

FIGURE 3–2. Comparison of the gram-positive and gram-negative bacterial cell walls. *A,* A gram-positive bacterium has a thick peptidoglycan layer that contains teichoic and lipoteichoic acids. *B,* A gram-negative bacterium has a thin peptidoglycan layer and an outer membrane that contains lipopolysaccharide, phospholipids, and proteins. The periplasmic space between the cytoplasmic and outer membranes contains transport, degradative, and cell wall synthetic proteins. The outer membrane is joined to the cytoplasmic membrane at adhesion points and is attached to the peptidoglycan by lipoprotein links.

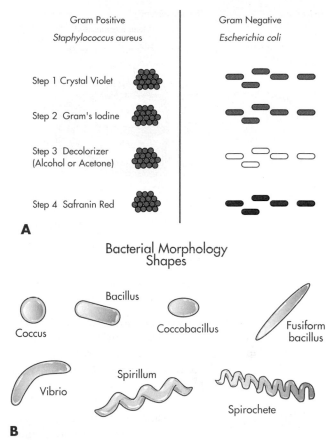

FIGURE 3–3. Gram-stain morphology of bacteria. *A,* The crystal violet of Gram stain is precipitated by Gram iodine and is trapped in the thick peptidoglycan layer in gram-positive bacteria. The decolorizer disperses the gram-negative outer membrane and washes the crystal violet from the thin layer of peptidoglycan. Gram-negative bacteria are visualized by the red counterstain. *B,* Bacterial morphologies.

The lack of a nuclear membrane simplifies the requirements and control mechanisms for the synthesis of proteins. Without a nuclear membrane, transcription and translation are coupled; in other words, ribosomes can bind to the mRNA, and protein can be made as the mRNA is being synthesized and still attached to the DNA.

The **bacterial ribosome consists of 30S + 50S subunits, forming a 70S ribosome**. This is unlike the eukaryotic 80S (40S + 60S) ribosome. The proteins and RNA of the bacterial ribosome are significantly different from those of eukaryotic ribosomes and are major targets for antibacterial drugs.

The **cytoplasmic membrane** has a lipid bilayer structure similar to the structure of the eukaryotic membranes, but it contains no steroids (e.g., cholesterol); mycoplasmas are the exception to this rule. The cytoplasmic membrane is responsible for many of the functions attributable to organelles in eukaryotes. These tasks include electron transport and energy production, which are normally achieved in the mitochondria (Fig. 3–5). In addition, the membrane contains transport proteins that allow the uptake of metabolites and the release of other substances, ion pumps to maintain a membrane potential, and enzymes. A coiled cytoplasmic membrane, the **mesosome,** acts as an anchor to bind and pull apart daughter chromosomes during cell division.

Cell Wall

The structure (Table 3–2), components, and functions (Table 3–3) of the cell wall distinguish gram-positive

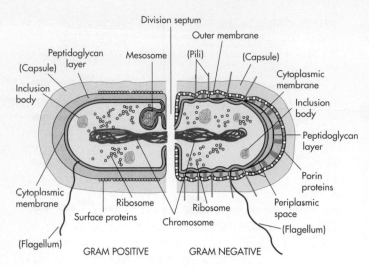

FIGURE 3–4. Gram-positive and gram-negative bacteria. A gram-positive bacterium has a thick layer of peptidoglycan (*left*). A gram-negative bacterium has a thin peptidoglycan layer and an outer membrane (*right*). Structures in ( ) are not found in all bacteria.

from gram-negative bacteria. The important differences in membrane characteristics are outlined in Table 3–4. The cytoplasmic membranes of most prokaryotes are surrounded by rigid **peptidoglycan** (**murein**) layers. The exceptions are *Archaeobacteria* organisms (which contain pseudoglycans or pseudomureins related to peptidoglycan) and mycoplasmas (which have no cell walls at all). Because the peptidoglycan provides rigidity, it also determines the shape of the particular bacterial cell. Gram-negative bacteria are also surrounded by outer membranes.

Gram-Positive Bacteria

A gram-positive bacterium has a *thick, multilayered cell wall consisting mainly of peptidoglycan* (150 to 500 Å) surrounding the cytoplasmic membrane (Fig. 3–6). The peptidoglycan is a meshlike exoskeleton similar in function to the exoskeleton of an insect. Unlike the exoskeleton of the insect, however, the peptidoglycan of the cell is sufficiently porous to allow diffusion of metabolites to the plasma membrane. The *peptidoglycan is essential* for the structure, for replication, and for survival in the normally hostile conditions in which

---

TABLE 3–2. Bacterial Membrane Structures

Structure	Chemical Constituents
Plasma membrane	Phospholipids, proteins, and enzymes involved in generation of energy, membrane potential, and transport
Cell wall	
Gram-positive bacteria	
Peptidoglycan	Glycan chains of GlcNAc and MurNAc cross-linked by peptide bridge
Teichoic acid	Polyribitol phosphate or glycerol phosphate cross-linked to peptidoglycan
Lipoteichoic acid	Lipid-linked teichoic acid
Gram-negative bacteria	
Peptidoglycan	Thinner version of that found in gram-positive bacteria
Periplasmic space	Enzymes involved in transport, degradation, and synthesis
Outer membrane	Phospholipids with saturated fatty acids
Proteins	Porins, lipoprotein, transport proteins
LPS	Lipid A, core polysaccharide, O antigen
Other structures	
Capsule	Polysaccharides (disaccharides and trisaccharides) and polypeptides
Pili	Pilin, adhesins
Flagellum	Motor proteins, flagellin
Proteins	M protein of streptococci (as an example)

GlcNAc = *N*-Acetylglucosamine; MurNAc = *N*-acetylmuramic acid; LPS = lipopolysaccharide.

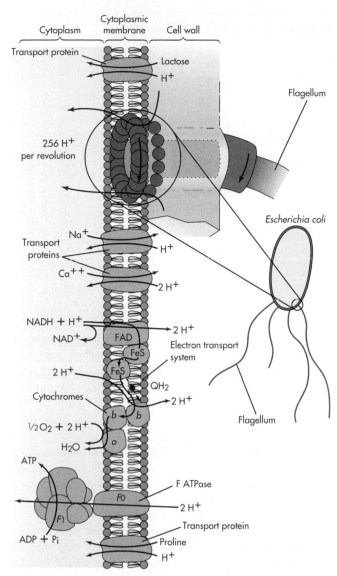

FIGURE 3–5. The cytoplasmic membrane contains the machinery for the production of adenosine triphosphate (ATP) (electron transport system, cytochromes, F1-adenosine triphosphatase [F1-ATPase]) and membrane potential. The membrane potential provides electrochemical energy for transport proteins and the flagellum "motor." ADP = adenosine diphosphate; NAD = nicotine adenine dinucleotide; NADH = reduced form of nicotine adenine dinucleotide; FAD = flavin adenine dinucleotide; Pi = phosphate.

teria succumb to the large osmotic pressure differences across the cytoplasmic membrane and lyse. Removal of the cell wall produces a **protoplast** that lyses unless it is osmotically stabilized.

The gram-positive cell wall may also include other components such as teichoic and lipoteichoic acids and complex polysaccharides (usually called C polysaccharides). Proteins such as the M protein of streptococci and R protein of staphylococci also associate with the peptidoglycan. **Teichoic acids** are water-soluble polymers of polyol phosphates, which are covalently linked to the peptidoglycan. **Lipoteichoic acids** have a fatty acid and are anchored in the cytoplasmic membrane. These molecules are common surface antigens that distinguish bacterial serotypes and promote attachment to other bacteria as well as to specific receptors on mammalian cell surfaces (adherence). Teichoic acids are important factors in virulence. Lipoteichoic acids are shed into the media and host and, although weaker, can initiate endotoxic-like activities (see later section).

Gram-Negative Bacteria

Gram-negative cell walls are more complex than are gram-positive cell walls, both structurally and chemically (see Fig. 3–2). Structurally, a gram-negative cell wall contains two layers external to the cytoplasmic membrane. Immediately external to the cytoplasmic

bacteria grow. During infection, the peptidoglycan can interfere with phagocytosis, is mitogenic (stimulates mitosis of lymphocytes), and has pyrogenic activity (induces fever).

The peptidoglycan can be degraded by treatment with **lysozyme**. Lysozyme, an enzyme in human tears and mucus, is also produced by bacteria and other organisms. Lysozyme degrades the glycan backbone of the peptidoglycan. Without the peptidoglycan, the bac-

TABLE 3–3. Functions of the Bacterial Envelope

Function	Component
Structural rigidity	All
Packaging of internal contents	All
Permeability barrier	Outer membrane or plasma membrane
Metabolic uptake	Membranes and periplasmic transport proteins, porins, permeases
Energy production	Plasma membrane
Adhesion to host cells	Pili, proteins, teichoic acid
Immune recognition by host	All outer structures
Escape from host immune recognition	Capsule, M protein
Antibiotic sensitivity	Peptidoglycan synthetic enzymes
Antibiotic resistance	Outer membrane
Motility	Flagella
Mating	Pili
Adhesion	Pili

TABLE 3–4. Membrane Characteristics of Gram-Positive and Gram-Negative Bacteria

Characteristic	Gram-Positive	Gram-Negative
Outer membrane	—	+
Cell wall	Thicker	Thinner
LPS	—	+
Endotoxin	—	+
Teichoic acid	Often present	Absent
Sporulation	Some strains	None
Capsule	Sometimes present	Sometimes present
Lysozyme	Sensitive	Resistant
Antibacterial activity of penicillin	More susceptible	More resistant
Exotoxin production	Some strains	Some strains

LPS = Lipopolysaccharide.

membrane is a *thin peptidoglycan layer*, which accounts for only 5% to 10% of the gram-negative cell wall by weight. There are *no teichoic or lipoteichoic acids* in the gram-negative cell wall. External to the peptidoglycan layer is the **outer membrane**, which is unique to gram-negative bacteria. The area between the external surface of the cytoplasmic membrane and the internal surface of the outer membrane is referred to as the **periplasmic space**. This space is actually a compartment containing a variety of hydrolytic enzymes, which are important to the cell for the breakdown of large macromolecules for metabolism. These enzymes typically include proteases, phosphatases, lipases, nucleases, and carbohydrate-degrading enzymes. In the case of pathogenic gram-negative species, many of the lytic virulence factors such as collagenases, hyaluronidases, proteases, and β-lactamase are in the periplasmic space. This space also contains components of the sugar transport systems and other binding proteins to facilitate the uptake of different metabolites and other compounds. Some binding proteins can be components of a chemotaxis system, which senses the external environment of the cell.

As mentioned previously, outer membranes (see Fig. 3–2) are unique to gram-negative prokaryotes. The outer membrane is like a stiff canvas sack around the bacteria. *The outer membrane maintains the bacterial structure and is a permeability barrier to large molecules* (e.g., proteins such as lysozyme*) and hydrophobic molecules.* It also provides protection from adverse environmental conditions such as the digestive system of the host (important for Enterobacteriaceae organisms). The outer membrane has an asymmetric bilayer structure that differs from any other biologic membrane in the structure of the outer leaflet of the membrane. The inner leaflet contains phospholipids normally found in

bacterial membranes. However, the outer leaflet is composed primarily of an amphipathic molecule (meaning that it has both hydrophobic and hydrophilic ends) called **lipopolysaccharide** (**LPS**). Except for those LPS molecules in the process of synthesis, the outer leaflet of the outer membrane is the only location where LPS molecules are found.

LPS is also called **endotoxin**, a powerful stimulator of immune responses. LPS activates B cells and induces macrophage and other cells to release interleukin-1 and interleukin-6, tumor necrosis factor, and other factors. LPS causes fever and can cause shock. The **Shwartzman reaction** (disseminated intravascular coagulation) follows the release of large amounts of endotoxin into the blood stream. LPS is shed from the bacteria into the media and host. *Neisseria meningitidis* sheds large amounts of a related compound, lipooligosaccharide (**LOS**), resulting in fever and symptoms.

The variety of proteins found in gram-negative outer membranes is limited, but several of the proteins are present in high concentration, resulting in a total protein content higher than that of the cytoplasmic membrane. Many of the proteins traverse the entire lipid bilayer and are thus transmembrane proteins. A group of these proteins is known as **porins** because they form pores **that allow the diffusion of hydrophilic molecules less than 700 Da in mass through the membrane**. *The outer membrane and the porin channel allow passage of metabolites and small hydrophilic antibiotics, but the outer membrane is a barrier for large or hydrophobic antibiotics and proteins such as lysozyme.*

The outer membrane also contains structural proteins and receptor molecules for bacteriophages and other ligands. The outer membrane is connected to the cytoplasmic membrane at **adhesion sites** and is tied to the peptidoglycan by **lipoprotein**. The lipoprotein is

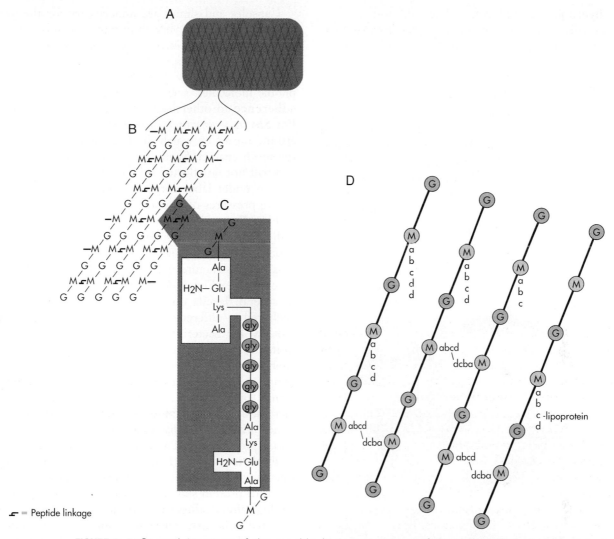

FIGURE 3–6. General structure of the peptidoglycan component of the cell wall. *A,* The peptidoglycan forms a meshlike layer around the cell. *B,* The peptidoglycan mesh consists of a polysaccharide polymer that is cross-linked by peptide bonds. *C,* Peptides are cross-linked through a peptide bond between the terminal D-alanine (D-ala) from one chain and a lysine (lys) (or another diamino amino acid) from the other chain. A pentaglycine bridge (gly₅) expands the cross-link in *Staphylococcus aureus* (as shown). *D,* Representation of the *Escherichia coli* peptidoglycan structure. Diaminopimelic acid, the diamino amino acid in the third position of the peptide, is directly linked to the terminal alanine of another chain to cross-link the peptidoglycan. Lipoprotein anchors the outer membrane to the peptidoglycan. M = *n*-Acetylmuramic acid; G = *N*-acetylglucosamine; Glu = glucosamine; gly = glycine. (*A* to *C* redrawn from Talaro K, Talaro AI, editors: *Foundations in microbiology,* ed 2, Dubuque, Iowa, 1996, Wm C Brown; *D* redrawn from Joklik KJ et al, editors: *Zinsser microbiology,* Norwalk, Conn, 1988, Appleton & Lange.)

covalently attached to the peptidoglycan and is anchored in the outer membrane. The adhesion sites provide a membranous route for the delivery of newly synthesized outer membrane components to the outer membrane.

The outer membrane is held together by divalent cation (Mg^{+2} and Ca^{+2}) linkages between phosphates on LPS molecules and hydrophobic interactions between the LPS and proteins. These interactions produce a stiff, strong membrane that can be disrupted by antibiotics (e.g., polymyxin) or by the removal of Mg and Ca ions (chelation with ethylenediaminetetraacetic acid [EDTA]). Disruption of the outer membrane weakens the bacteria and allows the permeability of large, hydrophobic molecules. The addition of lysozyme to cells treated in this manner produces **spheroplasts**, which, like protoplasts, are osmotically sensitive.

External Structures

Some bacteria (gram-positive or gram-negative) are closely surrounded by loose polysaccharide or protein layers called **capsules** (Fig. 3–7). In cases in which it is loosely adherent and nonuniform in density or thickness, the material is referred to as a **slime layer**. The capsule and slime layers are also called the **glycocalyx**. *Bacillus anthracis*, the exception to this rule, produces a polypeptide capsule. The capsule is hard to see in a microscope but can be visualized by the exclusion of India ink particles.

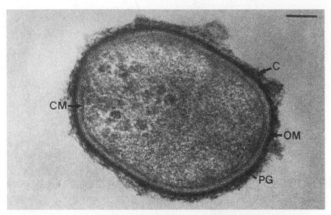

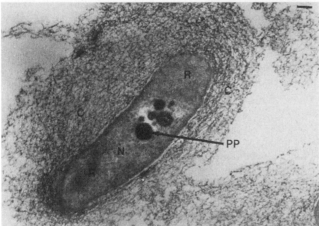

FIGURE 3–7. Transmission electron photomicrographs of *Porphyromonas* (formerly *Bacteroides*) gingivalis and *Pseudomonas aeruginosa* revealing the surface-associated capsule. Both strains were isolated from human patients, *P. gingivalis* from an adult with periodontitis and *P. aeruginosa* from a patient with cystic fibrosis. C = capsule; OM = outer membrane; PG = peptidoglycan; CM = cytoplasmic membrane; R = ribosome; PP = polyphosphate. Bar = 0.1 μm. (From Slots J, Taubman MA, editors: *Contemporary oral microbiology and immunology*, St Louis, 1992, Mosby.)

Capsules and slimes are unnecessary for the growth of bacteria but are very important for survival in the host. *The capsule is poorly antigenic and antiphagocytic and is a major virulence factor* (e.g., *Streptococcus pneumoniae*). The capsule can also act as a barrier to toxic hydrophobic molecules, such as detergents, and can promote **adherence** to other bacteria or to host tissue surfaces. For *Streptococcus mutans*, the dextran and levan capsules are the means by which the bacteria attach and stick to the tooth enamel. Synthesis of the capsule takes energy and will not be effected by the bacteria after continued growth under laboratory conditions away from the selective pressures of the host.

Flagella are ropelike propellers composed of helically coiled protein subunits (**flagellin**) that are anchored in the bacterial membranes through hook and basal body structures and that are driven by membrane potential (see Fig. 3–5). Bacterial species may have one or several flagella on their surfaces, and they may be anchored at different parts of the cell. Flagella provide motility for bacteria, allowing the cell to swim (**chemotaxis**) toward food and away from poisons. Bacteria approach food by swimming straight and then tumbling in a new direction. The swimming period becomes longer as the concentration of chemoattractant increases. The direction of flagellar spinning determines whether the bacteria swim or tumble. Flagella also express antigenic and strain determinants.

Fimbriae (**pili**) (Latin for "fringe") are hairlike structures on the outside of bacteria; they are composed of protein subunits (**pilin**). Fimbriae can be morphologically distinguished from flagella because they are smaller in diameter (3 to 8 nm versus 15 to 20 nm) and usually are not coiled in structure. Generally, several hundred fimbriae are arranged peritrichously (uniformly) over the entire surface of the bacterial cell. They may be as long as 15 to 20 μm, or many times the length of the cell.

Fimbriae promote adherence to other bacteria or to the host (alternative names are adhesins, lectins, evasins, and aggressins). As an adherence factor (**adhesin**), fimbriae are an important virulence factor for *E. coli* colonization and infection of the urinary tract, for *Neisseria gonorrhoeae* and other bacteria. The tips of the fimbriae may contain proteins (lectins) that bind to specific sugars (e.g., mannose). **F pili** (**sex pili**) promote the transfer of large segments of bacterial chromosomes between bacteria. These pili are encoded by a plasmid (F).

Bacterial Exceptions

Mycobacteria have a peptidoglycan layer (slightly different structure), which is intertwined with and covalently attached to an arabinogalactan polymer and surrounded by a waxlike lipid coat of mycolic acid (large α-branched β-hydroxy fatty acids), cord factor (glycolipid of trehalose and two mycolic acids), waxD (glycolipid of 15 to 20 mycolic acids and sugar), and sulfolipids. These bacteria are described as **acid-fast staining**. The coat is responsible for virulence and is antiphagocytic. *Corynebacterium* and *Nocardia* organisms also produce mycolic acid lipids. The **mycoplasmas** are also exceptions in that they have no peptidoglycan cell wall and they incorporate steroids from the host into their membranes.

Structure and Biosynthesis of the Major Components of the Bacterial Cell Wall

The cell wall components are large structures made up of polymers of subunits. This type of structure facilitates their synthesis. Like astronauts building a space station in space, bacteria face problems assembling their cell walls. Synthesis of the peptidoglycan, LPS, teichoic acid, and capsule occurs on the outside of the bacteria, away from the synthetic machinery and energy sources of the cytoplasm and in an inhospitable environment. For both the space station and the bacteria, prefabricated precursors and subunits of the final structure are assembled in a factory-like setting on the inside, attached to a conveyor belt–like structure, brought to the surface, and then attached to the preexisting structure. For bacteria, the molecular conveyor belt–like structure is a large hydrophobic phospholipid called **bactoprenol** (**undecaprenol, C_{55} isoprenoid**). The prefabricated precursors must also be activated with high energy bonds (e.g., phosphates) or other means to power the attachment reactions occurring outside the cell. For gram-negative bacteria, the outer membrane components are delivered through adhesion sites.

Peptidoglycan (Mucopeptide, Murein)

The peptidoglycan is a rigid mesh made up of ropelike linear polysaccharide chains cross-linked by peptides. The polysaccharide is made up of repeating disaccharides of **N-acetylglucosamine** (**GlcNAc, NAG, G**) and **N-acetylmuramic acid** (**MurNAc, NAM, M**) (Figs. 3–6 and 3–8).

A tetrapeptide is attached to the MurNAc. The peptide is unusual because it contains both D and L amino acids (D amino acids are not normally used in nature) and the peptide is produced enzymatically. The first two amino acids attached to the MurNAc may vary for different organisms.

The diamino amino acids in the third position are essential for the cross-linking of the peptidoglycan chain. Examples of diamino amino acids include lysine

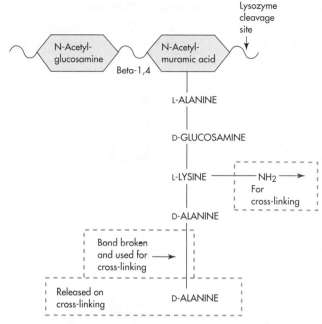

FIGURE 3–8. Precursor of peptidoglycan. The peptidoglycan is built from prefabricated units that contain a pentapeptide attached to the MurNAc. The pentapeptide contains a terminal D-alanine-D-alanine unit. This dipeptide is required for cross-linking the peptidoglycan and is the basis for the action of β-lactam and vancomycin antibiotics.

and diaminopimelic and diaminobutyric acids. The peptide cross-link is formed between the free amine of the diamino amino acid in the third position of the peptide and the D-alanine in the fourth position of another chain. *S. aureus* and other gram-positive bacteria use an amino acid bridge (e.g. a glycine$_5$ peptide) between these amino acids to lengthen the cross-link. The precursor form of the peptide has an extra D-alanine, which is released during the cross-linking step.

The peptidoglycan in gram-positive bacteria forms multiple layers and is often cross-linked in three dimensions, providing a very strong, rigid cell wall. In contrast, the peptidoglycan in gram-negative cell walls is usually only one molecule (layer) thick. The rigidity of the peptidoglycan mesh is determined by the number of cross-links and the length of the cross-link. The site where lysozyme cleaves the glycan of the peptidoglycan is shown in Figure 3–8.

Peptidoglycan Synthesis

Peptidoglycan synthesis occurs in four steps (Fig. 3–9). First, inside the cell, glucosamine is enzymatically converted into MurNAc and then energetically activated by a reaction with uridine triphosphate (UTP) to produce uridine diphosphate-N-acetylmuramic acid (UDP-MurNAc). Next, the UDP-MurNAc-pentapeptide pre-

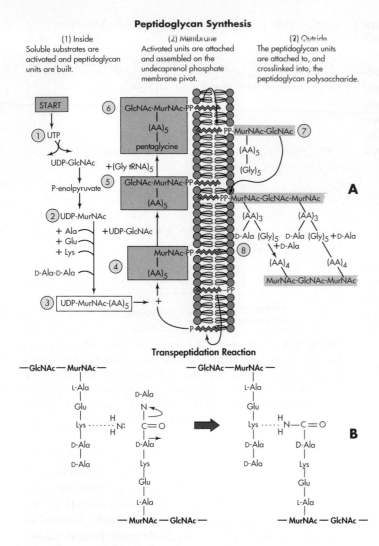

FIGURE 3–9. Peptidoglycan synthesis. *A,* Peptidoglycan synthesis occurs in three phases. (1) Peptidoglycan is synthesized from prefabricated units constructed and activated for assembly and transport inside the cell. (2) At the membrane, the units are assembled onto the undecaprenol phosphate conveyor belt, and assembly is completed. (3) The unit is translocated to the outside of the cell, where it is attached to the polysaccharide chain, and the peptide is cross-linked to finish the construction. Such a construction can be compared with the assembly of a space station. *B,* The cross-linking reaction is a transpeptidation. One peptide bond (produced inside the cell) is traded for another (outside the cell) with the release of D-alanine. The enzymes that catalyze the reaction are called D-*alanine,* D-*alanine transpeptidase-carboxypeptidases.* These enzymes are the targets of β-lactam antibiotics and are called *penicillin-binding proteins.*

cursor is assembled in a series of enzymatic steps (see Fig. 3–9).

Second, the UDP-MurNAc pentapeptide is attached to the **bactoprenol** "conveyor belt" in the cytoplasmic membrane through a pyrophosphate link with the release of uridine monophosphate (UMP). GlcNAc is added to make the disaccharide building block of the peptidoglycan. Some bacteria (e.g., *S. aureus*) add a pentaglycine or another chain to the diamino amino acid at the third position of the peptide chain to lengthen the cross-link. Third, the bactoprenol molecule translocates the disaccharide pentapeptide precursor to the outside of the cell. The GlcNAc-MurNAc disaccharide is then attached to a peptidoglycan chain using the pyrophosphate link between itself and the bactoprenol as energy to drive the reaction. The pyrophosphobactoprenol is converted back to a phosphobactoprenol and recycled. Fourth, outside the cell but near the membrane surface, peptide chains from adjacent glycan chains are cross-linked to each other by a peptide bond exchange (**transpeptidation**) between the free amine of the amino acid in the third position of

the pentapeptide (e.g., lysine) or the *N*-terminus of the attached pentaglycine chain and the D-alanine at the fourth position of the other peptide chain, releasing the terminal D-alanine of the precursor. This step requires no additional energy because peptide bonds are "traded."

The cross-linking reaction is catalyzed by membrane-bound **transpeptidases**. Related enzymes, **DD-carboxypeptidases**, remove extra terminal D-alanines, which limit the extent of cross-linking. These enzymes are called **penicillin-binding proteins (PBPs)** because they are targets for penicillin and other β-lactam antibiotics. Penicillin and related β-lactam antibiotics resemble the "transition state" conformation of the D-ALA-D-ALA unit when bound to these enzymes. Different PBPs are used for extending the peptidoglycan, creating a septum for cell division, and curving the peptidoglycan mesh (cell shape).

The peptidoglycan is constantly being synthesized and degraded. **Autolysins** such as lysozyme are important for determining bacterial shape. Inhibition of synthesis or the cross-linking of the peptidoglycan does not stop the autolysins, and their action weakens the mesh and the bacterial structure and leads to lysis and cell death. New peptidoglycan synthesis does not occur during starvation, which leads to a weakening of the peptidoglycan and a loss in the dependability of Gram stain.

An understanding of the biosynthesis of peptidoglycan is essential in medicine because these reactions are unique to bacterial cells and hence can be inhibited with little or no adverse effect on host (human) cells. A number of antibiotics target one or more steps in this pathway (see Chapter 20).

Teichoic Acid

Teichoic and lipoteichoic acid are polymers of chemically modified ribose or glycerol connected by phosphates (Fig. 3–10). Sugars, choline, or D-alanine may be attached to the hydroxyls of the ribose or glycerol, providing antigenic determinants. These can be distinguished by antibodies and may determine the bacterial serotype. Lipoteichoic acid has a fatty acid and is anchored in the membrane. Teichoic acid is synthesized

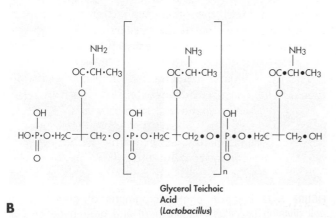

A

Ribitol-Teichoic Acid (*Staphylococcus*)

B

Glycerol Teichoic Acid (*Lactobacillus*)

FIGURE 3–10. Teichoic acid. Teichoic acid is a polymer of chemically modified ribitol (*A*) or glycerol phosphate (*B*). The nature of the modification (e.g., sugars, amino acids) can define the serotype of the bacteria. Teichoic acid may be covalently attached to the peptidoglycan. Lipoteichoic acid is anchored in the cytoplasmic membrane by a covalently attached fatty acid.

from building blocks in a manner similar to that of peptidoglycan. Teichoic acid and some **surface proteins** (e.g., protein A from *S. aureus*) are secreted from the cells and then enzymatically attached to the *N*-terminus of the peptide of peptidoglycan.

Lipopolysaccharide

LPS (**endotoxin**) *consists of three structural sections: Lipid A, core polysaccharide (rough core), and O antigen* (Fig. 3–11). Lipid A is a basic component of LPS and is essential for bacterial viability. *Lipid A is responsible for the endotoxin activity of LPS.* It has a phosphorylated glucosamine disaccharide backbone with fatty acids attached to anchor the structure in the outer membrane. The phosphates connect LPS units into aggregates. One carbohydrate chain is attached to the disaccharide backbone and extends away from the bacteria. The core polysaccharide is a branched polysaccharide of 9 to 12 sugars. Most of the core region is also essential for LPS structure and bacterial viability. The core region contains an unusual sugar, 2-keto-3-deoxy-octanoate (KDO), and is phosphorylated. The O antigen is attached to the core and extends away from the bacteria. It is a long, linear polysaccharide consisting of 50 to 100 repeating saccharide units of 4 to 7 sugars per unit.

LPS structure is used to classify bacteria. The basic structure of lipid A is identical for related bacteria and is similar for all gram-negative Enterobacteriaceae. The core region is the same for a species of bacteria. The O antigen distinguishes serotypes (strains) of a bacterial species. For example, the O157:H7 serotype identifies the *E. coli* agent of hemolytic-uremic syndrome.

The lipid A and core portions are enzymatically synthesized in a sequential manner on the inside surface of the cytoplasmic membrane. The repeat units of the O antigen are assembled on a bactoprenol molecule and then transferred to a growing O antigen chain. The finished O antigen chain is transferred to the core lipid A structure. The LPS molecule is translocated through adhesion sites to the outer surface of the outer membrane.

Cell Division

The replication of the bacterial chromosome also triggers the initiation of cell division (Fig. 3–12). The production of two daughter bacteria requires the growth and extension of the cell wall components followed by the production of a septum (cross wall) to divide the daughter bacteria into two cells. The septum consists of two membranes separated by two layers of peptidoglycan. Septum formation is initiated at the cell membrane; the septum grows from opposite sides toward the center of the cell, causing cleavage of the daughter cells. This process requires special transpepti-

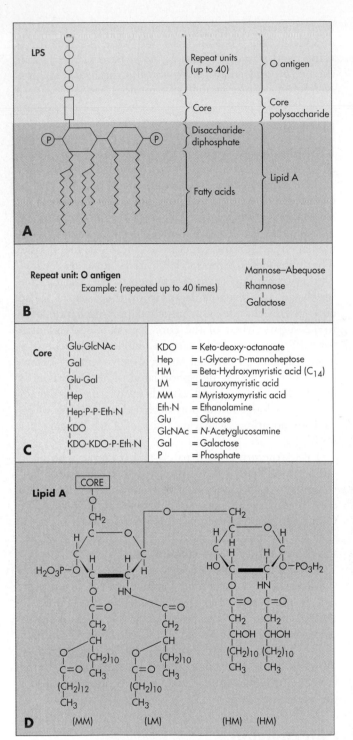

FIGURE 3–11. The lipopolysaccharide of the gram-negative cell envelope. *A,* Segment of the polymer showing the arrangements of the major constituents. *B,* Stucture of lipid A of *Salmonella typhimurium. C,* Polysaccharide core. *D,* Typical repeat unit (*S. typhimurium*). (Redrawn from Brooks GF, Butel JS, Ornston LN, editors: *Jawetz, Melnick and Aldenberg's medical microbiology,* ed 19, Norwalk, Conn, 1991, Appleton & Lange.)

dases and other enzymes. New peptidoglycan is synthesized in a defined growth zone, usually in a ring on either side of the growing septum. For streptococci, the growth zone is at 180 degrees from each other, producing linear chains of bacteria. In contrast, the growth zone of staphylococci is at 90 degrees. Incomplete cleavage of the septum can cause the bacteria to remain linked, forming chains (e.g., streptococci) or clusters (e.g., staphylococci).

Spores

Some gram-positive, but never gram-negative, bacteria such as members of the genera *Bacillus* and *Clostridium* (soil bacteria) are spore formers. Under harsh environmental conditions, such as the loss of a nutritional requirement, these bacteria can convert from a **vegetative state** to a **dormant state**, or **spore.** The location of the spore within a cell is a characteristic of the

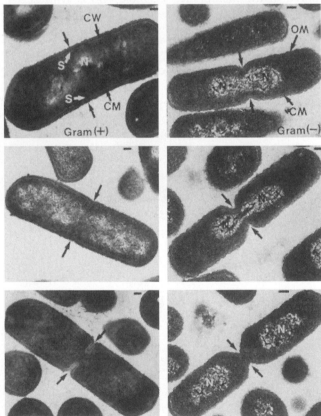

FIGURE 3–12. Electron photomicrographs of gram-positive cell division (*Bacillus subtilis*) (*left*) and gram-negative cell division (*Escherichia coli*) (*right*). *A* to *C* represent a progression in cell division. CW = Cell wall; CM = cytoplasmic membrane; S = septum; N = nucleoid; OM = outer membrane. Bar = 0.2 μm. (From Slots J, Taubman MA, editors: *Contemporary oral biology and immunology,* St Louis, 1992, Mosby.)

bacteria and can assist in identification of the bacterium.

The spore is a dehydrated, multishelled structure that protects and allows the bacteria to exist in "suspended animation" (Fig. 3–13). It contains a complete copy of the chromosome, the bare minimum concentrations of essential proteins and ribosomes, and a high concentration of **calcium bound to dipicolinic acid.** The spore has an inner membrane, two peptidoglycan layers, and an outer keratin-like protein coat. The spore looks refractile (bright) in the microscope. The structure of the spore protects the genomic DNA from desiccation, intense heat, radiation, and attack by most enzymes and chemical agents. In fact, bacterial spores are so resistant to environmental factors that they can exist for centuries as viable spores. Spores are also difficult to decontaminate with standard disinfectants.

Depletion of specific nutrients (e.g., alanine) from the growth medium triggers a cascade of genetic events (comparable to differentiation) leading to the produc-

tion of a spore. Spore mRNA are transcribed and other mRNA are turned off. Dipicolinic acid is produced, and antibiotics and toxins are often excreted. After duplication of the chromosome, one copy of DNA and cytoplasmic contents (**core**) are surrounded by its cytoplasmic membrane, the peptidoglycan, and the membrane of the septum. This wraps the DNA in the two layers of membrane and peptidoglycan that would normally divide the cell. This is surrounded by the **cortex**, which is made up of a thin inner layer of tightly crosslinked peptidoglycan surrounding a membrane (which used to be the cytoplasmic membrane) and a loose outer peptidoglycan layer. The cortex is surrounded by the tough, **keratin-like protein coat** which protects the spore. The process requires 6 to 8 hours for completion.

The germination or transformation of spores into the vegetative state is stimulated by disruption of the outer coat by mechanical stress, pH, heat, or another stressor and requires water and a triggering nutrient

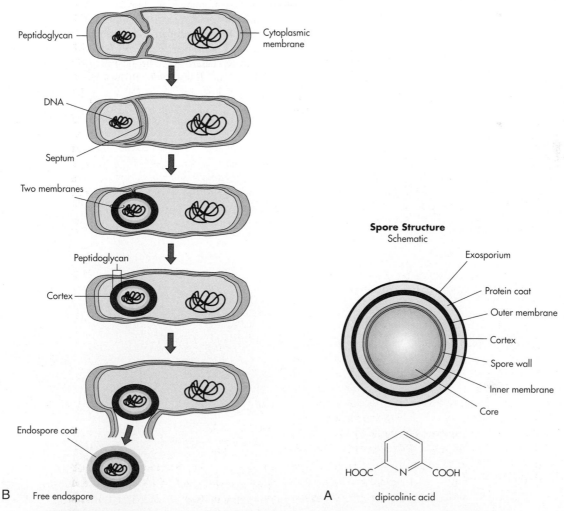

FIGURE 3–13. Endospores. *A,* Structure of a spore. *B,* Sporogenesis, the process of endospore formation.

(e.g., alanine). The process takes about 90 minutes. Once the germination process has begun, the spore will take up water, swell, shed its coats, and produce one new vegetative cell identical to the original vegetative cell, thus completing the entire cycle. Once germination has begun and the spore coat has been compromised, the spore is weakened and can be inactivated like other bacteria.

QUESTIONS

1. How does each of the differences between prokaryotes and eukaryotes (see Table 3–1) influence bacterial infection and treatment?

2. How do the differences between gram-positive and gram-negative cell walls influence the cells' clinical behavior? Detection? Treatment?

3. List the cell wall components that contribute to virulence by protecting the bacteria from immune responses. List those that contribute to virulence by eliciting toxic responses in the human host.

4. When peptidoglycan synthesis is inhibited, what processes kill the bacteria? List the precursors that would build up within the bacteria if recycling of bactoprenol were inhibited by vancomycin or bacitracin.

5. Why are spores more resistant to environmental stresses?

6. The laboratory would like to eliminate gram-positive bacteria from a mixture of gram-positive and gram-negative bacteria. Which of the following procedures would be more appropriate and why? Or why not?

   a. Treatment with ethylenediaminetetraacetic acid (a divalent cation chelator)
   b. Treatment with mild detergent
   c. Treatment with lysozyme
   d. Treatment with transpeptidase
   e. Treatment with ampicillin (a hydrophilic β-lactam antibiotic)

BIBLIOGRAPHY

Davis BD et al, editors: *Microbiology*, ed 4, Philadelphia, 1990, Lippincott.

Slots J, Taubman MA, editors: *Contemporary oral microbiology and immunology*, St Louis, 1992, Mosby.

Stanier RY, Doudoroff M, Adelberg EA: *The microbial world*, ed 4, Englewood Cliffs, NJ, 1976, Prentice-Hall.

Talaro K, Talaro AI, editors: *Foundations in microbiology*, ed 2, Dubuque, Iowa, 1996, Brown.

C H A P T E R 4

Bacterial Metabolism and Growth

Metabolic Requirements

Bacterial growth requires a source of energy and the raw materials to build the proteins, structures, and membranes that make up the structure and biochemical machines of the cell. Bacteria must obtain or synthesize the amino acids, carbohydrates, and lipids used as building blocks of the cell.

The minimum requirement for growth is a source of carbon and nitrogen, an energy source, water, and various ions. The essential elements and their functions are listed in Table 4–1. **Iron** is so important that many bacteria secrete special proteins (siderophores) to sequester iron from dilute solutions.

Oxygen (O_2 gas), although essential for the human host, is actually a poison for many bacteria. Some organisms, such as *Clostridium perfringens*, which causes gas gangrene, cannot grow in the presence of oxygen. Such bacteria are referred to as **obligate anaerobes.** Other organisms, such as *Mycobacterium tuberculosis*, which causes tuberculosis, require the presence of molecular oxygen for growth and are therefore referred to as **obligate aerobes.** Most bacteria, however, grow in either the presence or the absence of oxygen. These bacteria are referred to as **facultative anaerobes.**

Although some bacteria (such as chemotrophs) can derive energy directly from the oxidation of metal ions, such as iron, and other bacteria (such as blue-green algae) are capable of photosynthesis, pathogenic bacteria derive their energy by metabolizing sugars, fats, and proteins. Some bacteria, such as certain strains of *Escherichia coli* (a member of the intestinal flora), can synthesize all the amino acids, nucleotides, lipids, and carbohydrates necessary for growth and division when provided with the inorganic nutrients listed in Table 4–1 plus a simple source of carbon, such as glucose. At the other extreme are bacteria, such as the causative agent of syphilis, *Treponema pallidum*, whose growth requirements are so complex that a defined laboratory medium capable of supporting its growth has yet to be developed.

Growth requirements and metabolic byproducts may be used as a convenient means of classifying different bacteria. Those that can rely entirely on inorganic chemicals for their energy and source of carbon (CO_2) are referred to as autotrophs (lithotrophs), whereas many bacteria and animal cells that require organic carbon sources are known as heterotrophs (organotrophs).

Metabolism and the Conversion of Energy

All cells require a constant supply of energy to survive. This energy, typically in the form of adenosine triphosphate (ATP), is derived from the controlled breakdown of various organic substrates (carbohydrates, lipids, and proteins). This process of substrate breakdown and conversion into usable energy is known as **catabolism.** The energy produced may then be used in the synthesis of cellular constituents (cell walls, proteins, fatty acids, and nucleic acids), a process known as **anabolism.** Together these two processes, which are interrelated and tightly integrated, are referred to as **intermediary metabolism.**

The metabolic process generally begins with hydrolysis of large macromolecules in the external cellular environment by specific enzymes or exoenzymes (Fig. 4–1). The small subunit molecules produced (monosaccharides, short peptides, and fatty acids) are transported across the cell membranes into the cytoplasm by active or passive transport mechanisms specific for the metabolite. These mechanisms may use specific carrier or membrane transport proteins to help concentrate metabolites from the medium. The metabolites are converted by one or more pathways to one common universal intermediate, **pyruvic acid.** From pyruvic acid the carbons may be channeled toward energy production or the synthesis of new carbohydrates, amino acids, lipids, and nucleic acids.

Metabolism of Glucose

For the sake of simplicity, this section presents an overview of the pathways by which the model carbohy-

TABLE 4–1. Essential Elements, Their Sources, and Functions in Prokaryotes

Element	Source	Function in Metabolism
Major Essential Elements		
C	Organic compounds, CO_2	Major components of cellular material
O	O_2, H_2O, organic compounds	
H	H_2, H_2O, organic compounds	
N	NH_4^+, NO_3^-, N_2, organic compounds	
S	SO_4^{-2}, HS^-, S^0, organic sulfur compounds	Constituent of S-containing amino acids, cysteine, methionine, thiamine pyrophosphate, coenzyme A, biotin, and α-lipoic acid
P	HPO_4^{-2}	Constituent of nucleic acids, phospholipids, nucleotides
K	K^+	Major inorganic cation, co-factor (e.g., pyruvate kinase)
Mg	Mg^{2+}	Cofactor of many enzymes (e.g., kinases); component of cell walls, membranes, ribosomes, and phosphate esters
Ca	Ca^{2+}	Component of exoenzymes (amylases, proteases) and cell walls; major component of endospores as Ca-dipicolinate
Fe	Fe^{2+}, Fe^{3+}	Present in cytochromes, ferredoxins, and other iron-sulfur proteins; co-factor (dehydratases)
Na	Na^+	Transport
Cl	Cl^-	Important inorganic anion
Minor Essential Elements		
Zn	Zn^{2+}	Component of the enzymes alcohol dehydrogenase, alkaline phosphatase, aldolase, RNA and DNA polymerase
Mn	Mn^{2+}	Present in superoxide dismutase; co-factor of the enzymes PEP carboxykinase, isocitrate synthase
Mo	MoO_4^{-2}	Present in nitrate reductase, nitrogenase, xanthine dehydrogenase, and formate dehydrogenase
Se	SeO_3^{-2}	Component of glycine reductase and formate dehydrogenase
Co	Co^{2+}	Required element in coenzyme B_{12}–containing enzymes (glutamate mutase, methylmalonyl coenzyme A mutase)
Cu	Cu^{2+}	Present in cytochrome oxidase and nitrite reductase
Ni	Ni^{2+}	Present in urease, hydrogenase, and factor F_{430}
W	WO_4^{-2}	Present in some formate dehydrogenases

Modified from Gottschalk E: *Bacterial metabolism*, ed 2, New York, 1985, Springer-Verlag.

drate glucose is metabolized to produce energy or other usable substrates. Instead of releasing all the molecule's energy as heat (as for burning), the bacteria break down the glucose in discrete steps to allow the energy to be captured in usable forms. *Bacteria can produce energy from glucose by—in order of increasing efficiency—fermentation or anaerobic respiration (both of which occur in the absence of oxygen) or aerobic respiration.* For a discussion of the metabolism of other organic compounds, including proteins and lipids, see a textbook on biochemistry.

Embden-Meyerhof-Parnas Pathway

Bacteria use three major metabolic pathways in the catabolism of glucose. Most common among these is the **glycolytic,** or Embden-Meyerhof-Parnas (EMP), pathway (Fig. 4–2). This pathway represents the pri-

mary means in both bacteria and eukaryotic cells for the conversion of glucose to pyruvate, which as noted previously is central to various other cellular metabolic pathways. These reactions, which occur under both **aerobic and anaerobic** conditions, begin with activation of glucose to form glucose-6-phosphate. This reaction, as well as the third reaction in the series, in which fructose-6-phosphate is converted to fructose-1,6-diphosphate, requires 1 mole of ATP per mole of glucose and represents an initial investment of cellular energy stores.

Energy is produced during glycolysis in two different forms, chemical and electrochemical. In the first, the high-energy phosphate group of one of the intermediates in the pathway is used under the direction of the appropriate enzyme (a **kinase**) to generate **ATP** from adenosine diphosphate (ADP). This type of reaction, termed **substrate-level phosphorylation,** occurs

Catabolism

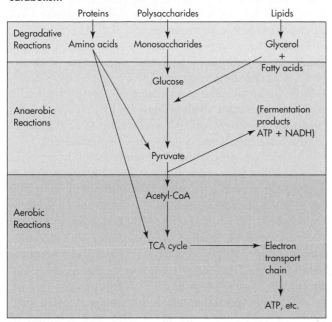

FIGURE 4–1. Catabolism of proteins, polysaccharides, and lipids produces glucose, pyruvate, or intermediates of the tricarboxylic acid (TCA) cycle and ultimately energy in the forms of adenosine triphosphate (ATP) or the reduced form of nicotinamide-adenine dinucleotide (NADH).

at two different points in the glycolytic pathway (i.e., conversion of 3-phosphoglycerol phosphate to 3-phosphoglycerate and 2-phosphoenolpyruvic acid to pyruvate). Four ATP molecules per molecule of glucose are produced in this manner. Two ATP molecules are consumed in the initial reactions, and glycolytic conversion of glucose to two molecules of pyruvic acid results in the net production of two molecules of ATP. The reduced form of **nicotinamide-adenine dinucleotide (NADH)** that is produced represents the second form of energy, which may then be converted to ATP in the presence of oxygen by a series of oxidation reactions.

In the absence of oxygen, substrate-level phosphorylation represents the primary means of energy production. The pyruvic acid produced from glycolysis is then converted to various end products depending on the bacterial species in question in a process known as **fermentation.** Many bacteria are identified on the basis of their fermentative end products, which are distinguished by gas chromatography (Fig. 4–3). These organic molecules, rather than oxygen, are used as electron acceptors to recycle NADH, which is produced during glycolysis, to NAD. In yeast, fermentative metabolism results in the conversion of pyruvate to ethanol. Alcoholic fermentation is uncommon in bacteria, which most commonly use the one-step conversion of pyruvic acid to lactic acid. This process is

responsible for making milk into yogurt and cabbage into sauerkraut. Other bacteria use more complex fermentative pathways, producing various acids, alcohols, and often gases (many of which have vile odors). These products lend flavors to various cheeses and wines.

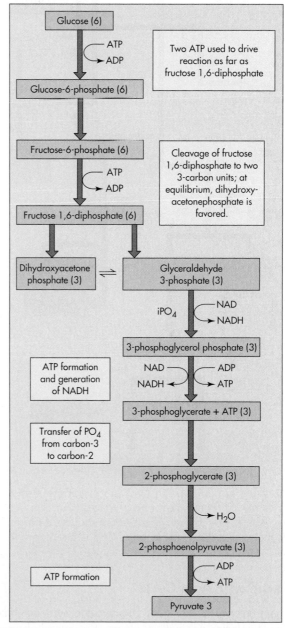

FIGURE 4–2. Embden-Meyerhof-Parnas (EMP) glycolytic pathway results in conversion of glucose to pyruvate. The sum of glucose + 2 ADP + 2 Pi + 2 NAD → 2 pyruvate + 4 ATP + 2 NADH + 2 H⁺. *Double arrows* denote 2 moles reacting per mole of glucose. ADP = adenosine diphosphate; iPO₄ = inorganic phosphate; Pi = phosphate; ATP = adenosine triphosphate; NAD = nicotinamide adenine dinucleotide; NADH = reduced form of NAD.

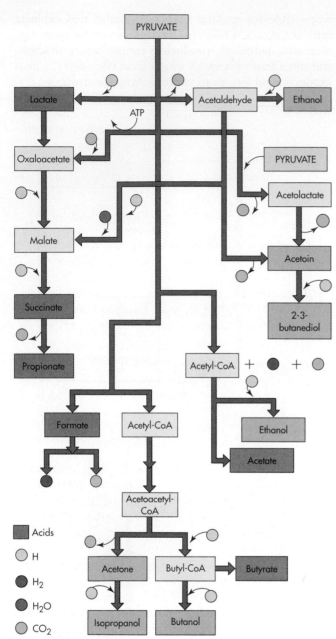

FIGURE 4–3. Fermentation of pyruvate by different microorganisms results in different end products. The clinical laboratory uses these pathways and end products as a means of distinguishing different bacteria. CoA = coenzyme A.

Tricarboxylic Acid Cycle

In the presence of oxygen, the pyruvic acid produced from glycolysis, as well as from the metabolism of other substrates, may be completely oxidized (controlled burning) to water and CO_2 using the tricarboxylic acid (TCA) cycle (Fig. 4–4), which results in production of additional energy. The process begins with the oxidative decarboxylation (release of CO_2) of pyruvate to the high-energy intermediate, acetyl coenzyme A (acetyl CoA); this reaction also produces NADH.

The two remaining carbons derived from pyruvate then enter the TCA cycle in the form of acetyl CoA by condensation with oxaloacetate, with the formation of citrate. In a stepwise series of oxidative reactions, the citrate is converted back to oxaloacetate, with the net production of 2 moles of CO_2, 3 moles of NADH, 1 mole of flavin adenine dinucleotide ($FADH_2$), and 1 mole of guanosine triphosphate (GTP). GTP is produced via substrate-level phosphorylation in a reaction in which succinyl CoA is converted to succinate.

The TCA cycle allows the organism to generate substantially more energy per mole of glucose than is possible with glycolysis alone. In addition to the GTP (an ATP equivalent) produced by substrate-level phosphorylation, the NADH and $FADH_2$ may enter the electron transport chain. In this chain, the electrons carried by NADH (or $FADH_2$) are passed in a stepwise fashion through a series of donor-acceptor pairs and ultimately to oxygen (Fig. 4–5). This process, known as **aerobic respiration,** results in the generation of 3 moles of ATP per mole of NADH and 2 moles of ATP per mole of $FADH_2$. The energetics of aerobic glucose metabolism are depicted in Fig. 4–5.

Some bacteria can use compounds other than oxy-

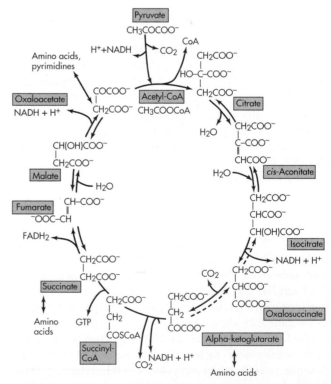

FIGURE 4–4. Tricarboxylic acid cycle occurs in aerobic conditions and is an amphibolic cycle. Precursors for the synthesis of amino acids and nucleotides are also shown. CoA = coenzyme A; GTP = guanosine triphosphate; $FADH_2$ = flavin adenine dinucleotide.

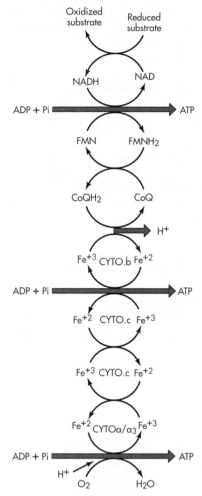

FIGURE 4–5. Electron transport chain, showing sequential oxidation and energy-generating steps. Electron transfer is accompanied by the flow of protons (H^+) from NADH through coenzyme Q (CoQ) and electrons through the cytochromes (CYTO). Three ATPs are formed per molecule of NADH reoxidized, but only two ATPs are formed per molecule of $FADH_2$ reoxidized. FMN = flavin mononucleotide. (Modified from Slots J, Taubman MA, editors: *Contemporary oral microbiology and immunology,* St Louis, 1992, Mosby.)

gen (e.g., NO_3^-, SO_4^{-2}, CO_2) as terminal electron acceptors during **anaerobic respiration.** Although this approach is more efficient than fermentation, which uses organic molecules as electron acceptors, it is less efficient than aerobic respiration because it produces less ATP.

Anaerobic organisms have neither aerobic electron transport nor a complete TCA cycle and therefore are less efficient at energy production than aerobic organisms. Fermentation produces 2 ATP molecules per glucose glycolysis, whereas aerobic metabolism can generate 19 times more energy (38 ATP molecules) from the same starting material (and it is much less smelly) (Fig. 4–6).

In addition to the efficient generation of ATP from glucose (and other carbohydrates), the TCA cycle represents a means by which carbons derived from **lipids** (in the form of acetyl CoA) may be shunted toward either energy production or the generation of biosynthetic precursors. Similarly, the cycle includes several points at which **deaminated amino acids** may enter (see Fig. 4–4). For example, deamination of glutamic acid yields α-ketoglutarate, whereas deamination of aspartic acid yields oxaloacetate, both of which are TCA cycle intermediates. The TCA cycle therefore serves the following functions:

1. It is the major mechanism for the generation of ATP.
2. It serves as the final common pathway for the complete oxidation of amino acids, fatty acids, and carbohydrates.
3. It supplies key intermediates (i.e., α-ketoglutarate, succinyl CoA, oxaloacetate) for the ultimate synthesis of amino acids (Fig. 4–7), lipids, purines, and pyrimidines.

The last two functions make the TCA cycle a so-called **amphibolic cycle** (i.e., it may function in the anabolic and the catabolic functions of the cell).

Pentose Phosphate Pathway

The final pathway of glucose metabolism considered here is known as the pentose phosphate pathway, or the **hexose monophosphate shunt** (Fig. 4–8). The function of this pathway is to provide precursors and reducing power in the form of nicotinamide-adenine dinucleotide phosphate (reduced form) (**NADPH**) for use in biosynthesis. In the first half of the pathway, glucose is converted to ribulose-5-phosphate, with consumption of 1 mole of ATP and generation of 2 moles of NADPH per mole of glucose. The ribulose-5-phosphate may then be converted to ribose-5-phosphate (a precursor in nucleotide biosynthesis) or alternatively to xylulose-5-phosphate. The remaining reactions in the pathway use enzymes known as **transketolases** and **transaldolases** to generate various sugars, which may function as biosynthetic precursors or may be shunted back to the glycolytic pathway for use in energy generation.

Biosynthesis

We have thus far discussed primarily the catabolic pathways of the bacterial cell, pathways that result in the generation of ATP, NADH, NADPH, and various chemical intermediates. These products may be used for synthesizing major cellular constituents (i.e., peptidoglycan, lipopolysaccharide, proteins, nucleic acids).

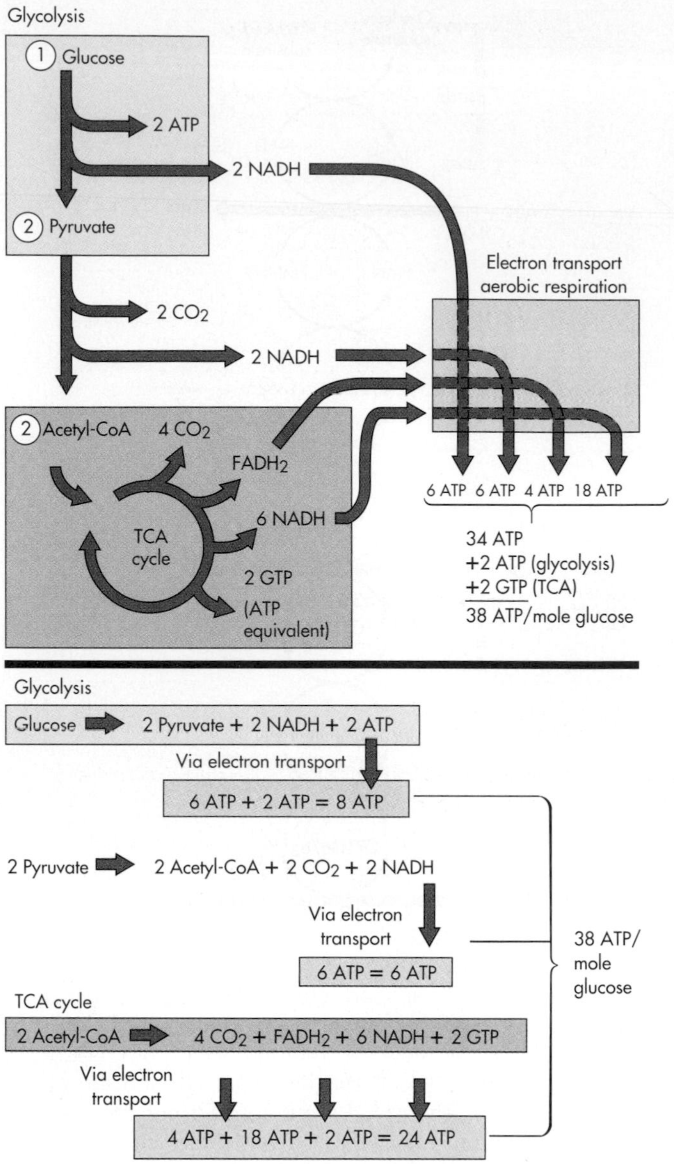

FIGURE 4–6. Aerobic glucose metabolism.

The following sections describe the important points of the synthesis of each macromolecule from component subunits. DNA and RNA are discussed more fully in Chapter 5.

Nucleic Acid Synthesis

As already discussed, nucleotides not only serve as components of DNA and RNA but also are crucial in the biosynthetic reactions in the growing cell by serving as activators of precursors in the synthesis of polysaccharides, including lipopolysaccharide and peptidoglycan. In addition, nucleotides serve as a usable form of metabolic energy.

The synthesis of the purine nucleotides (adenosine monophosphate and guanosine monophosphate) begins with ribose-5-phosphate formed as a product of the pentose monophosphate shunt. The bicyclic purine ring system is constructed in a stepwise fashion on the sugar phosphate moiety. The product of this series of reactions is the purine nucleotide, inosine monophosphate, which may then be converted to guanosine or adenosine monophosphate. In contrast, the pyrimidine nucleotides are produced by the synthesis of the pyrimidine orotate, which is then attached to the ribose phosphate, forming orotidine monophosphate. This nucleotide may then be converted to cytidine monophosphate or uridine monophosphate. The corresponding deoxynucleotides for use in DNA are synthesized by direct reduction at the 2' carbon atom of the sugar portion of the ribonucleotide. Production of thymine, a unique nucleotide for DNA, requires the tetrahydrofolate pathway, which makes this pathway a target for antibiotic action.

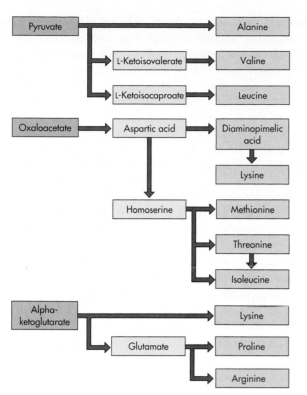

FIGURE 4–7. Examples of amino acids derived from the intermediates of the tricarboxylic acid cycle.

Transcription

The information carried in the genetic memory of the DNA is transcribed into a useful messenger RNA (mRNA) for subsequent translation into protein. RNA synthesis occurs in a manner similar to that of DNA replication, using a specific **DNA-dependent RNA polymerase.**

The process begins when **sigma factor** recognizes a particular sequence of nucleotides in the DNA (the **promoter;** see Chapter 5) and binds tightly to this site. Promoter sequences occur just before the start of the DNA that actually encodes a protein. Sigma factors bind to these promoters to provide a docking site for the RNA polymerase. Some bacteria encode several sigma factors to allow transcription of a group of genes under special conditions such as heat shock, starvation, special nitrogen metabolism, or sporulation. Once the polymerase has bound to the appropriate site on the DNA, RNA synthesis proceeds with the sequential addition of ribonucleotides complementary to the sequence in the DNA. Once an entire gene or group of genes (**operon;** see Chapter 5) has been transcribed, the RNA polymerase dissociates from the DNA, a process mediated by signals within the DNA. The bacterial DNA-dependent RNA polymerase is inhibited by rifampin, an antibiotic often used in the treatment of tuberculosis. The transfer RNA (tRNA), which is used in protein synthesis, and ribosomal RNA (rRNA), a component of the ribosomes, are also transcribed from the DNA.

Translation

Translation is the process by which the **genetic code,** in the form of mRNA, is converted into a sequence of amino acids, the protein product. For the purposes of translation, the nucleotide sequence of the mRNA is divided into groups of three consecutive nucleotides.

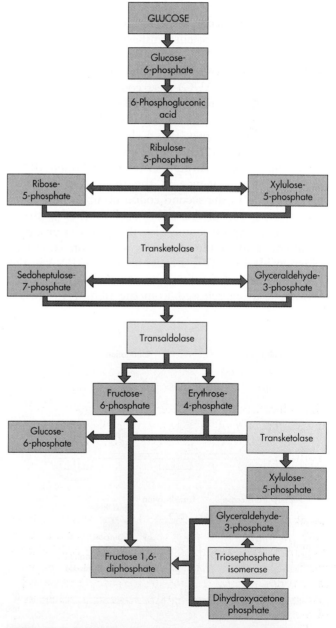

FIGURE 4–8. Pentose phosphate cycle or hexose monophosphate pathway. The enzymes transketolase and transaldolase are central to the cycle's activity.

Each set of three nucleotides is known as a **codon** and encodes a particular amino acid. Because there are four different nucleotides, 4^3, or 64, combinations of 3 are possible, each codon coding for only a single amino acid (or termination signal). However, because there are only 20 amino acids, each may be encoded by many triplet codons. This feature is known as the *degeneracy of the genetic code* and may function in protecting the cell from the effects of minor mutations in the DNA or mRNA. Each tRNA molecule contains a three-nucleotide sequence complementary to one of the codon sequences. This tRNA sequence is known as the **anticodon;** it allows base pairing and binds to the codon sequence on the mRNA. Attached to the opposite end of the tRNA is the amino acid that corresponds to the particular codon-anticodon pair.

The process of protein synthesis (Fig. 4–9) begins with the binding of the 30S ribosomal subunit and a special initiator tRNA for formyl methionine at the methionine codon (AUG) start codon to form the so-called **initiation complex.** The 50S ribosomal subunit binds to the complex to initiate mRNA synthesis. The ribosome contains two tRNA binding sites, the **A (aminoacyl) site** and the **P (peptidyl) site,** each of which allows base pairing between the bound tRNA and the codon sequence in the mRNA. The tRNA corresponding to the second codon occupies the A site. The amino group of the amino acid attached to the A site forms a peptide bond with the carboxyl group of the amino acid in the P site in a reaction known as **transpeptidation.** This process leaves the tRNA in the P site uncharged (without an attached amino acid), allowing it to be released from the ribosome. The ribosome then moves down the mRNA exactly three nucleotides, thereby transferring the tRNA with attached nascent peptide to the P site and bringing the next codon into the A site. The appropriate charged tRNA is brought into the A site, and the process is then repeated. Translation continues until the new codon in the A site is one of the three termination codons, for which there is no corresponding tRNA. At that point, the new protein is released to the cytoplasm and the translation complex may be disassembled, or the ribosome shuffles to the next start codon and starts a new protein. The 80S eukaryotic ribosome cannot start a new protein while still attached to the mRNA. This has implications for the synthesis of proteins for some viruses.

The process of protein synthesis represents an important target of antimicrobial action. The aminoglycosides (e.g., streptomycin and gentamicin), as well as the tetracyclines, act by binding to the small ribosomal subunit and inhibiting normal ribosomal function. Similarly, the macrolide and lincosamide groups of antibiotics (e.g., erythromycin and clindamycin) act by binding to the large ribosomal subunit.

Bacterial Growth

Bacterial replication is a coordinated process in which two equivalent daughter cells are produced. For growth to occur, there must be sufficient metabolites to support the synthesis of the bacterial components and especially the nucleotides for DNA synthesis. A cascade of regulatory events (synthesis of key proteins and RNA), much like a countdown at the Kennedy Space

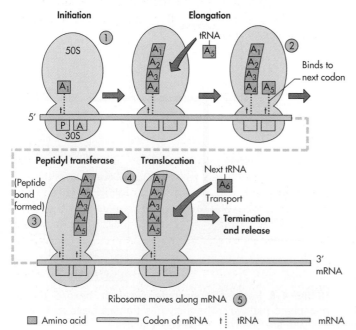

FIGURE 4–9. Bacterial protein synthesis. 1, Binding of the 30S subunit to the messenger RNA (mRNA) with the formylmethionine transfer RNA (fmet-tRNA) at the AUG start codon allows assembly of the 70S ribosome. The fmet-tRNA binds to the peptidyl site (P). 2, The next tRNA binds to its codon at the A site and, 3, "accepts" the growing peptide chain. 4, Before translocation to the peptidyl site. The process is repeated until a stop codon and the protein are released.

Center, must occur on schedule to initiate a replication cycle. *However, once it is initiated, DNA synthesis must run to completion, even if all nutrients have been removed from the medium.*

Chromosome replication is initiated at the membrane, and each daughter chromosome is anchored to a different portion of membrane. In some cells, the DNA associates with mesosomes. As the bacterial membrane grows, the daughter chromosomes are pulled apart. Commencement of chromosome replication also initiates the process of cell division, which can be visualized by the start of septum formation between the two daughter cells (Fig. 4–10; see also Chapter 3). New initiation events may occur before completion of chromosome replication and cell division.

Depletion of metabolites (starvation) or a buildup of toxic byproducts (e.g., ethanol) triggers the production of chemical **alarmones,** which cause synthesis to stop, but degradative processes continue. DNA synthesis continues until all initiated chromosomes are completed, despite the detrimental effect on the cell. Ribosomes are cannibalized for deoxyribonucleotide precursors, peptidoglycan and proteins are degraded for metabolites, and the cell shrinks. Septum formation may be initiated, but cell division may not occur. Many

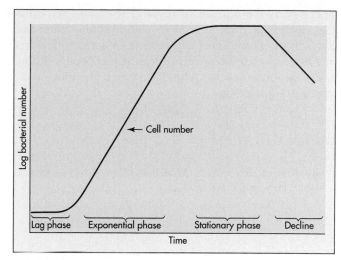

FIGURE 4–11. Phases of bacterial growth, starting with an inoculum of stationary-phase cells.

cells die. Similar signals may initiate **sporulation** in species capable of this process (see Chapter 3).

Population Dynamics

When bacteria are added to a medium, they require time to adapt to the new environment before they begin dividing (Fig. 4–11). This hiatus is known as the **lag phase** of growth. The bacteria will grow and divide at a **doubling time** characteristic of the strain and determined by the conditions during the **log or exponential phase.** During the log phase, the number of bacteria will increase to 2^n, in which n is the number of generations (doublings). The culture eventually runs out of metabolites, or a toxic substance builds up in the medium; the bacteria then stop growing and enter the **stationary phase.**

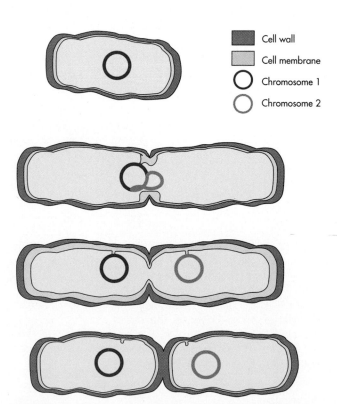

FIGURE 4–10. Bacterial cell division. Replication requires extension of the cell wall as well as replication of the chromosome and septum formation. Membrane attachment of the DNA pulls each daughter strand into a new cell.

■	Cell wall
▨	Cell membrane
○	Chromosome 1
○	Chromosome 2

QUESTIONS

1. How many moles of ATP are generated per mole of glucose in glycolysis, the TCA cycle, and electron transport? Which of these occur in anaerobic and which in aerobic conditions? Which is most efficient?

2. What products of anaerobic fermentation would be detrimental to host (human) tissue (e.g., *C. perfringens*)?

3. If the number of bacteria during log phase growth can be calculated by the following equation:

$$N_t = N_0 \times 2^{t/d}$$

where N_t is the number of bacteria after time (t), t/d is the amount of time divided by the doubling time, and N_0 is the initial number of bacteria, how many bacteria will be in the culture after 4 hours if the doubling time is 20 minutes and the initial bacterial inoculum contained 1000 bacteria?

BIBLIOGRAPHY

Davis BD et al, editors: *Microbiology*, ed 4, Philadelphia, 1990, JB Lippincott.

Jawetz E et al: *Review of medical microbiology*, ed 16, Los Altos, Calif, 1984, Lange.

Lehninger AL: *Principles of biochemistry*, New York, 1982, Worth.

Mandell GL et al, editors: *Principles and practice of infectious diseases*, ed 3, New York, 1990, Churchill Livingstone.

Slots J, Taubman MA, editors: *Contemporary oral microbiology and immunology*, St Louis, 1992, Mosby.

C H A P T E R 5

Bacterial Genetics

DNA: The Genetic Material

The bacterial genome is the total collection of genes carried by a bacterium both on its chromosome and on its extrachromosomal genetic elements, if any. The bacterial chromosome differs in several ways from the human chromosome. The chromosome of a typical bacterium such as *Escherichia coli* is a single, double-stranded, circular molecule of DNA containing approximately 5 million base pairs (or 5000 kilobase [kb] pairs), an approximate length of 1.3 mm (i.e., about 1000 times the diameter of the cell). The smallest bacterial chromosomes (from mycoplasmas) are about one-quarter this size. In comparison, humans have two copies of 23 chromosomes, which represent 2.9×10^9 base pairs 990 mm in length. Each genome contains many **operons,** which are made up of **genes.** Eukaryotes usually have two distinct copies of each chromosome (they are therefore diploid). Bacteria usually have only one copy of their chromosomes (they are therefore **haploid**). Because bacteria have only one chromosome, alteration of a gene (mutation) will have a more obvious effect on the cell. In addition, the structure of the bacterial chromosome is maintained by polyamines, such as spermine and spermidine, rather than by histones.

Bacteria may also contain **extrachromosomal genetic elements** such as **plasmids** or **bacteriophages** (bacterial viruses). These elements are independent of the bacterial chromosome and in most cases can be transmitted from one cell to another.

Genes are sequences of nucleotides that have a biologic function; examples are protein-structural genes (**cistrons,** which are coding genes), ribosomal RNA genes, and recognition and binding sites for other molecules (promoters and operators). **Promoters and operators** are nucleotide sequences that control the expression of a gene by influencing which sequences will be transcribed into messenger RNA (mRNA) (more discussion follows).

Operons are groups of one or more structural genes expressed from a particular promoter and ending at a transcriptional terminator. Thus, all the genes coding for the enzymes of a particular pathway can be coordinately regulated. Operons with many structural genes are **polycistronic.** The *E. coli lac* operon includes all the genes necessary for lactose metabolism, as well as the control mechanisms for turning off (in the presence of glucose) or turning on (in the presence of galactose or an inducer) these genes only when they are needed. The *lac* operon includes a repressor sequence, a promoter sequence and structural genes for the β-galactosidase enzyme, a permease, and an acetylase (Fig. 5–1). The *lac* operon is discussed later in this chapter.

Replication of DNA

The bacterial chromosome is a storehouse of information by which the characteristics of the cell are defined and by which all cellular processes are carried out. It is therefore essential that this molecule be duplicated without errors. Replication of the bacterial genome is triggered by a cascade of events linked to the growth rate of the cell. Replication of bacterial DNA is initiated at a specific sequence in the chromosome called OriC. The replication process requires an enzyme **(helicase)** to unwind the DNA at the origin to expose the DNA, an enzyme **(primase)** to synthesize primers to start the process, the enzyme or enzymes **(DNA-dependent DNA polymerases)** that copy the DNA but only in the 5' to 3' direction, and other enzymes.

New DNA is synthesized **semiconservatively,** using both strands of the parental DNA as templates. New DNA synthesis occurs at **growing forks** and proceeds **bidirectionally.** One strand (the leading strand) is copied continuously in the 5' to 3' direction, whereas the other strand (the lagging strand) must be synthesized as many pieces of DNA using RNA primers (Okazaki's fragments). The lagging strand DNA must be extended in the 5' to 3' direction as its template becomes available. Then the pieces are ligated together by the enzyme DNA ligase (Fig. 5–2). To maintain the high degree of accuracy required for replication, the DNA polymerases possess "proofreading" functions, which

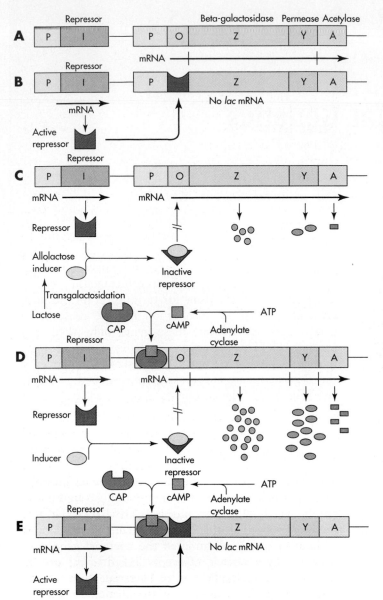

FIGURE 5–1. *A,* The lactose operon is transcribed as a polycistronic messenger RNA (mRNA) from the promoter (P) and translated into three proteins: *β*-galactosidase (Z), permease (Y), and acetylase (A). The *lac I* gene encodes the repressor protein. *B,* The lactose operon is not transcribed in the absence of an allolactose inducer, because the repressor competes with the RNA polymerase at the operator site (O). *C,* The repressor, complexed with the inducer, does not recognize the operator because of a conformation change in the repressor. The *lac* operon is thus transcribed at a low level. *D, Escherichia coli* is grown in a poor medium in the presence of lactose as the carbon source. Both the inducer and the CAP-cAMP complex are bound to the promoter, which is fully "turned on," and a high level of *lac* mRNA is transcribed and translated *E,* Growth of *E. coli* in a poor medium without lactose results in the binding of the CAP-cAMP complex to the promoter region and binding of the active repressor to the operator sequence, because no inducer is available. The result will be that the *lac* operon will not be transcribed. CAP = catabolite gene-activator protein; cAMP = cyclic adenosine monophosphate; ATP = adenosine triphosphate.

allow the enzyme to confirm that the appropriate nucleotide was inserted and to correct any errors that were made. During log-phase growth in rich medium, many initiations of chromosomal replication may occur before cell division. This process produces a series of nested bubbles of new daughter chromosomes, each with its pair of growth forks of new DNA synthesis. The polymerase moves down the DNA strand, incorporating the appropriate (complementary) nucleotide at each position. Replication is complete when the two replication forks meet 180 degrees from the origin. The process of DNA replication puts great torsional strain on the chromosomal circle of DNA; this strain is relieved by **topoisomerases** (e.g., gyrase). The topoisomerase is essential to the bacteria and is a target for the quinolone antibiotics.

Transcriptional Control

Regulation of Gene Expression

Bacteria have developed mechanisms to adapt quickly and efficiently to changes in concentrations of nutrients in their environment. The bacteria turn on a complete set of enzymes when necessary and avoid making the enzyme or enzymes of a pathway when the substrate is absent.

First, the organization of the genes of a biochemical pathway into an **operon,** with appropriate genetic control mechanisms, allows coordinated production of the necessary enzymes in response to a nutritional stimulus. Second, the transcription of the gene is regulated directly by repressor proteins (which bind to operators) in response to nutritional signals within the cell. Third,

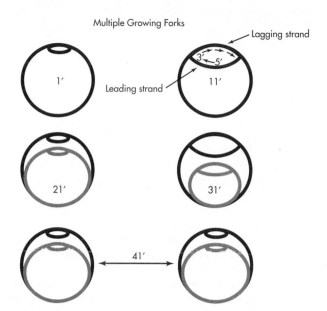

Multiple Growing Forks

Lagging strand

Leading strand

FIGURE 5–2. Assuming 40 minutes to complete one round of replication and assuming new initiation every 20 minutes, initiation of DNA synthesis precedes cell division. Multiple growing forks may be initiated in a cell before complete septum formation and cell division. The daughter cells are "born pregnant."

the rate of protein synthesis by the ribosome can regulate transcription in prokaryotes. The absence of a nuclear membrane in prokaryotes to separate the two processes allows the ribosome to bind to the mRNA as it is being transcribed from the DNA.

Transcriptional Regulation

Initiation of transcription may be under positive or negative control. Genes under **negative control** are expressed unless they are switched off by a **repressor protein.** This repressor protein prevents gene expression by binding to a specific DNA sequence, called the **operator,** making it impossible for the RNA polymerase to initiate transcription at the promoter. Inversely, genes whose expression is under **positive control** are not transcribed unless an active regulator protein, called an **apoinducer,** is present. The apoinducer binds to a specific DNA sequence and assists the RNA polymerase in the initiation steps by an unknown mechanism.

Operons can be **inducible or repressible.** Introduction of a substrate **(inducer)** into the growth medium may induce an operon to increase the expression of the enzymes necessary for its metabolism. The end products **(co-repressors)** of a pathway may signal that a pathway should be shut down or repressed by reducing the synthesis of its enzymes.

The lactose *(lac)* operon responsible for the degra-

dation of the sugar lactose is an inducible operon under positive and negative regulation (see Fig. 5–1). Normally the bacteria use glucose and not lactose. In the absence of lactose, the operon is repressed by the binding of the repressor protein to the operator sequence, thus impeding the RNA polymerase function. In the absence of glucose, however, the addition of lactose reverses this repression. Full expression of the *lac* operon also requires a protein-mediated, positive-control mechanism. In *E. coli,* a protein called the catabolite gene-activator protein (CAP) forms a complex with cyclic adenosine monophosphate (cAMP), acquiring the ability to bind to a specific DNA sequence present in the promoter. The CAP-cAMP complex enhances binding of the RNA polymerase to the promoter, thus allowing an increase in the frequency of transcription initiation. The CAP-cAMP complex may increase the operon transcription by protein-protein interaction with the RNA polymerase or by protein-DNA interaction.

The tryptophan operon **(trp operon)** contains the structural genes necessary for tryptophan biosynthesis and is under dual transcriptional control mechanisms (Fig. 5–3). Although tryptophan is essential for protein synthesis, too much tryptophan in the cell can be toxic; therefore, its synthesis must be regulated. At the DNA level, the repressor protein is activated by an increased intracellular concentration of tryptophan to prevent transcription. At the protein synthesis level, rapid translation of a "test peptide" at the beginning of the mRNA in the presence of tryptophan promotes the formation of a double-stranded loop in the RNA, which terminates transcription. The same loop is formed if no protein synthesis is occurring, a situation in which tryptophan synthesis would similarly not be required. This regulates tryptophan synthesis at the mRNA level in a process termed **attenuation,** in which mRNA synthesis is prematurely terminated.

Post-transcriptional or Translational Regulation

The rate and efficiency of protein synthesis can be controlled by other factors. These may include the structure of the mRNA or the concentrations of transfer RNA (tRNA) and amino acids in the cell. With polycistronic mRNAs, translational control may result in differences in the quantity of each protein expressed from each gene. For example, for the *lac* operon, β-galactosidase, galactoside permease, and acetylase are produced at a ratio of 10:5:2.

Mutation, Repair, and Recombination

DNA conveys genetic information; therefore, cells must be able to replicate DNA accurately. Further-

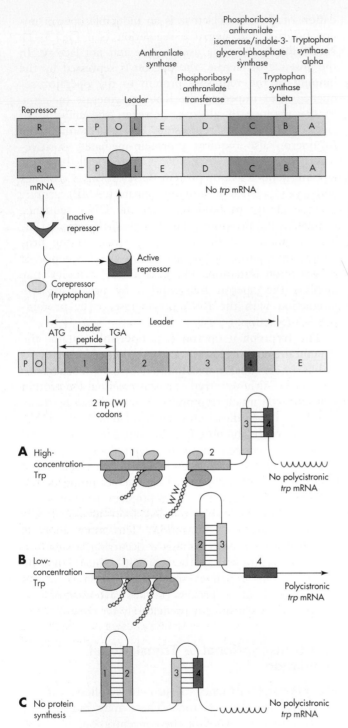

FIGURE 5–3. Regulation of the tryptophan *(trp)* operon. *A,* The *trp* operon encodes the five enzymes necessary for tryptophan biosynthesis. This *trp* operon is under dual control. *B,* The conformation of the inactive repressor protein is changed after its binding by the co-repressor tryptophan. The resulting active repressor (R) binds to the operator (O), blocking any transcription of the *trp* mRNA by the RNA polymerase. *C,* The *trp* operon is also under the control of an attenuation-antitermination mechanism. Upstream of the structural genes are the promoter (P), the operator, and a leader (L), which can be transcribed into a short peptide containing two tryptophans (W), near its distal end. The leader mRNA possesses four repeats (1, 2, 3, and 4), which can pair differently according to the tryptophan availability, leading to an early termination of transcription of the *trp* operon or its full transcription. In the presence of a high concentration of tryptophan, regions 3 and 4 of the leader mRNA can pair, forming a terminator hairpin, and no transcription of the *trp* operon occurs. However, in the presence of little or no tryptophan, the ribosomes stall in region 1 when translating the leader peptide because of the tandem of tryptophan codons. Then regions 2 and 3 can pair, forming the antiterminator hairpin and leading to transcription of the *trp* genes. Finally, the regions 1:2 and 3:4 of the free leader mRNA can pair, also leading to cessation of transcription before the first structural gene *trpE.* A = adenine; G = guanine; T = thymine.

more, accidental damage to DNA must be minimized by the elaboration of efficient DNA repair systems. These damage-containment systems are so important for the life of a cell that a bacterium may devote a large percentage of its genome to specify and control the enzymes involved.

Mutations Affecting the DNA

A mutation is any change in the base sequence of the DNA. A single base change can result in a **transition,** in which one purine is replaced by another purine or in which a pyrimidine is replaced by another pyrimidine. A **transversion,** in which, for example, a purine is replaced by a pyrimidine and vice versa, may also result. A **silent mutation** is a change at the DNA level that does not result in any change of amino acid in the encoded protein. This type of mutation occurs because more than one codon may encode an amino acid. A **missense mutation** results in a different amino acid being inserted in the protein, but this may be a **conservative mutation** if the new amino acid has similar properties (e.g., valine replacing alanine). Finally, a **nonsense mutation** changes a codon encoding an amino acid to a stop codon (e.g., TAG [thymidine-adenine-guanine]), which will cause the ribosome to fall off the mRNA and end the protein prematurely.

More drastic changes can occur in proteins when numerous bases are involved. For example, a small deletion or insertion that *is not in multiples of three* produces a **frameshift mutation.** This results in a change in the reading frame, usually leading to a nonsense peptide and premature truncation of the protein. **Null mutations,** which completely destroy gene function, arise when there is an extensive insertion, deletion, or gross rearrangement of the chromosome structure. Insertion of long sequences of DNA (many thousands of base pairs) by recombination, by transposition, or during genetic engineering can produce **null mutations** by separating the parts of a gene and inactivating the gene.

Many mutations occur spontaneously in nature (e.g., by polymerase mistakes); however, mutations can also be induced by physical or chemical agents. Among the physical agents used to induce mutations in bacteria are heat, which results in deamination of nucleotides; ultraviolet light, which causes pyrimidine dimer formation; and ionizing radiation, such as x-rays, which produce very reactive hydroxyl radicals that may be responsible for opening a ring of a base or causing single- or double-stranded breaks in the DNA.

Chemicals that are mutagens can be grouped into three classes. The first class is **nucleotide-base analogues;** they are incorporated into the DNA during replication and lead to mispairing and frequent mistakes during DNA replication. The similarity of 5-bromouracil to thymidine allows the former's incorporation into DNA. However, a structural rearrangement of the molecule allows 5-bromouracil to bind to guanine instead of adenine, changing a T-A base pair to a G-C base pair.

The second class is polycyclic flat molecules, such as ethidium bromide or acridine derivatives; they are examples of **frameshift mutagens.** They insert (or intercalate) between the bases as they stack with each other in the double helix and cause the addition or deletion of a single base. These intercalating agents increase the spacing of successive base pairs, destroying the regular

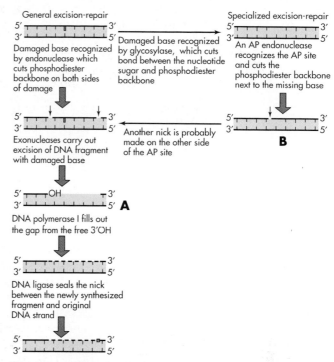

FIGURE 5–4. *A,* Generalized excision repair mechanism. *B,* Specialized excision repair mechanism. AP = apurinic (endonuclease).

sugar-phosphate backbone and decreasing the pitch of the helix. These changes lead to frequent mistakes during DNA replication.

The third class is **DNA-reactive chemicals;** they act directly on the DNA, resulting in a modification of the normal base into a chemically different structure. The modified bases may pair abnormally or may not pair at all. The damage may cause the removal of the base from the DNA backbone. These include nitrous acid (HNO_2) and alkylating agents, including nitrosoguanidine and ethyl methane sulfonate, which are known to add methyl or ethyl groups to the rings of the DNA bases.

Repair Mechanisms of DNA

A number of repair mechanisms have evolved in bacterial cells to minimize damage to DNA. These repair mechanisms can be divided into five groups:

1. **Direct DNA repair** is the enzymatic removal of damage, such as pyrimidine dimers and alkylated bases.
2. **Excision repair** is the excision of a DNA segment containing the damage, followed by synthesis of a new DNA strand (Fig. 5–4). Two types of excision-repair mechanisms, generalized and specialized, exist.

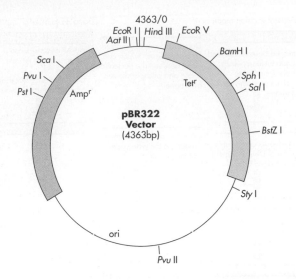

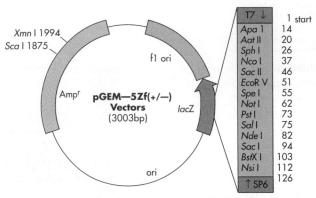

FIGURE 5–5. Plasmids. The pBR322 plasmid is one of the plasmids used for cloning DNA. This plasmid encodes resistance to ampicillin (Amp) and tetracycline (Tet) and an origin of replication (ori). The multiple cloning site in the pGEM plasmid provides different restriction enzyme cleavage sites for insertion of DNA within the β-galactosidase gene (*lacZ*). This is flanked by bacteriophage promoters to allow directional messenger RNA expression of the cloned sequence.

3. Recombinational or **postreplication repair** is the retrieval of missing information by genetic recombination when both DNA strands are damaged.
4. The **SOS response** is the induction of many genes (approximately 15) after DNA damage or interruption of DNA replication.
5. **Error-prone repair** is the last resort of a bacterial cell before it dies. It is used to fill in gaps when a DNA template is not available for directing an accurate repair.

Gene Exchange in Prokaryotic Cells

Many bacteria, especially many pathogenic bacterial species, are promiscuous with their DNA. The ex-

change of DNA between cells allows the exchange of genes and characteristics between cells, thus producing new strains of bacteria. This exchange may be advantageous for the recipient, especially if the exchanged DNA encodes antibiotic resistance. The transferred DNA can be integrated into the recipient chromosome or stably maintained as an extrachromosomal element **(plasmid)** or a bacterial virus **(bacteriophage)** and passed on to daughter bacteria as an autonomously replicating unit.

Plasmids are small genetic elements that replicate independently of the bacterial chromosome. Most plasmids are circular, double-stranded DNA molecules varying from 1500 to 400,000 base pairs. However, *Borrelia burgdorferi*, the causative agent of Lyme disease, and the related *Borrelia hermsii* are unique among all eubacteria because they possess linear plasmids. Like the bacterial chromosomal DNA, they can autonomously replicate and as such are referred to as **replicons.** Some plasmids, such as the *E. coli* F plasmid, are **episomes,** which means that they can integrate into the host chromosome.

Plasmids carry genetic information, which may not be essential but can provide a selective advantage to the bacteria. For example, plasmids may confer high levels of antibiotic resistance, encode the production of bacteriocins or toxins, and contain genes that may provide the bacteria with a unique advantage in metabolizing some substrates (Fig. 5–5). The number of copies of plasmid produced by a cell is determined by the particular plasmid. The copy number is the ratio of copies of the plasmid to the number of copies of the chromosome. This may be as few as 1 in the case of large plasmids or as many as 50 in smaller plasmids.

Large plasmids (20 to 120 kb), such as the **fertility factor F** found in *E. coli* or the resistance transfer factor (80 kb), can often mediate their own transfer from one cell to another by a process called **conjugation** (see the later section on conjugation). These conjugative plasmids encode all the necessary factors for their transfer. Other plasmids can be transferred into a bacterial cell by means other than conjugation, such as transformation or transduction. These terms are discussed later in the chapter.

Bacteriophages are bacterial viruses. These extrachromosomal genetic elements can survive outside of a host cell because the nucleic acid genome (which may be DNA or RNA) is protected by a protein coat (Fig. 5–6).

Bacteriophages infect bacterial cells and either repli-

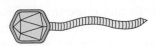

FIGURE 5–6. Bacteriophage λ.

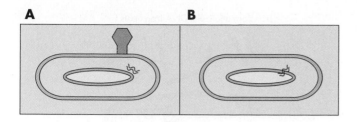

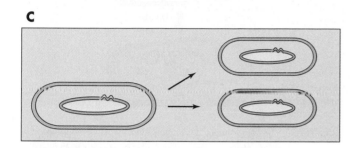

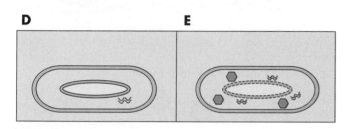

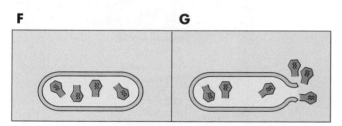

FIGURE 5–7. Lysogenic infection of bacterium with temperate bacteriophage. *A,* The phage infects a sensitive bacterium, and the phage DNA is injected. *B,* The phage DNA becomes integrated into the bacterial chromosome. *C,* The bacterium multiplies, apparently unaffected by the infection. It has been lysogenized. *D,* Occasionally the phage DNA is excised from the bacterial chromosome, takes control of the cell, and replicates. *E,* An individual cell (or, by induction, all the cells) produces phage components. *F,* The components are then later assembled into phage particles. *G,* Ultimately the cell lyses and releases mature phage particles.

cate to large numbers and cause the cell to lyse **(lytic infection)** or in some cases integrate into the host genome without killing the host (the **lysogenic state**), such as the *E. coli* bacteriophage λ (Fig. 5–7). Some lysogenic bacteriophages carry toxin genes (e.g., corynephage β carries the gene for the diphtheria toxin). Bacteriophage λ remains lysogenic as long as a repres-

sor protein is synthesized and prevents the phage from becoming unintegrated and replicating independently of the host chromosome. This reaction can be triggered if the host cell DNA is damaged by radiation or by another means or if the cell can no longer make the repressor protein, a signal that the host cell is unhealthy and is no longer a good place for "freeloading."

Transposons are mobile genetic elements (Fig. 5–8) that can move from one position to another in the genome or between different molecules of DNA. The simplest transposons are called insertion sequences. Complex transposons carry other genes, such as genes that provide resistance against antibiotics. Transposons sometimes insert into genes and inactivate those genes. If insertion and inactivation occur in a gene that encodes an essential protein, the cell dies.

Some pathogenic bacteria use a similar mechanism

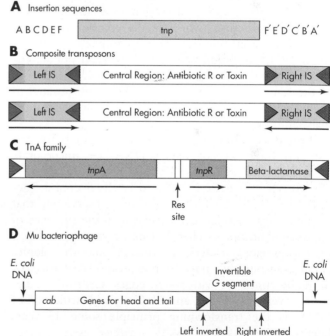

FIGURE 5–8. Transposons. *A,* The insertion sequences code only for a transposase (*tnp*) and possess inverted repeats (15 to 40 base pairs) at each end. *B,* The composite transposons contain a central-region coding for antibiotic resistances or toxins, flanked by two insertion sequences (IS), which can be either directly repeated or reversed. *C,* Tn3, a member of the TnA transposon family. The central region encodes three genes—a transposase (tnpA), a resolvase (tnpR), and a β-lactamase—conferring resistance to ampicillin. A resolution site (Res site) is used during the replicative transposition process. This central region is flanked on both ends by direct repeats of 38 base pairs. *D,* Phage-associated transposon is exemplified by the bacteriophage μ.

to coordinate the expression of a system of virulence factors. The genes for the activity may be grouped together in a **pathogenicity or virulence island,** which is surrounded by transposon-like mobile elements allowing them to move within the chromosome and to other bacteria. The entire genetic unit can be triggered by an environmental stimulus (e.g., pH, heat, contact with the host cell surface) as a way to coordinate the expression of a complex process. For example, the SPI-1 island of *Salmonella* encodes 25 genes that allow the bacteria to enter nonphagocytic cells.

Mechanisms of Genetic Transfer

The exchange of genetic material between bacterial cells may occur by one of three mechanisms: (1) **conjugation,** which is the mating or quasisexual exchange of genetic information from one bacterium (the donor) to another bacterium (the recipient); (2) **transformation,** which results in acquisition of new genetic markers by the incorporation of exogenous or foreign DNA; or (3) **transduction,** which is the transfer of genetic information from one bacterium to another by a bacteriophage. Conjugation occurs with most, if not all, eubacteria. Conjugation usually occurs between members of the same species but has also been demonstrated to occur between prokaryotes and cells from plants, animals, and fungi.

Transformation is the process by which bacteria take up fragments of naked DNA and incorporate them into their genomes. Transformation was the first mechanism of genetic transfer to be discovered in bacteria. In 1928, Griffith made the observation that pneumococcus virulence was related to the presence of a surrounding polysaccharide capsule and that extracts of encapsulated bacteria producing smooth colonies could transmit this trait to nonencapsulated bacteria, normally appearing with rough edges. Griffith's studies led to Avery, MacLeod, and McCarty's identification of DNA as the transforming principle some 15 years later.

Gram-positive and gram-negative bacteria can take up and stably maintain exogenous DNA (Fig. 5–9). Certain species are naturally capable of taking up exogenous DNA (such species are then said to be competent), including *Haemophilus influenzae, Streptococcus pneumoniae, Bacillus* species, and *Neisseria* species. Competence develops toward the end of logarithmic growth, some time before a population enters the stationary phase. Most bacteria do not exhibit a natural ability for DNA uptake. Chemical methods or electroporation (the use of high-voltage pulses) is used to introduce plasmid and other DNA into *E. coli* and other bacteria.

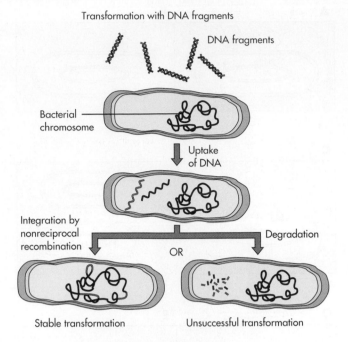

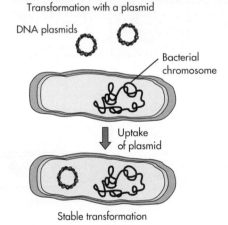

FIGURE 5–9. Bacterial transformation. Foreign DNA can be taken up or forced into bacteria and incorporated into the chromosome or maintained as a plasmid. This "transforms" the bacterium into a new organism.

Conjugation

Genetic transfer in *E. coli* was first reported by Lederberg and Tatum in 1946, when they observed sexlike exchange between two mutant strains of *E. coli* K12. Conjugation is the process by which DNA is passed directly by cell-to-cell contact during the mating of the bacteria. Conjugation results in one-way transfer of DNA from a donor (or male) cell to a recipient (or female) cell through the **sex pilus.** The mating type (sex) of the cell depends on the presence (male) or absence (female) of a conjugative plasmid, such as the

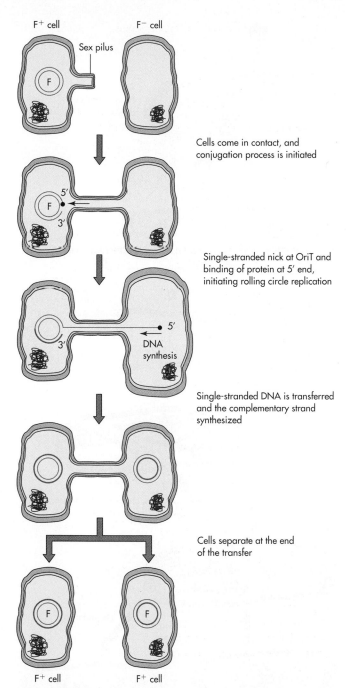

FIGURE 5–10. Genetic transfer of the F plasmid by conjugation.

F⁺ cell   F⁻ cell

Sex pilus

Cells come in contact, and conjugation process is initiated

Single-stranded nick at OriT and binding of protein at 5′ end, initiating rolling circle replication

DNA synthesis

Single-stranded DNA is transferred and the complementary strand synthesized

Cells separate at the end of the transfer

F⁺ cell   F⁺ cell

F plasmid of *E. coli*. The F plasmid is defined as conjugative because it carries all the genes necessary for its own transfer including the ability to make sex pili and to initiate DNA synthesis at the transfer origin (OriT) of the plasmid. In addition to *E. coli*, conjugation occurs for bacteroides, streptococci, streptomyces, and clostridia. Many of the large conjugative plasmids specify colicins or antibiotic resistance.

The F plasmid transfers itself, converting recipients into F⁺ male cells (Fig. 5–10). If a fragment of chromosomal DNA has been incorporated into the plasmid, it is designated an F prime (F′) plasmid. When it transfers into the recipient cell, it carries that fragment with it and converts it into an F′ male. If the F plasmid sequence is integrated into the bacterial chromosome, the cell is designated an Hfr cell. Hfr stands for high frequency of recombination.

The DNA that is transferred by conjugation is not a double helix but a single-stranded molecule. Mobilization begins when a plasmid-encoded protein makes a single-stranded, site-specific cleavage at the OriT. The nick initiates rolling circle replication, and the displaced linear strand is directed to the recipient cell. The transferred, single-stranded DNA is recircularized and its complementary strand synthesized.

An important property of the F plasmid is its ability to integrate into the bacterial chromosome, generating an Hfr cell. Such integration of the F plasmid involves breakage and rejoining of both molecules of DNA. In Hfr cells, the genes involved in mobilization and transfer are still expressed. Thus, conjugation can still be initiated by a nick at the OriT site within the chromosome to transfer a part of the plasmid sequence followed by chromosomal DNA and sometimes, but only rarely, the remainder of the F plasmid at the other end of the chromosome. It would take 100 minutes at 37°C to transfer the complete male genome to the female recipient. However, the fragile connection between the mating pairs is usually broken and the transfer aborted before being completed, explaining why only the chromosomal sequences adjacent to the integrated F are usually transferred. Artificial interruption of a mating between an Hfr and an F⁻ pair has been helpful in constructing a consistent map of the *E. coli* chromosomal DNA. In such maps, the position of each gene is given in minutes according to its time of entry into a recipient cell in relation to a fixed origin (Fig. 5–11).

Conjugative R (antibiotic resistance) plasmids have been found in gram-positive bacteria such as streptococci, streptomyces, and clostridia. Instead of using pili, the mating pair is brought together by the presence of an adhesin molecule on the surface of the donor cell.

Transduction

Genetic transfer by transduction is mediated by bacterial viruses (bacteriophages) (Fig. 5–12), which pick up fragments of DNA and package them into bacteriophage particles. The DNA is delivered to infected cells and becomes incorporated into the bacterial genomes. Transduction can be classified as **specialized** if the phages in question transfer particular genes (usually

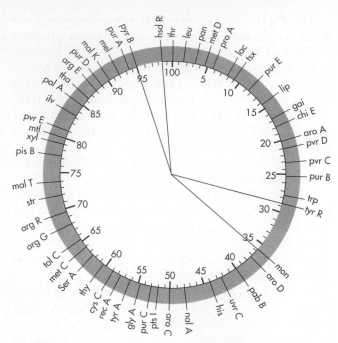

FIGURE 5–11. Chromosomal map of *Escherichia coli* genes. The time (minutes) to transfer DNA segments from the origin of the first Hfr strain is represented by the numbers. (Modified from Bachmann BJ, Low KB, Taylor AL: *Bacteriol Rev* 40:116–167, 1976.)

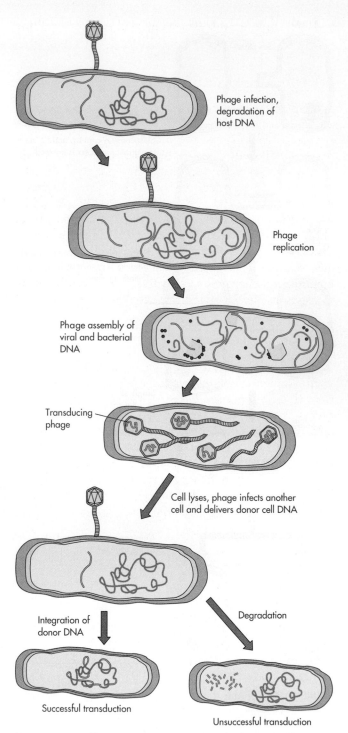

FIGURE 5–12. Transduction by bacteriophages. Bacteriophage infection can deliver genes into the target cell if the cell survives.

those adjacent to their integration sites in the genome) or **generalized** if the selection of the sequences is random because of accidental packaging of host DNA into the phage capsid.

Generalized transducing particles should contain primarily bacterial DNA and little or no phage DNA. For example, the P1 phage of *E. coli* encodes a nuclease that degrades the host *E. coli* chromosomal DNA. A small percentage of the resultant phage particles packages the DNA fragments into their capsids. The encapsulated DNA instead of phage DNA is injected into a new host cell, where it can recombine with the homologous host DNA. Generalized transducing particles are valuable in the **genetic mapping** of bacterial chromosomes. The closer two genes are within the bacterial chromosome, the more likely it is that they will be co-transduced.

Conjugative Transposons

Transposons can transfer DNA within a cell from one position to another in the genome or from the chromosomal DNA to a plasmid or the reverse. The transposons found in bacteria can be divided into three classes: insertion sequences, complex transposons, and phage-associated transposons. The **insertion-sequence** elements are the simplest transposons; they range in length from 150 to 1500 base pairs and possess inverted repeats of 15 to 40 base pairs at their ends (see Fig. 5–8). The insertion sequences carry only the genetic information necessary for their own transfer (i.e., the gene coding for the transposase). The insertion sequences can be detected if they insert into a gene and interrupt or inactivate the gene or turn on the expression of adjacent genes.

Recombination

Incorporation of the DNA into the chromosome occurs by recombination. There are two types of recombination: homologous and nonhomologous. **Homologous (legitimate) recombination** occurs between closely related DNA sequences and generally substitutes one sequence for another. The process requires a set of enzymes produced (in *E. coli*) by the *rec* genes. **Nonhomologous (illegitimate) recombination** occurs between dissimilar DNA sequences and generally produces insertions or deletions or both. This process usually requires specialized (sometimes site-specific) recombination enzymes, such as those produced by many transposons and lysogenic bacteriophages.

Genetic Engineering

Genetic engineering, also known as recombinant DNA technology, uses the techniques and tools developed by the bacterial geneticists to purify, amplify, modify, and express specific gene sequences. The use of genetic engineering and "cloning" has revolutionized biology and medicine. The basic tools of genetic engineering are (1) **cloning vectors,** which can be used to deliver the DNA sequences into receptive bacteria and amplify the desired sequence; (2) **restriction enzymes,** which are used to cleave DNA reproducibly at defined sequences (Table 5–1); and (3) **DNA ligase,** the enzyme that links the fragment to the cloning vector.

Cloning vectors must allow foreign DNA to be inserted into them but still must be able to replicate normally in the bacterial host. Many types of vectors are currently used. Plasmid vectors, such as pUC, pBR322, and pGEM (see Fig. 5–5), are used for DNA fragments up to 20 kb. Bacteriophages, such as λ, are used for larger fragments up to 25 kb. More recently, **cosmid** vectors have combined some of the advantages of plasmids and phages for fragments up to 45 kb.

Most cloning vectors have been "engineered" to have a site for insertion of foreign DNA; a means of selection, such as antibiotic resistance, for bacteria that have incorporated the vector; and a means of distinguishing the bacteria that have incorporated plasmids containing inserted DNA. Some plasmid vectors contain special sequences that aid in sequencing the cloned DNA or that promote expression of the gene or genes contained within the cloned DNA, either in prokaryotic or eukaryotic cells (e.g., prokaryote or eukaryote promoter sequences to precede the cloned DNA).

For cloning a foreign piece of DNA, both the vector and the DNA must be cleaved with restriction enzymes (Fig. 5–13). Restriction enzymes recognize a specific palindromic sequence and make a staggered cut, which generates sticky ends, or a blunt cut, which generates blunt ends (see Table 5–1). Most cloning vectors have a sequence that can be cleaved by many restriction enzymes, called the **multiple cloning site.** Ligation of the vector with the DNA fragments gener-

---

TABLE 5–1. Common Restriction Enzymes Used in Molecular Biology

Microorganism	Enzyme	Recognition Site
Acinetobacter calcoaceticus	AccI	⁵' G T ⎣(ᴬ/c) (ᴳ/ᴛ)⎤ A C C A (ᵀ/ᴳ) (c/ᴀ) ⎦T G
Bacillus amyloliquefaciens H	BamHI	⁵' G ⎣G A T C C C C T A G⎦ G
Escherichia coli RY13	EcoRI	⁵' G ⎣A A T T C C T T A A⎦ G
Haemophilus influenzae Rd	HindIII	⁵' A ⎣A G C T⎤ T T T C G A⎦ A
H. influenzae serotype c, 1160	HincII	⁵' G T (c/ᴛ) ⎪ (ᴳ/ᴀ) A C C A (ᴳ/ᴀ) ⎪ (c/ᴛ) T G
Providencia stuartii 164	PstI	⁵' C T G C A ⎤ G G ⎣A C G T C
Serratia marcescens	SmaI	⁵' C C C ⎪ G G G G G G ⎪ C C C
Staphylococcus aureus 3A	Sau3AI	⁵' ⎣G A T C C T A G⎦
Xanthomonas malvacearum	XmaI	⁵' C ⎣C C G G⎤ G G G G C C⎦ C

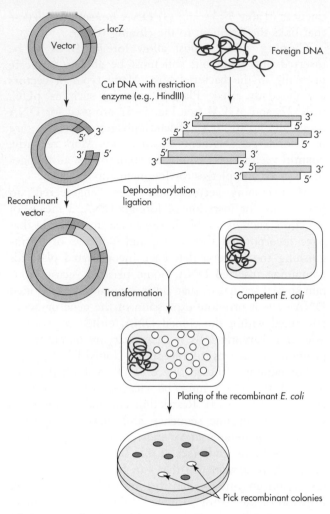

FIGURE 5–13. Cloning of foreign DNA in vectors. The vector and the foreign DNA are first digested by a restriction enzyme. Insertion of foreign DNA into the *lacZ* gene inactivates the β-galactosidase gene, allowing subsequent selection. The vector is then ligated to the foreign DNA, using bacteriophage T4 DNA ligase. The recombinant vectors are transformed into competent *Escherichia coli* cells. The recombinant *E. coli* cells are plated onto agar containing antibiotic, an inducer of the *lac* operon, and a chromophoric substrate that turns blue in cells having plasmid but not insert; but those cells with plasmid containing the insert remain white.

DNA. A **complementary DNA library** represents the genes that are expressed in a cell.

The recombinant DNA is then transformed into a bacterial host, usually *E. coli*, and the plasmid-containing bacteria are selected for antibiotic resistance (e.g., ampicillin resistance). The library can then be screened to find an *E. coli* clone possessing the desired DNA fragment. Various screening techniques can be used to identify the bacteria containing the appropriate recombinant DNA. The multiple cloning site used for inserting the foreign DNA is often part of the *lacZ* gene of the *lac* operon. Insertion of the foreign DNA into the *lacZ* gene inactivates the gene (acting almost like a transposon) and prevents the plasmid-directed synthesis of β-galactosidase in the recipient cell and also its cleavage of a chromophore to produce blue colonies. Recombinant plasmid-containing bacteria would produce normal white colonies.

Genetic engineering has been used to isolate and express the genes for useful proteins in bacteria, yeast, or even insect cells such as insulin, interferon, growth hormones, and interleukin. Large amounts of pure immunogen for a vaccine can be prepared without the need to work with the intact disease organisms.

The development of a vaccine against hepatitis B virus represents the first success of recombinant DNA vaccines approved for human use by the U.S. Food and Drug Administration. The hepatitis B surface antigen is produced by the yeast *Saccharomyces cerevisiae*. In the future, it may be sufficient to inject plasmid DNA capable of expressing the desired immunogen (DNA vaccine) into an individual to let the host cells express the immunogen and generate the immune response. Recombinant DNA technology has also become essential to laboratory diagnosis, forensic science, agriculture, and many other disciplines.

ates a molecule capable of replicating the inserted sequence called **recombinant DNA** (see Fig. 5–9). The total number of recombinant vectors obtained when cloning chromosomal DNA is known as a **genomic library** because there should be at least one representative of each gene in the library. An alternative approach to cloning the gene for a protein is to convert the mRNA for the protein into DNA using a retrovirus enzyme called reverse transcriptase (RNA-dependent DNA polymerase) to produce a complementary

---

QUESTIONS

1. What are the principal properties of a plasmid?
2. Give two mechanisms of regulation of bacterial gene expression. Use specific examples.
3. What types of mutations affect DNA and what agents are responsible for such mutations?
4. What mechanisms may be used by a bacterial cell for the exchange of genetic material? Briefly explain each mechanism.
5. Discuss the applications of molecular biotechnology to medicine, including contributions and uses in diagnosis.

BIBLIOGRAPHY

Alberts B et al: *Molecular biology of the cell*, ed 3, New York, 1994, Garland.

Cooper GM: *The cell: a molecular approach*, Washington, DC, 1997, American Society for Microbiology.

Lehninger AL, Nelson DL, Fox MM: *Principles of biochemistry*, ed 2, New York, 1993, Worth.

Lewin B: *Genes VI*, Oxford, England, 1997, Oxford University.

Lodish H et al: *Molecular cell biology*, ed 4, New York, 2000, WH Freeman.

Stryer L: *Biochemistry*, ed 4, New York, 1995, Freeman.

Voet D, Voet JG: *Biochemistry*, ed 2, New York, 1995, Wiley.

Watson JD et al: *Molecular biology of the gene*, ed 4, Menlo Park, Calif, 1987, Benjamin-Cummings.

CHAPTER 6

Viral Classification, Structure, and Replication

Viruses were first described as "filterable agents." Their small size allows them to pass through filters that are designed to retain bacteria. Unlike most bacteria, fungi, and parasites, **viruses are obligate intracellular parasites** that depend on the biochemical machinery of the host cell for replication. In addition, *reproduction of viruses occurs by assembly of the individual components rather than by binary fission* (Boxes 6–1 and 6–2).

The simplest viruses consist of a genome of DNA or RNA packaged in a protective shell of protein and, for some viruses, a membrane (Fig. 6–1). Viruses lack the capacity to make energy or substrates, cannot make their own proteins, and cannot replicate their genome independently of the host cell. To use the cell's biosynthetic machinery, the virus must be adapted to the biochemical rules of the cell.

The physical structure and genetics of viruses have been optimized by mutation and selection to infect humans and other hosts. To do this, the virus must be capable of transmission through potentially harsh environmental conditions, must traverse the skin or other protective barriers of the host, must be adapted to the biochemical machinery of the host cell for replication, and must escape elimination by the host immune response.

Knowledge of the structural (size and morphology) and genetic (type and structure of nucleic acid) features of a virus provides insight into how the virus replicates, spreads, and causes disease. The concepts presented in this chapter are repeated in greater detail in the discussions of specific viruses in later chapters.

Classification

Viruses range from the structurally simple and small parvoviruses and picornaviruses to the large and complex poxviruses and herpesviruses. Their names may describe viral characteristics, the diseases they are associated with, or even the tissue or geographic locale

where they were first identified. Names such as *picornavirus* (*pico*, "small"; *rna*, "ribonucleic acid") or *togavirus* (*toga*, Greek for "mantle," referring to a membrane envelope surrounding the virus) describe the structure of the virus, whereas the name *papovavirus* describes the members of its family (*pa*pilloma, *po*lyoma, and *va*cuolating viruses). The name *retrovirus* (*retro*, "reverse") refers to the virus-directed synthesis of DNA from an RNA template, whereas the *poxviruses* are named for the disease smallpox, caused by one of its members. The *adenoviruses* (*adeno*ids) and the *reoviruses* (*r*espiratory, *e*nteric, *o*rphan) are named for the body site from which they were first isolated. Reovirus was discovered before it was associated with a specific disease, and thus it was designated an "orphan" virus. Norwalk virus is named for Norwalk, Ohio; coxsackievirus is named for Coxsackie, New York; and many of the togaviruses, arenaviruses, and bunyaviruses are named after African places where they were first isolated.

Viruses can be grouped by characteristics such as disease (e.g., hepatitis), target tissue, means of transmission (e.g., enteric, respiratory), or vector (arboviruses; arthropod-borne virus) (Box 6–3). *The most consistent and current means of classification is by physical and biochemical characteristics such as size, morphology (e.g., presence or absence of a membrane envelope), type of genome, and means of replication* (Figs. 6–2 and 6–3). DNA viruses associated with human disease are divided into six families (Tables 6–1 and 6–2). The RNA viruses may be divided into at least 13 families (Tables 6–3 and 6–4).

Virion Structure

The units for measurement of virion size are nanometers (nm). The clinically important viruses range from 18 nm (parvoviruses) to 300 nm (poxviruses) (Fig. 6–4). The latter are almost visible with a light microscope and are approximately one fourth the size of a *Staphy-*

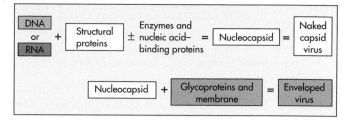

FIGURE 6–1. Components of the basic virion.

lococcus organism. *Larger virions can hold a larger genome that can encode more proteins, and they are generally more complex.*

The **virion** (the virus particle) consists of a nucleic acid **genome** packaged into a protein coat (**capsid**) or a membrane (**envelope**) (Fig. 6–5). The virion may also contain certain essential or accessory enzymes or other proteins. Capsid or nucleic acid–binding proteins may associate with the genome to form a **nucleocapsid,** which may be the same as the virion or surrounded by an envelope.

The genome of the virus consists of either DNA or RNA. *The DNA can be single-stranded or double-stranded, linear or circular. The RNA can be either positive sense (+) (like messenger RNA [mRNA]) or negative sense (−) (analogous to a photographic negative), double-stranded (+/−) or ambisense (containing + and − regions of RNA attached end to end). The RNA genome may also be segmented into pieces, with each piece encoding an individual gene.* Just as there are many different types of computer memory devices, all of these forms of nucleic acid can maintain and transmit the genetic information of the virus.

The outer layer of the virion is the **capsid** or **envelope.** These structures are the package, protection, and delivery vehicle during transmission of the virus from one host to another and for spread within the host to the target cell. The surface structures of the capsid and envelope mediate the interaction of the virus with the target cell. Removal or disruption of the outer package inactivates the virus. Antibodies generated against the components of these structures prevent virus infection.

The **capsid** is a rigid structure able to withstand harsh environmental conditions. Viruses with naked capsids are generally resistant to drying, acid, and detergents, including the acid and bile of the enteric tract. Many of these viruses are transmitted by the fecal-oral route and can endure transmission even in sewage.

The **envelope** is a membrane composed of lipids, proteins, and glycoproteins. The membranous structure of the envelope can be maintained only in aqueous solutions. It is readily disrupted by drying, acidic conditions, detergents, and solvents such as ether, resulting in inactivation of the virus. As a result, enveloped viruses must remain wet and are generally transmitted in fluids, respiratory droplets, blood, and tissue. Most cannot survive the harsh conditions of the gastrointestinal tract. The influence of virion structure on viral properties is summarized in Boxes 6–4 and 6–5.

Capsid Viruses

The viral capsid is assembled from individual proteins associated into progressively larger units. All of the

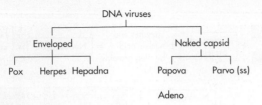

FIGURE 6–2. The DNA viruses and their morphology. The viral families are determined by the structure of the genome and the morphology of the virion.

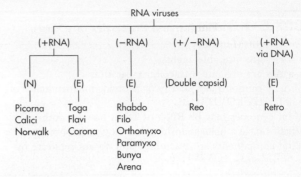

FIGURE 6–3. The RNA viruses, their genome structure, and their morphology. The viral families are determined by the structure of the genome and the morphology of the virion.

TABLE 6–1. Families of DNA Viruses and Some Important Members

Family	Members*
POXVIRIDAE†	*Smallpox virus*, vaccinia virus
Herpesviridae	*Herpes simplex virus* types 1 and 2, varicella-zoster virus, Epstein-Barr virus, cytomegalovirus, human herpesviruses 6, 7, and 8
Adenoviridae	*Adenovirus*
Hepadnaviridae	*Hepatitis B virus*
Papovaviridae	JC virus, BK virus, SV40, *papillomavirus*
Parvoviridae	*Parvovirus B19*, adeno-associated virus

*The italicized virus is the important or prototype virus for the family.

†The size of type is indicative of the relative size of the virus.

components of the capsid have chemical features that allow them to fit together and to assemble into a larger unit. Individual structural proteins associate into **subunits,** which associate into **protomers, capsomeres** (distinguishable in electron micrographs), and finally a recognizable **procapsid** or **capsid** (Fig. 6–6). A procapsid requires further processing to the final, transmissible capsid. For some viruses, the capsid forms around the genome; for others, the capsid forms as an empty shell (procapsid) to be filled by the genome.

The simplest viral structures that can be built stepwise are symmetrical and include **helical** and **icosahedral** structures. Helical structures appear as rods, whereas the icosahedron is an approximation of a sphere assembled from symmetrical subunits (Fig. 6–7). Nonsymmetrical capsids are complex forms and are associated with certain bacterial viruses (phages).

The classic example of a virus with helical symmetry is the tobacco mosaic plant virus. Its capsomeres self-

TABLE 6–2. Properties of Virions of Human DNA Viruses

Family	Genome* Molecular Mass × 10⁶ Daltons	Nature	Viron Shape	Size (nm)	DNA Polymerase†
Poxviridae	85–140	ds, linear	Brick-shaped, enveloped	300 × 240 × 100	+‡
Herpesviridae	100–150	ds, linear	Icosahedral, enveloped	Capsid, 100–110 Envelope, 120–200	+
Adenoviridae	20–25	ds, linear	Icosahedral	70–90	+
Hepadnaviridae	1.8	ds, circular§	Spherical, enveloped	42	+‡ ‖
Papovaviridae	3–5	ds, circular	Icosahedral	45–55	−
Parvoviridae	1.5–2.0	ss, linear	Icosahedral	18–26	−

*Genome invariably a single molecule.

†Polymerase encoded by virus.

‡Polymerase carried in the virion.

§Circular molecule is double-stranded for most of its length but contains a single-stranded region.

‖Reverse transcriptase.

ds = Double-stranded; ss = single-stranded.

TABLE 6-3. Families of RNA Viruses and Some Important Members

Family	Members*
Paramyxoviridae†	Parainfluenza virus, Sendai virus, *measles virus*, mumps virus, respiratory syncytial virus
Orthomyxoviridae	*Influenza virus* types A, B, and C
Coronaviridae	*Coronavirus*
Arenaviridae	*Lassa fever virus*, Tacaribe virus complex (Junin and Machupo viruses), lymphocytic choriomeningitis virus
Rhabdoviridae	*Rabies virus*, vesicular stomatitis virus
Filoviridae	*Ebola virus*, Marburg virus
Bunyaviridae	*California encephalitis virus*, LaCrosse virus, sandfly fever virus, hemorrhagic fever virus, Hanta virus
Retroviridae	Human T-cell leukemia virus types I and II, *human immunodeficiency virus*, animal oncoviruses
Reoviridae	*Rotavirus*, Colorado tick fever virus
Picornaviridae	Rhinoviruses, *poliovirus*, echoviruses, coxsackievirus, hepatitis A virus
Togaviridae	*Rubella virus*; western, eastern, and Venezuelan equine encephalitis virus; Ross River virus; Sindbis virus; Semliki Forest virus
Flaviviridae	*Yellow fever virus*, dengue virus, St. Louis encephalitis virus, hepatitis C virus
Caliciviridae	Norwalk virus
Delta	Delta agent

*The italicized virus is the important or prototype virus for the family.

†The size of the type is indicative of the relative size of the virus.

assemble on the RNA genome into rods extending to the length of the genome. The capsomeres cover and protect the RNA. Helical nucleocapsids are observed within the envelope of most negative-strand RNA viruses (see Fig. 55–1).

Simple icosahedrons are used by small, simple viruses such as the picornaviruses and parvoviruses. The icosahedron is made of 12 capsomeres, each with five-fold symmetry (**pentamer** or **penton**). For the picornaviruses, every pentamer is made up of five proto-

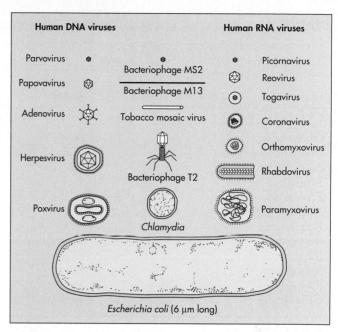

FIGURE 6-4. Relative sizes of viruses and bacteria. (Courtesy the Upjohn Company, Kalamazoo, Mich.)

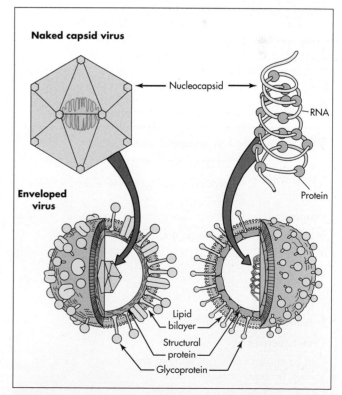

FIGURE 6-5. The structures of a naked capsid virus *(top left)* and enveloped viruses with an icosahedral *(left)* nucleocapsid or a helical *(right)* ribonucleocapsid. The helical ribonucleocapsid is formed by viral proteins associated with an RNA genome.

TABLE 6–4. Properties of Virions of Human RNA Viruses

Family	Genome* Molecular Mass × 10⁶ Daltons	Nature	Virion Shape*	Size (nm)	Polymerase in Virion	Envelope
Paramyxoviridae	5–7	ss, −	Spherical	150–300	+	+
Orthomyxoviridae	5	ss, −, seg	Spherical	80–120	+	+
Coronaviridae	6	ss, +	Spherical	80–130	−	+†
Arenaviridae	3–5	ss, −, seg	Spherical	50–300	+	+†
Rhabdoviridae	4	ss, −	Bullet-shaped	180 × 75	+	+
Filoviridae	4	ss, −	Filamentous	800 × 80	+	+
Bunyaviridae	4–7	ss, −	Spherical	90–100	+	+†
Retroviridae	2 × (2–3)‡	ss, +	Spherical	80–110	+§	+
Reoviridae	11–15	ds, seg	Icosahedral	60–80	+	−
Picornaviridae	2.5	ss, +	Icosahedral	25–30	−	−
Togaviridae	4	ss, +	Icosahedral	60–70	−	+
Flaviviridae	4	ss, +	Spherical	40–50	−	+
Caliciviridae	2.6	ss, +	Icosahedral	35–40	−	−

* Some enveloped viruses are very pleomorphic (sometimes filamentous).
  † No matrix protein.
  ‡ Genome has two identical single-stranded RNA molecules.
  § Reverse transcriptase.
  ss = Single-stranded; ds = double-stranded; seg = segmented; + or − = polarity of single-stranded nucleic acid.

mers, each of which is composed of three subunits of four separate proteins (see Fig. 6–6). X-ray crystallography and image analysis of cryoelectron microscopy have defined the structure of the picornavirus capsid to the molecular level. These studies have depicted a canyon-like cleft, which is a "docking site" to bind to the receptor on the surface of the target cell (see Fig. 54–2).

BOX 6–4. Viral Structure: Naked Capsid

Component

Protein.

Properties

Is environmentally stable to the following:
  Temperature
  Acid
  Proteases
  Detergents
  Drying
Is released from cell by lysis.

Consequences

Can be spread easily (on fomites, from hand to hand, by dust, by small droplets).
Can dry out and retain infectivity.
Can survive the adverse conditions of the gut.
Can be resistant to detergents and poor sewage treatment.
Antibody may be sufficient for immunoprotection.

BOX 6–5. Virus Structure: Envelope

Components

Membrane.
Lipids.
Proteins.
Glycoproteins.

Properties

Is environmentally labile—is disrupted by the following:
  Acid
  Detergents
  Drying
  Heat
Modifies cell membrane during replication.
Is released by budding and cell lysis.

Consequences

Must stay wet.
Cannot survive the gastrointestinal tract.
Spreads in large droplets, secretions, organ transplants, and blood transfusions.
Does not need to kill the cell to spread.
May need antibody and cell-mediated immune response for protection and control.
Elicits hypersensitivity and inflammation to cause immunopathogenesis.

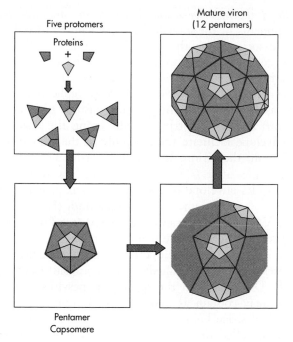

FIGURE 6-6. Capsid assembly of the icosahedral capsid of a picornavirus. Individual proteins associate into subunits, which associate into protomers, capsomeres, and an empty procapsid. Inclusion of the (+) RNA genome triggers its conversion to the final capsid form.

Larger capsid virions are constructed by inserting structurally distinct capsomeres between the pentons at the vertices. These capsomeres have six nearest neighbors **(hexons).** This extends the icosahedron and is called an **icosadeltahedron,** and its size is determined by the number of hexons inserted along the edges and planes between the pentons. *A soccer ball is an icosadeltahedron.* For example, the herpesvirus nucleocapsid has 12 pentons and 150 hexons. The herpesvirus nucleocapsid is also surrounded by an envelope. The adenovirus capsid is composed of 252 capsomeres, with 12 pentons and 240 hexons. A long fiber is attached to each penton of adenovirus to serve as the **viral attachment protein (VAP)** to bind to target cells, and it also contains the type-specific antigen (see Fig. 50–1). The reoviruses have an icosahedral double capsid with fiberlike proteins partially extended from each vertex. The outer capsid protects the virus and promotes its uptake across the gastrointestinal tract and into target cells, whereas the inner capsid contains enzymes for the synthesis of RNA (see Figs. 6–7 and 57–2).

Enveloped Viruses

The virion envelope is composed of lipids, proteins, and glycoproteins (see Fig. 6–5 and Box 6–5). It has a membrane structure similar to cellular membranes. Cellular proteins are rarely found in the viral envelope,

FIGURE 6-7. Cryoelectron microscopy and computer-generated three-dimensional image reconstructions of several icosahedral capsids. These images show the symmetry of capsids and the individual capsomeres. During assembly, the genome may fill the capsid through the holes in the herpesvirus and papovavirus capsomeres. 1, Equine herpesvirus nucleocapsid; 2, simian rotavirus; 3, reovirus type 1 (Lang) virion; 4, intermediate subviral particle (reovirus); 5, core (inner capsid) particle (reovirus); 6, human papillomavirus type 19 (papovavirus); 7, mouse polyomavirus (papovavirus); 8, cauliflower mosaic virus. (Bar = 50 nm.) (Courtesy Dr. Tim Baker, Purdue University.)

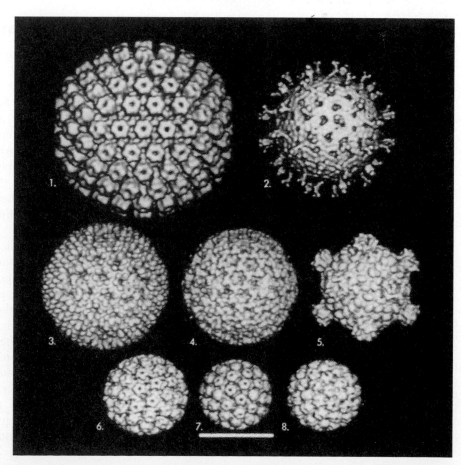

even though the envelope is obtained from cellular membranes. Most enveloped viruses are round or pleomorphic. (See Figs. 6–2 and 6–3 for the complete listing of enveloped viruses.) Two exceptions are the poxvirus, which has a complex internal and a bricklike external structure, and the rhabdovirus, which is bullet-shaped.

Most viral glycoproteins have asparagine-linked (*N*-linked) carbohydrate and extend through the envelope and away from the surface of the virion. For many viruses, these can be observed as spikes (Fig. 6–8). Most glycoproteins act as **VAPs** capable of binding to structures on target cells. VAPs that also bind to erythrocytes are termed **hemagglutinins (HAs)**. Some glycoproteins have other functions, such as the neuraminidase of orthomyxoviruses (influenza) and the Fc receptor and the C3b receptor associated with herpes simplex virus glycoproteins or the fusion glycoproteins of paramyxoviruses. Glycoproteins are also major antigens for protective immunity.

The envelope of the togaviruses surrounds an icosahedral nucleocapsid containing a positive-strand RNA genome. The envelope contains spikes consisting of two or three glycoprotein subunits anchored to the virion's icosahedral capsid. This causes the envelope to adhere tightly and conform (shrink-wrap) to an icosahedral structure discernible by cryoelectron microscopy.

All of the negative-strand RNA viruses are enveloped. Components of the viral RNA-dependent RNA polymerase associate with the (−) RNA genome of the orthomyxoviruses, paramyxoviruses, and rhabdoviruses to form helical nucleocapsids (see Fig. 6–5). These enzymes are required to initiate virus replication, and their association with the genome ensures their delivery into the cell. Matrix proteins lining the inside of the envelope facilitate the assembly of the ribonucleocapsid into the virion. Influenza A (orthomyxovirus) is an example of a (−) RNA virus with a segmented genome. Its envelope is lined with matrix proteins and has two glycoproteins: the hemagglutinin (HA), which is the VAP, and a neuraminidase (NA) (see Fig. 56–1). Bunyaviruses do not have matrix proteins.

The herpesvirus envelope is a baglike structure that encloses the icosadeltahedral nucleocapsid (see Fig. 51–1). Depending on the specific herpesvirus, the envelope may contain as many as 11 glycoproteins. The interstitial space between the nucleocapsid and the envelope is called the *tegument*, and it contains enzymes and proteins that facilitate the viral infection.

The poxviruses are enveloped viruses with large, complex, bricklike shapes (Fig. 52–1). The envelope encloses a dumbbell-shaped, DNA-containing nucleoid structure; lateral bodies; fibrils; and many enzymes and proteins, including the enzymes and transcriptional factors required for mRNA synthesis.

Viral Replication

The major steps in viral replication are the same for all viruses (Fig. 6–9 and Box 6–6). The cell acts as a factory, providing the substrates, energy, and machinery necessary for the synthesis of viral proteins and replication of the genome. Processes not provided by the cell must be encoded in the genome of the virus. The manner in which each virus accomplishes these steps and overcomes the cell's biochemical limitations is determined by the structure of the genome and of the virion (whether it is enveloped or has a naked capsid). This is illustrated in the examples in Figures 6–12 to 6–14.

The viral replication cycle can be separated into several phases. During the **early phase** of infection, the virus must recognize an appropriate target cell, attach to the cell, penetrate the plasma membrane and be taken up by the cell, release (uncoat) its genome into the cytoplasm, and if necessary deliver the genome to the nucleus. The **late phase** begins with the start of genome replication and viral macromolecular synthesis and proceeds through viral assembly and release. Uncoating of the genome from the capsid or envelope during the early phase abolishes its infectivity and identifiable structure, thus initiating the eclipse period. The **eclipse period**, like a solar eclipse, ends with the

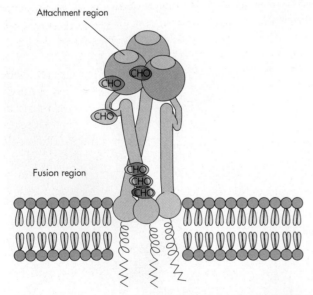

FIGURE 6–8. Diagram of the hemagglutinin glycoprotein trimer of influenza A virus, a representative spike protein. The region for attachment to the cellular receptor is exposed on the spike protein's surface. Under mild acidic conditions, the hemagglutinin changes conformation to expose a hydrophobic sequence at the "fusion region." CHO, *N*-linked carbohydrate attachment sites. (Modified from Schlesinger MJ, Schlesinger S: Domains of virus glycoproteins *Adv Virus Res* 33:1–44, 1987.)

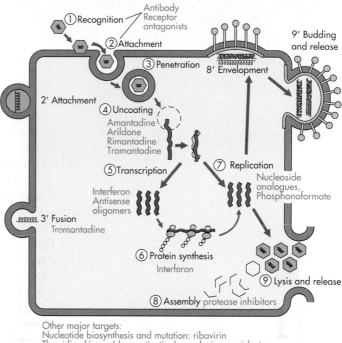

FIGURE 6–9. A general scheme of viral replication. Enveloped viruses have alternative means of entry (3) assembly, and exit from the cell (8′ and 9′). The steps in viral replication susceptible to antiviral drugs are listed in magenta.

appearance of new virions after virus assembly. The **latent period,** during which extracellular infectious virus is not detected, includes the eclipse period and ends on release of the virus (Fig. 6–10). Each infected cell may produce as many as 100,000 particles; however, only 1% to 10% of these particles may be infectious. The noninfectious particles **(defective particles)** result from mutations and errors in the manufacture and assembly of the virion. The yield of infectious virus per cell, or **burst size,** and the time required for a single cycle of virus reproduction are determined by the properties of the virus and the target cell.

BOX 6–6. **Steps in Viral Replication**

1. Recognition of the target cell
2. Attachment
3. Penetration
4. Uncoating
5. Macromolecular synthesis
   a. Early mRNA and nonstructural protein synthesis: genes for enzymes and nucleic acid–binding proteins
   b. Replication of genome
   c. Late mRNA and structural protein synthesis
   d. Post-translational modification of protein
6. Assembly of virus
7. Budding of enveloped viruses
8. Release of virus

mRNA = messenger RNA.

Recognition of and Attachment to the Target Cell

The binding of the **VAPs,** or structures on the surface of the virion capsid (Table 6–5), to **receptors on the cell** (Table 6–6) initially determines which cells can be infected by a virus. *The receptors for the virus on the cell may be proteins or carbohydrates on glycoproteins or glycolipids.*

The viral attachment structure for a capsid virus may be part of the capsid or a protein that extends from the capsid. A canyon on the surface of rhinovirus 14, a picornavirus, serves as a "keyhole" for the insertion of a portion of the intercellular adhesion molecule (ICAM-1) from the cell surface. The fibers of the adenoviruses and the σ-1 proteins of the reoviruses at the vertices of the capsid interact with receptors expressed on specific target cells.

Specific glycoproteins of enveloped viruses are the VAPs. The HA of influenza A virus binds to sialic acid expressed on many different cells and has a broad host range and tissue tropism. Similarly, the α-togaviruses and the flaviviruses are able to bind to receptors expressed on cells of many animal species, including arthropods, reptiles, amphibians, birds, and mammals. This allows them to infect animals, mosquitoes, and other insects and to be spread by them.

Viruses that bind to receptors expressed on specific cell types may be restricted to certain species **(host range)** (e.g., human, mouse) or specific cell types. The susceptible target cell defines the tissue **tropism** (e.g.,

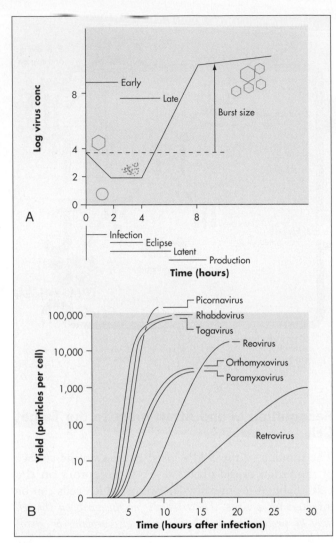

FIGURE 6–10. *A,* Single-cycle growth curve of a virus that is released on cell lysis. The different stages are defined by the presence or absence of visible viral components (eclipse period), infectious virus in the media (latent period), or macromolecular synthesis (early/late phases). *B,* Growth curve and burst size of representative viruses. (*A* modified from Davis BD et al: *Microbiology,* ed 4, Philadelphia, 1990, JB Lippincott; *B* modified from White DO, Fenner F: *Medical virology,* ed 3, New York, 1986, Academic Press.)

neurotropic, lymphotropic). Epstein-Barr virus, a herpesvirus, has a very limited host range and tropism because it binds to the C3d receptor (CR2) expressed on human B cells. The B19 parvovirus binds to globoside (blood group P antigen) expressed on erythroid precursor cells.

Penetration

Many interactions between the VAPs and the cellular receptors initiate the internalization of the virus into the cell. The mechanism of internalization depends on the virion structure and cell type. Most nonenveloped

viruses enter the cell by receptor-mediated endocytosis or by viropexis. **Endocytosis** is a normal process used by the cell for the uptake of receptor-bound molecules such as hormones, low-density lipoproteins, and transferrin. Picornaviruses and papovaviruses may enter by **viropexis.** Hydrophobic structures of capsid proteins may be exposed after viral binding to the cells, and these structures help the virus or the viral genome slip through (direct penetration) the membrane.

Enveloped viruses fuse their membranes with cellular membranes to deliver the nucleocapsid or genome directly into the cytoplasm. The optimum pH for fusion determines whether penetration occurs at the cell surface at neutral pH or whether the virus must be internalized by endocytosis and fusion occurs in an endosome at acidic pH. The fusion activity may be provided by the VAP or another protein. The HA of influenza A (see Fig. 6–8) binds to sialic acid receptors on the target cell. Under the mild acidic conditions of the endosome, the HA undergoes a dramatic conformational change to expose hydrophobic portions capable of promoting membrane fusion. Paramyxoviruses have a fusion protein that is active at neutral pH to promote virus-cell fusion. Paramyxoviruses can also promote cell-cell fusion to form multinucleated giant cells **(syncytia).** Some herpesviruses and retroviruses fuse with cells at a neutral pH and induce syncytia after replication.

Uncoating

Once internalized, the nucleocapsid must be delivered to the site of replication within the cell and the capsid or envelope removed. The genome of DNA viruses, except for poxviruses, must be delivered to the nucleus, whereas most RNA viruses remain in the cytoplasm. The uncoating process may be initiated by attachment to the receptor or promoted by the acidic environment or proteases found in an endosome or lysosome. Picornavirus capsids are weakened by the release of the VP4 capsid protein to allow uncoating. VP4 is released by insertion of the receptor into the keyhole-like canyon attachment site of the capsid. Enveloped viruses are uncoated on fusion with cell membranes. Fusion of the herpesvirus envelope with the plasma membrane releases its nucleocapsid, which then "docks" with the nuclear membrane to deliver its DNA genome directly to the site of replication. The release of the influenza nucleocapsid from its matrix and envelope is facilitated by protons from inside the endosome, which passes through the ion pore formed by the influenza M2 matrix protein.

The reovirus and poxvirus are only partially uncoated on entry. The outer capsid of reovirus is removed, but the genome remains in an inner capsid,

FIGURE 6–11. Viral macromolecular synthesis steps: The mechanism of viral mRNA and protein synthesis and genome replication are determined by the structure of the genome. 1. Double-stranded DNA (DS DNA) utilizes host machinery in the nucleus (except poxviruses) to make mRNA, which is translated by host cell ribosomes into proteins. Replication of viral DNA occurs by semiconservative means, by rolling circle, linear, and in other ways. 2. Single-stranded DNA (SS DNA) is converted into DS DNA and replicates like DS DNA. 3. +RNA resembles an mRNA that binds to ribosomes to make a polyprotein that is cleaved into individual proteins. One of the viral proteins is an RNA polymerase that makes a (−)RNA template and then more +RNA genome progeny and mRNAs. 4. −RNA is transcribed into mRNAs and a full-length +RNA template by an RNA polymerase carried in the virion. The (+)RNA template is used to make (−)RNA genome progeny. 5. DS RNA acts like −RNA. The (−) strands are transcribed into mRNAs by an RNA polymerase in the capsid. +RNAs get encapsidated and −RNAs are made in the capsid. 6. Retroviruses are +RNA that are converted to DNA (cDNA) by reverse transcriptase carried in the virion. cDNA integrates into the host chromosome, and the host makes mRNAs, proteins, and full-length RNA genome copies.

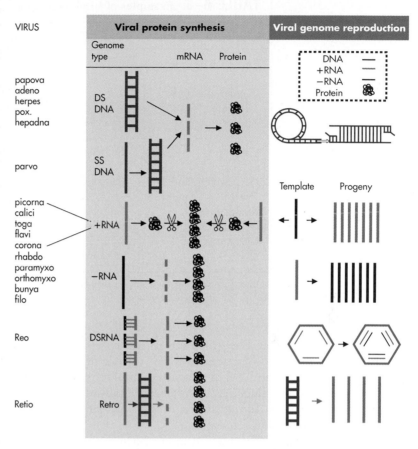

which contains the polymerases necessary for RNA synthesis. The initial uncoating of the poxviruses exposes a subviral particle to the cytoplasm, allowing synthesis of mRNA by virion-contained enzymes. An uncoating enzyme can then be synthesized to release the DNA-containing core into the cytoplasm.

Macromolecular Synthesis

Once inside the cell, the genome must direct the synthesis of viral mRNA, protein, and generate identical copies of itself. *Transcription, translation, and replication of the genome are therefore probably the most important*

TABLE 6–5. Examples of Viral Attachment Proteins

Virus Family	Virus	VAP
Picornaviridae	Rhinovirus	VP1-VP2-VP3 complex
Adenoviridae	Adenovirus	Fiber protein
Reoviridae	Reovirus	σ-1
	Rotavirus	VP7
Togaviridae	Semliki Forest virus	E1-E2-E3 complex
Rhabdoviridae	Rabies virus	G Protein
Orthomyxoviridae	Influenza A virus	HA
Paramyxoviridae	Measles virus	HA
Herpesviridae	Epstein-Barr virus	gp350 and gp220
Retroviridae	Murine leukemia virus	gp70
	Human immunodeficiency virus	gp120

gp = glycoprotein; VAP = viral attachment proteins.

TABLE 6–6. Examples of Viral Receptors

Virus	Target Cell	Receptor*
Epstein-Barr virus	B cell	C3d complement receptor CR2 (CD21)
Human immuno-deficiency virus	Helper T cell	CD4 molecule and chemokine co-receptor
Rhinovirus	Epithelial cells	ICAM-1 (immunoglobulin superfamily protein)
Poliovirus	Epithelial cells	Immunoglobulin superfamily protein
Herpes simplex virus	Many cells	Immunoglobulin superfamily protein
Rabies virus	Neuron	Acetylcholine receptor
Influenza A virus	Epithelial cells	Sialic acid
B19 parvovirus	Erythroid precursors	Erythrocyte P antigen (globoside)

* Other receptors for these viruses may also exist.
ICAM-1 = Intercellular adhesion molecule.

steps in viral multiplication. The genome is useless unless it can be transcribed into functional mRNAs capable of binding to ribosomes and being translated into proteins. The means by which each virus accomplishes these steps depends on the structure of the genome (Fig. 6–11) and the site of replication.

The cell's machinery for transcription and mRNA processing is found in the nucleus. *Most DNA viruses use the cell's DNA-dependent RNA polymerase* II *and other enzymes to make mRNA.* For example, eukaryotic mRNAs acquire a 3′ polyadenylated (poly A) tail and a 5′ methylated cap (for binding to the ribosome) and are processed to remove introns before being exported to the cytoplasm. Viruses that replicate in the cytoplasm must provide these functions or an alternative. Although poxviruses are DNA viruses, they replicate in the cytoplasm and therefore must encode enzymes for all these functions. *Most RNA viruses replicate and produce mRNA in the cytoplasm,* except for orthomyxoviruses and retroviruses. *RNA viruses must encode the necessary enzymes for transcription and replication because the cell has no means of replicating RNA.* The mRNAs for

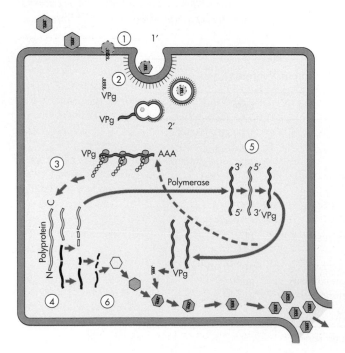

FIGURE 6–12. Replication of picornaviruses: a simple (+) RNA virus. (1) Interaction of the picornaviruses with receptors on the cell surface defines the target cell and weakens the capsid. (2) The genome is injected through the virion and across the cell membrane. 2′, The virion is endocytosed, and then the genome is released. (3) Alternatively, the genome is used as mRNA for protein synthesis. One large polyprotein is translated from the virion genome. (4) Then the polyprotein is proteolytically cleaved into individual proteins, including an RNA-dependent RNA polymerase. (5) The polymerase makes a (−) strand template from the genome and replicates the genome. A protein (VPg) is covalently attached to the 5′ end of the viral genome. (6) The structural proteins associate into the capsid structure, the genome is inserted, and the virions are released on cell lysis.

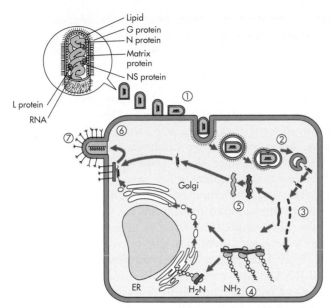

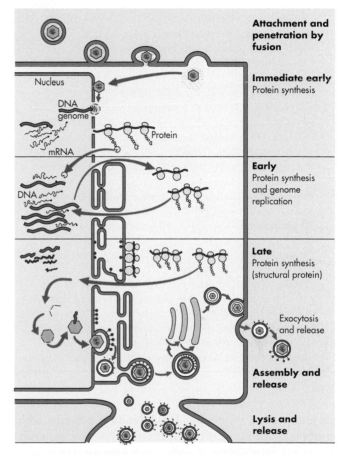

cleotides, polymerases, and other materials required for DNA virus replication. As a result, many DNA viruses encode proteins, which promote the growth of the host cell.

Transcription of the DNA virus genome (except for poxviruses) occurs in the nucleus, using host cell polymerases and other enzymes for viral mRNA synthesis. Transcription of the viral genes is regulated by

FIGURE 6–13. Replication of rhabdoviruses: a simple enveloped (−) RNA virus. (1) Rhabdoviruses bind to the cell surface and are (2) endocytosed. The envelope fuses with the endosome vesicle membrane to deliver the nucleocapsid to the cytoplasm. The virion must carry a polymerase, which (3) produces five individual messenger RNAs (mRNAs) and a full-length (+) RNA template. (4) Proteins are translated from the mRNAs, including one glycoprotein (G), which is co-translationally glycosylated in the endoplasmic reticulum (ER), processed in the Golgi apparatus, and delivered to the cell membrane. (5) The genome is replicated from the (+) RNA template, and N, L, and NS proteins associate with the genome to form the nucleocapsid. (6) The matrix protein associates with the G protein–modified membrane, which is followed by assembly of the nucleocapsid. (7) The virus buds from the cell in a bullet-shaped virion.

RNA viruses may or may not acquire a 5′ cap or poly A tail.

The naked genome of DNA viruses (except poxviruses) and the positive-sense RNA viruses (except retroviruses) are sufficient for initiating replication on injection into a cell. These genomes can interact directly with host machinery to promote mRNA or protein synthesis or both.

DNA Viruses

The smaller the DNA virus, the more dependent the virus is on the host cell (Box 6–7). The larger DNA viruses encode a DNA polymerase and proteins to enhance and control transcription and genome replication. Viral DNA and mRNA synthesis can be enhanced by speeding up the growth of the cell or by increasing the number of DNA templates for transcription after the replication of the genome. A growing cell provides deoxyribonu-

FIGURE 6–14. Replication of herpes simplex virus, a complex enveloped DNA virus. The virus binds to specific receptors and fuses with the plasma membrane. The nucleocapsid then delivers the DNA genome to the nucleus. Transcription and translation occur in three phases: immediate early, early, and late. Immediate early proteins promote the takeover of the cell; early proteins consist of enzymes, including the DNA-dependent DNA polymerase; and the late proteins are structural proteins, including the viral capsid and glycoproteins. The genome is replicated before transcription of the late genes. Capsid proteins migrate into the nucleus, assemble into icosadeltahedral capsids, and are filled with the DNA genome. The viral glycoproteins are inserted into the endoplasmic reticulum, and carbohydrate is attached. The glycoproteins diffuse to the contiguous nuclear envelope. The capsids filled with genomes bud through these modified membranes and are transferred to the Golgi apparatus; the glycoproteins are processed, and the virus is released by exocytosis. Alternatively, the virus may be released on cell lysis.

BOX 6–7. **Properties of DNA Viruses**

DNA is not transient or labile.
  Viral genomes remain in the infected cell.
  Many DNA viruses establish persistent infections (e.g., latent, immortalizing).
DNA genomes reside in the nucleus (except for poxviruses).
Viral DNA resembles host DNA for transcription and replication.
Viral genes must interact with host transcriptional machinery (except for poxviruses).
  Viral gene transcription is temporally regulated.
  Early genes encode DNA-binding proteins and enzymes.
  Late genes encode structural proteins.
DNA polymerases require a primer to replicate the viral genome.
The larger DNA viruses have more control over the replication of their genome.
  Parvovirus: requires cells undergoing DNA synthesis to replicate.
  Papovavirus: stimulates cell growth and DNA synthesis.
  Hepadnavirus: stimulates cell growth (?) and encodes its own polymerase.
  Adenovirus: stimulates cellular DNA synthesis and encodes its own polymerase.
  Herpesvirus: stimulates cell growth, encodes its own polymerase and encodes enzymes to provide deoxyribonucleotides for DNA synthesis.
  Poxvirus: encodes its own polymerase and enzymes to provide deoxyribonucleotides for DNA synthesis, replication machinery, and transcription machinery.

---

the interaction of specific DNA-binding proteins with promoter and enhancer elements in the viral genome. The viral promoter and enhancer elements are similar in sequence to those of the host cell to allow binding of the cell's transcriptional activation factors and DNA-dependent RNA polymerase. Cells from some tissues do not express the DNA-binding proteins necessary for activating the transcription of viral genes, and replication of the virus in that cell is thus prevented or limited. For example, neurons transcribe only one gene for herpes simplex virus unless activated by stress, and as a result, the virus remains in latency in the cell. Transcription is also a factor in determining the tissue tropism and host range of the virus.

Different DNA and RNA viruses control the duration, sequence, and quantity of viral gene and protein synthesis in different ways. The more complex viruses encode their own transcriptional activators, which enhance or regulate the expression of viral genes. For example, the herpes simplex virus encodes many proteins that regulate the kinetics of viral gene expression, including the VMW 65 (α-TIF protein, VP16). VMW 65 is carried in the virion, binds to the host cell transcription-activating complex (Oct-1), and enhances its ability to stimulate transcription of the immediate early genes of the virus.

In general, mRNA for nonstructural proteins is transcribed first (see Fig. 6–14). **Early gene products** (nonstructural proteins) are often DNA-binding proteins and enzymes, including virus-encoded polymerases. These proteins are catalytic, and only a few are required. *Replication of the genome usually initiates the transition to transcription of late gene products.* **Late viral genes** encode structural proteins. Many copies of these proteins are required to package the virus but are generally not required before the genome is replicated. Newly replicated genomes also provide new templates for more late gene mRNA synthesis. Different DNA and RNA viruses control the time and amount of viral gene and protein synthesis in different ways.

Genes may be transcribed from either DNA strand of the genome and in opposite directions. For example, the early and late genes of the SV40 papovavirus are on opposite, nonoverlapping DNA strands. Viral genes may have introns requiring post-transcriptional processing of the mRNA by the cell's nuclear machinery (splicing). The late genes of papovaviruses and adenoviruses are initially transcribed as a large RNA from a single promoter and then processed to produce several different mRNAs after removal of different intervening sequences (introns).

Replication of viral DNA follows the same biochemical rules as for cellular DNA. Replication is initiated at a unique DNA sequence of the genome, called the **origin (ori).** This is a site recognized by cellular or viral nuclear factors and the **DNA-dependent DNA polymerase.** Viral DNA synthesis is semiconservative, and viral and cellular *DNA polymerases require a primer* to initiate synthesis of the DNA chain. The parvoviruses have DNA sequences that are inverted and repeated to allow the DNA to fold back and hybridize with itself to provide a primer. Replication of the adenovirus genome is primed by deoxycytidine monophosphate attached to a terminal protein. A cellular enzyme (primase) synthesizes an RNA primer to start the replication of the papovavirus genome while the herpesviruses encode a primase.

Replication of the genome of the simple DNA viruses (e.g., parvoviruses, papovaviruses) uses the host DNA-dependent DNA polymerases, whereas the larger, more complex viruses (e.g., adenoviruses, herpesviruses, poxviruses) encode their own polymerases. Viral polymerases are usually faster but less precise than host cell polymerases, causing a higher mutation rate in viruses, as well as providing a target for antiviral drugs.

Hepadnavirus replication is unique in that a circular, positive-strand RNA intermediate is first synthesized by the cell's DNA-dependent RNA polymerase. The

RNA is surrounded by viral proteins, an RNA-dependent DNA polymerase (reverse transcriptase) in this virion core makes a negative-strand DNA, and then the RNA is degraded. Positive-strand DNA synthesis is initiated but stops when the genome and core are enveloped, yielding a partially double-stranded circular DNA genome.

Major limitations for replication of a DNA virus include availability of the DNA polymerase and deoxyribonucleotide substrates. Most cells in the resting phase of growth are not undergoing DNA synthesis, and deoxythymidine pools are limited. The parvoviruses are the smallest DNA viruses and are dependent on the host cell. They replicate only in growing cells such as erythroid precursor cells or fetal tissue. The larger DNA viruses are more independent. They may provide enzymes and other proteins that stimulate cell growth, and they may scavenge for deoxyribonucleotides (see Box 6–7). The T antigen of SV40, the E7 of papillomavirus, and the E1a protein of adenovirus bind to and prevent the function of growth-inhibitory proteins (p53 and the retinoblastoma gene product), resulting in cell growth. Herpes simplex virus encodes scavenging enzymes such as deoxyribonuclease, ribonucleotide reductase, and thymidine kinase to generate the necessary deoxyribonucleotide substrates for replication of its genome.

RNA Viruses

Replication and transcription of RNA viruses are similar processes because the viral genomes are usually either an mRNA (positive-strand RNA) (see Fig. 6–12) or a template for mRNA (negative-strand RNA) (Box 6–8; see Fig. 6–13). During replication and transcription, a double-stranded RNA replicative intermediate, a structure not normally found in uninfected cells, is formed.

The RNA virus genome must code for **RNA-dependent RNA polymerases (replicases and transcriptases)** because the cell has no means of replicating RNA. Because RNA is degraded relatively quickly, the RNA-dependent RNA polymerase must be provided or synthesized soon after uncoating to generate more viral RNA, or the infection will be aborted. Replication of the genome also provides new templates for production of more mRNA, which amplifies and accelerates virus replication.

The **positive-strand RNA viral genomes** of the picornaviruses, caliciviruses, coronaviruses, flaviviruses, and togaviruses act as mRNA, bind to ribosomes, and direct protein synthesis. *The naked positive-strand RNA viral genome is sufficient to initiate infection by itself.* After the virus-encoded, RNA-dependent RNA polymerase is produced, a negative-strand RNA template is synthesized. The template can then be used to generate more mRNA and to replicate the genome. For the togavi-

---

BOX 6–8. Properties of RNA Viruses

RNA is labile and transient.
Most RNA viruses replicate in the cytoplasm.
Cells cannot replicate RNA. RNA viruses must encode an RNA-dependent RNA polymerase.
The genome structure determines the mechanism of transcription and replication.
RNA viruses are prone to mutation.
The genome structure and polarity determine how viral mRNA is generated and proteins are processed.
RNA viruses, except (+) RNA genome, must carry polymerase

Picornaviruses, Togaviruses, Flaviviruses, Caliciviruses, and Coronaviruses

(+) RNA genome resembles mRNA and is translated into a polyprotein, which is proteolyzed. A (−) RNA template is used for replication.

Orthomyxoviruses, Paramyxoviruses, Rhabdoviruses, Filoviruses, and Bunyaviruses

(−) RNA genome is a template for individual mRNAs, but full-length (+) RNA template required for replication.

Reoviruses

(+/−) segmented RNA genome is a template for mRNA. (+) RNA may also be encapsulated to generate the (+/−) RNA and then more mRNA.

Retroviruses

(+) retrovirus RNA genome is converted into DNA, which is integrated into the host chromatin and transcribed as a cellular gene.

mRNA = messenger RNA.

---

ruses, the negative-sense RNA template is also used to produce a smaller RNA for the structural proteins (late genes). The mRNAs for these viruses are not capped at the 5′ end, but the genome encodes a short poly A sequence. Transcription and replication of coronaviruses share many of these aspects but are more complex.

The **negative-strand RNA virus genomes** of the rhabdoviruses, orthomyxoviruses, paramyxoviruses, filoviruses, and bunyaviruses are the templates for production of mRNA. The negative-strand RNA genome is not infectious by itself, and *a polymerase must be carried into the cell with the genome* (associated with the genome as part of the nucleocapsid) to make individual mRNA for the different viral proteins. As a result, a full-length positive-strand RNA must also be produced by the viral polymerase to act as a template to generate more copies of the genome. The (−)RNA genome is like a roll of 35-mm film negatives: Each frame encodes a photo/mRNA, but a full-length positive is required for replicating the roll. *Except for influenza viruses, transcription and replication of negative-strand RNA viruses occur in the cytoplasm.* The influenza transcriptase requires a primer to produce mRNA. It uses the 5' ends of cellular mRNA in the nucleus as primers for its polymerase and in the process steals the 5' cap from the cellular mRNA. The influenza genome is also replicated in the nucleus.

The reoviruses have a **segmented, double-stranded RNA genome** and undergo a more complex means of replication and transcription. The reovirus RNA polymerase is part of the inner capsid core. mRNA units are transcribed from each of the 10 or more segments of the genome while they are still in the core. The negative strands of the genome segments are used as templates for mRNA in a manner similar to that of the negative-strand RNA viruses. Reovirus-encoded enzymes contained in the inner capsid core add the 5' cap to viral mRNA. The mRNA does not have poly A. The mRNAs are released into the cytoplasm, where they direct protein synthesis or are sequestered into new cores. The positive-strand RNA in the new cores acts as a template for negative-strand RNA, and the core polymerase produces the progeny double-stranded RNA.

The arenaviruses have an **ambisense circular genome** with (+) sequences adjacent to (−) sequences. The early genes of the virus are transcribed from the negative-sense portion of the genome, and the late genes of the virus are transcribed from the full-length replicative intermediate.

Although the **retroviruses** have a positive-strand RNA genome, the virus provides no means for replication of the RNA in the cytoplasm. Instead, the retroviruses carry two copies of the genome, two transfer RNA (tRNA) molecules, and an RNA-dependent DNA polymerase **(reverse transcriptase)** in the virion. The tRNA is used as a primer for synthesis of a DNA copy **(cDNA)** of the genome. The cDNA is synthesized in the cytoplasm, travels to the nucleus, and is then integrated into the host chromatin. The viral genome becomes a cellular gene. Promoters at the end of the integrated viral genome enhance the transcription of the viral DNA sequences by the cell. Full-length RNA transcripts are used as new genomes, and individual mRNAs are generated by differential splicing of this RNA.

The most unusual mode of replication is reserved for the **deltavirus.** The deltavirus resembles a viroid. The genome is a circular, rod-shaped, single-stranded (1) RNA, which is extensively hybridized to itself. As the exception, the deltavirus RNA genome is replicated by the host cell DNA-dependent RNA polymerase II in the nucleus. The genome forms an RNA structure called a ribozyme, which cleaves the RNA circle to produce an mRNA.

Viral Protein Synthesis

All viruses depend on the host cell ribosomes, tRNA, and mechanisms for post-translational modification to produce their proteins. Unlike bacterial ribosomes, which can bind to a polycistronic mRNA and translate several gene sequences into separate proteins, the eukaryotic ribosome binds to mRNA and can make only one continuous protein and then it falls off the mRNA. Each virus deals with this limitation differently, depending on the structure of the genome. For example, the entire genome of a positive-strand RNA virus is read by the ribosome and translated into one giant **polyprotein.** The polyprotein is subsequently cleaved by cellular and viral proteases into functional proteins. DNA viruses, retroviruses, and most negative-strand RNA viruses transcribe separate mRNA for smaller polyproteins or individual proteins. The orthomyxovirus and reovirus genomes are segmented, and most of the segments code for single proteins for this reason.

Viruses use different tactics to promote preferential translation of their viral mRNA instead of cellular mRNA. In many cases, the concentration of viral mRNA in the cell is so large that it occupies most of the ribosomes, preventing translation of cellular mRNA. Adenovirus infection blocks the egress of cellular mRNA from the nucleus. Herpes simplex virus and other viruses inhibit cellular macromolecular synthesis and induce degradation of the cell's DNA and mRNA. To promote selective translation of its mRNA, poliovirus uses a virus-encoded protease to inactivate the 200,000-Da cap-binding protein of the ribosome to prevent binding and translation of 5' capped cellular mRNA. Togaviruses and many other viruses increase the permeability of the cell's membrane; thus, the ribosomal affinity for most cellular mRNA is decreased. All these actions also contribute to the cytopathology of the virus infection. The pathogenic consequences of these actions are discussed further in Chapter 46.

Some viral proteins require **post-translational modifications** such as phosphorylation, glycosylation, acylation, or sulfation. Protein phosphorylation is accomplished by cellular or viral protein kinases and is a means of modulating, activating, or inactivating proteins. Several herpesviruses and other viruses encode their own protein kinase. *Viral glycoproteins are synthesized on membrane-bound ribosomes and have the amino acid sequences to allow insertion into the rough endoplasmic reticulum and N-linked glycosylation.* The high-mannose precursor form of the glycoproteins progresses from the endoplasmic reticulum through the vesicular transport system of the cell and is processed through the Golgi apparatus. The sialic acid–containing mature glycoprotein is expressed on the plasma membrane of the cell unless the glycoprotein expresses protein sequences for retention in an intracellular organelle. The presence of the glycoproteins determines where the virion will assemble. Other modifications, such as *O*-glycosylation, acylation, and sulfation of the proteins, can also occur during progression through the Golgi apparatus.

Assembly

Virion assembly is analogous to a three-dimensional interlocking puzzle that puts itself together in the box. The virion is built from small, easily manufactured parts that enclose the genome in a functional package. Each part of the virion has recognition structures that allow the virus to form the appropriate protein-protein, protein–nucleic acid, and (for enveloped viruses) protein-membrane interactions needed to assemble into the final structure. The assembly process begins when the necessary pieces are synthesized and the concentration of structural proteins in the cell is sufficient to drive the process thermodynamically, much like a crystallization reaction. The assembly process may be facilitated by scaffolding proteins or other proteins that are activated or release energy on proteolysis. For example, cleavage of the VP0 protein of poliovirus releases the VP4 peptide, which solidifies the capsid.

The site and mechanism of virion assembly in the cell depend on where genome replication occurs and whether the final structure is a naked capsid or an enveloped virus. Assembly of the DNA viruses, other than poxviruses, occurs in the nucleus and requires transport of the virion proteins into the nucleus. RNA virus and poxvirus assembly occurs in the cytoplasm.

Capsid viruses may be assembled as empty structures (procapsids) to be filled with the genome (e.g., picornaviruses), or they may be assembled around the genome. Nucleocapsids of the retroviruses, togaviruses, and the negative-strand RNA viruses assemble around the genome and are subsequently enclosed in an envelope. The helical nucleocapsid of negative-strand RNA viruses includes the RNA-dependent RNA polymerase necessary for mRNA synthesis in the target cell.

For enveloped viruses, newly synthesized and processed viral glycoproteins are delivered to cellular membranes by vesicular transport. Acquisition of an envelope occurs after association of the nucleocapsid with the viral glycoprotein-containing regions of host cell membranes in a process called **budding.** Matrix proteins for negative-strand RNA viruses line and promote the adhesion of nucleocapsids with the glycoprotein-modified membrane. As more interactions occur, the membrane surrounds the nucleocapsid and the virus buds from the membrane.

The site of budding is determined by the type of genome and the protein sequence of the glycoproteins. Most RNA viruses bud from the plasma membrane, and the virus is released from the cell at the same time. The flaviviruses, coronaviruses, and bunyaviruses acquire their envelope by budding into the endoplasmic reticulum and Golgi membranes and may remain cell-associated in these organelles. The herpes simplex virus nucleocapsid assembles in the nucleus and buds at the nuclear membrane into the endoplasmic reticulum. The nucleocapsid may be dumped into the cytoplasm to reacquire its envelope from a Golgi membrane, or an enveloped herpesvirus may be transported to the Golgi apparatus. In either case, the virion is released by exocytosis, on cell lysis or transmitted through cell-cell bridges.

Viruses use different tricks to ensure that all the parts of the virus are assembled into complete virions. The RNA polymerase required for infection by negative-strand RNA viruses is carried on the genome as a helical nucleocapsid. The human immunodeficiency virus and other retrovirus genomes are packaged in a procapsid consisting of a polyprotein containing the protease, polymerase, integrase, and structural proteins. This procapsid binds to viral glycoprotein-modified membranes, and the virion buds from the membrane. The virus-encoded protease is activated within the virion and cleaves the polyprotein to produce the final, infectious nucleocapsid and the required proteins within the envelope.

Assembly of a complete, functional influenza or reovirus virion requires accumulation of at least one copy of each gene segment. Although the influenza virus has only 8 genome segments, virions can randomly package 10 to 11 segments. Statistically, this yields approximately 1 complete set of genomes and functional virus per 20 defective viruses. Reovirus genomes are likely to assemble in a similar manner.

Errors are made during viral assembly. Empty virions and virions containing defective genomes are produced. As a result, the particle–to–infectious virus ratio, also called particle–to–plaque-forming unit ratio, is high, usually greater than 10 and during rapid viral replication can even be 10^4. Defective viruses can occupy the machinery required for normal virus replication to prevent (interfere with) virus production **(defective interfering particles).**

Release

Viruses can be released from cells after lysis of the cell, by exocytosis, or by budding from the plasma membrane. Naked capsid viruses are generally released after lysis of the cell. Release of many enveloped viruses occurs after budding from the plasma membrane without killing the cell. Lysis and plasma membrane budding are efficient means of release. Viruses that bud or acquire their membrane in the cytoplasm (e.g., flaviviruses, poxviruses) remain cell-associated and are released by exocytosis or cell lysis. Viruses that bind to sialic acid receptors may also have a neuraminidase (e.g., orthomyxoviruses, certain paramyxoviruses). The neuraminidase removes potential sialic acid receptors on the glycoproteins of the virion and the host cell to prevent clumping and facilitate release.

Reinitiation of the Replication Cycle

The virus released to the extracellular medium is usually responsible for initiating new infections; however, **traversal of cell-cell bridges, virus-induced cell-cell fusion, or vertical transmission** of the genome to daughter cells can also spread the infection. The latter means allow the virus to escape antibody detection. Some herpesviruses, retroviruses, and paramyxoviruses can induce cell-cell fusion to create multinucleated giant cells (syncytia). The retroviruses and some DNA viruses can transmit their integrated copy of the genome vertically to daughter cells on cell division.

Viral Genetics

Mutations spontaneously and readily occur in viral genomes, creating new virus strains with properties differing from the **parental,** or **wild-type, virus.** These variants can be identified by their nucleotide sequences, antigenic differences (serotypes), or differences in functional or structural properties. Most mutations have no effect or are detrimental to the virus. Mutations in essential genes inactivate the virus, but mutations in other genes can produce antiviral drug resistance or alter the antigenicity or pathogenicity of the virus.

Errors in copying the viral genome during virus replication produce many mutations. This is because of the *poor fidelity of the viral polymerase and the rapid rate of genome replication.* In addition, *RNA viruses do not have a genetic error-checking mechanism.* As a result, the rates of mutation for RNA viruses are usually greater than for DNA viruses.

Mutations in essential genes are termed **lethal mutations.** These mutants are difficult to isolate because the virus cannot replicate. A **deletion mutant** results from the loss or selective removal of a portion of the genome and the function that it encodes. Other mutations may produce **plaque mutants,** which differ from the wild type in the size or appearance of the infected cells; **host range mutants,** which differ in the tissue type or species of target cell that can be infected; or **attenuated mutants,** which are variants that cause less serious infections in animals or humans. **Conditional mutants,** such as **temperature-sensitive (ts)** or **cold-sensitive mutants,** have a mutation in a gene for an essential protein that allows virus production only at certain temperatures. ts mutants generally grow well or relatively better at 30°C to 35°C, whereas elevated temperatures of 38°C to 40°C inactivate the mutated, essential gene product and prevent virus production.

New virus strains can also arise by genetic interac-

tions between viruses or between the virus and the cell (Fig. 6–15). Intramolecular genetic exchange between viruses or the virus and the host is termed **recombination.** Recombination can occur readily between two related DNA viruses. For example, co-infection of a cell with the two closely related herpesviruses (herpes simplex virus types 1 and 2) yields intertypic recombinant strains. These new hybrid strains have genes from both types 1 and 2. Integration of retroviruses into host cell chromatin is a form of recombination. Recombination of two related RNA viruses, Sindbis and eastern equine encephalitis virus, resulted in creation of another togavirus, western equine encephalitis virus.

Viruses with segmented genomes (such as influenza viruses and reoviruses) form hybrid strains on infection of one cell with more than one virus strain. This process, termed **reassortment,** is analogous to picking 10 marbles out of a box containing 10 black and 10 white marbles. New strains of influenza A virus are created on co-infection with a virus from different species (see Fig. 56–5).

In some cases, a defective viral strain can be rescued by the replication of another mutant, by the wild-type virus, or by a cell line bearing a replacement viral gene. Replication of the other virus provides the missing function required by the mutant **(complementation),** allowing replication to occur. A herpes simplex disabled infectious single cycle (DISC) vaccine virus is deleted in an essential gene and grown in a cell line that expresses that gene product to "complement" the virus. The virus that is produced can infect the normal cells of the vaccinated individual, but the virions that

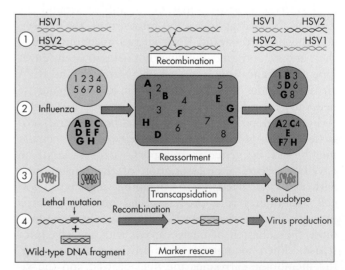

FIGURE 6–15. Genetic exchange between viral particles can give rise to new viral types, as illustrated. Representative viruses include the following: 1, intertypic recombination of herpes simplex virus type 1 *(HSV1)* and type 2 *(HSV2);* 2, reassortment of two strains of influenza virus; 3, rescue of a papovavirus defective in assembly by a complementary defective virus (transcapsidation); and 4, marker rescue of a lethal or conditional mutation.

are produced cannot replicate in the normal cells of a vaccinated individual. Rescue of a lethal or conditional-lethal mutant with a defined genetic sequence, such as a restriction endonuclease DNA fragment, is called **marker rescue.** Marker rescue is used to map the genomes of viruses such as herpes simplex virus. Virus produced from cells infected with different virus strains may be phenotypically mixed and have the proteins of one strain but the genome of the other **(transcapsidation). Pseudotypes** are generated when transcapsidation occurs between different types of virus, but this is rare.

Individual virus strains or mutants are **selected** by their ability to use the host cell machinery and to withstand the conditions of the body and the environment. Cellular properties that can act as selection pressures include the growth rate of the cell and tissue-specific expression of certain proteins required by the virus (e.g., enzymes, glycoproteins, transcription factors). The conditions of the body, its elevated temperature, natural and immune defenses, and tissue structure are also selection pressures for viruses. The viruses that cannot endure these conditions or evade the host defenses are eliminated. A small selective advantage in a mutant virus can shortly lead to its becoming the predominant viral strain. The high mutation rate of the human immunodeficiency virus promotes a switch in target cell tropism from macrophage to T cell, the development of antiviral drug-resistant strains after treatment, and the generation of antigenic variants during a patient's course of infection.

The growth of virus under benign laboratory conditions allows weaker strains to survive because of the absence of the selective pressures of the body. This process is used to develop attenuated virus strains for use in vaccines.

Viral Vectors for Therapy

Genetically manipulated viruses can be excellent delivery systems for foreign genes. Viruses can provide gene replacement therapy, can be used as vaccines to promote immunity to other agents or tumors, or can act as targeted killers of tumors. The advantages of using viruses are that they can be readily amplified by replication in appropriate cells and they target specific tissues and deliver the DNA or RNA into the cell. Viruses that are being developed as vectors include retroviruses, adenoviruses, herpes simplex virus, adeno-associated virus (parvovirus), poxviruses such as vaccinia and canarypox (see Fig. 52–3), and even some togaviruses. The viral vectors are usually defective or attenuated viruses in which the foreign DNA replaces a virulence or unessential gene. The foreign gene may be under the control of a viral promoter or even a tissue-specific promoter. Defective virus vectors are grown in cell lines that express the missing viral functions "com-plementing" the virus. The progeny can deliver their nucleic acid but not produce infectious virus. Retroviruses and adeno-associated viruses can integrate into cells and permanently deliver a gene into the chromosome. Adenovirus and herpes simplex virus promote targeted delivery of the foreign gene to receptor-bearing cells. Genetically attenuated herpes simplex viruses are being developed specifically to kill the growing cells of glioblastomas while sparing the surrounding neurons. Some day, virus vectors may be routinely used to treat cystic fibrosis, Duchenne's muscular dystrophy, lysosomal storage diseases, and immunologic disorders.

QUESTIONS

1. What features of these viruses are similar and what are different?
    a. Poliovirus and rhinovirus
    b. Poliovirus and rotavirus
    c. Poliovirus and western equine encephalitis virus
    d. Yellow fever virus and dengue virus
    e. Epstein-Barr virus and cytomegalovirus

2. Match the characteristics from column A with the appropriate viral families in column B based on your knowledge of their physical and genome structure and their implications.

A	B
1. Are resistant to detergents	Picornaviruses
2. Are resistant to drying	Togaviruses
3. Replication in the nucleus	Orthomyxoviruses
4. Replication in the cytoplasm	Paramyxoviruses
5. Can be released from the cell without cell lysis	Rhabdoviruses / Reoviruses
6. Provide a good target for antiviral drug action	Retroviruses / Herpesviruses
7. Undergo reassortment on co-infection with two strains	Papovaviruses / Adenoviruses
8. Make DNA from an RNA template	Poxviruses
9. Use a (+) RNA template to replicate the genome	Hepadnaviruses
10. Genome translated into a polyprotein	

3. Based on structural considerations, which of the virus families listed in question 2 should be able to endure fecal-oral transmission?

4. List the essential enzymes encoded by the virus families listed in question 2.

5. A mutant defective in the herpes simplex virus type 1 DNA polymerase gene replicates in the presence of herpes simplex virus type 2. The progeny virus contains the herpes simplex virus type 1 genome but is recognized by antibodies to herpes simplex virus type 2. Which genetic mechanisms may be occurring?

6. How are the early and late genes of the togaviruses, papovaviruses, and herpesviruses distinguished and how is the time of their expression regulated?

7. What are the consequences (no effect, decreased efficiency, or inhibition of replication) of a deletion mutation in the following viral enzymes?

    a. Epstein-Barr virus polymerase
    b. Herpes simplex virus thymidine kinase
    c. Human immunodeficiency virus reverse transcriptase
    d. Influenza B virus neuraminidase
    e. Rabies virus (rhabdovirus) G protein

BIBLIOGRAPHY

Belshe RB, editor: *Textbook of human virology*, ed 2, St Louis, 1991, Mosby.

Electron microscopic images of viruses, by Linda Stannard, University of Capetown, S.A. Available at http://www.uct.ac.za/depts/mmi/stannard/linda.html

Fields BN, Knipe DM, Howley PM, editors: *Virology*, ed 3, New York, 1996, Lippincott-Raven.

Flint SJ et al: *Principles of virology. Molecular biology, pathogenesis, and control*, Washington, DC, 2000, ASM Press.

Richman DD, Whitley RJ, Hayden FG: *Clinical virology*, New York, 1997, Churchill Livingstone.

Robbins PD, Ghivizzani SC: Viral vectors for gene therapy. *Pharmacol Ther* 80:35–47, 1998.

Specter S, Hodinka RL, Young SA: *Clinical virology manual*, ed 3, Washington, DC, 2000, ASM Press.

White DO, Fenner FJ: *Medical virology*, ed 4, Orlando, Fla, 1994, Academic Press.

Viruses in cell culture. Available at http://www.uct.ac.za/depts/mmi/stannard/linda.html

C H A P T E R 7

Fungal Classification, Structure, and Replication

The branch of biology that deals with the study of fungi is called mycology. Whereas the practical manifestations of these organisms have been known since antiquity, the systematic study of these organisms is approximately 150 years old. In addition to their disease-producing potential in humans, fungi are directly or indirectly harmful in many other ways. They contribute to food spoilage, are the major cause of plant diseases, and destroy timber, textiles, and several synthetic materials. As saprobes, however, they share with bacteria (particularly organisms such as the *Streptomyces*) a role in the decay of complex plant and animal remains in the soil, breaking them down into simpler molecules to be absorbed by future generations of plants. Without this essential decay process, the growth of plants, on which life depends, would eventually cease for lack of basic materials. Fungi are also specifically beneficial to humans. They are used in the production of antibiotics, organic acids, steroids, and products of fermentation, such as alcoholic beverages and soy sauce. The carbon dioxide produced by fungi makes dough rise in breadmaking, and the various ketones, aldehydes, and organic acids that result from the metabolic activities of fungi on milk curd and the juice of grapes provide the unique cheeses and wines we enjoy. Furthermore, fungi serve as scientific models to study genetics, biochemical processes, and relationships involving parasites and hosts.

Fungi are a diverse group of organisms that occupy many niches in the environment. In general, they are free living and abundant in nature; only a few live in the normal flora of humans. Although numerous species have been described, fewer than 100 are routinely associated with human diseases. Unlike viruses, protozoan parasites, and some species of bacteria, fungi do not need to colonize or infect the tissues of humans or animals to preserve or perpetuate the species. With only two major exceptions (candidiasis and tinea versicolor), virtually all fungal infections originate from an exogenous source, either by inhalation or by traumatic implantation.

Fungi are **eukaryotic organisms**. Most important, they possess a nucleus enclosed by a nuclear membrane. Unlike plant cells and some bacteria, fungi do not contain chlorophyll and cannot synthesize macromolecules from carbon dioxide and energy derived from light rays. Therefore, all fungi lead a heterotrophic existence in nature as **saprobes** (organisms that live on dead or decaying organic matter), **symbionts** (organisms that live together and in which the association is of mutual advantage), **commensals** (two organisms living in a close relationship in which one benefits by the relationship and the other neither benefits nor is harmed), or **parasites** (organisms that live on or within a host from which they derive benefits without making any useful contributions in return; in the case of pathogens, the relationship is harmful to the host).

Classification

Conflicts often arise in considering relationships between certain fungi, and no universal consensus may be possible concerning the classification or even the nomenclature of a given organism. Differences of opinion occasionally arise, because one taxonomist may place greater emphasis on certain phenotypic features of an isolate than on criteria deemed more important by other individuals. Another difficulty is the conflict between those who group many organisms and those who prefer to emphasize minor phenotype differences and split them into many groups. The result of these conflicting opinions is the controversy that frequently arises about the proper names of individual fungi. As a practical matter, the use of multiple names for the same organism has created a great deal of confusion in the medical literature.

Organisms are classified for convenience of reference; thus, the scheme of classification should reflect natural relationships between them. Biochemical, ultra-

TABLE 7–1. Taxonomic Classification of the Fungi Kingdom

Classification	Sexual Characteristics	Medically Important Genera
Phylum Zygomycota	Sexual reproduction occurs through fusion of two compatible gametangia to produce zygote. Asexual reproduction is characterized by production of sporangiospores.	Agents causing zygomycosis
Phylum Dikaryomycota	Dikaryotic life cycle includes extended dikaryotic phase after sexual conjugation; that is, haploid nuclei do not fuse immediately.	—
Subphylum Ascomycotina	Sexual reproduction occurs through fusion of two compatible nuclei to form diploid nucleus followed by meiosis to yield haploid progeny; entire process occurs within sac called *ascus,* and resultant spores are called *ascospores.*	Agents causing ringworm, histoplasmosis, and blastomycosis
Subphylum Basidiomycotina	Sexual reproduction takes place in sac called *basidium,* where two compatible nuclei fuse to form diploid nucleus, followed by meiosis to yield haploid progeny. These then mature on outer surface of basidium. Haploid progeny are called *basidiospores.*	Agent causing cryptococcosis
Form-class Deuteromycotina (Fungi imperfecti)	Sexual stage has not been observed in fungi classified in this category	*Candida, Trichosporon, Torulopsis, Pityrosporum, Epidermophyton, Coccidioides,* and *Paracoccidioides* species

structural, molecular biologic, and genetic studies support the concept that at least five kingdoms are necessary to accommodate all living things. These are the Monera (prokaryotes), Protista (protozoa), Fungi, Plantae, and Animalia. The Fungi kingdom is composed of two phyla (Table 7–1), the Zygomycota (organisms that produce a zygote during their sexual cycle) and the Dikaryomycota (organisms that have an extended state in which nuclei of different genotypes replicate autonomously in the same protoplasm as a result of sexual conjugation). The phylum Dikaryomycota is divided into two subphyla, the Ascomycotina and the Basidiomycotina, which are defined according to the type of structure that forms and houses the haploid progeny. Those organisms for which a sexual phase has not been observed are classified in the form-class Deuteromycotina or Fungi imperfecti.

Structure

Fungi have structures typical of eukaryotic cells. Figure 7–1 illustrates a section of a model fungal cell with its component parts. In contrast to bacterial cells, fungal cells possess a complex cytosol that contains microvesicles, microtubules, ribosomes, mitochondria, Golgi apparatus, nuclei, a double-membraned endoplasmic reticulum, and other structures. The nuclei of fungi are enclosed by a membrane and contain virtually all of the cellular DNA. They have a true nucleolus rich in RNA. An interesting and unique property of this membrane is that during the mitotic cycle it persists throughout metaphase, in contrast to the nuclear membrane of plant and animal cells, which dissolves and then reforms after the chromosomes segregate to their centromeres.

Enclosing the complex cytosol is another membrane called the **plasmalemma** that is composed of glycoproteins, phospholipids, and ergosterol. The fact that fungi possess ergosterol in contrast to cholesterol, which is the major sterol found in tissues of mammals, is important because most antifungal strategies are based on the presence of ergosterol in fungal membranes. (Antifungal agents are discussed in Chapter 67.)

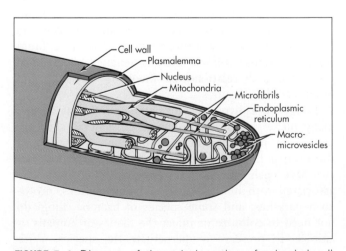

FIGURE 7–1. Diagram of the apical portion of a hyphal cell illustrating its component parts.

Unlike mammalian cells, fungi possess a multilayered rigid cell wall immediately exterior to the plasmalemma. The cell wall is structurally and biochemically complex, containing **chitin**, a homopolymer of β-(1,4)-linked *N*-acetylglucosamine residues, as its structural foundation. Layered on the chitin are glucans, mannoproteins, and other complex polysaccharides in association with polypeptides. In filamentous fungi, the biosynthesis of chitin occurs at the growing tip. The synthesis of chitin is controlled by the activity of three chitin synthases. These enzymes exist in the cytosol in discrete membrane-bound packets called **chitosomes**. The active form of chitin synthase is found in the plasmalemma, and polymerization of chitin microfibrils occurs outside this membrane.

In addition to the cell wall, some fungi produce a capsular polysaccharide. This structure isolates the organism from its surrounding environment and at the same time is in direct communication with that environment; in the case of pathogens, this environment is host tissue. The cell wall and structures such as the capsular material determine virulence and play a role in eliciting host immune responses. (See Chapter 70 for a discussion of *Cryptococcus neoformans*.)

Most fungi respire aerobically, but some have a limited capacity for anaerobiosis (fermentation), and others are strict anaerobes. Metabolically, they are heterotrophic and biochemically versatile, producing primary (e.g., citric acid, ethanol, glycerol) and secondary (e.g., penicillin, amanitins, aflatoxins) metabolites. The division time for these organisms is long (hours) compared with that of bacteria (minutes).

Fungi are gram-positive, and the vegetative cells are not acid-fast. In histopathologic sections, fungi can be stained by special procedures because of the glucans and other complex polysaccharides that make up the cell wall (methenamine-silver or periodic acid-Schiff staining methods).

Whereas the ability of fungi to cause disease in humans or animals appears to be accidental, most disease-producing fungi have developed characteristics that enable them to adapt to hostile tissue environments and grow. Fungi that colonize the cutaneous layers of the epidermis or invade hair and nails metabolize **keratin**, the tough, fibrous, insoluble protein that forms the principal matter of these tissues. Other fungi, such as *Histoplasma capsulatum*, *Blastomyces dermatitidis*, *Paracoccidioides brasiliensis*, and *Coccidioides immitis* have developed the capacity to overcome various host cellular defense mechanisms, can grow at the higher temperatures of the host (37°C) as well as the temperatures found in natural environments (about 25°C), and can survive in a lowered oxidation-reduction state (a situation found in damaged tissues).

Fungi can be divided into two basic morphologic forms: yeast and hyphae. Their developmental histories encompass both vegetative and reproductive phases. These phases are frequently present simultaneously in growing cultures and may not be easily separated.

Yeasts are unicellular and reproduce asexually by processes termed blastoconidia formation (budding) (Fig. 7–2*A*) or fission (Fig. 7–2*B*).

Most fungi have branching, threadlike tubular filaments called hyphae (Fig. 7–2*C* to *F*) that elongate at their tips by a process called apical extension. These filamentous structures are either coenocytic (hollow and multinucleate) (Fig. 7–2*D*) or septate (divided by partitions) (Fig. 7–2*E* and *F*). The collective term for a mass of hyphae is **mycelium** (synonymous with mold). Hyphae that grow submerged or on the surface of a culture medium are called **vegetative hyphae** because they are responsible for absorbing nutrients. Those

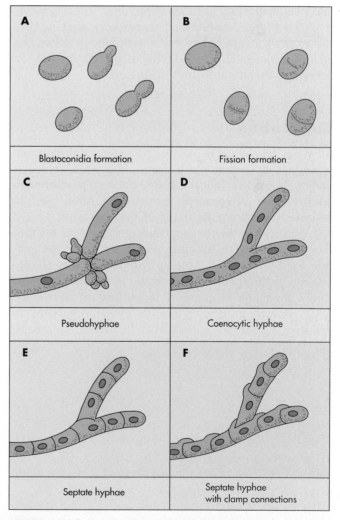

FIGURE 7–2. Fungal cell morphology. *A*, Yeast cells reproducing by blastoconidia formation. *B*, Yeast cells dividing by fission. *C*, Pseudohyphal development. *D*, Coenocytic hyphae. *E*, Septate hyphae. *F*, Septate hyphae with clamp connections.

that project above the surface of the medium are called **aerial hyphae**. Aerial hyphae often produce specialized structures called conidia (i.e., asexual reproductive elements also called propagules) that are easily airborne and disseminated into the environment. The shape, size, and certain developmental features of conidia are useful to the mycologist in identifying the specific species. This is illustrated in Chapters 69 to 71.

The morphology of *Candida albicans*, part of the normal flora of the mouth, gastrointestinal tract, and membranes lining the mucosa of other cavities and tissues, is unique. In addition to being yeastlike or filamentous, this organism can assume a pseudohyphal morphology wherein the cells are elongated and linked like sausages (see Fig. 7–2*C*). Pseudohyphal development is an exaggerated form of budding; the newly formed cells do not take on an oval shape and pinch off from the parent but rather remain attached and continue to elongate. The morphology of fungi is not fixed because some are dimorphic (e.g., *H. capsulatum*, *B. dermatitidis*, *C. immitis*, *P. brasiliensis*); that is, they can exist in a mycelial or yeast morphology depending on the environmental conditions of growth (in soil, on decaying vegetation, or in host tissues).

Replication

All fungi reproduce by asexual processes, and most can reproduce by sexual mechanisms. If a sexual phase is observed for any fungal isolate, the terms **anamorph** (asexual) and **teleomorph** (sexual) are often used to describe the taxonomic status of the organism. This is reflected mostly in the nomenclature used to refer to that organism. For example, the anamorphic designation for the organism causing histoplasmosis is *H. capsulatum*; if the specific isolate exists in the teleomorphic state, the name is changed to *Ajellomyces capsulatum*. This convention is used for all fungal organisms to maintain taxonomic consistency. In clinical situations,

however, it is common to refer to the organisms by their asexual designations, because the anamorphic state is isolated from clinical specimens and the sexual phase occurs only under the extremely controlled conditions of a culture.

QUESTIONS

1. How do fungi differ from bacteria (size, nucleus, cytosol, cytosolic membrane, cell wall, physiology, staining properties, generation time)?

2. What is the basic difference between the cell membrane (plasmalemma) of fungal and mammalian cells?

3. How do yeasts differ from molds, and what does the term dimorphism mean when it is applied to fungi?

4. What do the terms anamorph and teleomorph mean, and of what importance are they?

BIBLIOGRAPHY

Dixon DM, Rhodes JC, Fromtling RA: Taxonomy, classification, and morphology of fungi. In Murray PR et al, editors: *Manual of clinical microbiology*, ed 7, Washington, DC, 1999, American Society for Microbiology.

Evans EGV, Gentles JC: *Essentials of medical mycology*, New York, 1985, Churchill Livingstone.

Lehman PF: Fungal structure and morphology. In Ajello L, Hay RJ, editors: *Topley and Wilson's Microbiology and microbial diseases*, vol. 4, *Medical mycology*. London 1998, Arnold.

Lipke PN, Ovalle R: Yeast cell walls: new structures, new challenges, *J Bacteriol* 180:3735–3740, 1998.

Margulis L, Schwartz KV: *Five kingdoms*, ed 2, New York, 1988, WH Freeman.

Moore-Landecker E: *Fundamentals of the fungi*, ed 3, Englewood Cliffs, NJ, 1990, Prentice-Hall.

CHAPTER 8

Parasitic Classification, Structure, and Replication

T his chapter provides an introduction to parasite classification and physiology. The brief review is intended to enhance the reader's comprehension of the interrelationships among parasitic organisms, their epidemiology and transmission of disease, the specific disease processes involved, and the possibilities for prevention and control of maladies. We have deliberately attempted to simplify the taxonomy by using it to address the major divisions involved in medical parasitology: specifically, intestinal and urogenital protozoa, blood and tissue protozoa, nematodes, trematodes, and cestodes.

The Importance of Parasites

Medical parasitology is the study of invertebrate animals capable of causing disease in humans and other animals. Although parasitic diseases are frequently considered "tropical" and thus of little importance to physicians practicing in the more temperate, developed countries of the world, it is clear that the world has become a very small place and that physician knowledge of parasitic diseases is essential. The global impact of parasitic infections and the number of parasite-associated deaths is staggering and must be of concern to all health care workers (Table 8–1). Increasingly, tourists, missionaries, Peace Corps volunteers, and others are visiting and working for extended periods of time in exotic, remote parts of the world. Thus, they are at risk for parasitic and other infections that are rare in the United States and other developed countries. Another source of infected patients is the ever-increasing number of refugees from developing countries. Finally, the profound immunosuppression problems that accompany advances in medical therapy (e.g., organ transplantation), as well as those associated with persons infected with the human immunodeficiency virus, place a growing number of individuals at risk for developing infections caused by certain parasites. Given these considerations, clinicians and laboratory workers should be aware of the possibility of parasitic disease and should be trained in ordering, performing, and interpreting the appropriate laboratory tests to aid in the diagnosis and therapy.

Classification and Structure

The parasites of humans are classified within the kingdom Animalia and are separated into two subkingdoms, Protozoa and Metazoa (Table 8–2). Parasite classification takes into account the morphology of intracytoplasmic structures, such as the nucleus, the type of locomotive organelles, and the mode of reproduction (Table 8–3). The Protozoa are animals in which all life functions occur in a single cell. The Metazoa are multicellular animals in which life functions occur in cellular structures organized as tissue and organ systems.

Protozoa

Protozoa are simple microorganisms that range in size from 2 to 100 μm. Their protoplasm is enclosed by a cell membrane and contains numerous organelles, including a membrane-bound nucleus, an endoplasmic reticulum, food-storage granules, and contractile and digestive vacuoles. The nucleus contains clumped or dispersed chromatin and a central karyosome. Organs of motility vary from simple cytoplasmic extrusions or pseudopods to more complex structures such as flagella or cilia. The subkingdom Protozoa comprises seven major subgroups or phyla, four of which are the concern of medical parasitology.

Sarcomastigophora

Phylum Sarcomastigophora consists of the amebae (subphylum Sarcodina) and the flagellates (subphylum Mastigophora). Locomotion of amebae is accomplished by the extrusion of pseudopodia ("false feet"), whereas

TABLE 8–1. Estimated Worldwide Prevalence of Parasitic Infections

Infection	Number of Infected	Annual Deaths*
Amebiasis	1% of world population	40,000–110,000
Giardiasis	200 million	—
Malaria	400–490 million	2.2–2.5 million
African trypanosomiasis	100,000 new cases/yr	5000
American trypanosomiasis	24 million	60,000
Leishmaniasis	1.2 million	—
Schistosomiasis	150 million	0.5 million
Opisthorchiasis	13.5 million	—
Paragonimiasis	2.1 million	—
Fasciolopsiasis	10 million	—
Filariasis	128 million	—
Onchocerciasis	17.7 million	—
Dracunculiasis	<100,000	—
Ascariasis	1.3 billion	1550†
Hookworm	1.3 billion	—
Trichuriasis	900 million	—
Strongyloidiasis	35 million	—
Cestodiasis	65 million	—

*Mortality data included where available.
†From intestinal obstruction.
Modified from Markell EK, John DT, Krotoski WA, editors: *Markell and Voge's medical parasitology*, ed 8, Philadelphia, 1999, WB Saunders.

flagellates move by the lashing of their whiplike flagella. The number and position of flagella can vary in different species. In addition, specialized structures associated with the flagella may produce a characteristic morphologic appearance that may be useful in species identification.

Ciliophora

Phylum Ciliophora consists of the ciliates, which include a variety of free-living and symbiotic species. Ciliate locomotion involves the coordinated movement of rows of hairlike structures, or cilia. Cilia are structurally similar to flagella but are usually shorter and more numerous. Some ciliates are multinucleate. The only ciliate parasite of humans, *Balantidium coli*, contains two nuclei: a large macronucleus and a small micronucleus.

Apicomplexa

Phylum Apicomplexa organisms are often referred to as *sporozoa* or *coccidia*. These unicellular organisms have a system of organelles at their apical end that produces substances to help the organism penetrate host cells and thus become an intracellular parasite.

Microspora

Phylum Microspora organisms were formerly classified with the Sporozoa. The Microspora are small intracellular parasites that differ significantly in structure from the Apicomplexa. These parasites are characterized by the structure of their spores, which have a complex tubular extrusion mechanism (polar tubule) used to inject the infective material (sporoplasm) into host cells.

Metazoa

The subkingdom Metazoa includes all animals that are not Protozoa. This text discusses two groups of organisms of major importance: the helminths ("worms") and the arthropods (crabs, insects, ticks, and the like).

Helminths

The helminths are complex, multicellular organisms that are elongated and bilaterally symmetrical. They are considerably larger than the protozoan parasites and generally are macroscopic, ranging in size from less than 1 mm to 1 m or more. The external surface of some worms is covered with a protective cuticle, which is acellular and may be smooth or possess ridges, spines, or tubercles. The protective covering of flatworms is known as a tegument. Frequently, helminths

TABLE 8–2. Medically Important Parasites (Kingdom, Animalia)

Subkingdom	Phylum	Organisms
Protoza	Sarcomastigophora	Ameba, flagellates
	Ciliophora	Ciliates
	Apicomplexa	Sporozoa, Coccidia
	Microspora	Microsporidia
Metazoa	Nematoda	Roundworms
	Platyhelminthes	Flatworms
	Trematodes	Flukes
	Cestodes	Tapeworms
	Arthropoda	
	Chilopoda	Centipedes
	Pentastomida	Tongue worms
	Crustacea	Crabs, crayfish, shrimp, copepods
	Arachnida	Mites, ticks, spiders, scorpions
	Insecta	Mosquitoes, flies, lice, fleas, wasps, ants, beetles, moths, roaches, true bugs

possess elaborate attachment structures such as hooks, suckers, teeth, or plates. These structures are usually located anteriorly and may be useful in classifying and identifying the organisms (see Table 8–3). Helminths typically have primitive nervous and excretory systems. Some have alimentary tracts; however, none has a circulatory system (see Table 8–3). The helminths are separated into two phyla, the Nematoda and the Platyhelminthes.

Nematoda. Phylum Nematoda consists of the roundworms, which have cylindrical bodies. The sexes of roundworm are separate, and these organisms have a complete digestive system. The nematodes may be intestinal parasites or may infect the blood and tissue.

Platyhelminthes. Phylum Platyhelminthes consists of the flatworms, which have flattened bodies that are leaflike or resemble ribbon segments. Platyhelminthes can be further separated into trematodes and cestodes.

Trematodes, or flukes, have leaf-shaped bodies. Most are hermaphroditic, with male and female sex organs in a single body. Their digestive systems are incomplete and have only saclike tubes. Their life cycle is complex; snails serve as first intermediate hosts and other aquatic animals or plants as second intermediate hosts.

Cestodes, or tapeworms, have bodies composed of ribbons of proglottids, or segments. All are hermaphro-

ditic, and all lack digestive systems; nutrition is absorbed through the body walls. The life cycles of some cestodes are simple and direct, whereas those of others are complex and require one or more intermediate hosts.

Arthropods

Phylum Arthropoda is the largest group of animals in the kingdom Animalia. Arthropods are complex, multicellular organisms that may be involved directly in causing an invasive or a superficial (infestation) disease process or indirectly as intermediate hosts and vectors of many infectious agents, including protozoan and metazoan parasites (Table 8–4). In addition, envenomization by biting and stinging arthropods can result in adverse reactions in humans that range from local allergic and hypersensitivity reactions to severe anaphylactic shock and death. There are five major classes of arthropods (see Table 8–2).

Chilopoda. Class Chilopoda consists of terrestrial forms, such as centipedes. These organisms are of medical importance because of their poison claws, which may produce a painful "bite."

Pentastomida. The pentastomids, or tongue worms, are bloodsucking endoparasites of reptiles, birds, and mammals. Adult pentastomids are white and cylindrical or flattened parasites that possess two distinct body regions: an anterior cephalothorax and an abdomen. Humans may serve as intermediate hosts for these parasites.

Crustacea. Class Crustacea consists of familiar aquatic forms, such as crabs, crayfish, shrimp, and copepods. Several are involved as intermediate hosts in life cycles of various intestinal or blood and tissue helminths.

Arachnida. Class Arachnida consists of familiar terrestrial forms, such as mites, ticks, spiders, and scorpions. Unlike insects, these animals have no wings or antennae, and adults have four pairs of legs, compared with three pairs for insects. Of medical importance are those serving as vectors for microbial diseases (mites and ticks) or as venomous animals that bite (spiders) or sting (scorpions).

Insecta. Class Insecta consists of familiar aquatic and terrestrial forms, such as mosquitoes, flies, midges, fleas, lice, bugs, wasps, and ants. Wings and antennae are present, and adult forms have three pairs of legs. Of medical importance are the many insects that serve as vectors for microbial diseases (mosquitoes, fleas, flies, lice, and bugs) or as venomous animals that sting (bees, wasps, and ants).

TABLE 8–3. Biologic, Morphologic, and Physiologic Characteristics of Pathogenic Parasites

Organism Class	Morphology	Reproduction	Organelles of Locomotion	Respiration	Nutrition
Protozoa					
Ameba	Unicellular; cyst and trophocyte forms	Binary fission	Pseudopods	Facultative anaerobe	Assimilation by pinocytosis or phagocytosis
Flagellates	Unicellular; cyst and trophozoite forms; possibly intracellular	Binary fission	Flagella	Facultative anaerobe	Simple diffusion or ingestion via cytostome, pinocytosis, or phagocytosis
Ciliates	Unicellular; cysts and trophozoite	Binary fission or conjugation	Cilia	Facultative anaerobe	Ingestion via cytostome, food vacuole
Coccidia	Unicellular, frequently intracellular; multiple forms, including trophozoites, sporozoites, cysts (oocysts), gametes	Schizogony and sporogony	None	Facultative anaerobe	Simple diffusion
Microsporidia	Obligate intracellular forms; small, simple cells and spores	Binary fission, schizogony and sporogony	None	Facultative anaerobe	Simple diffusion
Helminths					
Nematodes	Multicellular; round, smooth, spindle shaped, tubular alimentary tract; possibility of teeth or plates for attachment	Separate sexes	No single organelle; active muscular motility	Adults: usually anaerobic, larvae: possibly aerobic	Ingestion or absorption of body fluids, tissue, or digestive contents
Trematodes	Multicellular; leaf shaped with oral and ventral suckers, blind alimentary tract	Hermaphroditic (*Schistosoma* group has separate sexes)	No single organelle; muscle-directed motility	Adults: usually anaerobic	Ingestion or absorption of body fluids, tissue, or digestive contents
Cestodes	Multicellular; head with segmented body (proglottids); lack of alimentary tract; head equipped with hood and/or suckers for attachment	Hermaphroditic	No single organelle; usually, attachment to mucosa, possible muscular motility (proglottids)	Adults: usually anaerobic	Absorption of nutrients from intestine
Arthropods					
Chilopoda	Elongated; many legs; distinctive head and trunk; poison claws on first segment	Separate sexes	Legs	Aerobic	Carnivore
Pentastomida	Wormlike; cylindrical, or flattened; two distinct body regions; digestive and reproductive organs; lack of circulatory and respiratory systems	Separate sexes	Muscle-directed motility	Aerobic	Ingestion of body fluids and tissue
Crustacea	Hard external carapace; one pair of maxillae; five pairs of biramous legs	Separate sexes	Legs	Aerobic	Ingestion of body fluids and tissue, carnivorous
Arachnida	Body divided into cephalothorax and abdomen; eight legs and poisoning fangs	Separate sexes	Legs	Aerobic	Carnivore
Insecta	Body: head, thorax, and abdomen; one pair of antennae; three pairs of appendages, up to two pairs of wings	Separate sexes	Legs, wings	Aerobic	Ingestion of fluids and tissues

TABLE 8–4. **Transmission and Distribution of Pathogenic Parasites**

Organism	Infective Form	Mechanism of Spread	Distribution
Intestinal Protozoa			
Entamoeba histolytica	Cyst/trophozoite	Indirect (fecal-oral) Direct (venereal)	Worldwide
Giardia lamblia	Cyst	Fecal-oral route	Worldwide
Dientamoeba fragilis	Trophozoite	Fecal-oral route	Worldwide
Balantidium coli	Cyst	Fecal-oral route	Worldwide
Isospora belli	Oocyst	Fecal-oral route	Worldwide
Cryptosporidium species	Oocyst	?Fecal-oral route	Worldwide
Enterocytozoon bieneusi	Spore	?Fecal-oral route	North America, Europe
Urogenital Protozoa			
Trichomonas vaginalis	Trophozoite	Direct (venereal) route	Worldwide
Blood and Tissue Protozoa			
Naegleria and *Acanthamoeba* species	Cyst/trophozoite	Direct inoculation, inhalation	Worldwide
Plasmodium species	Sporozoite	*Anopheles* mosquito	Tropical and subtropical areas
Babesia species	Pyriform body	*Ixodes* trick	North America, Europe
Toxoplasma gondii	Oocysts and tissue cysts	Fecal-oral route, carnivorism	Worldwide
Leishmania species	Promastigote	*Phlebotomus* sandfly	Tropical and subtropical areas
Trypanosoma cruzi	Trypomastigote	Reduviid bug	North, Central, and South America
Trypanosoma brucei	Trypomastigote	Tsetse fly	Africa
Nematodes			
Enterobius vermicularis	Egg	Fecal-oral route	Worldwide
Ascaris lumbricoides	Egg	Fecal-oral route	Areas of poor sanitation
Toxocara species	Egg	Fecal-oral route	Worldwide
Trichuris trichiura	Egg	Fecal-oral route	Worldwide
Ancylostoma duodenale	Filariform larva	Direct skin penetration from contaminated soil	Tropical and subtropical areas
Necator americanus	Filariform larva	Direct skin penetration, autoinfection	Tropical and subtropical areas
Strongyloides stercoralis	Filariform larva	Direct skin penetration, autoinfection	Tropical and subtropical areas
Trichinella spiralis	Encysted larva in tissue	Carnivorism	Worldwide
Wuchereria bancrofti	Third-stage larva	Mosquito	Tropical and subtropical areas
Brugia malayi	Third-stage larva	Mosquito	Tropical and subtropical areas
Loa loa	Filariform larva	*Chrysops* fly	Africa
Mansonella species	Third-stage larva	Biting midges or black flies	Africa, Central and South America
Onchocerca volvulus	Third-stage larva	*Simulium* black fly	Africa, Central and South America
Dracunculus medinensis	Third-stage larva	Ingestion of infected cyclops	Africa, Asia
Dirofilaria immitis	Third-stage larva	Mosquito	Japan, Australia, United States
Trematodes			
Fasciolopsis buski	Metacercaria	Ingestion of metacercaria encysted on aquatic plants	China, Southeast Asia, India
Fasciola hepatica	Metacercaria	Metacercaria on water plants	Worldwide
Opisthorchis (Clonorchis) sinensis	Metacercaria	Metacercaria encysted in freshwater fish	China, Japan, Korea, Vietnam
Paragonimus westermani	Metacercaria	Metacercaria encysted in freshwater crustaceans	Asia, Africa, India, Latin America
Schistosoma species	Cercaria	Direct penetration of skin by free-swimming cercaria	Africa, Asia, India, Latin America

Continued on following page

TABLE 8–4 *Continued*

Organism	Infective Form	Mechanism of Spread	Distribution
Cestodes			
Taenia solium	Cysticercus, embryonated egg or proglottid	Ingestion of infected pork Ingestion of egg (cysticercosis)	Pork-eating countries: Africa, Southeast Asia, China, Latin America
Taenia saginata	Cysticercus	Ingestion of cysticercus in meat	Worldwide
Diphyllobothrium latum	Sparganum	Ingestion of sparganum in fish	Worldwide
Echinococcus granulosus	Embryonated egg	Ingestion of eggs from infected canines	Sheep-raising countries: Europe, Asia, Africa, Australia, United States
Echinococcus multilocularis	Embryonated egg	Ingestion of eggs from infected animals, fecal-oral route	Canada, Northern United States, Central Europe
Hymenolepis nana	Embryonated egg	Ingestion of eggs, fecal-oral route	Worldwide
Hymenolepis diminuta	Cysticercus	Ingestion of infected beetle larvae in contaminated grain products	Worldwide
Dipylidium caninum	Cysticercoid	Ingestion of infected fleas	Worldwide

Physiology and Replication

Protozoa

The nutritional requirements of the parasitic protozoa are generally simple and require the assimilation of organic nutrients. The amebae, ameboflagellates, and certain other protozoa accomplish this assimilation by the rather primitive process of pinocytosis or phagocytosis of soluble or particulate matter (see Table 8–3). The engulfed material is enclosed in digestive vacuoles. The flagellates and ciliates generally ingest food at a definitive site or structure, the peristome or cytostome. Other protozoan parasites, such as the intracellular microsporidia, assimilate nutrients by simple diffusion. The ingested food material may be retained in intracytoplasmic granules or in vacuoles. The undigested particles and waste may be eliminated from the cell by extrusion of the material at the cell surface. Respiration in most parasitic protozoa is accomplished by facultatively anaerobic processes.

To ensure survival under harsh or unfavorable environmental conditions, many parasitic protozoa develop into a cyst form that is less metabolically active. This cyst is surrounded by a thick external cell wall capable of protecting the organism from otherwise lethal physical and chemical insults. The cyst form is an integral part of the life cycle of many protozoan parasites and facilitates the transmission of the organism from host to host in the external environment (see Table 8–4). Parasites that cannot form cysts must rely on direct transmission from host to host or require an arthropod vector to complete their life cycles (see Table 8–4).

In addition to cyst formation, many protozoan parasites have developed elaborate immunoevasive mechanisms that allow them to respond to attack by the host immune system by continuously changing their surface antigens, thus ensuring continued survival within the host. Reproduction among the protozoa is generally by simple binary fission (**merogony**), although the life cycle of some protozoa, such as the sporozoans, includes cycles of multiple fission (**schizogony**) alternating with a period of sexual reproduction (**sporogony or gametogony**).

Metazoa

Helminths

The nutritional requirements of helminthic parasites are met by active ingestion of host tissue, fluids, or both, with resultant tissue destruction, or by more passive absorption of nutrients from the surrounding fluids and intestinal contents (see Table 8–3). The muscular motility of many helminths expends considerable energy, and the worms rapidly metabolize carbohydrates. Nutrients are stored in the form of glycogen, the content of which is high in most helminths. Similar to respiration in protozoa, respiration in helminths is primarily anaerobic, although the larval forms may require oxygen.

A significant proportion of the energy requirement of helminths is dedicated to supporting the reproductive process. Many worms are quite prolific, producing as many as 200,000 offspring each day. In general, helminthic parasites are egg laying (oviparous), although a few species may bear live young (viviparous). The resulting larvae are always morphologically distinct from the adult parasites and must undergo several developmental stages or molts before attaining adulthood.

The major protective barrier for most helminths is the tough external layer (cuticle or tegument). Worms may also secrete enzymes that destroy host cells and neutralize immunologic and cellular defense mechanisms. Similar to protozoan parasites, some helminths possess the ability to alter the antigenic properties of their external surfaces and thus evade the host immune response. This is accomplished in part by incorporating host antigens into their external cuticular layer. In this way, the worm avoids immunologic recognition, and in some diseases (e.g., schistosomiasis), it allows the parasite to survive within the host for decades.

Arthropods

Arthropods have segmented bodies, paired jointed appendages, and well-developed digestive and nervous systems. Sexes are separate. Respiration by aquatic forms is via gills and by terrestrial forms is via tubular body structures. All have a hard chitin covering as an exoskeleton.

Summary

Physician awareness of parasitic diseases is undoubtedly more critical now than at any time in the history of medical practice. Physicians today must be prepared to answer questions from patients about protection from malaria and the risks of drinking water and eating fresh fruits and vegetables in remote areas where they may be traveling. With this knowledge of parasitic diseases, the physician can also evaluate signs, symptoms, and incubation periods in returning travelers and make a diagnosis and begin treatment for a patient with a possible parasitic disease. The risks of parasitic diseases in immunosuppressed individuals and in those with the acquired immunodeficiency syndrome must also be understood and taken into account.

Proper education regarding parasitic diseases in medical curricula cannot be overemphasized as a requirement for physicians whose practice includes travelers to foreign countries and refugee populations. Many of the important parasites responsible for human diseases are transmitted by arthropod vectors or are acquired by the consumption of contaminated food or water. The various modes of transmission and distribution of parasitic diseases are presented in appropriate detail in the following chapters; however, the data in Table 8–4 are provided as an outline.

QUESTIONS

1. How do protozoa adapt to harsh environmental conditions?
2. Which morphologic form is important in the transmission of protozoa from host to host?
3. How do helminths, such as schistosomes, avoid the host immune response?
4. How do arthropods cause human disease?

BIBLIOGRAPHY

Garcia LS, editor: *Diagnostic medical parasitology*, ed. 4, Washington, DC, 2001, American Society for Microbiology.

Markell EK, John DT, Krotoski WA, editors: *Markell and Voge's medical parasitology*, ed 8, Philadelphia, 1999, WB Saunders.

Murray PR et al, editors: *Manual of clinical microbiology*, ed 7, Washington, DC, 1999, American Society for Microbiology.

Strickland GT, editors: *Hunter's tropical medicine and emerging infectious disease*, ed 8, Philadelphia, 2000, WB Saunders.

C H A P T E R 9

Commensal and Pathogenic Microbial Flora in Humans

Medical microbiology is the study of the interactions between animals (primarily humans) and microorganisms such as bacteria, viruses, fungi, and parasites. Although the primary interest is in diseases caused by these interactions, it must also be appreciated that microorganisms play a critical role in human survival. The normal commensal population of microbes participates in the metabolism of food products, provides essential growth factors, protects against infections with highly virulent microorganisms, and stimulates the immune response. In the absence of these organisms, life as we know it would be impossible.

The microbial flora in and on the human body is in a continual state of flux determined by a variety of factors, such as age, diet, hormonal state, health, and personal hygiene. Whereas the human fetus lives in a protected, sterile environment, the newborn is exposed to microbes from the mother and environment. The infant's skin is colonized first, followed by the oropharynx, gastrointestinal tract, and other mucosal surfaces. Throughout the life of an individual, this microbial population continues to change. Changes in health can drastically disrupt the delicate balance that is maintained among the heterogeneous organisms coexisting within us. For example, hospitalization can lead to the replacement of normally avirulent organisms in the oropharynx with gram-negative bacilli (e.g., *Klebsiella*, *Pseudomonas*) that can invade the lungs and cause pneumonia. Likewise, the growth of *Clostridium difficile* in the gastrointestinal tract is controlled by the indigenous bacteria present in the intestines. In the presence of antibiotics, however, this indigenous flora is eliminated, and *C. difficile* is able to proliferate and produce gastrointestinal disease.

Exposure of an individual to an organism can lead to one of three outcomes. The organism can (1) transiently colonize the person, (2) permanently colonize the person, or (3) produce disease. It is important to understand the distinction between colonization and disease. (NOTE–many people use the term **infection** inappropriately as a synonym for both terms.) Organisms that colonize humans (whether for a short period [transient] or permanently) do not disrupt normal body functions. In contrast, disease occurs when the interaction between microbe and human leads to a pathologic process characterized by damage to the human host. This process can result from microbial factors (e.g., damage to organs caused by the proliferation of the microbe or the production of toxins or cytotoxic enzymes) or the host's immune response to the organism.

An understanding of medical microbiology requires knowledge not only of the different classes of microbes but also of their propensity for causing disease. A few infections are caused by **strict pathogens** (i.e., organisms always associated with human disease). Some examples of strict pathogens and the diseases they cause include *Mycobacterium tuberculosis* (tuberculosis), *Neisseria gonorrhoeae* (gonorrhea), *Francisella tularensis* (tularemia), *Plasmodium* spp. (malaria), and rabies virus (rabies). Most infections are caused by **opportunistic pathogens**, organisms that are typically members of the patient's normal microbial flora (e.g., *Staphylococcus aureus*, *Escherichia coli*, *Candida albicans*). These organisms do not produce disease in their normal setting but establish disease when they are introduced into unprotected sites (e.g., blood stream, tissues). The factors responsible for the virulence of strict and opportunistic pathogens are discussed in later chapters.

The microbial population that colonizes the human body is numerous and diverse. The most common organisms that form the commensal flora and their propensity to cause disease are summarized in this chapter.

Respiratory Tract and Head

Mouth, Oropharynx, and Nasopharynx

The upper respiratory tract is colonized with numerous organisms, with 10 to 100 anaerobes for every aerobic bacterium (Box 9–1). The most common anaerobic bacteria are *Peptostreptococcus, Veillonella, Actinomyces,* and *Fusobacterium* spp.; the most common aerobic bacteria are *Streptococcus, Haemophilus,* and *Neisseria* spp. The relative proportion of these organisms varies at different anatomic sites; for example, the microbial flora on the surface of a tooth is quite different from the flora in saliva or in the subgingival spaces. Most of the common organisms in the upper respiratory tract are relatively avirulent and are rarely associated with disease unless they are introduced into normally sterile sites (e.g., sinuses, middle ear, brain). Potentially pathogenic organisms can also be found in the upper airways, including group A *Streptococcus, Streptococcus pneumoniae, S. aureus, Neisseria meningitidis, Haemophilus influenzae, Moraxella catarrhalis,* and Enterobacteriaceae. Isolation of these organisms from an upper respiratory tract specimen does not define their pathogenicity. Their involvement with a disease process must be demonstrated to the exclusion of other pathogens. For example, with the exception of group A *Streptococcus,* these organisms are rarely responsible for pharyngitis, even though they can be isolated from patients with this disease.

Ear

The most common organism colonizing the outer ear is coagulase-negative *Staphylococcus.* Other organisms colonizing the skin have been isolated from this site, as well as potential pathogens such as *S. pneumoniae, Pseudomonas aeruginosa,* and the Enterobacteriaceae. The pathogenic organisms have also been associated with disease at this site.

Eye

The surface of the eye is colonized with coagulase-negative staphylococci as well as rare numbers of organisms found in the nasopharynx (e.g., *Haemophilus* spp., *Neisseria* spp., viridans streptococci). Disease is typically associated with *S. pneumoniae, S. aureus, H. influenzae, N. gonorrhoeae, Chlamydia trachomatis, P. aeruginosa,* and *Bacillus* spp.

Lower Respiratory Tract

The larynx, trachea, bronchioles, and lower airways are generally sterile, although transient colonization with secretions of the upper respiratory tract may occur after aspiration. Acute disease of the lower airway is usually caused by the more virulent bacteria present in the mouth (e.g., *S. pneumoniae, S. aureus, H. influenzae,* members of the family Enterobacteriaceae such as *Klebsiella*). Chronic aspiration may lead to a polymicrobial disease in which anaerobes are the predominant pathogens, particularly *Peptostreptococcus* and anaerobic gram-negative bacilli. Fungi such as *Candida albicans* can cause disease of the lower airway, but invasion of these organisms into tissue must be demonstrated to exclude simple colonization. In contrast, the presence of the dimorphic fungi (e.g., *Histoplasma, Coccidioides,* and *Blastomyces* spp.) is diagnostic because colonization with these organisms never occurs.

Gastrointestinal Tract

The gastrointestinal tract is colonized with microbes at birth and remains the home for a diverse population of organisms throughout the life of the host (Box 9–2). Although the opportunity for colonization with new organisms occurs daily with the ingestion of food and water, the population remains relatively constant unless exogenous factors such as antibiotic treatment disrupt the balanced flora.

Esophagus

Oropharyngeal bacteria and yeast, as well as the bacteria that colonize the stomach, can be isolated from the esophagus; however, most organisms are believed to be transient colonizers that do not establish permanent residence. Bacteria rarely cause disease of the esophagus (esophagitis); most infections are caused by *Candida* spp. and viruses such as herpes simplex virus and cytomegalovirus.

Stomach

Because the stomach contains hydrochloric acid and pepsinogen (secreted by the parietal and chief cells lin-

---

BOX 9–1. **Most Common Microbes Colonizing the Respiratory Tract**

Bacteria

Acinetobacter
Actinobacillus
Actinomyces
Cardiobacterium
Corynebacterium
Eikenella
Enterobacteriaceae
Eubacterium
Fusobacterium
Haemophilus
Kingella
Moraxella
Mycoplasma
Neisseria
Peptostreptococcus
Porphyromonas
Prevotella
Propionibacterium
Staphylococcus
Streptococcus
Stomatococcus
Treponema
Veillonella

Fungi

Candida

Parasites

Entamoeba
Trichomonas

BOX 9-2. **Most Common Microbes Colonizing the Gastrointestinal Tract**

Bacteria	*Porphyromonas*
Acinetobacter	*Prevotella*
Actinomyces	*Propionibacterium*
Bacteroides	*Pseudomonas*
Bifidobacterium	*Staphylococcus*
Campylobacter	*Streptococcus*
Clostridium	*Veillonella*
Corynebacterium	**Fungi**
Eubacterium	*Candida*
Enterobacteriaceae	
Enterococcus	**Parasites**
Fusobacterium	*Blastocystis*
Haemophilus	*Chilomastix*
Helicobacter	*Endolimax*
Lactobacillus	*Entamoeba*
Mobiluncus	*Iodamoeba*
Peptostreptococcus	*Trichomonas*

---

ing the gastric mucosa), the only organisms present are small numbers of acid-tolerant bacteria such as the lactic acid–producing bacteria (*Lactobacillus* and *Strepto-coccus* spp.) and *Helicobacter pylori*. *H. pylori* is a cause of gastritis and ulcerative disease. The microbial population can dramatically change in numbers and diversity in patients receiving drugs that neutralize or reduce the production of gastric acids.

Small Intestine

In contrast with the anterior portion of the digestive tract, the small intestine is colonized with many different bacteria, fungi, and parasites. Most of these organisms are anaerobes, such as *Peptostreptococcus*, *Porphyromonas*, and *Prevotella*. Common causes of gastroenteritis (e.g., *Salmonella* and *Campylobacter* spp.) can be present in small numbers as asymptomatic residents; however, their detection in the clinical laboratory generally indicates disease. If the small intestine is obstructed, such as after abdominal surgery, then a condition called blind loop syndrome can occur. In this case, stasis of the intestinal contents leads to the colonization and proliferation of the organisms typically present in the large intestine, with a subsequent malabsorption syndrome.

Large Intestine

More microbes are present in the large intestine than anywhere else in the human body. It is estimated that more than 10^{11} bacteria per gram of feces can be found, with anaerobic bacteria in excess by more than 1000-fold. Various yeasts and nonpathogenic parasites

can also establish residence in the large intestine. The most common bacteria include *Bifidobacterium*, *Eubacterium*, *Bacteroides*, *Enterococcus*, and the Enterobacteriaceae. *E. coli* is present in virtually all humans from birth until death. Although this organism represents less than 1% of the intestinal population, it is the most common aerobic organism responsible for intra-abdominal infections. Likewise, *Bacteroides fragilis* is a minor member of the intestinal flora but the most common anaerobe responsible for intra-abdominal disease. In contrast, *Eubacterium* and *Bifidobacterium* are the most common bacteria in the large intestine but are rarely responsible for disease.

Antibiotic treatment can rapidly alter the population, causing the proliferation of antibiotic-resistant organisms such as enterococci, *Pseudomonas*, and fungi. *C. difficile* can also grow rapidly in this situation, leading to disease ranging from diarrhea to pseudomembranous colitis. Exposure to other enteric pathogens, such as *Shigella*, enterohemorrhagic *E. coli*, and *Entamoeba histolytica*, can also disrupt the colonic flora and produce significant intestinal disease.

Genitourinary System

In general, the anterior urethra and vagina are the only anatomic areas of the genitourinary system permanently colonized with microbes (Box 9–3). Although the urinary bladder can be transiently colonized with bacteria migrating upstream from the urethra, these should be cleared rapidly by the bactericidal activity of the uroepithelial cells and the flushing action of voided urine. The other structures of the urinary system should be sterile except when disease or an anatomic abnormality is present. Likewise, the uterus should also remain free of organisms.

BOX 9-3. **Most Common Microbes Colonizing the Genitourinary Tract**

Bacteria	*Mobiluncus*
Actinomyces	*Mycoplasma*
Bacteroides	*Peptostreptococcus*
Bifidobacterium	*Porphyromonas*
Clostridium	*Prevotella*
Corynebacterium	*Propionibacterium*
Enterococcus	*Staphylococcus*
Enterobacteriaceae	*Streptococcus*
Eubacterium	*Treponema*
Fusobacterium	*Ureaplasma*
Gardnerella	
Haemophilus	**Fungi**
Lactobacillus	*Candida*

Anterior Urethra

The commensal population of the urethra consists of a variety of organisms, with lactobacilli, streptococci, and coagulase-negative staphylococci the most numerous. These organisms are relatively avirulent and are rarely associated with human disease. In contrast, the urethra can be colonized transiently with fecal organisms such as *Enterococcus*, Enterobacteriaceae, and *Candida*—all of which can invade the urinary tract, multiply in urine, and lead to significant disease. Pathogens such as *N. gonorrhoeae* and *C. trachomatis* are common causes of urethritis and can persist as asymptomatic colonizers of the urethra. The isolation of these two organisms in clinical specimens should always be considered significant, regardless of the presence or absence of clinical symptoms.

Vagina

The microbial population of the vagina is more diverse and is dramatically influenced by hormonal factors. Newborn girls are colonized with lactobacilli at birth, and these bacteria predominate for approximately 6 weeks. After that time, the levels of maternal estrogen have declined, and the vaginal flora changes to include staphylococci, streptococci, and Enterobacteriaceae. When estrogen production is initiated at puberty, the microbial flora again changes. Lactobacilli reemerge as the predominant organisms, and many other organisms are also isolated, including staphylococci (*S. aureus* less commonly than the coagulase-negative species), streptococci (including group B *Streptococcus*), *Enterococcus*, *Gardnerella*, *Mycoplasma*, *Ureaplasma*, Enterobacteriaceae, and a variety of anaerobic bacteria. *N. gonorrhoeae* is a common cause of vaginitis. In the absence of this organism, significant numbers of cases develop when the balance of vaginal bacteria is disrupted, resulting in decreases in the number of lactobacilli and increases in the number of *Mobiluncus* and *Gardnerella*. *Trichomonas vaginalis*, *C. albicans*, and *Candida glabrata* are also important causes of vaginitis. Although herpes simplex virus and papillomavirus would not be considered normal flora of the genitourinary tract, these viruses can establish persistent infections.

Cervix

Although the cervix is not normally colonized with bacteria, *N. gonorrhoeae* and *C. trachomatis* are important causes of cervicitis. *Actinomyces* can also produce disease at this site.

Skin

Although many organisms come into contact with the skin surface, this relatively hostile environment does

---

BOX 9–4. **Most Common Microbes Colonizing the Skin**

Bacteria	*Propionibacterium*
Acinetobacter	*Staphylococcus*
Aerococcus	*Streptococcus*
Bacillus	**Fungi**
Clostridium	*Candida*
Corynebacterium	*Malassezia*
Micrococcus	
Peptostreptococcus	

---

not support the survival of most organisms (Box 9–4). Gram-positive bacteria (e.g., coagulase-negative *Staphylococcus* and, less commonly, *S. aureus*, corynebacteria, and propionibacteria) are the most common organisms found on the skin surface. *Clostridium perfringens* is isolated on the skin of approximately 20% of healthy individuals, and the fungi *Candida* and *Malassezia* are also found on skin surfaces, particularly in moist sites. Streptococci can colonize the skin transiently, but the volatile fatty acids produced by the anaerobe propionibacteria are toxic for these organisms. Gram-negative bacilli do not permanently colonize the skin surface (with the exception of *Acinetobacter* and a few other less common genera) because the skin is too dry.

QUESTIONS

1. What is the distinction between *colonization* and *disease*?
2. Give examples of strict pathogens and opportunistic pathogens.
3. What factors regulate the microbial populations of organisms that colonize humans?

BIBLIOGRAPHY

Balows A, Truper H: *The prokaryotes*, ed 2, New York, 1992, Springer-Verlag.

Murray P: Human microbiota. In Balows A et al: *Topley and Wilson's microbiology and microbial infections*, ed 9, London, 1999, Edward Arnold.

Murray P: *Pocket guide to clinical microbiology*, ed 2, Washington, DC, 1998, American Society for Microbiology.

Sharp S: Commensal and pathogenic microorganisms of humans. In Murray P et al, editors: *Manual of clinical microbiology*, ed 7, Washington, DC, 1999, American Society for Microbiology.

CHAPTER 10

Sterilization, Disinfection, and Antisepsis

Medical microbiology involves the study of the pathogenesis and chemotherapy of infectious diseases, as well as the examination of how diseases can be prevented. An important aspect of the control of infections is an understanding of the principles of sterilization, disinfection, and antisepsis (Box 10–1).

Sterilization

Sterilization is the total destruction of all microbes, including the more resilient forms such as bacterial spores, mycobacteria, nonenveloped (nonlipid) viruses, and fungi. This can be accomplished using physical, gas vapor, or chemical sterilants (Table 10–1).

Physical sterilants such as **moist** and **dry heat** are the most common sterilizing methods used in hospitals and are indicated for most materials except those that are heat-sensitive or consist of toxic or volatile chemicals. **Filtration** is useful for removing bacteria and fungi from air (with high-efficiency particulate air [HEPA] filters) or from solutions. These filters are unable to remove viruses and some small bacteria. Sterilization by **ultraviolet** or **ionizing radiation** (e.g., microwave or gamma rays) is also commonly used. The limitation of ultraviolet radiation is that direct exposure is required.

The gas vapor sterilant most commonly used is **ethylene oxide**. Although it is highly efficient, strict regulations limit its use because ethylene oxide is extremely toxic. Sterilization with **formaldehyde gas** is also limited because the chemical is carcinogenic. Its use is restricted primarily to sterilization of HEPA filters. **Hydrogen peroxide** vapors are effective sterilants because of the oxidizing nature of the gas. It is used for the sterilization of instruments. A variation is **plasma gas sterilization**, in which hydrogen peroxide is vaporized, and then reactive free radicals are produced with either microwave-frequency or radio-frequency energy. Because this is an efficient sterilizing method that does not produce toxic byproducts, it is anticipated that plasma gas sterilization will replace many of the applications for ethylene oxide. One additional gas vapor sterilant is **chlorine dioxide gas**, which denatures proteins by oxidation. Although further work with this method is required, the lack of toxicity also makes chlorine dioxide gas sterilization an attractive alternative to ethylene oxide sterilization.

Two chemical sterilants have also been used: **peracetic acid** and **glutaraldehyde**. Peracetic acid, an oxidizing agent, has excellent activity, and the end products (i.e., acetic acid and oxygen) are nontoxic. In contrast, safety is a concern with glutaraldehyde, and care must be used when handling this chemical.

Disinfection

Microbes are also destroyed by disinfection procedures, although more resilient organisms can survive. Unfortunately, the terms *disinfection* and *sterilization* are casually interchanged, which can result in some confusion. This occurs because disinfection processes have been categorized as high level, intermediate level, and low level. High-level disinfection can generally approach sterilization in effectiveness, whereas spore forms can survive intermediate-level disinfection, and many microbes can remain viable when exposed to low-level disinfection.

Even the classification of disinfectants (Table 10–2) by their level of activity is misleading. The effectiveness of these procedures is influenced by the nature of the item to be disinfected, number and resilience of the contaminating organism or organisms, amount of organic material present (which can inactivate the disinfectant), type and concentration of disinfectant, and duration and temperature of exposure.

High-level disinfectants are used for items involved with invasive procedures that cannot withstand sterilization procedures (e.g., certain types of endoscopes, surgical instruments with plastic or other com-

---

BOX 10–1. Definitions

Sterilization—Use of physical procedures or chemical agents to destroy all microbial forms, including bacterial spores.

Disinfection—Use of physical procedures or chemical agents to destroy most microbial forms; bacterial spores and other relatively resistant organisms (e.g., mycobacteria, viruses, fungi) may remain viable; disinfectants are subdivided into high-, intermediate-, and low-level agents.

Antisepsis—Use of chemical agents on skin or other living tissue to inhibit or eliminate microbes; no sporicidal action is implied.

Germicide—Chemical agent capable of killing microbes; spores may survive.

Sporicide—Germicide capable of killing bacterial spores.

TABLE 10–2. Methods of Disinfection

Method	Concentration (Level of Activity)
Heat	
Moist heat	75°C to 100°C for 30 min (high)
Liquid	
Glutaraldehyde	2% (high)
Hydrogen peroxide	3% to 25% (high)
Formaldehyde	3% to 8% (high/intermediate)
Chlorine dioxide	Variable (high)
Peracetic acid	Variable (high)
Chlorine compounds	100 to 1000 ppm of free chlorine (high)
Alcohol (ethyl, isopropyl)	70% to 95% (intermediate)
Phenolic compounds	0.4% to 5.0% (intermediate/low)
Iodophor compounds	30 to 50 ppm of free iodine/L (intermediate)
Quaternary ammonium compounds	0.4% to 1.6% (low)

---

ponents that cannot be autoclaved). Disinfection of these and other items is most effective if treatment is preceded by cleaning the surface to remove organic matter. Examples of high-level disinfectants include treatment with moist heat and use of liquids such as glutaraldehyde, hydrogen peroxide, peracetic acid, chlorine dioxide, and other chlorine compounds.

Intermediate-level disinfectants (i.e., alcohols, iodophor compounds, phenolic compounds) are used to clean surfaces or instruments in which contamination with bacterial spores and other highly resilient organisms is unlikely. These have been referred to as semicritical instruments and devices and include flexible fiberoptic endoscopes, laryngoscopes, vaginal specula, anesthesia breathing circuits, and other items. **Low-level disinfectants** (i.e., quaternary ammonium compounds) are used to treat noncritical instruments and devices such as blood pressure cuffs, electrocardiogram electrodes, and stethoscopes. Although these items come into contact with patients, they do not penetrate through mucosal surfaces or into sterile tissues.

The level of disinfectants used for environmental surfaces is determined by the relative risk these surfaces pose as a reservoir for pathogenic organisms. For example, a higher level of disinfectant should be used to clean the surface of instruments contaminated with blood than that used to clean surfaces that are "dirty," such as floors, sinks, and countertops. The exception to this rule is if a particular surface has been implicated in a nosocomial infection, such as a bathroom contaminated with *Clostridium difficile* (spore-forming anaerobic bacterium) or a sink contaminated with *Pseudomonas aeruginosa*. In these cases, a disinfectant with appropriate activity against the implicated pathogen should be selected.

TABLE 10–1. Methods of Sterilization

Method	Concentration or Level
Physical Sterilants	
Steam under pressure	121°C or 132°C for various time intervals
Dry heat	1 hr at 171°C; 2 hr at 160°C; 16 hr at 121°C
Filtration	0.22- to 0.45-μm pore size; HEPA filters
Ultraviolet radiation	Variable exposure to 254-nm wavelength
Ionizing radiation	Variable exposure to microwave or gamma radiation
Gas Vapor Sterilants	
Ethylene oxide	450 to 1200 mg/L at 29°C to 65°C for 2 to 5 hr
Formaldehyde vapor	2% to 5% at 60°C to 80°C
Hydrogen peroxide vapor	30% at 55°C to 60°C
Plasma gas	Highly ionized hydrogen peroxide gas
Chlorine dioxide gas	Variable
Chemical Sterilants	
Peracetic acid	0.2%
Glutaraldehyde	2%

HEPA = high-efficiency particulate air.

Antisepsis

Antiseptic agents (Table 10–3) are used to reduce the number of microbes on skin surfaces. These com-

TABLE 10–3. Antiseptic Agents

Antiseptic Agent	Concentration
Alcohol (ethyl, isopropyl)	70% to 90%
Iodophors	1 to 2 mg of free iodine/L; 1% to 2% available iodine
Chlorhexidine	0.5% to 4%
Parachlorometaxylenol	0.5% to 3.75%
Triclosan	0.3% to 2%

pounds are selected for their safety and efficacy. A summary of their germicidal properties is presented in Table 10–4. **Alcohols** have excellent activity against all groups of organisms except spores and are nontoxic, although they tend to dry the skin surface because they remove lipids. They also do not have residual activity and are inactivated by organic matter. Thus, the surface of the skin should be cleaned before alcohol is applied. **Iodophors** are also excellent skin antiseptic agents, having a range of activity similar to that of alcohols. They are slightly more toxic to the skin than is alcohol, have limited residual activity, and are inactivated by organic matter. Iodophors and iodine preparations are frequently used with alcohols for disinfecting the skin surface. **Chlorhexidine** has broad antimicrobial activity, although it kills organisms at a much slower rate than does alcohol. Its activity persists, although organic material and high pH levels decrease its effectiveness. The activity of **parachlorometaxylenol** (PCMX) is limited primarily to gram-positive bacteria. Because it is nontoxic and has residual activ-

ity, it has been used in handwashing products. **Triclosan** is active against bacteria but not against other organisms. It is a common antiseptic agent in deodorant soaps and some toothpastes.

Mechanisms of Action

The following section briefly reviews the mechanisms by which the most common sterilants, disinfectants, and antiseptics work.

Moist Heat

Attempts to sterilize items using boiling water are inefficient because only a relatively low temperature (100°C) can be maintained. Indeed, spore formation by a bacterium is commonly demonstrated by boiling a solution of organisms and then subculturing the solution. Vegetative organisms are killed by boiling, but the spores remain viable. If organisms grow on the subculture plate, the bacteria are capable of sporulating. In contrast, steam under pressure in an autoclave is a very effective form of sterilization; the higher temperature causes denaturation of microbial proteins. The rate of killing organisms during the autoclave process is rapid but is influenced by the temperature and duration of autoclaving, size of the autoclave, flow rate of the steam, density and size of the load, and placement of the load in the chamber. Care must be used to avoid creating air pockets, which inhibit penetration of the steam into the load. In general, most autoclaves are operated at 121°C to 132°C for 15 minutes or longer. The effectiveness of sterilization can be monitored by including commercial preparations of *Bacillus stearother-*

TABLE 10–4. Germicidal Properties of Disinfectants and Antiseptic Agents

Agent	Bacteria	Mycobacteria	Bacterial Spores	Fungi	Viruses
Disinfectants					
Alcohol	+	+	–	+	+/–
Hydrogen peroxide	+	+	+/–	+	+
Formaldehyde	+	+	+	+	+
Phenolics	+	+	–	+	+/–
Chlorine	+	+	+/–	+	+
Iodophors	+	+/–	–	+/–	1/
Glutaraldehyde	+	+	+	+	+
Quaternary ammonium compounds	+/–	–	–	+/–	–
Antiseptic Agents					
Alcohol	+	+	–	+	+
Iodophors	+	+	–	+	+
Chlorhexidine	+	+	–	+/–	+
Parachlorometaxylenol	+/–	+/–	–	+/–	–
Triclosan	+	+/–	–	–	?

mophilus spores. An ampule of these spores is placed in the center of the load, is removed at the end of the autoclave process, and is incubated at 37°C. If the sterilization process is successful, the organisms fail to sporulate and do not grow.

Dry Heat

Hot air can also be used to sterilize items such as glassware. This method is not as efficient as the moist air method because diffusion and penetration of heat is slow, long sterilization periods and high temperatures are required, materials can be damaged by the oxidation process of this prolonged heating, and dry heat tends to stratify in the processing chamber. Sterilization requires processing for 1 hour at 171°C, 2 hours at 160°C, or 16 hours at 121°C. The effectiveness is monitored with spore tests using *Bacillus subtilis*, which is relatively resistant to killing by dry air (in contrast with *B. stearothermophilus*).

Ethylene Oxide

Ethylene oxide is a colorless gas, soluble in water and common organic solvents, that is used to sterilize heat-sensitive items. The sterilization process is relatively slow and is influenced by the concentration of gas, relative humidity and moisture content of the item to be sterilized, exposure time, and temperature. The exposure time is reduced by 50% for each doubling of ethylene oxide concentration. Likewise, the activity of ethylene oxide approximately doubles with each temperature increase of 10°C. Sterilization with ethylene oxide is optimal in a relative humidity of approximately 30%, with decreased activity at higher or lower humidity. This is particularly problematic if the contaminated organisms are dried onto a surface or lyophilized. Ethylene oxide exerts its sporicidal activity through the alkylation of terminal hydroxyl, carboxyl, amino, and sulfhydryl groups. This process blocks the reactive groups required for many essential metabolic processes. Examples of other strong alkylating gases used as sterilants are formaldehyde and β-propiolactone. Because ethylene oxide can damage viable tissues, the gas must be dissipated before the item can be used. This aeration period is generally 24 hours or longer. The effectiveness of sterilization is monitored with the *B. subtilis* spore test.

Aldehydes

As with ethylene oxide, the aldehydes exert their effect through alkylation. The two best known aldehydes are **formaldehyde** and **glutaraldehyde**, both of which can be used as sterilants or high-level disinfectants. Formaldehyde gas can be dissolved in water (called *formalin*) at a final concentration of 37%. Stabilizers such as methanol are added to formalin. Low concentrations of formalin are bacteriostatic (inhibit but do not kill organisms), whereas higher concentrations (e.g., 20%) can kill all organisms. This microbicidal activity can be enhanced by combining formaldehyde with alcohol (e.g., 20% formalin in 70% alcohol). Exposure of skin or mucous membranes to formaldehyde can be toxic. Glutaraldehyde is less toxic for viable tissues, but it can still cause burns on the skin or mucous membranes. Glutaraldehyde is more active at alkaline pH levels ("activated" by sodium hydroxide) but is less stable. Glutaraldehyde is also inactivated by organic material, so items to be treated must first be cleaned.

Oxidizing Agents

Examples of oxidants include ozone, peracetic acid, and hydrogen peroxide, with the last used most commonly. **Hydrogen peroxide** effectively kills most bacteria at a concentration of 3% to 6% and kills all organisms, including spores, at higher concentrations (10% to 25%). The active oxidant form is not hydrogen peroxide but rather the free hydroxyl radical formed by the decomposition of hydrogen peroxide. Hydrogen peroxide is used to disinfect plastic implants, contact lenses, and surgical prostheses.

Halogens

Halogens, such as compounds containing iodine or chlorine, are used extensively as disinfectants. **Iodine compounds** are the most effective halogens available for disinfection. Iodine is a highly reactive element that precipitates proteins and oxidizes essential enzymes. It is microbicidal against virtually all organisms, including spore-forming bacteria and mycobacteria. Neither the concentration nor the pH of the iodine solution affects the microbicidal activity, although the efficiency of iodine solutions is increased in acid solutions because more free iodine is liberated. Iodine acts more rapidly than do other halogen compounds or quaternary ammonium compounds. However, the activity of iodine can be reduced in the presence of some organic and inorganic compounds, including serum, feces, ascitic fluid, sputum, urine, sodium thiosulfate, and ammonia. Elemental iodine can be dissolved in aqueous potassium iodide or alcohol, or it can be complexed with a carrier. The latter compound is referred to as an *iodophor* (iodo, "iodine"; phor "carrier"). Povidone iodine (iodine complexed with polyvinylpyrrolidone) is used most commonly, is relatively stable and nontoxic to tissues and metal surfaces, but is expensive compared with other iodine solutions.

Chlorine compounds are also used extensively as disinfectants. Aqueous solutions of chlorine are rapidly bactericidal, although their mechanisms of action are not defined. Three forms of chlorine may be present in water: elemental chlorine (Cl_2), which is a very strong oxidizing agent; hypochlorous acid (HOCl); and hypochlorite ion (OCl_2). Chlorine also combines with ammonia and other nitrogenous compounds to form chloramines or *N*-chloro compounds. Chlorine can exert its effect by the irreversible oxidation of SH groups of essential enzymes. Hypochlorites are believed to interact with cytoplasmic components to form toxic *N*-chloro compounds, which interfere with cellular metabolism. The efficacy of chlorine is inversely proportional to the pH, with greater activity observed at acid pH levels. This is consistent with greater activity associated with hypochlorous acid rather than with hypochlorite ion concentration. The activity of chlorine compounds also increases with concentration (e.g., a twofold increase in concentration results in a 30% decrease in time required for killing) and temperature (e.g., a 50% to 65% reduction in killing time with a 10°C increase in temperature). Organic matter and alkaline detergents can reduce the effectiveness of chlorine compounds. These compounds demonstrate good germicidal activity, although spore-forming organisms are 10- to 1000-fold more resistant to chlorine than are vegetative bacteria.

Phenolic Compounds

Phenolic compounds (germicides) are rarely used as disinfectants. They are, however, of historical interest because they were used as a comparative standard for assessing the activity of other germicidal compounds. The ratio of germicidal activity by a test compound to that by a specified concentration of phenol yielded the phenol coefficient. A value of 1 indicated equivalent activity, greater than 1 indicated activity less than phenol, and less than 1 indicated activity greater than phenol. These tests are limited because phenol is not sporicidal at room temperature (but is sporicidal at temperatures approaching 100°C) and has poor activity against non–lipid-containing viruses. This is understandable because phenol is believed to act by disrupting lipid-containing membranes, resulting in leakage of cellular contents. Phenolic compounds are active against the normally resilient mycobacteria because the cell wall of these organisms has a very high concentration of lipids. Exposure of phenolics to alkaline compounds significantly reduces their activity, whereas halogenation of the phenolics enhances their activity. The introduction of aliphatic or aromatic groups into the nucleus of halogen phenols also increases their activity. Bis-phenols are two phenol compounds linked together. The activity of these compounds can also be potentiated by halogenation. One example of a halogenated bis-phenol is **hexachlorophene,** an antiseptic with activity against gram-positive bacteria.

Quaternary Ammonium Compounds

Quaternary ammonium compounds consist of four organic groups covalently linked to nitrogen. The germicidal activity of these cationic compounds is determined by the nature of the organic groups, with the greatest activity observed with compounds with 8 to 18 carbon long groups. Examples of quaternary ammonium compounds include **benzalkonium chloride** and **cetylpyridinium chloride**. These compounds act by denaturing cell membranes to release the intracellular components. Quaternary ammonium compounds are bacteriostatic at low concentrations and bactericidal at high concentrations. However, organisms such as *Pseudomonas*, *Mycobacterium*, and the fungus *Trichophyton*, among others, are resistant to these compounds. Indeed, some *Pseudomonas* strains can grow readily in quaternary ammonium solutions. Many viruses and all bacterial spores are also resistant. Quaternary ammonium compounds are neutralized by ionic detergents, organic matter, and dilution.

Alcohols

The germicidal activity of alcohols increases with increasing chain length (maximum of 5 to 8 carbons). The two most commonly used alcohols are **ethanol** and **isopropanol**. These are rapidly bactericidal against vegetative bacteria, mycobacteria, some fungi, and lipid-containing viruses. Unfortunately, alcohols have no activity against bacterial spores and have poor activity against some fungi and non–lipid-containing viruses. Activity is greater in the presence of water. Thus, 70% alcohol is more active than is 95% alcohol. Alcohol is a common disinfectant for skin surfaces and, when followed by treatment with an iodophor, is extremely effective for this purpose. Alcohols are also used to disinfect items such as thermometers.

QUESTIONS

1. Define the following terms and give three examples of each: *sterilization*, *disinfection*, and *antisepsis*.

2. Define the three levels of disinfection and give examples of each. When would each type of disinfectant be used?

3. What factors influence the effectiveness of sterilization with moist heat, dry heat, and ethylene oxide?

4. Give examples of each of the following disinfectants and their mode of action: iodine compounds, chlorine compounds, phenolic compounds, and quaternary ammonium compounds.

BIBLIOGRAPHY

Block SS: *Disinfection, sterilization, and preservation*, ed 2, Philadelphia, 1977, Lea and Febiger.

Brody TM, Larner J, Minneman KP: *Human pharmacology: molecular to clinical*, ed 3, St Louis, 1998, Mosby.

Widmer A, Frei R: Decontamination, disinfection, and sterilization. In Murray P et al, editors: *Manual of clinical microbiology*, ed 7, Washington, DC, 1999, American Society for Microbiology.

Basic Concepts in the Immune Response

CHAPTER 11

Elements of Host Protective Responses

We live in a microbial world, and our bodies are constantly being exposed to bacteria, fungi, parasites, and viruses. Our bodies' defenses to this onslaught are similar to a military defense. The initial defense mechanisms are **barriers**, such as the skin, that prevent entry of the foreign agents. If these barriers are compromised or the agent gains entry in another way, the local militia of **innate responses** (complement, natural killer cells, neutrophils, macrophages) must quickly rally to the challenge and prevent expansion of the invasion. Finally, if this step is not effective, a major campaign must be specifically directed against the invader by **immune responses** (antibody and T cells) at whatever cost (immunopathogenesis). Similarly, knowledge of the characteristics (antigens) of the enemy through immunization enables the body to mount a faster, more effective response (activation of memory B and T cells on rechallenge).

The different elements of the immune system interact and communicate with soluble molecules and by direct cell-to-cell interaction. These interactions provide the mechanisms for activation and control of the protective responses. Unfortunately, the protective responses to some infectious agents are insufficient; in other cases, the response to the challenge is excessive. In either case, disease occurs.

Activators and Stimulators of Immune Function

Immune cells communicate by direct cell-to-cell interactions (touch) and by the sensing of soluble molecules (similar to taste or smell), including proteins such as cytokines, chemokines, and interferons and lipids such as steroids and prostaglandins. **Cytokines** are proteins produced by lymphoid and other cells that stimulate and regulate the immune response (Table 11–1 and Box 11–1). **Interferons** are low-molecular-weight proteins produced in response to viral infections (interferon-α and interferon-β) or on activation of the immune response (interferon-γ) that promote antiviral

and antitumor responses and stimulate immune responses (see Chapter 14). **Chemokines** are small proteins ($\approx$ 8000 Da) that are associated with inflammatory responses. Neutrophils, basophils, monocytes, and T cells express receptors and can be activated by specific chemokines. The chemokines and other proteins (e.g., the C3a and C5a products of the complement cascade) are chemotactic factors that establish a chemical path to attract phagocytic and inflammatory cells to the site of infection.

Cells of the Immune Response

Immune responses are mediated by specific cells with defined functions. The characteristics of the most important cells of the immune system and their appearances are presented in Figure 11–1, Table 11–2, and Table 11–3.

The white blood cells can be distinguished morphologically, on the basis of (1) histologic staining, (2) immunologic functions, and (3) intracellular and cell surface markers. Monoclonal antibodies are used to distinguish subsets of the different types of cells according to their cell surface markers. These markers have been defined within clusters of differentiation and the markers indicated by "**CD**" numbers (Table 11–4).

BOX 11–1. Major Cytokine-Producing Cells

Innate

Macrophages: IL-1, TNF-α, TNF-β, IL-6, IL-12, GM-CSF

Immune: T cells

CD4 TH1 cells: IL-2, interferon-γ TNF-β, IL-3, GM-CSF, TNF-α

CD4 TH2 cells: IL-4, Il-5, IL-10, IL-3, IL-9, IL-13, GM-CSF, TNF-α

GM-CSF = granulocyte-macrophage colony-stimulating factor; IL = interleukin; TNF = tumor necrosis factor.

TABLE 11–1. Cytokines and Chemokines

Factor	Source	Major Target	Function
Interferon-α, interferon-β	Leukocytes, fibroblasts	Virally infected cells, tumor cells NK cells	Induction of antiviral state; activation of NK cells, enhancement of cell-mediated immunity
Interferon-γ	CD4 TH1 cells, NK cells	Macrophages,* T cells	Activation of macrophage, promotion of inflammation, promotion of TH1 and inhibition of TH2 responses
IL-1α, IL-1β	Macrophage, fibroblasts, epithelial cells, endothelial cells	T cells, B cells, PMN, tissue, central nervous system	Many actions: promotion of inflammatory and acute phase responses, fever, activation of T cells
TNF-α (cachectin)	Similar to IL-1	—	Similar to IL-1, antitumor and wasting (cachexia–weight loss) functions
TNF-β	T cells	PMN, tumors	Lymphotoxin: tumor killing, activation of PMN
Colony-stimulating factors (e.g., GM-CSF)	T cells, stromal cells	Stem cells	Growth and differentiation of specific cell types
IL-2	CD4 T cells (TH0, TH1)	T cells, B cells, NK cells	T- and B-cell growth
IL-3	CD4 T cells, keratinocytes	Stem cells	Differentiation
IL-4	CD4 (TH0, TH2), T cells	B and T cells	B-cell growth and differentiation; Ig production; TH2 responses
IL-5	CD4 TH2 cells	B cells, eosinophils	B-cell growth and differentiation, IgA and IgE production, eosinophil production, allergic responses
IL-6	Macrophages, T and B cells, fibroblasts, epithelial cells, endothelial cells	T cells and B cells, hepatocytes	Stimulation of acute-phase and inflammatory responses, fever, Ig secretion, B-cell growth and development
IL-7	Bone marrow, stroma	Precursor cells and stem cells	Growth of pre-B cell, thymocyte, T cell, and cytotoxic lymphocyte
IL-10	CD4 TH2 cells	B cells, CD4 TH1 cells	B-cell growth, inhibition of TH1 response
IL-12	Macrophage	NK cells, CD4 TH1 cells	Activation
TGF-β	CD4 TH3 cells	B cells	IgA production; immunosuppression of B, T, and NK cells and macrophages; promotion of oral tolerance, wound healing
α-chemokines: C-X-C chemokines—two cysteines separated by one amino acid (IL-8; IP-10; GRO-α, GRO-β, GRO-γ)	Many cells	Neutrophils, T cells, macrophages	Chemotaxis, activation
β-chemokines: C-C chemokines—two adjacent cysteines (MCP-1; MIP-α; MIP-β; RANTES)	Many cells	T cells, macrophages, basophils	Chemotaxis, activation

*Applies to one or more cells of the monocyte-macrophage lineage.

GM-CSF = granulocyte-macrophage colony-stimulating factor; GRO = growth related oncogene; Ig = immunoglobulin; IL = interleukin; IP = interferon-α protein; MCP = monocyte chemoattractant protein; MIP = macrophage inflammatory protein; NK = natural killer; PMN = polymorphonuclear leukocytes; RANTES = regulated on activation, normal T expressed and secreted; TNF = tumor necrosis factor.

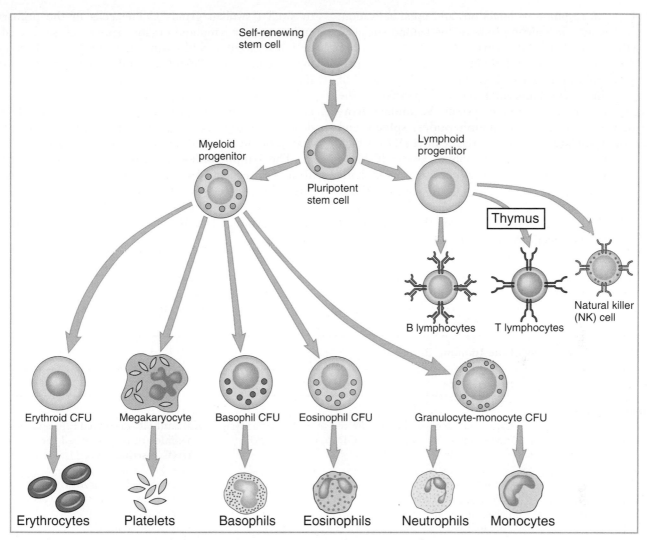

FIGURE 11-1. Morphology and lineage of cells involved in the immune response. Mononuclear cells include lymphocytes, monocytes, and macrophages. Polymorphonuclear leukocytes include neutrophils, eosinophils, basophils, and mast cells. (From Abbas K et al: *Cellular and molecular immunology,* ed 4, Philadelphia, 2000, WB Saunders.)

A special class of cells that are **antigen-presenting cells (APCs) express class II major histocompatibility complex (MHC) antigens** (HLA-DR, HLA-DP, HLA-DQ). APCs include B cells, macrophages family cells and a limited number of other cell types. In addition, these and **all nucleated cells express class I MHC (MHC I) antigens** (HLA-A, HLA-B, HLA-C).

Hematopoietic Cell Differentiation

Differentiation of a common progenitor cell, termed the pluripotent **stem cell**, gives rise to all blood cells. Differentiation of these cells begins during development of the fetus and continues throughout life. The

pluripotent stem cell differentiates into stem cells (sometimes referred to as colony-forming units) for different lineages of blood cells, including the lymphoid (T and B cells), myeloid, erythrocytic, and megakaryoblastic (source of platelets) lineages (see Fig. 11-1). The stem cells reside primarily in the bone marrow but can also be isolated from the fetal blood in umbilical cords and as rare cells in adult blood. Differentiation of stem cells into the functional blood cells is triggered by specific cell surface interactions with the stromal cells of the marrow and specific cytokines produced by these and other cells. The **thymus and the "bursal equivalent" in the Peyer's patches promote development of T cells and B cells, respectively.** Helper T cells, macrophages, and other cells release cytokines in response to infections and upon activation; the cytokines in turn promote hematopoietic cell growth and terminal differentiation.

The bone marrow and thymus are considered **primary lymphoid organs** (Fig. 11–2). These sites of initial lymphocyte differentiation are essential to the development of the immune system. **Secondary lymphoid organs** include the **lymph nodes, spleen,** and **mucosa-associated lymphoid tissues** (**MALT**), which also include gut-associated lymphoid tissue (GALT) (e.g., Peyer's patches) and bronchus-associated lymphoid tissue (BALT) (e.g., tonsils, appendix). These sites are where B and T cells reside and respond to antigenic challenges. Proliferation of the lymphocytes in response to infectious challenge causes these tissues

to swell ("swollen glands"). The cells of the primary and secondary lymphoid organs express cell surface adhesion molecules (**addressins**) that interact with homing receptors (**cell adhesion molecules**) expressed on B and T cells.

The spleen and lymph nodes are capsulated organs in which the macrophages and B and T cells reside in defined regions. Their location facilitates interactions that promote immune responses to antigen (Fig. 11–3). The **lymph nodes** are kidney-shaped organs 2 to 10 mm in diameter that filter the fluid that passes from intercellular spaces into the lymphatic system and then through the lymph nodes, almost like a sewage processing plant. A lymph node consists of the following three layers:

TABLE 11–2. Cells of the Immune Response

Cells	Characteristics	Markers	Functions
Natural Cytolytic Cells			
Natural killer cells	Large granular lymphocytes	Fc receptors for antibody; CD16, CD56, CD57	Kill antibody-decorated cells and virus-infected or tumor cell (**no MHC restriction**)
Phagocytic Cells			
Neutrophils (polymorphonuclear leukocytes)	Granulocytes with short life span, multilobed nucleus and granules, segmented band forms (more immature)	—	*Phagocytose* and kill *bacteria*
Eosinophils	Bilobed nucleus, heavily granulated cytoplasm	Staining with eosin	Are involved in parasite defense and allergic response
Macrophages	See below	—	—
Antigen-Presenting Cells (APCS)		***Class II MHC Expressing Cells***	***Present Antigen to CD4 T cells***
Monocytes*	Found in lymphocytes, blood, lungs, and other organs	Horseshoe-shaped nucleus, lysosomes, granules	*Are precursors to macrophage-lineage,* cytokine release
Macrophages*	Possible residence in tissue, spleen, lymph nodes, and other organs; activated by interferon-γ and TNF	Large, granular cells; Fc and C3 receptors	Initiate inflammatory and acute phase response; activated cells are antibacterial and have antiviral and antitumor activities
Langerhans' cells*	Presence in skin	—	Transport antigen to lymph nodes
Dendritic cells*	Lymph nodes, tissue	—	Are efficient antigen presenters
Microglial cells*	CNS and brain	—	Produce cytokines
Kupffer cells*	Presence in liver	—	Filter particles from blood (e.g., viruses)
B cells	See below	—	
Antigen-Responsive Cells			
T cells (all)	Mature in thymus; large nucleus, small cytoplasm	CD2, CD3, T-cell receptor	

TABLE 11–2. Cells of the Immune Response *(Continued)*

Cells	Characteristics	Markers	Functions
CD4 T cells	Helper/DTH cells; **activation** by APCs through **class II MHC antigen presentation**	CD2, CD3, T-cell receptor, CD4	Produce IL-2, other cytokines; stimulate T- and B-cell growth; promote B-cell differentiation (class-switching), antibody production
	TH1 subtype	IL-2, Ifn-γ, LT production	Promote initial defenses (local), DTH, T killer cells
	TH2 subtype	IL-4, IL-5, IL-6, IL-10 production	Promote later humoral responses
CD8 T killer cells	**Recognition** of antigen presented by **class I MHC antigens**	CD2, CD3, T-cell receptor, CD8	Kill viral, tumor, non-self (transplant) cells; secrete TH1 lymphokines
CD8 T cells (suppressor cells)	**Recognition** of antigen presented by **class I MHC antigens**	CD2, CD3, T-cell receptor, CD8	Suppress T- and B-cell response
Antibody-Producing Cells			
B cells	Mature in Peyer's patches, bone marrow, bursal equivalent; large nucleus, small cytoplasm; activation by antigens and T-cell factors	Surface antibody, **class II MHC antigens**	Produce antibody and present antigen
Plasma cells	Small nucleus, large cytoplasm	—	Are terminally differentiated, antibody factories
Other Cells			
Basophils/mast cells	Granulocytic	Fc receptors for IgE	Release histamine, provide allergic response, are antiparasitic

*Monocyte = macrophage lineage.

APCs = antigen-presenting cells; CNS = central nervous system; DTH = delayed-type hypersensitivity; Ig = immunoglobulin; IL = interleukin; LT = lymphotoxin; MHC = major histocompatibility complex; TNF = tumor necrosis factor.

1. The cortex, the outer layer that contains mainly B cells and macrophages arranged in clusters called follicles.
2. The paracortex, which contains dendritic cells that bring antigens from the tissues to be presented to the T cells to initiate immune responses.
3. The medulla, which contains B and T cells and antibody-producing plasma cells.

The **spleen** is a large organ that filters antigens from blood and removes aged blood cells and platelets (Fig. 11–4). The spleen consists of two types of tissue, the white pulp and the red pulp. The white pulp consists of arterioles surrounded by lymphoid cells (periarteriolar lymphoid sheath) in which the T cells surround the central arteriole. B cells are organized into primary unstimulated or secondary stimulated follicles that have a germinal center. The germinal center contains memory cells, macrophages, and follicular dendritic cells (APCs of lymphoid origin). The red pulp is a storage site for blood cells and the site of turnover of aged platelets and erythrocytes. **MALT** contains less structured aggregates of lymphoid cells (Fig. 11–5). For example, the **Peyer's patches** along the intestinal wall have special cells in the epithelium (M cells) that deliver antigens to the lymphocytes contained

TABLE 11–3. Normal Blood Cell Counts

	Mean Number per Microliter	Normal Range
White blood cells (leukocytes)	7,400	4,500–11,000
Neutrophils	4,400	1,800–7,700
Eosinophils	200	0–450
Basophils	40	0–200
Lymphocytes	2,500	1,000–4,800
Monocytes	300	0–800

From Abbas AK, Lichtman AH, Pober JS: *Cellular and molecular immunology,* ed 4, Philadelphia, 2000, WB Saunders.

TABLE 11–4. Selected CD Markers of Importance

CD Markers	Identity and Function	T Cell	B Cell	NK	Monocyte	Macrophage
CD2 (LFA-3R)	Erythrocyte receptor	**				
CD3	TCR subunit (γ, δ, ϵ, ζ, η); activation	**				
CD4	Class II MHC receptor	**				
CD5						
CD8	Class I MHC receptor	**				
CD11b (CR3)	C3b complement receptor 3 (α chain)					
CD14	LPS-binding protein receptor					
CD16 (Fc-γ RIII)	Mediation of phagocytosis and ADCC			**		
CD21 (CR2)	C3d complement receptor, EBV receptor		**			
CD25 (TAC)	IL-2 receptor (α chain), early activation marker	*	*		*	*
CD28	Receptor for B-7 costimulation: activation	**	*			
CD32 (Fc-γ RII)	Low-affinity receptor for immune complexes					**
CD35 (CR1)	C3b and C4b complement receptor					
CD40	Stimulation of B cell		**			
CD40 L	Receptor for CD40	**				
CD45 (LCA)	Augments activation of B and T cells			•		
CD45RO	Isoform (on memory cells)					
CD56 (NKH1)	Adhesion molecule	•		**		
CD57 (leu-7)	Adhesion molecule		•	**		
CD64 (Fc-γ RI)	High-affinity IgG receptor					
CD70	CD27-ligand: costimulation of B and T cells	*	*			
CD80	B 7-1: costimulation of T cells on APCs		+			+
CD86	B 7-2: costimulation of T cells on APCs		+			+
CD152 (CTLA-4)	Receptor for B-7; tolerance	**				

TABLE 11–4. Selected CD Markers of Importance *(Continued)*

CD Markers	Identity and Function	T Cell	B Cell	NK	Monocyte	Macrophage
Adhesion Molecules						
CD11a	LFA-1 (α chain)					
CD29	VLA (β chain)					
VLA-1, VLA-2, VLA-3	α integrins	*				
VLA-4	α_4 integrin homing receptor	+	+		+	
CD50	ICAM-3	+	+	+	+	+
CD54	ICAM-1					
CD58	LFA-3					

This table shows the recognized CD markers of hemopoietic cells and their distribution. A filled rectangle or + means cell population present; a half-filled triangle is subpopulation. *, activated cells only; **, markers that identify or are critical to the cell type.

ADCC = antibody-dependent cellular cytotoxicity; APCs = antigen-presenting cells; CTLA = cytotoxic T-lymphocyte associated protein; EBV = Epstein Barr virus; ICAM = intercellular adhesion molecule; Ig = immunoglobulin; IL = interleukin; LCA = leukocyte common antigen; LFA = leukocyte function–associated antigen; LPS = lipopolysaccharide; MHC = major histocompatibility complex; TAC = T-cell activation complex; T-cell antigen receptor; VLA = very late activation (antigen).

Modified from Male D et al: *Advanced immunology*, ed 3, St. Louis, 1996, Mosby.

in defined regions (T [interfollicular] and B [germinal]).

Polymorphonuclear Leukocytes

Polymorphonuclear leukocytes (**neutrophils**) constitute 50% to 70% of circulating white blood cells (see Fig. 11–1) and are a primary **phagocytic defense** against bacterial infection. These short-lived cells circulate in the blood for 7 to 10 hours and then migrate into the tissue, where they live for 3 days longer. Neutrophils are 11 to 14 μm in diameter, lack mitochondria, have a granulated cytoplasm in which granules stain with both acidic and basic stains, and have a multilobed nucleus. Neutrophils leave the blood and concentrate at the site of infection in response to chemotactic factors. During infection, the neutrophils in the blood increase in number and include precursor forms. These precursors are termed **band forms**, in contrast to the terminally differentiated and **segmented neutrophils**. The finding of such an increase and change in neutrophils by a blood count is sometimes termed *a left shift with an increase in bands vs. segs.* Neutrophils ingest bacteria by phagocytosis and expose the bacteria to antibacterial substances and enzymes contained in **primary** (**azurophilic**) and **secondary** (**specific**) **granules**. Azurophilic granules are reservoirs for enzymes such as myeloperoxidase, β-glucuronidase,

elastase, and cathepsin G. Specific granules serve as reservoirs for lysozyme and lactoferrin.

Eosinophils are heavily granulated cells (11 to 15 μm in diameter) with a bilobed nucleus that stain with the acid dye eosin Y. They are also phagocytic, motile, and granulated. The granules contain acid phosphatase, peroxidase, and eosinophilic basic proteins. Eosinophils play a role in the defense against **parasitic infections**. The eosinophilic basic proteins are toxic to many parasites. **Basophils**, another type of granulocyte, are not phagocytic but release the contents of their granules during allergic responses (type 1 hypersensitivity).

Mononuclear Phagocyte System

The **mononuclear phagocyte system** (previously called the *reticuloendothelial system*) consists of monocytes (see Fig. 11–1) in the blood and cells derived from monocytes, such as **macrophages, alveolar macrophages in the lungs, dendritic cells, Kupffer cells in the liver, intraglomerular mesangial cells in the kidney, histiocytes in connective tissue, synovial A cells, and microglial cells in the brain. Alveolar and serosal (e.g., peritoneal) macrophages** are examples of "wandering" macrophages. **Brain microglia** are cells that enter the brain around the time of birth and differentiate into fixed cells.

Monocytes are 10 to 18 μm in diameter with a

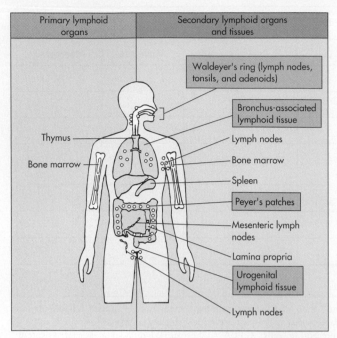

Primary lymphoid organs	Secondary lymphoid organs and tissues

Waldeyer's ring (lymph nodes, tonsils, and adenoids)

Bronchus-associated lymphoid tissue

Thymus

Lymph nodes

Bone marrow

Bone marrow

Spleen

Peyer's patches

Mesenteric lymph nodes

Lamina propria

Urogenital lymphoid tissue

Lymph nodes

FIGURE 11–2. Thymus and bone marrow are primary lymphoid organs. They are sites of maturation for T and B cells, respectively. Cellular and humoral immune responses occur in the secondary (peripheral) lymphoid organs and tissues; effector and memory cells are generated here. The spleen responds predominantly to blood-borne antigens. Lymph nodes mount immune responses to antigens in intercellular fluid and in the lymph, absorbed either through the skin (superficial nodes) or from internal viscera (deep nodes). Tonsils, Peyer's patches, and other mucosa-associated lymphoid tissues (*blue boxes*) respond to antigens that have penetrated the surface mucosal barriers. (From Roitt I et al: *Immunology*, ed 4, St Louis, 1996, Mosby.)

single-lobed, kidney bean–shaped nucleus. They represent 3% to 8% of peripheral blood leukocytes. Different cytokines or tissue environments promote myeloid stem cells and monocytes to differentiate into the various macrophages and dendritic cells. These mature forms have different morphologies corresponding to their ultimate tissue location and function and may not express all of the macrophage activities or cell surface markers.

Macrophages are long-lived cells that are phagocytic, contain lysosomes and, unlike neutrophils, have mitochondria. Macrophages have the following basic functions: (1) phagocytosis, (2) antigen presentation to T cells to initiate specific immune responses, and (3) secretion of cytokines to activate and promote innate and immune responses (Fig. 11–6). Macrophages express cell surface receptors for the Fc portion of immunoglobulin (Ig) G (**Fc-γ RI, Fc-γ RII, Fc-γ RIII**) and for the C3b product of the complement cascade

(**CR1, CR3**). These receptors facilitate the phagocytosis of antigen, bacteria, or viruses coated with these proteins. Toll-like and other pattern-recognition receptors recognize pathogen associated molecular patterns (PAMPs) and activate protective responses. Macrophages also express the **class II MHC antigen**, which allows these cells to present antigen to CD4 helper T cells to initiate the immune response. Macrophages secrete **interleukin-1, interleukin-6, tumor necrosis factor,** and **interleukin-12** in response to bacterial interaction, which stimulate immune and inflammatory responses, including fever. A T-cell–derived lymphokine, **interferon-γ**, activates macrophages. **Activated macrophages** have enhanced phagocytic, killing, and antigen-presenting capabilities.

Dendritic cells (DCs) are professional APCs that can also produce cytokines. Different immature dendritic cells are found in tissue and blood; they include **Langerhans cells** in the skin, **dermal interstitial**

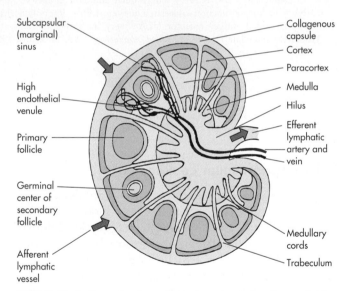

Subcapsular (marginal) sinus

Collagenous capsule

Cortex

Paracortex

Medulla

High endothelial venule

Hilus

Efferent lymphatic artery and vein

Primary follicle

Germinal center of secondary follicle

Medullary cords

Afferent lymphatic vessel

Trabeculum

FIGURE 11–3. Organization of the lymph node. Beneath the collagenous capsule is the subcapsular sinus, which is lined with phagocytic cells. Lymphocytes and antigens from surrounding tissue spaces or adjacent nodes pass into the sinus via the afferent lymphatic system. The cortex contains aggregates of B cells (primary follicles), most of which are stimulated (secondary follicles) and have a site of active proliferation or germinal center. The paracortex contains mainly T cells, many of which are associated with the interdigitating cells (antigen-presenting cells). Each lymph node has its own arterial and venous supplies. Lymphocytes enter the node from the circulation through the specialized high endothelial venules in the paracortex. The medulla contains both T and B cells as well as most of the lymph node plasma cells organized into cords of lymphoid tissue. Lymphocytes can leave the node only through the efferent lymphatic vessel. (From Roitt I et al: *Immunology*, ed 4, St Louis, 1996, Mosby.)

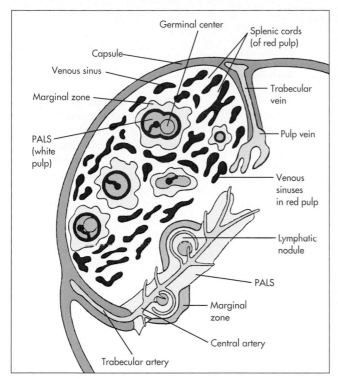

FIGURE 11–4. Organization of lymphoid tissue in the spleen. The white pulp contains germinal centers and is surrounded by the marginal zone, which contains numerous macrophages, antigen-presenting cells, slowly recirculating B cells, and natural killer cells. The red pulp contains venous sinuses separated by splenic cords. Blood enters the tissues via the trabecular arteries, which give rise to the many-branched central arteries. Some end in the white pulp, supplying the germinal centers and mantle zones, but most empty into or near the marginal zones. PALS = periarteriolar lymphoid sheath. (From Roitt I et al: *Immunology,* ed 4, St Louis, 1996, Mosby.)

cells, **splenic marginal dendritic** cells, and dendritic cells in the **liver, thymus, germinal centers of the lymph nodes,** and **blood**. These cells capture and phagocytose antigen efficiently. On doing so, they mature into dendritic cells and move to T-cell–rich regions of lymph nodes to present antigen on class I and class II MHC antigens.

Lymphocytes

The lymphocytes are 6 to 10 μm in diameter, smaller than leukocytes. The two major classes of lymphocytes, **B cells** and **T cells**, have a large nucleus and smaller, agranular cytoplasm. Although B and T cells are indistinguishable by morphologic features, they can be distinguished on the basis of function and surface markers (Table 11–5). Lymphoid cells that are not B or T cells

(non-B/non-T cells, or null cells) are large granular lymphocytes (LGLs) also known as **natural killer (NK) cells**.

The primary function of **B cells** is to **make antibody**, but they also internalize antigen, process the antigen, and present the antigen to T cells to initiate or enhance the immune response. B cells can be identified by the presence on their cell surfaces of immunoglobulins, class II MHC molecules, and receptors for the C3b and C3d products of the complement cascade (CR1, CR2) (Fig. 11–7). The B-cell name is derived from its site of differentiation in birds, the *b*ursa of Fabricius and the *b*one marrow of mammals. B-cell differentiation also takes place in the fetal liver and fetal spleen. Activated B cells either develop into **memory cells**, which express the CD45RO cell surface marker and circulate until activated by specific antigen, or terminally differentiate into plasma cells. **Plasma cells**, which have small nuclei and large cytoplasm, are factories for antibody production.

T cells acquired their name because they develop in the *t*hymus. T cells have the following two major functions in response to foreign antigen:

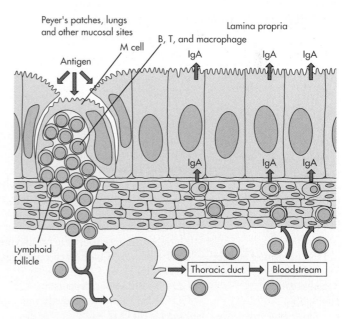

FIGURE 11–5. Lymphoid cells stimulated with antigen in Peyer's patches (or the lungs or another mucosal site) migrate via the regional lymph nodes and thoracic duct into the blood stream and then to the lamina propria of the gut and probably other mucosal surfaces. Thus, lymphocytes stimulated at one mucosal surface may become distributed throughout the MALT (mucosa-associated lymphoid tissue) system. IgA = immunoglobulin A. (From Roitt I et al: *Immunology,* ed 4, St Louis, 1996, Mosby.)

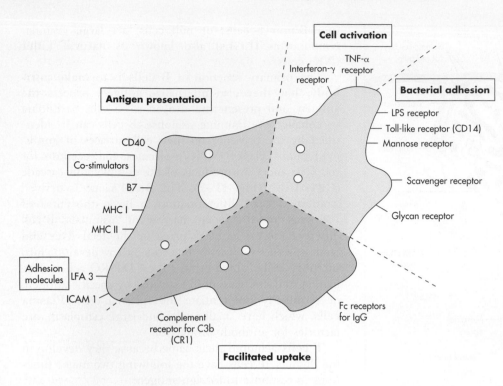

FIGURE 11–6. Macrophage surface structures mediate cell function. Bacteria and antigens either bind directly to receptors or bind through antibody or complement receptors (opsonization) and can then be phagocytized; the cell is activated and presents antigen to T cells. The dendritic cell shares many of these characteristics.

TABLE 11–5. Comparison of B and T Cells

Property	T Cells	B Cells
Origin	Bone marrow	Bone marrow
Maturation	Thymus	Bursal equivalent: bone marrow, Peyer's patches
Functions	Helper: initiation and promotion of immune response	**Antibody production**
	DTH: promotion and amplification of inflammatory response	Antigen presentation to T cells
	CTL: class I MHC–restricted cytolysis	—
Protective response	Resolution of intracellular and fungal infections	Protection against rechallenge, block spread of agent in blood, opsonize, etc.
Products*	Cytokines, interferon-γ, growth factors, cytolytic substances (perforin, granzymes)	IgM, IgD, IgG, IgA, or IgE
Distinguishing surface markers	CD2 (sheep red blood cell receptor), TCR, CD3, CD4, or CD8	Surface antibody, complement receptors, class II MHC antigens
Subsets	CD4 TH0: helper precursor	B cells: antibody, antigen presentation
	CD4 TH1: activates growth, macrophage, and CTLs (DTH)	Plasma cell: terminally differentiated antibody factories
	CD4 TH2: B-cell growth, class switching	
	CD4 TH3: class switching-IgA, suppression	Memory cells: long-lived, anamnestic response
	CD8: cytotoxic T cells (CTL)	
	CD8: suppressor cells	
	Memory cells: long-lived, anamnestic response	

*Depending on subset.

CTL = cytotoxic lymphocyte; DTH = delayed-type hypersensitivity; Ig = immunoglobulin; MHC = major histocompatibility complex; TCR = T-cell receptor.

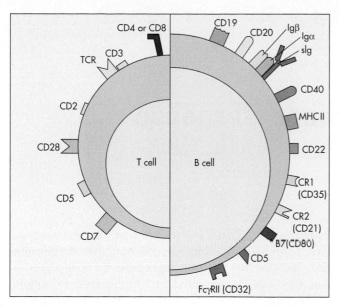

FIGURE 11–7. Surface markers of human B and T cells.

responses. T cells also produce **memory cells** that express CD45RO. Terminally differentiated CD4 and CD8 T cells express the class II MHC antigen. A smaller number of T cells ($\approx$ 5%) express the $\gamma\delta$ **TCR** but do not express CD4 or CD8. These cells generally reside in skin and mucosa and are important for innate immunity.

The **large granular lymphocyte NK cells** resemble the CD8 T cells in cytolytic function toward virally infected and tumor cells but differ in the mechanism for identifying the target cell. NK cells also have Fc receptors, which are used in antibody-dependent killing, and hence are also called **antibody-dependent cellular cytotoxicity (ADCC or K) cells**. The cytoplasmic granules contain cytolytic proteins to mediate the killing.

1. Control, suppress (when necessary) and activate immune and inflammatory responses by releasing cytokines.
2. Directly kill virally infected cells, foreign cells (e.g., tissue grafts), and tumors.

T cells make up 60% to 80% of peripheral blood lymphocytes.

T cells were initially distinguished from B cells on the basis of their ability to bind and surround themselves (forming rosettes) with sheep erythrocytes through the CD2 molecule. All T cells express an antigen-binding **T-cell receptor (TCR)**, which resembles but differs from antibody, and **CD2-** and **CD3-associated** proteins on their cell surface (see Fig. 11–7). T cells are divided into three major groups on the basis of the type of TCR and the cell surface expression of two proteins, CD4 and CD8. Most lymphocytes express the $\alpha\beta$ **TCR**. **CD4-expressing T cells** include the helper cells and the cells that induce delayed-type hypersensitivity (DTH). These T cells produce and secrete cytokines that stimulate and activate other immune responses. The CD4 T cells can be further divided into TH0, TH1, TH2, and TH3 subgroups according to the spectrum of cytokines they secrete. TH1 cells promote inflammatory and DTH responses, whereas TH2 cells promote antibody production. TH3 cells promote IgA production and T-cell tolerance. The **CD8 T cells** also release cytokines but are better known for their ability to recognize and kill virally infected cells, foreign tissue transplants (non-self grafts), and tumor cells as cytotoxic killer T cells. CD8 T cells are also responsible for suppressing immune

QUESTIONS

A professor was teaching an introductory course and described the different immune cells with the following nicknames. Describe why the nicknames are appropriate or why they are not.

1. Macrophage: Pac man (a computer game character that eats dots but eats bad guys when activated).
2. T cells: Police department.
3. CD4 T cell: Desk sergeant/dispatch officer.
4. CD8 T cell: "Cop on the beat"/patrol officer.
5. B cell: Product design and building company.
6. Plasma cell: Factory.
7. Mast cell: Activatable chemical warfare unit.
8. Neutrophil: Trash collector and disinfector.
9. Dendritic cell: Billboard display.

BIBLIOGRAPHY

Abbas AK, Lichtman AH, Pober JS: *Cellular and molecular immunology*, ed 4, Philadelphia, 2000, WB Saunders.
Goldsby RA, Kindt TJ, Osborne BA: *Kuby immunology*, ed 4, New York, 2000, WH Freeman.
Immunology Today: Issues contain understandable reviews on current topics in immunology.
Janeway CA et al: *Immunobiology: the immune system in health and disease*, ed 4, New York, 1999, Current Biology Publications and Garland Press.
Male D et al: *Advanced immunology*, ed 3, St Louis, 1996, Mosby.
Roitt I, Brostoff J, Male D: *Immunology*, ed 4, St Louis, 1996, Mosby.
Sompayrac L: *How the immune system works*, Malden, Mass, 1999, Blackwell Scientific.

CHAPTER 12

The Humoral Immune Response

The primary molecular component of the humoral immune response is antibody. Antibody molecules are synthesized by B cells and plasma cells in response to challenge by antigen. Antibodies provide protection from rechallenge by an infectious agent, block spread of the agent in the blood, and facilitate elimination of the infectious agent. To accomplish these tasks, an incredibly large repertoire of antibody molecules must be available to recognize the tremendous number of infectious agents and molecules that challenge our bodies. In addition to interacting specifically with foreign structures, antibody must interact with host systems and cells (e.g., complement, macrophages) to promote clearance of antigen and activation of subsequent immune responses (Box 12–1). Antibody molecules also serve as the cell surface receptors on the B cell to stimulate these antibody factories to grow and produce more antibody in response to antigenic challenge.

Immunogens, Antigens, and Epitopes

Almost all of the proteins and carbohydrates associated with an infectious agent, whether a bacterium, fungus, virus, or parasite, are considered foreign to the human host and have the potential to induce an immune response. A protein or carbohydrate that challenges the immune system and that can initiate an immune response is called an **immunogen** (Box 12–2). Immunogens may contain more than one antigen (e.g., bacteria). An **antigen** is a molecule that is recognized by specific antibody or T cells. An **epitope (antigenic determinant)** is the actual molecular structure that interacts with a single antibody molecule. Within a protein, an epitope may be formed by a specific sequence **(linear epitope)** or a three-dimensional structure **(conformational epitope)**. Antigens and immunogens usually contain several epitopes, each capable of binding to a different antibody molecule. As described later, a **monoclonal antibody** recognizes a single epitope.

Not all molecules are immunogens. In general, *proteins are the best immunogens, carbohydrates are weaker immunogens, and lipids and nucleic acids are poor immunogens.* In general, the immunogen must be of sufficient size, and proteins must be degradable by phagocytes so that they can be presented to lymphocytes, to initiate an immune response. **Haptens (incomplete immunogens)** cannot initiate but can be recognized by an immune response. The hapten often is too small to immunize an individual but can be recognized by antibody. Haptens can be made immunogenic by attachment to a **carrier molecule,** such as a protein. For example, dinitrophenol conjugated to bovine serum albumin is an immunogen for the dinitrophenol hapten.

During artificial immunization (e.g., vaccines), an adjuvant is used to enhance the response to antigen. **Adjuvants** usually prolong the presence of antigen in the tissue and activate or promote uptake of the immunogen by macrophages and lymphocytes. Most vaccines are precipitated onto alum to promote the slow release of antigen and the uptake by macrophages. Cells are stimulated and antigen is released slowly when emulsified in complete Freund's adjuvant (consisting of heat-killed mycobacteria in mineral oil). Complete Freund's adjuvant is not for human use, but newer, less toxic adjuvants are being tested for use with human vaccines. These include liposomes (defined lipid complexes), bacterial cell wall components, molecular cages for antigen, and polymeric surfactants. Cholera toxin and *Escherichia coli* lymphotoxin are potent adjuvants for secretory antibody (immunoglobulin [Ig] A).

Some molecules will not elicit an immune response in an individual. During growth of the fetus, the body develops **immune tolerance** toward self-antigens as well as any foreign antigens that may be introduced before maturation of the immune system. Later in life, tolerance may develop under special conditions; for example, ingestion of high concentrations of bovine myelin can cause an individual to develop tolerance to myelin. This has been proposed as a potential therapy for the autoimmunopathogenesis that causes multiple sclerosis.

The type of immune response initiated by an immunogen is dependent on its molecular structure. A prim

---

BOX 12–1. Antimicrobial Action of Antibodies

Are opsonic: promote ingestion and killing by phagocytic cells (IgG)

Neutralize (block attachment) toxins and virus

Agglutinate bacteria: may aid in clearing

Render motile organisms nonmotile

Combine with antigens on the microbial surface, activate the complement cascade, thus inducing an inflammatory response, bringing fresh phagocytes and serum antibodies into the site

Combine with antigens on the microbial surface, activate the complement cascade, anchor the membrane attack complex involving C5b to C9

---

itive but rapid antibody response can be initiated toward *bacterial polysaccharides, peptidoglycan, or flagellin.* These molecules have a large, repetitive structure, which is sufficient to activate B cells directly to make antibody without the participation of T-cell help and are termed **T-independent antigens.** In these cases, the response is limited to production of **IgM** antibody and fails to stimulate an anamnestic (memory) response. In most cases, B-cell production of antibody requires help, in the form of cytokines, from T cells; therefore, the antigen must be recognized and stimulate both T and B cells. **T-dependent antigens** are usually proteins; they stimulate all five classes of immunoglobulins and elicit an anamnestic response. In addition to the structure of the antigen, the amount, route of administration, and other factors influence the type of immune response, including the types of antibody produced. These factors influence the activation of different subclasses of helper T cells (TH1, TH2, and TH3) to produce different cytokines, which promote production of different types of antibody. For example, oral or nasal administration of a vaccine promotes production of a secretory form of **IgA** (sIgA) that would not be produced on intramuscular challenge.

Immunoglobulin Types and Structures

Immunoglobulins are subdivided into classes and subclasses based on the structure and antigenic distinction of their heavy chains. IgG, IgM, and IgA are the major antibody forms, whereas IgD and IgE make up less than 1% of the total immunoglobulins. The IgA and IgG classes of immunoglobulin are divided further into subclasses based on differences in the Fc portion. There are four subclasses of IgG, designated as IgG1 through IgG4, and two IgA subclasses (IgA1 and IgA2) (Fig. 12–1).

Antibody molecules are Y-shaped molecules with two major structural regions that mediate the two major functions of the molecule (Fig. 12–1 and Table 12–1). The **variable-region/antigen-combining site** must be able to identify and specifically interact with an epitope on an antigen. A large number of different antibody molecules, each with a different variable region, is produced in every individual to recognize the seemingly infinite number of different antigens in nature. The **Fc portion** (stem of the antibody Y) interacts with host systems and cells (e.g., complement, macrophages) to promote clearance of antigen and activation of subsequent immune responses. For IgG and IgA, the Fc portion interacts with other proteins to promote transfer across the placenta and the mucosa, respectively (Table 12–2).

IgG and IgA have a flexible **hinge region** rich in proline and susceptible to cleavage by proteolytic enzymes. Digestion of IgG molecules with **papain** yields two **Fab** and one **Fc** fragments (Fig. 12–2). Each Fab fragment has one antigen-binding site. By contrast, the Fc fragment has no antigen-binding site but is responsible for fixation of complement and attachment of the molecule to cell surface immunoglobulin receptors **(FcR)** on macrophages, natural killer, and T cells. **Pepsin** cleaves the molecule, producing an **F(ab′)$_2$** fragment with two antigen-binding sites and a **pFc′** fragment.

The different types and parts of immunoglobulin can also be distinguished using antibodies directed against different portions of the molecule. **Isotypes (IgM, IgD, IgG, IgA, IgE)** are determined by antibodies directed against the Fc portion of the molecule. *(Iso is the same for each person.)* **Allotypic** differences occur for antibody molecules with the same isotype but contain protein sequences that differ from one person to another (in addition to the antigen-binding region).

BOX 12–2. Definitions

Immunogen—Substance capable of *eliciting* an immune response

Antigen—Substance *recognized* by immune response

Epitope—Molecular structure recognized by immune response

Hapten—Incomplete immunogen that cannot initiate response but that can be recognized by antibody

Carrier—Protein modified by hapten to elicit response

Adjuvant—Substance that promotes immune response to immunogen

T-independent antigens—Antigens with large, repetitive structures (e.g., bacteria, flagellin, lipopolysaccharide, polysaccharide)

T-dependent antigens—Antigens that must be presented to T and B cells for antibody production

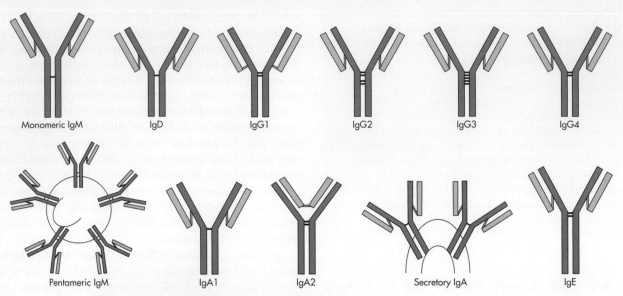

FIGURE 12–1. Comparative structures of the immunoglobulin (Ig) classes and subclasses in humans. IgA and IgM are held together in multimers by the J chain. IgA can acquire the secretory component for the traversal of epithelial cells.

TABLE 12–1. Immunoglobulins

Ig	IgG	IgM	IgA	IgD	IgE
CD4 T-helper subclass association	TH1, TH2	T independent and TH1	TH2, TH3	—	TH2
Total Ig (%)	85	5–10	5–15	<1	<1
Molecular mass (kDa)	154	900	160 (+ dimer)	185	190
H-chain class	γ	μ	α	δ	ϵ
Subclass	γ-1, γ-2, γ-3, γ-4	—	α-1, α-2	—	—
Serum half-life (days)	23	5	6	2–3	2–3
Principal site of action	Serum and tissue	Serum	Secretions	Receptor for B cells	Mast cells
Principal biologic effect	Resistance: opsonin, secondary response	Resistance: precipitin, primary response	Resistance: protection of mucous membranes	B-cell activation	Anaphylaxis
Complement fixation	+++	++++	+	−	−
Opsonin for macrophage, PMN	+				
Mucosal secretion	−	−	+	−	−
Crossing of placenta	+	−	−	−	−

PMN = polymorphonuclear neutrophil (leukocyte); +/− = relative activity.

TABLE 12–2. Fc Interactions with Immune Components

Immune Component	Interaction	Function
Fc receptor	Macrophages	Opsonization
	PMNs	Opsonization
	T cells	Activation
	NK cells (antibody-dependent cellular cytotoxicity)	Killing
	Mast cells for immunoglobulin E	Allergic reactions, antiparasitic
Complement	Complement system	Opsonization, killing (especially bacteria)

PMN = Polymorphonuclear neutrophils.

(Every one ["allo"] of them cannot have the same IgG.) The **idiotype** refers to the protein sequences in the variable region that generate the large number of antigen-binding regions. *(There are many different idiots.)*

On a molecular basis, each antibody molecule is made up of heavy and light chains encoded by separate genes. The basic immunoglobulin unit consists of **two heavy (H)** and **two light (L) chains.** IgM and IgA consist of multimers of this basic structure. The heavy and light chains of immunoglobulin are fastened to- gether by **interchain disulfide bonds.** Two types of light chains—**κ and λ**—are present in all five immu- noglobulin classes, although only one type is present in an individual molecule. Approximately 60% of human immunoglobulin molecules have κ light chains, and 40% have λ light chains. There are **five types of heavy chains,** one for each isotype of antibody **(IgM, μ; IgG, γ; IgD, δ; IgA, α; and IgE, ε).** Intrachain disulfide bonds define molecular domains within each chain. Light chains have a variable and a constant do- main. The heavy chains have a variable and three (IgG, IgA) or four (IgM, IgE) constant domains. The vari- able domains on the heavy and light chains interact to form the antigen-binding site. The constant domains from each chain provide the molecular structure to the immunoglobulin and define the interaction of the anti- body molecule with host systems and hence its ulti- mate function. The heavy chain of the different anti- body molecules can also be synthesized with a membrane-spanning region to make the antibody an antigen-specific receptor for the B cell.

Immunoglobulin D

IgD, which has a molecular mass of 185 kDa, accounts for less than 1% of serum immunoglobulins. IgD exists primarily as membrane IgD, which serves with IgM as an antigen receptor on early B-cell membranes to help initiate antibody responses by activating B-cell growth.

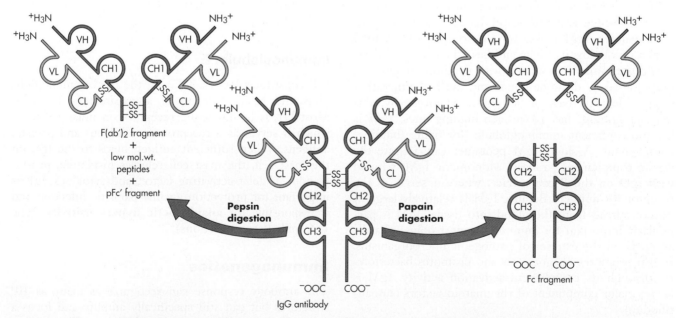

FIGURE 12–2. Proteolytic digestion of immunoglobulin G (IgG). Pepsin treatment produces a dimeric F(ab')₂ fragment. Papain treatment produces monovalent Fab fragments and an Fc fragment. The F(ab')₂ and the Fab fragments bind antigen but lack a functional Fc region. *Blue* = heavy chain; *orange* = light chain.

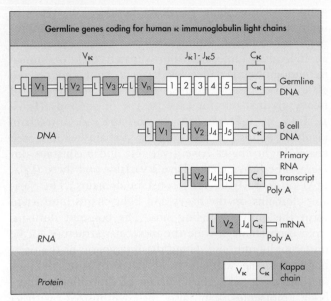

FIGURE 12–3. Rearrangement of the germline genes to produce the human immunoglobulin κ light chains. Genetic recombination juxtaposes one of the 100 V-region genes with a J-region gene and a Cκ gene during differentiation into a pre-B cell. The remaining intervening sequences are removed by splicing the messenger RNA. L = leader sequence.

IgD and IgM are the only isotypes expressed by the same cell.

Immunoglobulin M

IgM is the first antibody produced in response to antigenic challenge and can be produced in a T-independent manner. IgM makes up 5% to 10% of the total immunoglobulins in adults and has a half-life of 5 days. It is a **pentameric molecule** with five immunoglobulin units joined by disulfide bonds and the **J chain,** with a total molecular mass of 900 kDa. Theoretically, this immunoglobulin has 10 antigen-binding sites. IgM is the most efficient immunoglobulin for fixing (binding) complement. A single IgM pentamer can activate the classic complement pathway. Monomeric IgM is found with IgD on the B-cell surface, where it serves as the receptor for antigen. Because IgM is relatively large, it cannot spread from the blood into tissue. IgM is particularly important for immunity against polysaccharide antigens on the exterior of pathogenic microorganisms. It also promotes phagocytosis and promotes bacteriolysis through its complement-activation activity. IgM is also a major component of rheumatoid factors (autoantibodies).

Immunoglobulin G

IgG composes approximately 85% of the immunoglobulins in adults. It has a molecular mass of 154 kDa based on two L chains of 22,000 Da each and two H chains of 55,000 Da each. The four subclasses of IgG differ in structure (see Fig. 12–1), relative concentration, and function. Production of IgG requires T-cell help. IgG, as a class of antibody molecules, has the longest half-life (23 days) of the five immunoglobulin classes, crosses the placenta, and is the principal antibody in the anamnestic or booster response. IgG shows high avidity or binding capacity for antigens, fixes complement, stimulates chemotaxis, and acts as an opsonin to facilitate phagocytosis.

Immunoglobulin A

IgA composes 5% to 15% of the serum immunoglobulins and has a half-life of 6 days. It has a molecular mass of 160 kDa and a basic four-chain monomeric structure. However, it can occur as monomers, dimers, trimers, and multimers combined by the J chain (similar to IgM). In addition to serum IgA, a **secretory IgA** appears in body secretions and provides localized immunity. IgA production requires specialized T-cell help as well as mucosal stimulation. Adjuvants, such as cholera toxin and attenuated *Salmonella* bacteria, can promote an IgA response. IgA binds to a **poly-Ig receptor** on epithelial cells for transport across the cell. The poly-Ig receptor remains bound to IgA and is then cleaved to become the **secretory component** when secretory IgA is secreted from the cell. An adult secretes approximately 2 g of IgA per day. Secretory IgA appears in colostrum, intestinal and respiratory secretions, saliva, tears, and other secretions. IgA-deficient individuals have an increased incidence of respiratory tract infections.

Immunoglobulin E

IgE constitutes less than 1% of the total immunoglobulins and has a half-life of approximately 2.5 days. Most IgE is bound to Fc receptors on **mast cells,** on which it serves as a receptor for allergens and parasite antigens. When sufficient antigen binds to the IgE on the mast cell, the mast cell releases histamine, prostaglandin, platelet-activating factor, and cytokines. IgE is important for protection against parasitic infection and is responsible for **anaphylactic hypersensitivity** (type 1) (rapid allergic reactions).

Immunogenetics

The antibody response can recognize as many as 10^8 structures but can still specifically amplify and focus a response directed to a specific challenge. The mechanisms for generating this antibody repertoire and the different immunoglobulin subclasses are tied to the genetic events that accompany the development (differentiation) of the B cell (Figs. 12–3 and 12–4).

Human chromosomes 2, 22, and 14 contain immunoglobulin genes for κ, λ, and H chains, respectively. The **germline form** of these genes consists of different and separate sets of genetic building blocks for the light **(V and J gene segments)** and heavy chains **(V, D, and J gene segments),** which are genetically recombined to produce the immunoglobulin variable regions. These variable regions are then associated with the constant-region C gene segments. For the κ light chain, there are 300 V gene segments, 5 J gene segments, and 1 C gene segment. The number of λ gene segments for V and J is more limited. For the heavy chain, there are 300 to 1000 V genes, 12 D genes, 6 (heavy-chain) J genes, but only 9 C genes (one for each class and subclass of antibody [μ; δ; γ₃, γ₁, γ₂, and γ₄; ε; α₁ and α₂]). In addition, gene segments for membrane-spanning peptides can be attached to the heavy-chain genes to allow the antibody molecule to insert into the B-cell membrane as an antigen-activation receptor.

Production of the final antibody molecule in the pre-B and B cell requires genetic recombination at the DNA level and post-transcriptional processing at the RNA level to assemble the immunoglobulin gene and messenger RNA (mRNA) (Fig. 12–5). Each of the V, D, and J segments is surrounded by DNA sequences that promote **directional recombination and loss of the intervening DNA sequences.** Juxtaposition of randomly chosen V and J gene segments of the light chains and the V, D, and J gene segments of the heavy chains produces the variable region of the immunoglobulin chains. **Somatic mutation** of the immuno-

globulin gene occurs later in activated B cells to add to the enormous number of possible coding sequences for the variable region and to fine-tune a specific immune response. Attachment of the variable-region sequences (VDJ) to the beginning of the C gene segments by recombination produces a heavy-chain gene containing the μ; δ; γ₃, γ₁, γ₂, and γ₄; ε; and α₁ and α₂ sequences in the indicated order. In the pre–B and immature B cells, mRNAs are produced and contain the variable-region gene segments connected to the C gene sequences for μ and δ. Processing of the mRNA removes either the μ or δ, as if it were an intron, to produce the final immunoglobulin. The pre-B cell expresses cytoplasmic IgM, whereas the B cell expresses cytoplasmic and cell surface IgM and cell surface IgD. IgM and IgD are the only pair of isotypes that can be expressed on the same cell.

Class switching (IgM to IgG, IgE, or IgA) occurs in mature B cells in response to different cytokines produced by TH1, TH2, or TH3 CD4 helper T cells. Genetic recombination juxtaposes the appropriate constant-region sequence with the variable-region sequences and in the process deletes the intervening C-region gene segments (see Fig. 12–5). Each of the C gene segments, except for δ, is preceded by a DNA sequence called the **switch site.** After the appropriate cytokine signal, the switch in front of the μ sequence recombines with the switch in front of the γ₃, γ₁, γ₂, or γ₄; ε; or α₁, or α₂ sequences, creating a DNA loop that is subsequently removed. Processing of the RNA transcript yields the final mRNA for the immunoglobulin heavy-chain protein. For example, IgG1 production would result from excision of DNA containing the C gene segments C μ, C δ, and C γ₃ to attach the variable region to the γ₁ C gene segment. **Class switching does not change the variable region.**

The final steps in B-cell differentiation to memory cells or plasma cells do not change the antibody gene. **Memory cells** are long-lived, antigen-responsive B cells expressing the CD45RO surface marker. Memory cells can be activated in response to antigen later in life to grow and produce specific antibody. **Plasma cells** are terminally differentiated B cells with a small nucleus but a large cytoplasm filled with endoplasmic reticulum. Plasma cells are antibody factories.

Antibody Response

An initial repertoire of IgM and IgD immunoglobulins is generated in pre-B cells by the genetic events previously described (Fig. 12–6). Differentiation of the pre-B cell to the B cell is accompanied by expression of cell surface IgM and IgD. Cell surface antibody is associated with signal transduction receptors, Ig-α (CD79a) and Ig-β (CD79b), in the membrane through which antigen binding initiates an activation signal. The activation signal is mediated by a cascade of pro-

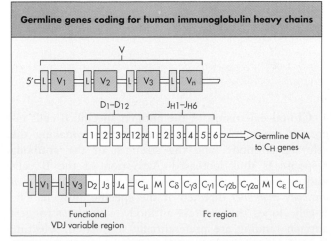

FIGURE 12–4. Rearrangement of the germline genes to produce the human immunoglobulin (Ig) heavy chains. A V-region gene (of 100 possible) combines with a D-region gene (of 12 possible) and a J-region gene (of 6 possible). Constant-region genes (corresponding to IgM [μ], IgD [δ], IgG [γ], IgE [ε], and IgA [α]) are attached to the VDJ region. M = membrane-spanning segment.

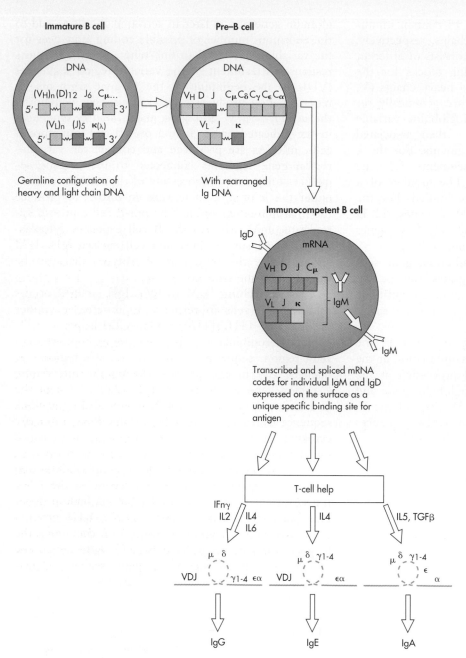

FIGURE 12–5. Differentiation of the B cell promotes genetic recombination and class switching. Switch regions in front of the constant-region genes (including immunoglobulin [Ig] G subclasses) allow attachment of a preformed VDJ region with different heavy-chain constant-region genes, genetically removing the μ, δ, and other intervening genes. This produces an immunoglobulin gene with the same VDJ region (except for somatic mutation) but different heavy-chain genes. Splicing of messenger RNA (mRNA) produces the final IgM RNA.

tein tyrosine kinases, phospholipase C, and calcium fluxes that activate transcription and cell growth. The activation signal is amplified by other surface molecules, including the CR2 (CD21) complement (C3d) receptor. T-independent antigens cross link sufficient numbers of surface antibody to promote growth of the antigen-specific B cells. In this manner, each of the B cells that recognizes the different epitopes of the antigen will increase in number in a process termed **clonal expansion.** Production of antibody to T-dependent antigens requires interaction of the B cell with the helper T cell through CD40 (on the B cell), CD40L (T cell), and the action of cytokines (interleukin-4 [IL-4], IL-5, IL-2, or interferon-γ).

Clonal expansion of the antigen-specific B cells increases the number of antibody factories making the relevant antibody, and the strength of the antibody response is thus increased. Activation of the B cells also promotes *somatic mutation, increasing the diversity of antibody molecules* directed at the specific antigen. The B-cell clones that express antibody with the strongest antigen binding are preferentially stimulated, selecting for a better antibody response.

Class switching is induced by the different combinations of cytokines produced by helper T cells. **TH1-helper responses (IL-2, interferon-γ) promote production of IgM and IgG. TH2-helper responses (IL-4, IL-5, IL-6, IL-10) promote production of**

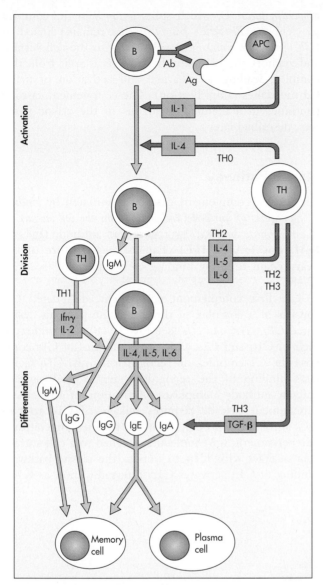

FIGURE 12–6. B-cell activation. Binding of antigen, cross-linking of cell surface receptors, the C3d product of complement, endotoxin, and cytokines activate the growth and differentiation of B cells. IFNγ = interferon-γ; APC = antigen-presenting cell; Ig = immunoglobulin; IL = interleukin; TGF-β = transforming growth factor-β.

cleared. After the initial lag phase, however, the antibody titer increases logarithmically to reach a plateau.

Reexposure to an immunogen, a **secondary response,** induces a heightened antibody response (also termed **anamnestic response**). The antibodies develop more rapidly, last longer, and reach a higher titer. The antibodies in a secondary response are principally of the IgG class, although IgM antibodies can also be detected in response to some infections.

During an immune response, antibodies are made against different epitopes of the foreign object, protein, or infectious agent. *Specific antibody is a mixture of many different immunoglobulin molecules made by many different B cells* **(polyclonal antibody),** each immunoglobulin molecule differing in the epitope that it recognizes and the strength of the interaction. Different antibody molecules are made to different epitopes on the antigen, and each binds with different strengths (**avidity,** multivalent binding of antibody to antigen; **affinity,** monovalent binding to an epitope) for the same antigen.

Monoclonal antibodies are identical antibodies produced by a single clone of cells or by myelomas (cancers of plasma cells) or hybridomas. Hybridomas are cloned, laboratory-derived cells obtained by the fusion of antibody-producing spleen cells and a myeloma cell. In 1975, Kohler and Millstein developed the technique for producing monoclonal antibodies from B-cell hybridomas. The hybridoma is immortal and produces a single (monoclonal) antibody. This technique has revolutionized the study of immunology because it allows selection (cloning) of individual antibody-producing cells and their development into cellular factories for production of large quantities of that antibody. Monoclonal antibodies have been commercially produced for both diagnostic reagents and therapeutic purposes.

IgM, IgG, IgE, and IgA. IgA production is especially promoted by IL-5 and transforming growth factor-β (TGF-β), a TH3 response. All three types of responses promote the development of memory cells. Terminal differentiation produces the plasma cell.

The primary antibody response is characterized by the initial production of IgM, and then as the response matures, IgG antibodies rapidly increase in concentration (Fig. 12–7). IgM antibodies appear in the blood within 3 days to 2 weeks after exposure to a novel immunogen. The first antibodies that are produced react with residual antigen and therefore are rapidly

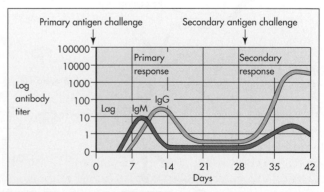

FIGURE 12–7. Time course of immune responses. The primary response occurs after a lag period. The immunoglobulin (Ig) M response is the earliest response. The secondary immune response (anamnestic response) reaches a higher titer, lasts longer, and consists predominantly of IgG.

Complement

The complement system is an alarm and a weapon against infection, especially bacterial infection. The complement system is activated directly by bacteria and bacterial products **(alternate or properdin pathway)**, by lectin binding to sugars on the bacterial cell surface **(mannose-binding protein)**, or by complexes of antibody and antigen **(classic pathway)** (Fig. 12–8). Activation by either pathway initiates a cascade of proteolytic events that produce chemotactic factors to attract phagocytic and inflammatory cells to the site, increase vascular permeability to allow access to the site of infection, bind to the agent to promote their phagocytosis **(opsonization)** and elimination, and directly kill the infecting agent. The three activation pathways of complement coalesce at a common junction point, the activation of the **C3 component.**

Alternate Pathway

The alternate pathway is activated directly by bacterial cell surfaces and their components (e.g., endotoxin, microbial polysaccharides) as well as other factors. This pathway can be activated before the establishment of an immune response to the infecting bacteria because it does not depend on antibody and does not involve the early complement components (C1, C2, and C4). The initial activation of the alternate pathway is mediated by *properdin factor B* binding to C3b and then with *properdin factor D*, which splits *factor B* in the complex to yield the *Bb active fragment* that remains linked to *C3b (activation unit)*. The C3b sticks to the cell surface and anchors the complex. Inactive *Ba* is split from this complex, leading to cleavage and activation of many C3 molecules (amplification). The complement cascade continues in a manner analogous to the classic pathway, described later.

Classic Pathway

The classic complement cascade is initiated by *binding to aggregates of antibody and antigen on the cell surface or in an immune complex.* Aggregation of antibody **(IgG or IgM, not IgA or IgE)** changes the structure of the heavy chain to allow binding to complement (see Fig. 12–8).

The first complement component, designated *C1,* consists of a complex of three separate proteins designated *C1q, C1r, and C1s* (see Fig. 12–8). One molecule each of C1q and C1s with two molecules of C1r compose the C1 complex or **recognition unit.** C1q facilitates binding of the recognition unit to cell surface antigen-antibody complexes. Activation of the classic complement cascade requires linkage of C1q to two IgG antibodies through their Fc regions. In contrast, one pentameric IgM molecule attached to a cell surface may interact with C1q to initiate the classic pathway. Binding of C1q activates C1r (referred to now as C1r*)

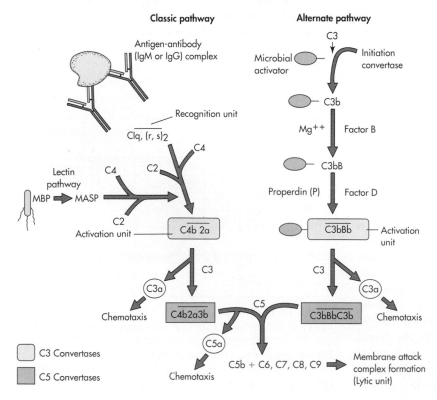

FIGURE 12–8. The classic and alternate complement pathways. Despite different activators, both pathways promote cleavage and activation of C3 and C5, which may be followed by construction of the membrane attack complex. Cleavage of C3 produces C3b, C3d, and C3a. MBP = mannose-binding protein; MASP = MBP-associated serine protease.

and in turn C1s (C1s*). C1s* then cleaves *C4* to C4a and C4b and *C2* to C2a and C2b. The ability of a single recognition unit to split numerous C2 and C4 molecules represents an amplification mechanism in the complement cascade. The union of *C4b* and *C2a* produces **C4b2a**, which is known as **C3 convertase**. This complex binds to the cell membrane and cleaves *C3* into *C3a* and *C3b* fragments. The C3b protein has a unique thioester bond that will covalently attach C3b to a cell surface or be hydrolyzed. The C3 convertase amplifies the response by splitting many C3 molecules. The interaction of C3b with C4b2a bound to the cell membrane produces **C4b3b2a**, which is termed **C5 convertase**. This activation unit splits *C5* into *C5a* and *C5b* fragments and represents yet another amplification step.

Lectin Pathway

Mannose-binding protein (previously known as RaRF) is a large serum protein that binds to nonreduced mannose, fucose, and glucosamine on bacterial and other cell surfaces. Mannose-binding protein resembles and replaces the C1q component and on binding to bacterial surfaces activates the cleavage of mannose-binding protein–associated serine protease. Mannose-binding protein–associated serine protease cleaves the C4 and C2 components to produce the C3 convertase, the junction point of the complement cascade.

Biologic Activities of Complement Components

Cleavage of the C3 and C5 components produces important factors that enhance clearance of the infectious agent by promoting access to the infection site and by attracting the cells that mediate protective inflammatory reactions. **C3b** is an **opsonin**, which promotes clearance of bacteria by binding directly to the cell membrane to make the cell more attractive to phagocytic cells such as neutrophils and macrophages, which have receptors for C3b. C3b can be cleaved further to generate **C3d**, which is an activator of B lymphocytes. Complement fragments **C3a** and **C5a** serve as powerful **anaphylatoxins** that stimulate mast cells to release histamine, which *enhances vascular permeability and smooth muscle contraction*. **C3a** and **C5a** also act as attractants **(chemotactic factors)** for neutrophils and macrophages. These cells also express receptors for C3b, are phagocytic, and promote inflammatory reactions.

Membrane Attack Complex

The terminal stage of the classic pathway involves creation of the **membrane attack complex**, which is also called **the lytic unit** (Fig. 12–9). The five terminal complement proteins (C5 through C9) associate into a membrane attack complex on target cell membranes to mediate injury. Initiation of membrane attack complex assembly begins with C5 cleavage into C5a and C5b fragments. A $(C5b,6,7,8)_1(C9)_n$ complex forms and drills a hole in the membrane, leading to the hypotonic lysis of cells. The C9 component is similar to perforin, which is produced by cytolytic T cells and NK cells.

Regulation of Complement Activation

Humans have several mechanisms for preventing generation of the C3 convertase to protect against inappropriate complement activation. These include C1 inhibitor, C4 binding protein, Factor H, Factor I, and the cell surface proteins, decay-accelerating factor (DAF) and membrane co-factor protein. In addition, CD59 (protectin) prevents formation of the membrane attack complex. Most infectious agents lack these pro-

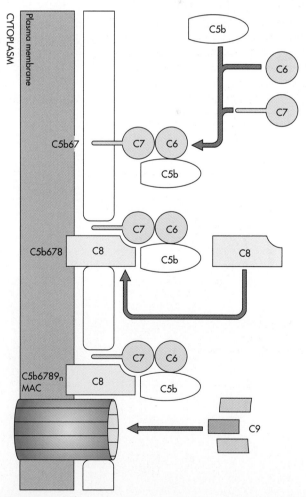

FIGURE 12–9. Cell lysis by complement. Activation of C5 initiates the molecular construction of an oil-well–like membrane attack complex (MAC).

tective mechanisms and remain susceptible to complement. A genetic deficiency in these protection systems can result in disease.

QUESTIONS

What is wrong with each of these statements and why?

1. The laboratory tested a baby for IgM maternal antibodies.

2. An investigator attempted to use fluorescent-labeled F(ab')$_2$ fragments to locate class II major histocompatibility complex molecules on the cell surface of antigen-presenting cells without cross-linking (binding two molecules together) these cell surface molecules.

3. A patient is diagnosed as having been infected with a specific strain of influenza A (A/Bangkok/1/79/H3N2) on the basis of the presence of anti-influenza IgG in serum taken from the patient at the initial visit (within 2 days of symptoms).

4. A patient with a T-cell deficiency, unable to promote class switching of B cells, was also considered unable to use the complement systems.

5. Analysis of immunoglobulin genes from B cells taken from the patient described in question 4 did not contain recombined VDJ variable-region gene sequences.

6. A patient was considered to have a B-cell deficiency because serum levels of IgE and IgD were undetectable despite proper concentrations of IgG and IgM.

BIBLIOGRAPHY

Abbas AK, Lichtman AH, Pober JS: *Cellular and molecular immunology*, ed 4, Philadelphia, 2000, WB Saunders.

Goldsby RA, Kindt TJ, Osborne BA: *Kuby immunology*, ed 4, New York, 2000, WH Freeman.

Immunology Today: Issues contain understandable reviews on current topics in immunology.

Janeway CA et al: *Immunobiology: the immune system in health and disease*, ed 4, New York, 1999, Current Biology/Garland Publishing.

Male D et al: *Advanced immunology*, ed 3, St Louis, 1996, Mosby.

Roitt I, Brostoff J, Male D: *Immunology*, ed 5, St Louis, 1997, Mosby.

Sompayrac L: *How the immune system works*, Malden, Mass, 1999, Blackwell Science.

C H A P T E R   1 3

Cellular Immune Responses

Cellular immune responses are mediated by monocyte-macrophage lineage cells, large granular lymphocytes (LGLs) (natural killer [NK] cells), and T cells. The LGLs provide early responses to infection, releasing cytokines (soluble messengers) and killing virally infected and tumor (NK) cells and antibody-decorated cells (antibody-dependent cellular cytotoxicity [ADCC]). Cells of the monocyte-macrophage lineage bridge the gap between the innate and the antigen-specific protective responses as phagocytic, killer, cytokine-producing, and antigen-presenting cells (APCs). The T cell plays a central role in activating and controlling (helping) immune and inflammatory responses through the release of cytokines. T cells are also very important for eliminating (killing) tumor cells and virally infected cells. T cells are morphologically similar to B cells but can be distinguished from B cells by specific cell surface antigenic markers. These markers include the antibody-like T-cell receptor (TCR) and its associated components (CD3 [CD for cluster of differentiation]) and a receptor for sheep red blood cells (CD2). These cells communicate through direct cell-to-cell interactions and with cytokines.

Development of T Cells

T-cell precursors develop into T cells in the thymus (Fig. 13–1). Contact with the thymic epithelium and hormones such as thymosin, thymulin, and thymopoietin II in the thymus promote extensive proliferation and differentiation of the individual's T-cell populations during fetal development. While T cell precursors are in the thymus, genetic events generate numerous TCRs, each expressed on a different T-cell clone. T cells that react with the host (self-reactive) are forced into committing suicide (apoptosis), and the remaining T cells differentiate into the subpopulations of T cells.

The helper T cells (CD4) activate and control immune and inflammatory responses by releasing cytokines (soluble messengers). Helper T cells interact with peptide antigens presented on class II major histocom-patibility complex (MHC) molecules expressed on APCs (macrophages and B cells) (Fig. 13–2). The vocabulary of cytokines secreted by a specific CD4 T cell in response to antigenic challenge further distinguishes the CD4 T cell as a TH1 or TH2 cell. **TH1 cells** promote inflammatory responses, which are especially important for controlling intracellular (mycobacterial and viral) and fungal infections, as well as certain types of antibody production. TH2 cells promote antibody and memory responses. A TH3 subtype has also been described; it is involved in production of immunoglobulin (Ig) A. The TH1 and TH2 responses are antagonistic and TH3 responses suppress TH1 and TH2 responses.

Cytolytic and suppressor T cells (CD8) "patrol" the body for cells expressing virus or tumor-like abnormal proteins presented by the class I MHC molecules. Class I MHC molecules are found on all nucleated cells.

Natural Killer Cells

NK cells are an important part of the natural immune (innate) system. NK cells are often the first cellular response to a viral infection, are important for their antitumor activity, and amplify inflammatory reactions after bacterial infection. NK cells are also responsible for **ADCC**, in which they bind and kill antibody-coated cells.

NK cells are LGLs that share many characteristics with T cells except the mechanism for target cell recognition. NK cells are stimulated by (1) the interferons IFN-α and IFN-β (produced early in response to a viral infection), (2) tumor necrosis factor-α (TNF-α), and (3) interleukins IL-12, IL-15 (both produced by activated macrophages), and IL-2 (produced by CD4 TH1 cells). The NK cells express many of the same cell surface markers as T cells (e.g., CD2, CD7, IL-2 receptor [IL-2R], and **FasL** [Fas ligand]) as well as the **Fc receptor for IgG (CD16)**, and complement receptors for ADCC. Activated NK cells produce IFN-γ, IL-1, and granulocyte-macrophage colony-stimulating

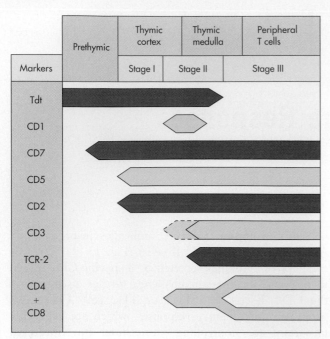

Markers	Prethymic	Thymic cortex	Thymic medulla	Peripheral T cells
		Stage I	Stage II	Stage III
Tdt				
CD1				
CD7				
CD5				
CD2				
CD3				
TCR-2				
CD4 + CD8				

FIGURE 13–1. Human T-cell development. T-cell markers are useful for the identification of the differentiation stages of the T cell and for characterizing T-cell leukemias and lymphomas. Tdt = Cytoplasmic terminal deoxynucleotide transferase.

factor (GM-CSF), which stimulate the macrophage to promote the initial response. The granules in an NK cell contain toxic molecules **perforin,** a pore-forming protein, and **granzymes** (esterases), which are similar to the granules in a CD8 cytotoxic T lymphocyte (CTL).

Unlike T cells, NK cells do not express TCR or CD3. Also, they neither recognize a specific antigen nor require presentation of antigen by MHC molecules. The NK system does not involve memory or require sensitization and cannot be enhanced by specific immunization.

The NK cell binds to carbohydrates and other cell surface proteins on target cells and will kill a target cell unless it receives an inhibitory signal upon binding its **killer-cell inhibitory receptors** to a class I MHC molecule on the target cell. The proper expression of class I MHC on the cell surface is like a secret password that sends an inhibitory signal to prevent NK killing of the target cell. Binding of the NK cell to antibody-coated target cells (ADCC) also initiates killing but without control by the inhibitory signal. The **killing mechanisms** are similar to those of CTLs, including **perforin** disruption of the target cell membrane, the toxic effects of the **granzymes**, and **the FasL-Fas** protein induction of apoptosis (see later discussion of CD8 T cells).

Cytokine-Activated Killer Cells

Cytokine-activated killer (**LAK** [L from earlier term "lymphokine"]) cells are IL-2–activated effectors that are able to bind and kill many types of tumor and virally infected cells. Most LAK cell activity is derived from NK cells, but some T cells also become LAK cells.

Cells of the Monocyte-Macrophage Lineage

Monocytes are myeloid cells that develop from the same lineage as polymorphonuclear granulocytes. Monocytes mature into macrophages and cells of the macrophage lineage that differ in function and tissue location. **Dendritic cell precursors** and **dendritic cells** also develop from the monocyte or from stem cells and are excellent APCs.

The surface markers on monocyte-macrophages correspond to the cells' functions. These cells express the following substances:

1. **Receptors for opsonins** (e.g., immunoglobulin Fc receptors [Fc-γ RI, Fc-γ RII, Fc-γ RIII] and **complement receptors** [CR1, CR3]).
2. **Lectins** (specific sugar-binding proteins such as mannosyl-fucosyl receptors).
3. A **receptor for the lipopolysaccharide-binding**

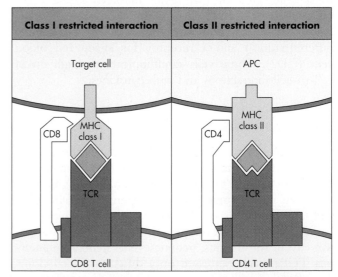

FIGURE 13–2. MHC restriction and antigen presentation to T cells. *Left,* Antigenic peptides bound to class I MHC molecules are presented to the T-cell receptor (TCR) on CD8 T killer/suppressor cells. *Right,* Antigenic peptides bound to class II MHC molecules on the antigen-presenting cell (APC) (B cell, dendritic cell or macrophage) are presented to CD4 helper and delayed-type hypersensitivity T cells.

protein (CD14) to facilitate bacterial uptake and promote activation.

4. Adhesion molecules to promote cell-to-cell interactions; for example, leukocyte function–associated (antigen)-1 (LFA-1).
5. The B7 and class II MHC proteins to allow **antigen presentation** to T cells.

Macrophages are activated to different functional levels by different stimuli. Ingestion of microbes promotes the release of IL-1, IL-12, and TNF, which initiate inflammatory reactions and activate the CD4 TH1 immune responses. In turn, sufficient levels of TNF or IFN-γ, produced by NK and CD4 TH1 cells, activate killing mechanisms in the macrophage (activated/angry macrophage) to reinforce local responses. The **activated macrophage** can kill phagocytosed microbes, virally infected cells, and tumor cells. Continuous stimulation of macrophages by T cells, as in the case of an unresolved mycobacterial infection, promotes the fusion of macrophages into **multinucleate giant cells** and large macrophages called epithelioid cells that surround the infection and form a **granuloma**.

Dendritic cells (DCs) are professional APCs that can also produce cytokines. Precursor DCs and monocytes circulate in the blood and then differentiate into immature DCs in tissue. The various immature DCs that are found in tissue and blood include (1) **Langerhans cells** in the skin, (2) **dermal interstitial cells**, (3) **follicular DCs** (lymph node and spleen), (4) **interdigitating cells** (lymph node and spleen), (5) **splenic marginal DCs**, and (6) DCs in the **liver, thymus, germinal centers of the lymph nodes** and **blood**. These cells are efficient at capturing and phagocytosing antigen; upon doing so, they mature into DCs. Mature DCs lose phagocytic abilities, upregulate class II MHC and B7-1 and B7-2 (costimulatory) molecules to facilitate antigen presentation, and move to T cell areas of lymph nodes. DCs can present antigen through class I MHC to CD8 T cells and through class II MHC to CD4 T cells and even to B cells to promote antibody production. DCs are so effective at presenting antigen that 10 cells loaded with antigen are sufficient to initiate protective immunity in a mouse to a lethal bacterial challenge.

Characteristics of T Cells

T cells were initially distinguished from B cells on the basis of their ability to bind sheep red blood cells and form rosettes. T cells are defined through the use of antibodies that distinguish their cell surface molecules. The T-cell surface proteins include (1) the T cell receptor (TCR), (2) the CD4 and CD8 coreceptors, (3) accessory proteins that promote recognition and activa-

tion, (4) cytokine receptors, and (5) adhesion proteins. All of these proteins determine the types of cell-to-cell interactions for the T cell and therefore the functions of the cell.

The **TCR complex** is a combination of the antigen recognition structure (TCR) and cell-activation machinery (**CD3**) (Fig. 13–3). There are two types of T-cell antigen receptors, the **TCR1**, consisting of γ **and** δ **chains**, and the **TCR2**, consisting of α **and** β **chains**. T cells expressing TCR1 (γ/δ**T cells**) are more primitive T cells, are generally restricted to mucosal epithelium and other tissue locations, and are important for stimulating innate and mucosal immunity. TCR2 is expressed on most T cells (α/β **T cells**), and these cells are primarily responsible for antigen-activated immune responses.

As for the B cell, each T-cell clone recognizes and responds to a different antigen, as defined by its TCR. Each TCR molecule is made up of two different polypeptide chains. As with antibody, each TCR chain has a constant region and a variable region. The repertoire of T-cell antigen receptors is very large and can identify a tremendous number of antigenic specificities (estimated to be able to recognize 10^{15} separate epitopes). The genetic mechanisms for the development of this diversity are similar to those for antibody (Fig. 13–4). The TCR gene is made up of multiple V, D, and J segments, similar to the antibody gene. Different V, D, and J segments recombine to form different TCR genes. Unlike antibody genes, however, TCR genes

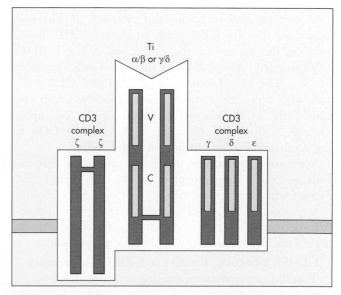

FIGURE 13–3. T-cell receptor (TCR). The TCR consists of different subunits. Antigen recognition occurs through the α/β or γ/δ subunits. The CD3 complex of γ, δ, ε, and ζ subunits promotes T-cell activation. V = Variable region; C = constant region.

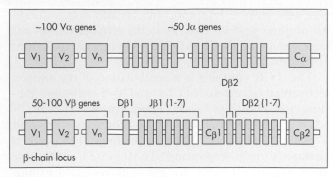

FIGURE 13–4. Structure of the T-cell receptor (TCR) gene. Note the similarity to immunoglobulin genes.

can contain more than one D segment, increasing the potential for diversity. However, somatic mutation does not occur for the TCR gene.

The **CD3 complex** is found on all T cells and consists of the γ, ϵ_2, δ, and ζ_2 polypeptide chains. The CD3 complex is the **signal transduction unit** for the TCR. **Tyrosine protein kinases** associate with the CD3 complex when antigen is bound to the TCR complex, promoting a cascade of protein phosphorylations and other events that lead to activation of the T cell and production of IL-2 and IL-2R.

The **CD4 and CD8 proteins** are coreceptors for the TCR, because they facilitate the interaction of the TCR with the antigen-presenting MHC molecule and can enhance the activation response. The **CD4** molecule is present on and identifies the helper or delayed-type hypersensitivity (DTH) T cells. CD4 binds to class II MHC molecules on the surface of APCs. **CD8** is present on and identifies the cytotoxic (CTL) and suppressor T cells. CD8 binds to class I MHC molecules on the surface of the target cell. Class I MHC molecules are expressed on all nucleated cells (see later section). The cytoplasmic tails of CD4 and CD8 associate with a protein tyrosine kinase (p56[lck]), which enhances the TCR-induced activation of the cell upon binding to the APC or target cell. CD4 or CD8 is found on α/β T cells but not on γ/δ T cells.

Accessory molecules expressed on the T cell include several protein receptors on the cell surface that interact with proteins on APCs and target cells, leading to activation of the T cell, promoting tighter interactions between the cells, or facilitating the killing of the target cell. These accessory molecules are as follows:

1. **CD45RA (native T cells)** or **CD45RO (memory T cells)**, a transmembrane protein tyrosine phosphatase.
2. **CD28** or cytotoxic T lymphocyte associated protein–4 (**CTLA-4**) (on activated T cells), which binds to the B7 protein on APCs to deliver a costimulation or inhibitory signal to the T cell.

3. **CD5**, which is present on all T cells and promotes activation on binding to its ligand on B cells.
4. **FasL**, which initiates apoptosis in a target cell that expresses Fas on its cell surface.

Adhesion molecules tighten the interaction of the T cell with the APC or target cell and may also promote activation. Adhesion molecules include **LFA-1**, which interacts with the **intercellular adhesion molecules (ICAM-1, ICAM-2, and ICAM-3)** on the target cell. **CD2** was originally identified by its ability to bind to sheep red blood cells (**erythrocyte receptor**). CD2 binds to LFA-3 on the target cell and promotes cell-to-cell adhesion and T-cell activation. **Very late antigens (VLA-4 and VLA-5)** are expressed on activated cells later in the response and bind to fibronectin on target cells to enhance the interaction.

T cells express receptors for many cytokines that activate and regulate T-cell function. The **cytokine receptors** activate protein kinase cascades upon binding of cytokine to deliver their signal to the nucleus. *IL-1 and IL-2 receptors are activation receptors.* **IL-2R** is composed of three subunits. β/γ subunits are on most T cells (also NK cells) and have intermediate affinity for IL-2. The α subunit (CD25) is synthesized in response to cell activation (a marker of activation), forming high-affinity $\alpha/\beta/\gamma$ IL-2R. Binding of IL-2 to the IL-2R initiates a growth-stimulating signal to the T cell, which also promotes the production of more IL-2 and IL-2R. Other cytokine receptors regulate the growth and cytokine expression of the T cell.

Antigen Presentation to T Cells

Unlike cell surface immunoglobulin on the B cell, which senses ("tastes" or "sniffs") the presence of soluble foreign molecules floating past the cell, the TCR on the T cell must be presented with the relevant epitope, which is cleaved from the protein and cradled in a molecular holder on the surface of APCs for the T cell to "touch" and respond to. **Class I** and **II MHC** molecules provide the molecular cradle for the peptide. The **CD8** molecule on cytolytic/suppressor T cells binds to and promotes the interaction with class I MHC molecules on target cells. This allows the T cells to sense the presence of self-antigenic and non–self-antigenic peptides. The **CD4** molecule on helper/DTH T cells binds to and promotes interactions with class II MHC molecules on APCs.

Class I MHC molecules are found on all nucleated cells and are the major determinant of "self." The class I MHC molecule, also known as **HLA** for human and H-2 for mouse, consists of two chains, a **variable heavy chain** and a **light chain (β_2-microglobulin)** (Fig. 13–5). Differences in the heavy chain of the HLA molecule among individuals (*allotypic differences*)

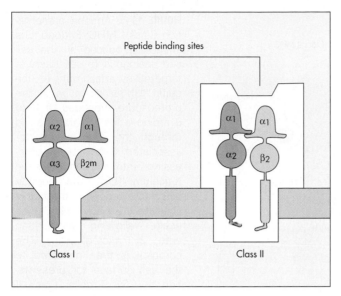

FIGURE 13–5. Structure of class I and class II MHC molecules. The class I MHC molecules consist of two subunits, the heavy chain and β_2-microglobulin. Class II MHC molecules consist of two subunits, α and β.

elicit the T-cell response that prevents graft (tissue) transplantation. There are three major HLA genes and proteins: HLA-A, HLA-B, and HLA-C (Fig. 13–6). Each cell expresses a pair of different **HLA-A, HLA-B**, and **HLA-C** genes, one from each parent. *The class I MHC molecule binds an antigenic peptide of eight or nine amino acids in a cleft formed by the heavy chain.* The class I MHC molecule presents antigenic peptides from within the cell (**endogenous)** to CD8-expressing T cells. Upregulation of class I MHC molecules makes the cell a better target for T cell action. Some cells (brain) and some virus infections (cytomegalovirus) downregulate the expression of MHC I antigens to reduce their potential as targets for T cells.

Class II MHC molecules are found almost exclusively on APCs, cells that interact with CD4 T cells (e.g., macrophages, dendritic cells, B cells). The class II MHC molecule (once known as **HLA-D**) is encoded by the **DP, DQ**, and **DR** loci. The class II MHC molecule is a dimer of α **and** β **subunits** (see Fig. 13–5). The class II MHC molecule binds an antigenic peptide of 11 or more amino acids in a cleft formed by the α and β subunits. The class II MHC molecule presents ingested (**exogenous**) antigenic peptides to CD4-expressing T cells.

Peptide Presentation by Class I and Class II MHC Molecules

Unlike antibodies that can recognize conformational epitopes, T-cell antigenic peptides must be linear epitopes. A T-cell antigen must be a peptide of 8 to 11

amino acids that is able to bind to the molecular cleft of the class I or class II MHC molecule and still expose a T-cell epitope to the TCR. Because of these constraints, a protein may have only one T-cell antigenic peptide. The routes of proteolysis producing the antigenic peptide differ for cells expressing peptides from cellular proteins ("self" and "non-self") (**endogenous route of antigen presentation**) to CD8 T cells in contrast to APCs, which present foreign antigens to CD4 T cells (**exogenous route of antigen presentation**) (Fig. 13–7).

Class I MHC molecules bind and present peptides from **endogenous** proteins (proteins synthesized within a cell). Class I MHC molecules present peptides, which are degraded from cellular proteins (trash) by the **proteosome** (a protease machine) and then shuttled into the endoplasmic reticulum (ER) through the **TAP** (transporter associated with antigen processing). These peptides are often from nuclear proteins and glycoproteins or have been marked by attachment of the **ubiquitin** protein. An antigenic peptide, which binds to the heavy chain of the class I MHC molecule as the molecule is being assembled, is required for the class I MHC molecule to assemble properly with β_2-microglobulin, exit the ER, and proceed to the cell membrane. The peptide binding cleft of the class I MHC molecule is closed-ended, like a pita pocket bread, and holds a peptide of 8 to 9 amino acids. During a **viral infection**, large quantities of viral proteins are produced and degraded into peptides, which occupy many of the class I MHC molecules to be presented to CD8 T cells. **Transplanted cells** (**grafts**) express peptides on their MHC molecules that differ from those in the host and therefore may be recog-

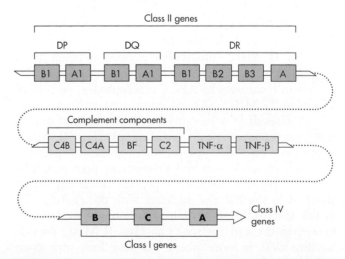

FIGURE 13–6. Genetic map of the major histocompatability complex (MHC). Genes for class I and class II molecules as well as complement components and tumor necrosis factor (TNF) are within the MHC gene complex.

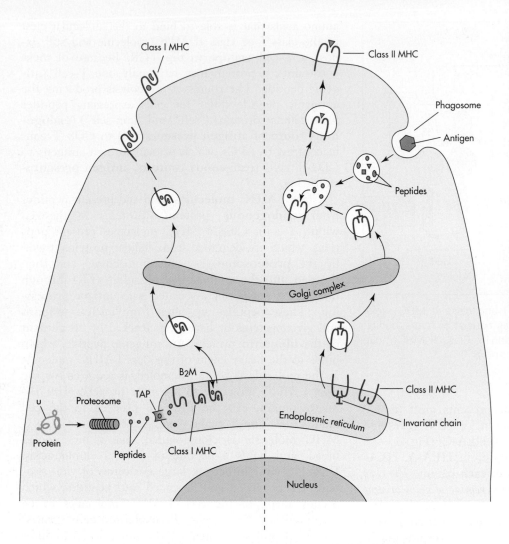

FIGURE 13–7. Antigen presentation Class I MHC: Endogenous antigen (produced by the cell and analogous to cell trash) is targeted by attachment of ubiquitin (U) for digestion in the proteosome. Peptides of 8 to 9 amino acids are transported through the TAP (transporter associated with antigen processing) into the endoplasmic reticulum (ER). The peptide binds to a groove in the heavy chain of the class I MHC molecule, allowing association with β_2 microglobulin. The complex is then delivered to the cell surface for presentation to CD8 T cells. Class II MHC: Class II MHC molecules assemble in the ER. Upon acquisition of the invariant chain, they are transported in a vesicle. Exogenous antigen (phagocytosed) is degraded in lysosomes, which then fuse with a vesicle containing the class II MHC molecules. The invariant chain is degraded, and peptides of 11 to 13 amino acids bind to the class II MHC molecule. The complex is then delivered to the cell surface for presentation to CD4 T cells.

nized as foreign. **Tumor cells** often express peptides derived from abnormal or embryonic proteins, which may elicit responses in the host because the host was not tolerized to these proteins.

Class II MHC molecules present peptides from exogenous proteins that were phagocytosed and degraded in lysosomes by APCs, macrophages, or B cells. The class II MHC protein acquires its antigenic peptide as a result of a merging of the vesicular transport pathway (carrying newly synthesized class II MHC molecules) and the lysosomal degradation pathway (carrying phagocytosed and proteolysed proteins). The antigenic peptides displace a peptide (invariant chain) attached in the ER and associate with the cleft formed in the class II MHC protein; the complex is then delivered to the cell surface. The class II MHC peptide binding cleft is more like a hot dog bun with open ends and holds a peptide of 11 to 12 amino acids.

The following analogy might aid the understanding of this process: All cells degrade their protein "trash" and then display it on the cell surface on class I MHC

trash cans. CD8 T cells "policing" the neighborhood are not alarmed by the normal, everyday peptide trash. A viral intruder would produce large amounts of viral peptide trash (e.g., beer cans, pizza boxes) displayed on class I MHC molecular garbage cans, which would alert the policing CD8 T cells. APCs (dendritic cells, macrophages, and B cells) are similar to garbage collectors; they gobble up the neighborhood trash, degrade it, display it on class II MHC molecules, and then move to a lymph node to present the antigenic peptides to the CD4 T cells in the "police station." Foreign antigens would alert the CD4 T cells to release cytokines and activate an immune response.

Activation of CD4 T Cells and Their Response to Antigen

CD4 helper T cells are activated by the interaction of the TCR with antigenic peptide in the context of class II MHC molecules (Fig. 13–8). The interaction is strengthened by the binding of CD4 to the class II

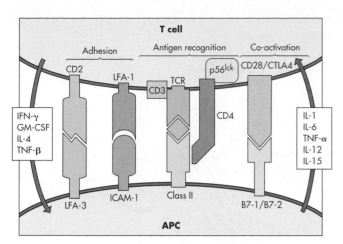

FIGURE 13–8. The molecules involved in the interaction between T cells and antigen-presenting cells (APCs). The various cytokines and their direction of action are also shown. GM-CSF = granulocyte-macrophage colony-stimulating factor; ICAM-1 = intercellular adhesion molecule 1, IFN-γ = interferon-γ; TNF = tumor necrosis factor. (From Roitt I et al: *Immunology*, ed 4, St Louis, 1996, Mosby.)

MHC molecule and the linkage of adhesion proteins on the T cell and the APC. The signal is transmitted to the nucleus through the CD3 complex through activation of phospholipase C and protein kinase C, release of intracellular calcium, and the activation of specific protein kinase cascades. Several tyrosine protein kinase cascades are also activated by the CD3 complex. The result is the activation of specific transcription factors in the nucleus.

A **costimulatory signal** is required, however, to induce growth of the T cell as a fail-safe mechanism to ensure legitimate activation. Costimulatory signals are generated by the interaction of CD28 on the T cell, with the B7-1 and B7-2 molecules on the macrophage, dendritic, or B cell APC, or by cytokines binding to their receptors. Resting T cells require cytokine signals (e.g., IL-1, IL-2) to initiate growth of the cell. Proper activation of the helper T cell promotes production of IL-2 to activate other T cells and increases expression of IL-2Rs on the cell surface, enhancing the cell's own ability to bind and maintain activation by IL-2. Once activated, the IL-2 sustains the growth of the cell, and other cytokines influence whether the helper T cell matures into a TH1 or TH2 helper cell (see following section).

Partial activation (T-cell receptor interaction with MHC peptide) without appropriate cytokine or CD28-B7 costimulation leads to **anergy** (unresponsiveness) or apoptotic death (cell suicide) of the T cell. This is a mechanism for (1) eliminating self-reactive immature and other T cells in the developing thymus and (2) promoting the development of **tolerance** to self pro-

teins. In addition, binding of the CTLA-4 costimulator molecule on T cells with B7 on target or APC cells can result in anergy toward the antigen.

TH1 and TH2 Cells

The CD4 T cells are divided into TH0, TH1, TH2, and TH3 classes, depending on the cytokines that they secrete and, thus, the responses that they induce (Fig. 13–9 and Table 13–1). Understanding the TH0, TH1, TH2 division of cytokine production is the basis for understanding the generation of immune responses. TH0 cells produce IL-2, IFN-γ, and IL-4. TH0 cells mature into either TH1 or TH2 cells, depending on the antigen, concentration of antigen, APC, and cytokine stimulation. Once activated, the TH1 and TH2 cells produce cytokines that stimulate their own growth (autocrine) but inhibit the growth of the other type of CD4 T cell.

TH1 cells are activated by IL-12 and IL-15 and antigen presentation, which are from macrophages and dendritic cells. TH1 cells are characterized by secretion of **IL-2, IFN-γ,** and **TNF-β (lymphotoxin)**. These cytokines stimulate inflammatory responses and the production of IgM and specific subclasses of IgG that can fix complement. **IFN-γ**, also known as **macrophage activation factor**, reinforces TH1 responses by promoting more IL-12 production. TH1 cells are inhibited by IL-10, which is produced by TH2 cells.

TABLE 13–1. Cytokines Produced by TH0, TH1, and TH2 Cells*

Cytokine	TH0	TH1	TH2
IFN-γ	+	+ +	−
IL-2	+	+ +	−
TNF-β (LT)	+	+ +	−
Chemokines	+	+	−
GM-CSF	+	+ +	+
TNF-α	+	+ +	+
IL-3	+	+ +	+ +
IL-4	+	−	+ +
IL-5	+	−	+ +
IL-6	+	−	+ +
IL-10	+	−	+ +

*The relative ability of TH0, TH1, and TH2 cells to produce different cytokines after activation. The cytokines that differentiate TH1 and TH2 cells are boxed.

GM-CSF = granulocyte-macrophage colony-stimulating factor; IFN = interferon; IL = interleukin; LT = lymphotoxin; TNF = tumor necrosis factor; + = minor product; + + = major product; − = no product.

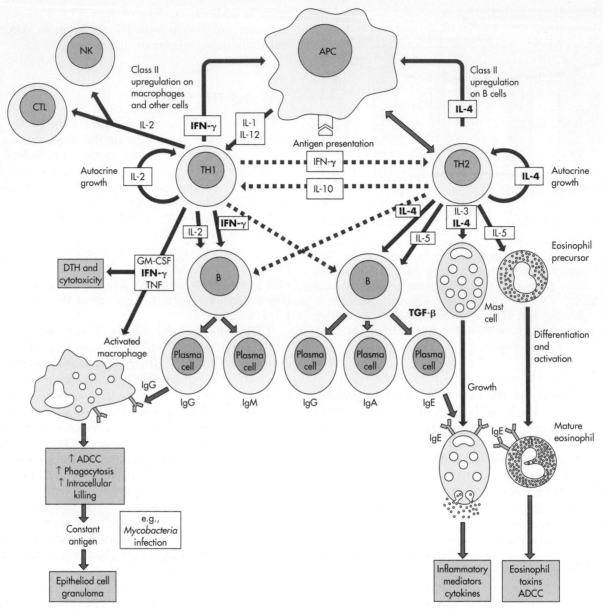

FIGURE 13–9. Cytokines produced by TH1 and TH2 cells and their effects on the immune system. TH1 responses are initiated by IL-12 and interferon-γ and TH2 responses by IL-4. TH1 cells promote inflammation and the production of complement and macrophage-binding antibody (*solid blue lines*) and inhibit TH2 responses (*dotted blue lines*). TH2 cells promote humoral response (*solid red lines*) and inhibit TH1 responses (*dotted red lines*). ADCC = antibody-dependent cellular cytotoxicity; APC = antigen-presenting cell; CTL = cytotoxic T cell; DTH = delayed-type hypersensitivity; GM-CSF = granulocyte-macrophage colony-stimulating factor; TNF = tumor necrosis factor. Colored square denotes end result.

Activated TH1 cells also express the **FasL,** which can interact with **Fas on target cells** to promote apoptosis (killing) of the target cell.

The **TH1 response** (**1 meaning first**) *usually occurs first and is a local response.* It often occurs early in an infection. The TH1 responses amplify local inflammatory reactions and DTH reactions by activating macrophages, NK, and CD8 cytotoxic T cells and also ex-

pand the immune response by stimulating growth of B and T cells with IL-2. The inflammatory responses and complement-binding antibody stimulated by TH1 responses are important for eliminating intracellular infections (e.g., viruses, bacteria, and parasites) and fungi but are also associated with autoimmune inflammatory diseases (e.g., multiple sclerosis, Crohn's disease, rheumatoid arthritis).

TH2 cells are activated by B-cell, dendritic cell, or macrophage presentation of antigen in the lymph nodes, usually later in an immune response. TH2 cells release IL-4, IL-5, IL-6, and IL-10, cytokines that promote humoral (systemic) responses by stimulating B-cell differentiation, resulting in immunoglobulin class switching and memory B cell and plasma cell production. TH2 cells are stimulated by IL-4 and inhibited by IFN-γ. The **TH2 response (2 meaning second)** *results later and acts systemically.* The TH2 response may be stimulated later in an infection, when antigen reaches the B cells in lymph nodes, and the B cells expressing specific cell surface antibody can capture, process, and present it. B-cell presentation of antigen to TH2 cells initiates an activation circuit, stimulating the growth of and clonally expanding the helper T cells and B cells, which are specific for the same antigen. The TH2 response results in maturation of the immune response to the antigen as well as production of IgG, IgE, IgA, and memory B cells for future protection. Stimulation of TH2 responses against intracellular infections can exacerbate these infectious diseases by prematurely shutting off the TH1 responses but can modulate inflammatory and autoimmune diseases.

Some cytokines are secreted by both TH1 and TH2 cells. Examples are IL-3, TNF-α, GM-CSF, and chemokines.

TH3 cells are characterized by their production of IL-5 and TGF-β, which are important for promoting B-cell differentiation to produce IgA. TGF-β inhibits TH1 and TH2 cell action to promote tolerance.

CD8 T Cells

CD8 T cells include **CTLs** and **suppressor cells**. CTLs are part of the TH1 response and are important for eliminating virally infected cells and tumor cells. CD8 T cells can also secrete TH1-like cytokines. Less is known about suppressor cells.

The CTL response is initiated when CTL precursors are stimulated by binding of the TCR and CD8 to the antigenic peptide on class I MHC molecules and a costimulatory signal from IL-2 or a CD28-B7 interaction with dendritic cells or macrophages (Fig. 13–10). The activated CD8 T cells divide and differentiate into mature CTLs. During a viral challenge of mice, specific CTL numbers are observed to increase up to 100,000 times. When the activated CTL finds a target cell, it binds tightly through interactions of the TCR with antigen-bearing class I MHC proteins and adhesion molecules on both cells (similar to the closing of a zipper). **Granules** containing toxic molecules, **granzymes (esterases)**, and a pore-forming protein (perforin) move to the site of interaction and release their contents into the pocket formed between the T cell and target cell. **Perforin** generates holes in the target cell membrane to allow the granule contents to enter

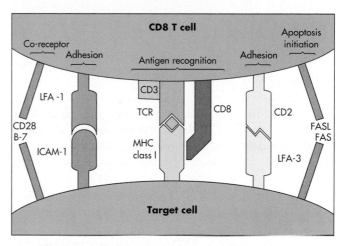

FIGURE 13–10. Interactions between CD8 cytotoxic T lymphocyte (Tc cell) and target cells. The Fas-FasL interaction promotes apoptosis. ICAM-1 = intercellular adhesion molecule 1. (From Roitt I et al: *Immunology*, ed 4, St Louis, 1996, Mosby.)

and induce **apoptosis (programmed cell death)** in the target cell. T cells can also initiate apoptosis in target cells through the interaction of the **FasL on the T cell with the Fas protein on the target cell surface.** FasL is a member of the TNF family of proteins and Fas is a member of the TNF receptor family of proteins. Apoptosis is characterized by degradation of the target cell DNA into discrete fragments of multiples of approximately 200 base pairs and disruption of internal membranes. The cells shrink into apoptotic bodies, which are readily phagocytosed by macrophages and dendritic cells. Apoptosis is a clean method of cell death, unlike necrosis, which signals neutrophil action and further tissue damage. TH1 CD4 T cells also express FasL and can initiate apoptosis in target cells.

Suppressor T cells provide antigen-specific regulation of helper T cell function through inhibitory cytokines and other means. Like CTLs, suppressor T cells interact with class I MHC (class I MHC restricted).

QUESTIONS

1. The importance of specific molecules can be determined through development of genetically deficient strains of mice (knockout mice) and then testing the immune systems of these mice. Describe the immune functions that should be missing and the cell types that should be affected for the mice deficient in the following molecules:

    a. Class I MHC.
    b. Class II MHC.

   c. TCR γ/δ.
   d. IL-2 receptor.
   e. CD4.
   f. B7-1 and B7-2.
   g. IFN-γ.
   h. IL-1.

2. The division of helper T cell responses into TH1, TH2 and TH3 subsets provides one of the most useful approaches to understanding immune responses to challenge. What would be the consequence of each of the following?

   a. Initiation of TH2 response to an intracellular infection (e.g., *Mycobacterium leprae*) before a TH1 response.

   b. Uncontrolled TH1 response to a vaginal yeast infection (e.g., *Candida albicans*).

   c. Insufficient TH1 response to viral infection of neonate due to low levels of IFN-γ (e.g., herpes simplex virus).

   d. Immunization with a mixture of IL- 2, GM-CSF, and IFN-γ and human immunodeficiency virus glycoprotein 120 antigen rather than the antigen alone.

BIBLIOGRAPHY

Abbas AK et al: *Cellular and molecular immunology*, ed 4, Philadelphia, 2000, WB Saunders.

Goldsby RA et al: *Kuby immunology*, ed 4, New York, 2000, WH Freeman.

Immunology Today: Issues contain understandable reviews on current topics in immunology.

Janeway CA et al: *Immunobiology: the immune system in health and disease*, ed 4, New York, 1999, Current Biology Publications and Garland Press.

Male D et al: *Advanced immunology*, ed 3, St Louis, 1996, Mosby.

Roitt I et al: *Immunology*, ed 5, St Louis, 1997, Mosby.

Sompayrac L: *How the immune system works*, Malden, Mass, 1999, Blackwell Scientific.

CHAPTER 14

Immune Responses to Infectious Agents

The previous chapters in this section introduced the different components of host protection. This chapter describes how the different components interact to produce a protective response and the immunopathogenic consequences that may arise as a result of the response. The importance of any one of these protective responses becomes obvious when it is genetically deficient or is blocked by chemotherapy, disease, or infection (e.g., acquired immunodeficiency syndrome [AIDS]).

We have three basic lines of protection against invasion by infectious agents; they are:

1. **Natural barriers,** which restrict entry of the agent (e.g., skin, mucus, ciliated epithelium, gastric acid, bile).
2. **Innate, antigen-nonspecific immune defenses**, which provide rapid, local responses to challenge by an invader (e.g., fever, interferon, complement, neutrophils, macrophages, natural killer [NK] cells).
3. **Antigen-specific immune responses**, which specifically target, attack, and eliminate the invaders that succeed in passing the first two defenses (e.g., antibody, T cells).

The importance of each of the mechanisms for combating an infection differs for infectious agents (Table 14–1). Phagocytic cells, the alternative pathway of complement and antibody, are most important for resolving bacterial infections, except for intracellular bacteria. Intracellular bacteria (i.e., mycobacteria) are inaccessible to antibody and therefore require TH1, delayed-type hypersensitivity (DTH) responses involving T cells and macrophages. Interferon, NK, and T-cell responses are most important for viral infections. Antibody also plays a role in antiviral immunity, especially in restricting the spread of virus by viremia. TH1-DTH responses are especially important for antifungal protection. Activated macrophage, T-cell, eosinophil, and immunoglobulin (Ig) E–mast cell responses are important for protection against parasitic infections.

The protections initiated by TH1-type immune responses (interferon-γ, cytolytic and inflammatory responses) are especially important for resolving infections by intracellular bacteria, viruses, fungi, and parasites. TH2 responses (humoral) are most important for resolving bacterial and parasitic infections and for the establishment of future antibody responses (mem-

TABLE 14–1. Antimicrobial Defenses for Infectious Agents

	Bacteria	Intracellular Bacteria	Viruses	Fungi	Parasites
Neutrophils	+ +	−	−	−	−
Macrophages	+	+ +	+	+	−
Complement	+	−	−	−	−
NK cells	−	−	+	−	−
CD4 TH1—DTH	−*	+ +	+ +	−	−
CD8—CTL	−	−	+ +	−	−
Antibody	+ +	+	+	+	+ + (IgE)†

* DTH (delayed-type hypersensitivity) is important for intracellular infections.
† Immunoglubulin E and mast cells are especially important for worm infections.
CTL = cytotoxic T lymphocytes; NK = natural killer.

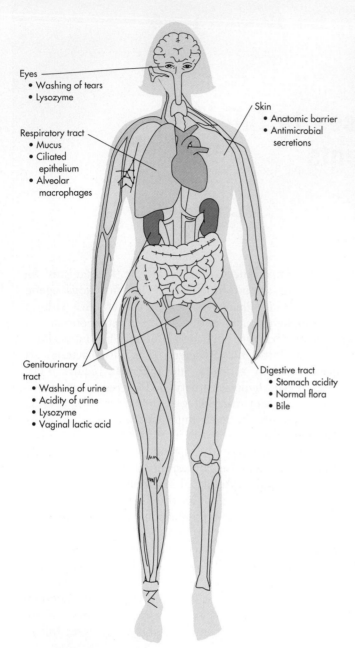

Eyes
• Washing of tears
• Lysozyme

Respiratory tract
• Mucus
• Ciliated
  epithelium
• Alveolar
  macrophages

Skin
• Anatomic barrier
• Antimicrobial
  secretions

Genitourinary
tract
• Washing of urine
• Acidity of urine
• Lysozyme
• Vaginal lactic acid

Digestive tract
• Stomach acidity
• Normal flora
• Bile

FIGURE 14–1. Barrier defenses of the human body.

ory) and production of secretory IgA for the protection of mucosal surfaces.

Barriers to Infection

The **skin** and **mucous membranes** serve as barriers to most infectious agents (Fig. 14–1 and Table 14–2), with few exceptions (e.g., papillomavirus, dermatophytes ["skin-loving" fungi]). Free fatty acids produced in sebaceous glands and by organisms on the skin surface, lactic acid in perspiration, and the low pH and relatively dry environment of the skin all form unfavorable conditions for the survival of most organisms.

The mucosal epithelium covering the orifices of the body is protected by mucus secretions and cilia. For example, pulmonary airways are coated with mucus, which is continuously transported toward the mouth by ciliated epithelial cells. Large airborne particles get caught in the mucus, whereas small particles (0.05 to 3 microns (μm), the size of viruses or bacteria) that reach the alveoli are phagocytosed by macrophages and transported out of the airspaces. Cigarette smoke or other pollutants as well as some bacteria and viruses (e.g., *Bordetella pertussis*, influenza virus), can interfere with this clearance mechanism by damaging the ciliated epithelial cells, thus rendering the patient susceptible to secondary bacterial pneumonia. Antimicrobial substances (lysozyme, lactoferrin, and secretory IgA) found in secretions at mucosal surfaces (e.g., tears, mucus, saliva) also provide protection. Lysozyme induces lysis of bacteria by cleaving the polysaccharide backbone of the peptidoglycan of gram-positive bacteria. Lactoferrin, an iron-binding protein, deprives microbes of the free iron they need for growth.

The **acidic environment** of the stomach, bladder, and kidneys and the **bile** of the intestines inactivate many viruses and bacteria. **Urinary flow** also limits the establishment of infection.

Body temperature and especially **fever** limit or prevent the growth of many microbes. In addition, the immune response is more efficient at elevated temperatures.

Antibacterial Responses

Figure 14–2 illustrates the progression of protective responses to a bacterial challenge. Protection is initiated on activation of innate responses on a local basis and progresses to acute-phase and antigen-specific responses on a systemic scale. A summary of antibacterial responses is presented in Box 14–1.

Acute inflammation is an early defense mechanism to contain an infection, prevent its spread from the initial focus, and signal subsequent specific immune responses. Inflammatory responses are beneficial but can also cause tissue damage and, as a result, contribute to the symptoms of disease. The three major events in acute inflammation are (1) expansion of capillaries to increase blood flow (seen as blushing or a rash), (2) increase in permeability of the microvasculature structure to allow escape of fluid, plasma proteins, and leukocytes from the circulation (source of edema), and (3) exit of leukocytes from the capillaries and their accumulation at the site of injury.

Activation of Response

Bacterial components are excellent activators of the innate antigen-nonspecific protective responses (Box

TABLE 14–2. Nonspecific Humoral Defense Mechanisms

Factor	Function	Source
Lysozyme	Catalyzes hydrolysis of bacterial peptidoglycan	Tears, saliva, nasal secretions, body fluids, lysosomal granules
Lactoferrin, transferrin	Bind iron and compete with microorganisms for it	Specific granules of PMNs
Lactoperoxidase	May be inhibitory to many microorganisms	Milk and saliva
β-lysin	Is effective mainly against gram-positive bacteria	Thrombocytes, normal serum
Chemotactic factors	Induce directed migration of PMNs, monocytes, and other cells	Bacterial substances, products of cell injury, denatured proteins, complement, and chemokines
Properdin	Activates complement in the absence of antibody-antigen complex	Normal plasma
Defensins	Block cell-transport activities	Polymorphonuclear granules

PMNs = Polymorphonuclear leukocytes (neutrophils).

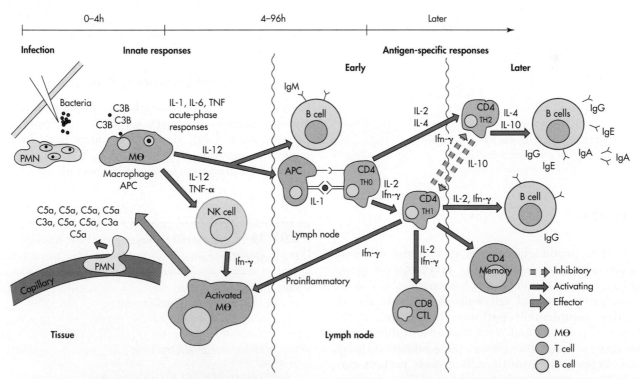

FIGURE 14–2. Antibacterial responses. First, innate antigen-nonspecific responses attract and promote polymorphonuclear neutrophil (PMN) and macrophage (Mθ) responses. Antigen-presenting cells (APCs) and antigen reach the lymph node to activate early immune responses (TH1 and immunoglobulin [Ig] M). Later, TH2 systemic antibody responses and memory cells are developed. CTL = cytotoxic T lymphocyte; Ifn = interferon; IL = interleukin, TNF = tumor necrosis factor.

BOX 14–1. **Summary of Antibacterial Responses**

Complement

Alternative and Lectin pathways activated by bacterial surfaces.
    Classic pathway activated later by antibody-antigen complexes.
    Production of chemotactic and anaphylotoxic proteins (C3a, C5a).
    Opsonization of bacteria (C3b).
    Promotion of killing of gram-negative bacteria.
    Activation of B cells (C3d).

Neutrophils

Important antibacterial phagocytic cell.
    Killing by oxygen-dependent and oxygen-independent mechanisms.

Macrophages

Important antibacterial phagocytic cell.
    Killing by oxygen-dependent and oxygen-independent mechanisms.
    Production of IL-1, IL-6, and IL-12; TNF-α and TNF-β, and interferon-α.
    Activation of acute-phase and inflammatory responses.
    Presentation of antigen to CD4 T cell.

T Cells

TH1 CD4 responses important for intracellular bacterial infections.
    TH2 CD4 response important for all bacterial infections.
    CD8 cytolytic T cells not very important.

Antibody

Binding to surface structures of bacteria (fimbriae, lipoteichoic acid, capsule).
    Blocking of attachment.
    Opsonization of bacteria for phagocytosis.
    Promotion of complement action.
    Promotion of clearance of bacteria.
    Neutralization of toxins and toxic enzymes.

native pathway or via the mannose-binding protein (see Chapter 12) is a very early and important antibacterial defense. Complement activates inflammatory responses and can also directly kill gram-negative bacteria and, to a much lesser extent, gram-positive bacteria (the thick peptidoglycan of gram-positive bacteria shields them from lysis). Activation of the complement cascade by gram-positive or gram-negative bacteria provides the following protective factors:

1. Chemotactic factors (**C5a**) to attract neutrophils and macrophages to the site of infection.
2. **Anaphylotoxins** (**C3a** and **C5a**) to stimulate mast cell release of histamine and thereby increase vascular permeability, allowing access to the infection site.
3. **Opsonins** (**C3b**), which bind to bacteria and promote their phagocytosis.
4. A **B-cell activator** (**C3d**).

Antibody (**IgM or IgG**), which is present later in an infection, enhances the complement response through activation of the **classic complement cascade**.

Kinins and clotting factors induced by tissue damage are also involved in inflammation (e.g., factor XII [Hageman factor], bradykinin, fibrinopeptides). These factors increase vascular permeability and are chemotactic for leukocytes. Products of arachidonic acid metabolism also affect inflammation. These products include prostaglandins and leukotrienes, which can mediate essentially every aspect of acute inflammation.

Chemotaxis and Leukocyte Migration

Chemotactic factors produced in response to infection and inflammatory responses, such as complement components (C3a, C5a), bacterial products (e.g., formyl-methionyl-leucyl-phenylalanine [f-met-leu-phe), and chemokines, are powerful chemoattractants for neutro-

14–2). The peptidoglycan layer in bacterial cell walls (teichoic acid and peptidoglycan fragments of gram-positive bacteria) and lipopolysaccharide (LPS) in gram-negative bacterial cell walls can activate the **alternative complement pathway** (**properdin**) in the absence of antibody and, with **mannose-binding protein,** can activate the classic complement pathway. Macrophages and dendritic cells express **pattern-recognition receptors,** including the Toll-like receptors, which recognize these bacterial structures and activate protective responses. **LPS (endotoxin)** is a very strong activator of macrophages, B cells, and selected other cells (e.g., endothelial cells).

Activation of the **complement system** by the alter-

BOX 14–2. **Bacterial Components That Activate Protective Responses**

Direct activation:
    Lipopolysaccharide (endotoxin)
    Lipoteichoic acid
    Lipoarabinomannan
    Glycolipids and glycopeptides
    Polyanions
    N-Formyl peptides (formyl-methionyl-leucyl-phenylalanine)
Chemotactic:
    Peptidoglycan fragments
    Cell surface activation of alternative pathways of complement (C3a, C5a)

FIGURE 14–3. Neutrophil diapedesis in response to inflammatory signals. Tumor necrosis factor-α (TNF-α) and chemokines activate the expression of selectins and intercellular P⁻ and E⁻ adhesion molecules (ICAM-1) on the endothelium, near the inflammation, and their ligands integrins, L-selectin and LFA-1 (leukocyte function-associated antigen) on the neutrophil. The neutrophil binds progressively tighter to the endothelium until it finds its way through the endothelium.

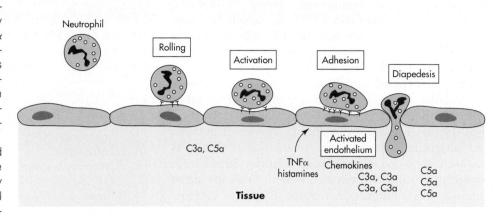

phils, macrophages, and, later in the response, lymphocytes. **Chemokines** are sticky proteins that establish a chemically lighted "runway" to guide these cells to the site of an infection and also activate them. The chemokines and tumor necrosis factor-α (TNF-α) cause the endothelial cells lining the capillaries near the inflammation and the leukocytes passing by to express complementary adhesion molecules (molecular "Velcro"). The leukocytes slow, roll, attach to the lining, and then extravasate across (pass through) (**diapedesis**) the capillary wall to the site of inflammation (Fig. 14–3).

Phagocytes and Phagocytosis

Polymorphonuclear neutrophils (PMNs), monocytes, and occasionally eosinophils are the first cells to appear in response to acute inflammation; they are followed later by macrophages.

Neutrophils are PMNs that provide a major antibacterial response. They are attracted to the site of infection, where they phagocytose and then kill the internalized bacteria. An increased number of neutrophils in the blood, body fluids (e.g., cerebrospinal fluid), or tissue indicates a bacterial infection. The mobilization of neutrophils is accompanied by a "left shift," an increase in the number of immature **band forms** released from the bone marrow (*left* refers to the beginning of a chart of neutrophil development).

Phagocytosis of bacteria by macrophages and neutrophils involves the steps attachment, internalization, and digestion. **Attachment of the bacteria** to the macrophage is mediated by receptors for bacterial carbohydrates (lectins [specific sugar-binding proteins]), **receptors for opsonins** (e.g., complement [C3b], mannose-binding protein receptors), fibronectin receptors (especially for *Staphylococcus aureus*), and Fc receptors for antibody. After attachment, the particle is surrounded by a portion of plasma membrane, which

forms a **phagocytic vacuole** around the microbe. This vacuole fuses with the **primary lysosomes** (macrophages) or **granules** (PMNs) to allow inactivation and digestion of the vacuole contents. Phagocytic killing may be oxygen-dependent or oxygen-independent, depending on the antimicrobial chemicals produced by the granules (Fig. 14–4). Activation of macrophages is promoted by interferon-γ (IFN-γ) (best), granulocyte-

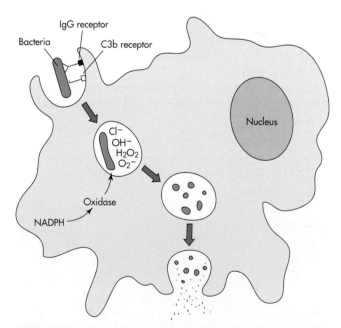

FIGURE 14–4. Phagocytosis and killing of bacteria. Bacteria are bound directly or are opsonized by mannose-binding protein, immunoglobulin G (IgG) and/or C3b receptors promoting their adherence and uptake by phagocytes. Within the phagosome, oxygen-dependent and oxygen-independent mechanisms kill and degrade the bacteria. NADPH = reduced form of nicotinamide-adenine dinucleotide phosphate.

macrophage colony-stimulating factor (GM-CSF), TNF-α, and lymphotoxin (TNF-β), which are produced earlier in the infection by NK cells or later by CD4 T cells. Activation of macrophages is required for macrophages to kill internalized microbes.

Oxygen-dependent killing is activated by a powerful oxidative burst that culminates in the formation of hydrogen peroxide and other antimicrobial substances (Box 14–3). The fusion of specific lysosomal granules and phagosomes permits the interaction of NADPH (reduced form of nicotinamide adenine dinucleotide phosphate) oxidase with cytochrome b. With the aid of quinone, this combination reduces oxygen to superoxide anion (O_2^-), which in the presence of a catalyst (e.g., superoxide dismutase) is converted to hydrogen peroxide. In the neutrophil, hydrogen peroxide with myeloperoxidase (released by primary granules during fusion to the phagolysosome) transforms chloride ions into hypochlorous ions that kill the microorganisms. **Nitric oxide** produced during this response has antimicrobial activity and is also a major second messenger molecule (like cyclic AMP), which enhances the inflammatory and other responses by activating guanylate cyclase.

The **neutrophil** can also mediate **oxygen-independent killing** upon fusion of the phagosome with azurophilic granules containing cationic proteins (e.g., cathepsin G) and specific granules containing lysozyme and lactoferrin. These proteins kill gram-negative bacteria by disrupting their cell membrane integrity, but they are far less effective against gram-positive bacteria, which are killed principally through the oxygen-dependent mechanism.

LPS and other bacterial cell wall components stimulate macrophages to release interleukins IL-1 and IL-6,

---

BOX 14–4. **Secreted Products of Macrophages with a Protective Effect on the Body**

Hematopoietic factors IL-6, IL-12, GM-CSF, G-CSF, M-CSF
Cytotoxic factors
   Oxygen metabolites:
     Hydrogen peroxide
     Superoxide anion
     Nitric oxide
   Hydrolytic enzymes:
     Collagenase
     Lipase
     Phosphatase
Endogenous pyrogen IL-1
Tumor necrosis factor (TNF)
Interferon-α
Complement components:
   C1 through C5
   Properdin
   Factors B, D, I, and H
Coagulation factors
Plasma proteins
Arachidonic acid metabolites:
   Prostaglandin
   Thromboxane
   Leukotrienes

CSF = colony-stimulating factor; G = granulocyte; IL = interleukin; M = macrophage.

TNF-α, and chemokines. These cytokines are **endogenous pyrogens** because they promote fever production and enhance the inflammatory response by further activating macrophages and promoting the acute-phase response. Unfortunately, the cytotoxins, cytokines, and other molecules (Box 14–4) that are released can also injure endothelium and tissue.

The **acute-phase response** is triggered by inflammation, tissue injury, IL-1, IL-6, TNF-α (produced by macrophages), prostaglandin E_1, and interferons associated with infection (Box 14–5). Acute-phase proteins that are produced and released into the serum include complement, coagulation proteins, LPS-binding proteins, transport proteins, protease inhibitors, and adherence proteins. **Fever** is triggered by IL-1, TNF-α, and interferons. IL-1 stimulation of the liver promotes production of **C-reactive protein.** C-reactive protein complexes with the polysaccharides of numerous bacteria and fungi and activates the alternate complement pathway, facilitating removal of these organisms from the body through greater phagocytosis. The acute-phase proteins reinforce the innate defenses against infection, but their excessive production during sepsis (induced by endotoxin) can cause serious problems, such as shock.

BOX 14–3. **Antibacterial Compounds of the Phagolysosome**

Oxygen-Dependent Compounds

Hydrogen peroxide: NADPH oxidase and NADH oxidase
Superoxide
Hydroxyl radicals (OH)
Activated halides (Cl$^-$, I$^-$, Br$^-$): myeloperoxidase
Nitrous oxide

Oxygen-Independent Compounds

Acids
Lysosome (degrades bacterial peptidoglycan)
Lactoferrin (chelates iron)
Defensins and other cationic proteins (damage membranes)
Proteases, elastase, cathepsin G

BOX 14–5. Acute-Phase Reactants

α_1-antitrypsin
α_1-glycoprotein
Amyloid A and P
Antithrombin III
C-reactive protein
C1 esterase inhibitor
C3 complement
Ceruloplasmin
Fibrinogen
Haptoglobin
Orosomucoid
Plasminogen
Transferrin
Lypopolysaccharide-binding proteins

Macrophages and cells of the macrophage lineage play many roles in addition to the phagocytosis of bacteria and antigen (Fig. 14–5), including a major role in the transition between the antigen-nonspecific and antigen-specific responses. The macrophages produce IL-12, which activates NK cells at the site of infection and initiates the TH1 response. The NK cells, and later the CD4 T cells, produce IFN-γ to

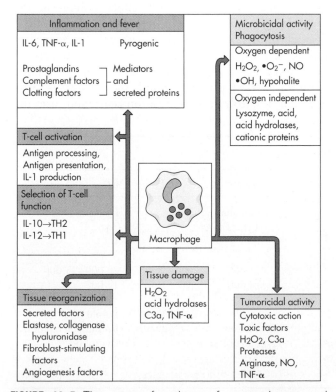

FIGURE 14–5. The many functions of macrophages and members of the macrophage family. IL = Interleukin; TNF = tumor necrosis factor. (From Roitt et al: *Immunology*, ed 4, St Louis, 1996, Mosby.)

further activate macrophages. Macrophages, and especially dendritic cells, deliver antigen to the lymph nodes for presentation to CD4 T cells and also stimulate the T cells with IL-1 in addition to IL-12.

Specific Immune Responses to Bacteria

Ingestion of bacteria or bacterial antigens mobilizes the macrophages and dendritic cells to move to the lymph nodes and interact with CD4 T cells (see Fig. 14–2). The initial interaction occurs with CD4 TH0 cells. Antigenic peptides (having more than 11 amino acids) produced from phagocytosed proteins (exogenous route) are bound to class II major histocompatibility complex (MHC) molecules and presented by these antigen-presenting cells (APCs) to the TH0 cells. The TH0 cells are activated by (1) a combination of antigenic peptide in the MHC II complex with the T-cell antigen receptor and CD4, (2) costimulatory signals provided by the interaction of CD28 molecules on the T cells with the B7 molecule on the macrophage, and (3) IL-1 and IL-12. The TH0 cells produce IL-2, IFN-γ, and IL-4. Simultaneously, B cells expressing surface IgM and IgD specific for the bacterial antigens are activated and produce IgM. Microbial cell wall polysaccharides, especially LPS, activate B cells and promote the specific IgM antibody responses. Swollen lymph nodes are an indication of lymphocyte activation in response to antigenic challenge.

The conversion of TH0 cells to TH1 cells is promoted by IL-12 and reinforced by IFN-γ. **TH1 CD4 T cells** (1) promote and reinforce inflammatory responses (e.g., IFN-γ activation of macrophage) as well as growth of T and B cells (IL-2) to expand the immune response and (2) promote B cells to produce complement-binding antibodies (IgM and, upon class switching, IgG). These responses are important for the early phases of an antibacterial defense. TH1 responses are also essential for combating intracellular infections with bacteria such as mycobacteria, which are protected from antibody. IFN-γ activates macrophage and other inflammatory processes (DTH) to kill the infected cell. Alternatively, the continuous stimulation induced by a chronic infection (e.g., tuberculosis) can promote fusion of macrophage to giant cells and epithelioid cells, forming a granuloma around the infection. CD8 T cells are not very important for antibacterial immunity.

CD4 TH2 T-cell responses occur later and are often initiated by the B-cell presentation of antigen. Binding of antigen to the cell surface antibody on B cells activates the B cells and also promotes uptake, and processing of the antigen, and presentation of antigenic peptides on class II MHC molecules to the CD4 TH2 cell. The TH2 cell produces IL-4, IL-5, IL-6, and IL-10, which enhance IgG production and, depending on other factors, production of IgE or IgA. The TH2 response also promotes terminal differentiation of B cells to plasma-cell antibody factories or production of memory B cells.

Antibodies are the primary protection against extracellular bacteria and reinfection. Antibody is important for promoting complement activation, opsonizing the bacteria for phagocytosis, blocking bacterial adhesion, and neutralizing (inactivating) exotoxins (e.g., tetanospasmin, botulinum toxin) and other cytotoxic proteins produced by bacteria (e.g., degradative enzymes). Vaccine immunization with inactivated exotoxins (toxoids) is the primary means of protection against the potentially lethal effects of exotoxins.

IgM antibodies are produced early in the antibacterial response. IgM bound to bacteria activates the classic complement cascade, promoting both the direct killing of gram-negative bacteria and the inflammatory responses. The large size of IgM limits its ability to spread into the tissue. Later in the immune response, T-cell help promotes differentiation of the B-cell and immunoglobulin class switching to produce IgG. **IgG** antibodies are the predominant antibody, especially on rechallenge. IgG antibodies, except IgG4, fix complement and promote phagocytic uptake of the bacteria through Fc receptors on macrophages. The production of **IgA** requires TH2 and TH3 (transforming growth factor-β [TGF-β]) cytokines. IgA is the primary secretory antibody and is important for protecting mucosal membranes. Secretory IgA contains the secretory component that promotes interaction and passage of IgA through mucosal epithelial cells. IgA neutralizes the binding of bacteria and their toxins at epithelial cell surfaces.

Bacterial Immunopathogenesis

Activation of the inflammatory and acute-phase responses can initiate significant tissue and systemic damage. Although IL-1, IL-6, and TNF-α promote protective responses to a local infection, these same responses can be life-threatening when activated by systemic infection. Activation of macrophages in the liver and spleen by endotoxin can promote release of TNF-α into the blood, causing many of the symptoms of **sepsis,** including hemodynamic failure, shock, and death (see Chapter 19). Antibodies produced against bacterial antigens that share determinants with human proteins can initiate tissue destruction (e.g., antibodies produced in post-streptococcal glomerulonephritis and rheumatic fever). Nonspecific activation of CD4 T cells by **superantigens** (e.g., toxic shock syndrome toxin of *S. aureus*) promotes the production of large amounts of cytokines and eventually the death of the activated T cell. The sudden, massive release of cytokines can cause shock and severe tissue damage (e.g., toxic shock syndrome) (see Chapter 19).

Bacterial Evasion of Protective Responses

The mechanisms used by bacteria to evade host protective responses are discussed in Chapter 19 as virulence factors. These mechanisms include (1) the inhibition of phagocytosis and intracellular killing in the phagocyte, (2) inactivation of complement function, (3) cleavage of IgA, (4) intracellular growth (avoidance of antibody), and (5) change in bacterial antigenic appearance. Some microorganisms, including but not limited to mycobacteria (also *Listeria* and *Brucella* species), survive and multiply within macrophages and use the

TABLE 14–3. Basic Properties of Human Interferons (IFNs)

Property	IFN-α	IFN-β	IFN-γ
Previous designations	Leukocyte-IFN	Fibroblast-IFN	Immune IFN
	Type I	Type I	Type II
Genes	>20	1	1
Molecular mass (Da)*			
Major subtypes	16,000–23,000	23,000	20,000–25,000
Cloned†	19,000	19,000	16,000
Glycosylation	No‡	Yes	Yes
pH 2 stability	Stable‡	Stable	Labile
Induction	Viruses	Viruses	Immune activation
Principal source	Epithelium, leukocytes	Fibroblast	Lymphocyte
Introns in gene	No	No	Yes
Homology with human IFN-α	100%	30%–50%	<10%

* Molecular mass of monomeric form. Interferons often occur as polymers.
† Nonglycosylated form, as produced in bacteria by recombinant DNA technology.
‡ Most subtypes, but not all.

From White DO: *Antiviral chemotherapy, interferons and vaccines,* Basel, 1984, Karger; and Samuel CE: Antiviral actions of interferon: interferon-regulated proteins and their surprisingly selective antiviral activities. *Virology* 183:1–11, 1991.

macrophages as a protective reservoir or transport system to help spread the organisms throughout the body. However, activated macrophages can kill the intracellular pathogens.

Specific Immune Responses to Viruses

Host Defenses Against Viral Infection

The immune response is the best and, in most cases, the only means of controlling a viral infection (Fig. 14–6). The humoral and cellular immune responses are important for antiviral immunity. Unlike its goal in a bacterial infection, the ultimate goal of the immune response in a viral infection is to eliminate both the virus and the host cells harboring or replicating the virus. Interferon, NK cells, CD4 DTH responses, and CD8 cytotoxic killer cells are more important for viral infections than for bacterial infections. Failure to resolve the infection may lead to persistent or chronic infection or death.

Nonspecific Immune Defenses

Body temperature, fever, interferons, other cytokines, the mononuclear phagocyte system, and NK cells provide a local, rapid response to viral infection and also activate the specific immune defenses. Often, the nonspecific defenses are sufficient to control a viral infection, thus preventing the occurrence of symptoms.

Viral infection can induce the release of cytokines (e.g., TNF, IL-1) and interferon from infected cells and macrophages. These soluble protein factors trigger local and systemic responses. Induction of fever and stimulation of the immune system are two of these systemic effects.

Body temperature and fever can limit the replication of or destabilize some viruses. Many viruses are less stable (e.g., herpes simplex virus) or cannot replicate (rhinoviruses) at 37°C or higher.

Cells of the **mononuclear phagocyte system** phagocytose the viral and cell debris from virally infected cells. Macrophages in the liver (Kupffer cells) and spleen rapidly filter many viruses from the blood. Antibody and complement bound to a virus facilitate its uptake by macrophages (opsonization). Macrophages also present antigen to T cells and release IL-1 and interferon to initiate the antigen-specific immune response. Activated macrophages can also distinguish and kill infected target cells.

NK cells are activated by interferon and specific cytokines to kill virally infected cells. Viral infection may reduce the expression of MHC antigens or may alter the carbohydrates on cell surface proteins to provide cytolytic signals to the NK cell.

Interferon

Interferon was first described by Isaacs and Lindemann as a factor that "interferes with" the replication of many different viruses. Interferon is the body's *first* active defense against a viral infection, an "early warning system" at the local and systemic levels. *In addition to activating a target cell antiviral defense to block viral replication, interferons activate the immune response and enhance T-cell recognition of the infected cell.* Interferon is a very important defense against infection but is also a cause of the systemic symptoms associated with many viral infections, such as malaise, myalgia, chills, and fever (nonspecific "flu"-like symptoms).

IFN comprises a family of proteins that can be subdivided according to several properties, including size, stability, cell of origin, and mode of action (Table 14–3). **IFN-α** and **IFN-β** share many properties, including structural homology and mode of action. **IFN-α** is made by B cells, monocytes, macrophages, and a rare blood cell (possibly a pre-dendritic cell). **IFN-β** is made by fibroblasts and other cells in response to viral infection and other stimuli. **IFN-γ** is produced by activated T and NK cells later in the infection. Although IFN-γ inhibits viral replication, its structure and mode of action differ from those of the other interferons. IFN-γ is also known as **macrophage activation factor** and is the defining component of the TH1 response.

The best inducer of IFN-α and IFN-β production is **double-stranded RNA**, *such as the replicative intermediates of RNA viruses* (Box 14–6). One double-stranded RNA molecule per cell is sufficient to induce the production of interferon. Interaction of some enveloped

---

BOX 14–6. Interferons

Induction

Interferon production is stimulated by viral infection:
   Double-stranded RNA (e.g., RNA virus intermediate).
   Viral inhibition of cellular protein synthesis.
   Enveloped virus interaction with rare blood leukocyte.

Mechanism of Action

Release from an initial infected cell occurs.
   Interferon binds to a specific cell surface receptor on another cell.
   Interferon induces the "antiviral state": synthesis of protein kinase, 2′–5′ oligoadenylate synthetase, and ribonuclease L.
   Viral infection of the cell activates these enzymes.
   Enzymes stop protein synthesis that blocks viral replication.

viruses (e.g., herpes simplex virus and human immuno-deficiency virus) with a rare blood cell can promote production of *IFN-α*. Inhibition of protein synthesis in a virally infected cell can decrease the production of a repressor protein of the interferon gene, allowing expression of the interferon gene. Nonviral interferon inducers include the following:

1. Intracellular microorganisms (e.g., mycobacteria, fungi, and protozoa).
2. Immune stimulators or mitogens (e.g., endotoxins, phytohemagglutinin).
3. Double-stranded polynucleotides (e.g., poly I:C, poly dA:dT).
4. Synthetic polyanion polymers (e.g., polysulfates, polyphosphates, and pyran).
5. Antibiotics (e.g., kanamycin, cycloheximide).
6. Low-molecular-weight synthetic compounds (e.g., tilorone, acridine dyes).

IFN-α and IFN-β can be induced and released within hours of infection (Fig. 14–7). The interferon binds to specific receptors on the neighboring cells and induces the production of antiviral proteins—**the antiviral state**. However, these antiviral proteins are not activated until they bind double-stranded RNA. The major antiviral effects of interferon are produced by two enzymes, $2'-5'$ oligoadenylate synthetase (an unusual polymerase) and a protein kinase specific for an important ribosomal factor (eukaryotic initiation factor [eIF-2]). Viral infection of the cell and production of double-stranded RNA activate these enzymes and trigger a cascade of biochemical events that leads to the inhibition of protein synthesis, the degradation of messenger RNA (preferentially viral mRNA), and other activities. This process essentially puts the cellular protein synthesis factory "on strike" and prevents viral replication (Fig. 14–8). It must be stressed that interferon induces an antiviral state but does not directly block viral replication. The antiviral state lasts for 2 to 3 days, which may be sufficient for the cell to degrade and eliminate the virus without being killed.

Interferons stimulate cell-mediated immunity by activating effector cells and enhancing recognition of the virally infected target cell. Interferons stimulate pre-NK cells to differentiate to NK cells to *activate an early, local, natural defense against infection*. Activation of macrophages by IFN-γ promotes production of more interferon, secretion of other biologic response modifiers, phagocytosis, recruitment, and inflammatory responses. All interferon types stimulate the expression of class I MHC (human leukocyte antigen) and class II MHC antigens on the cell surface. IFN-γ increases the expression of class II MHC antigens on the macrophage to help promote antigen presentation to T cells. IFN-α and IFN-β increase the expression of class I MHC antigens, enhancing the cell's ability to present antigen and making the cell a better target for cytotoxic T cells (CTLs).

Interferon also has widespread regulatory effects on cell growth, protein synthesis, and the immune re-

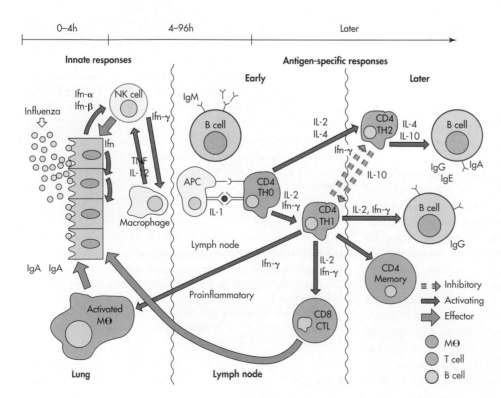

FIGURE 14–6. Antiviral responses. The response to a virus (e.g., influenza virus) initiates with interferon production and action and NK cells. Activation of antigen-specific immunity resembles the antibacterial response except that CD8 cytotoxic T lymphocytes (CTLs) are important antiviral responses. APC = antigen-presenting cell; HLA = human leukocyte antigen; Ifn = interferon, Mθ = macrophage; TNF = tumor necrosis factor.

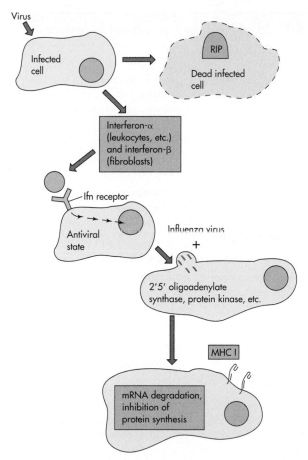

FIGURE 14–7. Induction of the antiviral state by interferon-α or interferon-β. Interferon is produced in response to viral infection but does not affect the initially infected cell. The interferon binds to a cell surface receptor on other cells and induces production of antiviral enzymes (antiviral state). The infection and production of double-stranded RNA activates the antiviral activity. MHCl = major histocompatability antigen type 1.

BOX 14–7. Activities of Interferons

Antiviral Actions

Interferons initiate an antiviral state in cells.
  Interferons block viral protein synthesis.
  Interferons inhibit cell growth.

Immunomodulatory Actions

Interferon-α and interferon-β activate NK cells.
  Interferon-α activates macrophages.
  Interferon-γ activates macrophages.
  Interferons increase expression of major histocompatibility (MHC) antigens.
  Interferons regulate the activities of T cells.

Other Actions

Interferons regulate inflammatory processes.
  Interferons regulate tumor growth.

---

sponse (Box 14–7). All three interferon types block cell proliferation at appropriate doses.

Genetically engineered recombinant interferon is being used as an antiviral therapy for some viral infections (e.g., condyloma acuminata, hepatitis C). Effective treatment requires the use of the correct interferon subtype(s) and its prompt delivery at the appropriate concentration. Interferons have also been used in clinical trials for the treatment of certain cancers. Interferon treatment has "flu"-like side effects, such as chills, fever, and fatigue.

Antigen-Specific Immunity

Humoral immunity and cell-mediated immunity play different roles in resolving viral infections (eliminating the virus from the body). Humoral immunity (antibody) acts mainly on extracellular virions, whereas cell-mediated immunity (T cells) is directed at the virus-producing cell (see Fig. 14–6).

Humoral Immunity

Practically all viral proteins are foreign to the host and are immunogenic (capable of eliciting an antibody response). However, not all immunogens elicit protective immunity. *The best protective antibody response is generated toward the viral proteins that interact with cell surface receptors (viral attachment proteins).* These antigens include the viral capsid proteins of naked viruses and the glycoproteins of enveloped viruses. Antibodies to other viral antigens may be useful for serologic analysis of the viral infection (Box 14–8).

Antibody blocks the progression of disease through the **neutralization and opsonization** of cell-free virus. Antibody can neutralize the virus by binding to the viral attachment proteins, thus preventing their interaction with target cells, or by destabilizing the virus, thus initiating its degradation. Binding of antibody to the virus also opsonizes the virus, promoting its uptake and clearance by macrophages. Antibody recognition of infected cells can also promote antibody-dependent cellular cytotoxicity (ADCC) by NK cells.

The major antiviral role of antibody is to *prevent the spread of extracellular virus to other cells*, which is especially important in limiting the spread of the virus by **viremia**. *Antibody is most effective at resolving cytolytic infections.* Resolution occurs because the virus kills the cell factory and the antibody eliminates the extracellular virus. Antibody is the primary defense initiated by vaccination.

T-Cell Immunity

T cell–mediated immunity promotes antibody and inflammatory responses (CD4 helper T cells) and kills

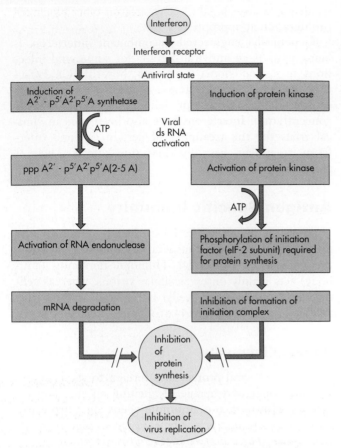

FIGURE 14–8. The two major routes for interferon inhibition of viral protein synthesis. One mechanism involves the induction of an unusual polymerase (2′–5′ oligoadenylate synthetase [2–5A]) that is activated by double-stranded RNA (ds RNA). The activated enzyme synthesizes an unusual adenine trinucleotide with a 2′, 5′-phosphodiester linkage. The trinucleotide activates an endonuclease that degrades (messenger RNA (mRNA). The other mechanism involves the induction of a protein kinase that inactivates the eukaryotic initiation factor (eIF-2α) by phosphorylating one of the subunits to prevent initiation of protein synthesis. ATP = adenosine triphosphate.

infected cells (CD8 CTLs) (see Box 14–8). The **CD4 TH1** response is generally more important than TH2 responses for controlling a viral infection, especially noncytolytic and enveloped viruses. Cytokines produced by CD4 TH1 cells activate **CTLs (CD8)**, which can then kill cells expressing the appropriate complex of viral peptide with class I MHC protein. The CTL response probably evolved as a defense against virus infection. The peptides expressed on class I MHC antigens are obtained from viral proteins synthesized within the infected cell (endogenous route). *CTL targets include peptides derived from viral proteins that may not elicit protective antibody* (e.g., intracellular or internal

---

BOX 14–8. **Summary of Antiviral Responses**

Interferon

Interferon is induced by double-stranded RNA, inhibition of cellular protein synthesis, or enveloped virus.

Interferon initiates the antiviral state in surrounding cells.

Interferon blocks local viral replication.

Interferon initiates systemic antiviral responses.

Natural Killer (NK) Cells

NK cells are activated by interferon-α and IL-12 and activate macrophages (interferon-γ).

NK cells target and kill virus-infected cells (especially enveloped viruses).

Macrophage and Dendritic Cells

Macrophages filter viral particles from blood.

Macrophages inactivate opsonized virus particles.

Macrophages and dendritic cells present viral antigen to CD4 T cells.

T Cells

T cells are essential for controlling enveloped and noncytolytic viral infections.

T cells recognize viral peptides presented by major histocompatibility (MHC) molecules on cell surfaces.

Antigenic viral peptides (linear epitopes) can come from any viral protein (e.g., glycoproteins, nucleoproteins).

TH1 CD4 responses are more important than TH2 responses.

CD8 cytotoxic T cells respond to viral peptide–class I MHC protein complexes on the cell surface.

TH2 CD4 responses are important for the maturation of antibody response.

TH2 CD4 responses may be detrimental if they prematurely limit the TH1 inflammatory and cytolytic responses.

Antibody

Antibody neutralizes extracellular virus:

It blocks viral attachment proteins (glycoproteins, capsid proteins).

It destabilizes viral structure.

Antibody opsonizes virus for phagocytosis.

Antibody promotes killing of target cell by the complement cascade and antibody-dependent cellular cytotoxicity.

Antibody resolves lytic viral infections.

Antibody blocks viremic spread to target tissue.

Immunoglobulin (Ig) M is an indicator of recent or current infection.

IgG is more effective antiviral than IgM.

Secretory IgA is important for protecting mucosal surfaces.

virion proteins, nuclear proteins, improperly folded or processed proteins [cell trash]) in addition to viral glycoproteins. For example, the matrix and nucleoproteins of the influenza virus and the ICP4 (nuclear) protein of herpes simplex virus are targets for CTL lysis but do not elicit protective antibody.

Cell-mediated immunity is especially important for resolving infections by syncytia-forming viruses, which can spread from cell to cell without exposure to antibody (e.g., measles, herpes simplex, and varicella-zoster viruses), and noncytolytic viruses (e.g., hepatitis A and measles viruses) and for controlling latent viruses (herpes viruses and papillomaviruses). *CTLs kill infected cells and, as a result, eliminate the source of new virus.*

TABLE 14–4. Examples of Viral Evasion of Immune Responses

Mechanism	Viral Examples	Action
Humoral Response		
Hidden from antibody	Herpesviruses, retroviruses	Latent infection
	Herpes simplex virus, varicella-zoster virus, paramyxoviruses, human immunodeficiency virus	Cell-to-cell infection (syncytia formation)
Antigenic variation	Lentiviruses (human immunodeficiency virus)	Genetic change after infection
	Influenza virus	Annual genetic changes
Secretion of blocking antigen	Hepatitis B virus	Hepatitis B surface antigen
Decay of complement	Herpes simplex virus	Glycoprotein C, which binds and promotes C3 decay
Interferon		
Block production	Hepatitis B virus	Inhibition of interferon transcription
	Epstein-Barr virus	IL-10 analogue (BCRF-1) blocks interferon-γ production
Block action	Adenovirus	Inhibits upregulation of MHC expression VA1 RNA, blocks double-stranded RNA activation of interferon-induced protein kinase
Immune Cell Function		
Impairment of lymphocyte function	Herpes simplex virus	Prevention of CD8 T-cell killing
	Human immunodeficiency virus	Kills CD4 T cells and alteration of macrophages
	Measles virus	Suppression of NK, T, and B cells
Immunosuppressive factors	Esptein-Barr virus	BCRF, BCRF-1 (similar to IL-10) suppression of TH1 CD4 helper T-cell responses
Decreased Antigen Presentation		
Reduced MHCI expression	Adenovirus 12	Inhibition of class I MHC transcription
		19-kDa protein (E3 gene) binds class I MHC heavy chain, blocking translocation to surface
	Cytomegalovirus	H301 protein blocks surface expression of β_2-microglobulin and class I MHC molecules
	Herpes simplex virus	ICP47 blocks TAP, preventing peptide binding to class I MHC molecules
Inhibition of Inflammation		
—	Poxvirus, adenovirus	Blocking of action of IL-1 or tumor necrosis factor

IL = interleukin; MHCI = major histocompatibility complex antigen type 1; NK = natural killer; PMN = polymorphonuclear neutrophil; TAP = transporter associated with antigen production.

Immune Response to Viral Challenge

Primary Viral Challenge

The nonspecific immune responses are the earliest responses to viral challenge and are often sufficient to limit viral spread (see Fig. 14–6). The **interferon** produced in response to most viral infections initiates the protection of adjacent cells, enhances antigen presentation by increasing the expression of MHC antigens, and initiates the clearance of infected cells by activating NK cells and antigen-specific responses. Virus and viral components released from the infected cells are phagocytosed by resident **macrophages** and **dendritic cells** that mobilize and move to the lymph nodes. Macrophages in the liver and spleen are especially important for clearing virus from the blood stream (filters). These cells degrade and process the viral antigens and express on their cell surface appropriate peptide fragments bound to class II MHC antigens. Macrophages also release IL-1, IL-6, and TNF to induce fever and, with IL-12, promote activation of helper T cells (TH1).

Antiviral antigen–specific responses are similar to antibacterial antigen–specific responses, except that the CD8 T cell plays a more important role. **IgM** is the first anti-viral antibody produced, and its production indicates a primary infection. **IgG** and **IgA** are produced 2 to 3 days after IgM. Secretory IgA is made in response to a viral challenge through the natural openings of the body, that is, the eyes, mouth, and respiratory and gastrointestinal systems. **CD8 killer/suppressor** T cells are present at approximately the same time as serum IgG. During infection, the number of CD8 T cells specific for antigen may increase 50,000 to 100,000 times. The CD8 T cells move to the site of infection and kill virally infected cells. Recognition and binding to class I MHC viral peptide–expressing target cells promotes apoptotic killing of the target cells either through the release of perforin and granzymes to disrupt the cell membrane or through the binding of the Fas ligand with Fas on the target cell. Resolution of the infection occurs later, when sufficient antibody is available to neutralize all virus progeny or when cellular immunity has been able to reach and eliminate the infected cells. For the resolution of most enveloped and noncytolytic viral infections, DTH and CTL responses are required (in addition to antibody) to kill the viral factory. In many cases, IgG and CTLs in the blood are detected after viral replication has been controlled.

Secondary Viral Challenge

In any war, it is easier to eliminate an enemy if its identity and origin are known and if establishment of its foothold can be prevented. Similarly, in the body, prior immunity allows rapid, specific mobilization of defenses to prevent disease symptoms, promote rapid clearance of the virus, and block viremic spread from the primary site of infection to the target tissue to prevent disease. As a result, most secondary viral challenges are asymptomatic. Antibody and memory B and T cells are present in an immune host to generate a more rapid and extensive anamnestic response to the virus. Secretory IgA is produced quickly to provide an

---

TABLE 14–5. Examples of Antiparasitic Immune Responses

Parasite	Habitat	Main Host Effector Mechanism*	Method of Avoidance
Trypanosoma brucei	Blood stream	Antibody + complement	Antigenic variation
Plasmodium species	Hepatocyte, blood cell	Antibody, cytokines (TH1)	Intracellular, antigenic variation
Toxoplasma gondii	Macrophage	O_2 metabolites, NO, lyso-somal enzymes (TH1)	Inhibition of fusion with lysosomes
Trypanosoma cruzi	Many cells	O_2 metabolites, NO, lyso-somal enzymes (TH1)	Escape into cytoplasm, thus avoiding digestion in lysosome
Leishmania species	Macrophage	O_2 metabolites, NO, lyso-somal enzymes (TH1)	Impairment of O_2 burst and scavenging of products; avoidance of digestion
Trichinella spiralis	Gut, blood, muscle	Myeloid cells, antibody + complement (TH2)	Encystment in muscle
Schistosoma mansoni	Skin, blood, lungs, portal vein	Myeloid cells, antibody + complement (TH2)	Acquisition of host antigens, blockade by antibody; soluble antigens and immune complexes; antioxidants
Wuchereria bancrofti	Lymphatic system	Myeloid cells, antibody + complement (TH2)	Thick extracellular cuticle; antioxidants

*Antibody is most important for extracellular pathogens. Cell-mediated immunity (TH1 response) is most important for intracellular pathogens.

From Roitt, et al. *Immunology*, ed 4, St Louis, 1996, Mosby.

important defense to reinfection through the natural openings of the body, but it is produced only transiently.

The nature of the immune response to a viral infection is determined by host, viral, and other factors. Host factors include genetic background, immune status, age, and the general health of the individual. In addition, **immunologically privileged sites** in the body (e.g., brain, eyes) have unique approaches to combating infections, because they suppress T-cell responses to prevent the serious tissue destruction that accompanies inflammation. Viral factors include viral strain, infectious dose, and route of entry. The time required to initiate immune protection, the extent of the response, the level of control of the infection, and the potential for immunopathology (see Chapter 46) resulting from the infection differ after a primary infection and after a rechallenge.

Viral Mechanisms for Escaping the Immune Response

A major factor in the virulence of a virus is its ability to escape immune resolution. Viruses may escape immune resolution by evading detection, preventing activation, or blocking the delivery of the immune response. Specific examples are presented in Table 14–4. Some viruses even encode special proteins that suppress the immune response.

Specific Immune Responses to Fungi

The primary protective responses to fungal infection are promoted by **TH1-mediated inflammatory reactions.** Patients deficient in these responses (e.g., patients with AIDS) are most susceptible to fungal infections. **Macrophages activated by IFN-γ** are important for killing the fungi. Neutrophil production of cationic proteins may be important for some fungal infections (e.g., mucormycosis), and nitric oxide may be important against *Cryptococcus* and other fungi. Antibody, as an opsonin, may facilitate clearance of the fungi.

Specific Immune Responses to Parasites

It is difficult to generalize about the mechanisms of antiparasite immunity, because there are many different parasites that have different forms and reside in different tissue locations during their life cycles (Table 14–5). In general, stimulation of *CD4 TH1, CD8 T-cell, and macrophage responses are important for intracellular infections, and TH2 antibody responses are important for extracellular parasites in blood and fluids.* **IgE** and **eosinophil** and **mast cell** action are especially important for eliminating worm (cestodes and nematodes) infections.

Control of the infection may depend on which response is initiated in the host. For example, initiation of a TH2 response to *Leishmania* species is detrimental, because it prevents the generation of protective TH1 responses. Parasites have developed sophisticated mechanisms for avoiding immune clearance and often establish chronic infections.

Extracellular parasites, such as *Trypanosoma cruzi, Toxoplasma gondii,* and *Leishmania* species, are phagocytosed by **macrophage. Antibody** may promote the uptake of (opsonize) the parasites. Killing of the parasites follows activation of the macrophage by IFN-γ (produced by NK or CD4 TH1 cells) or TNF-α (produced by other macrophages) and induction of **oxygen-dependent killing mechanisms** (peroxide, superoxide, nitric oxide). In the absence of macrophage activation, the parasites may replicate in the macrophage. The observation that IL-4 and antibody production in response to *Leishmania* infection correlated with the inhibition of protective inflammatory responses and poor outcome provided the basis for the discovery that TH1 and TH2 responses are separate and antagonistic.

CD4 TH1 production of IFN-γ and activation of

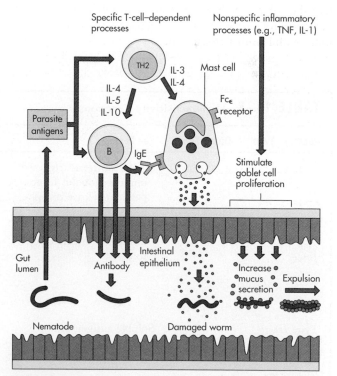

FIGURE 14–9. Elimination of nematodes from the gut. TH2 responses are important for stimulating the production of antibody. Antibody can damage the worm. Immunoglobulin (Ig) E is associated with mast cells, the release of histamine, and toxic substances. Increased mucus secretion also promotes expulsion. IL = interleukin; TNF = tumor necrosis factor. (From Roitt I et al: *Immunology,* ed 4, St Louis, 1996, Mosby.).

macrophages are also essential for protection against intracellular protozoa and for the development of **granulomas** around *Schistosoma mansoni* eggs and worms in the liver. The granuloma, formed by layers of inflammatory cells, protects the liver from toxins produced by the eggs but also causes fibrosis. The development of fibrosis interrupts the venous blood supply to the liver, leading to hypertension and cirrhosis.

Neutrophils act much like macrophages: They phagocytose and kill extracellular parasites through both oxygen-dependent and oxygen-independent mechanisms. **Eosinophils** localize near parasites, bind to IgG or IgE on the surface of larvae or worms (e.g., helminths, *S. mansonii*, *Trichinella spiralis*), degranulate by fusing their intracellular granules with the plasma membrane, and release the **major basic protein** into the intercellular space. The major basic protein is toxic to the parasite.

For parasitic worm infections, cytokines produced by CD4 TH2 responses are very important for stimulating the production of IgE and the activation of mast cells (Fig. 14–9). IgE bound to Fc receptors on mast cells targets the cells to antigens of the infecting parasite. In the lumen of the intestine, antigen binding and cross-linking of the IgE on the mast cell surface stimulate the release of histamine and substances toxic to the parasite and promote mucus secretion to coat and promote expulsion of the worm.

IgG antibody also plays an important role in antiparasite immunity as an opsonin and by activating complement on the surface of the parasite.

Evasion of Immune Mechanisms by Parasites

Animal parasites have developed remarkable mechanisms for establishing chronic infections in the vertebrate host (see Table 14–5). These mechanisms include intracellular growth, inactivation of phagocytic killing, release of blocking antigen (e.g., *Trypanosoma brucei*, *Plasmodium falciparum*), and development of cysts (e.g., protozoa: *Entamoeba histolytica*; helminths: *T. spiralis*) to limit access by the immune response. The African trypanosomes can reengineer the genes for their surface antigen (variable surface glycoprotein) and therefore change their antigenic appearance. Schistosomes can coat themselves with host antigens, including MHC molecules.

Other Immune Responses

Antitumor responses and **rejection of tissue transplants** are primarily mediated by T cells. CD8 cytolytic T cells recognize and kill tumors expressing peptides from embryologic proteins, mutated proteins, or other proteins on class I MHC molecules (endogenous route of peptide presentation). These proteins may be expressed in an illegitimate manner in the tumor cell,

---

TABLE 14–6. Hypersensitivity Reactions

Reaction Type	Onset Time	Key Features	Beneficial Effects	Pathologic Effects
Type I	<30 min	Soluble antigen–triggered, immunoglobulin E–dependent release of vasoactive mediators	Antiparasitic responses and toxin neutralization	Localized allergies (e.g., hay fever, asthma) Systemic anaphylaxis
Type II	<8 h	Cell-bound antibody–promoting C'-mediated cytotoxicity	Direct lysis and phagocytosis of extracellular bacteria and other susceptible microbes	Destruction of red blood cells (e.g., transfusion reactions, Rh disease) Organ-specific tissue damage in some autoimmune diseases (e.g., Goodpasture's syndrome)
Type III	<8 h	Soluble antigen-antibody complexes activate C'	Acute inflammatory reaction at site of extracellular microbes and their clearance	Arthus reaction (localized) Serum sickness and drug reactions (generalized) Systemic autoimmune diseases
Type IV	24–72 h (acute) >1 week (chronic)	Soluble antigen presented to CD4 T cells by MHCII leads to release of TH1 cytokines, activating macrophages and cytotoxic T lymphocytes	Protection against infection by fungi, intracellular bacteria, and viruses	Acute: contact dermatitis, tuberculosis skin test Chronic: granuloma formation, graft rejection

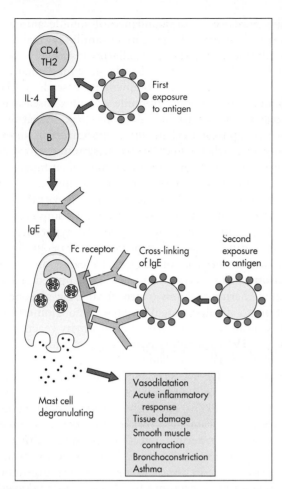

FIGURE 14–10. Type I hypersensitivity: Immunoglobulin (Ig) E–mediated atopic and anaphylactic reactions. IgE produced in response to the initial challenge binds to Fc receptors on mast cells and basophils. Allergen binding to the cell surface IgE promotes the release of histamine and prostaglandins from granules to produce symptoms. Examples are hay fever, asthma, penicillin allergy, and reaction to bee stings. IL = interleukin.

Immunopathogenesis

Hypersensitivity Responses

Once activated, the immune response is sometimes difficult to control and causes tissue damage. Hypersensitivity reactions are responsible for many of the symptoms associated with microbial infections, especially viral infections. The four types of hypersensitivity responses are distinguished primarily by the mechanism of initiation and the time course (Table 14–6).

Type I hypersensitivity is caused by **IgE** and is associated with **allergic, atopic**, and **anaphylactic reactions** (Fig. 14–10). IgE binds to Fc receptors on mast cells and becomes the cell surface receptor for antigens (**allergens**). Cross-linking of the IgE triggers degranulation, releasing **chemoattractants** (cytokines, leukotrienes) to attract eosinophils, neutrophils, and mononuclear cells; **activators** (histamine, platelet-activating factor, tryptase, kininogenase) to promote vasodilatation and edema; and **spasmogens** (histamine, prostaglandin D_2, leukotrienes), to directly affect bronchial smooth muscle and promote mucus secretion. IgE allergic reactions are rapid-onset reactions. Desensitization (allergy shots) produces IgG to bind the allergen and prevent allergen binding to IgE.

Type II hypersensitivity is caused by **antibody binding** to cell surface molecules and the subsequent activation of *cytolytic responses by the* **classic complement cascade** *or by cellular mechanisms* (Fig. 14–11). Examples of these reactions are (1) myasthenia gravis (because of antibodies to acetylcholine receptors on

and the host immune response may not be tolerized to them. IL-2 treatment in vitro generates lymphokine-activated killer (LAK cells) and NK cells that target tumor cells, possibly a result of a reduction in class I MHC molecules on the tumor cell surface. IFN-γ–activated ("angry") macrophages can also distinguish and kill tumor cells.

Rejection of allografts used for tissue transplants results from the expression of foreign peptides on foreign class I MHC antigens. In addition to host rejection of the transplanted tissue, cells from the donor of a blood transfusion or a tissue transplant can react against the new host in a **graft versus host (GVH) response**. An in vitro test of T-cell activation and growth in a GVH-like response is the **mixed lymphocyte reaction**. Activation is usually measured as DNA synthesis (radioactive thymidine uptake).

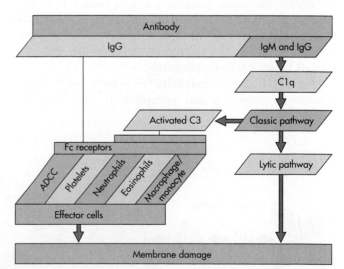

FIGURE 14–11. Type II hypersensitivity: mediated by antibody and complement. Complement activation promotes direct cell damage through the complement cascade and by the activation of effector cells. Examples are Goodpasture's syndrome, the response to Rh factor in newborns, and autoimmune endocrinopathies. ADCC = antibody-dependent cellular cytotoxicity; Ig = immunoglobulin.

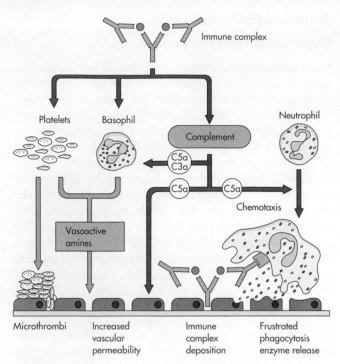

FIGURE 14–12. Type III hypersensitivity: immune complex deposition. Immune complexes can be trapped in the kidney and elsewhere in the body, can activate complement, and cause other damaging responses. Examples are serum sickness, nephritis associated with chronic hepatitis B infection, and Arthus reaction.

neurons), (2) autoimmune hemolytic anemia, and (3) Goodpasture's syndrome (lung and kidney basement membrane damage). Another example is hemolytic disease of the newborn (blue babies), which is caused by the reaction of maternal antibody generated during the first pregnancy to Rh factors on fetal erythrocytes of a second baby (Rh incompatibility).

Type III hypersensitivity responses result from **immune complexes** and **complement** (Fig. 14–12).

In the presence of an abundance of soluble antigen in the blood stream, large antigen-antibody complexes form, become trapped in capillaries (especially in the kidney), and then initiate the classic complement cascade. Activation of the complement cascade initiates inflammatory reactions. Immune complex disease may be caused by persistent infections (e.g., hepatitis B, malaria, staphylococcal infective endocarditis), autoimmunity (e.g., rheumatoid arthritis, systemic lupus erythematosus), or consistent inhalation of antigen (e.g., mold, plant, or animal antigens). For example, hepatitis B infection produces large amounts of hepatitis B surface antigen, which may form immune complexes that lead to glomerulonephritis. Type III hypersensitivity reactions can be induced in presensitized people by the intradermal injection of antigen to cause an **Arthus reaction**, a skin reaction characterized by redness and swelling. Serum sickness, extrinsic allergic alveolitis (a reaction to inhaled fungal antigen), and glomerulonephritis result from type III hypersensitivity reactions.

Type IV hypersensitivity responses are CD4 T cell–induced DTH inflammatory responses (Fig. 14–13 and Table 14–7). Although essential for the control of fungal infections and intracellular bacteria (e.g., mycobacteria), DTH is also responsible for **contact dermatitis** (e.g., cosmetics, nickel) and the response to poison ivy. Intradermal injection of **tuberculin antigen** (purified protein derivative) elicits firm swelling that is maximal 48 to 72 hours after injection and is indicative of prior exposure to *Mycobacterium tuberculosis* (Fig. 14–14). **Granulomas** form in response to the intracellular growth of *M. tuberculosis*. These structures consist of an epithelioid (Langhans cells) created from chronically activated macrophages, fused epithelioid cells (giant cells) surrounded by lymphocytes, and fibrosis caused by the deposition of collagen from fibroblasts. Granulomatous hypersensitivity occurs with tuberculosis, leprosy, schistosomiasis, sarcoidosis, and Crohn's disease.

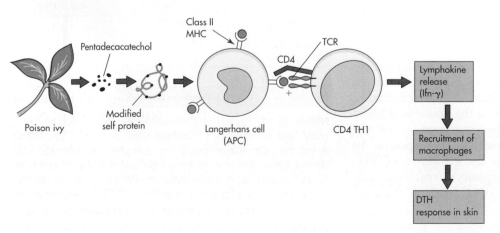

FIGURE 14–13. Type IV hypersensitivity delayed-type hypersensitivity (DTH) mediated by CD4 T cells (TH1). In this case, chemically modified self-proteins are processed and presented to CD4 T cells, which release cytokines, including interferon-γ (Ifn-γ), which promote inflammation. Other examples of DTH are the tuberculin response (purified protein derivative test) and reaction to metals such as nickel. APC = antigen presenting cell; TCR = T-cell receptor.

TABLE 14–7. **Important Characteristics of Four Types of Delayed-Type Hypersensitivity Reactions**

Type	Reaction Time	Clinical Appearance	Histologic Appearance	Antigen
Jones-Mote	24 hours	Skin swelling	Basophils, lymphocytes, mononuclear cells	Intradermal antigen: ovalbumin
Contact	48 hours	Eczema	Mononuclear cells, edema, raised epidermis	Epidermal: nickel, rubber, poison ivy
Tuberculin	48 hours	Local induration and swelling with or without fever	Mononuclear cells, lymphocytes and monocytes, reduced macrophages	Dermal: tuberculin, mycobacterial, and leishmanial
Granulomatous	4 weeks	Skin induration	Epithelioid cell granuloma, giant cells, macrophages, fibrosis with or without necrosis	Persistent antigen or antigen-antibody complexes in macrophages or "nonimmunologic" (e.g., talcum powder)

Autoimmune Responses

Normally, a person is tolerized to self-antigens during the development of the immune system as a fetus and later in life by other mechanisms (e.g., oral tolerization). However, deregulation of the immune response may be initiated by cross-reactivity with microbial antigens (e.g., group A streptococcal infection, rheumatic fever), polyclonal activation of lymphocytes induced by tumors or infection (e.g., malaria, Epstein-Barr virus infection), or a genetic predisposition caused by lack of tolerization to specific antigens.

Autoimmune reactions result from the presence of autoantibodies, activated T cells, and hypersensitivity reactions. People with certain MHC antigens are at higher risk for autoimmune responses (e.g., HLA-B27

and juvenile rheumatoid arthritis and ankylosing spondylitis). Many of these responses are associated with inflammatory TH1-type responses. Multiple sclerosis, an inflammatory response directed against myelin basic protein, may be triggered by immune responses to one or more viruses, such as human herpes virus 6 or measles. Activation of TH2 responses to counteract the TH1 inflammation may provide a therapeutic approach for these diseases.

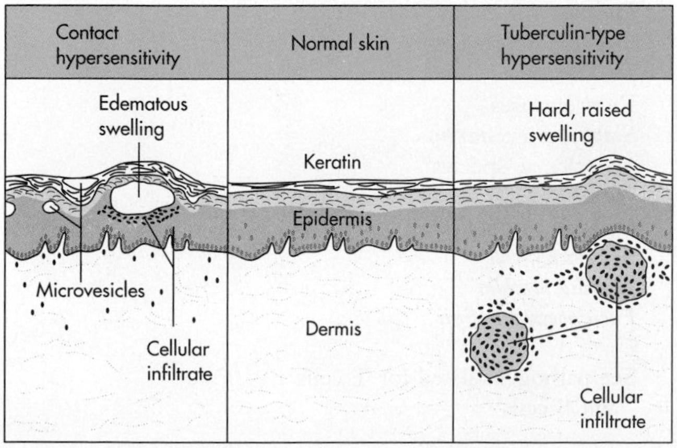

Immunodeficiency

Immunodeficiency may result from genetic deficiencies, starvation, drug-induced immunosuppression (e.g., steroid treatment, cancer chemotherapy, chemotherapeutic suppression of tissue graft rejection), cancer (especially of immune cells), or disease (e.g., AIDS) and may naturally occur in neonates and pregnant women. Deficiencies in specific protective responses put a patient at high risk for serious disease due to the infectious agents that would be controlled by that response (Table 14–8). These "natural experiments" illustrate the importance of specific responses in controlling specific infections.

Immunosuppression

Immunosuppressive therapy is important for reducing excessive inflammatory or immune responses of macrophages and T cells or for preventing the rejection of tissue transplants by T cells. **Anti-inflammatory treatments** primarily target the production of TNF and IL-1 by mononuclear cells. Corticosteroids prevent their production by macrophages and may be toxic to T cells. Antibody to TNF and soluble forms of the TNF receptor block the binding of TNF and prevent its action. **Immunosuppressive therapy for transplantation** generally inhibits the action or causes the

FIGURE 14–14. Contact and tuberculin hypersensitivity responses. These type IV responses are cell-mediated but differ in the site of cell infiltration and in the symptoms. Contact hypersensitivity occurs in the epidermis and leads to the formation of blisters; tuberculin-type hypersensitivity occurs in the dermis and is characterized by swelling.

TABLE 14–8. Infections Associated with Defects in Immune Responses

Defect	Pathogen
Induction by physical means (e.g., burns, trauma)	*Pseudomonas aeruginosa* *Staphylococcus aureus* *Staphylococcus epidermidis* *Streptococcus pyogenes* *Aspergillus* species *Candida* species
Granulocyte and monocyte defects in movement, phagocytosis, or killing or decreased number of cells (neutropenia)	*Staphylococcus aureus* *Streptococcus pyogenes* *Haemophilus influenzae* Gram-negative bacilli *Escherichia coli* *Klebsiella* species *Pseudomonas aeruginosa* *Nocardia* species *Aspergillus* species *Candida* species
Individual components of complement system	*Staphylococcus aureus* *Streptococcus pneumoniae* *Pseudomonas* species *Proteus* species *Neisseria* species *Neisseria meningitidis*
T cells	Cytomegalovirus Herpes simplex virus Herpes zoster virus *Listeria monocytogenes* *Mycobacterium* species *Nocardia* species *Aspergillus* species *Candida* species *Cryptococcus neoformans* *Histoplasma capsulatum* *Pneumocystis carinii* *Strongyloides stercoralis*
B cells	Enteroviruses *Staphylococcus aureus* *Streptococcus* species *Haemophilus influenzae* *Neisseria meningitidis* *Escherichia coli* *Giardia lamblia* *Pneumocystis carinii*
Combined immunodeficiency	See pathogens listed for T cells and B cells

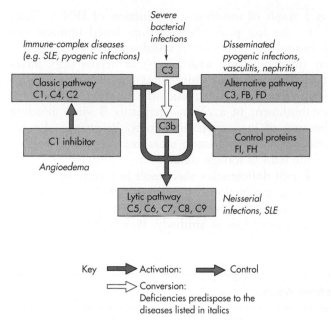

FIGURE 14–15. Consequences of deficiencies in the complement pathways. Factors B binds to C3b on cell surfaces, and the plasma serine protease D cleaves and activates B-C3b as part of the alternative pathway. Factors FI and FH limit the inappropriate activation of complement. FH binds to C3b and prevents activation and is a co-factor for FI. FI is a serine protease that cleaves C3b and C4b. C1 inh = C1 inhibitor; SLE = systemic lupus erythematosus.

Defects in Phagocyte Action

People with defective phagocytic function are more susceptible to bacterial infections but not to viral or protozoal infections (Fig. 14–16). The clinical relevance of oxygen-dependent killing is illustrated by **chronic granulomatous disease** in children who have diminished levels of cytochrome b and fail to form superoxide anions. Even though phagocytosis is normal, these children have an impaired ability to oxidize NADPH and destroy bacteria through the oxidative pathway. In patients with **Chédiak-Higashi syndrome**, the neutrophil granules fuse when the cells are immature in the bone marrow. Thus, neutrophils from these patients can phagocytose bacteria but have greatly diminished ability to kill them. **Asplenic individuals** are at risk for infection with encapsulated organisms because such people lack the filtration mechanism of spleen macrophages. Other deficiencies are shown in Figure 14–16.

Deficiencies in Antigen-Specific Immune Responses

People deficient in **T-cell function** are susceptible to opportunistic infections by (1) viruses, especially envel-

lysis of T cells. Cyclosporin, tacrolimus (FK-506), and rapamycin prevent the activation of T cells. Anti-CD3 and anti-CD25 prevent activation of, and may promote killing of, T cells to prevent a response. Administration of antibody to costimulatory molecules such as B7 or CD40 ligand at the time of transplant can block proper T-cell activation and promote anergy rather than responsiveness.

Hereditary Complement Deficiencies and Microbial Infection

Inherited **deficiencies of C1q, C1r, C1s, C4,** and **C2** components are associated with defects in activation of the classic complement pathway that lead to greater susceptibility to pyogenic (pus-producing) staphylococcal and streptococcal infections (Fig. 14–15). A **deficiency of C3** leads to a defect in activation of both the classic and alternative pathways, which also results in an higher incidence of pyogenic infections. **Defects of the properdin factors** impair activation of the alternative pathway, which also results in an increased susceptibility to pyogenic infections. Finally, **deficiencies of C5 through C9** are associated with defective cell killing, which raises the susceptibility to disseminated neisserial infections.

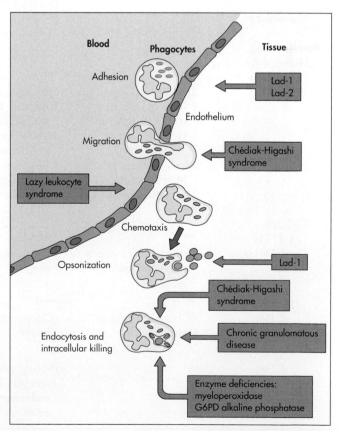

FIGURE 14–16. Consequences of phagocyte dysfunction. G6PD = glucose-6-phosphate dehydrogenase; Lad = leukocyte adhesion deficiency.

oped and noncytolytic viruses and viruses that establish latent or recurrent infections, (2) intracellular bacteria, and (3) fungi (Table 14–9). T-cell deficiencies can also prevent the maturation of B-cell antibody responses. T-cell deficiencies can arise from genetic disorders (e.g., X-linked immunodeficiency syndrome, Duncan's disease, DiGeorge syndrome) (Table 14–10), infection (e.g., human immunodeficiency virus and AIDS), cancer chemotherapy, or immunosuppressive therapy for tissue transplantation.

The immaturity of the immune system of **neonates** increases their susceptibility to infections resolved by TH1-associated responses, including infections by herpes viruses. Neonates are deficient in TH1 responses

as a result of insufficient production of IFN-γ. Similarly, the less pronounced cell-mediated immune and inflammatory responses of **children** decrease the severity (in comparison with adults) of herpes (e.g., infectious mononucleosis, chickenpox) and hepatitis B infections but also increase the potential for the establishment of a chronic hepatitis B virus infection because of incomplete resolution. Pregnancy also induces immunosuppressive measures to prevent rejection of the fetus (a foreign tissue).

B-cell deficiencies may result in a complete lack of antibody production (hypogammaglobulinemia), inability to undergo class switching, or inability to produce specific subclasses of antibody. People deficient in anti-

---

TABLE 14–9. Comparison of Immune Responses to Infectious Agents

	Bacteria	Viruses	Fungi	Parasites
Natural				
Interferon (α, β)		****		
Neutrophils	**** Phagocytosis/killing	*	**	*
Eosinophil				***
Natural Killer Cells		*** (Virally infected cells)		
Macrophages	*** Phagocytosis, APC	*** Phagocytosis, APC	**	**
Specific				
Humoral:				
Antibody	***** IgM and IgG + C′: lysis, opsonization secretory IgA, etc., block adherence	**** IgM, IgG, IgA and C′ Especially for cytolytic viruses, and VIREMIA Neutralization and opsonization	*** IgM, IgG, IgA	** IgE
Complement	Opsonization, lysis of gram-negatives bacteria, chemotaxis	Opsonization, disruption of enveloped viruses and infected cells	Opsonization and chemotaxis	Opsonization and chemotaxis
Cellular:				

T-DTH
   (CD4) (also
   IFN-γ)
	****
	 (Intracellular bacteria only) *(via macrophage)*
		******
		 All viruses *(Via macrophage)*
			*****
			 (Via macrophage)	

T-helper (CD4)	***** (Class-switching of antibody)	***** (Class-switching of antibody)	***** (Class-switching of antibody)	***** (Class-switching of antibody)
T-cytolytic (CD8)		**** (Virally infected cells) Especially for enveloped and noncytolytic viruses		

Number of asterisks indicates importance of response.
APC = antigen-presenting cell; C′ = complement system; DTH = delayed-type hypersensitivity; Ig = immunoglobulin.

TABLE 14–10. Immunodeficiencies of Lymphocytes

Condition	T Cell No.	T Cell Function	B Cell No.	Serum Antibodies	Incidence*
XLA, Bruton's syndrome	√	√	↓↓	IgG, IgA, IgM ↓↓	Rare
X-SCID	↓↓	↓	√	↓	Rare
XLP, Duncan's syndrome	√	↓	√	√ or ↓	Rare
X-hyper IgM	√	↓	√	IgG ↓↓, IgA ↓↓, IgM ↑	Rare
Wiskott-Aldrich syndrome	√	↓	√	IgA ↑, IgE ↑, IgM ↓	Rare
ADA deficiency (SCID)	↓↓	↓↓	↓	↓	Very rare
PNP deficiency (SCID)	↓	↓	√	√	Very rare
HLA deficiency	√	↓	√	Poor Ag response	Very rare
Ataxia telangiectasia	↓	↓	√	IgE ↓, IgA ↓, IgG2 ↓	Uncommon
DiGeorge syndrome	↓↓	↓	√	√	Very rare
IgA deficiency	√	√	√	IgA ↓	Common

*Approximate incidence: Very rare = <10⁻⁶; rare = 10⁻⁵ to 10⁻⁶; common = 10⁻² to 10⁻³.

ADA = adenosine deaminate; Ag = antigen; HLA = human leukocyte antigen; Ig = immunoglobulin; PNP = purine nucleoside phosphorylase; XLA = X-linked agammaglobulinemia; XLP = X-linked lymphoproliferative (syndrome); X-SCID = X-linked severe combined immunodeficiency disease; √ = normal; ↑ = increased; ↓ = decreased or defective.

From Brostoff J, Male DK: *Clinical immunology: an illustrated outline,* St Louis, 1994, Mosby.

body production are very susceptible to **bacterial infection.** IgA deficiency, which occurs in 1 of 700 white people, results in a greater susceptibility to **respiratory infections.** A deficiency in IgG₂ antibodies raises the risk for capsular bacterial infections, since IgG₂ antibodies constitute the primary anticapsule response.

tation of the antigens and the cells and cytokines involved in generating each response.

a. Tetanus toxoid: intramuscular injection of formalin-fixed, heat-inactivated tetanus toxin protein.
b. Inactivated polio vaccine: intramuscular injection of chemically inactivated polio virus incapable of replication.
c. Live, attenuated measles vaccine: intramuscular injection of virus that replicates in cells and expresses antigen in cells and on cell surfaces.

QUESTIONS

1. Describe the types of immune responses that would be generated to the following different types of vaccines. Consider the route of processing and presen-

2. Reproduce (photocopy or write out on separate paper) the table that follows and fill in the appropriate columns:

Immunodeficiency Disease	Immune Defect	Susceptibility to Specific Infections
Chédiak-Higashi syndrome		
Chronic granulomatous disease		
Complement C5 deficiency		
Complement C3 deficiency		
Complement C1 deficiency		
IgA deficiency		
X-linked agammaglobulinemia		
X-linked T-cell deficiency		
AIDS		
DiGeorge syndrome		
IgE deficiency		

BIBLIOGRAPHY

Abbas AK, Lichtman AH, Pober JS: *Cellular and molecular immunology*, ed 4, Philadelphia, 2000, WB Saunders.

Alcami A, Koszinowski UH: Viral mechanisms of immune evasion, *Trends Microbiol* 8:410–418, 2000.

Goldsby RA, Kindt TJ, Osborne BA: *Kuby immunology*, ed 4, New York, 2000, WH Freeman.

Immunology Today: Issues contain understandable reviews on current topics in immunology.

Janeway CA et al: *Immunobiology: the immune system in health and disease*, ed 4, New York, 1999, Current Biology Publications and Garland Press.

Male D et al: *Advanced immunology*, ed 3, St Louis, 1996, Mosby.

Roitt I, Brostoff J, Male D: *Immunology*, ed 4, St Louis, 1996, Mosby.

Sompayrac L: *How the immune system works*, Malden, Mass, 1999, Blackwell Scientific.

CHAPTER 15

Antimicrobial Vaccines

Immune responses, whether generated in reaction to immunization or administered as therapy, can prevent or lessen the serious symptoms of disease by **blocking the spread** of a bacterium, bacterial toxin, or virus to its target organ or by acting rapidly at the site of infection. The immunization of a population, like personal immunity, stops the spread of the infectious agent by reducing the number of susceptible hosts (**herd immunity**). Immunization programs, on national and international levels, have achieved the following goals:

1. Protection of population groups from the symptoms of pertussis, diphtheria, tetanus, and rabies.
2. Control of the spread of measles, mumps, and rubella.
3. Elimination of wild-type poliomyelitis in the Western Hemisphere and smallpox in the world.

In conjunction with immunization programs, measures can be taken to prevent disease by limiting the exposure of healthy people to infected people (**quarantine**) and by eliminating the source (e.g., water purification) or means of spread (e.g., mosquito eradication) of the infectious agent. Smallpox is an example of an infection that was controlled by such means. As of 1977, it has been eliminated through a successful World Health Organization (WHO) program combining vaccination and quarantine.

Vaccine-preventable diseases still occur, however, where immunization programs (1) are unavailable or too expensive (Third World countries) or (2) are neglected (e.g., the United States). An example is measles, which causes 2 million deaths annually worldwide for the first reason and outbreaks of which are becoming more common in the United States for the second reason.

Types of Immunization

The injection of purified antibody or antibody-containing serum for the rapid, temporary protection or treatment of a person is termed **passive immunization**. Newborns receive natural passive immunity from maternal immunoglobulin that crosses the placenta or is present in the mother's milk.

Active immunization occurs when an immune response is stimulated in response to challenge with an immunogen such as exposure to an infectious agent (**natural immunization**) or through exposure to microbes or their antigens in **vaccines**. Upon subsequent challenge with the virulent agent, a secondary immune response is activated that is faster and more effective at protecting the individual or antibody is present to block the spread or function of the agent.

Passive Immunization

Passive immunization may be used as follows:

1. To prevent disease after a known exposure (e.g., needlestick injury with hepatitis B virus–contaminated blood).
2. To ameliorate the symptoms of an ongoing disease.
3. To protect immunosuppressed patients.
4. To block the action of bacterial toxins and prevent the diseases they cause (i.e., as therapy).

Immune serum globulin preparations derived from seropositive humans or animals (e.g., horses) are available as prophylaxis for several bacterial and viral diseases (Table 15–1). Human serum globulin is prepared from pooled plasma and contains the normal repertoire of antibodies for an adult. Special high-titer immune globulin preparations are available for hepatitis B virus (HBIg), varicella zoster virus (VZIg), rabies (RIg), and tetanus (TIg). Human immunoglobulin is preferable to animal immunoglobulin, because there is little risk of a hypersensitivity reaction (serum sickness).

Monoclonal antibody preparations are being developed for protection against various agents and diseases. Also in development are monoclonal antibodies that can block the pathogenic mechanisms associated with infection, such as neutrophil adherence and septic shock.

TABLE 15–1. Immune Globulins Available for Postexposure Prophylaxis*

Disease	Source
Hepatitis A	Human
Hepatitis B	Human†
Measles	Human
Rabies	Human†
Chickenpox, zoster	Human†
Cytomegalovirus	Human
Tetanus	Human,† equine
Botulism	Equine
Diphtheria	Equine

* Immune globulins to other agents may also be available.

† Specific, high-titer antibody is available and is the preferred therapy.

Active Immunization

The term *vaccine* is derived from vaccinia virus, a less virulent member of the poxvirus family that was used to immunize people against smallpox. Vaccines can be subdivided into two groups on the basis of whether they infect the person (**live vaccines** such as vaccinia) or not (**inactivated/subunit/killed vaccines**) (Fig. 15–1). DNA vaccines represent a new potential means of immunization. In this approach, plasmid DNA is injected into muscle or skin, after which it expresses the gene for the immunogen.

Inactivated Vaccines

Inactivated vaccines provide a large amount of antigen to produce a protective antibody response without the risk of infection by the agent. Inactivated vaccines can be produced through the chemical (e.g., formalin) or heat inactivation of bacteria, bacterial toxins, or viruses or through the purification of the components or subunits of the infectious agents.

These vaccines are usually administered with an adjuvant, such as alum, which boosts their immunogenicity. Better adjuvants are being developed that use bacterial cell wall components, synthetic polymers, or liposomes. The adjuvant also influences the type of immune response induced by the vaccine (TH1 or TH2). Attenuated forms of cholera toxin (CT) and *Escherichia coli* lymphotoxin (LT) are being developed as potent adjuvants that promote production of secretory immunoglobulin (Ig) A after intranasal or oral immunization.

Inactivated rather than live vaccines are used to confer protection against most bacteria and viruses that cannot be attenuated, may cause recurrent infection, or have oncogenic potential. Inactivated vaccines are generally safe, except in people who have allergic reactions

to vaccine components. For example, many vaccines are produced in eggs and so cannot be administered to people who are allergic to eggs. The immune response evoked by inactivated vaccines is predominantly a TH2 (antibody) immune response and is more limited than that evoked by live vaccines. The disadvantages of inactivated vaccines in comparison with live vaccines are as follows (Table 15–2):

1. Immunity is not usually lifelong.
2. Immunity may be only humoral and not cell-mediated.
3. The vaccine does not elicit a local IgA response.
4. Booster shots are required.
5. Larger doses must be used.

There are three major types of inactivated bacterial vaccines: **toxoid** (inactivated toxins), **inactivated (killed)** bacteria, and **capsule or protein subunits** of the bacteria. The bacterial vaccines currently available are listed in Table 15–3. Most antibacterial vaccines protect against the pathogenic action of toxins.

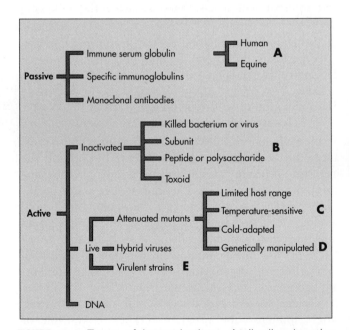

FIGURE 15–1. Types of immunizations. Antibodies (passive immunization) can be provided to block the action of an infectious agent, or an immune response can be elicited (active immunization) by natural infection or vaccination. The different forms of passive and active immunization are indicated. *A,* Equine antibodies can be used if human antibody is not available. *B,* Vaccine can consist of components purified from the infectious agent or can be developed through genetic engineering. *C,* Vaccine selected by passage in animals, embryonated eggs, or tissue culture cells. *D,* Deletion, insertion, reassortment, and other laboratory-derived mutants. *E,* Vaccine composed of a virus from a different species, which has a common antigen with the human virus.

TABLE 15–2. Advantages and Disadvantages of Live Versus Inactivated Vaccines

Property	Live	Inactivated
Route of administration	Natural[a] or injection	Injection
Dose of virus, cost	Low	High
Number of doses	Single[b]	Multiple
Need for adjuvant	No	Yes[c]
Duration of immunity	Long-term	Short-term
Antibody response	IgG, IgA[d]	IgG
Cell-mediated immune response	Good	Poor
Heat lability in tropics	Yes[e]	No
Interference[f]	Occasional	None
Side effects	Occasional mild symptoms[g]	Occasional sore arm
Reversion to virulence	Rarely	None

[a] Oral or respiratory, in certain cases.

[b] A single booster may be required (yellow fever, measles, rubella) after 6–10 years.

[c] However, no satisfactory adjuvants other than alum are licensed for human use.

[d] IgA if delivered via the oral or respiratory route. Oral polio vaccine can prevent wild-type poliovirus from multiplying in the gut and thus facilitate near eradication of the virus from the community.

[e] Magnesium chloride and other stabilizers and cold storage assist preservation.

[f] Interference from other viruses or diseases.

[g] Especially rubella and measles.

Ig = immunoglobulin.

From White DO, Fenner FJ: *Medical virology*, ed 3, New York, 1986, Academic.

Inactivated viral vaccines are available for **polio, hepatitis A, influenza, rabies,** and other viruses. The Salk polio (inactivated poliomyelitis vaccine or IPV) and the influenza vaccines are prepared through the formaldehyde inactivation of virions. The influenza vaccine, which is formulated annually, is a mixture of viruses predicted to threaten the population for the coming year. In the past, a rabies vaccine was prepared by means of formalin inactivation of infected rabbit neurons or duck embryos. Now, however, it is prepared through the chemical inactivation of virions grown in human diploid tissue culture cells. Because of the slow course of rabies, the vaccine can be adminis-

tered immediately after a person is exposed to the virus and still elicit a protective antibody response.

A **subunit vaccine** can be developed after identification of the bacterial or viral components that elicit a protective immune response. Surface structures of bacteria and the viral attachment proteins (capsid or glycoproteins) elicit protective antibodies. T-cell epitopes may also be included in a subunit vaccine. The immunogenic component can be isolated from the bacterium, virus, or virally infected cells by biochemical means, or the vaccine can be prepared through genetic engineering by the expression of cloned viral genes in bacteria or eukaryotic cells. For example, the hepatitis B virus subunit vaccine was initially prepared from surface antigen obtained from human sera of chronic carriers of the virus. The form of vaccine used in the United States is now purified from yeast bearing the gene for the antigen. The antigen is purified, chemically treated, and absorbed onto alum to be used as a vaccine.

Vaccines against *Haemophilus influenzae B, Neisseria meningitidis, Salmonella typhi,* and *Streptococcus pneumoniae* are prepared from **capsular polysaccharides**. Unfortunately, **polysaccharides are generally poor immunogens**. The meningococcal vaccine contains the polysaccharides of four major serotypes (A/C/Y/W-135). The pneumococcal vaccine contains polysaccharides from 23 serotypes. The immunogenicity of polysaccharides can be enhanced by chemical linkage to a protein carrier (**conjugate vaccine**)(e.g., diphtheria toxoid, *N. meningitidis* outer membrane protein, or *Corynebacterium diphtheriae* protein). The *H. influenzae B* polysaccharide–diphtheria toxoid carrier complex (Hib) is approved for administration to infants. An *S. pneumoniae* "pneumococcal" conjugate vaccine has been developed in which polysaccharide from the seven most prevalent strains in the United States is attached to a nontoxic form of the diphtheria toxin (CRM197). This vaccine is available for infants and young children. The other polysaccharide vaccines are less immunogenic and should be administered only to children older than 2 years.

The Lyme disease (*Borrelia burgdorferi*) vaccine is a subunit vaccine that initiates protection in a unique manner. The immunogen consists of an outer membrane protein (OspA) of the bacteria that is expressed while the bacteria is in the vector (deer tick). The antibodies generated in the human are ingested by the tick when it takes its blood meal, and these antibodies inactivate the bacteria to prevent infection and disease.

Live Vaccines

Live vaccines are prepared with organisms limited in their ability to cause disease (**avirulent** or **attenuated**). Live vaccines are especially useful for protection against infections caused by enveloped viruses, which

TABLE 15–3. Bacterial Vaccines*

Bacteria (Disease)	Vaccine Components	Who Should Receive Vaccinations
Corynebacterium diphtheriae (diphtheria)	Toxoid	Children and adults
Clostridium tetani (tetanus)	Toxoid	Children and adults
Bordetella pertussis (pertussis)	Killed cell or acellular	Children
Haemophilus influenzae B (Hib)	Capsule polysaccharide; capsule polysaccharide–protein conjugate	Children
Neisseria meningitidis A and C (meningococcal disease)	Capsule polysaccharide	People at high risk (e.g., those with asplenia), travelers to epidemic areas (e.g., military personnel), children
Streptococcus pneumoniae (pneumococcal disease; meningitis)	Capsule polysaccharides; capsule polysaccharide–protein conjugate	People at high risk (e.g., those with asplenia), children, the elderly
Vibrio cholerae (cholera)	Killed cell	Travelers at risk to exposure
Salmonella typhi (typhoid)	Killed cell, polysaccharide	Travelers at risk to exposure, household contacts, sewage workers
Bacillus anthracis (anthrax)	Killed cell	Handlers of imported fur, military personnel
Yersinia pestis (plague)	Killed cell	Veterinarians, animal handlers
Francisella tularensis (tularemia)	Live attenuated	Animal handlers in endemic areas
Coxiella burnetii (Q fever)	Inactivated	Sheep handlers, laboratory personnel working with *C. burnetii*
Mycobacterium tuberculosis (TB)	Live attenuated bacille Calmette-Guérin *(Mycobacterium bovis)*	Not recommended in United States
Borrelia burgdorferi (Lyme disease)	Subunit	People in endemic regions

*Listed in order of frequency of use.

require T-cell immune responses for resolution of the infection. Immunization with a live vaccine resembles the natural infection, the immune response progresses through TH1 and then TH2 immune responses, and humoral, cellular, and memory immune responses are developed. Immunity is generally long-lived and, depending on the route of administration, can mimic the normal immune response to the infecting agent. However, there are two problems with live vaccines, as follows:

1. The vaccine virus may still be dangerous for immunosuppressed people or pregnant women, who do not have the immunologic resources to resolve even a weakened virus infection.
2. The vaccine may revert to a virulent viral form.

Live bacterial vaccines include the orally administered live, attenuated *S. typhi* strain Ty2la vaccine for typhoid; the Calmette-Guérin bacillus vaccine for tuberculosis, which consists of an attenuated strain of *Mycobacterium bovis*; and an attenuated tularemia vaccine. The antibody and cell-mediated immune responses elicited by a live vaccine may be required

against intracellularly growing bacteria. The Calmette-Guérin bacillus vaccine is not routinely used in the United States because people vaccinated with it show a false-positive reaction to the purified protein derivative (PPD) test, which is the screening test used to control tuberculosis in the United States.

Live virus vaccines consist of less virulent mutants (**attenuated**) of the wild-type virus, viruses from other species that share antigenic determinants, or genetically engineered viruses lacking virulence properties (see Fig. 15–1). Wild-type viruses are attenuated by growth in embryonated eggs or tissue culture cells, at nonphysiologic temperatures (32°C to 34°C), and away from the selective pressures of the host immune response. These conditions **select** for, or allow the growth of, viral strains (mutants) that (1) are less virulent because they grow poorly at 37°C (**temperature-sensitive strains** [e.g., measles vaccine] and cold-adapted strains), (2) do not replicate well in any human cell (**host-range mutants**), (3) cannot escape immune control, or (4) can replicate at a benign site but do not disseminate, bind, or replicate in the target tissue characteristically affected by the disease (e.g., polio vaccine replicates in the gastrointestinal tract but does not reach or infect the brain). Examples of attenuated live virus vaccines currently in use are listed in Table 15–4.

The first vaccine, that for smallpox, was developed by Jenner. The idea for the vaccine came to him when he noted that cowpox (vaccinia), a virulent virus from another species that shares antigenic determinants with smallpox, caused benign infections in humans but conferred protective immunity against smallpox. Similarly, the vaccine for the first tumor virus, Marek's disease virus of chickens, consists of the turkey herpesvirus. In addition, vaccines consisting of bovine, simian, or a reassortment of these rotaviruses have shown success in protecting infants against human rotavirus in clinical trials.

Sabin developed the first live oral polio vaccine (OPV) in the 1950s. The attenuated virus vaccine is obtained by multiple passage of the three types of poliovirus through monkey kidney tissue culture cells. At least 57 mutations are accumulated in the polio type 1 vaccine strain. When this vaccine is administered orally, IgA is secreted in the gut and IgG in the serum, providing protection along the normal route of infec-

tion by the wild-type virus. The vaccination program has been so successful that wild-type polio has been eliminated in the Western Hemisphere. Unfortunately, because of the risk of vaccine virus–induced polio disease, the IPV is favored over the OPV for routine well-baby immunizations (Fig. 15–2).

Live vaccines for measles, mumps, rubella (administered together as the MMR vaccine) and now varicella-zoster have been developed. Protection against these infections requires a potent cellular immune response, so the vaccine is administered at 2 years of age, late enough to prevent interference by maternal antibodies and to elicit a mature T-cell response. A killed measles vaccine proved to be a failure because it conferred an incomplete immunity that induced more serious symptoms (atypical measles) on challenge with wild-type measles virus than the symptoms associated with the natural infection.

The initial live measles vaccine consisted of the Edmonston B strain, which was developed by Enders and colleagues. This virus underwent extensive passage at 35°C through primary human kidney cells, human amnion cells, and chicken embryo cells. The currently used Moraten (United States) and Schwarz (other

---

TABLE 15–4. Viral Vaccines*

Virus	Vaccine Components	Who Should Receive Vaccinations
Polio	Inactivated (IPV, Salk vaccine)	Children
	Attenuated (oral polio vaccine, Sabin vaccine)	Children
Measles	Attenuated	Children
Mumps	Attenuated	Children
Rubella	Attenuated	Children
Varicella-zoster	Attenuated	Children
Influenza	Inactivated	Adults, especially medical personnel and the elderly
Hepatitis B	Subunit	Newborns, health care workers, high-risk groups (e.g., promiscuous people, intravenous drug users)
Hepatitis A	Inactivated	Children, child-care workers, travelers to endemic areas, Native Americans and Alaskans
	Live (China)	
Adenovirus	Attenuated	Military personnel
Yellow fever	Attenuated	Travelers at risk to exposure, military personnel
Rabies	Inactivated	Anyone exposed to virus
		Preexposure: veterinarians, animal handlers
Rotavirus	Rhesus/bovine/human hybrids	In development
Smallpox	Live vaccinia virus	No longer necessary
Japanese encephalitis	Inactivated	Travelers at risk to exposure
Eastern, Western, Russian spring-summer encephalitis viruses	Inactivated	Military personnel

*Listed in order of frequency of use.

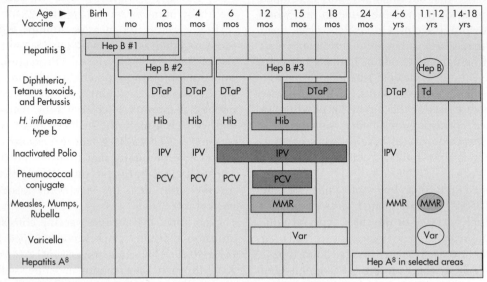

Recommended Childhood Immunization Schedule
United States, January - December 2000

Vaccines are listed under routinely recommended ages. Bars indicate range of recommended ages for immunization. Any dose not given at the recommended age should be given as a "catch-up" immunization at any subsequent visit when indicated and feasible. Ovals indicate vaccines to be given if previously recommended doses were missed or given earlier than the recommended minimum age.

Age ▶ Vaccine ▼	Birth	1 mo	2 mos	4 mos	6 mos	12 mos	15 mos	18 mos	24 mos	4-6 yrs	11-12 yrs	14-18 yrs
Hepatitis B		Hep B #1										
			Hep B #2			Hep B #3					Hep B	
Diphtheria, Tetanus toxoids, and Pertussis			DTaP	DTaP	DTaP		DTaP			DTaP	Td	
H. influenzae type b			Hib	Hib	Hib	Hib						
Inactivated Polio			IPV	IPV		IPV				IPV		
Pneumococcal conjugate			PCV	PCV	PCV	PCV						
Measles, Mumps, Rubella						MMR				MMR	MMR	
Varicella						Var					Var	
Hepatitis A⁸									Hep A⁸ in selected areas			

Approved by the Advisory Committee on Immunization Practices (ACIP), the American Academy of Pediatrics (AAP), and the American Academy of Family Physicians (AAFP).

FIGURE 15–2. Recommended immunization schedule from the Centers for Disease Control and Prevention. Vaccines are listed at the ages routinely recommended for their administration. *Bars* indicate the range of acceptable ages for vaccination. For example, hepatitis B vaccine should be administered to children at 11 to 12 years of age who have not been previously vaccinated; varicella-zoster virus vaccine should be administered to children who were not previously vaccinated and who lack a reliable history of chickenpox. DTaP = diphtheria and tetanus toxoids and acellular pertussis vaccines; Td = tetanus and diphtheria toxoids, absorbed, for adult use.

countries) vaccine strains of measles were obtained by further passage of the Edmonston B strain in chick embryos at 32°C.

The mumps vaccine (Jeryl Lynn strain) and rubella vaccine (Wistar RA 27/3) viruses were also attenuated by extensive passage of the virus in cell culture. The varicella-zoster vaccine uses the Oka strain, an attenuated virus. The varicella-zoster vaccine requires a mature T-cell response, and is administered along with the MMR vaccine.

Future Directions for Vaccination

Molecular biology techniques are being used to develop new vaccines. New live vaccines can be created by genetic engineering mutations to inactivate or delete a virulence gene instead of through random attenuation of the virus by passage through tissue culture. Genes from infectious agents that cannot be properly attenuated can be inserted into safe viruses (e.g., vaccinia, canarypox) to form **hybrid virus vaccines**. This

approach holds the promise of allowing the development of a polyvalent vaccine to many agents in a single, safe, inexpensive, and relatively stable vector. Upon infection, the hybrid virus vaccine need not complete a replication cycle but will express and initiate an immune response to the inserted antigens. The vaccinia and canarypox virus vector systems have been used in several experimental hybrid vaccines and for the rabies vaccine for forest animals. Other vectors that have been considered are retroviruses, adenovirus, and herpes simplex virus.

A new **defective infectious single-cycle virus (DISC)** vaccine would immunize an individual but could proceed through only one round of virus replication. A virus with a deletion of an essential gene is grown in a tissue culture cell that expresses the gene to "complement" the defect in the virus. Upon vaccination, the progeny virus infects the host and produces only one round of virus, sufficient for immunization, but the new virus cannot replicate.

Genetically engineered **subunit vaccines** are being

developed through cloning of genes encoding immunogenic proteins into bacterial and eukaryotic vectors. The greatest difficulties in the development of such vaccines are (1) identifying the appropriate subunit or peptide immunogen that can elicit protective antibody and, ideally, T-cell responses and (2) presenting the antigen in the correct conformation. Once identified, the gene can be isolated, cloned, and expressed in bacteria or yeast cells, and then large quantities of these proteins can be produced. Genes for protective immunogens such as the surface antigen of hepatitis B (*in use*), the glycoprotein 120 of the human immunodeficiency virus (HIV), the hemagglutinin of influenza, the G antigen of rabies, and the glycoprotein D of herpes simplex virus have been cloned and their proteins generated in bacteria or eukaryotic cells for use or potential use as subunit vaccines. Use of a virus-like particle (VLP), assembled from the genetically engineered capsid proteins of papillomavirus, has shown promise in animal trials.

Peptide subunit vaccines consist of *specific epitopes* of microbial proteins that elicit neutralizing antibody or desired T-cell responses. To generate such a response, the peptide must contain sequences that allow it to be processed by an antigen-presenting cell, to bind to a major histocompatibility complex (MHC) antigen for presentation to T cells, and to be recognized by helper T cells to facilitate antibody production. The immunogenicity of the peptide can be enhanced by its covalent attachment to a carrier protein (such as tetanus toxoid or keyhole limpet hemocyanine) or an immunologic peptide that can specifically present the epitope to the appropriate immune response. Better vaccines will be developed as the mechanisms of antigen presentation and T-cell receptor–specific antigens become better understood.

Anti-idiotype antibodies are also being investigated as potential vaccines. Such antibodies recognize the variable region of a monoclonal antiviral antibody, which is like a cast of the viral epitope. The anti-idiotype antibody resembles the original viral epitope, as if it were molded in the cast. Immunization with an anti-idiotype antibody or the viral peptide would therefore elicit the production of similar antibodies.

DNA vaccines offer great potential for immunization against infectious agents that require T-cell and antibody responses but that are not appropriate for use in live vaccines. For these vaccines, the gene for a protein that elicits protective responses is cloned into a plasmid that allows the protein to be expressed in eukaryotic cells. The naked DNA is injected into the muscle or skin of the vaccine recipient, where the DNA is taken up by cells, the gene is expressed, and the protein is produced and presented to the immune response to elicit TH1 and TH2 responses. It is easier to develop a DNA vaccine than other types of vaccines.

With the advent of new technology, it should be possible to develop vaccines against infectious agents such as *Streptococcus mutans* (to prevent tooth decay), the herpesviruses, HIV, and parasites such as *Plasmodium falciparum* (malaria) and *Leishmania*. In fact, it should be possible to produce a vaccine to almost any infectious agent once the appropriate protective immunogen is identified and its gene isolated.

Immunization Programs

An effective vaccine program can save millions of dollars in health care costs. Such a program not only protects each vaccinated person against infection and disease but also reduces the number of susceptible people in the population, thereby preventing the spread of the infectious agent within the population. Although immunization may be the best means of protecting people against infection, vaccines cannot be developed for all infectious agents. One reason is that it is very time-consuming and costly to develop vaccines. Considerations that are weighed in the choice of a candidate for a vaccine program are listed in Box 15–1.

Smallpox was eliminated by means of an effective vaccine program because it was a good candidate for such a program; the virus existed in only one serotype, symptoms were always present in infected people, and the vaccine was relatively benign and stable. However, its elimination came about only as the result of a concerted, cooperative effort on the part of the WHO and local health agencies worldwide. Rhinovirus is an example of a poor candidate for vaccine development, because the viral disease is not serious and there are too many serotypes for vaccination to be successful. Practical aspects of and problems with vaccine development are listed in Box 15–2.

From the standpoint of the individual, the ideal vaccine should elicit dependable, lifelong immunity to infection without serious side effects. Factors that influence the success of an immunization program include not only the composition of the vaccine but also the timing, site, and conditions of its administration.

The recommended schedules of vaccinations for children are given in Figure 15–2. Infants are immu-

---

BOX 15–1. **Properties of a Good Candidate for Vaccine Development**

Organism causes significant illness.
  Organism exists as only one serotype.
  Antibody blocks infection or systemic spread.
  Organism does not have oncogenic potential.
  Vaccine is heat-stable so that it can be transported to endemic areas.

BOX 15–2. Problems with Vaccine Use

Live vaccine can occasionally revert to virulent forms.

Interference by other organisms may prevent the infection produced by a live virus vaccine; for example, rubella prevents replication of polio virus.

Vaccination of an immunocompromised person with a live vaccine can be life-threatening.

Side effects to vaccination can occur; these include hypersensitivity and allergic reactions to the antigen, to nonmicrobial material in the vaccine, and to contaminants (e.g., eggs).

Vaccine development and liability insurance for the manufacturer are very expensive.

Organisms with many serotypes are difficult to control with vaccination.

---

nized with the diphtheria, tetanus, pertussis, (DTP), and Hib inactivated vaccines as well as the inactivated or live oral polio vaccine. The inactivated hepatitis A vaccine can also be administered on this schedule or to adults at risk of infection. The hepatitis B vaccine is suggested for the first year of life as well as later in life. The live MMR and varicella-zoster vaccines are administered at 2 years of age, after the baby's immune response has matured and maternal antibodies have dissipated. Booster immunizations of inactivated vaccines and the live measles vaccine are required later in life. Adults should be immunized with vaccines for *S. pneumoniae* (pneumococcus), influenza, rabies, hepatitis B virus, and other diseases, depending on their jobs, the type of traveling they do, and other risk factors that may make them particularly susceptible to specific infectious agents.

QUESTIONS

1. Why is an inactivated rather than a live vaccine used for the following immunizations: rabies, influenza, tetanus, hepatitis B virus, *H. influenzae* B, diphtheria, and pertussis?

2. Tetanus is treated with passive immunization and prevented by active immunization. Compare the nature and function of each of these therapies.

3. The inactivated polio vaccine is administered intramuscularly, whereas the live polio vaccine is administered as an oral vaccine. How do the course of the immune response and the immunoglobulins produced in response to each vaccine differ? What step in poliovirus infection is blocked in a person vaccinated by each vaccine?

4. Why have large-scale vaccine programs not been developed for rhinovirus, herpes simplex virus, and respiratory syncytial virus?

5. Describe the public or personal health benefits that justify the development of the following major vaccine programs: measles, mumps, rubella, polio, smallpox, tetanus, and pertussis.

BIBLIOGRAPHY

Advisory Committee on Immunization Practices (ACIP): Statements [on line]. Available at http://www2.cdc.gov/mmwr

Centers for Disease Control and Prevention: Immunization information page [on line]. (1997). Available at http://www.cdc.gov/diseases/immuni.html

Conrad DA, Jensen HB: New and improved vaccines, *Postgrad Med* 100:113–127, 1996.

Hill DR: Immunizations, *Infect Dis Clin North Am* 6:291, 1992.

National Coalition for Adult Immunization [on line]. Available at http://www.nfid.org/ncai/

Plotkin SA, Orenstein WA: *Vaccines*, ed 3, Philadelphia, 1999, WB Saunders.

Vaccination information sheets [on line]. Available at http://www.immunize.org/vis

Vaccines: NIAID fact sheet [on line]. Available at http://www.niaid.nih.gov/publications/vaccine.htm

World Health Organization: Diseases and vaccines [on line]. Available at http://www.who.int/vaccines-diseases/index.html

General Principles of Laboratory Diagnosis

CHAPTER 16

Microscopic Principles and Applications

The true complexity of our surroundings was unappreciated until microorganisms were revealed with the microscope. Indeed, the use of microscopy has helped define the relationships among a diversity of organisms, ranging from the smallest viruses consisting of a few proteins and minimal genetic information to multicellular parasites almost 10 m long.

In general, microscopy is used in microbiology for two basic purposes: the initial detection of microbes and the preliminary or definitive identification of microbes. The microscopic examination of clinical specimens is used to detect bacterial cells, fungal elements, parasites (eggs, larvae, or adult-forms), and viral inclusions present in infected cells. Characteristic morphologic properties can be used for the preliminary identification of most bacteria and are used for the definitive identification of many fungi and parasites. The microscopic detection of organisms stained with antibodies labeled with fluorescent dyes or other markers has proved to be very useful for the specific identification of many viruses and bacteria. Five general microscopic methods have been used (Box 16–1).

Microscopic Methods

Brightfield (Light) Microscopy

The basic components of light microscopes consist of a light source used to illuminate the specimen positioned on a stage, a condenser used to focus the light on the specimen, and two lens systems (**objective lens** and **ocular lens**) used to magnify the image of the specimen. In brightfield microscopy, the specimen is visualized by transillumination, with light passing up through the condenser to the specimen. The image is then magnified first by the objective lens and then by the ocular lens. The total magnification of the image is the product of the magnifications of the objective and ocular lenses. Three different objective lenses are commonly used: low power ($\times 10$), which can be used to scan a specimen; high dry ($\times 40$), which is used to look for large microbes such as parasites and filamentous fungi; and oil immersion ($\times 100$), which is used to observe bacteria, yeasts (single-cell stage of fungi), and the morphologic details of larger organisms and cells. Ocular lenses can further magnify the image (generally, 10- to 15-fold).

The limitation of brightfield microscopy is the resolution of the image (i.e., the ability to distinguish that two objects are separate and not one). The **resolving power** of a microscope is determined by the wavelength of light used to illuminate the subject and the angle of light entering the objective lens (referred to as the **numerical aperture**). The best brightfield microscopes have a resolving power of approximately 0.2 μm, which allows most bacteria but not viruses to be visualized. Although most bacteria and larger microorganisms can be seen with brightfield microscopy, the **refractive indices** of the organisms and background are similar. Thus, organisms must be stained with a dye so that they can be observed, or an alternative method must be used.

Darkfield Microscopy

The same objective and ocular lenses used in brightfield microscopes are used in darkfield microscopes; however, a special **condenser** is used that prevents transmitted light from directly illuminating the specimen. Only oblique, scattered light reaches the specimen and passes into the lens systems, which causes the specimen to be brightly illuminated against a black background. The advantage of this method is that the resolving power of darkfield microscopy is significantly improved compared with that of brightfield microscopy (i.e., 0.02 μm versus 0.2 μm), which makes it possible for extremely thin bacteria such as *Treponema pallidum* (etiologic agent of syphilis), *Borrelia burgdorferi* (Lyme disease), and *Leptospira* spp. (leptospirosis) to be de-

BOX 16–1. Microscopic Methods

Brightfield (light) microscopy
Darkfield microscopy
Phase-contrast microscopy
Fluorescent microscopy
Electron microscopy

tected. The disadvantage of this method is that because light passes around rather than through organisms, their internal structure cannot be studied.

Phase-Contrast Microscopy

Phase-contrast microscopy enables the internal details of microbes to be examined. In this form of microscopy, as parallel beams of light are passed through objects of different densities, the wavelength of one beam moves out of "phase" relative to the other beam of light (i.e., the beam moving through the more dense material is retarded more than the other beam). Through the use of **annular rings** in the condenser and the objective lens, the differences in phase are amplified so that in-phase light appears brighter than out-of-phase light. This creates a three-dimensional image of the organism or specimen, which permits more detailed analysis of the internal structures.

Fluorescent Microscopy

Some compounds called **fluorochromes** can absorb short-wavelength ultraviolet or ultrablue light and emit energy at a higher visible wavelength. Although some microorganisms show natural fluorescence (**autofluorescence**), fluorescent microscopy typically involves staining organisms with fluorescent dyes and then examining them with a specially designed fluorescent microscope. The microscope uses a high-pressure mercury, halogen, or xenon vapor lamp that emits a shorter wavelength of light than that emitted by traditional brightfield microscopes. A series of filters are used to block the heat generated from the lamp, eliminate infrared light, and select the appropriate wavelength for exciting the fluorochrome. The light emitted from the fluorochrome is then magnified through traditional objective and ocular lenses. Organisms and specimens stained with fluorochromes appear brightly illuminated against a black background, although the colors vary depending on the fluorochrome selected. The contrast between the organism and background is great enough that the specimen can be screened rap-

idly under low magnification and then the material examined under higher magnification once fluorescence is detected.

Electron Microscopy

Unlike other forms of microscopy, **magnetic coils** (rather than lenses) are used in electron microscopes to direct a beam of electrons from a tungsten filament through a specimen and onto a screen. Because a much shorter wavelength of light is used, magnification and resolution are improved dramatically. Individual viral particles (as opposed to viral inclusion bodies) can be seen with electron microscopy. Samples are usually stained or coated with metal ions to create contrast. There are two types of electron microscopes: **transmission electron microscopes**, in which electrons like light pass directly through the specimen, and **scanning electron microscopes**, in which electrons bounce off the surface of the specimen at an angle and a three-dimensional picture is produced.

Examination Methods

Clinical specimens or suspensions of microorganisms can be placed on a glass slide and examined under the microscope (i.e., direct examination of a wet mount). Although large organisms and cellular material can be seen using this method, analysis of the internal detail is frequently difficult. Phase-contrast microscopy can overcome some of these problems; alternatively, the specimen or organism can be stained by a variety of methods (Table 16–1).

Direct Examination

Direct examination methods are the simplest for preparing samples for microscopic examination. The sample can be suspended in water or saline (**wet mount**), mixed with alkali to dissolve background material (**potassium hydroxide [KOH] method**), or mixed with a combination of alkali and a contrasting dye (e.g., **lactophenol cotton blue, iodine**). The dyes nonspecifically stain the cellular material, increasing the contrast with the background, and permit examination of the detailed structures. A variation is the **India ink method**, in which the ink darkens the background rather than the cell. This method is used to detect capsules surrounding organisms such as the yeast *Cryptococcus* (the dye is excluded by the capsule, creating a clear halo around the yeast cell) and is a rapid method for the preliminary detection and identification of this important fungus.

TABLE 16–1. Microscopic Preparations and Stains Used in the Clinical Microbiology Laboratory

Staining Method	Principle and Applications
Direct Examination	
Wet mount	Unstained preparation examined by brightfield, darkfield, or phase-contrast microscopy.
10% KOH	KOH used to dissolve proteinaceous material and facilitate detection of fungal elements that are not affected by strong alkali solution. Dyes such as lactophenol cotton blue can be added to increase contrast between fungal elements and background.
India ink	Modification of KOH procedure in which ink is added as contrast material. Dye primarily used to detect *Cryptococcus* species in cerebrospinal fluid and other body fluids. Polysaccharide capsule of *Cryptococcus* species excludes ink, creating halo around yeast cell.
Lugol's iodine	Iodine is added to wet preparations of parasitology specimens to enhance contrast of internal structures. Facilitates differentiation of ameba and host white blood cells.
Differential Stains	
Gram stain	Most commonly used stain in microbiology laboratory, forming basis for separating major groups of bacteria (e.g., gram-positive, gram-negative). After fixation of specimen to glass slide (by heating or alcohol treatment), specimen is exposed to crystal violet, and then iodine is added to form complex with primary dye. During decolorization with alcohol or acetone, complex is retained in gram-positive bacteria but lost in gram-negative organisms; counterstain safranin is retained by gram-negative organisms (hence, their red color). Degree to which organism retains stain is function of organism, culture conditions, and staining skills of microscopist.
Iron hematoxylin stain	Used for detection and identification of fecal protozoa. Helminth eggs and larvae retain too much stain and are more easily identified with wet-mount preparation.
Methenamine silver stain	Generally performed in histology laboratories rather than in microbiology laboratories. Used primarily for detection of fungal elements in tissue, although other organisms, such as bacteria, can be detected. Silver staining requires skill because nonspecific staining can render slides uninterpretable.
Toluidine blue O stain	Used primarily for detection of *Pneumocystis* organisms in respiratory specimens. Cysts stain reddish blue to dark purple on light-blue background. Background staining is removed by sulfation reagent. Yeast cells stain and are difficult to distinguish from *Pneumocystis* cells. Trophozoites do not stain. Many laboratories have replaced this stain with specific fluorescent stains.
Trichrome stain	Alternative to iron hematoxylin for staining protozoa. Protozoa have bluish-green to purple cytoplasms with red or purplish-red nuclei and inclusion bodies; specimen background is green.
Wright-Giemsa stain	Used to detect blood parasites; viral and chlamydial inclusion bodies; and *Borrelia*, *Toxoplasma*, *Pneumocystis*, and *Rickettsia* species. Polychromatic stain that contains mixture of methylene blue, azure B, and eosin Y. Giemsa stain combines methylene blue and eosin. Eosin ions are negatively charged and stain basic components of cells orange to pink, whereas other dyes stain acidic cell structures various shades of blue to purple. Protozoan trophozoites have red nucleus and grayish-blue cytoplasm; intracellular yeasts and inclusion bodies typically stain blue; rickettsiae, chlamydiae, and *Pneumocystis* species stain purple.
Acid-Fast Stains	
Ziehl-Neelsen stain	Used to stain mycobacteria, as well as other acid-fast organisms. Organisms are stained with basic carbolfuchsin and resist decolorization with acid-alkali solutions. Background is counterstained with methylene blue. Organisms appear red against light-blue background. Uptake of carbolfuchsin requires heating specimen (hot acid-fast stain).
Kinyoun stain	Cold acid-fast stain (does not require heating). Same principle as Ziehl-Neelsen stain.
Auramine-rhodamine stain	Same principle as other acid-fast stains except that fluorescent dyes (auramine and rhodamine) are used for primary stain and potassium permanganate (strong oxidizing agent) is the counterstain and inactivates unbound fluorochrome dyes. Organisms fluoresce yellowish green against black background.

(continued)

Staining Method	Principle and Applications
TABLE 16–1. *continued*	
Modified acid-fast stain	Weak decolorizing agent is used with any of three acid-fast stains listed. Whereas mycobacteria are strongly acid-fast, other organisms stain more weakly (e.g., *Nocardia, Rhodococcus, Tsukamurella, Gordona, Cryptosporidium, Isospora, Sarcocystis,* and *Cyclospora*). These organisms can be stained more efficiently by using weak decolorizing agent. Organisms that retain this stain are referred to as partially acid-fast.
Fluorescent Stains	
Acridine orange stain	Used for detection of bacteria and fungi in clinical specimens. Dye intercalates into nucleic acid (native and denatured). At neutral pH, bacteria, fungi, and cellular material stain reddish orange. At acid pH (4.0), bacteria and fungi remain reddish orange, but background material stains greenish yellow.
Auramine-rhodamine stain	Same as acid-fast stains.
Calcofluor white stain	Used to detect fungal elements and *Pneumocystis* species. Stain binds to cellulose and chitin in cell walls; microscopist can mix dye with KOH. (Many laboratories have replaced traditional KOH stain with this stain.)
Direct fluorescent antibody stain	Antibodies (monoclonal or polyclonal) are complexed with fluorescent molecules. Specific binding to an organism is detected by presence of microbial fluorescence. Technique has proved useful for detecting or identifying many organisms (e.g., *Streptococcus pyogenes; Bordetella, Francisella, Legionella, Chlamydia, Cryptosporidium,* and *Giardia;* influenza virus; herpes simplex virus). Sensitivity and specificity of the test are determined by the number of organisms present in the test sample and quality of antibodies used in reagents.

KOH = potassium hydroxide.

Differential Stains

A variety of differential stains are used to stain specific organisms or components of cellular material. The **Gram stain** is the best known and most widely used stain and forms the basis for the phenotypic classification of bacteria. Yeasts can also be stained with this method (yeasts are gram-positive). The **iron hematoxylin** and **trichrome** stains are invaluable for the identification of protozoan parasites, and the **Wright-Giemsa** stain is used to identify blood parasites and other selected organisms. Stains such as methenamine silver and toluidine blue O have largely been replaced by more sensitive or technically easier to use differential or fluorescent stains.

Acid-Fast Stains

At least three different acid-fast stains are used, each exploiting the fact that some organisms retain a primary stain even when exposed to strong decolorizing agents such as mixtures of acids and alcohols. The **Ziehl-Neelsen** is the oldest method used but requires heating the specimen during the staining procedure. Many laboratories have now replaced this method with either the cold acid-fast stain (**Kinyoun method**) or the fluorochrome stain (**auramine-rhodamine method**).

The fluorochrome method is preferred, however, because a large area of the specimen can be examined rapidly by simply searching for fluorescing organisms against a black background. Some organisms are "partially acid-fast," retaining the primary stain only when they are decolorized with a weakly acidic solution. This property is characteristic of a only a few organisms (see Table 16–1), making it quite valuable for their preliminary identification.

Fluorescent Stains

The auramine-rhodamine acid-fast stain is a specific example of a fluorescent stain. Numerous other fluorescent dyes have also been used to stain specimens. For example, the **acridine orange stain** can be used to stain bacteria and fungi, and **calcofluor white** stains the chitin in fungal cell walls. Although the acridine orange stain is rather limited in its applications, the calcofluor white stain has replaced the potassium hydroxide stains. Another procedure is the examination of specimens with specific antibodies labeled with fluorescent dyes (**fluorescent antibody stains**). The presence of fluorescing organisms is a rapid method for both the detection and identification of the organism.

QUESTIONS

1. Explain the principles underlying brightfield, darkfield, phase-contrast, fluorescent, and electron microscopy. Give one example in which each method would be used.

2. List three examples of direct microscopic examinations, differential stains, acid-fast stains, and fluorescent stains.

BIBLIOGRAPHY

Chapin K, Murray P: Reagents, stains, and media. In Murray P et al, editors: *Manual of clinical microbiology*, ed 7, Washington, DC, 1999, American Society for Microbiology.

Murray P: *ASM pocket guide to clinical microbiology*, ed. 2, Washington, DC, 1998, American Society for Microbiology.

CHAPTER 17

Molecular Diagnosis

Like the evidence left at the scene of a crime, the DNA, RNA, or proteins of an infectious agent in a clinical sample can be used to help identify the agent. In many cases, the agent can be detected and identified in this way even if it cannot be isolated or detected by immunologic means. New techniques and applications of the techniques are being developed for the analysis of infectious agents.

The advantages of molecular techniques are their sensitivity, specificity, and safety. From the standpoint of their safety, these techniques do not require isolation of the infectious agent and can be performed on chemically fixed (inactivated) samples or extracts. Because of their sensitivity, very dilute samples of microbial DNA can be detected in a tissue even if the agent is not replicating or producing other evidence of infection. The potential specificity of these techniques allows strains to be distinguished on the basis of differences in their genotype (i.e., mutants). This is especially useful for distinguishing antiviral drug-resistant strains, which may differ by a single nucleotide.

Detection of Microbial Genetic Material

Electrophoretic Analysis of DNA and Restriction Fragment Length Polymorphism

The genome structure and genetic sequence are major distinguishing characteristics of the family, type, and strain of microorganism. Specific strains of microorganisms can be distinguished on the basis of their DNA or RNA or by the DNA fragments produced when the DNA is cleaved by specific restriction endonucleases (**restriction enzymes**). Restriction enzymes recognize specific DNA sequences that have a palindromic structure; an example follows:

$\rightarrow$

G AATTC   EcoR1 recognition sequence

CTTAA G   and cleavage

$\leftarrow$

The DNA sites recognized by restriction endonucleases differ in their sequence, length, and frequency of occurrence. As a result, different restriction endonucleases cleave the DNA of a sample in different places, yielding fragments of different lengths. The cleavage of different DNA samples with one restriction endonuclease can also yield fragments of many different lengths. The differences in the length of the DNA fragments among the different strains of a specific organism produced on cleavage with one or more restriction endonucleases is termed **restriction fragment length polymorphism** (RFLP).

DNA or RNA fragments of different sizes or structures can be distinguished by their electrophoretic mobility in an agarose or polyacrylamide gel. Different forms of the same DNA sequence and different lengths of DNA move through the mazelike structure of an agarose gel at different speeds, allowing their separation. The DNA can be visualized by staining with ethidium bromide. Smaller fragments (fewer than 20,000 base pairs), such as those from bacterial plasmids or from viruses, can be separated and distinguished by normal electrophoretic methods. Larger fragments, such as those from whole bacteria, can be separated only by using a special electrophoretic technique called pulsed-field gel electrophoresis.

RFLP is useful, for example, for distinguishing different strains of herpes simplex virus (HSV). Comparison of the electrophoretic analysis of the restriction endonuclease cleavage patterns of DNA from different isolates can identify a pattern of virus transmission from one person to another or can distinguish HSV-1 from HSV-2. RFLP has also been used to show, for example, the spread of a strain of *Streptococcus* producing necrotizing fasciitis from one patient to other patients, an emergency medical technician, and the emergency department and attending physicians (Fig. 17–1).

Genetic Probes

DNA probes can be used like antibodies as sensitive and specific tools to detect, locate, and quantitate spe-

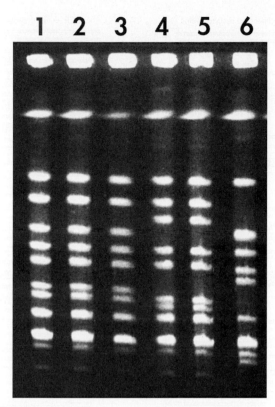

FIGURE 17–1. Restriction fragment length polymorphism distinction of DNA from bacterial strains separated by pulsed-field gel electrophoresis. Lanes *1* to *3* show Sma1–digested DNA isolated from two family members with necrotizing fasciitis and from their physician (pharyngitis). Lanes *4* to *6* are from unrelated *Streptococcus pyogenes* strains. (Courtesy of Dr. Joe DiPersio, Akron, Ohio.)

DNA probe allows the use of a fluorescent- or enzyme-labeled avidin or streptavidin (a protein that binds tightly to biotin) molecule to detect viral nucleic acids in a cell in a way similar to the way in which indirect immunofluorescence or an enzyme immunoassay localizes an antigen.

The DNA probes can detect specific genetic sequences in fixed, permeabilized tissue biopsy specimens

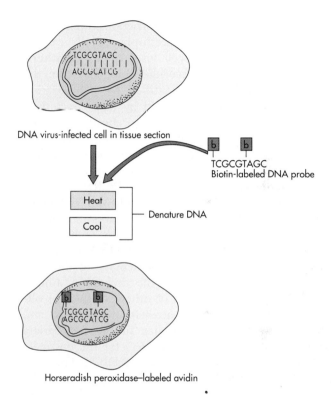

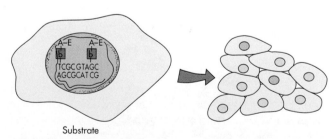

FIGURE 17–2. DNA probe analysis of virus-infected cells. Such cells can be localized in histologically prepared tissue sections using DNA probes consisting of as few as nine nucleotides or bacterial plasmids containing the viral gene. A tagged DNA probe is added to the sample. In this case, the DNA probe is labeled with biotin-modified thymidine, but radioactive agents can also be used. The sample is heated to denature the DNA and cooled to allow the probe to hybridize to the complementary sequence. Horseradish peroxidase–labeled avidin is added to bind to the biotin on the probe. The appropriate substrate is added to color the nuclei of virally infected cells. *b*, biotin; *C*, cytosine; *G*, guanine; *A*, adenine.

cific nucleic acid sequences in clinical specimens (Fig. 17–2). Because of the specificity and sensitivity of DNA probe techniques, individual species or strains of an infectious agent can be detected even if they are not growing or replicating.

DNA probes are chemically synthesized or obtained by cloning specific genomic fragments or an entire viral genome into bacterial vectors (plasmids, cosmids). DNA copies of RNA viruses are made with the retrovirus reverse transcriptase and then cloned into these vectors. After chemical or heat treatments to melt (separate) the DNA strands in the sample, the DNA probe is added and allowed to **hybridize** (bind) with the identical or nearly identical sequence in the sample. The **stringency** (the requirement for an exact sequence match) of the interaction can be varied so that related sequences can be detected or different strains (mutants) can be distinguished. The DNA probes are labeled with radioactive or chemically modified nucleotides (e.g., biotinylated uridine) so that they can be detected and quantitated. The use of a biotin-labeled

by **in situ hybridization**. The localization of cytomegalovirus- (Fig. 17–3) or papillomavirus-infected cells by in situ hybridization is preferable to an immunologic means of doing so and is the only commercially available means of localizing papillomavirus. There are now many commercially available viral probes and kits for detecting viruses.

Specific nucleic acid sequences in extracts from a clinical sample can be detected by applying a small volume of the extract to a nitrocellulose filter (**dot blot**) and then probing the filter with labeled, specific viral DNA. Alternatively, the restriction endonuclease cleavage pattern separated electrophoretically can be transferred onto a nitrocellulose filter (**Southern blot**—DNA:DNA probe hybridization), and then the specific sequence can be identified by hybridization with a specific genetic probe and by its characteristic electrophoretic mobility. Electrophoretically separated RNA (**Northern blot**—RNA:DNA probe hybridization) blotted onto a nitrocellulose filter can be detected in a similar manner.

The **polymerase chain reaction** (**PCR**) can detect single copies of viral DNA by amplifying the DNA many million-fold and is one of the newest techniques of genetic analysis (Fig. 17–4). In this technique, a sample is incubated with two short DNA oligomers, termed **primers**, that are complementary to the ends of a known genetic sequence of the viral DNA, a heat-stable DNA polymerase (Taq or other polymerases obtained from thermophilic bacteria), nucleotides, and buffers. The oligomers hybridize to the appropriate sequence of DNA and act as primers for the polymerase, which copies that segment of the DNA. The sample is then heated to denature the DNA (separating the

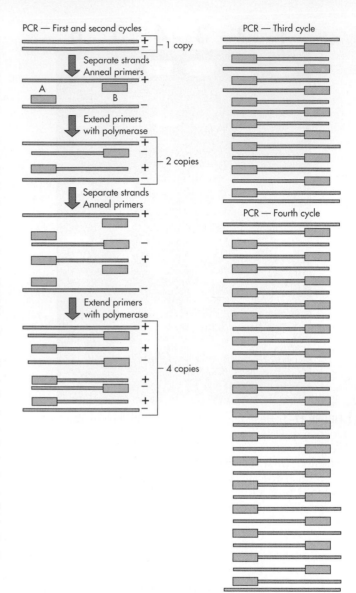

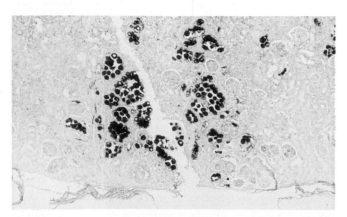

FIGURE 17–3. In situ localization of cytomegalovirus (CMV) infection using a genetic probe. CMV infection of the renal tubules of a kidney is localized with a biotin-labeled, CMV-specific DNA probe and is visualized by means of the horseradish peroxidase–conjugated avidin conversion of substrate, in a manner similar to enzyme immunoassay. (Courtesy of Donna Zabel, Akron, Ohio.)

FIGURE 17–4. Polymerase chain reaction (PCR). This technique is a rapid means of amplifying a known sequence of DNA. A sample is mixed with a heat-stable DNA polymerase, excess deoxyribonucleotide triphosphates, and two DNA oligomers (**primers**), which complement the ends of the target sequence to be amplified. The mixture is heated to denature the DNA and then cooled to allow binding of the primers to the target DNA and extension of the primers by the polymerase. The cycle is repeated 20 to 40 times. After the first cycle, only the sequence bracketed by the primers is amplified. In the **RT-PCR** technique, RNA can also be amplified after its conversion to DNA by reverse transcriptase. *A* and *B*, DNA oligomers used as primers; + and −, DNA strands. (Modified from Blair GE, Blair Zajdel ME: *Biochem Educ* 20:87–90, 1992.)

TABLE 17–1. Molecular Techniques

Technique	Purpose	Clinical Examples
RFLP	Comparison of DNA	Molecular epidemiology, HSV-1 strains
DNA electrophoresis	Comparison of DNA	Viral strain differences (up to 20,000 bases)
Pulsed-field gel electrophoresis	Comparison of DNA (large pieces of DNA)	Streptococcal strain comparisons
In situ hybridization	Detection and localization of DNA sequences in tissue	Detection of nonreplicating DNA virus (e.g., cytomegalovirus, human papillomavirus)
Dot blot	Detection of DNA sequences in solution	Detection of viral DNA
Southern blot	Detection and characterization of DNA sequences by size	Identification of specific viral strains
Northern blot	Detection and characterization of RNA sequences by size	Identification of specific viral strains
PCR	Amplification of very dilute DNA samples	Detection of DNA viruses
RT-PCR	Amplification of very dilute RNA samples	Detection of RNA viruses
Branched-chain DNA	Amplification of very dilute DNA or RNA samples	Quantitation of DNA and RNA viruses
SDS-PAGE	Separation of proteins by molecular weight	Molecular epidemiology of HSV

HSV = herpes simplex virus; PCR = polymerase chain reaction; RFLP = restriction fragment length polymorphism; RT-PCR = reverse transcriptase polymerase chain reaction; SDS-PAGE = sodium dodecyl sulfate–polyacrylamide gel electrophoresis.

strands of the double helix) and cooled to allow hybridization of the primers to the new DNA. Each copy of DNA becomes a new template. The process is repeated many (20 to 40) times to amplify the original DNA sequence in an exponential manner. A target sequence can be amplified a million-fold in a few hours using this method. This technique is especially useful for detecting latent and integrated virus sequences, such as is the case for retroviruses, herpesviruses, papillomaviruses, and other papovaviruses.

The **RT-PCR** technique is a variation of the PCR, and it involves the use of the reverse transcriptase of retroviruses to convert viral RNA or messenger RNA to DNA before PCR amplification. In 1993, hantavirus sequences were used as primers for RT-PCR to identify the agent causing an outbreak of hemorrhagic pulmonary disease in the Four Corners area of New Mexico. It showed the infectious agent to be a hantavirus.

The **branched-chain DNA assay** is a new alternative to PCR and RT-PCR for detecting small amounts of specific RNA or DNA sequences. This technique is especially useful for quantitating plasma levels of HIV RNA. In this case, plasma is incubated in a special tube that is lined with a short complementary DNA sequence to capture the viral RNA. Another complementary DNA sequence is added to bind to the sample, but this DNA is attached to an artificially branched chain of DNA. On development, each branch is capable of initiating a detectable signal. This amplifies the signal from the original sample.

Detection of Proteins

In some cases, viruses and other infectious agents can be detected on the basis of the finding of certain characteristic enzymes or specific proteins. For example, the detection of reverse transcriptase in serum or cell culture indicates the presence of a retrovirus. The pattern of proteins from a virus or another agent after sodium dodecyl sulfate–polyacrylamide gel electrophoresis (SDS-PAGE) can also be used to identify and distinguish different strains of viruses or bacteria. In the SDS-PAGE technique, SDS binds to the backbone of the protein to generate a uniform peptide structure and protein length-to-charge ratio, such that the mobility of the protein in the gel is inversely related to the logarithm of its molecular weight. For example, the patterns of electrophoretically separated HSV proteins can be used to distinguish different types and strains of HSV-1 and HSV-2. Antibody can be used to identify specific proteins separated by SDS-PAGE using a Western blot technique (see Chapters 48 and 61). The molecular techniques used to identify infectious agents are summarized in Table 17–1.

BIBLIOGRAPHY

DiPersio JR et al: Spread of serious disease-producing M3 clones of group A *Streptococcus* among family members and health care workers, *Clin Infect Dis* 22:490–495, 1996.

Forbes BA, Weissfeld AS, Sahm DF: *Baily and Scott's diagnostic microbiology*, ed 10, St. Louis, 1998, Mosby.

Fredericks DN, Relman DA: Application of polymerase chain reaction to the diagnosis of infectious diseases, *Clin Infect Dis* 29:475–486, 1999.

Murray PR: *ASM pocket guide to clinical microbiology*, ed 2, Washington, DC, 1998, American Society for Microbiology.

Specter S, Hodinka RL, Young SA: *Clinical virology manual*, ed 3, Washington, DC, 2000, ASM Press.

C H A P T E R 1 8

Serologic Diagnosis

Immunologic techniques are used to detect, identify, and quantitate antigen in clinical samples as well as to evaluate the antibody response to infection and a person's history of exposure to infectious agents. The specificity of the antibody-antigen interaction and the sensitivity of many of the immunologic techniques make them powerful laboratory tools (Table 18–1). In most cases, the same technique can be used to evaluate antigen and antibody.

Antibodies

Antibodies can be used as sensitive and specific tools to detect, identify, and quantitate the antigens from a virus, bacterium, fungus, or parasite. Specific antibodies may be obtained from convalescent patients (e.g., antiviral antibodies) or prepared in animals. These antibodies are **polyclonal**; that is, they are heterogeneous antibody preparations that can recognize many epitopes on a single antigen. **Monoclonal** antibodies recognize individual epitopes on an antigen. Monoclonal antibodies for some antigens are commercially available, especially for lymphocyte cell surface antigens.

The development of monoclonal antibody technology revolutionized the science of immunology. For example, because of the specificity of these antibodies, lymphocyte subsets (e.g., CD4 and CD8 T cells) and lymphocyte cell surface antigens were identified. Monoclonal antibodies are the products of hybrid cells generated by the fusion and cloning of splenocytes from an immunized mouse and a myeloma cell line, which produces a hybridoma. The myeloma provides immortalization to the antibody-producing splenocytes. *Each hybridoma clone is a factory for one antibody molecule, yielding a monoclonal antibody that recognizes only one epitope.* In the near future, monoclonal antibodies will be prepared through genetic engineering.

The advantages of monoclonal antibodies are that their specificity can be confined to a single epitope on an antigen and that they can be prepared in "industrial-sized" tissue culture preparations. A major disadvantage of monoclonal antibodies is that they are often too specific, such that a monoclonal antibody specific for one epitope on a viral antigen of one strain may not be able to detect different strains of the same virus.

Methods of Detection

Antibody-antigen complexes can be detected directly, by precipitation techniques or labeling of the antibody with a radioactive, fluorescent, or enzyme probe, or indirectly, through measurement of an antibody-directed reaction, such as complement fixation. *Most of the procedures for detecting and identifying antigen can also be used for serologically evaluating antibody levels.*

Precipitation and Immunodiffusion Techniques

Specific antigen-antibody complexes and cross-reactivity can be distinguished by immunoprecipitation techniques. Within a limited concentration range for both antigen and antibody, termed the **equivalence zone,** the antibody cross-links the antigen into a complex that is too large to stay in solution and therefore precipitates. This technique is based on the multivalent nature of antibody molecules (e.g., immunoglobulin [Ig] G has two antigen binding domains). The antigen-antibody complexes are soluble at concentration ratios of antigen to antibody that are above and below the equivalence concentration.

Various immunodiffusion techniques make use of the equivalence concept to determine the identity of an antigen or the presence of antibody. **Single radial immunodiffusion** can be used to detect and quantify an antigen. In this technique, antigen is placed into a well and allowed to diffuse into antibody-containing agar. The higher the concentration of antigen, the farther it diffuses before it reaches equivalence with the antibody in the agar and precipitates as a ring around the well.

The **Ouchterlony immunodouble diffusion** technique is used to determine the relatedness of different

TABLE 18–1. Selected Immunologic Techniques

Technique	Purpose	Clinical Examples
Ouchterlony immunodouble diffusion	Detect and compare antigen and antibody	Fungal antigen and antibody
Immunofluorescence	Detection and localization of antigen	Viral antigen in biopsy (e.g., rabies, herpes simplex virus)
Enzyme immunoassay (EIA)	Same as immunofluorescence	Same as for immunofluorescence
Immunofluorescence flow cytometry	Population analysis of antigen-positive cells	Immunophenotyping
Enzyme-linked immunosorbent assay (ELISA)	Quantitation of antigen and antibody	Viral antigen (rotavirus), viral antibody (anti-HIV)
Western blot	Detection of antigen-specific antibody	Confirmation of anti-HIV seropositivity
Radioimmunoassay (RIA)	Same as ELISA	Same as for ELISA
Complement fixation	Quantitate specific antibody titer	Fungal, viral antibody
Hemagglutination inhibition	Antiviral antibody titer, serotype of virus strain	Seroconversion to current influenza strain, identification of influenza
Latex agglutination	Quantitation and detection of antigen and antibody	Rheumatoid factor, fungal antigens, streptococcal antigens

HIV = Human immunodeficiency virus.

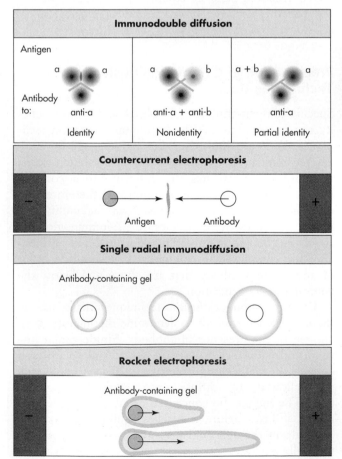

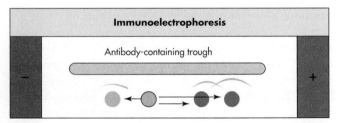

FIGURE 18–1. Analysis of antigens and antibodies by immunoprecipitation. The precipitation of protein occurs at the equivalence point, at which multivalent antibody forms large complexes with antigen. *A,* Ouchterlony immunodouble diffusion. Antigen and antibody diffuse from wells, meet, and form a precipitin line. If identical antigens are placed in adjacent wells, the concentration of antigen between them is doubled, and precipitation does not occur in this region. If different antigens are used, two different precipitin lines are produced. If one sample shares antigen (1/2) but is not identical, then a single spur results for the complete antigen. *B,* Countercurrent electrophoresis. This technique is similar to the Ouchterlony method, but antigen movement is facilitated by electrophoresis. *C,* Single radial immunodiffusion. This technique involves the diffusion of antigen into an antibody-containing gel. Precipitin rings indicate an immune reaction, and the area of the ring is proportional to the concentration of antigen. *D,* Rocket electrophoresis. Antigens are separated by electrophoresis into an agar gel that contains antibody. The length of the "rocket" indicates concentration of antigen. *E,* Immunoelectrophoresis. Antigen is placed in a well and separated by electrophoresis. Antibody is then placed in the trough, and precipitin lines form as antigen and antibody diffuse toward each other.

antigens, as shown in Figure 18–1. In this technique, solutions of antibody and antigen are placed in separate wells cut into agar, and the antigen and antibody are allowed to diffuse toward each other to establish concentration gradients of each substance. A visible precipitin line occurs where the concentrations of antigen and antibody reach equivalence (see Fig. 18–1). On the basis of the pattern of the precipitin lines, this technique can also be used to determine whether samples are identical, share some but not all epitopes (partial identity), or are distinct. This technique is used to detect antibody to fungal antigens (e.g., *Histoplasma* species, *Blastomyces* species, coccidioidomycoses).

In other immunodiffusion techniques the antigen may be separated by electrophoresis in agar and then reacted with antibody (immunoelectrophoresis), it may be transferred by means of electrophoresis into agar that contains antibody (rocket electrophoresis), or antigen and antibody may be placed in separate wells and allowed to move electrophoretically toward each other (countercurrent immunoelectrophoresis).

Immunoassays for Cell-Associated Antigen (Immunohistology)

Antigens on the cell surface or within the cell can be detected by **immunofluorescence** and **enzyme immunoassay (EIA)**. In **direct immunofluorescence**, a fluorescent molecule is covalently attached to the antibody (e.g., fluorescein isothiocyanate–labeled rabbit antiviral antibody). In **indirect immunofluorescence**, a second fluorescent antibody specific for the primary antibody (e.g., fluorescein isothiocyanate–labeled goat anti-rabbit antibody) is used to detect the primary antiviral antibody and locate the antigen (Figs. 18–2 and 18–3). In EIA, an enzyme such as horseradish peroxidase or alkaline phosphatase is conjugated to the antibody and converts a substrate into a chromophore to mark the antigen. These techniques are useful for the analysis of tissue biopsy specimens, blood cells, and tissue culture cells.

The **flow cytometer** can be used to analyze the immunofluorescence of cells in suspension and is especially useful for identifying and quantitating lympho-

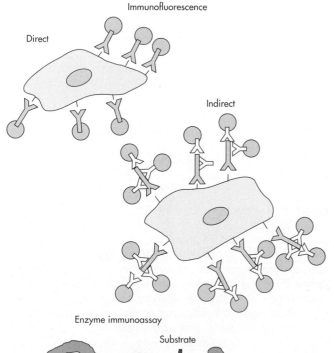

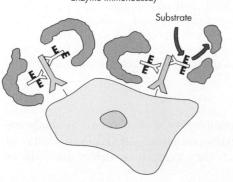

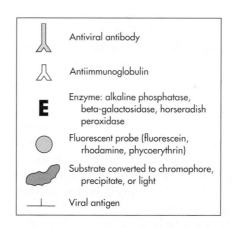

FIGURE 18–2. Immunofluorescence and enzyme immunoassays for antigen localization in cells. Antigen can be detected by *direct* assay with antiviral antibody modified covalently with a fluorescent or enzyme probe or by *indirect* assay using antiviral antibody and chemically modified antiimmunoglobulin. The enzyme converts substrate to a precipitate, chromophore, or light.

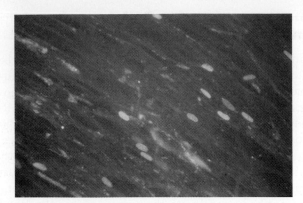

FIGURE 18–3. Immunofluorescence localization of herpes simplex virus–infected nerve cells in a brain section from a patient with herpes encephalitis. (From Emond RT, Rowland HAK: *A color atlas of infectious diseases,* ed 2, London, 1987, Wolfe.)

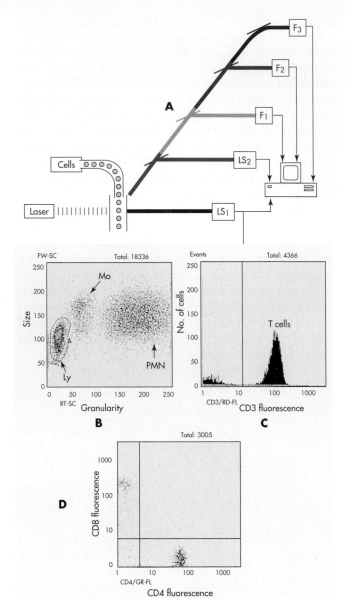

cytes (immunophenotyping). A laser is used in the flow cytometer to excite the fluorescent antibody attached to the cell and to determine the size of the cell by means of light-scattering measurements. The cells flow past the laser at rates of more than 5000 cells per second, and analysis is performed electronically. The **fluorescence-activated cell sorter** (**FACS**) is a flow cytometer that can also isolate specific subpopulations of cells for tissue culture growth on the basis of their size and immunofluorescence.

The data obtained from a flow cytometer are usually presented in the form of a histogram, with the fluorescence intensity on the x-axis and the number of cells on the y-axis, or in the form of a dot plot, in which more than one parameter is compared for each cell. The flow cytometer can perform a differential analysis of white blood cells and compare CD4 and CD8 T-cell populations simultaneously (Fig. 18–4). Flow cytometry is also useful for analyzing cell growth after the fluorescent labeling of DNA and other fluorescent applications.

Immunoassays for Antibody and Soluble Antigen

The **enzyme-linked immunosorbent assay** (**ELISA**) uses antigen immobilized on a plastic surface, bead, or filter to capture and separate the specific antibody from other antibodies in a patient's serum (Fig. 18–5). The affixed patient antibody is then detected by an anti-human antibody with a covalently linked enzyme (e.g., horseradish peroxidase, alkaline phosphatase, β-galactosidase). It is quantitated spectrophotometrically according to the intensity of the color produced in response to the enzyme conversion of an appropriate substrate. The actual concentration of antibody can be

FIGURE 18–4. Flow cytometry. *A,* The flow cytometer evaluates individual cell parameters as the cells flow past a laser beam at rates of more than 5000 per second. Cell size and granularity are determined by light scattering (LS), and antigen expression is evaluated by immunofluorescence (F) using antibodies labeled with different fluorescent probes. *B* to *D,* T-cell analysis of a normal patient. *B,* Light-scatter analysis was used to define the lymphocytes (Ly), monocytes (Mo), and polymorphonuclear leukocytes (PMN). *C,* The lymphocytes were analyzed for CD3 expression to identify T cells (presented in a histogram). *D,* CD4 and CD8 T cells were identified. Each dot represents one T cell. (Data proved by Dr. Tom Alexander, Akron, Ohio.)

determined by comparison with standard antibody solutions. The many variations of ELISAs differ in the way in which they capture or detect antibody or antigen.

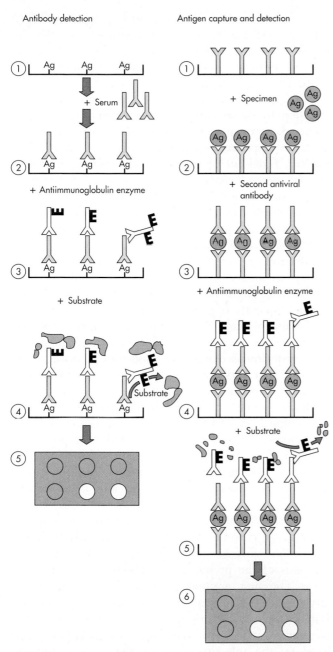

FIGURE 18–5. Enzyme immunoassays for quantitation of antibody or antigen. *A,* Antibody detection. *1,* Viral antigen obtained from infected cells, virions, or genetic engineering is affixed to a surface. *2,* Patient serum is added and is allowed to bind to the antigen. Unbound antibody is washed away. *3,* Enzyme-conjugated antihuman antibody is added, and unbound antibody is washed away. *4,* Substrate is added and, *5,* converted into chromophore, precipitate, or light. *B,* Antigen capture and detection. *1,* Antiviral antibody is affixed to a surface. *2,* A specimen containing antigen is added, and unbound antigen is washed away. *3,* A second antiviral antibody is added to detect the captured antigen. *4,* Enzyme-conjugated antihuman antibody is added, washed, and followed by, *5,* substrate, which is, *6,* converted into chromophore, precipitate, or light.

ELISAs can also be used to quantitate the soluble antigen in a patient's sample. In these assays, soluble antigen is captured and concentrated by an immobilized antibody and then detected with a different antibody labeled with the enzyme. An example of a commonly used ELISA is the home pregnancy test for the human chorionic gonadotropin hormone.

Western blot analysis is a variation of an ELISA. In this technique, viral proteins separated by electrophoresis according to their molecular weight or charge are transferred (blotted) onto a filter paper (e.g., nitrocellulose, nylon). When exposed to a patient's serum, the immobilized proteins capture virus-specific antibody and are visualized with an enzyme-conjugated anti-human antibody. This technique shows the proteins recognized by the patient serum. Western blot analysis is used to confirm ELISA results in patients suspected to be infected with the human immunodeficiency virus (HIV) (Figs. 18–6 and 48–7).

In **radioimmunoassay** (**RIA**), radiolabeled (e.g., with iodine 125) antibody or antigen is used to quantitate antigen-antibody complexes. RIA can be performed as a capture assay, as described previously for ELISA, or as a competition assay. In a competition assay, antibody in a patient's serum is quantitated according to its ability to compete with and replace a laboratory-prepared radiolabeled antibody from antigen-antibody complexes. The antigen-antibody complexes are precipitated and separated from free antibody, and the radioactivity is measured for both fractions. The amount of the patient's antibody is then quantitated from standard curves prepared with use of known quantities of competing antibody. The radioallergosorbent assay is a variation of an RIA capture assay in which radiolabeled anti-IgE is used to detect allergen-specific responses.

Complement fixation is a standard but technically difficult serologic test (Box 18–1). In this test, the patient's serum sample is reacted with laboratory-de-

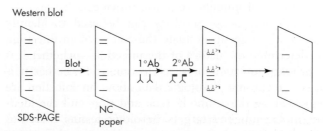

FIGURE 18–6. Western blot. Proteins are separated by sodium dodecyl sulfate–polyacrylamide gel electrophoresis (SDS-PAGE), electroblotted onto nitrocellulose (NC) paper, and incubated with antigen-specific or patient's antisera (1°Ab) and then enzyme-conjugated anti-human serum (2°Ab). Enzyme conversion of substrate identifies the antigen.

rived antigen and extra complement. Antibody-antigen complexes bind, activate, and fix (use up) the complement. The residual complement is then assayed through the lysis of red blood cells coated with antibody. Antibodies measured by this system generally develop slightly later in an illness than those measured by other techniques.

Antibody inhibition assays make use of the specificity of an antibody to prevent infection (**neutralization**) or other activity (**hemagglutination inhibition**) to identify the strain of the infecting agent, usually a virus, or to quantitate antibody responses to a specific strain of virus. For example, hemagglutination inhibition is used to distinguish different strains of influenza A. These tests are discussed further in Chapter 48.

Latex agglutination is a rapid, technically simple assay for detecting the antibody or soluble antigen. Virus-specific antibody causes latex particles coated with viral antigens to clump. Conversely, antibody-coated latex particles are used to detect soluble viral antigen. In passive hemagglutination, antigen-modified erythrocytes are used as indicators instead of latex particles.

Serology

The humoral immune response provides a history of a patient's infections. Serology can be used to identify the infecting agent, evaluate the course of an infection, or determine the nature of the infection—whether it is a primary infection or a reinfection and whether it is acute or chronic. Serologic data about an infection are provided by the antibody type and titer and the identity of the antigenic targets. Serologic testing is used to identify viruses and other agents that are difficult to isolate and grow in the laboratory or that cause diseases with slower courses (Box 18–2).

The relative antibody concentration is reported as a titer. A **titer** is the inverse of the greatest dilution, or lowest concentration (e.g., dilution of 1:64 = titer of 64), of a patient's serum that retains activity in the

assays just described. The patient's specific IgG, IgA, IgE, or IgM can be evaluated separately through the use of a labeled second anti-human antibody specific for the antibody isotype by indirect immunofluorescence, latex agglutination, ELISA, or RIA.

Serology is used to determine the time course of an infection by determining whether **seroconversion** has occurred. Seroconversion occurs when antibody is produced in response to a primary infection. *Specific IgM antibody, found during the first 2 to 3 weeks of a primary infection, generally indicates a recent primary infection.* Seroconversion is indicated by the finding *of at least a fourfold increase in the antibody titer between serum obtained during the acute phase of disease and that obtained at least 2 to 3 weeks later, during the convalescent phase.* Reinfection or recurrence later in life causes an **anamnestic** (secondary or booster) response. Antibody titers may remain high, however, in patients whose disease recurs frequently (e.g., herpesviruses).

Because of the inherent imprecision of serologic assays based on twofold serial dilutions, confirmation of seroconversion is defined as a fourfold increase in the antibody titer between acute and convalescent sera. For example, samples with 512 units and 1023 units of antibody, which are extremely different, would both give a signal on a 512-fold dilution but not on a 1024-fold dilution, and both results would be reported as titers of 512. On the other hand, samples with 1020 units and 1030 units are not significantly different but would be reported as titers of 512 and 1024, respectively.

Serology can also be used to determine the stage of a slower or chronic infection (e.g., hepatitis B, infectious mononucleosis caused by Epstein-Barr virus) on the basis of the presence of antibody to specific antigens. The first antibodies to be detected are those directed against antigens most available to the immune system (e.g., on the virion, on surfaces of infected cells, secreted). Later in the infection, when cells have been lysed by the infecting virus or the cellular immune response, antibodies directed against the intracellular proteins and enzymes are detected.

QUESTIONS

Describe the diagnostic procedure or procedures (molecular or immunologic) that would be appropriate for each of the following applications:

1. Determination of the apparent molecular weights of the HIV proteins.
2. Detection of human papillomavirus 16 (a nonreplicating virus) in a Papanicolaou (Pap) smear.
3. Detection of herpes simplex virus (a replicating virus) in a Pap smear.
4. Presence of *Histoplasma* fungal antigens in a patient's serum.
5. CD4 and CD8 T-cell concentrations in blood from a patient infected with HIV.
6. The presence of antibody and the titer of anti-HIV antibody.
7. Genetic differences between two herpes simplex viruses (DNA virus).
8. Genetic differences between two parainfluenza viruses (RNA virus).
9. Amount of rotavirus antigen in stool.
10. Detection of group A streptococci and their distinction from other streptococci.

BIBLIOGRAPHY

Forbes BA, Weissfeld AS, Sahm DF, editors: *Bailey and Scott's diagnostic microbiology*, ed 10, St. Louis, 1998, Mosby.

Murray PR: *ASM pocket guide to clinical microbiology*, Washington, DC, 1996, American Society for Microbiology.

Specter S et al: *Clinical virology manual*, ed 3, Washington, DC, 2000, ASM Press.

Bacteriology

CHAPTER 19

Mechanisms of Bacterial Pathogenesis

To a bacterium, the human body is a collection of environmental niches that provide the warmth, moisture, and food necessary for growth. Bacteria have acquired genetic traits that enable them to enter (invade) the environment, remain in a niche (adhere or colonize), gain access to food sources (degradative enzymes), and escape clearance by host immune and nonimmune protective responses (e.g., **capsule**). Unfortunately, many of the mechanisms that bacteria use to maintain their niche and the by-products of bacterial growth (e.g., acids, gas) cause damage and problems for the human host. Many of these genetic traits are **virulence factors,** which enhance the ability of bacteria to cause disease. Although many bacteria cause disease by directly destroying tissue, some release toxins, which are then disseminated by the blood to cause system-wide pathogenesis (Box 19–1). The surface structures of bacteria are powerful stimulators of host responses (acute phase: interleukin-1, interleukin-6, tumor necrosis factor), which can be protective but are often the significant causes of the disease symptoms (e.g., sepsis).

Not all bacteria cause disease, but some always cause disease once infection occurs. The human body is colonized with numerous microbes (**normal flora**), many of which serve important functions for their hosts, such as aiding in the digestion of food, producing vitamins (e.g., vitamin K), and protecting the host from colonization with pathogenic microbes. Although many of these endogenous bacteria can cause disease, they normally reside in locations such as the gastrointestinal (GI) tract, skin, and upper respiratory tract, which are technically outside the body (Fig. 19–1). Normal flora bacteria cause disease if they enter normally sterile sites of the body. **Virulent bacteria** have mechanisms that promote their growth in the host at the expense of the host's tissue or organ function. Symptoms result from the damage or loss of tissue or organ function or the development of host inflammatory responses. **Opportunistic bacteria** cause disease only in people with preexisting conditions that enhance their susceptibility. For example, *Pseudomonas aeruginosa* infects burn vic-

tims and the lungs of patients with cystic fibrosis, and patients with the acquired immunodeficiency syndrome are very susceptible to infection by intracellularly growing bacteria such as the mycobacteria.

The **symptoms of a disease** are determined by the function of the tissue affected, although **systemic responses,** produced by toxins, and host defense responses may also occur. The seriousness of the symptoms depends on the importance of the organ affected and the extent of the damage caused by the infection. Infections of the central nervous system are always serious. The bacterial strain and **inoculum size** are also major factors in determining whether disease occurs; however, this can vary from a relatively small inoculum (e.g., fewer than 200 *Shigella* for shigellosis) to a very large inoculum (e.g., 10^8 *Vibrio cholerae* or *Campylobacter* organisms for GI tract infections). Host factors can also have a role. For example, although a million or more *Salmonella* organisms are necessary for gastroenteritis to become established in a healthy person, only a few thousand organisms are necessary in a person whose gastric pH is neutral. Congenital defects, immunodeficiency states (see Chapter 14), and other disease-related conditions may also increase a person's susceptibility to infection.

Entry into the Human Body

For infection to become established, bacteria must first gain entry into the body (Fig. 19–1 and Table 19–1). Natural defense mechanisms and barriers, such as skin, mucus, ciliated epithelium, and secretions containing antibacterial substances (e.g., lysozyme), make it difficult for bacteria to gain entry into the body. However, these barriers are sometimes broken (e.g., a cut in the skin, a tumor or ulcer in the bowel), providing a portal of entry for the bacteria, or the bacteria may have the means to compromise the barrier and invade the body. On invasion, the bacteria can travel in the blood stream to other sites in the body.

The **skin** has a thick, horny layer of dead cells that protects the body from infection. However, cuts in the

BOX 19–1. **Bacterial Virulence Mechanisms**

Adherence
Invasion
Byproducts of growth (gas, acid)
Toxins
    Degradative enzymes
    Cytotoxic proteins
Endotoxin
Superantigen
Induction of excess inflammation
Evasion of phagocytic and immune clearance
Capsule
Resistance to antibiotics

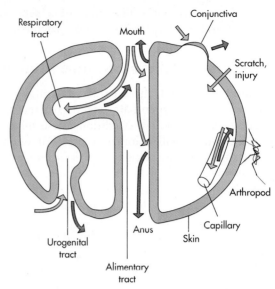

FIGURE 19–1. Body surfaces as sites of microbial infection and shedding. *Green arrows,* infection; *purple arrows,* shedding. (Redrawn from Mims C et al: *Medical microbiology,* London, 1993, Mosby-Wolfe.)

skin, produced accidentally or surgically or kept open with catheters or other surgical appliances, provide a means for the bacteria to gain access to the susceptible tissue underneath. For example, *Staphylococcus aureus* and *Staphylococcus epidermidis,* which are a part of the normal flora on skin, can enter the body through breaks in the skin and pose a major problem for people with indwelling catheters and intravenous lines.

The *mouth, nose, respiratory tract, ears, eyes, urogenital tract, and anus are sites through which bacteria can enter the body.* These natural openings in the skin and their associated body cavities are protected by natural defenses such as the mucus and ciliated epithelium that line the upper respiratory tract, the lysozyme and other antibacterial secretions in tears and mucus, and the acid and bile in the GI tract. However, many bacteria are unaffected or have the means to evade these defenses. For example, the outer membrane of the gram-

negative bacteria makes these bacteria more resistant to lysozyme, acid, and bile. The enterobacteria are thus enabled to colonize the GI tract, where they serve the beneficial function of producing the vitamin K that the body needs. These endogenous bacteria are normally benign and restricted to the body cavities that they colonize. However, these bacteria can enter normally sterile sites of the body, such as the peritoneum and the blood stream, through a break in the normal barrier. An example of this is the patient whose colon

TABLE 19–1. **Bacterial Port of Entry**

Route	Examples
Ingestion	*Salmonella* species, *Shigella* species, *Yersinia enterocolitica,* enterotoxigenic *Escherichia coli, Vibrio* species, *Campylobacter* species, *Clostridium botulinum, Bacillus cereus, Listeria* species, *Brucella* species
Inhalation	*Mycobacterium* species, *Nocardia* species, *Mycoplasma pneumoniae, Legionella* species, *Bordetella, Chlamydia psittaci, Chlamydia pneumoniae, Streptococcus* species
Trauma	*Clostridium tetani*
Needlestick	*Staphylococcus aureus, Pseudomonas* species
Arthropod bite	*Rickettsia* species, *Ehrlichia* species, *Coxiella* species, *Francisella* species, *Borrelia* species, *Yersinia pestis*
Sexual transmission	*Neisseria gonorrhoeae, Chlamydia trachomatis, Treponema pallidum*

tumor was diagnosed after detection of a septicemia (blood-borne infection) caused by enteric bacteria.

Colonization, Adhesion, and Invasion

As previously mentioned, the GI tract is naturally colonized by benign and potentially beneficial bacteria. In some cases, environmental conditions determine the bacteria that can or will colonize a site. For example, *Legionella* grows in the lungs but does not readily spread because it cannot tolerate high temperatures (35°C). Colonization of sites that are normally sterile, such as the lung, implies the existence of a defect in a natural defense mechanism or a new portal of entry. Patients with cystic fibrosis have such defects because of the reduction in their ciliary mucoepithelial function and altered mucosal secretions; as a result, they suffer from colonization by *S. aureus* and *P. aeruginosa*.

Bacteria may use specific mechanisms to adhere to and colonize different body surfaces (Table 19–2). If the bacteria can adhere to epithelial or endothelial cell linings of the bladder, intestine, and blood vessels, they cannot be washed away, and this adherence allows them to colonize the tissue. For example, natural bladder function eliminates any bacteria not affixed to the bladder wall. *Escherichia coli* and other bacteria have **adhesins** that bind to specific receptors on the tissue surface, and these keep them from being washed away.

Many of these adhesin proteins are present at the tips of **fimbriae (pili)** and bind tightly to specific sugars on the target tissue. (This sugar-binding activity defines these proteins as lectins.) For example, most *E. coli* strains that cause pyelonephritis produce a fimbrial adhesin termed P fimbriae. This adhesin can bind to receptors for α-D-galactosyl-β-D-galactoside (Gal-Gal), which is part of the P blood group antigen structure on human erythrocytes and uroepithelial cells. *Neisseria gonorrhoeae* pili are also important virulence factors; they bind to oligosaccharide receptors on epithelial cells. *Yersinia* organisms, *Bordetella pertussis*, and *Mycoplasma pneumoniae* express adhesin proteins that are not on fimbriae. *Streptococcus pyogenes* uses **lipoteichoic acid** and the F protein (binds to fibronectin) to bind to epithelial cells.

A special bacterial adaptation that facilitates colonization, especially of surgical appliances such as artificial valves or indwelling catheters, is a **biofilm** produced by the bacteria. Bacteria in biofilms are bound within a sticky web of polysaccharide that binds the cells together and to the surface. Dental plaque is an example of a biofilm. The biofilm matrix can also protect the bacteria from host defenses and antibiotics.

Although bacteria do not have mechanisms that enable them to cross skin, several bacteria can cross mucosal membranes and other tissue barriers to enter normally sterile sites and more susceptible tissue.

TABLE 19–2. **Examples of Bacterial Adherence Mechanisms**

Microbe	Adhesin	Receptor
Staphylococcus aureus	Lipoteichoic acid	Unknown
Staphylococcus species	Slime	Unknown
Streptococcus, group A	LTA-M protein complex	Fibronectin
Streptococcus pneumoniae	Protein	*N*-acetylhexosamine-gal
Escherichia coli	Type 1 fimbriae	D-Mannose
	Colonization factor antigen 1 fimbriae	GM ganglioside
	P fimbriae	P blood group glycolipid
Other Enterobacteriaceae	Type 1 fimbriae	D-Mannose
Neisseria gonorrhoeae	Fimbriae	GD$_1$ ganglioside
Treponema pallidum	P$_1$, P$_2$, P$_3$	Fibronectin
Chlamydia species	Cell surface lectin	*N*-acetylglucosamine
Mycoplasma pneumoniae	Protein P1	Sialic acid
Vibrio cholerae	Type 4 pili	Fucose and mannose

LTA = lipoteichoic acid.

These invasive bacteria either destroy the barrier or penetrate into the cells of the barrier. *Shigella, Salmonella,* and *Yersinia* organisms are enteric bacteria that produce an invasin protein that promotes the binding of the bacteria to M cells of the colon, which in turn stimulates the cell to invaginate and take in the bacteria. *Shigella* can then spread to adjacent cells, whereas *Salmonella* can pass through to the other side and initiate systemic infection. *Salmonella* species and enteropathogenic strains of *E. coli* encode the protein machinery for invasion within a pathogenicity island of DNA. **Pathogenicity islands** are large chromosomal regions that contain sets of genes encoding numerous virulence factors. In many cases, a virulence process requiring coordinated expression of several genes is encoded in a pathogenicity island. These genes may be turned on by a single stimulus (e.g., the temperature of the gut) and can be transferred as a unit to different sites within a chromosome or to other bacteria. Pathogenicity islands found in other bacteria encode different sets of virulence genes.

Pathogenic Actions of Bacteria

Tissue Destruction

Byproducts of bacterial growth, especially fermentation, result in the production of acids, gas, and other substances that are toxic to tissue. In addition, **many bacteria release degradative enzymes** to break down tissue, thereby providing food for the growth of the organisms and promoting the spread of the bacteria, especially if blood vessels are involved. For example, *Clostridium perfringens* organisms are part of the normal flora of the GI tract but are also opportunistic pathogens that can establish infection in oxygen-depleted tissues and cause gas gangrene. These anaerobic bacteria produce enzymes (e.g., phospholipase C, collagenase, protease, hyaluronidase), several toxins, and acid and gas from bacterial metabolism, which destroy the tissue. Staphylococci produce many different enzymes that modify the tissue environment. These enzymes include hyaluronidase, fibrinolysin, and lipases. Streptococci also produce enzymes, including streptolysins S and O, hyaluronidase, and streptokinases; these enzymes facilitate the development of infection and its spread.

Toxins

Toxins are bacterial components that directly harm tissue or trigger destructive biologic activities. Toxin and toxin-like activities are caused by cell wall components, degradative enzymes that cause lysis of cells, and specific receptor-binding proteins that initiate toxic reactions in a specific target tissue or initiate a systemic response (such as fever) by promoting the inappropriate release of cytokines. In many cases, the toxin is completely responsible for causing the characteristic symptoms of the disease. For example, the **preformed toxin** present in food mediates the food poisoning caused by *S. aureus* and *Bacillus cereus* and the botulism caused by *Clostridium botulinum.* The symptoms caused by preformed toxin occur much sooner than for other forms of gastroenteritis because the effect is like eating a food poison and the bacteria do not need to grow for the symptoms to occur. Because a toxin can be spread systemically through the blood stream, symptoms may arise at a site distant from the site of infection, such as occurs in tetanus, which is caused by *Clostridium tetani,* or the toxin can be disseminated throughout the body, as occurs in the staphylococcal scalded skin syndrome.

Endotoxin and Other Cell Wall Components

The presence of bacterial cell wall components is a powerful multi-alarm warning to the body to signal infection and activate the host's protective systems. In some cases, the host response is excessive and may even be life-threatening. On infection with gram-positive bacteria, **peptidoglycan** and its breakdown products, as well as **teichoic** and **lipoteichoic acids,** are released, and these stimulate toxin-like **pyrogenic acute-phase responses.** The **lipopolysaccharide** produced by gram-negative bacteria is an even more powerful activator of acute-phase and inflammatory reactions. **The lipid A portion of lipopolysaccharide** is responsible for **endotoxin** activity. It is important to appreciate that endotoxin is not the same as exotoxin and that *only gram-negative bacteria make endotoxin.*

Gram-negative bacteria release endotoxin during infection. Endotoxin binds to specific receptors on macrophages, B cells, and other cells and stimulates the production and release of **acute-phase cytokines,** such as interleukin-1, tumor necrosis factor–α, interleukin-6, and prostaglandins (Fig. 19–2). Endotoxin also stimulates the growth (mitogenic) of B cells. At low concentrations, endotoxin stimulates the mounting of protective responses such as fever, vasodilatation, and the activation of the immune and inflammatory responses (Box 19–2). However, the endotoxin levels in the blood of patients with **gram-negative bacterial sepsis** (bacteria in the blood) can be very high, and the response to these can be overpowering, resulting in shock and possibly death. High concentrations of endotoxin activate the alternative pathway of complement and promote high fever, hypotension, shock produced by vasodilatation and capillary leakage, and disseminated intravascular coagulation stemming from the activation of the blood coagulation pathways. The high fever, petechiae (skin lesions resulting from the capillary leakage), and potential symptoms of shock (result-

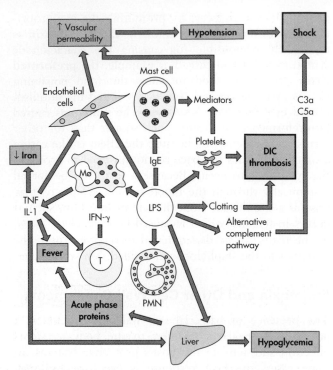

FIGURE 19–2. The many activities of lipopolysaccharide (LPS). This bacterial endotoxin activates almost every immune mechanism as well as the clotting pathway, which together make lipopolysaccharide one of the most powerful immune stimuli known. DIC = disseminated intravascular coagulation; IFN-γ = interferon-γ; IgE = immunoglobulin E; IL-1 = interleukin-1; PMN = polymorphonuclear neutrophil leukocytes; TNF = tumor necrosis factor. (Redrawn from Mims C et al: *Medical microbiology,* London, 1993, Mosby-Wolfe.)

ing from increased vascular permeability) associated with *Neisseria meningitidis* infection can be related to the large amounts of endotoxin released during infection.

Exotoxins

Exotoxins are proteins that can be produced by grampositive or gram-negative bacteria and include cytolytic enzymes and receptor-binding proteins that alter the function or kill the cell. In many cases, the toxin gene is encoded on a plasmid (tetanus toxin of *C. tetani*, LT and ST toxins of enterotoxigenic *E. coli*) or a lysogenic phage (*Corynebacterium diphtheriae* and *C. botulinum*). An example of a cytolytic enzyme is the α-toxin (phospholipase C) produced by *C. perfringens*, which breaks down sphingomyelin and other membrane phospholipids, resulting in cell lysis.

Many toxins are dimeric with A and B subunits (**A-B toxins**). The B portion of the A-B toxins binds to a specific cell surface receptor, and then the A subunit is

transferred into the interior of the cell, where cell injury is induced. The tissues targeted by these toxins are very defined and limited (Fig. 19–3 and Table 19–3). The biochemical targets of A-B toxins include ribosomes, transport mechanisms, and intracellular signaling (cyclic adenosine monophosphate production, G protein function) with effects ranging from diarrhea to loss of neuronal function to death. The functional properties of cytolytic and other exotoxins are discussed in greater detail in the chapters dealing with the specific diseases involved.

Superantigens are a special group of toxins (Fig. 19–4). These molecules activate T cells by binding simultaneously to a T-cell receptor and a major histocompatibility complex class II (MHC II) molecule on another cell without requiring antigen. *This nonspecific means of activating T cells can trigger life-threatening autoimmune-like responses by stimulating the release of large amounts of interleukins,* such as interleukin-1 and interleukin-2. This superantigen stimulation of T cells can also lead to death of the activated T cells, resulting in the loss of specific T-cell clones and the loss of their immune responses. Superantigens include the toxic shock syndrome toxin of *S. aureus*, staphylococcal enterotoxins, and the erythrogenic toxin A or C of *S. pyogenes*.

Immunopathogenesis

In many cases, the symptoms of a bacterial infection are produced by excessive immune and inflammatory responses triggered by the infection. As described earlier, the acute-phase response to cell wall components, especially endotoxin, is an initial phase of the protective antibacterial response but can also cause the life-threatening symptoms associated with sepsis and meningitis (see Fig. 19–2). Tissue damage induced by neutrophils, macrophage, and complement at the site of the infection and granuloma formation induced by CD4 T cells and macrophages for *Mycobacterium tuberculosis* can lead to tissue destruction. The bacterial M protein of *S. pyogenes* antigenically mimics heart tissue

---

BOX 19–2. **Endotoxin-Mediated Toxicity**

Fever
Leukopenia followed by leukocytosis
Activation of complement
Thrombocytopenia
Disseminated intravascular coagulation
Decreased peripheral circulation and perfusion to major
    organs
Shock
Death

A   **Inhibition of protein synthesis**

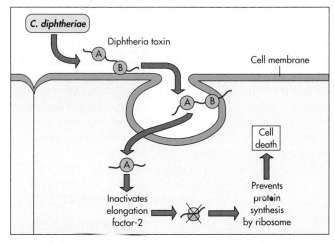

B   **Hyperactivation**

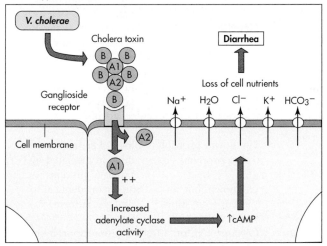

C   **Effects on nerve–muscle transmission**

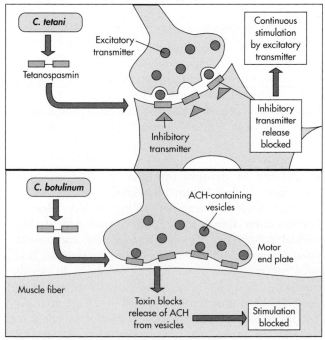

such that anti-M protein antibodies cross react with and can initiate damage to the heart to cause rheumatic fever. Immune complexes deposited in the glomeruli of the kidney, cause poststreptococcal glomerulonephritis. For *Chlamydia, Treponema* (syphilis), *Borrelia* (Lyme disease), and other bacteria, the host immune response is an important cause of disease symptoms in patients.

Mechanisms for Escaping Host Defenses

Logically, the longer a bacterial infection remains in a host, the more time the bacteria have to cause damage. Therefore, bacteria that can evade or incapacitate the host defenses have a greater potential for causing disease. Bacteria have developed ways to avoid the major antibacterial defenses by evading recognition and killing by phagocytic cells, by inactivating or evading the complement system and antibody, and even by growing inside cells to hide from these host responses (Box 19–3).

The capsule is one of the most important virulence factors (Box 19–4). These slime layers function by shielding the bacteria from immune and phagocytic responses. Capsules are usually made of polysaccharides, which are usually poor immunogens. The *S. pyogenes* capsule, for example, is made of hyaluronic acid, which mimics human connective tissue, thereby masking the bacteria and keeping them from being recognized by the immune system. The capsule also acts like a slimy football jersey, in that it is hard to grasp and tears away when grabbed by a phagocyte. The capsule also protects a bacterium from the environment of a phagolysosome within the macrophage or leukocyte. All of these properties can extend the time bacteria spend in blood (bacteremia) before being eliminated by host responses. Mutants of normally encapsulated bacteria that lose the ability to make a capsule also lose their virulence; examples of such bacteria are *Streptococcus pneumoniae* and *N. meningitidis.*

Bacteria can hide from antibody responses by **intracellular growth** *or by* **antigenic variation.** Bacteria that grow intracellularly include mycobacteria, francisellae, brucellae, chlamydiae, and rickettsiae. Unlike most bac-

FIGURE 19–3. The mode of action of dimeric A-B exotoxins. The bacterial A-B toxins often consist of a two-chain molecule. The B chain promotes entry of the bacteria into cells, and the A chain has inhibitory activity against some vital function. cAMP = cyclic adenosine monophosphate; ACH = acetylcholine. (Redrawn From Mims C et al: *Medical microbiology,* London, 1993, Mosby-Wolfe.)

TABLE 19–3. Properties of A-B Type Bacterial Toxins

Toxin	Organism	Gene Location	Subunit Structure	Target Cell Receptor	Biologic Effects
Anthrax toxins	*Bacillus anthracis*	Plasmid	Three separate proteins (EF, LF, PA)	Unknown, probably glycoprotein	EF + PA: increase in target cell cAMP level, localized edema; LF + PA: death of target cells and experimental animals
Bordetella adenylate cyclase toxin	*Bordetella* species	Chromosomal	A-B	Unknown, probably glycolipid	Increase in target cell cAMP level, modified cell function or cell death
Botulinum toxin	*Clostridium botulinum*	Phage	A-B	Possibly ganglioside (GD_{1b})	Decrease in peripheral, presynaptic acetylcholine release, flaccid paralysis
Cholera toxin	*Vibrio cholerae*	Chromosomal	A-5B	Ganglioside (GM_1)	Activation of adenylate cyclase, increase in cAMP level, secretory diarrhea
Diphtheria toxin	*Corynebacterium diphtheriae*	Phage	A-B	Probably glycoprotein	Inhibition of protein synthesis, cell death
Heat-labile enterotoxins	*Escherichia coli*	Plasmid		Similar or identical to cholera toxin	
Pertussis toxin	*Bordetella pertussis*	Chromosomal	A-5B	Unknown, probably glycoprotein	Block of signal transduction mediated by target G proteins
Pseudomonas exotoxin A	*Pseudomonas aeruginosa*	Chromosomal	A-B	Unknown, but different from diphtheria toxin	Similar or identical to diphtheria toxin
Shiga toxin	*Shigella* dysenteriae	Chromosomal	A-5B	Glycoprotein or glycolipid	Inhibition of protein synthesis, cell death
Shiga-like toxins	*Shigella* species, *E. coli*	Phage		Similar or identical to Shiga toxin	
Tetanus toxin	*Clostridium tetani*	Plasmid	A-B	Ganglioside (GT_1) and/or GD_{1b}	Decrease in neurotransmitter release from inhibitory neurons, spastic paralysis

cAMP = cyclic adenosine monophosphate.

Modified from Mandell G, Douglas G, Bennett J: *Principles and practice of infectious disease*, ed 3, New York, 1990, Churchill Livingstone.

teria, control of these infections requires TH1 immune reactions in which CD4 T cells activate macrophages and result in inflammatory reactions. *N. gonorrhoeae* can vary the structure of surface antigens to evade antibody responses.

Phagocytes (neutrophil, macrophage) are an important antibacterial defense, but many bacteria can circumvent phagocytic killing in various ways. They can produce enzymes capable of lysing phagocytic cells (e.g., the streptolysin produced by *S. pyogenes* or the α-toxin produced by *C. perfringens*). They can inhibit phagocytosis (e.g., the effect of the **capsule** surround-

ing and the **M protein** produced by *S. pyogenes*) or block intracellular killing. Bacterial mechanisms for protection from intracellular killing include blocking phagolysosome fusion to prevent contact with its bactericidal contents (*Mycobacterium* species), capsule-mediated or enzymatic resistance to the bactericidal lysosomal enzymes or substances, and the ability to exit the phagosome into the host cytoplasm before being exposed to lysosomal enzymes (Table 19–4 and Fig. 19–5). For example, staphylococci produce catalase, an enzyme that makes the myeloperoxidase system less effective. Many of the bacteria that are internalized but

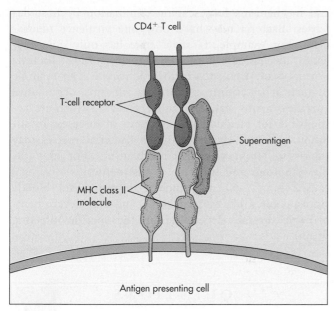

FIGURE 19–4. Superantigen binding to the external regions of the T-cell receptor and the class II major histocompatibility complex (MHC) molecules.

survive phagocytosis can use the cell as a place to grow and to hide from immune responses and as a means of being disseminated throughout the body.

Other important host defenses subverted by bacteria include the alternate pathway of complement and antibody. Bacteria evade complement action by masking themselves and by inhibiting activation of the cascade. The long O antigen of lipopolysaccharide prevents the complement from gaining access to the membrane and protects gram-negative bacteria from damage. Immunoglobulin A antibody is inactivated by an immunoglobulin A–specific protease made by *N. gonorrhoeae*. *S. aureus* makes an immunoglobulin G–binding protein,

protein A, which masks the bacteria and thereby prevents antibody action.

S. aureus can also escape host defenses by walling off the site of infection. *S. aureus* can produce coagulase, an enzyme that promotes the conversion of fibrin to fibrinogen to produce a clotlike barrier; this feature distinguishes *S. aureus* from *S. epidermidis*. *M. tuberculosis* is able to survive in a host by promoting the development of a granuloma, within which viable bacteria may reside for the life of the infected person. The bacteria may resume growth if there is a decline in the immune status of the person.

Summary

The primary virulence factors of bacteria are the capsule, adhesins, invasins, degradative enzymes, toxins,

---

BOX 19–4. **Examples of Encapsulated Microorganisms**

Staphylococcus aureus
Streptococcus pneumoniae
Streptococcus pyogenes (group A)
Streptococcus agalactiae (group B)
Bacillus anthracis
Bacillus subtilis
Neisseria gonorrhoeae
Neisseria meningitidis
Haemophilus influenzae
Escherichia coli
Klebsiella pneumoniae
Salmonella species
Yersinia pestis
Campylobacter fetus
Pseudomonas aeruginosa
Bacteroides fragilis
Cryptococcus neoformans (yeast)

BOX 19–3. **Microbial Defenses Against Host Immunologic Clearance**

Encapsulation
Antigenic mimicry
Antigenic masking
Antigenic shift
Production of anti-immunoglobulin proteases
Destruction of phagocyte
Inhibition of chemotaxis
Inhibition of phagocytosis
Inhibition of phagolysosome fusion
Resistance to lysosomal enzymes
Intracellular replication

TABLE 19–4. **Methods That Circumvent Phagocytic Killing**

Method	Example
Inhibition of phagolysome fusion	*Legionella* species, *Mycobacterium tuberculosis*, *Chlamydia* species
Resistance to lysosomal enzymes	*Salmonella typhimurium*, *Coxiella* species, *Ehrlichia* species, *Mycobacterium leprae*, *Leishmania* species
Adaptation to cytoplasmic replication	*Listeria* species, *Francisella* species, *Rickettsia* species

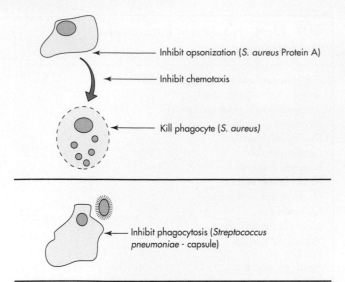

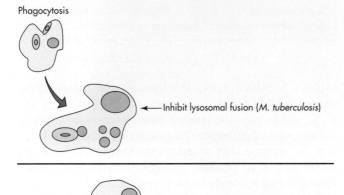

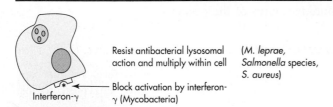

FIGURE 19–5. Bacterial mechanisms for escaping phagocytic clearance. Selected examples of bacteria that use the indicated antiphagocytic mechanisms are given.

and mechanisms for escaping elimination by host defenses. Bacteria may have only one virulence mechanism. For example, *C. diphtheriae* has only one virulence mechanism: diphtheria toxin. Other bacteria express many virulence factors. *S. aureus* is an example of such a bacterium; it expresses adhesins, degradative enzymes, toxins, catalase, and coagulase, which are responsible for producing a spectrum of diseases. In addition, different strains within a bacterial species may express different virulence mechanisms. For example, the symptoms and sequelae of gastroenteritis (diarrhea) caused by *E. coli* may include invasion and bloody stools, cholera-like watery stools, and even severe hemorrhagic disease, depending on the specific infecting strain.

QUESTIONS

1. Name three routes by which exogenous pathogens can infect a person. List five examples of organisms that use each route.

2. How are microbes able to resist immunologic clearance? Give at least one specific example of each mechanism.

3. What are the two general types of exotoxins? List examples of each type.

BIBLIOGRAPHY

Finlay BB, Falkow S: Common themes in microbial pathogenicity revisited, *Microbiol Mol Biol Rev* 61:136–169, 1997.

Gorbach SL, Bartlett JG, Blacklow NR: *Infectious diseases*, ed 2, Philadelphia, 1997, WB Saunders.

Groisman EA, Ochman H: How *Salmonella* became a pathogen, *Trends Microbiol* 5:343–349, 1997.

Lee CA: Pathogenicity islands and the evolution of bacterial pathogens, *Infect Agents Dis* 5:1–7, 1996.

Mandell GJ et al: *Mandell, Douglas and Bennett's principles and practice of infectious diseases*, ed 5, New York, 2000, Churchill Livingstone.

McClane BA, Mietzner TA, Dowling JN et al: *Microbial pathogenesis: a principles-oriented approach*, Madison, Conn., 1999, part of Blackwell Science, Inc. Fence Creek Publishing.

McGee J et al: *Oxford textbook of pathology*, vol 1, Oxford, 1992, Oxford University Press.

Papageorgiou AC, Acharya KR: Microbial superantigens: from structure to function, *Trends Microbiol* 8:369–375, 2000.

CHAPTER 20

Antibacterial Agents

This chapter provides an overview of the mechanisms of action and antibacterial spectrum of the most commonly used antibiotics as well as a description of the common mechanisms of bacterial resistance. The terminology appropriate for this discussion is summarized in Box 20–1.

The year 1935 was an important one for the chemotherapy of systemic bacterial infections. Although antiseptics had been applied topically to prevent the growth of microorganisms, systemic bacterial infections had not as yet responded to any existing agents. In this year, the red azo dye protosil was shown to protect mice against systemic streptococcal infection and to be curative in patients suffering from such infections. It was soon found that protosil was cleaved in the body to release *p*-aminobenzene sulfonamide, or sulfanilamide, which was subsequently shown to have antibacterial activity. These observations regarding the first "sulfa" drug ushered in a new era in medicine. Compounds (antibiotics) produced by microorganisms were eventually discovered to inhibit the growth of other microorganisms. For example, Fleming first noted that the mold *Penicillium* prevented the multiplication of staphylococci. A concentrate from a culture of this mold was prepared, and the remarkable antibacterial activity and lack of toxicity of the first antibiotic, penicillin, were demonstrated. Streptomycin and the tetracyclines were developed in the 1940s and 1950s, followed rapidly by the development of additional aminoglycosides, semisynthetic penicillins, cephalosporins, quinolones, and other antimicrobials. All these antibacterial agents greatly increased the range of infectious diseases that could be prevented or cured.

Despite the rapidity with which new chemotherapeutic agents are introduced, bacteria have shown a remarkable ability to develop resistance to these agents. Thus, antibiotic therapy will not be the predicted magical cure for all infections; rather, it is only one weapon, albeit an important one, against infectious diseases. It is also important to recognize that because resistance to antibiotics is frequently not predictable, physicians must rely on their clinical experience for the initial selection of empirical therapy. Guidelines for the management of infections caused by specific organisms are discussed in the relevant chapters of this text.

The results of in vitro antimicrobial susceptibility testing are valuable for selecting chemotherapeutic agents active against the infecting organism. Extensive work has been performed in an effort to standardize the testing methods and improve the clinical predictive value of the results. Despite these efforts, the in vitro tests are simply a measurement of the effect of the antibiotic against the organism under specific conditions. The selection of an antibiotic and the patient's outcome are influenced by a variety of interrelated factors, including the pharmacokinetic properties of the antibiotic, drug toxicity, the clinical disease, and the patient's general medical status.

The basic mechanisms and sites of antibiotic activity are summarized in Table 20–1 and Figure 20–1 respectively.

Inhibition of Cell Wall Synthesis

By far, the most common mechanism of antibiotic activity is interference with bacterial cell wall synthesis. Most of the cell wall–active antibiotics are classified as β-lactam antibiotics (e.g., penicillins, cephalosporins, cephamycins, carbapenems, monobactams, β-lactamase inhibitors), so named because they share a common β-lactam ring structure. Other antibiotics that interfere with construction of the bacterial cell wall include vancomycin, bacitracin, and the antimycobacterial agents isoniazid, ethambutol, cycloserine, and ethionamide.

Beta-Lactam Antibiotics

The major structural component of bacterial cell walls is the peptidoglycan layer. The basic structure is a chain of 10 to 65 disaccharide residues consisting of alternating molecules of *N*-acetylglucosamine and *N*-acetylmuramic acid. These chains are then cross-linked with peptide bridges that create a rigid mesh coating for the bacteria. The building of the chains and cross-

BOX 20-1. Terminology

Antibacterial spectrum—range of activity of an antimicrobial against bacteria. A **broad-spectrum** antibacterial drug can inhibit a wide variety of gram-positive and gram-negative bacteria, whereas a **narrow-spectrum** drug is active only against a limited variety of bacteria.

Bacteriostatic activity—level of antimicrobial activity that **inhibits** the growth of an organism. This is determined in vitro by testing a standardized concentration of organisms against a series of antimicrobial dilutions. The lowest concentration that inhibits the growth of the organism is referred to as the **minimum inhibitory concentration (MIC).**

Bactericidal activity—level of antimicrobial activity that **kills** the test organism. This is determined in vitro by exposing a standardized concentration of organisms to a series of antimicrobial dilutions. The lowest concentration that kills 99.9% of the population is referred to as the **minimum bactericidal concentration (MBC).**

Antibiotic combinations—combinations of antibiotics that may be used (1) to broaden the antibacterial spectrum for empirical therapy or the treatment of polymicrobial infections, (2) to prevent the emergence of resistant organisms during therapy, and (3) to achieve a synergistic killing effect.

Antibiotic synergism—combinations of two antibiotics that have enhanced bactericidal activity when tested together compared with the activity of each antibiotic.

Antibiotic antagonism—combination of antibiotics in which the activity of one antibiotic interferes with the activity of the other (e.g., the sum of the activity is less than the activity of the individual drugs).

β-lactamase—an enzyme that hydrolyzes the β-lactam ring in the β-lactam class of antibiotics, thus inactivating the antibiotic. The enzymes specific for penicillins and cephalosporins are the **penicillinases** and **cephalosporinases,** respectively.

---

cause they have an outer membrane that overlies the peptidoglycan layer. Penetration of β-lactam antibiotics into gram-negative bacilli requires transit through the **outer membrane pores.** Changes in the proteins **(porins)** that form the walls of the pores can alter the size or charge of these channels and result in the exclusion of the antibiotic. Bacteria can also acquire a **modified PBP** that fails to bind to β-lactam antibiotics but contributes to the synthesis of the peptidoglycan layer. The modified PBP can originate either from a mutation in the PBP gene (e.g., *Streptococcus pneumoniae* resistant to penicillins) or through the acquisition of a new PBP (e.g., *Escherichia coli* PBP introduced into *Staphylococcus aureus* confers resistance to oxacillin). Finally, bacteria can produce **β-lactamases** that inactivate the β-lactam antibiotics. More than 200 different β-lactamases have been described. Some are specific for penicillins (i.e., penicillinases) or cephalosporins (i.e., cephalosporinases), whereas others have a broad range of activity including some that are capable of inactivating most β-lactam antibiotics. This latter group of β-lactamases **(extended-spectrum β-lactamases [ESBLs])** is particularly troublesome because they are commonly encoded on plasmids and can be transferred from organism to organism. This has severely limited the empirical use of β-lactam antibiotics in some hospitals.

Penicillins

Penicillin antibiotics (Box 20–2) are highly effective antibiotics with an extremely low toxicity. The basic

links is catalyzed by specific enzymes (e.g., transpeptidases, carboxypeptidases, endopeptidases). These regulatory enzymes are also called **penicillin-binding proteins (PBPs)** because they can be bound by β-lactam antibiotics. When growing bacteria are exposed to these antibiotics, the antibiotic binds to the PBPs in the growing bacterial cell wall, thereby inhibiting synthesis but not turnover (degradation) of peptidoglycan and resulting in bacterial cell death. Thus, the β-lactam antibiotics generally act as bactericidal agents.

Bacteria can become resistant to β-lactam antibiotics by three general mechanisms: (1) prevention of the interaction between the antibiotic and the target PBP, (2) decreased binding of the antibiotic to the PBP, and (3) hydrolysis of the antibiotic by β-lactamases. The first mechanism of resistance is seen only in gram-negative bacteria (particularly *Pseudomonas* species) be-

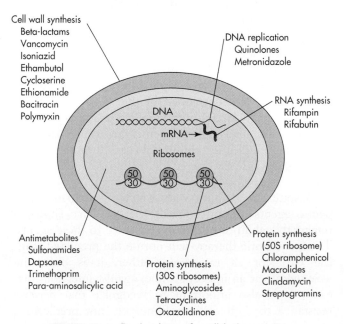

FIGURE 20–1. Basic sites of antibiotic activity.

TABLE 20–1. Basic Mechanisms of Antibiotic Action

Antibiotic	Action
Disruption of Cell Wall	
Penicillin	Binds PBPs and enzymes responsible for peptidoglycan synthesis
Cephalosporin	Binds PBPs and enzymes responsible for peptidoglycan synthesis
Cephamycin	Binds PBPs and enzymes responsible for peptidoglycan synthesis
Carbapenem	Binds PBPs and enzymes responsible for peptidoglycan synthesis
Monobactam	Binds PBPs and enzymes responsible for peptidoglycan synthesis
β-lactamase inhibitor/β-lactam	Binds β-lactamases and prevents enzymatic inactivation of β-lactam
Vancomycin	Inhibits cross-linkage of peptidoglycan layers
Isoniazid	Inhibits mycolic acid synthesis
Ethionamide	Inhibits mycolic acid synthesis
Ethambutol	Inhibits arabinogalactan synthesis
Cycloserine	Inhibits cross-linkage of peptidoglycan layers
Polymyxin	Inhibits bacterial membranes
Bacitracin	Inhibits bacterial cytoplasmic membrane and movement of peptidoglycan precursors
Inhibition of Protein Synthesis	
Aminoglycoside	Produces premature release of aberrant peptide chains from 30S ribosome
Tetracycline	Prevents polypeptide elongation at 30S ribosome
Oxazolidinone	Prevents initiation of protein synthesis at 30S ribosome
Macrolide	Prevents polypeptide elongation at 50S ribosome
Clindamycin	Prevents polypeptide elongation at 50S ribosome
Streptogramins	Prevents polypeptide elongation at 50S ribosome
Inhibition of Nucleic Acid Synthesis	
Quinolone	Binds α subunit of DNA gyrase
Rifampin	Prevents transcription by binding DNA-dependent RNA polymerase
Rifabutin	Prevents transcription by binding DNA-dependent RNA polymerase
Metronidazole	Disrupts bacteria DNA (is cytotoxic compound)
Antimetabolite	
Sulfonamides	Inhibit dihydropteroate synthase and disrupt folic acid synthesis
Dapsone	Inhibits dihydropteroate synthase
Trimethoprim	Inhibits dihydrofolate reductase and disrupts folic acid synthesis

PBPs = penicillin-binding proteins.

BOX 20–2. Penicillins

Antibiotics	Spectrum of Activity
Natural penicillins (penicillin G, penicillin V)	Active against all β-hemolytic and most other streptococci; limited activity against staphylococci; active against meningococci and most gram-positive anaerobes; poor activity against aerobic and anaerobic gram-negative bacilli
Penicillinase-resistant penicillins (nafcillin, methicillin, oxacillin, cloxacillin, dicloxacillin)	Similar to natural penicillins except enhanced activity against staphylococci
Extended-spectrum penicillins (ampicillin, amoxicillin, carbenicillin, ticarcillin, mezlocillin, piperacillin)	Activity against gram-positive cocci equivalent to natural penicillins; active against some gram-negative bacilli
β-lactam with β-lactamase inhibitor (amoxicillin/clavulanic acid, ampicillin/sulbactam, ticarcillin/clavulanic acid, piperacillin/tazobactam)	Activity similar to β-lactam plus improved activity against β-lactamase–producing staphylococci and selected gram-negative bacilli; not all β-lactamases are inhibited; piperacillin/tazobactam is the most active

---

BOX 20−3. Selected Examples of Cephalosporins and Cephamycins

Antibiotics	Spectrum of Activity
Narrow-spectrum (cephalexin, cephalothin, cefazolin, cephapirin, cephradine)	Activity equivalent to oxacillin against gram-positive bacteria; some gram-negative activity (e.g., *E. coli, Klebsiella, P. mirabilis*)
Expanded spectrum (cefaclor, cefamandole, cefuroxime, cefotetan, cefoxitin)	Activity equivalent to oxacillin against gram-positive bacteria; improved gram-negative activity to include *Enterobacter, Citrobacter,* and additional *Proteus* species
Broad spectrum (cefixime, cefotaxime, ceftriaxone, ceftazidime)	Activity equivalent to oxacillin against gram-positive bacteria; improved gram-negative activity to include *Pseudomonas*
Extended spectrum (cefepime, cefpirome)	Activity equivalent to oxacillin against gram-positive bacteria; marginally improved gram-negative activity

---

compound is an organic acid with a β-lactam ring obtained from culture of the mold *Penicillium chrysogenum.* If the mold is grown by a fermentation process, large amounts of a key intermediate, 6-aminopenicillanic acid (the β-lactam ring is fused with a thiazolidine ring), are produced. The biochemical modification of this intermediate yields derivatives that have decreased acid lability and increased absorption in the gastrointestinal tract, resistance to destruction by penicillinase, or a broader spectrum of activity that includes gram-negative bacteria.

Penicillin G is incompletely absorbed because it is inactivated by gastric acid. Thus, it is used mainly as an intravenous drug for the treatment of infections caused by the limited number of susceptible organisms. Penicillin V is more resistant to acid and is the preferred oral form for the treatment of susceptible bacteria. **Penicillinase-resistant penicillins,** such as nafcillin and oxacillin, are used to treat infections caused by susceptible staphylococci. Ampicillin was the first **extended-spectrum penicillin,** although the spectrum of activity was limited primarily to *Escherichia* and *Proteus* species. However, other extended-spectrum penicillins (e.g., carbenicillin, ticarcillin, piperacillin) that have been developed are effective against a broader range of gram-negative bacteria, including *Klebsiella, Enterobacter,* and *Pseudomonas* species.

A novel class of penicillins are those that have been combined with β-**lactamase inhibitors.** The β-lactamase inhibitors (e.g., clavulanic acid, sulbactam, tazobactam) are relatively inactive by themselves but, when combined with some penicillins (e.g., ampicillin, amoxicillin, ticarcillin, piperacillin), are effective in treating some infections caused by β-lactamase−producing bacteria. The inhibitors irreversibly bind and inactivate susceptible bacterial β-lactamases (although not all are bound by these inhibitors), permitting the companion drug to disrupt bacterial cell wall synthesis.

Cephalosporins and Cephamycins

The cephalosporins (Box 20−3) are β-lactam antibiotics derived from 7-aminocephalosporanic acid (the β-lactam ring is fused with a dihydrothiazine ring) that was originally isolated from the mold *Cephalosporium.* The cephamycins are closely related to the cephalosporins, except that they contain oxygen in place of sulfur in the dihydrothiazine ring, rendering them more stable to β-lactamase hydrolysis. The cephalosporins and cephamycins have the same mechanism of action as the penicillins but have a wider antibacterial spectrum, are resistant to many β-lactamases, and have improved pharmacokinetic properties.

Biochemical modifications in the basic antibiotic molecule resulted in the development of antibiotics with improved activity and pharmacokinetic properties. The activity of **narrow-spectrum,** first-generation antibiotics is primarily restricted to *Escherichia coli, Klebsiella* species, *Proteus mirabilis,* and oxacillin-susceptible gram-positive cocci. Many of the **expanded-spectrum,** second-generation antibiotics are also active against *Haemophilus influenzae, Enterobacter* species, *Citrobacter* species, *Serratia* species, and some anaerobes, such as *Bacteroides fragilis.* The **broad-spectrum,** third-generation antibiotics and **expanded spectrum,** fourth-generation antibiotics are active against most Enterobacteriaceae and *Pseudomonas aeruginosa.* Expanded-spectrum antibiotics offer the advantage of increased stability to β-lactamases. Unfortunately, gram-negative bacteria have rapidly developed resistance to most cephalosporins and cephamycins (primarily as the result of β-lactamase production), which has significantly compromised the use of all these agents.

Other Beta-Lactam Antibiotics

Other classes of β-lactam antibiotics (Box 20−4) are the **carbapenems** (e.g., imipenem, meropenem) and

BOX 20–4. Other Beta-Lactam Antibiotics	
Antibiotics	**Spectrum of Activity**
Carbapenems (imipenem, meropenem)	Broad spectrum antibiotics active against most aerobic and anaerobic gram-positive and gram-negative bacteria except oxacillin-resistant staphylococci, most *Enterococcus faecium*, and selected gram-negative bacilli (e.g., some *Burkholderia, Stenotrophomonas*, some *Pseudomonas*)
Monobactam (aztreonam)	Active against selected aerobic gram-negative bacilli but inactive against anaerobes or gram-positive cocci

monobactams (e.g., aztreonam). The carbapenems are broad-spectrum antibiotics that are active against virtually all groups of organisms, with only a few exceptions (e.g., resistance has been reported for all oxacillin-resistant staphylococci, selected Enterobacteriaceae and *Pseudomonas*, and other gram-negative bacilli). In contrast, the monobactams are narrow-spectrum antibiotics that are active only against aerobic, gram-negative bacteria. Anaerobic bacteria and gram-positive bacteria are resistant. The advantage of narrow spectrum antibiotics is that they can be used to treat specific infections without disrupting the patient's normal, protective bacterial population.

Glycopeptides

Vancomycin, originally obtained from *Streptomyces orientalis*, is a complex glycopeptide that disrupts cell wall peptidoglycan synthesis in growing gram-positive bacteria. Vancomycin interacts with the D-alanine–D-alanine termini of the pentapeptide side chains, which interferes sterically with the formation of the bridges between the peptidoglycan chains. Vancomycin is used for the management of infections caused by oxacillin-resistant staphylococci and other gram-positive bacteria resistant to β-lactam antibiotics. Vancomycin is inactive against gram-negative bacteria because the molecule is too large to pass through the outer membrane and reach the peptidoglycan target site. In addition, some organisms are intrinsically resistant to vancomycin (e.g., *Leuconostoc, Lactobacillus, Pediococcus*, and *Erysipelothrix*) because the pentapeptide terminates in D-alanine–D-lactate, which does not bind vancomycin. Intrinsic resistance is also found in some species of enterococci that contain a D-alanine–D-serine terminus (i.e., *Enterococcus gallinarum, Enterococcus casseliflavus*). Finally, some species of enterococci (particularly *Enterococcus faecium* and *Enterococcus faecalis*) have acquired resistance to vancomycin. The genes for this resistance, which is also related to changes in the pentapeptide terminus, are carried on plasmids and have seriously compromised the usefulness of vancomycin for the treatment of enterococcal infections. There is

appropriate concern that if these genes are transferred to staphylococci (this has been done in laboratory experiments), then a highly resistant and virulent organism will emerge.

Polypeptides

Bacitracin, which was isolated from *Bacillus licheniformis*, is a mixture of polypeptides used in topically applied products (e.g., creams, ointments, sprays) for the treatment of skin infections caused by gram-positive bacteria (particularly those caused by *Staphylococcus* and group A *Streptococcus*). Gram-negative bacteria are resistant to this agent. Bacitracin inhibits cell wall synthesis by interfering with dephosphorylation and the recycling of the lipid carrier responsible for moving the peptidoglycan precursors through the cytoplasmic membrane to the cell wall. It may also damage the bacterial cytoplasmic membrane and inhibit RNA transcription. Resistance to the antibiotic is most likely due to failure of the antibiotic to penetrate into the bacterial cell.

The **polymyxins** are a group of cyclic polypeptides derived from *Bacillus polymyxa*. These antibiotics insert into bacterial membranes by interacting with lipopolysaccharides and the phospholipids in the outer membrane, producing increased cell permeability and eventual cell death. Polymyxin B and E (colistin) are capable of causing serious nephrotoxicity. Thus, their use has been limited chiefly to the external treatment of localized infections such as external otitis, eye infections, and skin infections caused by sensitive organisms. Oral administration is used to sterilize the gut. These antibiotics are most active against gram-negative bacilli because gram-positive bacteria do not have an outer membrane.

Isoniazid, Ethionamide, Ethambutol, and Cycloserine

Isoniazid, ethionamide, ethambutol, and cycloserine are cell wall–active antibiotics used for the treatment of mycobacterial infections. **Isoniazid** (isonicotinic acid hydrazide [INH]) is bactericidal against actively replicating mycobacteria. Although the exact mechanism of action is unknown, the synthesis of mycolic acid is affected (the desaturation of the long-chain fatty acids and the elongation of fatty acids and hydroxy lipids are disrupted). **Ethionamide,** a derivative of INH, also blocks mycolic acid synthesis. **Ethambutol** interferes with the synthesis of arabinogalactan in the cell wall, and **cycloserine** inhibits two enzymes, D-alanine–D-alanine synthetase and alanine racemase, that catalyze cell wall synthesis. Resistance to these four antibiotics results primarily from reduced drug uptake into the bacterial cell or alteration of the target sites.

Inhibition of Protein Synthesis

The primary action of the agents in the second largest class of antibiotics is the inhibition of protein synthesis (see Table 20–1).

Aminoglycosides

The aminoglycoside antibiotics (Box 20–5) consist of amino sugars linked through glycosidic bonds to an aminocyclitol ring. Streptomycin, neomycin, kanamycin, and tobramycin were originally isolated from *Streptomyces* species, and gentamicin and sisomicin were isolated from *Micromonospora* species. Amikacin and netilmicin are synthetic derivatives of kanamycin and sisomicin, respectively. These antibiotics exert their effort by passing through the bacterial outer membrane (in gram-negative bacteria), cell wall, and cytoplasmic membrane to the cytoplasm, where they inhibit bacterial protein synthesis by irreversibly binding to the 30S ribosomal proteins. This attachment to the ribosomes has two effects: production of aberrant proteins as the result of misreading of the messenger RNA (mRNA), and interruption of protein synthesis by causing the premature release of the ribosome from mRNA.

The aminoglycosides are bactericidal because of their ability to bind irreversibly to ribosomes and are commonly used to treat serious infections caused by many gram-negative bacilli and some gram-positive organisms. Penetration through the cytoplasmic membrane is an aerobic, energy-dependent process, so anaerobes are resistant to aminoglycosides. Streptococci and enterococci are resistant to aminoglycosides because the aminoglycosides fail to penetrate through the cell wall of these bacteria. Treatment of these organisms requires coadministration of an aminoglycoside with an inhibitor of cell wall synthesis (e.g., penicillin, ampicillin, vancomycin).

The most commonly used antibiotics in this class are **gentamicin** and **tobramycin,** both of which have a broad spectrum of activity. **Netilmicin** is reported to be less ototoxic than gentamicin or tobramycin, but netilmicin also has less antibacterial activity. All three aminoglycosides are used to treat systemic infections caused by susceptible gram-negative bacteria, including the Enterobacteriaceae and *Pseudomonas* species. **Amikacin** is frequently used to treat infections caused by gram-negative bacteria that are resistant to other aminoglycosides, and **streptomycin** has been used for the treatment of tuberculosis, tularemia, and streptococcal or enterococcal infections (in combination with a penicillin). Although **kanamycin** was one of the first aminoglycosides with a broad activity against gram-negative bacteria, it is now rarely used because it is inactive against *Pseudomonas* species.

Resistance to the antibacterial action of aminoglycosides can develop in one of three ways: mutation of the ribosomal binding site, decreased uptake of the antibiotic into the bacterial cell, or enzymatic modification of the antibiotic. Resistance caused by alteration of the bacterial ribosome is relatively uncommon, except in members of the genus *Enterococcus*. Because these important gram-positive cocci can be killed only with the synergistic combination of an aminoglycoside with a cell wall antibiotic, this resistance is clinically signifi-

BOX 20–5. Aminoglycosides and Aminocyclitols	
Antibiotics	**Spectrum of Activity**
Aminoglycosides (streptomycin, kanamycin, gentamicin, tobramycin, amikacin)	Primarily used to treat infections with gram-negative bacilli; kanamycin with limited activity; tobramycin slightly more active than gentamicin vs. *Pseudomonas;* amikacin most active; streptomycin and gentamicin combined with cell wall–active antibiotic to treat enterococcal infections; streptomycin active vs. mycobacteria and selected gram-negative bacilli
Aminocyclitol (spectinomycin)	Active vs. *Neisseria gonorrhoeae*

cant. Resistance caused by inhibited transport of the antibiotic into the bacterial cell is occasionally observed with *Pseudomonas* but more commonly seen with anaerobic bacteria. Enzymatic modification of aminoglycosides by phosphorylation, adenylation, and acetylation of the amino and hydroxyl groups of the antibiotic is the most common mechanism of resistance. The differences in the antibacterial activity among the aminoglycosides are determined by their relative susceptibility to these enzymes.

Tetracyclines

The tetracylines (Box 20–6) are broad-spectrum, bacteriostatic antibiotics that inhibit protein synthesis in bacteria by binding reversibly to the 30S ribosomal subunits, thus blocking the binding of aminoacyl-transfer RNA (tRNA) to the 30S ribosome–mRNA complex. Tetracyclines (i.e., **tetracycline, doxycycline, minocycline)** are effective in the treatment of infections caused by *Chlamydia, Mycoplasma, Rickettsia,* and other selected gram-positive and gram-negative bacteria. All tetracyclines have a similar spectrum of activity, with the primary difference among the antibiotics in their pharmacokinetic properties. Resistance to the tetracyclines can stem from decreased penetration of the antibiotic into the bacterial cell, active efflux of the antibiotic out of the cell, alteration of the ribosomal target site, or enzymatic modification of the antibiotic. Mutations in the chromosomal gene encoding the outer membrane porin protein, OmpF, can lead to low-level resistance to the tetracyclines, as well as to other antibiotics (e.g., β-lactams, quinolones, chloramphenicol).

Researchers have identified a variety of genes in different bacteria that control the active efflux of the tetracyclines from the cell. This is the most common cause of resistance. Resistance to the tetracyclines can also result from the production of proteins similar to elongation factors that protect the 30S ribosome.

When this happens, the antibiotic can still bind to the ribosome, but protein synthesis is not disrupted.

Oxazolidinones

The oxazolidinones are a narrow-spectrum class of antibiotics that block initiation of protein synthesis by interfering with the formation of the initiation complex at the 30S ribosomal subunit. Because of this unique mechanism, cross-resistance with other protein inhibitors does not occur. The current representative of this class is **linezolid,** which has activity against all staphylococci, streptococci, and enterococci (including those strains resistant to penicillins, vancomycin, and the aminoglycosides). Because the multidrug-resistant enterococci are difficult to treat, use of linezolid is generally reserved for these infections.

Chloramphenicol

Chloramphenicol has a broad antibacterial spectrum similar to that of tetracycline but is the drug of choice only for the treatment of typhoid fever. The reason for its limited use is that besides interfering with bacterial protein synthesis, it disrupts protein synthesis in human bone marrow cells and can produce blood dyscrasias such as aplastic anemia (1 per 24,000 treated patients). Chloramphenicol exerts its bacteriostatic effect by binding reversibly to the peptidyl transferase component of the 50S ribosomal subunit, thus blocking peptide elongation. Resistance to chloramphenicol is observed in bacteria producing plasmid-encoded chloramphenicol acetyltransferase, which catalyzes the acetylation of the 3-hydroxy group of chloramphenicol. The product is incapable of binding to the 50S subunit. Less commonly, chromosomal mutations alter the outer membrane porin proteins, causing the gram-negative bacilli to be less permeable.

BOX 20–6. **Macrolides and Tetracyclines**

Antibiotics	Spectrum of Activity
Macrolides (erythromycin, clarithromycin, azithromycin)	Broad-spectrum antibiotics active against gram-positive and some gram-negative bacteria, *Neisseria, Legionella, Mycoplasma, Chlamydia, Chlamydophila, Treponema,* and *Rickettsia;* clarithromycin and azithromycin active against some mycobacteria
Tetracyclines (tetracycline, doxycycline, minocycline)	Broad-spectrum antibiotics with activity similar to that of macrolides.

Macrolides

Erythromycin, derived from *Streptomyces erythreus,* is the model macrolide antibiotic (see Box 20–6). The basic structure of this class of antibiotics is a macrocyclic lactone ring bound to two sugars, desosamine and cladinose. Modification of the macrolide structure has led to the development of newer agents, including **azithromycin** and **clarithromycin.** Macrolides are bacteriostatic antibiotics with a broad spectrum of activity. They have been used to treat pulmonary infections caused by *Mycoplasma, Legionella,* and *Chlamydia* species, as well as to treat infections caused by *Campylobacter* species and gram-positive bacteria in patients allergic to penicillin. Azithromycin and clarithromycin have also been used to treat infections caused by mycobacteria (e.g., *Mycobacterium avium* complex). Macrolides exert their effect by their reversible binding to the 50S ribosome, which blocks polypeptide elongation. Resistance to the macrolides stems from the methylation of the 23S ribosomal RNA, which prevents binding by the antibiotic. Destruction of the lactone ring by an erythromycin esterase or the active efflux of the antibiotic from the bacterial cell can also be the source of resistance.

Clindamycin

Clindamycin (in the family of lincosamide antibiotics) is a derivative of lincomycin, which was originally isolated from *Streptomyces lincolnensis.* Like chloramphenicol and the macrolides, clindamycin blocks protein elongation by binding to the 50S ribosome. It inhibits peptidyl transferase by interfering with the binding of the amino acid–acyl-tRNA complex. Clindamycin is active against staphylococci and anaerobic gram-negative bacilli but is generally inactive against aerobic gram-negative bacteria. Methylation of the 23S ribosomal RNA is the source of bacterial resistance. Because both erythromycin and clindamycin can induce

this enzymatic resistance (also plasmid mediated), cross-resistance between these two classes of antibiotics is observed.

Streptogramins

The streptogramins are a class of cyclic peptides produced by *Streptomyces* species. These antibiotics are administered as a combination of two components, group A and group B streptogramins, that act synergistically to inhibit protein synthesis. The antibiotic currently available in this class is **quinupristin-dalfopristin** (known by the trade name Synercid). Dalfopristin binds to the 50S ribosomal subunit and induces a conformational change that facilitates binding of quinupristin. Dalfopristin prevents peptide chain elongation, and quinupristin initiates premature release of peptide chains from the ribosome. This combination drug is active against staphylococci, streptococci, and *E. faecium* (but not *E. faecalis*). Use of the antibiotic has been restricted primarily to treating vancomycin-resistant *E. faecium* infections.

Inhibition of Nucleic Acid Synthesis

Quinolones

The quinolones (Box 20–7) are synthetic chemotherapeutic agents that inhibit bacterial DNA gyrases or topoisomerases, which are required for DNA replication, recombination, and repair. **Nalidixic acid** was used to treat urinary tract infections caused by a variety of gram-negative bacteria, but resistance to the drug developed rapidly, causing it to fall out of use. This drug has now been replaced by newer, more active quinolones, such as **ciprofloxacin, levofloxacin,** and **gatifloxacin.** The newer quinolones (referred to as fluoroquinolones) were made by modifying the two-ring quinolone nucleus. These antibiotics have excellent activity against gram-positive and gram-negative

---

BOX 2–7. Quinolones

Antibiotics	Spectrum of Activity
Narrow spectrum (nalidixic acid)	Active against selected gram-negative bacilli; no useful gram-positive activity
Broad spectrum (ciprofloxacin, levofloxacin, lomefloxacin, norfloxacin, ofloxacin)	Broad-spectrum antibiotics with activity against gram-positive and gram-negative bacteria
Expanded spectrum (gatifloxacin, grepafloxacin, clinafloxacin, moxifloxacin)	Broad-spectrum antibiotics with enhanced activity against gram-positive bacteria (particularly streptococci and enterococci) compared with early quinolones; activity against gram-negative bacilli similar to that of ciprofloxacin and related quinolones

bacteria, although resistance can develop rapidly in *Pseudomonas*, oxacillin-resistant staphylococci, and enterococci.

DNA gyrase consists of two α and two β subunits, with the quinolones binding to the α subunits. Alteration of this subunit is the principal mechanism of bacterial resistance, although decreased drug uptake has also been observed. Decreased uptake stems from changes in porin proteins on the bacterial surface. Both resistance mechanisms are chromosomally mediated.

Rifampin and Rifabutin

Rifampin, a semisynthetic derivative of rifamycin B produced by *Streptomyces mediterranei*, binds to DNA-dependent RNA polymerase and inhibits the initiation of RNA synthesis. Rifampin is bactericidal for *Mycobacterium tuberculosis* and is very active against aerobic gram-positive cocci, including staphylococci and streptococci.

Because resistance can develop rapidly, rifampin is usually combined with one or more other effective antibiotics. Rifampin resistance in gram-positive bacteria results from a mutation in the chromosomal gene that codes for the β subunit of RNA polymerase. Gram-negative bacteria are resistant intrinsically to rifampin as the result of decreased uptake of the hydrophobic antibiotic. **Rifabutin,** a derivative of rifamycin, has a similar mode of activity and spectrum of activity. It is particularly active against *M. avium*.

Metronidazole

Metronidazole was originally introduced as an oral agent for the treatment of *Trichomonas* vaginitis. However, it was also found to be effective in the treatment of amebiasis, giardiasis, and serious anaerobic bacterial infections (including those caused by *B. fragilis*). Metronidazole has no significant activity against aerobic or facultatively anaerobic bacteria. The antimicrobial properties of metronidazole stem from the reduction of its nitro group by bacterial nitroreductase, thereby producing cytotoxic compounds that disrupt the host DNA. Resistance results from either decreased uptake of the antibiotic or elimination of the cytotoxic compounds before they can interact with host DNA.

Antimetabolites

The **sulfonamides** are antimetabolites that compete with *p*-aminobenzoic acid, thereby preventing the synthesis of the folic acid required by certain microorganisms. Because mammalian organisms do not synthesize folic acid (required as a vitamin), sulfonamides do not interfere with mammalian cell metabolism. **Trimethoprim** is another antimetabolite that interferes with folic acid metabolism by inhibiting dihydrofolate reductase, thereby preventing the conversion of dihydrofolate to tetrahydrofolate. This inhibition blocks the formation of thymidine, some purines, methionine, and glycine. Trimethoprim is commonly combined with sulfamethoxazole to produce a synergistic combination active at two steps in the synthesis of folic acid. **Dapsone** and ***p*-aminosalicylic** acid are also antifolates that have proved to be useful for treating mycobacterial infections.

Sulfonamides are effective against a broad range of gram-positive and gram-negative organisms, such as *Nocardia*, *Chlamydia*, and some protozoa. Short-acting sulfonamides such as sulfisoxazole are among the drugs of choice for the treatment of acute urinary tract infections caused by susceptible bacteria such as *E. coli*. Trimethoprim-sulfamethoxazole is effective against a large variety of gram-positive and gram-negative microorganisms and is the drug of choice for the treatment of acute and chronic urinary tract infections. The combination is also effective in the treatment of infections caused by *Pneumocystis carinii*, bacterial infections of the lower respiratory tract, otitis media, and uncomplicated gonorrhea.

Resistance to these antibiotics can stem from a variety of mechanisms. Bacteria such as *Pseudomonas* are resistant as the result of permeability barriers. A decreased affinity of dihydrofolate reductase can be the source of trimethoprim resistance. In addition, bacteria that use exogenous thymidine (e.g., enterococci) are also intrinsically resistant.

Other Antibiotics

Clofazimine is a lipophilic antibiotic that binds to mycobacterial DNA. It is highly active against *M. tuberculosis*, is a first-line drug for the treatment of *Mycobacterium leprae* infections, and has been recommended as a secondary antibiotic for the treatment of infections caused by other mycobacterial species.

Pyrazinamide (PZA) is active against *M. tuberculosis* at a low pH, such as that found in phagolysosomes. The active form of this antibiotic is pyrazinoic acid, produced when PZA is hydrolyzed in the liver. The mechanism by which PZA exerts its effect is unknown.

QUESTIONS

1. Describe the mode of action of the following antibiotics: penicillin, vancomycin, isoniazid, gentamicin, tetracycline, erythromycin, polymyxin, ciprofloxacin, and sulfamethoxazole.

2. By what three mechanisms do bacteria become resistant to β-lactam antibiotics? What is the mechanism responsible for oxacillin resistance in *Staphylococcus*? Imipenem resistance in *Pseudomonas*? Penicillin resistance in *S. pneumoniae*?

3. By what three mechanisms have organisms developed resistance to aminoglycosides?

4. What mechanism is responsible for resistance to the quinolones?

5. How do trimethoprim and the sulfonamides differ in their mode of action?

BIBLIOGRAPHY

Kucers A, Bennett NM: *The use of antibiotics: a comprehensive review with clinical emphasis*, ed 4, Philadelphia, 1989, Lippincott.

Mandell GL, Bennett JE, Dolin R: *Principles and practice of infectious diseases*, ed 5, New York, 2000, Churchill Livingstone.

Murray P et al: *Manual of clinical microbiology*, ed 7, Washington, DC, 1999, American Society for Microbiology.

CHAPTER 21

Laboratory Diagnosis of Bacterial Diseases

Microbiology differs from all other specialties in clinical pathology in that the objective of many of the tests is to isolate viable organisms. This means that the proper specimen must be collected, delivered expeditiously to the laboratory in the appropriate transport system, and inoculated onto media that will support the growth of the most likely pathogens. Care must also be taken to keep the specimen from being contaminated with clinically insignificant organisms that are present in the environment or that colonize the patient's mucosal surfaces. Collection of the proper specimen and its rapid delivery to the clinical laboratory are primarily the responsibility of the patient's physician, whereas appropriate transport systems and culture methods are selected by the clinical microbiologist. These responsibilities are not mutually exclusive, however. The microbiologist should be prepared to instruct the physician about what specimens should be collected if a particular diagnosis is suspected and the physician must provide the microbiologist with information about the clinical diagnosis so that the right culture media and growth conditions are selected. The chapters and bibliographic citations that follow provide information about the selection of culture media for specific pathogens. The primary focus of this chapter, however, is to provide guidelines for the proper collection and transport of different specimens (Table 21–1) as well as general information about the laboratory processing of specimens. Whenever an unusual or fastidious pathogen is suspected (e.g., *Bordetella pertussis*, *Francisella tularensis*), the laboratory should be notified so that the appropriate transport system and culture media can be obtained.

Blood

The culture of blood is one of the most important procedures performed in the clinical microbiology laboratory. The success of this test is directly related to the methods used to collect the blood sample. The single most important factor that determines the success of a blood culture is the volume of blood processed. Specifically, there is a 40% increase in the rate of cultures positive for organisms if 20 mL rather than 10 mL of blood are cultured because more than half of all septic patients have fewer than one organism per milliliter of blood. Therefore, approximately 20 mL of blood should be collected from an adult for each blood culture and proportionally smaller volumes should be collected from children and neonates. Because many hospitalized patients are susceptible to infections with organisms colonizing their skin, careful disinfection of the patient's skin with alcohol followed by 2% iodine is important.

Bacteremia and fungemia are defined as the presence of bacteria and fungi, respectively, in the blood stream, and these infections are referred to collectively as septicemia. Clinical studies have shown that septicemia can be continuous or intermittent. **Continuous septicemia** occurs primarily in patients with intravascular infections (e.g., endocarditis, septic thrombophlebitis, intravascular catheter infections) or with overwhelming sepsis (e.g., septic shock). **Intermittent septicemia** occurs in patients with other infections in which the focus of the infection is at a distal site (e.g., lungs, urinary tract, soft tissues). The timing of blood collection is not important for patients with continuous septicemias, but it is critical for patients with intermittent septicemias. In addition, because clinical signs of sepsis (e.g., fever, chills, hypotension) are a response to the release of endotoxins or exotoxins from the organisms, these signs occur as long as 1 hour after the organisms have been cleared from the blood stream. Thus, the worst time to collect blood samples for culture is when the patient develops a fever. Two to three blood samples should be collected at random times during a 24-hour period; it is not necessary to collect any additional samples, even in patients receiving antibiotics.

TABLE 21–1. Bacteriology Specimen Collection for Bacterial Pathogens

Specimen	Transport System	Specimen Volume	Other Considerations
Blood—routine bacterial culture	Blood culture bottle with nutrient media	Adults: 20 mL/culture Children: 5–10 mL/culture Neonates: 1–2 mL/culture	Skin should be disinfected with 70% alcohol followed by 2% iodine; 2–3 cultures collected every 24 hr unless patient is in septic shock or antibiotics will be started immediately; blood collections should be separated by 30–60 min; blood is divided equally into two bottles of nutrient media.
Blood—intracellular bacteria (e.g. *Brucella*, *Francisella*, *Neisseria* species)	Same as that for routine blood cultures; lysis-centrifugation system	Same as that for routine blood cultures	Considerations are same as those for routine blood cultures; release of intracellular bacteria may improve organism's recovery; *Neisseria* species is inhibited by some anticoagulants (sodium polyanethoesulfonate).
Blood—*Leptospira* species	Sterile heparinized tube	1–5 mL	Specimen is useful only during the first week of illness; afterward, urine should be cultured.
Cerebrospinal fluid	Sterile screw-capped tube	Bacteria culture: 1–5 mL Mycobacterial culture: as large a volume as possible	Specimen must be collected aseptically and delivered immediately to laboratory; it should not be exposed to heat or refrigeration.
Other normally sterile fluids (e.g., abdominal, chest, synovial, pericardial)	Small volume: sterile screw-capped tube; large volume: blood culture bottle with nutrient medium	As large a volume as possible	Specimens are collected with needle and syringe; swab is not used because quantity of collected specimen is inadequate; air should not be injected into culture bottle because it will inhibit growth of anaerobes.
Catheter	Sterile screw-capped tube or specimen cup	N/A	The entry site should be disinfected with alcohol; catheter should be aseptically removed on receipt of specimen in laboratory; catheter is rolled across blood agar plate and then discarded.
Respiratory—throat	Swab immersed in transport medium	N/A	Area of inflammation is swabbed; exudate is collected if present; contact with saliva should be avoided because it can inhibit recovery of group A streptococci.
Respiratory—epiglottis	Collection of blood for culture	Same as for blood culture	Swabbing the epiglottis can precipitate complete airway closure; blood cultures should be collected for specific diagnosis.
Respiratory—sinuses	Sterile anaerobic tube or vial	1–5 mL	Specimens must be collected with needle and syringe; culture of nasopharynx or oropharynx has no value; specimen should be cultured for aerobic and anaerobic bacteria.
Respiratory—lower airways	Sterile screw-capped bottle; anaerobic tube or vial only for specimens collected by avoiding upper tract flora	1–2 mL	Expectorated sputum; if possible, patient rinses mouth with water before collection of the specimen; patient should cough deeply and expectorate lower airway secretions directly into sterile cup; collector should avoid contamination with saliva. Bronchoscopy specimen: anesthetics can inhibit growth of bacteria, so specimens should be processed immediately; if "protected" bronchoscope is used, anaerobic cultures can be performed. Transtracheal aspirate or direct lung aspirate: specimens can be processed for aerobic and anaerobic bacteria.

(continued)

Specimen	Transport System	Specimen Volume	Other Considerations
Ear	Capped, needleless syringe; sterile screw-capped tube	Whatever volume is collected	Specimen should be aspirated with needle and syringe; culture of external ear has no predictive value for otitis media.
Eye	Inoculate plates at bedside (seal and transport to laboratory immediately)	Whatever volume is collected	For infections on surface of eye, specimens are collected with swab or by corneal scrapings; for deep-seated infections, aspiration of aqueous or vitreous fluid is performed; all specimens should be inoculated onto appropriate media at collection; delays will result in significant loss of organisms.
Exudates (transudates, drainage, ulcers)	Swab immersed in transport medium; aspirate in sterile screw-capped tube	Bacteria: 1–5 mL Mycobacteria: 3–5 mL	Contamination with surface material should be avoided; specimens are generally unsuitable for anaerobic culture.
Wounds (abscess, pus)	Aspirate in sterile screw-capped tube or sterile anaerobic tube or vial	1–5 mL of pus	Specimens should be collected with sterile needle and syringe; curette is used to collect specimen at base of wound; swabbed specimens should be avoided.
Tissues	Sterile screw-capped tube; sterile anaerobic tube or vial	Representative sample from center and border of lesion	Specimen should be aseptically placed into appropriate sterile container; adequate quantity of specimen must be collected to recover small numbers of organisms.
Urine—midstream	Sterile urine container	Bacteria: 1 mL Mycobacteria: ≥10 mL	Contamination of specimen with bacteria from the urethra or vagina should be avoided; first portion of the voided specimen is discarded; organisms can grow rapidly in urine, so specimens must be transported immediately to laboratory, held in bacteriostatic preservative, or refrigerated.
Urine—catheterized	Sterile urine container	Bacteria: 1 mL Mycobacteria: ≥10 mL	Catheterization is not recommended for routine cultures (risk of inducing infection); first portion of collected specimen is contaminated with urethral bacteria, so it should be discarded (similar to midstream voided specimen); specimen must be transported rapidly to laboratory.
Urine—suprapubic aspirate	Sterile anaerobic tube or vial	Bacteria: 1 mL Mycobacteria: ≥10 mL	This is an invasive specimen, so urethral bacteria are avoided; it is only valid method available for collecting specimens for anaerobic culture; also useful for collection of specimens from children or adults unable to void uncontaminated specimens.
Genitals	Specially designed swabs for *Neisseria gonorrhoeae* and *Chlamydia* probes	N/A	Area of inflammation or exudate should be sampled; endocervix (not vagina) and urethra should be cultured for optimal detection.
Feces (stool)	Sterile screw-capped container	N/A	Rapid transport to laboratory is necessary to prevent production of acid (bactericidal for some enteric pathogens) by normal fecal bacteria; it is unsuitable for anaerobic culture; because large number of different media will be inoculated, swab should not be used for specimen collection.

N/A = Not applicable.

Most blood samples are inoculated into bottles filled with enriched nutrient broths. This should be done when the sample is collected. To ensure the maximal recovery of important organisms, two bottles of media should be inoculated for each culture. When these inoculated bottles of broth are received in the laboratory, they are incubated at 37°C and inspected at regular intervals for evidence of microbial growth. When growth is detected, the broths are subcultured to isolate the organism for identification and antimicrobial susceptibility testing. Most clinically significant isolates are detected within the first 2 days of incubation; however, all cultures should be incubated for a minimum of 5 to 7 days. More prolonged incubation is generally unnecessary, except for fastidious organisms. Because few organisms are typically present in the blood of a septic patient, it is not worthwhile to stain samples of blood (e.g., Gram stain) for microscopic analysis.

Cerebrospinal Fluid

Bacterial meningitis is a serious disease that is associated with high morbidity and mortality if the etiologic diagnosis is delayed. Because some common pathogens are labile (e.g., *Neisseria meningitidis*, *Streptococcus pneumoniae*), specimens of cerebrospinal fluid should be processed immediately after they are collected. Under no circumstance should the specimen be refrigerated or heated. The patient's skin is disinfected with alcohol and iodine before lumbar puncture, and the cerebrospinal fluid is collected into sterile screw-capped tubes. On receipt of the specimen in the microbiology laboratory, it is concentrated by centrifugation, and the sediment is used to inoculate bacteriologic media and prepare a Gram stain. Other stains are used if mycobacterial (acid-fast stain) infections are suspected. The laboratory technician should notify the physician immediately if a stain or culture is positive for organisms.

Other Normally Sterile Fluids

A variety of other normally sterile fluids may be collected for bacteriologic culture, including abdominal (peritoneal), chest (pleural), synovial, and pericardial fluids. If a large volume of fluid can be collected by aspiration (e.g., abdominal or chest fluids), it should be inoculated into blood culture bottles containing nutrient media. A small portion should also be sent to the laboratory in a sterile tube so that appropriately stained specimens (e.g., Gram, acid-fast) can be prepared. A large variety of organisms may be responsible for causing infections at these sites, including polymicrobial mixtures of aerobic and anaerobic organisms. For this reason, biologic staining is useful for identifying the organisms responsible for the infection. If only small

quantities of fluid are collected, the specimen can be inoculated directly onto agar media. Because relatively few organisms may be in the sample (as a result of the dilution of organisms or microbial elimination by the host immune response), it is important to culture as large a volume of fluid as possible. Because anaerobes may also be present in the sample (particularly samples obtained from patients with intra-abdominal or pulmonary infections), the specimen should not be exposed to oxygen.

Upper Respiratory Tract Specimens

Most bacterial infections of the pharynx are caused by group A *Streptococcus*. Other bacteria that can cause pharyngitis include *Corynebacterium diphtheriae*, *B. pertussis*, *Neisseria gonorrhoeae*, *Chlamydophila pneumoniae*, and *Mycoplasma pneumoniae*. These bacteria, however, are relatively uncommon, and special techniques must be used to isolate them. Other potentially pathogenic bacteria, such as *Staphylococcus aureus*, *S. pneumoniae*, *Haemophilus influenzae*, Enterobacteriaceae, and *Pseudomonas aeruginosa* may be present in the oropharynx, but they rarely cause pharyngitis.

A Dacron or calcium alginate swab should be used to collect pharyngeal specimens. The tonsillar areas, posterior pharynx, and any exudate or ulcerative area should be sampled. Contamination of the specimen with saliva should be avoided because bacteria in saliva can overgrow or inhibit the growth of group A streptococci. If a pseudomembrane is present (e.g., as with *C. diphtheriae* infections), a portion should be dislodged and submitted for culture. Group A streptococci and *C. diphtheriae* are very resistant to drying, so special precautions are not required for transport of the specimen to the laboratory. In contrast, specimens collected for the recovery of *B. pertussis* and *N. gonorrhoeae* should be inoculated onto culture media immediately after they are collected and before they are sent to the laboratory. Specimens obtained for the isolation of Chlamydiaceae and *M. pneumoniae* should be transported in a special transport medium.

Group A streptococci can be detected directly in the clinical specimen through the use of immunoassays for the group-specific antigen. Although these tests are very specific, they are insensitive and cannot be used to reliably exclude the diagnosis of group A streptococcal pharyngitis.

Other upper respiratory tract infections can involve the epiglottis and sinuses. Complete airway obstruction can be precipitated by attempts to culture the epiglottis (particularly in children). Thus, these cultures should never be performed. The specific diagnosis of a sinus infection requires (1) the direct aspiration of the sinus, (2) appropriate anaerobic transport of the specimen to the laboratory (using a system that avoids exposing anaerobes to oxygen and drying), and (3) prompt processing. Culture of the nasopharynx or oropharynx is not useful and should not be performed. *S. pneumoniae*, *H. influenzae*, *Moraxella catarrhalis*, *S. aureus*, and anaerobes are the most common pathogens that cause sinusitis.

Lower Respiratory Tract Specimens

A variety of techniques can be used to collect lower respiratory tract specimens; these include expectoration, induction with saline, bronchoscopy, transtracheal aspiration (rarely used today), and direct aspiration through the chest wall. Because upper airway bacteria may contaminate expectorated and induced sputa, the specimen should be inspected microscopically to assess the magnitude of oral contamination and the value of processing the specimen. Specimens containing many squamous epithelial cells and no predominant bacteria in association with leukocytes should not be processed for culture. The presence of squamous epithelial cells indicates that the specimen has been contaminated with saliva. Such contamination can be avoided by obtaining the specimen using a protected bronchoscope, transtracheal aspiration, or direct lung aspiration. These invasive procedures must be used to collect uncontaminated specimens from patients with anaerobic lung infections. Most lower respiratory tract pathogens grow within 2 to 3 days, although it may take additional time for the bacterium to be isolated and identified. If infection with a mycobacterium such as *Mycobacterium tuberculosis* is suspected, the laboratory should be notified so that special culture techniques and acid-fast stains can be used.

Ear and Eye

Tympanocentesis (the aspiration of fluid from the middle ear) is required to make the specific diagnosis of a middle ear infection. This is unnecessary in most patients, however, because the most common pathogens that cause these infections (*S. pneumoniae*, *H. influenzae*, and *M. catarrhalis*) can be treated empirically.

Outer ear infections are typically caused by *P. aeruginosa* ("swimmer's ear") or *S. aureus*. The proper specimen to be obtained for culture is a scraping of the involved area of the ear.

Collection of specimens for the diagnosis of ocular infections is difficult because the sample obtained is generally very small and relatively few organisms may be present. Samples of the eye surface should be collected by a swab before topical anesthetics are applied, followed by corneal scrapings whenever necessary. The eye must be directly aspirated to collect intraocular specimens. The culture media should be inoculated when the specimens are collected and before they are sent to the laboratory. Although most common ocular pathogens grow rapidly (e.g., *S. aureus*, *S. pneumoniae*, *H. influenzae*, *P. aeruginosa*, *Bacillus cereus*), some may require prolonged incubation (e.g., coagulase-negative staphylococci) or the use of specialized culture media (*N. gonorrhoeae*, *Chlamydia trachomatis*).

Wounds, Abscesses, and Tissues

Open, draining wounds can frequently be colonized with potentially pathogenic organisms unrelated to the specific infectious process. Therefore, it is important to collect samples from deep in the wound after the surface has been cleaned. Whenever possible, a swab should be avoided because it is difficult to obtain a representative sample without contamination with organisms colonizing the surface. Likewise, aspirates from a closed abscess should be collected from both the center and the wall of the abscess. Simply collecting pus from an abscess is generally nonproductive because most organisms actively replicate at the base of the abscess rather than in the center. Drainage from soft tissue infections can be collected by aspiration. If fluctuance is not obtained, a small quantity of saline can be infused into the tissue and then withdrawn for culture. Saline containing a bactericidal preservative should not be used.

Tissues should be obtained from representative portions of the infectious process, with multiple samples collected whenever possible. The tissue specimen should be transported in a sterile screw-capped container, and sterile saline should be added to prevent drying if a small sample (e.g., biopsy specimen) is collected. A sample of tissue should also be submitted for histologic examination. Because collection of tissue specimens requires invasive procedures, every effort should be made to collect the proper specimen and ensure that it is cultured for all clinically significant organisms that may be responsible for the infection. This requires close communication between the physician and microbiologist.

Urine

Urine is one of the most frequently submitted specimens for culture. Because potentially pathogenic bacteria colonize the urethra, the first portion of urine collected by voiding or catheterization should be discarded. Urinary tract pathogens can also grow in urine, so there should be no delay in the transport of specimens to the laboratory. If the specimen cannot be cultured immediately, it should be refrigerated or placed into a bacteriostatic **urine preservative**. Once the specimen is received in the laboratory, 1 to 10 μl is inoculated onto each culture medium (generally one nonselective agar medium and one selective medium).

This is done so that the number of organisms in the urine can be quantitated, which is useful for assessing the significance of an isolate, although small numbers of organisms in a patient with pyuria can be clinically significant. Numerous urine screening procedures (e.g., biochemical tests, microscopy stains) have been developed and are used widely; however, these procedures cannot be recommended because they are invariably insensitive in detecting a clinically significant, low-grade bacteriuria.

Genital Specimens

Despite the variety of bacteria associated with sexually transmitted diseases, most laboratories concentrate on detecting *N. gonorrhoeae* and *C. trachomatis*. This was done traditionally by inoculating the specimen onto media selective for these organisms. This is a slow process, however, taking 2 or more days for a positive culture to be obtained and more time for isolates to be identified definitively. Culture was also found to be insensitive because the organisms are extremely labile and die rapidly during transit under less than optimal conditions. For these reasons, researchers have developed a variety of nonculture methods. The most popular methods used today are nucleic acid amplification procedures (e.g., amplification of species-specific DNA sequences by the polymerase chain reaction, ligase chain reaction, and other methods) for both organisms. Detection of these amplified sequences with probes is both sensitive and specific.

The other major bacterium that causes sexually transmitted disease is *Treponema pallidum*, the etiologic agent of syphilis. This organism cannot be cultured in the clinical laboratory, so the diagnosis is made using microscopy or serology. Material from lesions must be examined using darkfield microscopy because the organism is too thin to be detected using brightfield microscopy. In addition, the organism dies rapidly when exposed to air and drying conditions, so the microscopic examination must be performed at the time the specimen is collected. The serologic diagnosis of syphilis is the method of choice and is discussed in Chapter 41.

Fecal Specimens

A large variety of bacteria can cause gastrointestinal infections. For these bacteria to be recovered in culture, an adequate stool sample must be collected (generally not a problem in a patient with diarrhea), transported to the laboratory in a manner that ensures the viability of the infecting organisms, and inoculated onto the appropriate selective media. Rectal swabs should not be submitted, because a variety of selective media must be inoculated for the various possible pathogens to be recovered. The quantity of feces collected on a swab would be inadequate.

Stool specimens should be collected in a clean pan and then transferred into a tightly sealed waterproof container. The specimens should be transported promptly to the laboratory to prevent acidic changes in the stool (caused by bacterial metabolism), which are toxic for organisms such as *Shigella*. If a delay is anticipated, the feces should be mixed with a preservative such as phosphate buffer mixed with glycerol or Cary-Blair transport medium (if *Campylobacter* infection is suspected). In general, however, rapid transport of the specimen to the laboratory is always superior to the use of any transport medium.

It is important to notify the laboratory if a particular enteric pathogen is suspected, because this will help the laboratory select the appropriate culture medium. For example, although *Vibrio* species can grow on the common media used for the culture of stool specimens, the use of media selective for *Vibrio* facilitates the rapid isolation and identification of this organism. In addition, some organisms are not isolated routinely by the laboratory procedures. For example, enterotoxigenic *Escherichia coli* can grow on routine culture media but would not be readily distinguished from nonpathogenic *E. coli*. Likewise, other organisms would not be expected to be in a stool sample because their disease is caused by toxin produced in the food and not by growth of the organism in the gastrointestinal tract (e.g., *S. aureus*). The microbiologist should be able to select the appropriate test (e.g., culture, toxin assay) if the specific pathogen is indicated. *Clostridium difficile* is a significant cause of antibiotic-associated gastrointestinal disease. Although the organism can be cultured from stool specimens if the specimens are delivered promptly to the laboratory, the most specific way to diagnose the infection is by detecting the *C. difficile* toxin in fecal extracts. The toxin is responsible for the disease.

Because many bacteria, both pathogenic and nonpathogenic, are present in fecal specimens, it frequently takes at least 3 days for the enteric pathogen to be isolated and identified. For this reason, stool cultures are used to confirm the clinical diagnosis, and therapy, if indicated, should not be delayed pending the culture results. Indeed, antimicrobial susceptibility testing is usually not performed with most enteric pathogens.

QUESTIONS

1. What is the most important factor that influences the recovery of microorganisms in blood collected from patients with sepsis?

2. Which organisms are important causes of bacterial pharyngitis?

3. What criteria should be used to assess the quality of a lower respiratory tract specimen?

4. What methods are used to detect the three most common bacteria that cause sexually transmitted diseases?

BIBLIOGRAPHY

Baron EJ, Peterson L, Finegold SM: *Bailey and Scott's diagnostic microbiology*, ed 9, St. Louis, 1995, Mosby.

Mandell G, Bennett JE, Dolin R: *Principles and practice of infectious diseases*, ed 5, New York, 2000, Churchill Livingstone.

Murray PR et al: *Manual of clinical microbiology*, ed 7, Washington, DC, 1999, American Society for Microbiology.

C H A P T E R   2 2

Staphylococcus and Related Organisms

The gram-positive cocci are a heterogeneous collection of approximately 21 genera that colonize humans. Features that they have in common are their spherical shape, their Gram-stain reaction, and an absence of endospores. The presence or absence of catalase activity is a simple test that is used to subdivide the various genera. The aerobic catalase-positive genera (*Staphylococcus*, *Micrococcus*, *Stomatococcus*, and *Alloiococcus*) are discussed in this chapter, the aerobic catalase-negative genera (*Streptococcus*, *Enterococcus*, and related organisms) are discussed in the next two chapters, and the anaerobic gram-positive cocci (*Peptostreptococcus*) are discussed in Chapter 36.

The name *Staphylococcus* is derived from the Greek term *staphylé*, meaning "a bunch of grapes." This name refers to the fact that the cells of these gram-positive cocci grow in a pattern resembling a cluster of grapes; however, organisms in clinical material may also appear as single cells, pairs, or short chains (Figure 22–1). Most staphylococci are 0.5 to 1 μm in diameter and are nonmotile, aerobic or facultatively anaerobic (i.e., able to grow both aerobically and anaerobically), and catalase-positive and grow in a medium containing 10% sodium chloride and at a temperature ranging from 18°C to 40°C. The organisms are present on the skin and mucous membranes of humans, other mammals, and birds. The genus currently comprises 32 species and 15 subspecies, many of which are found on humans (Table 22–1). *Staphylococcus* is an important pathogen in humans, causing a wide spectrum of life-threatening systemic diseases; infections of the skin, soft tissues, bones, and urinary tract; and opportunistic infections (Table 22–2). The species most commonly associated with human diseases are *Staphylococcus aureus* (the most virulent and best-known member of the genus), *Staphylococcus epidermidis*, *Staphylococcus saprophyticus*, *Staphylococcus capitis*, and *Staphylococcus haemolyticus*. *S. aureus* colonies are golden as the result of the carotenoid pigments that form during their growth, hence the species name. It is also the only species found in humans that produces the enzyme coagulase; thus, all other species are commonly referred to as coagulase-negative staphylococci.

The genus *Micrococcus* was recently reorganized with many species formerly classified as *Micrococcus* now placed in other genera. Only two species, *Micrococcus luteus* and *Micrococcus lylae*, remain in the genus. Both species are found in nature and can colonize humans, primarily on the surface of the skin. These cocci resemble staphylococci and can be confused with the coagulase-negative staphylococci; however, micrococci grow only aerobically, a feature that can help separate them from the staphylococci. Although micrococci may be found in patients with opportunistic infections, their isolation in clinical specimens usually represents clinically insignificant contamination with skin flora.

Stomatococcus mucilaginosus, the only species in this genus, is a commensal organism that resides in the oropharynx and upper respiratory tract. The organism resembles staphylococci; however, a prominent mucoid capsule is present, which allows the organism to adhere to the body surfaces and foreign material (e.g., catheters, shunts, prosthetic valves and joints). In recent years, this organism has been reported to be the cause of an increasing number of opportunistic infections (endocarditis, septicemia, and catheter-related infections) in immunocompromised patients.

Alloiococcus otitidis is the only species in this genus. It is an aerobic, gram-positive coccus that has been implicated in chronic middle ear infections in children. Because this organism grows slowly, its role in disease may be underappreciated.

The remainder of this chapter concentrates on a description of *Staphylococcus* and its role in human disease.

Physiology and Structure

The structure of the staphylococcal cell wall is illustrated in Figure 22–2.

Capsule

A loose-fitting, polysaccharide layer (**slime layer**) is only occasionally found on staphylococci cultured in

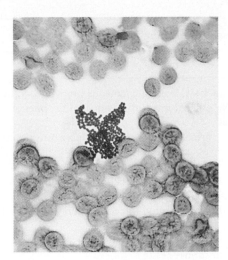

FIGURE 22–1. Gram stain of *Staphylococcus aureus*.

vitro, but it is believed to be more commonly present in vivo. Eleven capsular serotypes have been identified in *S. aureus*, with serotypes 5 and 7 associated with the majority of infections. The capsule protects the bacteria by inhibiting the chemotaxis and phagocytosis of the organisms by polymorphonuclear leukocytes, as well as by inhibiting the proliferation of mononuclear

cells after mitogen exposure. It also facilitates the adherence of bacteria to catheters and other synthetic material (e.g., grafts, shunts, prosthetic valves and joints). This property is particularly important for the survival of relatively avirulent coagulase-negative staphylococci.

Peptidoglycan

Half of the cell wall by weight is **peptidoglycan,** a feature common to gram-positive bacteria. The peptidoglycan consists of layers of glycan chains built with 10 to 12 alternating subunits of *N*-acetylmuramic acid and *N*-acetylglucosamine. Tetrapeptide side chains are attached to the *N*-acetylmuramic acid subunits and are then crosslinked with peptide bridges. For example, the glycan chains in *S. aureus* are cross-linked with pentaglycine bridges that are attached to L-lysine in one tetrapeptide chain and to D-alanine in an adjacent chain. Unlike gram-negative bacteria, the peptidoglycan layer in gram-positive organisms consists of many cross-linked layers, which makes the cell wall more rigid. The peptidoglycan has endotoxin-like activity, stimulating the production of endogenous pyrogens, activation of complement and the production of interleukin-1 from monocytes, and aggregation of polymor-

TABLE 22–1. Human Colonization and Disease Caused by
Staphylococcus, Micrococcus, Stomatococcus, and *Alloiococcus*

Species	Human Colonization	Human Disease
Staphylococcus spp.		
S. aureus	Common	Common
S. epidermidis	Common	Common
S. saprophyticus	Common	Common
S. capitis	Common	Common
S. haemolyticus	Common	Uncommon
S. lugdunensis	Common	Uncommon
S. saccharolyticus	Common	Rare
S. warneri	Common	Rare
S. hominis	Common	Rare
S. auricularis	Common	Rare
S. xylosus	Common	Rare
S. simulans	Common	Rare
S. cohnii	Common	Rare
S. caprae	Uncommon	Rare
S. pasteuri	Uncommon	Rare
S. schleiferi	Rare	Rare
Micrococcus spp.		
M. luteus	Common	Rare
M. lylae	Uncommon	Rare
Stomatococcus mucilaginosus	Common	Uncommon
Alloiococcus otitidis	Uncommon	Uncommon

TABLE 22–2. *Staphylococcus, Micrococcus, Stomatococcus,* and *Alloiococcus* and Their Diseases

Organism	Diseases
Staphylococcus aureus	Toxin-mediated (food poisoning, toxic shock syndrome); cutaneous (impetigo, folliculitis, furuncles, carbuncles, wound infections); other (bacteremia, endocarditis, pneumonia, empyema, osteomyelitis, septic arthritis)
Staphylococcus epidermidis	Bacteremia; endocarditis; surgical wounds; urinary tract infections; opportunistic infections of catheters, shunts, prosthetic devices, and peritoneal dialysates
Staphylococcus saprophyticus	Urinary tract infections, opportunistic infections
Staphylococcus capitis	Bacteremia, endocarditis, urinary tract infections, wound infections, pneumonia, bone and joint infections, opportunistic infections
Staphylococcus haemolyticus	Bacteremia, endocarditis, urinary tract infections, wound infections, and opportunistic infections
Micrococcus spp.	Opportunistic infections
Stomatococcus mucilaginosus	Bacteremia, endocarditis, opportunistic infections
Alloiococcus otitidis	Chronic middle ear infections

phonuclear leukocytes (a process responsible for abscess formation).

Teichoic Acids

Teichoic acids are species-specific, phosphate-containing polymers that are bound covalently to the peptidoglycan layer or through lipophilic linkage to the cytoplasmic membrane (lipoteichoic acids). Ribitol teichoic acid with *N*-acetylglucosamine residues (polysaccharide A) is present in *S. aureus,* and glycerol teichoic acid with glucosyl residues (polysaccharide B) is present in *S. epidermidis.* Teichoic acids mediate the attachment of staphylococci to mucosal surfaces through their specific binding to fibronectin. Although the teichoic acids are poor immunogens, a specific antibody response is stimulated when they are bound to peptidoglycan. The monitoring of this antibody response has been used to detect systemic staphylococcal disease although this is less sensitive than are other diagnostic tests.

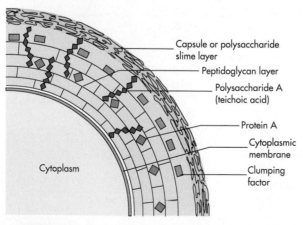

FIGURE 22–2. Structure of staphylococcal cell wall.

Capsule or polysaccharide slime layer
Peptidoglycan layer
Polysaccharide A (teichoic acid)
Protein A
Cytoplasmic membrane
Clumping factor
Cytoplasm

Protein A

The surface of most *S. aureus* strains (but not the coagulase-negative staphylococci) is uniformly coated with **protein A.** This protein is covalently linked to the peptidoglycan layer and has a unique affinity for binding to the Fc receptor of immunoglobulin (Ig)G_1, IgG_2, and IgG_4, thus effectively preventing the antibody-mediated immune clearance of the organism. Extracellular protein A can also bind antibodies, thereby forming immune complexes with the subsequent consumption of the complement.

The presence of protein A has been exploited in some serologic tests, in which protein A–coated *S. aureus* is used as a nonspecific carrier of antibodies directed against other antigens. Additionally, detection of protein A can be used as a specific identification test for *S. aureus.*

Coagulase and Other Surface Proteins

Numerous surface proteins have been identified in staphylococci. The outer surface of most strains of *S. aureus* contains **clumping factor** (also called **bound coagulase**). This protein binds fibrinogen, converts it to insoluble fibrin, causing the staphylococci to clump or aggregate. Detection of this protein is the primary test for identifying *S. aureus.* Other surface proteins that appear to be important for adherence to host tissues include collagen-binding protein, elastin-binding protein, and fibronectin-binding protein.

Cytoplasmic Membrane

The **cytoplasmic membrane** is made up of a complex of proteins, lipids, and a small amount of carbohydrates. It serves as an osmotic barrier for the cell and provides an anchorage for the cellular biosynthetic and respiratory enzymes.

Pathogenesis and Immunity

Staphylococcal Toxins

S. aureus produces many virulence factors (Table 22–3), including at least five cytolytic or membrane-damaging toxins (alpha, beta, delta, gamma, and Panton-Valentine [P-V] leukocidin); two exfoliative toxins; eight enterotoxins (A-E, G-I), and toxic shock syndrome toxin-1 (TSST-1). The cytolytic toxins have also been described as hemolysins, but this is a misnomer because the activities of the first four toxins are not restricted solely to red blood cells and P-V leukocidin is unable to lyse erythrocytes. The cytotoxins can lyse neutrophils, resulting in the release of the lysosomal enzymes that subsequently damage the surrounding tissues. One cytotoxin, P-V leukocidin, has been linked with severe cutaneous infections.

The enterotoxins and TSST-1 belong to a class of polypeptides known as **superantigens.** These toxins bind to class II major histocompatibility complex molecules on macrophages, which in turn interact with the β subunit of specific T-cell receptors, leading to the nonspecific proliferation of the T cells and the release of cytokines. The systemic effects of these diseases result from this process. Classification of the exfoliative toxins with these superantigens is controversial.

Alpha Toxin

α **Toxin,** which can be encoded on both the bacterial chromosome and a plasmid, is a 33,000-d polypeptide that is produced by most strains of *S. aureus*. The toxin disrupts the smooth muscle in blood vessels and is toxic to many types of cells, including erythrocytes, leukocytes, hepatocytes, platelets, and cultivated cells (e.g., human diploid fibroblasts, HeLa cells, Ehrlich ascites carcinoma cells). It becomes integrated in the hydrophobic regions of host cell membrane, leading to formation of 1- to 2-nm pores. The rapid efflux of K^+ and influx of Na^+, Ca^{2+}, and other small molecules

---

TABLE 22–3. *Staphylococcus aureus* Virulence Factors

Virulence Factors	Biologic Effects
Structural Components	
Capsule	Inhibits chemotaxis and phagocytosis; inhibits proliferation of mononuclear cells; facilitates adherence to foreign bodies
Peptidoglycan	Provides osmotic stability; stimulates production of endogenous pyrogen (endotoxin-like activity); leukocyte chemoattractant (abscess formation); inhibits phagocytosis
Teichoic acid	Regulates cationic concentration at cell membrane; binds to fibronectin
Protein A	Inhibits antibody-mediated clearance by binding IgG_1, IgG_2, and IgG_4 Fc receptors; leukocyte chemoattractant; anticomplementary
Cytoplasmic membrane	Osmotic barrier; regulates transport into and out of cell; site of biosynthetic and respiratory enzymes
Toxins	
Cytotoxins (α, β, δ, γ, P-V leukocidin)	Toxic for many cells, including leukocytes, erythrocytes, macrophages, platelets, and fibroblasts
Exfoliative toxins (ETA, ETB)	Serine proteases that split the intercellular bridges in the stratum granulosum epidermis
Enterotoxins (A–E, G–I)	Superantigens (stimulates proliferation of T cells and release of cytokines); stimulates release of inflammatory mediators in mast cells, increasing intestinal peristalsis and fluid loss, as well as nausea and vomiting
Toxic Shock Syndrome Toxin-1	Superantigen (stimulates proliferation of T cells and release of cytokines); produces leakage or cellular destruction of endothelial cells
Enzymes	
Coagulase	Converts fibrinogen to fibrin
Catalase	Catalyzes removal of hydrogen peroxide
Hyaluronidase	Hydrolyzes hyaluronic acids in connective tissue, promoting the spread of staphylococci in tissue
Fibrinolysin	Dissolves fibrin clots
Lipases	Hydrolyzes lipids
Nucleases	Hydrolyzes DNA
Penicillinase	Hydrolyzes penicillins

P-V = Panton-Valentine.

leads to osmotic swelling and cell lysis. The sensitivity to this varies for animal species (rabbit erythrocytes are 1000-fold more sensitive than are human cells) and cell type (e.g., fibroblasts can repair membrane damage more effectively than can erythrocytes). α Toxin is believed to be an important mediator of tissue damage in staphylococcal disease.

Beta Toxin

β **Toxin,** also called **sphingomyelinase C,** is a 35,000-d heat-labile protein produced by most strains of *S. aureus*. This enzyme has a specificity for sphingomyelin and lysophosphatidylcholine and is toxic to a variety of cells, including erythrocytes, leukocytes, macrophages, and fibroblasts. It catalyzes the hydrolysis of membrane phospholipids in susceptible cells, with lysis proportional to the concentration of sphingomyelin exposed on the cell surface. This is believed to be responsible for the differences in species susceptibility to the toxin. The role of β toxin in human disease remains to be proved; however, together with α toxin, it is believed to be responsible for the tissue destruction and abscess formation characteristic of staphylococcal diseases.

Delta Toxin

δ **Toxin** is a 3,000-d polypeptide produced by almost all *S. aureus* strains and the majority of other staphylococci. The toxin has a wide spectrum of cytolytic activity, affecting erythrocytes, many other mammalian cells, as well as intracellular membrane structures. This relatively nonspecific membrane toxicity is consistent with the belief that the toxin acts as a surfactant disrupting cellular membranes by means of a detergent-like action.

Gamma Toxin and Panton-Valentine Leukocidin

γ **Toxin** and **P-V leukocidin** are bicomponent toxins, composed of two polypeptide chains: the S (slow-eluting proteins) component and F (fast-eluting proteins) component. Three S proteins (HlgA [hemolysin γ A], HlgC, LukS-P-V) and two F proteins (HlgB, LukF-P-V) have been identified. Bacteria capable of producing both toxins can encode all these proteins with the potential for producing six distinct toxins. All six toxins can lyse neutrophils and macrophages, whereas the greatest hemolytic activity is associated with HlgA-HlgB, HlgC-HlgB, and HlgA-LukF-P-V. Cell lysis is mediated by pore formation with subsequent increased permeability to cations and osmotic instability.

Exfoliative Toxins

Staphylococcal scalded skin syndrome (SSSS), a spectrum of diseases characterized by exfoliative dermatitis, is mediated by exfoliative toxins. The prevalence of toxin production in *S. aureus* strains varies geographically but is generally less than 5% to 10%. Two distinct forms of exfoliative toxin (ETA and ETB) have been identified, and either can produce disease. ETA is heat-stable and the gene is chromosomal, whereas ETB is heat-labile and plasmid-mediated. Ultrastructural studies have shown that exposure to the toxins, which are serine proteases, is followed by the splitting of the intercellular bridges (desmosomes) in the stratum granulosum epidermis. The precise mechanism for this action is still unknown. The toxins are not associated with cytolysis or inflammation, so neither staphylococci nor leukocytes are typically present in the involved layer of the epidermis. After exposure of the epidermis to the toxin, protective neutralizing antibodies develop, leading to resolution of the toxic process. SSSS is seen mostly in young children and only rarely in older children and adults. One possible explanation for this is that ETA and ETB bind to GM_4-like glycolipids present in the epidermis of susceptible neonates but not in older children or adults.

Enterotoxins

Eight serologically distinct **staphylococcal enterotoxins** (A-E, G-I) and three subtypes of entertoxin C have been identified. The enterotoxins are stable to heating at 100°C for 30 minutes and are resistant to hydrolysis by gastric and jejunal enzymes. Thus, once a food product has been contaminated with enterotoxin-producing staphylococci and the toxins have been produced, neither reheating the food nor the digestive process will be protective. These toxins are produced by 30% to 50% of all *S. aureus* strains. Enterotoxin A is most commonly associated with disease. Enterotoxins C and D are found in contaminated milk products, and enterotoxin B causes staphylococcal pseudomembranous enterocolitis. Less is known about the prevalence of the other enterotoxins. The precise mechanism of toxin activity is not understood because a satisfactory animal model is not available. These toxins are superantigens, however, capable of inducing nonspecific activation of T cells and cytokine release. Characteristic histologic changes in the stomach and jejunum include infiltration of neutrophils into the epithelium and underlying lamina propria, with loss of the brush border in the jejunum. Stimulation of release of inflammatory mediators from mast cells is believed to be responsible for the emesis that is characteristic of staphylococcal food poisoning.

Toxic Shock Syndrome Toxin-1

TSST-1, formerly called pyrogenic exotoxin C and enterotoxin F, is a 22,000-d heat and proteolysis resistant, chromosomally mediated exotoxin. Virtually all *S. aureus* strains responsible for menstruation-associated toxic shock syndrome (TSS) and half of the strains responsible for other forms of TSS produce TSST-1. Enterotoxin B and, rarely, enterotoxin C are responsible for approximately half the cases of nonmenstruation-associated TSS. TSST-1 is a superantigen, capable of inducing nonspecific cytokine release from macrophages and T lymphocytes, and increased hypersensitivity to endotoxin. TSST-1 can also produce leakage of endothelial cells at low concentrations and a cytotoxic effect to the cells at high concentrations. The ability of TSST-1 to penetrate mucosal barriers, even though the infection remains localized in the vagina or at the site of a wound, is responsible for the systemic effects of TSS. Death in patients with TSS is due to hypovolemic shock leading to multiorgan failure.

Staphylococcal Enzymes

Coagulase

S. aureus strains possess two forms of **coagulase:** bound and free. Coagulase bound to the staphylococcal cell wall can directly convert fibrinogen to insoluble fibrin and cause the staphylococci to clump. The cell-free coagulase accomplishes the same result by reacting with a globulin plasma factor (coagulase-reacting factor) to form staphylothrombin, a thrombin-like factor. This factor catalyzes the conversion of fibrinogen to insoluble fibrin. The role of coagulase in the pathogenesis of disease is speculative, but coagulase may cause the formation of a fibrin layer around a staphylococcal abscess, thus localizing the infection and protecting the organisms from phagocytosis.

Catalase

All staphylococci produce **catalase,** which catalyzes the conversion of toxic hydrogen peroxide to water and oxygen. Hydrogen peroxide can accumulate during bacterial metabolism or after phagocytosis.

Hyaluronidase

Hyaluronidase hydrolyzes hyaluronic acids, the acidic mucopolysaccharides present in the acellular matrix of connective tissue. This enzyme facilitates the spread of *S. aureus* in tissues. More than 90% of *S. aureus* strains produce this enzyme.

Fibrinolysin

Fibrinolysin, also called **staphylokinase,** is produced by virtually all *S. aureus* strains and can dissolve fibrin clots. Staphylokinase is distinct from the fibrinolytic enzymes produced by streptococci.

Lipases

All strains of *S. aureus* and more than 30% of the strains of coagulase-negative *Staphylococcus* produce several different **lipases.** As their name implies, these enzymes hydrolyze lipids, an essential function to ensure the survival of staphylococci in the sebaceous areas of the body. It is believed that these enzymes must be present for staphylococci to invade cutaneous and subcutaneous tissues and for superficial skin infections (e.g., furuncles [boils], carbuncles) to develop.

Nuclease

A thermostable **nuclease** is another marker for *S. aureus*. The role of this enzyme in the pathogenesis of infection is unknown.

Penicillinase

More than 90% of staphylococcal isolates were susceptible to penicillin in 1941, the year the antibiotic was first used clinically. Resistance to penicillin quickly developed, however, primarily because the organisms could produce **penicillinase** (β-lactamase). The widespread distribution of this enzyme was ensured by its presence on transmissible plasmids.

Epidemiology

Staphylococci are ubiquitous. All persons have coagulase-negative staphylococci on their skin, and transient colonization of moist skin folds with *S. aureus* is common (Boxes 22–1 and 22–2). Colonization of the umbilical stump, skin, and perineal area of neonates with *S. aureus* is common. *S. aureus* and coagulase-negative staphylococci are also found in the oropharynx, gastrointestinal tract, and urogenital tract. Short-term or persistent *S. aureus* carriage in older children and adults is more common in the anterior nasopharynx than in the oropharynx. Approximately 15% of normal healthy adults are persistent nasopharyngeal carriers of *S. aureus*, with a higher incidence reported for hospitalized patients, medical personnel, persons with eczematous skin diseases, and those who regularly use needles either illicitly (e.g., drug abusers) or for medical reasons (e.g., patients with insulin-dependent diabetes, patients receiving allergy injections, those undergoing hemodialysis). Adherence of the organism to the mucosal epithelium is regulated by fibronectin receptors for staphylococcal teichoic acids

Because staphylococci are found on the skin and in the nasopharynx, shedding of the bacteria is common and is responsible for many hospital-acquired infections. Staphylococci are susceptible to high temperatures, as well as to disinfectants and antiseptic solu-

---

BOX 22–1. Summary of *Staphylococcus aureus* Infections

Physiology and Structure

Gram-positive cocci aranged in clusters.

Facultative anaerobe (capable of aerobic and anaerobic growth).

Coagulase ("clumping factor") positive (key identification test).

Species-specific teichoic acid.

Protein A (useful for identification).

Capsule.

Virulence

Virulence factors—see Table 22–3.

Epidemiology

Normal flora on human skin and mucosal surfaces.

Organisms can survive on dry surfaces for long periods (owing to thickened peptidoglycan layer and absence of outer membrane—characteristics of all gram-positive bacteria).

Person-to-person spread through direct contact or exposure to contaminated fomites (e.g., bed linens, clothing).

Risk factors include presence of a foreign body (e.g., splinter, suture, prosthesis, catheter), previous surgical procedure, use of antibiotics that suppress the normal microbial flora).

Patients at risk for specific diseases include menstruating women (toxic shock syndrome), infants (scalded skin syndrome), young children with poor personal hygiene (impetigo and other cutaneous infections), intravascular catheters (bacteremia and endocarditis); patients with compromised pulmonary function or an antecedent viral respiratory infection (pneumonia).

Infections are found worldwide and generally with no seasonal prevalence (except that food poisoning is more common in summer and during late-year holidays).

Diseases

Refer to Table 22–2.

Toxin-mediated diseases include food poisoning, toxic shock syndrome, and scalded skin syndrome.

Pyogenic diseases include impetigo, folliculitis, furuncles, carbuncles, and wound infections.

Other systemic diseases (frequently associated with bacteremia) include pneumonia (typically after viral respiratory infection), empyema (complication of pneumonia or surgical intervention), septic arthritis, osteomyelitis, acute endocarditis, and catheter-related bacteremia.

Diagnosis

Microscopy is useful for pyogenic infections but not blood stream infections or toxin-mediated infections.

Staphylococci grow rapidly when cultured on nonselective media.

Detection of staphylococcal antigens by serology are generally of low value.

Treatment, Control, and Prevention

The antibiotics of choice are oxacillin (or other penicillinase-resistant penicillin) or vancomycin for oxacillin-resistant strains.

The focus of infection (e.g., abscess) must be identified and drained.

Treatment is symptomatic for patients with food poisoning (although the source of infection should be identified so that appropriate preventive procedures can be enacted).

Proper cleansing of wounds and use of disinfectant help prevent infections.

Thorough hand washing and covering of exposed skin helps medical personnel prevent infection or spread to other patients.

---

tions; however, the organisms can survive on dry surfaces for long periods. The organisms can be transferred to a susceptible person either through direct contact or through contact with fomites (e.g., contaminated clothing, bed linens). Therefore, medical personnel must use proper hand-washing techniques to prevent the transfer of staphylococci from themselves to patients or among patients.

Clinical Diseases

Staphylococcus aureus

S. aureus causes disease through the production of toxin or through the direct invasion and destruction of tissue. The clinical manifestations of some staphylococcal diseases are almost exclusively the result of toxin activity (e.g., SSSS, staphylococcal food poisoning, and TSS), whereas other diseases result from the prolifera-

tion of the organisms, leading to abscess formation and tissue destruction (e.g., cutaneous infections, endocarditis, pneumonia, empyema, osteomyelitis, septic arthritis) (Fig. 22–3). In the presence of a foreign body (e.g., splinter, catheter, shunt, prosthetic valve or joint), significantly fewer staphylococci are necessary to establish disease. Likewise, patients with congenital diseases associated with an impaired chemotactic or phagocytic response (e.g., Job-Buckley syndrome, Wiskott-Aldrich syndrome, chronic granulomatous disease) are more susceptible to staphylococcal diseases.

Staphylococcal Scalded Skin Syndrome

In 1878, Gottfried Ritter von Rittershain described 297 infants younger than 1 month who had bullous exfoliative dermatitis. The disease he described, now called **Ritter's disease** or **SSSS,** is characterized by the abrupt

---

BOX 22−2. Summary of Coagulase-Negative Staphylococcal Infections

Physiology and Structure

Gram-positive cocci arranged in clusters.

Facultative anaerobe (capable of aerobic and anaerobic growth).

Catalase-positive but coagulase-negative.

Species-specific teichoic acid.

Capsule ("slime" layer) present.

Virulence

Refer to Table 22–3.

Epidemiology

Normal human flora on skin and mucosal surfaces.

Organisms can survive on dry surfaces for long periods.

Person-to-person spread through direct contact or exposure to contaminated fomites (although most infections are with the patient's own organisms).

Patients at risk are those with foreign bodies (e.g., suture, prosthesis, shunt, catheter).

The organisms are ubiquitous, so there are no geographic or seasonal limitations.

Diseases

Diseases—see Table 22–2.

Catheter-related bacteremia.

Subacute endocarditis associated with previously damaged or artificial heart valve.

Central nervous system shunt infection.

Surgical wound infection when a foreign body (e.g., suture, prosthesis, medical hardware) is present.

Diagnosis

As with *S. aureus* infections.

Treatment, Control, and Prevention

The antibiotics of choice are oxacillin (or other penicillinase-resistant penicillin) or vancomycin for oxacillin-resistant strains.

Removal of the foreign body is frequently required for successful treatment.

Prompt treatment for endocarditis or shunt infections is necessary to prevent further tissue damage or immune complex formation.

Maintenance of sterile intravascular catheters helps prevent infections.

---

onset of a localized perioral erythema (redness and inflammation around the mouth) that covers the entire body within 2 days. Slight pressure displaces the skin (a positive Nikolsky's sign), and large bullae or cutaneous blisters form soon thereafter and are followed by desquamation of the epithelium (Fig. 22–4). The blisters contain clear fluid but no organisms or leukocytes, a finding consistent with the fact that the disease is caused by the bacterial toxin. The epithelium becomes intact again within 7 to 10 days, when protective antibodies appear. Scarring does not occur because only the top layer of epidermis is sloughed. Although this is a disease primarily of neonates and young children, the mortality rate is low. When death does occur, it is a result of secondary bacterial infection of the denuded skin areas.

Bullous impetigo is a localized form of SSSS. Specific strains of toxin-producing *S. aureus* (e.g., phage type 71) are associated with the formation of superficial skin blisters (Fig. 22–5). Unlike patients with the disseminated manifestations of SSSS, patients with bullous impetigo have localized blisters that are culture-positive. The erythema does not extend beyond the borders of the blister, and Nikolsky's sign is not present. The disease occurs primarily in infants and young children and is highly communicable.

Staphylococcal Food Poisoning

Staphylococcal food poisoning, one of the most common foodborne illnesses, is an intoxication rather than

on infection. Disease is caused by bacterial toxin present in food rather than from a direct effect of the organisms on the patient. The most commonly contaminated foods are processed meats such as ham and salted pork, custard-filled pastries, potato salad, and ice cream. Growth of *S. aureus* in salted meats is consistent with the ability of this organism to replicate selectively in the presence of high salt concentrations. Unlike many other forms of food poisoning in which an animal reservoir is important, staphylococcal food poisoning results from contamination of the food by a human carrier. Although contamination can be prevented by not allowing individuals with an obvious staphylococcal skin infection to prepare food, approximately half of the infections originate from carriers with asymptomatic nasopharyngeal colonization. After the staphylococci have been introduced into the food, the food must remain at room temperature or warmer for the organisms to grow and release the toxin. The contaminated food will not appear or taste tainted. Subsequent heating of the food will kill the bacteria but not inactivate the heat-stable toxin.

After ingestion of contaminated food, the onset of disease is abrupt and rapid, with a mean incubation period of 4 hours, again consistent with a disease mediated by preformed toxin. Further toxin is not produced by ingested staphylococci, so the disease has a rapid course, with symptoms generally lasting fewer than 24 hours. Staphylococcal food poisoning is characterized by severe vomiting, diarrhea, and abdominal pain or nausea. Sweating and headache may occur, but

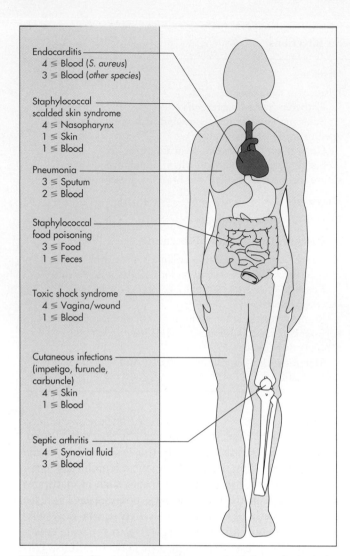

Endocarditis
4 ≤ Blood (*S. aureus*)
3 ≤ Blood (*other species*)

Staphylococcal
scalded skin syndrome
4 ≤ Nasopharynx
1 ≤ Skin
1 ≤ Blood

Pneumonia
3 ≤ Sputum
2 ≤ Blood

Staphylococcal
food poisoning
3 ≤ Food
1 ≤ Feces

Toxic shock syndrome
4 ≤ Vagina/wound
1 ≤ Blood

Cutaneous infections
(impetigo, furuncle,
carbuncle)
4 ≤ Skin
1 ≤ Blood

Septic arthritis
4 ≤ Synovial fluid
3 ≤ Blood

FIGURE 22–3. Staphylococcal diseases. Isolation of staphylococci from sites of infection. *1+*, less than 10% positive cultures; *2+*, 10% to 50% positive cultures; *3+*, 50% to 90% positive cultures; *4+*, more than 90% positive cultures.

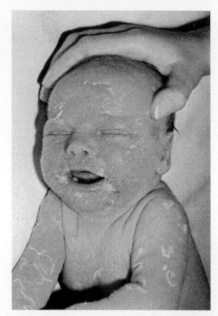

FIGURE 22–4. Staphylococcal scalded skin syndrome. (From Emond RT, Rowland HAK: *A color atlas of infectious diseases,* London, 1987, Wolfe.)

tion occurs among the different enterotoxins. Immunity is short-lived, however, and second episodes of staphylococcal food poisoning can occur, particularly with serologically distinct enterotoxins.

Certain strains of *S. aureus* can also cause enteroco-

fever is not seen. The diarrhea is watery and non-bloody, and dehydration may result from the considerable fluid loss.

The toxin-producing organisms can be cultured from the contaminated food if the organisms are not killed during food preparation. The enterotoxins are heat stable, so contaminated food can be tested for toxins at a public health facility (these tests are rarely performed).

Treatment is for the relief of the abdominal cramping and diarrhea and for the replacement of fluids. Antibiotic therapy is not indicated because as already noted, the disease is mediated by preformed toxin and not by replicating organisms. Neutralizing antibodies to the toxin can be protective and limited cross-protec-

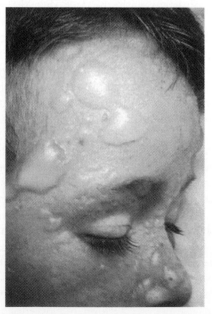

FIGURE 22–5. Bullous impetigo, a localized form of staphylococcal scalded skin syndrome. (From Emond RT, Rowland HAK: *A color atlas of infectious diseases,* London, 1987, Wolfe.)

litis, which is manifested clinically by watery diarrhea, abdominal cramps, and fever. Enterocolitis occurs primarily in patients who have received broad-spectrum antibiotics, which suppress the normal colonic flora and permit the growth of *S. aureus.* The diagnosis of staphylococcal enterocolitis can be confirmed only after other, more common causes of infection have been excluded (e.g., *Clostridium difficile* colitis). Abundant staphylococci are typically present in the stool of affected patients, and the normal gram-negative bacteria are absent. Fecal leukocytes are observed, and white plaques with ulceration are seen on the colonic mucosa.

Toxic Shock Syndrome

The first outbreak of **TSS** occurred in 1928 in Australia, where the disease developed in 21 children, 12 of whom died after an injection with an *S. aureus*–contaminated vaccine. Fifty years later, Todd observed what he called **toxic shock syndrome** in seven children with systemic disease, and the first reports of TSS in menstruating women were published in the summer of 1980. This was followed by a dramatic increase in the incidence of TSS, particularly in women. Subsequently, it was discovered that TSST-1-producing strains of *S. aureus* could multiply rapidly in hyperabsorbent tampons and release toxin. After the recall of these tampons, the incidence of disease, particularly in menstruating women, decreased rapidly. At present, it is estimated that 6000 cases of TSS occur annually in the United States. Although it was originally reported that coagulase-negative staphylococci could cause TSS, it is now believed that this disease is restricted to *S. aureus.*

The disease is initiated with the localized growth of toxin-producing strains of *S. aureus* in the vagina or a wound, followed by release of the toxin into the blood stream. Clinical manifestations start abruptly and include fever, hypotension, and a diffuse macular erythematous rash. Multiple organ systems (gastrointestinal, musculature, renal, hepatic, hematologic, central nervous) are also involved, and the entire skin including the palms and soles desquamates (Fig. 22–6). The initially high fatality rate has been decreased to approximately 5% as the etiology and epidemiology of this disease have become better understood. Unless the patient is specifically treated with an effective antibiotic, however, the risk of recurrent disease is as high as 65%. Serologic studies have demonstrated that more than 90% of adults have antibodies to TSST-1. These antibodies are protective because disease appears to be restricted to patients without detectable antibodies. Additionally, more than 50% of patients with TSS fail to develop protective antibodies after their disease resolves.

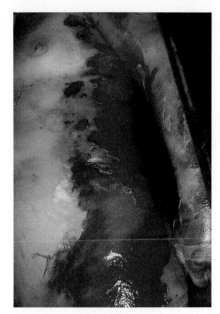

FIGURE 22–6. Toxic shock syndrome. A fatal infection with cutaneous and soft tissue involvement.

Cutaneous Infections

Localized, **pyogenic staphylococcal infections** include impetigo, folliculitis, furuncles, and carbuncles. **Impetigo,** a superficial infection affecting mostly young children, occurs primarily on the face and limbs. Initially, a small macule (flattened red spot) is seen, and then a pus-filled vesicle (pustule) on an erythematous base develops. Crusting occurs after the pustule ruptures. Multiple vesicles at different stages of development are common, owing to the secondary spread of the infection to adjacent skin sites (Fig. 22–7). Impetigo is usually caused by *S. aureus,* although group A streptococci, either alone or with *S. aureus,* are responsible for 20% of cases.

Folliculitis is a pyogenic infection in the hair follicles. The base of the follicle is raised and reddened, and there is a small collection of pus beneath the epidermal surface. If this occurs at the base of the eyelid, it is called a **stye. Furuncles** (boils), an extension of folliculitis, are large, painful, raised nodules with an underlying collection of dead and necrotic tissue. These can drain spontaneously or after surgical incision.

Carbuncles occur when furuncles coalesce and extend to the deeper subcutaneous tissue. Multiple sinus tracts are usually present. Unlike patients with folliculitis and furuncles, patients with carbuncles have chills and fevers, indicating the systemic spread of staphylococci via bacteremia to other tissues.

Staphylococcal **wound infections** can also occur in patients after a surgical procedure or after trauma, with organisms colonizing the skin introduced into the

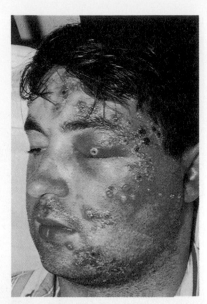

FIGURE 22–7. Pustular impetigo. Note the vesicles at different stages of development, including pus-filled vesicles on an erythematous base and dry, crusted lesions. (From Emond RT, Rowland HAK: *A color atlas of infectious diseases,* London, 1987, Wolfe.)

wound. The staphylococci are generally not able to establish an infection in an immunocompetent person unless a foreign body is present in the wound (e.g., stitches, a splinter, dirt). Infections are characterized by edema, erythema, pain, and an accumulation of purulent material. The infection can be easily managed if the wound is reopened, the foreign matter removed, and the purulence drained. If signs such as fever and malaise are observed or if the wound does not clear in response to localized management, antibiotic therapy directed against *S. aureus* is indicated.

Bacteremia and Endocarditis

S. aureus is a common cause of **bacteremia.** Although bacteremias caused by most other organisms originate from an identifiable focus of infection, such as an infection of the lungs, urinary tract, or gastrointestinal tract, the initial foci of infection in approximately one third of patients with *S. aureus* bacteremias are not known. Most likely, the infection spreads to the blood stream from an innocuous-appearing skin infection. More than 50% of the cases of *S. aureus* bacteremia are acquired in the hospital after a surgical procedure or result from the continued use of a contaminated intravascular catheter. *S. aureus* bacteremias, particularly prolonged episodes, are associated with dissemination to other body sites, including the heart.

Acute **endocarditis** caused by *S. aureus* is a serious disease, with a mortality rate approaching 50%. Al-

though patients with *S. aureus* endocarditis may initially have nonspecific influenza-like symptoms, their condition can deteriorate rapidly and include disruption of cardiac output and peripheral evidence of septic embolization (Fig. 22–8). Unless appropriate medical and surgical intervention is instituted immediately, the patient's prognosis is poor. An exception to this is *S. aureus* endocarditis in parenteral drug abusers, whose disease normally involves the right side of the heart (tricuspid valve) rather than the left. The initial symptoms may be mild, but fever, chills, and pleuritic chest pain caused by pulmonary emboli are generally present. Clinical cure of the endocarditis is the rule, although it is common for complications to occur as the result of secondary spread of the infection to other organs.

Pneumonia and Empyema

S. aureus respiratory disease can develop after the aspiration of oral secretions or from the hematogenous spread of the organism from a distant site. **Aspiration pneumonia** is seen primarily in the very young, the aged, and patients with cystic fibrosis, influenza, chronic obstructive pulmonary disease, and bronchiectasis. The clinical and radiographic presentations of the pneumonia are not unique. Radiographic examination reveals the presence of patchy infiltrates with consolidation or abscesses, the latter consistent with the organism's ability to secrete cytotoxic toxins and enzymes and to form localized abscesses. **Hematogenous pneu-**

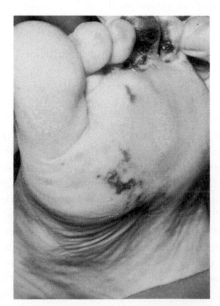

FIGURE 22–8. Septic embolization, caused by occlusion of capillaries with microcolonies of staphylococci, is common in bacteremic patients, particularly patients with endocarditis. (From Emond RT, Rowland HAK: *A color atlas of infectious diseases,* London, 1987, Wolfe.)

monia is common for patients with bacteremia or endocarditis.

Empyema occurs in 10% of patients with pneumonia, and *S. aureus* is responsible for one third of all cases. Because the organism can become consolidated in loculated areas, drainage of the purulent material is sometimes difficult.

Osteomyelitis and Septic Arthritis

S. aureus **osteomyelitis** can result from the hematogenous dissemination to bone, or it can be a secondary infection resulting from trauma or the extension of disease from an adjacent area. Hematogenous spread in children generally results from a cutaneous staphylococcal infection and usually involves the metaphyseal area of long bones, a highly vascularized area of bony growth. This infection is characterized by the sudden onset of localized pain over the involved bone and by high fever. Blood cultures are positive in about 50% of cases.

The hematogenous osteomyelitis that is seen in adults commonly occurs in the form of vertebral osteomyelitis and rarely in the form of an infection of the long bones. Intense back pain with fever is the initial symptom. Radiographic evidence of osteomyelitis in children and adults is not seen until 2 to 3 weeks after the initial symptoms appear. **Brodie's abscess** is a sequestered focus of staphylococcal osteomyelitis that arises in the metaphyseal area of a long bone and occurs only in adults. The staphylococcal osteomyelitis that occurs after trauma or a surgical procedure is generally accompanied by inflammation and purulent drainage from the wound or the sinus tract overlying the infected bone. Because the staphylococcal infection may be restricted to the wound, isolation of the organism from this site is not conclusive evidence of bony involvement. With appropriate antibiotic therapy and surgery, the cure rate for staphylococcal osteomyelitis is excellent.

S. aureus is the primary cause of **septic arthritis** in young children and in adults who are receiving intra-articular injections or who have mechanically abnormal joints. Secondary involvement of multiple joints is indicative of hematogenous spread from a localized focus. *S. aureus* is replaced by *Neisseria gonorrhoeae* as the most common cause of septic arthritis in sexually active persons. Staphylococcal arthritis is characterized by a painful, erythematous joint, with purulent material obtained on aspiration. Infection is usually demonstrated in the large joints (e.g., shoulder, knee, hip, elbow). The prognosis in children is excellent, but in adults, it depends on the nature of the underlying disease as well as the occurrence of any secondary infectious complications.

Staphylococcus epidermidis and Other Coagulase-Negative Staphylococci

Endocarditis

S. epidermidis and the related coagulase-negative staphylococci can infect native and prosthetic heart valves. Infections of native valves are believed to result from the inoculation of organisms onto a damaged heart valve (e.g., a congenital malformation, damage resulting from rheumatic heart disease). This form of staphylococcal endocarditis is relatively rare and is more commonly caused by streptococci.

In contrast, staphylococci are a major cause of endocarditis of artificial valves. The organisms are introduced at the time of valve replacement, and the infection characteristically has an indolent course, with clinical signs and symptoms not developing for as long as 1 year after the procedure. Although the heart valve can be infected, more commonly the infection occurs at the site where the valve is sewn to the heart tissue. Thus, infection with abscess formation can lead to separation of the valve at the suture line and to mechanical heart failure. Because of the nature and site of infection, septic embolization and persistent bacteremia are less common in patients with staphylococcal prosthetic valve endocarditis than in those with other forms of endocarditis. The prognosis is guarded for patients who have this infection, and prompt medical and surgical management is critical.

Catheter and Shunt Infections

From 20% to 65% of all infections of catheters and shunts are caused by coagulase-negative staphylococci. These infections have become a major medical problem because long-dwelling catheters and shunts are used commonly for the medical management of critically ill patients. The coagulase-negative staphylococci are particularly well adapted for causing these infections because they can produce a polysaccharide slime that bonds them to catheters and shunts and protects them from antibiotics and inflammatory cells. A persistent bacteremia is generally observed in patients with infections of shunts and catheters because the organisms have continual access to the blood stream. Immune complex–mediated glomerulonephritis occurs in patients with long-standing disease.

Prosthetic Joint Infections

Infections of artificial joints, particularly the hip, can be caused by coagulase-negative staphylococci. The patient usually only experiences localized pain and mechanical failure of the joint. Systemic signs such as fever and leukocytosis are not prominent, and blood cultures are usually negative. Treatment consists of joint replacement and antimicrobial therapy. The risk of reinfection of the new joint is considerably increased in such patients.

Urinary Tract Infections

S. saprophyticus has a predilection for causing urinary tract infections in young, sexually active women and is rarely responsible for infections in other patients. It is also infrequently found as an asymptomatic colonizer of the urinary tract. Infected women usually have dysuria (pain on urination), pyuria (pus in urine), and numerous organisms in the urine. Typically, patients respond rapidly to antibiotics, and reinfection is uncommon.

Laboratory Diagnosis

Microscopy

Staphylococci are gram-positive cocci that form clusters when grown on agar media but commonly appear as single cells or small groups of organisms in clinical specimens. The successful detection of organisms in a clinical specimen depends on the type of the infection (e.g., abscess, bacteremia, impetigo) and the quality of the material submitted for analysis. If the clinician scrapes the base of the abscess with a swab or curette, then an abundance of organisms should be observed in the Gram-stained specimen. Aspirated pus consists primarily of necrotic material with relatively few organisms, so these specimens are not as useful. Few organisms are generally present in the blood of bacteremic patients (an average of less than 1 organism per milliliter of blood), so blood specimens should be cultured but not stained. Staphylococci are seen in the nasopharynx of patients with SSSS and in the vagina of patients with TSS, but these staphylococci cannot be distinguished from the organisms that normally colonize these sites. Diagnosis of these diseases is made by the clinical presentation of the patient, with isolation of *S. aureus* in culture confirmatory. Staphylococci are implicated in food poisoning by the clinical presentation of the patient (e.g., rapid onset of vomiting and abdominal cramps) and a history of specific food ingestion (e.g., salted ham). Gram stains of the food or patient specimens are generally not indicated.

Culture

Clinical specimens should be inoculated onto nutritionally enriched agar media supplemented with sheep blood. If there is a mixture of organisms in the specimen (e.g., wound or respiratory specimen), *S. aureus* can be isolated selectively on agar media supplemented with 7.5% sodium chloride, which inhibits the growth of most other organisms, and mannitol, which is fermented by *S. aureus* but not by most other staphylococci. Staphylococci grow rapidly on nonselective media, both aerobically and anaerobically, with large, smooth colonies seen within 24 hours. As noted earlier, *S. aureus* colonies are commonly golden, particularly when the cultures are incubated at room temperature. Almost all isolates of *S. aureus* and some strains of coagulase-negative staphylococci produce hemolysis on sheep blood agar. The hemolysis is caused by cytotoxins, particularly α toxin.

Serology

Attempts to detect staphylococcal structural antigens in blood or clinical specimens have generally been unsuccessful. However, antibodies to cell wall teichoic acids are present in many patients with long-standing *S. aureus* infections. Antibodies develop within 2 weeks of the onset of disease and are detected in most patients with staphylococcal endocarditis. This test is less reliable, however, in the detection of antibodies in patients with staphylococcal osteomyelitis or wound infections because the focus of infection is sequestered in these settings and the organisms frequently do not stimulate a humoral immune response. The finding of elevated antibody titers in a bacteremic patient indicates the need for a prolonged course of antimicrobial therapy. The importance of negative serologic findings must be carefully weighed, however, because the test is relatively insensitive.

Identification

Relatively simple biochemical tests (e.g., positive reactions for coagulase [clumping factor], heat-stable nuclease, alkaline phosphatase, and mannitol fermentation) can be used to differentiate *S. aureus* and the other staphylococci. Differentiation of the coagulase-negative staphylococci is more complex, however, and is not routinely done in many clinical laboratories unless the isolates are demonstrated to be clinically significant.

Antibiotic susceptibility patterns (antibiograms), biochemical profiles (biotyping), susceptibility to bacteriophages (phage typing), and nucleic acid analysis can be used for the intraspecies characterization of isolates for epidemiologic purposes. Antibiograms and biotyping are performed in most laboratories as part of the routine identification of an isolate. The tests are not highly discriminatory, however, and are useful only if two isolates have a different antibiotic susceptibility pattern or biochemical profile. Phage typing differentiates among staphylococcal strains by their pattern of susceptibility to lysis by an international collection of specific bacteriophages. This testing is performed only by research laboratories and has now been replaced by nucleic acid analysis in epidemiologic studies. The analysis of plasmid and genomic DNA by pulsed-field gel electrophoresis or similar techniques has evolved rapidly to be the most sensitive way to characterize isolates at the species and subspecies level. These methods are currently used in many research and clinical laboratories.

Treatment, Prevention, and Control

Staphylococci quickly developed drug resistance after penicillin was introduced, and today less than 10% of the strains are susceptible to this antibiotic. This resistance is mediated by penicillinase (β-lactamase specific for penicillins), which hydrolyzes the β-lactam ring of penicillin. The genetic information encoding the production of this enzyme is carried on transmissible plasmids, which facilitated the rapid dissemination of resistance among staphylococci.

Because of the problems with penicillin-resistant staphylococci, semisynthetic penicillins resistant to β-lactamase hydrolysis (e.g., methicillin, nafcillin, oxacillin, dicloxacillin) were developed. Unfortunately, the staphylococci developed resistance to these antibiotics, as well. Currently, 30% to 50% of the strains of *S. aureus* and more than 50% of the coagulase-negative staphylococci are resistant to these semisynthetic penicillins. Resistance occurs as the result of acquisition of a gene, *mec*A, that codes for a novel penicillin-binding protein, PBP2'. The penicillins and other β-lactam antibiotics kill bacteria by their ability to bind to penicillin-binding proteins, which are enzymes responsible for construction of the cell wall peptidoglycan. PBP2' is not bound by penicillins but retains its enzymatic activity. Not all bacteria in a resistant population may express this penicillin-binding protein (**heterogeneous resistance**), so traditional susceptibility methods may not detect resistance. The definitive method for identifying a resistant isolate is detection of the PBP2' gene, a test that can now be performed in many clinical laboratories (Fig. 22–9). Expression of PBP2' renders the bacteria resistant to all β-lactam antibiotics (including the cephalosporins and carbapenems).

Staphylococci have demonstrated the remarkable ability to develop resistance to most antibiotics. Until recently, the one antibiotic that has remained uniformly active against staphylococci has been vancomycin, the current antibiotic of choice for treating staphylococci resistant to oxacillin. Unfortunately, isolates of *S. aureus* have now been found with decreased susceptibility to vancomycin, and frank resistance to vancomycin has been observed in coagulase-negative staphylococci. The mechanism of this resistance is unknown; however, there is evidence that changes in cell wall synthesis have led to reversible vancomycin binding that effectively prevents vancomycin from disrupting

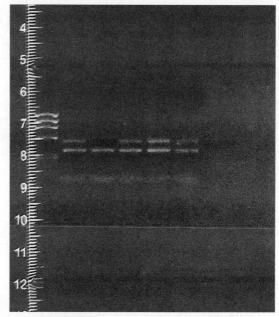

FIGURE 22–9. *mec*A gene analysis by pulsed-field gel electrophoresis (PFGE). After DNA amplification by polymerase chain reaction, the DNA preparation is exposed to a probe for the *mec*A gene. The presence of the gene is detected by PFGE. The first column is a size marker; the second and third columns are positive and negative controls, respectively; and the last three columns are *Staphylococcus aureus* isolates from three patients. All three patients had the *mec*A gene and are, therefore, resistant to oxacillin, other penicillins, all cephalosporins, carbapenems, and all other β-lactam antibiotics.

peptidoglycan synthesis. Although this form of resistance is troublesome, it is more alarming that the genes responsible for vancomycin resistance in enterococci can be artificially transferred to staphylococci. If this occurs in nature (an occurrence that seems unavoidable), then staphylococci will be highly resistant to vancomycin. This will create a highly virulent bacterium that is essentially untreatable.

Staphylococci are ubiquitous organisms present on the skin and mucous membranes, and their introduction through breaks in the skin occurs frequently. However, the number of organisms required to establish an infection (**infectious dose**) is generally large unless a foreign body is present in the wound (e.g., dirt, a splinter, stitches). Proper cleansing of the wound and the application of an appropriate disinfectant (e.g., germicidal soap, iodine solution, hexachlorophene) will prevent most infections in healthy individuals.

The spread of staphylococci from person to person is more difficult to prevent. An example of this is surgical wound infections, which can be caused by relatively few organisms because foreign bodies and devitalized tissue may be present. Although it is unrealistic to sterilize the operating room personnel and environment, the risk of contamination during an operative procedure can be minimized through proper hand washing and the covering of exposed skin surfaces. The spread of oxacillin-resistant organisms can also be difficult to control because asymptomatic nasopharyngeal carriage is the most frequent source of these organisms. However, some success in this regard has been achieved through the use of chemoprophylaxis consisting of vancomycin and rifampin.

CASE STUDY AND QUESTIONS

■ An 18-year-old man fell on his knee while playing basketball. The knee was painful, but the overlying skin was unbroken. The next day, the knee was swollen and remained painful, so he was taken to the local emergency department. Clear fluid was aspirated from the knee, and the physician prescribed symptomatic treatment. Two days later, the swelling returned, the pain increased, and erythema developed over the knee. Because the patient also felt systemically ill and had an oral temperature of 38.8°C, he returned to the emergency department. Aspiration of the knee yielded cloudy fluid, and cultures of the fluid and blood were positive for S. aureus.

1. Name two possible sources of this organism.

2. Staphylococci cause a variety of diseases, including SSSS, TSS, food poisoning, cutaneous infections, and endocarditis. How do the clinical symptoms of these diseases differ from the infection in this patient? Which of these diseases are intoxications?

3. What toxins have been implicated in staphylococcal diseases? Which staphylococcal enzymes have been proposed as virulence factors?

4. Which structures in the staphylococcal cell and which toxins protect the bacterium from phagocytosis?

5. What is the antibiotic of choice for treating staphylococcal infections? (Give two examples.)

6. If the patient returns in 2 weeks and the physician suspects osteomyelitis has developed, how should the clinical diagnosis be confirmed?

BIBLIOGRAPHY

Dinges MM et al: Exotoxins of *Staphylococcus aureus*, *Clin Microbiol Rev* 13:16–34, 2000.

Gravet A et al: Predominant *Staphylococcus aureus* isolated from antibiotic-associated diarrhea is clinically relevant and produces enterotoxin A and the biocomponent toxin LukE-LukD, *J Clin Microbiol* 37:4012–4019, 1999.

Holmberg SD, Blake PA: Staphylococcal food poisoning in the United States: new facts and old misconceptions, *JAMA* 251:487–489, 1984.

Hovelius B, Mardh PA: *Staphylococcus saprophyticus* as a common cause of urinary tract infections, *Rev Infect Dis* 6:328–337, 1984.

Kloos WE, Bannerman TL: Update on clinical significance of coagulase-negative staphylococci, *Clin Microbiol Rev* 7:117–140, 1994.

Ladhani S et al: Clinical, microbial, and biochemical aspects of the exfoliative toxins causing staphylococcal scalded skin syndrome, *Clin Microbiol Rev* 12:224–242, 1999.

Lowy FD: *Staphylococcus aureus* infections, *N Engl J Med* 339:520–532, 1998.

Mulligan ME et al: Methicillin-resistant *Staphylococcus aureus*: a consensus review of the microbiology, pathogenesis, and epidemiology with implications for prevention and management, *Am J Med* 94:313–323, 1993.

Murray PR et al: *Manual of clinical microbiology*, ed 7, Washington, DC, 1999, American Society for Microbiology.

Rupp ME, Archer GL: Coagulase-negative staphylococci: pathogens associated with medical progress, *Clin Infect Dis* 19:231–245, 1994.

Waldvogel FA: New resistance in *Staphylococcus aureus*, *N Engl J Med* 340:556–557, 1999.

C H A P T E R 2 3

Streptococcus

The genus *Streptococcus* is a diverse collection of gram-positive cocci typically arranged in pairs or chains. Most species are facultative anaerobes, and some grow only in an atmosphere enhanced with carbon dioxide (**capnophilic growth**). Their nutritional requirements are complex, necessitating the use of blood- or serum-enriched media for isolation. Carbohydrates are fermented, resulting in the production of lactic acid, and unlike *Staphylococcus* species, streptococci are catalase-negative.

The streptococci are important human pathogens (Box 23–1). Unfortunately, the differentiation of species within the genus is complicated, because three different schemes are used to classify the organisms, as follows (Table 23–1):

1. Serologic properties: Lancefield groupings A to H, K to M, and O to V.
2. Hemolytic patterns: complete (β) hemolysis, incomplete (α) hemolysis, and no (γ) hemolysis.
3. Biochemical (physiologic) properties.

The serologic classification scheme was developed by Lancefield in 1933 for differentiating β-hemolytic strains. Most β-hemolytic strains and some α-hemolytic and nonhemolytic strains possess group-specific antigens, most of which are cell wall carbohydrates. These antigens can be readily detected by immunologic assays and have been useful for the rapid identification of some streptococcal pathogens. For example, group A *Streptococcus* (*Streptococcus pyogenes*) is responsible for streptococcal pharyngitis. The group antigen for this organism can be detected by rapid immunoassays directly from throat swab specimens.

Most α-hemolytic and nonhemolytic streptococci do not possess the group-specific cell wall antigens. These organisms must be identified from their physiologic properties. Unfortunately, the classification schemes are not mutually exclusive. For example, *Streptococcus anginosus* strains may be nontypable (viridans group) or may react with the antisera for groups A, C, F, or G. Likewise, *Streptococcus agalactiae* (group B) is usually β-hemolytic but may also be nonhemolytic.

Streptococcus pyogenes

Two species of streptococci are classified in group A— *S. pyogenes* and *S. anginosus*. *S. pyogenes* is the more common pathogen and is discussed here, and *S. anginosus* will be discussed later in the chapter. *S. pyogenes* is an important cause of a variety of suppurative and nonsuppurative diseases (see Box 23–1). Although they are the most common cause of bacterial pharyngitis, these organisms have become notorious because they can cause dramatic, life-threatening diseases. Indeed, reports of these "flesh-eating" bacteria have flooded both the scientific literature and the tabloid press.

Physiology and Structure

Isolates of *S. pyogenes* are 0.5- to 1.0-μm, spherical cocci that form short chains in clinical specimens and longer chains when grown in liquid media (Fig. 23–1). Growth is optimal on enriched blood agar media but is inhibited if the medium contains a high concentration of glucose. After 24 hours of incubation, 1- to 2-mm white colonies with large zones of β-hemolysis are observed. Encapsulated strains may appear mucoid on freshly prepared media but wrinkled on dry media. Nonencapsulated colonies are smaller and glossy.

The antigenic structure of *S. pyogenes* has been extensively studied. The basic structural framework of the cell wall is the peptidoglycan layer, which is similar in composition to that found in other gram-positive bacteria. Within the cell wall are the group-specific and type-specific antigens.

Group-Specific Carbohydrate

The group-specific carbohydrate, which constitutes approximately 10% of the dry weight of the cell, is a dimer of *N*-acetylglucosamine and rhamnose. This antigen is used to classify group A streptococci and distinguish them from other streptococcal groups.

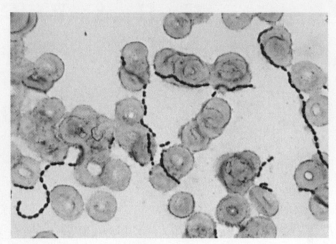

FIGURE 23–1. Gram stain of *Streptococcus pyogenes*.

Type-Specific Proteins

The **M protein** is a major type-specific protein associated with virulent streptococci. It consists of two polypeptide chains complexed in an α helix. The carboxyl terminus is anchored in the cytoplasmic membrane and is highly conserved among all group A streptococci. The amino terminus, which extends through the cell wall to the cell surface, is responsible for the antigenic variability observed among the more than 80 serotypes of M proteins. M proteins are subdivided into class I and class II molecules. The class I M proteins have the constant (C) region exposed, whereas antibodies do not develop against the C region of class II M proteins. This appears to be important for patients who develop rheumatic fever, because their disease is mediated by strains with the class I M proteins.

A secondary type-specific protein that is a useful epidemiologic marker for bacterial strains that fail to express the M protein is the **T (trypsin-resistant) protein.** The structural function of this protein is unknown. Although the epidemiologic classification of *S. pyogenes* has been based traditionally on identification of specific M or T types, it is likely that this procedure will be replaced by sequencing the *emm* gene that encodes the M protein.

Other Cell Surface Components

Other important components in the cell wall of *S. pyogenes* include **M-like proteins, lipoteichoic acid,** and **F protein.** The M-like proteins are encoded by a complex of more than 20 genes that comprise the *emm* gene superfamily. These genes are responsible for M proteins, M-like proteins, and other immunoglobulin

TABLE 23–1. Classification of Common Streptococcal Pathogens

Biochemical Classification	Serologic Classification	Hemolysis Patterns
S. pyogenes	A	Beta
S. anginosus group	A, C, F, G, nongroupable	Beta; occasionally alpha or nonhemolytic
S. agalactiae	B	Beta; occasionally nonhemolytic
S. dysgalactiae	C, G	Beta
S. bovis	D	Alpha; nonhemolytic; occasionally beta
Viridans group streptococci	Nongroupable	Alpha or nonhemolytic
S. pneumoniae	Nongroupable	Alpha

(Ig)-binding proteins. Lipoteichoic acid and F protein facilitate binding of host cells by complexing with fibronectin, which is present on the host cell surface.

Capsule

The outermost layer of the cell is the **capsule,** which is composed of hyaluronic acid containing repeating molecules of glucuronic acid and *N*-acetylglucosamine. The capsule prevents phagocytosis of the bacteria by providing a physical barrier between the opsonic complement proteins bound to the bacterial surface and phagocytic cells.

Pathogenesis and Immunity

The virulence of group A streptococci is determined by the ability of the bacteria to adhere to the surface of host cells, invade into the epithelial cells, avoid opsonization and phagocytosis, and produce a variety of toxins and enzymes (Table 23–2). More than 10 different bacterial antigens have been demonstrated to mediate adherence to host cells, with lipoteichoic acid, M proteins, and F protein the most important. The initial adherence is a weak interaction between lipoteichoic acid and fatty acid binding sites on fibronectin and epithelial cells. Subsequent adherence involves M protein, F protein, and other adhesins that interact with specific host cell receptors.

Recent evidence has demonstrated that *S. pyogenes* can invade into epithelial cells, a process that is mediated by M protein and F protein, as well as other bacterial antigens. This internalization is believed to be important for maintenance of persistent infections (e.g., recurrent streptococcal pharyngitis) as well as invasion into deep tissues.

S. pyogenes also has multiple mechanisms for avoiding opsonization and phagocytosis. The conserved region of M protein can bind the serum β-globulin, factor H, which is a regulatory protein for the alternative complement pathway. The complement component C3b, an important mediator of phagocytosis, is destabilized by factor H. Thus, when C3b binds to the cell surface in the region of the M protein, it is degraded by factor H, and phagocytosis is prevented. The effect is overcome only when the patient produces antibodies directed against the specific M protein type. The binding of fibrinogen to the surface of M protein also blocks activation of complement by the alternate pathway and reduces the amount of bound C3b. The M-related proteins interfere with phagocytosis. Finally, *S. pyogenes* can produce C5a peptidase that can inactivate C5a and, thus, block chemotaxis of neutrophils and mononuclear phagocytes.

Additionally, a number of enzymes and toxins can mediate the pathology observed with *S. pyogenes* infections.

Pyrogenic Exotoxins

The **streptococcal pyrogenic exotoxins (Spes),** originally called erythrogenic toxins, are produced by lysogenic strains of streptococci and are similar to the toxin produced in *Corynebacterium diphtheriae*. Three immunologically distinct heat-labile toxins (SpeA, SpeB, and SpeC) have been described in *S. pyogenes* and in rare strains of groups C and G streptococci. The toxins act as superantigens, interacting with both

TABLE 23–2. Virulence Factors of *Streptococcus pyogenes*

Virulence Factor	Biologic Effect
Capsule	Antiphagocytic
Lipoteichoic acid	Binds to epithelial cells
M protein	Adhesin; antiphagocytic; degrades complement component C3b
M-like proteins	Binds immunoglobulins M, and G and α_2-macroglobulin (protease inhibitor)
F protein	Mediates adherence to epithelial cells
Pyrogenic exotoxins	Mediate pyrogenicity, enhancement of delayed hypersensitivity and susceptibility to endotoxin, cytotoxicity, nonspecific mitogenicity for T cells, immunosuppression of B-cell function, and production of scarlatiniform rash
Streptolysin S	Lyses leukocytes, platelets, and erythrocytes; stimulates release of lysosomal enzymes; nonimmunogenic
Streptolysin O	Lyses leukocytes, platelets, and erythrocytes; stimulates release of lysosomal enzymes; immunogenic
Streptokinase	Lyses blood clots; facilitates spread of bacteria in tissues
DNase	Depolymerizes cell-free DNA in purulent material
C5a peptidase	Degrades complement component C5a

macrophages and helper T cells with the release of (1) interleukin-1 (IL-1), IL-2, and IL-6, (2) tumor necrosis factor-α (TNF-α) and TNF-β, and (3) interferon-γ. These cytokines mediate a variety of important effects, including the shock and the organ failure seen characteristically in patients with streptococcal toxic shock syndrome. The toxins are also responsible for the rash observed in patients with scarlet fever, although it is unclear whether the rash results from the direct effect of the toxin on the capillary bed or, more likely, is secondary to a hypersensitivity reaction.

Streptolysins S and O

Streptolysin S is an oxygen-stable, nonimmunogenic, cell-bound hemolysin that can lyse erythrocytes, leukocytes, and platelets. Streptolysin S can also stimulate the release of lysosomal contents after engulfment, with subsequent death of the phagocytic cell. Streptolysin S is produced in the presence of serum (the S indicates serum dependence) and is responsible for the characteristic β-hemolysis seen on blood agar media.

Streptolysin O is an oxygen-labile hemolysin capable of lysing erythrocytes, leukocytes, platelets, and cultured cells. Antibodies are readily formed against streptolysin O, a feature differentiating it from streptolysin S, and are useful for documenting recent group A streptococcal infection (**ASO test**). Because streptolysin O is irreversibly inhibited by cholesterol in skin lipids, however, patients with *S. pyogenes* skin infections do not develop anti-streptolysin O (ASO) antibodies. This hemolysin cross-reacts with similar oxygen-labile toxins produced by *S. pneumoniae* and *Clostridium* species.

Streptokinases

At least two forms of **streptokinase** (**A** and **B**) have been described. These enzymes can lyse blood clots and may be responsible for the rapid spread of *S. pyogenes* in infected tissues. Anti-streptokinase antibodies are also a useful marker for infection.

Deoxyribonucleases

Four immunologically distinct **deoxyribonucleases** (**DNases A** to **D**) have been identified. These enzymes are not cytolytic but can depolymerize free DNA present in pus. This process reduces the viscosity of the abscess material and facilitates spread of the organisms. Antibodies developed against DNase B are an important marker of cutaneous *S. pyogenes* infections.

C5a Peptidase

Complement component C5a mediates inflammation by recruiting and activating phagocytic cells. **C5a peptidase** disrupts this process by degrading C5a.

Other Enzymes

Other enzymes, including hyaluronidase ("spreading factor") and diphosphopyridine nucleotidase (DPNase), have been described for group A streptococci. The role of these enzymes in pathogenesis is unknown.

Epidemiology

Group A streptococci commonly colonize the oropharynx of healthy children and young adults (Box 23–2). Although the incidence of carriage is reported to be 15% to 20%, these figures are misleading. Highly selective culture techniques are necessary to detect small numbers of organisms in oropharyngeal secretions. Additionally, colonization with group A streptococci was assumed to be synonymous with colonization with *S. pyogenes*. It is now known, however, that *S. anginosus* can carry the group-specific A antigen and is present in the oropharynx. This species is not believed to cause pharyngitis.

Colonization with *S. pyogenes* is transient, regulated by the person's ability to mount specific immunity to the M protein of the colonizing strain and the presence of competitive organisms in the oropharynx. Untreated patients produce antibodies against the specific bacterial M protein that can result in long-lived immunity; however, this antibody response is diminished in treated patients. Bacteria such as the α-hemolytic and nonhemolytic streptococci are able to produce antibiotic-like substances called **bacteriocins,** which suppress the growth of group A streptococci.

In general, *S. pyogenes* disease is caused by recently acquired strains that can establish an infection of the pharynx or skin before specific antibodies are produced or competitive organisms are able to proliferate. Pharyngitis due to *S. pyogenes* is primarily a disease of children between the ages of 5 and 15 years, but infants and adults are also susceptible. The pathogen is spread from person to person through respiratory droplets. Crowding, such as in classrooms and daycare facilities, increases the opportunity for the organism to spread, particularly during the winter months. Soft tissue infections (i.e., pyoderma, erysipelas, cellulitis, fasciitis) are typically preceded by initial skin colonization with group A streptococci, after which the organisms are introduced into the superficial or deep tissues through a break in the skin.

Clinical Diseases

Suppurative Streptococcal Disease

Pharyngitis. **Pharyngitis** generally develops 2 to 4 days after exposure to the pathogen, with an abrupt onset of sore throat, fever, malaise, and headache. The posterior pharynx can appear erythematous with

---

BOX 23–2. Summary of *Streptococcus pyogenes* Infections

Physiology and Structure

Gram-positive cocci arranged in long chains.
    Facultative anaerobe.
    Beta-hemolytic, encapsulated colonies.
    Catalase-negative; PYR-positive; bacitracin-susceptible (important identification tests).
    Group-specific carbohydrate (A antigen) and type-specific antigen (M protein) in cell wall.
    Produce streptolysin O and DNase B (antibodies against these antigens [ASO, anti–DNase B] clinically important).

Virulence

Refer to Table 23–2.

Epidemiology

Asymptomatic colonization in upper respiratory tract and transient colonization of skin.
    Can survive on dry surfaces for long periods.
    Person-to-person spread by respiratory droplets (pharyngitis) or through breaks in skin after direct contact with infected person, fomite, or arthropod vector.
    Individuals at higher risk for disease include children 5 to 15 years old (pharyngitis); patients with extensive soft tissue infections and bacteremia (streptococcal toxic shock syndrome); children 2 to 5 years who have poor personal hygiene (pyoderma); young children and older adults with preexisting respiratory tract or skin infections caused by *S. pyogenes* (erysipelas, cellulitis); children with severe streptococcal disease (rheumatic fever, glomerulonephritis).
    Although the organism is ubiquitous, there are seasonal incidences of specific diseases: pharyngitis and associated rheumatic fever or glomerulonephritis (more common in cold months); pyoderma and associated glomerulonephritis (more common in warm months).

Diseases

Streptococcal pharyngitis ("strep" throat).
    Scarlet fever (complication of pharyngitis).
    Pyogenic cutaneous infections—impetigo, erysipelas, cellulitis.
    Necrotizing fasciitis involving deep subcutaneous tissues.
    Streptococcal toxic shock syndrome.
    Rheumatic fever and acute glomerulonephritis (complications of pharyngitis or cutaneous infections).

Diagnosis

Microscopy is useful in pyogenic infections.
    Direct antigen tests are useful for the diagnosis of streptococcal pharyngitis, but negative results must be confirmed by culture.
    Culture is highly sensitive.
    ASO test is useful for confirming rheumatic fever and acute glomerulonephritis. Anti–DNase B test should also be performed if acute glomerulonephritis is suspected.

Treatment, Control, and Prevention

Penicillin is drug of choice; erythromycin or oral cephalosporin is used for patients allergic to penicillin; antistaphylococcal antibiotics are given for mixed infections.
    Oropharyngeal carriage occurring after treatment can be re-treated; treatment is not indicated for prolonged asymptomatic carriage, because antibiotics disrupt normal protective flora.
    Starting antibiotic therapy within 10 days in patients with pharyngitis prevents rheumatic fever.
    For patients with a history of rheumatic fever, antibiotic prophylaxis is required before procedures (e.g., dental) that can induce bacteremias leading to endocarditis.
    For glomerulonephritis, no specific antibiotic treatment or prophylaxis is indicated.

---

an exudate, and cervical lymphadenopathy can be prominent. Despite these clinical signs and symptoms, differentiating streptococcal pharyngitis from viral pharyngitis is difficult. For example, only about 50% of patients with "strep throat" have pharyngeal or tonsillar exudates. Likewise, many young children with exudative pharyngitis have viral disease. The specific diagnosis can be made only with bacteriologic or serologic tests.

Scarlet fever is a complication of streptococcal pharyngitis that occurs when the infecting strain is lysogenized by a temperate bacteriophage that stimulates production of a pyrogenic exotoxin. Within 1 to 2 days after the initial clinical symptoms of pharyngitis develop, a diffuse erythematous rash initially appears on the upper chest and then spreads to the extremities. The area around the mouth is generally spared (circumoral pallor), as are the palms and soles. A yellowish white coating initially covers the tongue and is later shed, revealing a red, raw surface beneath ("strawberry tongue"). The rash, which blanches when pressed, is best seen on the abdomen and in skin folds (Pastia's lines). The rash disappears over the next 5 to 7 days and is followed by desquamation.

Suppurative complications of streptococcal pharyngitis have become rare since the advent of antimicrobial therapy. Abscesses of the peritonsillar and retropharyngeal areas are seen, however, as are disseminated infections to the brain, heart, bones, and joints.

Pyoderma. **Pyoderma (impetigo)** is a confined, purulent ("pyo") infection of the skin ("derma") that primarily affects exposed areas (i.e., face, arms, legs). Infection begins when the skin is colonized with *S. pyogenes* after direct contact with an infected person or a fomite. Then the organism is introduced into the subcutaneous tissues through a break in the skin (e.g., scratch, insect bite). Vesicles develop and then become pustules (pus-filled vesicles), which then rupture and crust over. The regional lymph nodes can become enlarged, but the systemic signs of infection (e.g., fever, sepsis, involvement of other organs) are uncommon. Secondary spread of the infection caused by scratching is typical.

Pyoderma is seen primarily in young children (2 to 5 years old) with poor personal hygiene and occurs primarily during the warm, moist summer months. Although *S. pyogenes* is responsible for most streptococcal skin infections, groups C and G streptococci have also been implicated. *Staphylococcus aureus* is also commonly present in the lesions. The strains of streptococci that cause skin infections are different from those that cause pharyngitis, although pyoderma serotypes can colonize the pharynx and establish a persistent carriage state.

Erysipelas. **Erysipelas** (*erythros*, "red"; *pella*, "skin") is an acute infection of the skin. Patients experience local pain and inflammation (erythema, warmth), lymph node enlargement, and systemic signs (chills, fever, leukocytosis). The involved skin area is typically raised and distinctly differentiated from the uninvolved skin (Fig. 23–2). Erysipelas occurs most commonly in young children or older adults, historically on the face but now more commonly on the legs, and usually is preceded by respiratory tract or skin infections with *S. pyogenes* (less commonly with group C or G streptococci).

Cellulitis. Unlike erysipelas, **cellulitis** typically involves the skin and deeper subcutaneous tissues, and the distinction between infected and noninfected skin is not as clear. As in erysipelas, local inflammation and systemic signs are observed. Precise identification of the offending organism is necessary, because many different microbes can cause cellulitis.

Necrotizing Fasciitis. **Necrotizing fasciitis**, an infection that occurs deep in the subcutaneous tissue, spreads along the fascial planes and is characterized by an extensive destruction of muscle and fat. The organism (referred to by the news media as "flesh-eating bacteria") is introduced into the tissue through a break in the skin (e.g., minor cut or trauma, vesicular viral infection, burn, surgery). Initially there is evidence of cellulitis, after which bullae form and gangrene and systemic symptoms develop. Systemic toxicity, multiorgan failure, and death (mortality exceeds 50%) are the hallmarks of this disease; thus, prompt medical intervention is necessary to prevent a poor prognosis. Unlike cellulitis, which can be treated with antibiotic therapy alone, fasciitis must also be treated aggressively with the surgical débridement of nonviable tissue.

Streptococcal Toxic Shock Syndrome. Although the incidence of severe *S. pyogenes* disease declined steadily after the advent of antibiotics, this trend changed dramatically in the late 1980s, when infections characterized by multisystem toxicity were reported. Most patients initially experience soft tissue inflammation at the site of the infection and pain as well as nonspecific symptoms, such as fever, chills, malaise, nausea, vomiting, and diarrhea. The pain intensifies as the disease progresses to shock and organ failure (e.g., kidney, lungs, liver, heart)—features similar to those of staphylococcal toxic shock syndrome. However, patients with streptococcal disease are bacteremic, and most have necrotizing fasciitis.

Although people of all age groups are susceptible to **streptococcal toxic shock syndrome**, patients with certain conditions are at increased risk, such as those with human immunodeficiency virus (HIV) infection, cancer, diabetes mellitus, heart or pulmonary disease, and varicella-zoster virus infection as well as intravenous drug abusers and those who abuse alcohol. The strains of *S. pyogenes* responsible for this syndrome differ from the strains causing pharyngitis, in that most of the former are M serotypes 1 or 3 and many have prominent mucopolysaccharide hyaluronic acid capsules (mucoid strains). The production of pyrogenic exotoxins, particularly SpeA, is also a prominent feature of these organisms.

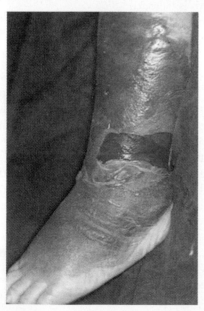

FIGURE 23–2. Acute stage of erysipelas of the leg. Note the erythema in the involved area and bullae formation. (From Emond RTD, Rowland HAK: *A color atlas of infectious diseases*, ed 2, London, 1989, Wolfe.)

Other Suppurative Diseases. *S. pyogenes* has been associated with a variety of other suppurative infections, including puerperal sepsis, lymphangitis, and pneumonia. Although these infections are still seen, they became less common after the introduction of antibiotic therapy.

Bacteremia. *S. pyogenes* is the second most common β-hemolytic *Streptococcus* isolated in blood cultures (Fig. 23–3). Patients with localized infections such as pharyngitis, pyoderma, and erysipelas rarely have bacteremia. The blood cultures in most patients with necrotizing fasciitis or toxic shock syndrome, however, are positive for the organism; the mortality in this population of patients approaches 40%.

Nonsuppurative Streptococcal Disease

Rheumatic Fever. **Rheumatic fever** is a nonsuppurative complication of *S. pyogenes* disease. It is characterized by inflammatory changes involving the heart, joints, blood vessels, and subcutaneous tissues. Involvement of the heart manifests as a pancarditis (endocarditis, pericarditis, myocarditis) and is frequently associated with subcutaneous nodules. Chronic, progressive damage to the heart valves may occur. Joint manifestations can range from arthralgias to frank arthritis, with multiple joints involved in a migratory pattern (i.e., involvement shifts from one joint to another).

The incidence of rheumatic fever has decreased from a peak of more than 10,000 cases per year reported in 1961 to 112 cases reported in 1994 (the last year of mandatory reporting). The disease is caused by specific M types (e.g., types 1, 3, 5, 6, and 18). Rheumatic fever is associated with streptococcal pharyngitis but not cutaneous streptococcal infections. As would be expected, the epidemiologic characteristics of the disease mimic those of streptococcal pharyngitis. It is most common in young school-age children, with no male or female predilection, and occurs primarily during the fall or winter. Although disease occurs most commonly in patients with severe streptococcal pharyngitis, as many as a third of patients have asymptomatic or mild infection. Rheumatic fever can recur with subsequent streptococcal infection if antibiotic prophylaxis is not used. The risk for recurrence decreases with time.

Because no specific diagnostic test can identify patients with rheumatic fever, the diagnosis is made on the basis of clinical findings and documented evidence of a recent *S. pyogenes* infection such as (1) culture results, (2) detection of the group A antigen, or (3) an elevation in anti–streptolysin O (ASO), anti–DNase B, or anti-hyaluronidase antibodies. The absence of an elevated or rising antibody titer would be strong evidence against rheumatic fever.

Acute Glomerulonephritis. The second nonsuppurative complication of streptococcal disease is **acute glomerulonephritis**, which is characterized by acute inflammation of the renal glomeruli with edema, hypertension, hematuria, and proteinuria. Specific nephritogenic strains of group A streptococci are associated with this disease. The pharyngeal and pyodermal strains differ. The epidemiologic characteristics of the disease are similar to those of the initial streptococcal infection (Table 23–3).

Diagnosis is determined on the basis of the clinical presentation and the finding of evidence of a recent *S. pyogenes* infection. Young patients generally have an uneventful recovery, but the long-term prognosis for adults is unclear. Progressive, irreversible loss of renal function has been observed in adults.

Laboratory Diagnosis

Microscopy

Gram stains of samples of affected tissue can be used to make a rapid, preliminary diagnosis of *S. pyogenes* soft issue infections or pyoderma. Because streptococci do not normally colonize the skin surface, the finding of gram-positive cocci in pairs and chains in association with leukocytes is important. In contrast, streptococci are part of the normal oropharyngeal flora, so their presence in a respiratory specimen from a patient with pharyngitis has poor predictive value.

Antigen Detection

A variety of immunologic tests using antibodies that react with the group-specific carbohydrate in the bacterial cell wall can be used to detect group A strepto-

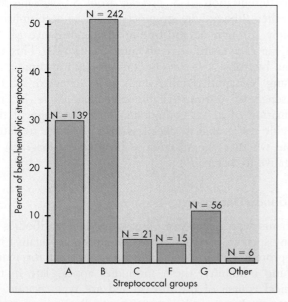

FIGURE 23–3. Distribution of streptococcal groups in bacteremic adults admitted to Barnes Hospital in St. Louis from 1986 to 2000. During this period, 479 patients with β-hemolytic streptococcal bacteremia were seen.

TABLE 23–3. Epidemiologic Features of Acute Streptococcal Glomerulonephritis

Feature	Pharyngitis Associated	Pyoderma Associated
Seasonal occurrence	Winter and spring	Late summer and early autumn
Geographical distribution	Temperate and cold climates	Hot and tropical climates
Age	School-age children	Preschool-age children
Familial occurrence	Common	Common
Attack rate after infection with nephritogenic strain (%)	10–15	10–15
Carrier state	Pharynx (common)	Skin (rare)
Serologic types	Limited to pharynx	Limited to skin
Anti–streptolysin O response	Common	Uncommon
Anti–DNase B response	Common	Common

cocci directly in throat swabs. The antigen is extracted through treatment of the specimen with nitrous acid or pronase for 5 minutes. The extract is then mixed with specific antibodies that are immobilized on a filter membrane (enzyme immunoassay [EIA]) or bound to latex particles. The development of a positive indicator in the EIA or the agglutination of the latex particles represents a positive result.

Although these assays are very specific, the sensitivity of the tests is low (probably no better than 90%), so all negative results must be confirmed by culture. A nucleic acid probe is also available for the direct detection of *S. pyogenes* in clinical specimens. Although this test is highly sensitive and specific, its cost may limit its usefulness.

Culture

Despite the difficulty of collecting throat swab specimens from children, specimens must be obtained from the posterior oropharynx (e.g., tonsils). Fewer bacteria are present in the anterior areas of the mouth, and the mouth (particularly saliva) is colonized with bacteria that inhibit the growth of *S. pyogenes*. Therefore, contamination of even a properly collected specimen may obscure or suppress the growth of *S. pyogenes*. The recovery of *S. pyogenes* from skin infections is not a problem. The crusted top of the lesion is raised, and the purulent material and base of the lesion are cultured. Culture specimens should not be obtained from open, draining skin pustules, because they might be superinfected with staphylococci.

As discussed previously, streptococci have fastidious growth requirements. Antibiotics (e.g., trimethoprim-sulfamethoxazole) can be added to blood agar plates to suppress the growth of oral bacterial flora. Although these selective plates have proved very useful, the growth of *S. pyogenes* on the plates is delayed, and prolonged incubation must be used (2 to 3 days). It is also unclear what atmosphere of incubation should be used. Because virtually all *S. pyogenes* produce streptolysin S, cultures can be incubated in air. They should not be incubated in air supplemented with carbon dioxide, however, because such an environment favors the growth of inhibitory bacteria.

Identification

S. pyogenes historically were identified from their susceptibility to **bacitracin** (Table 23–4). With this method, a disk saturated with bacitracin is placed onto a plate inoculated with group A streptococci, and after overnight incubation, strains inhibited by bacitracin are considered group A streptococci.

Group A streptococci are now identified definitively through the demonstration of the group-specific carbohydrate, a technique that was not practical until the introduction of direct antigen detection tests.

Differentiation of *S. pyogenes* from *S. anginosus* and all other β-hemolytic streptococci can be accomplished rapidly through demonstration of the presence of the enzyme **L-pyrrolidonyl arylamidase (PYR)**. This enzyme hydrolyzes *L*-pyrrolindonyl-β-naphthylamide, releasing β-naphthylamine, which is detected in the presence of p-dimethylaminocinnamaldehyde by the formation of a red compound. The advantage of this specific test is that it takes less than 1 minute to determine whether the reaction is positive (*S. pyogenes*) or negative (*S. anginosus*).

Antibody Detection

Patients with *S. pyogenes* disease produce antibodies to many specific enzymes. Although antibodies against the M protein are produced and are important for maintaining immunity, these antibodies appear late in the clinical course of the disease and are type-specific. In contrast, the measurement of antibodies against streptolysin O (the **ASO test**) is useful for confirming rheumatic fever or acute glomerulonephritis resulting from

TABLE 23–4. Biochemical Identification of Common Streptococci

| Organism | Susceptibility | | Hippurate Hydrolysis | CAMP Reaction | Bile Solubility |
	Bacitracin	Optochin			
*S. pyogenes**	S	R	–	–	–
S. agalactiae	R	R	+	+	–
S. anginosus†	R	R	–	–	–
S. dysgalactiae‡	R	R	–	–	–
S. pneumoniae	R	S	–	–	+
Viridans group	R	R	–	–	–

CAMP = Christie, Atkins, Mundi-Petersen (test); PYR = *L*-pyrrolidonyl arylamidase; R = resistant; S = susceptible.

  * *S. pyogenes* has a positive PYR reaction.

  † *S. angionosus* has negative PYR reaction and a positive Voges-Proskauer (VP) reaction.

  ‡ *S. dysgalactiae* has negative PYR and Voges-Proskauer (VP) reactions.

a recent streptococcal pharyngeal infection. These antibodies appear 3 to 4 weeks after the initial exposure to the organism and then persist.

An elevated ASO titer is not observed in patients with streptococcal pyoderma. The production of other antibodies against streptococcal enzymes, particularly DNase B, has been documented in patients with streptococcal pyoderma and pharyngitis. The **anti–DNase B test** should be performed if streptococcal glomerulonephritis is suspected.

Treatment, Prevention, and Control

S. pyogenes is very sensitive to penicillin. Erythromycin or an oral cephalosporin can be used in patients with a history of penicillin allergy. However, this therapy is ineffective in patients with mixed infections that involve *S. aureus*. Treatment in this case should include oxacillin or vancomycin. Newer macrolides (e.g., azithromycin, clarithromcyin) are not more effective than erythromycin, and resistance or poor clinical response has limited the usefulness of the tetracyclines and sulfonamides. Drainage and aggressive surgical débridement must be promptly initiated in patients with serious soft tissue infections.

Persistent oropharyngeal carriage of *S. pyogenes* can occur after a complete course of therapy. This state may stem from poor compliance with the prescribed course of therapy, reinfection with a new strain, or persistent carriage in a sequestered focus. Because penicillin resistance has not been observed in patients with oropharyngeal carriage, they can be given an additional course of treatment. If carriage persists, re-treatment is not indicated, because prolonged antibiotic therapy can disrupt the normal bacterial flora. Antibiotic therapy in patients with pharyngitis speeds the relief of symptoms and, if initiated within 10 days of the initial clinical disease, prevents rheumatic fever. Antibiotic therapy

does not appear to influence the progression to acute glomerulonephritis.

Patients with a history of rheumatic fever require long-term antibiotic prophylaxis to prevent recurrence of the disease. Because damage to the heart valve predisposes these patients to endocarditis, they also require antibiotic prophylaxis before they undergo procedures that can induce transient bacteremias (e.g., dental procedures). Specific antibiotic therapy does not alter the course of acute glomerulonephritis, however, and prophylactic therapy is not indicated because recurrent disease is not observed in these patients.

Streptococcus agalactiae (Group B)

S. agalactiae is the only species that carries the group B antigen. This organism was initially recognized as a cause of puerperal sepsis. Although still associated with the disease, *S. agalactiae* has become better known as an important cause of septicemia, pneumonia, and meningitis in newborn children as well as a cause of serious disease in adults (see Box 23–1).

Physiology and Structure

Group B streptococci are gram-positive cocci (0.6 to 1.2 μm) that form short chains in clinical specimens and longer chains in culture, features that make them indistinguishable on Gram stain from *S. pyogenes*. They grow well on nutritionally enriched media, and in contrast with the colonies of *S. pyogenes*, the colonies of *S. agalactiae* are buttery with a narrow zone of β-hemolysis. Some strains (1% to 2%) are nonhemolytic, although their prevalence may be underestimated because nonhemolytic strains are not commonly screened for the group B antigen.

Strains of *S. agalactiae* can be subdivided on the basis of three serologic markers:

1. The B antigen or group-specific cell wall polysaccharide antigen (composed of rhamnose, *N*-acetylglucosamine, and galactose).
2. Type-specific capsular polysaccharides (Ia, Ib, and II to VIII).
3. The surface protein, C protein.

Eleven immunologically distinct serotypes have been described: Ia, Ia/c, Ib/c, II, IIc, III, IV, V, VI, VII, and VIII. These serotypes are important epidemiologic markers, with serotypes Ia, III, and V being most commonly associated with colonization and disease. Knowledge of the specific serotypes associated with disease and of shifting patterns of serotype prevalence is also important for vaccine development.

Pathogenesis and Immunity

The following two questions about group B streptococcal disease can be posed:

1. Why are the very young at increased risk?
2. Why are certain serotypes more commonly associated with disease?

Antibodies developed against the type-specific capsular antigens of group B streptococci are protective, a factor that partly explains the predilection of this organism for neonates. Genital colonization with group B streptococci has been associated with increased risk of premature delivery. Premature infants are at greater risk of disease because they have lower levels of type-specific maternal antibodies.

Additionally, functional classical and alternative complement pathways are required for killing group B streptococci, particularly types Ia, III, and V. As a result, there is a greater likelihood of systemic spread of the organism in colonized premature infants with physiologically low complement levels or for infants in whom the receptors for complement or for the Fc fragment of IgG antibodies are not exposed on neutrophils. It has also been found that the type-specific capsular polysaccharides of types Ia, Ib, and II streptococci have a terminal residue of sialic acid. Sialic acid can inhibit activation of the alternative complement pathway, thus interfering with the phagocytosis of these strains of group B streptococci.

Group B streptococci produce several enzymes, including DNases, hyaluronidase, neuraminidase, proteases, hippurase, and hemolysins. Although these enzymes are useful for identifying the organism, their role in the pathogenesis of infection is unknown.

Epidemiology

Group B streptococci colonize the lower gastrointestinal tract and the genitourinary tract (Box 23–3). Tran-

---

BOX 23–3. **Summary of Group B Streptococcal Infections**

Physiology and Structure

Gram-positive cocci arranged in long chains.
　Facultative anaerobe.
　Catalase-negative; positive CAMP and hippurate hydrolysis reactions (important identification tests).
　Group-specific carbohydrate (B antigen) in cell wall and type-specific antigens in capsule.

Virulence

Thick peptidoglycan layer in cell wall permits survival on dry surfaces.
　Capsule interferes with phagocytosis.
　Hydrolytic enzymes may facilitate tissue destruction and systemic spread of the bacteria.

Epidemiology

Asymptomatic colonization of the upper respiratory tract and genitourinary tract.
　Most infections in newborns acquired from mother during pregnancy or at time of birth.
　Neonates are at higher risk for infection if (1) there is premature rupture of membranes, prolonged labor, preterm birth, or disseminated maternal group B streptococcal disease and (2) mother is without type-specific antibodies and has low complement levels.

Women with genital colonization are at risk for postpartum sepsis.
　Men and nonpregnant women with diabetes mellitus, cancer, or alcoholism are at increased risk for disease.
　No seasonal incidence.

Diseases

Two forms of neonatal disease: early-onset and late-onset; these diseases are characterized by meningitis, pneumonia, and bacteremia.
　Other infections with group B streptococci are endometritis, urinary tract infection, wound infection, and bacteremia.

Diagnosis

Antigen tests are too insensitive. Culture using a selective broth is the diagnostic test of choice.

Modes of Control

Penicillin G is the drug of choice; a combination of penicillin and aminoglycoside is used in patients with serious infections; vancomycin is used for patients allergic to penicillin.
　For high-risk babies, antibiotic therapy and passive immunization by transfusion with blood containing type-specific antibodies are performed.

sient vaginal carriage has been observed in 10% to 30% of pregnant women, although the incidence depends on the time during the gestation period when the sampling is done and the culture techniques used. A similar incidence has been observed in nonpregnant women.

Approximately 60% of infants born to colonized mothers become colonized with their mothers' organisms. The likelihood of colonization at birth is higher if the mother is heavily colonized. Other risk factors for neonatal colonization are premature delivery, prolonged membrane rupture, and intrapartum fever. The serotypes most commonly associated with neonatal disease are Ia (35% to 40%), III (30%), and V (15%). Serotypes Ia and V are the most common in adult disease, with serotype III less commonly isolated.

Colonization with subsequent development of disease in the neonate can occur in utero, at birth, or during the first few months of life. Disease in infants younger than 7 days of age is called **early-onset disease**; disease appearing between 1 week and 3 months of life is considered **late-onset disease**. The incidence of disease has declined dramatically in the 1990s through the use of intrapartum antibiotic prophylaxis. Despite this promising trend, approximately 2200 infections occurred in 1999 among children in their first week of life.

There are more group B streptococcal infections in adults than in neonates, but the overall incidence is higher in neonates. The risk of disease is greater in pregnant women than in men and nonpregnant women. Urinary tract infections, amnionitis, endometritis, and wound infections are the most common manifestations in pregnant women. Infections in men and nonpregnant women are primarily skin and soft tissue infections, bacteremia, urosepsis (urinary tract infection with bacteremia), and pneumonia. Group B streptococci are the most common β-hemolytic streptococci isolated in blood cultures (see Fig. 23-3). Conditions that predispose to the development of adult disease include diabetes mellitus, cancer, and alcoholism.

Clinical Diseases

Early-Onset Neonatal Disease

Clinical symptoms of group B streptococcal disease acquired in utero or at birth develop during the first week of life. Early-onset disease, which is characterized by bacteremia, pneumonia, or meningitis, is indistinguishable from sepsis caused by other organisms. Pulmonary involvement is observed in most infants, and meningeal involvement may be initially inapparent, so examination of cerebrospinal fluid is required for all infected children. The mortality rate has decreased to less than 5% as a result of rapid diagnosis and better supportive care; however, 15% to 30% of infants surviving meningitis have neurologic sequelae, including blindness, deafness, and severe mental retardation.

Late-Onset Neonatal Disease

Disease in older infants is acquired from an exogenous source (e.g., mother, another infant). The predominant manifestation is bacteremia with meningitis, which resembles disease caused by other bacteria. Although the survival rate is high, neurologic complications are common in children with meningitis.

Infections in Pregnant Women

Urinary tract infections frequently occur in women during and immediately after pregnancy. Because childbearing women are generally in good health, the prognosis is excellent for those who receive appropriate therapy. Secondary complications of bacteremia, such as endocarditis, meningitis, and osteomyelitis, are rare.

Infections in Men and Nonpregnant Women

Compared with pregnant women who acquire group B streptococcal infection, men and nonpregnant women with group B streptococcal infections are generally older and have debilitating underlying conditions. The most common presentations are bacteremia, pneumonia, bone and joint infections, and skin and soft tissue infections. Because these patients frequently have compromised immunity, mortality is higher in this population (i.e., between 15% and 32%).

Laboratory Diagnosis

Antigen Detection

Direct detection of the organism with antibodies prepared against the group-specific carbohydrate is useful for the rapid detection of group B streptococcal disease in neonates. A variety of methods are used, including staphylococcal coagglutination, latex agglutination, and EIA. Unfortunately, the direct antigen test is too insensitive to be used to screen mothers and predict which newborns are at increased risk for acquiring neonatal disease. Thus, use of the antigen test for this application is not recommended. Currently, culture is the only reliable method for determining whether a pregnant woman is colonized with group B streptococci.

Culture

Group B streptococci readily grow on a nutritionally enriched medium, producing large colonies after 24 hours of incubation. β-Hemolysis may be difficult to detect or absent, posing a problem in the detection of the organism when other organisms are present in the culture (e.g., vaginal culture). Thus, a selective broth medium, with antibiotics added to suppress the growth of other organisms, should be used to detect group B streptococcal carriage in pregnant women.

Identification

A preliminary identification of an isolate can be made by demonstration of a positive **CAMP** (Christie, Atkins, Munch-Petersen) **test** (Fig. 23–4) or by the **hydrolysis of hippurate**. Group B streptococci are identified definitively by the demonstration of the group-specific carbohydrate or the use of commercially prepared molecular probes.

Treatment, Prevention, and Control

Group B streptococci are generally susceptible to penicillin G, which is the drug of choice. However, the minimum inhibitory concentration (MIC) needed to inhibit the organism is approximately 10 times greater than that needed to inhibit *S. pyogenes*. In addition, tolerance to penicillin (the ability of the antibiotic to inhibit but not kill the organism) has been reported. For these reasons, a combination of penicillin and an aminoglycoside is frequently used in the management of serious infections. Vancomycin is an alternative therapy for patients allergic to penicillin. Antibiotic

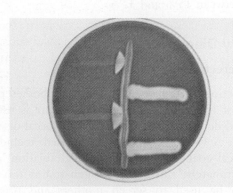

FIGURE 23–4. CAMP (Christie, Atkins, Mundi-Petersen) reaction with group B streptococci. Group B streptococci produce a diffusible, heat-stable protein (CAMP factor) that enhances β-hemolysis of *Staphylococcus aureus*. *S. aureus* (streaked from the top to the bottom of the agar plate) produces sphingomyelinase C, which can bind to erythrocyte membranes. When exposed to the group B CAMP factor, the cells undergo hemolysis (compare the two positive reactions of enhanced hemolysis to the left of the *S. aureus* streak with the two negative reactions to the right). (From Howard BJ: *Clinical and pathogenic microbiology,* St. Louis, 1987, Mosby.)

resistance to erythromycin and tetracycline has been observed.

In an effort to prevent neonatal disease, it is recommended that all pregnant women should be screened for colonization with group B streptococci at 35 to 37 weeks of gestation. Chemoprophylaxis should be used for all women who are either colonized or at high risk. A pregnant woman is considered to be at high risk to give birth to a baby with invasive group B disease if she has previously given birth to an infant with the disease or risk factors for the disease are present at birth. These risk factors are (1) intrapartum temperature of at least 38°C, (2) membrane rupture at least 18 hours before delivery, and (3) vaginal or rectal culture positive for organisms at 35 to 37 weeks of gestation. Intravenous penicillin G administered at least 4 hours before delivery is recommended; clindamycin or a cephalosporin is used for penicillin-allergic women. This approach ensures high protective antibiotic levels in the infant's circulatory system at the time of birth.

Because newborn disease is associated with decreased circulating antibodies in the mother, efforts have been directed at developing a polyvalent vaccine against serotypes Ia, Ib, II, III, and V. The capsular polysaccharides are poor immunogens; however, complexing them with tetanus toxoid has improved the immunogenicity of the vaccine. Clinical trials with this polyvalent vaccine are under way.

Other Beta-Hemolytic Streptococci

Among the other β-hemolytic streptococci, groups C, F, and G are the most commonly associated with human disease. The two species of particular importance are (1) *S. anginosus*, which can possess the group A, C, F, or G capsular polysaccharide, and (2) *S. dysgalactiae*, which has the group C or G antigen. It should be noted that an individual isolate possesses only one group antigen, a finding consistent with the belief that the species are actually a group of closely related species. Isolates of *S. anginosus* grow as small colonies (requiring 2 days of incubation) with a narrow zone of β-hemolysis (Fig. 23–5*A*). This species is primarily associated with abscess formation and not pharyngitis (in contrast with *S. pyogenes*). *S. dysgalactiae* produce large colonies with a large zone of β-hemolysis on blood agar media (Fig. 23–5*B*), a behavior similar to that of *S. pyogenes*. Like *S. pyogenes*, *S. dysgalactiae* causes pharyngitis, which is sometimes complicated by acute glomerulonephritis but never rheumatic fever.

Another groupable *Streptococcus* is *Streptococcus bovis*. Although the original β-hemolytic strain was classified by Lancefield as group D, most strains are α-hemolytic and have now been reclassified with the viridans streptococci. *S. bovis* is clinically significant, because strains

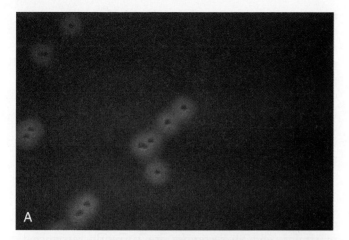

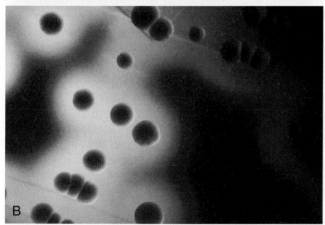

FIGURE 23–5. Group C *Streptococcus. A, S. anginosus,* small-colony species. *B, S. dysgalactiae,* large-colony species.

that cause bacteremia have a prominent association with occult malignancy of the colon.

Viridans Streptococci

The viridans group of streptococci are a heterogeneous collection of α-hemolytic and nonhemolytic streptococci. Their group name is derived from *viridis* (Latin for "green"), a reflection of the fact that many of these bacteria produce a green pigment on blood agar media. The taxonomic nomenclature for these species is confusing because European and American microbiologists have not reached a consensus on it. Thus, different species names are often used interchangeably in the literature. At least 24 species have been identified in the United States, and they are classified into five subgroups (Table 23–5). The precise classification of these bacteria can be problematic and is beyond the scope of this text.

Although most isolates of viridans streptococci do not possess a group-specific carbohydrate, their reactivity with some groups of carbohydrates has been re-

ported. This is particularly true for *S. anginosus* and *S. bovis*. It should also be noted that *Streptococcus pneumoniae* is a member of the *Streptococcus mitis* group. Although *S. pneumoniae* is discussed separately, it is important to realize that it is very closely related to streptococcal species in the viridans group.

Like most other streptococci, viridans species are nutritionally fastidious, requiring complex media supplemented with blood products and, frequently, an incubation atmosphere augmented with 5% to 10% carbon dioxide. Some strains are "nutritionally deficient," in that they can grow only in the presence of exogenously supplied pyridoxal, the active form of vitamin B_6. These organisms can usually grow initially in blood cultures but cannot grow when subcultured unless pyridoxal-supplemented media are used. These strains have been reclassified into a new genus, *Abiotrophia*, although most investigators still refer to them as nutritionally deficient streptococci.

The viridans streptococci colonize the oropharynx, gastrointestinal tract, and genitourinary tract. They are rarely found on the skin surface, because the surface fatty acids are toxic to them. Although these organisms can cause a variety of infections, they are most commonly associated with dental caries, subacute endocarditis, and suppurative intra-abdominal infections. *Streptococcus mutans* and *Streptococcus sanguis* adhere to tooth enamel or previously damaged heart valves, probably because of the insoluble dextran that they produce from glucose. *Streptococcus anginosus* is responsible for causing pyogenic infections, as was found with the groupable strains.

In the past, most strains of viridans streptococci were highly susceptible to penicillin, with MICs of less than 0.1 $\mu g/mL$. However, moderately resistant (penicillin MIC of 0.2 to 2 $\mu g/mL$) and highly resistant (MIC >2 $\mu g/mL$) streptococci have become common. Resistance is particularly common in the *S. mitis* group, which includes *S. pneumoniae*; this issue is discussed in greater detail in the next section. Infections

TABLE 23–5. Classification of Viridans Group of *Streptococcus*

Group	Species
S. anginosus	*S. anginosus, S. constellatus, S. intermedius*
S. bovis	*S. bovis, S. alactolyticus, S. equinus*
S. mitis	*S. mitis, S. pneumoniae, S. sanguis, S. parasanguis, S. gordonii, S. crista, S. oralis*
S. mutans	*S. mutans, S. sobrinus, S. cricetus, S. rattus, S. downei, S. macacae*
S. salivarius	*S. salivarius, S. vestibularis, S. thermophilus*
Ungrouped	*S. acidominimus, S. suis*

with isolates that are moderately resistant can generally be treated with a combination of penicillin and an aminoglycoside. However, alternative antibiotics, such as a broad-spectrum cephalosporin or vancomycin, must be used to treat serious infections caused by penicillin-resistant strains.

Streptococcus pneumoniae

S. pneumoniae was isolated independently by Pasteur and Steinberg more than a hundred years ago. Since that time, research with this organism has led to a greater understanding of molecular genetics, antibiotic resistance, and vaccine-related immunoprophylaxis. Unfortunately, pneumococcal disease is still a leading cause of morbidity and mortality.

Physiology and Structure

The pneumococcus is an encapsulated, gram-positive coccus. The cells are 0.5 to 1.2 μm in diameter, oval or lancet-shaped, and arranged in pairs or short chains (Fig. 23–6). Older cells decolorize readily and appear gram-negative. Colonial morphology varies. Colonies of encapsulated strains are generally large (1 to 3 mm in diameter on blood agar; smaller on chocolatized or heated blood agar), round, and mucoid; colonies of nonencapsulated strains are smaller and appear flat. All colonies undergo autolysis with aging—that is, the central portion of the colony dissolves, leaving a dimpled appearance. Colonies appear α-hemolytic on blood agar if incubated aerobically and may be β-hemolytic if grown anaerobically. The α-hemolytic appearance results from production of pneumolysin, an enzyme that degrades hemoglobin, producing a green product.

The organism has fastidious nutritional require-

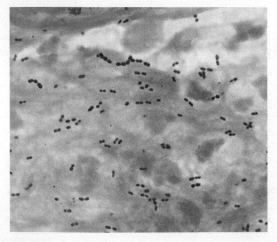

FIGURE 23–6. Gram stain of *Streptococcus pneumoniae.*

ments and can grow only on enriched media supplemented with blood products. *S. pneumoniae* can ferment several carbohydrates, with lactic acid the primary metabolic byproduct. *S. pneumoniae* grows poorly in media with high glucose concentrations because lactic acid rapidly reaches toxic levels in such preparations. Like all streptococci, the organism lacks catalase. Unless an exogenous source of catalase is provided (e.g., from blood), the accumulation of hydrogen peroxide inhibits the growth of *S. pneumoniae*, as observed on chocolatized blood agar.

Virulent strains of *S. pneumoniae* are covered with a complex polysaccharide capsule. The capsular polysaccharides have been used for the serologic classification of strains, and 90 serotypes are currently recognized. Purified capsular polysaccharides from the most commonly isolated serotypes are used in a polyvalent vaccine.

The peptidoglycan layer of the cell wall of the pneumococcus is typical of gram-positive cocci. Attached to alternating subunits of *N*-acetylglucosamine and *N*-acetylmuramic acid are oligopeptide chains, which in turn are cross-linked by pentaglycine bridges. The other major component of the cell wall is teichoic acid, which is rich in galactosamine, phosphate, and choline. The choline is unique to the cell wall of *S. pneumoniae* and plays an important regulatory role in cell wall hydrolysis. Choline must be present for activity of the pneumococcal autolysin, **amidase,** during cell division.

Two forms of **teichoic acid** exist in the pneumococcal cell wall, one exposed on the cell surface and a similar form covalently bound to the plasma membrane lipids. The exposed teichoic acid is linked to the peptidoglycan layer and extends through the overlying capsule. This species-specific structure, called the **C polysaccharide,** is unrelated to the group-specific carbohydrate observed by Lancefield in β-hemolytic streptococci. The C polysaccharide precipitates a serum globulin fraction (**C-reactive protein [CRP]**) in the presence of calcium. CRP is present in low concentrations in healthy people but in elevated concentrations in patients with acute inflammatory diseases. The lipid-bound teichoic acid in the bacterial cytoplasmic membrane is called the **F antigen** because it can cross-react with the Forssman surface antigens on mammalian cells.

Pathogenesis and Immunity

Although *S. pneumoniae* has been extensively studied, much remains to be learned about the pathogenesis of pneumococcal disease. The disease manifestations are caused primarily by the host response to infection rather than the production of organism-specific toxic factors. However, an understanding of how *S. pneumo-*

niae colonizes the oropharynx, spreads into normally sterile tissues, stimulates a localized inflammatory response, and evades being killed by phagocytic cells is crucial (Table 23–6).

Colonization and Migration

S. pneumoniae is a human pathogen that colonizes the oropharynx and then, in specific situations, is able to spread to the lungs, paranasal sinuses, or middle ear. It can also be transported in the blood stream to distal sites such as the brain. The initial colonization of the oropharynx is mediated by the binding of the bacteria to epithelial cells by means of **surface protein adhesins**. Subsequent migration of the organism to the lower respiratory tract can be prevented if the bacteria are enveloped in mucus and removed from the airways by the action of ciliated epithelial cells. The bacteria counteract this envelopment by producing **secretory IgA (sIgA) protease** and **pneumolysin**. Secretory IgA traps bacteria in mucin by attaching itself to the bacteria at the antigen-binding site and to mucin at the Fc region. The bacterial protease prevents this interaction. **Pneumolysin**, a cytotoxin similar to the streptolysin O in *S. pyogenes*, binds cholesterol in the host cell membrane and creates pores. This activity can destroy the ciliated epithelial cells as well as phagocytic cells.

Tissue Destruction

A characteristic of pneumococcal infections is the mobilization of inflammatory cells to the focus of infection. The process is mediated by pneumococcal teichoic acid, peptidoglycan fragments, and pneumolysin. **Teichoic acid** and the **peptidoglycan fragments** activate the alternative complement pathway, producing C5a, which mediates the inflammatory process. This activity is augmented by the bacterial amidase, which enhances release of the cell wall components. **Pneumolysin** activates the classic complement pathway, resulting in the production of C3a and C5a. In turn, cytokines such as IL-1 and TNF-α are produced by the activated leukocytes, leading to the further migration of inflammatory cells to the site of infection, fever, tissue damage, and other signs characteristic of pneumococcal infection. The production of **hydrogen peroxide** by *S. pneumoniae* can also lead to tissue damage caused by reactive oxygen intermediates.

Finally, **phosphorylcholine** present in the bacterial cell wall can bind to receptors for platelet-activating factor that are expressed on the surface of endothelial cells, leukocytes, platelets, and tissue cells such as those in the lungs and meninges. By binding these receptors, the bacteria can enter the cells, where they are protected from opsonization and phagocytosis, and pass into sequestered areas such as blood and the central nervous system. This activity facilitates the spread of disease.

Phagocytic Survival

S. pneumoniae survives phagocytosis because of the antiphagocytic protection afforded by its **capsule** and the pneumolysin-mediated suppression of the phagocytic cell oxidative burst, which is required for intracellular killing. The virulence of *S. pneumoniae* is a direct result of this capsule. Encapsulated (smooth) strains can cause disease in humans and experimental animals, whereas nonencapsulated (rough) strains are avirulent. Antibodies directed against the type-specific capsular polysaccharides protect against disease due to immunologically related strains. The capsular polysaccharides are soluble and have been called **specific soluble substances.** Free polysaccharides can protect viable organisms from phagocytosis by binding with opsonic antibodies.

Epidemiology

S. pneumoniae is a common inhabitant of the throat and nasopharynx in healthy people (Box 23–4). A 5% to 75% incidence of such carriage has been reported, but

TABLE 23–6. *Streptococcus pneumoniae* Virulence Factors

Virulence Factor	Biologic Effect
Colonization and Migration	
Surface protein adhesins	Binds to epithelial cells
Secretory IgA protease	Disrupts secretory IgA–mediated clearance
Pneumolysin	Possibly destroys ciliated epithelial cells
Tissue Destruction	
Teichoic acid	Activates alternative complement pathway
Peptidoglycan fragments	Activate alternative complement pathway
Pneumolysin	Activates classic complement pathway
Hydrogen peroxide	Allows reactive oxygen intermediates to cause damage
Phosphorylcholine	Binds phosphodiesterase-activating factor, allowing bacteria to enter host cells
Phagocytic Survival	
Capsule	Antiphagocytic
Pneumolysin	Suppresses phagocytic oxidative burst

BOX 23-4. Summary of *Streptococcus pneumoniae* Infections

Physiology and Structure

Elongated or "lancet-shaped," gram-positive cocci arranged in pairs (diplococci).

Facultative anaerobe.

Teichoic acid ("C polysaccharide") in cell wall is rich in choline that can react with a serum protein (referred to as the C-reactive protein)—this is a useful diagnostic test for systemic disease.

An autolytic enzyme (amidase) is present in the cell wall. Older cells undergo spontaneous autolysis, producing colonies with dimpled center. Detection of these colonies and demonstration that the colonies are lysed when exposed to bile constitute an important identification test.

Bacteria are inhibited by optochin (useful identification test).

Virulence

Refer to Table 23-6.

Epidemiology

Most infections are caused by endogenous spread from the colonized nasopharynx or oropharynx to distal site (e.g., lungs, sinuses, ears, blood, meninges).

Colonization is highest in young children.

Person-to-person spread through infectious droplets is rare.

Individuals with antecedent viral respiratory tract disease or other conditions that interfere with bacterial clearance from respiratory tract are at increased risk for pulmonary disease.

Children and the elderly are at risk for meningitis.

People with hematologic disorder (malignancy, sickle cell disease) or functional asplenia are at risk for fulminant sepsis.

Although the organism is ubiquitous, disease is more common in cool months.

Diseases

Pneumonia (one of the most common causes of community-acquired disease).

Meningitis (most common causes of bacterial meningitis in most age groups).

Common cause of sinusitis and otitis media.

Can cause a variety of systemic infections, including bacteremia and endocarditis.

Diagnosis

Microscopy is highly sensitive, as is culture, unless the patient has been treated with antibiotics.

Treatment, Prevention, and Control

Penicillin is the drug of choice for susceptible strains, although resistance is increasingly common.

Cephalosporins, erythromycin, chloramphenicol, or vancomycin are used for patients allergic to penicillin or for treatment of penicillin-resistant strains.

Immunization with 23-valent vaccine can prevent infection, although response to the vaccine is lowest in patients at greatest risk for serious disease, and the effectiveness of the vaccine is controversial.

---

the incidence is significantly affected by the methods used to detect the organism and the population studied. Colonization is more common in children than in adults, and common in adults living in a household with children. Colonization with *S. pneumoniae* initially occurs at about 6 months of age. Subsequently, the child is transiently colonized with other serotypes of the organism. The duration of carriage decreases with each successive serotype carried, in part because of the development of serotype-specific immunity. Although new serotypes are acquired throughout the year, the incidence of carriage and associated disease is highest during the cool months (Fig. 23-7). The strains of pneumococci that cause disease are the same as those associated with carriage. When infection occurs, generally the patient acquires a new serotype rather than one associated with prolonged carriage.

Pneumococcal disease occurs when organisms colonizing the nasopharynx and oropharynx spread to distal loci, such as the lungs (pneumonia), paranasal sinuses (sinusitis), ears (otitis media), and meninges (meningitis). Bacteremia, with subsequent spread of the disease

to other body sites, can occur with all of these infections.

S. pneumoniae is a common cause of bacterial pneumonia (an estimated 500,000 cases annually in the United States), meningitis (6000 cases annually), otitis media and sinusitis (more than 7 million cases annually), and bacteremia (55,000 cases annually). The incidence of disease is highest in children and the elderly, populations that have low levels of protective antibodies directed against the pneumococcal capsular polysaccharides.

Pneumonia occurs when the endogenous oral organisms are aspirated into the lower airways. Although strains can spread on airborne droplets from one person to another in a closed population, epidemics are rare. Disease occurs when the natural defense mechanisms (epiglottal reflex, trapping of bacteria by the mucus-producing cells lining the bronchus, removal of organisms by the ciliated respiratory epithelium, and cough reflex) are circumvented, permitting organisms colonizing the oropharynx to gain access to the lungs. Pneumococcal disease is most commonly associated

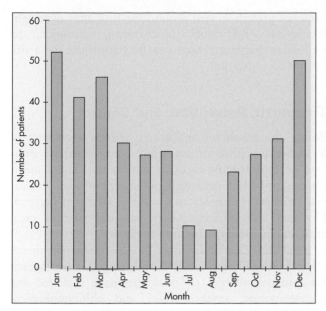

FIGURE 23–7. Seasonal incidence of *Streptococcus pneumoniae* invasive disease. Monthly incidence of bacteremia at Barnes Hospital in St. Louis from 1980 to 1995.

with an antecedent viral respiratory disease, such as influenza or measles, or with other conditions that interfere with bacterial clearance, such as chronic pulmonary disease, alcoholism, congestive heart failure, diabetes mellitus, and chronic renal disease.

Clinical Diseases

Pneumonia

Pneumococcal **pneumonia** develops when the bacteria multiply in the alveolar spaces. After aspiration, the bacteria grow rapidly in the nutrient-rich edema fluid. Erythrocytes, leaking from congested capillaries, accumulate in the alveoli, followed by the neutrophils and then the alveolar macrophages. Resolution occurs when specific anti-capsular antibodies develop, facilitating phagocytosis of the organism and microbial killing.

The onset of the clinical manifestations of pneumococcal pneumonia is abrupt, consisting of a severe shaking chill and sustained fever of 39°C to 41°C. The patient commonly has symptoms of a viral respiratory tract infection 1 to 3 days before the onset. Most patients have a productive cough with blood-tinged sputum, and they commonly have chest pain (pleurisy). Because the disease is associated with aspiration, it is generally localized in the lower lobes of the lungs (hence the name **lobar pneumonia**). However, children and the elderly can have a more generalized bronchopneumonia. Patients usually recover rapidly after the initiation of appropriate antimicrobial therapy, with complete radiologic resolution in 2 to 3 weeks.

The overall mortality rate is 5%, although the likelihood of death is influenced by the serotype of the organism and the age and underlying disease of the patient. The mortality rate is considerably higher in patients with disease caused by *S. pneumoniae* type 3 as well as in elderly patients and patients with documented bacteremia. Patients with splenic dysfunction or splenectomy can also have severe pneumococcal disease, as a result of decreased bacterial clearance from the blood stream and the defective production of early antibodies. In these patients, disease is associated with a fulminant course and high mortality rate.

Abscesses do not commonly form in patients with pneumococcal pneumonia, except in those infected with specific serotypes (e.g., serotype 3). Pleural effusions are seen in approximately 25% of patients with pneumococcal pneumonia, and empyema (purulent effusion) is a rare complication.

Sinusitis and Otitis Media

S. pneumoniae is a common cause of acute infections of the paranasal sinuses and ear. The disease is usually preceded by a viral infection of the upper respiratory tract, after which polymorphonuclear leukocytes infiltrate and obstruct the sinuses and ear canal. Middle ear infection (**otitis media**) is primarily seen in young children, but bacterial **sinusitis** can occur in patients of all ages.

Meningitis

S. pneumoniae can spread into the central nervous system after bacteremia, infections of the ear or sinuses, or head trauma that causes a communication between the subarachnoid space and the nasopharynx. Bacterial **meningitis** can occur in patients of all ages but is primarily a pediatric disease. Although pneumococcal meningitis is relatively uncommon in neonates, *S. pneumoniae* is now a leading cause of disease in children and adults. Mortality and severe neurologic deficits are 4 to 20 times more common in patients with meningitis due to *S. pneumoniae* than in those with meningitis due to other organisms.

Bacteremia

Bacteremia occurs in 25% to 30% of patients with pneumococcal pneumonia and in more than 80% of patients with meningitis. In contrast, bacteria are generally not present in the blood stream of patients with sinusitis or otitis media. Endocarditis can occur in patients with normal or previously damaged heart valves. Destruction of valve tissue is common.

Laboratory Diagnosis

Microscopy

Gram stain of sputum specimens is a rapid way to diagnose pneumococcal disease. The organisms characteristically appear as lancet-shaped, gram-positive diplococci surrounded by an unstained capsule; however, they may also appear to be gram-negative because they tend not to stain well (particularly older cultures). In addition, their morphology may be distorted in a patient receiving antibiotic therapy. Gram stain consistent with *S. pneumoniae* can be confirmed with the **quellung** (German for "swelling") reaction. In this test, polyvalent anti-capsular antibodies are mixed with the bacteria, and then the mixture is examined microscopically. A greater refractiveness around the bacteria is a positive reaction for *S. pneumoniae*.

Culture

Sputum specimens should be inoculated onto an enriched nutrient medium supplemented with blood. *S. pneumoniae* is recovered in the sputum cultures from only half of the patients who have pneumonia, because the organism has fastidious nutritional requirements and is rapidly overgrown by contaminating oral bacteria. A selective medium such as blood agar with 5 μg/mL of gentamicin has been used with some success to isolate the organism from sputum specimens, but it takes some technical skill to distinguish *S. pneumoniae* from the other α-hemolytic streptococci that are frequently present in the specimen.

For the organism responsible for sinusitis or otitis to be diagnosed definitively, an aspirate must be obtained from the sinus or middle ear. Culture should not be performed for specimens taken from the nasopharynx or outer ear. It is not difficult to isolate *S. pneumoniae* from specimens of cerebrospinal fluid unless antibiotic therapy has been initiated before the specimen is collected. Culture findings are negative in as many as half of infected patients who have received even a single dose of antibiotics.

Identification

Isolates of *S. pneumoniae* are lysed rapidly when the autolysins are activated after exposure to bile (**bile solubility test**). Thus, the organism can be identified by placement of a drop of bile on an isolated colony. Most colonies of *S. pneumoniae* are dissolved within a few minutes, whereas other α-hemolytic streptococci remain unchanged. *S. pneumoniae* can also be identified from its susceptibility to **optochin** (ethylhydrocupreine dihydrochloride). The isolate is streaked onto a blood agar plate, and a disk saturated with optochin is placed in the middle of the inoculum. A zone of inhibited

bacterial growth is seen around the disk after overnight incubation. Additional biochemical, serologic, or molecular diagnostic tests can be performed for a definitive identification.

Treatment, Prevention, and Control

Before the advent of antibiotics, specific treatment of *S. pneumoniae* infection was guided by the passive infusion of type-specific capsular antibodies. These opsonizing antibodies enhanced polymorphonuclear leukocyte–mediated phagocytosis and the killing of bacteria. However, this immunotherapy was discontinued once antimicrobial therapy became available.

Penicillin rapidly became the treatment of choice for pneumococcal disease. Alternative effective agents for patients allergic to penicillin have included the cephalosporins, erythromycin, and chloramphenicol (for meningitis). Resistance to tetracycline is well documented. In 1977, isolates of *S. pneumoniae* resistant to multiple antibiotics, including penicillin, were reported by researchers in South Africa. Until 1990, high-level resistance to penicillin (MIC of at least 2 μg/mL) was relatively uncommon, and only 5% of all strains of *S. pneumoniae* isolated in the United States were considered to be moderately resistant (MIC of 0.1 to 1.0 μg/mL). However, this situation has changed dramatically. Resistance to penicillin has now been observed for as many as a third of the strains isolated in the United States and in a higher number of those isolated in other countries. Greater resistance to penicillins is associated with a decreased affinity of the antibiotic for the penicillin-binding proteins present in the bacterial cell wall. Patients infected with resistant bacteria have an increased risk of an adverse outcome.

Efforts to prevent or control the disease have focused on the development of effective anticapsular vaccine. The current vaccine contains 23 different capsular polysaccharides. Approximately 94% of all strains isolated from infected patients either are included in the vaccine or are serologically related to the vaccine serotypes. Longitudinal studies have shown that the serotypes of *S. pneumoniae* associated with disease have not been influenced by the use of the vaccine. The vaccine is immunogenic in normal adults, and the immunity is long-lived. The vaccine is not as effective, however, in some patients at high risk for pneumococcal disease, as follows:

1. Patients with asplenia, sickle cell disease, hematologic malignancy, and human immunodeficiency virus infection.
2. Patients who have undergone renal transplant.
3. Young children.
4. The elderly.

This lack of effectiveness of the anticapsular vaccine

has led some to argue that the vaccine should not be used.

CASE STUDY AND QUESTIONS

■ A 62-year-old man with a history of chronic obstructive pulmonary disease (COPD) came to the emergency department because of a fever of 40°C, chills, nausea, vomiting, and hypotension. The patient also produced tenacious yellowish sputum that had increased in quantity over the preceding 3 days. His respiratory rate was 18 breaths/min, and his blood pressure was 94/52 mmHg. Chest radiographic examination showed extensive infiltrates in the left lower lung that involved both the lower lobe and the lingula. Multiple blood cultures and culture of the sputum yielded *S. pneumoniae*. The isolate was susceptible to cefazolin, vancomycin, and erythromycin but resistant to penicillin.

1. What predisposing condition made this patient more susceptible to pneumonia and bacteremia caused by *S. pneumoniae*? What other populations of patients are susceptible to these infections? What other infections are caused by this organism, and what populations are most susceptible?

2. What is the mechanism most likely responsible for this isolate's resistance to penicillin?

3. What infections are caused by *S. pyogenes*, *S. agalactiae*, *S. anginosus*, *S. dysgalactiae*, and viridans streptococci?

4. What are the major virulence factors of *S. pneumoniae*, *S. pyogenes*, and *S. agalactiae*?

5. *S. pyogenes* can cause streptococcal toxic shock syndrome. How does this disease differ from the disease produced by staphylococci?

6. What two nonsuppurative diseases can develop after localized *S. pyogenes* disease?

BIBLIOGRAPHY

Barry AL: Antimicrobial resistance among clinical isolates of *Streptococcus pneumoniae* in North America, *Am J Med* 107: 28S–33S, 1999.

Bisno AL, Stevens DL: Streptococcal infections of skin and soft tissues, *N Engl J Med* 334:240–245, 1996.

Blumberg HM et al: Invasive group B streptococcal disease: the emergence of serotype V, *J Infect Dis* 173:365–373, 1996.

Bruyn GAW et al: Mechanisms of host defense against infection with *Streptococcus pneumoniae*, *Clin Infect Dis* 14:251–262, 1992.

Cunningham M: Pathogenesis of group A streptococcal infections, *Clin Microbiol Rev* 13:470–511, 2000.

Fiore AE et al: Clinical outcomes of meningitis caused by *Streptococcus pneumoniae* in the era of antibiotic resistance, *Clin Infect Dis* 30:71–77, 2000.

Fiorentino M: The return of rheumatic fever, *Clin Microbiol Newsletter* 18:25–29, 1996.

Hausdorff WP et al: Which pneumococcal serogroups cause the most invasive disease: implications for conjugate vaccine formulation and use: Parts I and II, *Clin Infect Dis* 30: 100–121, 122–140, 2000.

Holm SE: Invasive group A *Streptococcus* infections, *N Engl J Med* 335:590–591, 1996 (editorial).

Jackson LA et al: Risk factors for group B streptococcal disease in adults, *Ann Intern Med* 123:415–420, 1995.

Katz AR, Morens DM: Severe streptococcal infections in historical perspective, *Clin Infect Dis* 14:298–307, 1992.

Kaul R et al: Population-based surveillance for group A streptococcal necrotizing fasciitis: clinical features, prognostic indicators, and microbiologic analysis of seventy-seven cases, *Am J Med* 103:18–24, 1997.

Metlay J et al: Impact of penicillin susceptibility on medical outcomes for adult patients with bacteremic pneumococcal pneumonia, *Clin Infect Dis* 30:520–528, 2000.

Schuchat A: Epidemiology of group B streptococcal disease in the United States: shifting paradigms, *Clin Microbiol Rev* 11:497–513, 1998.

Stevens DL: Streptococcal toxic shock syndrome: spectrum of disease, pathogenesis, and new concepts in treatment, *Emerging Infect Dis* 1:69–78, 1995.

Tuomanen EI, Austriah R, Masure HR: Pathogenesis of pneumococcal infection, *N Engl J Med* 332:1280–1284, 1995.

C H A P T E R 2 4

Enterococcus and Other Gram-Positive Cocci

Twelve genera of catalase-negative, gram-positive cocci are recognized as human pathogens (Table 24–1). *Streptococcus* (see Chapter 23) and *Enterococcus* are the genera most frequently isolated and most commonly responsible for human disease. The other genera (Table 24–2) are relatively uncommon and are discussed only briefly here.

Enterococcus

The enterococci ("enteric cocci") were previously classified as group D streptococci because they possess the group D cell wall antigen, a glycerol teichoic acid that is associated with the cytoplasmic membrane (Box 24–1). Despite this observation, it was recognized that these organisms were distinct from other group D streptococci (referred to as *nonenterococcal group D streptococci* [e.g., *Streptococcus bovis*]). The enterococcal and nonenterococcal groups were originally differentiated on the basis of their physiologic properties and with nucleic acid analysis. In 1984, the enterococci were reclassified into the new genus *Enterococcus*, and there are currently 16 species in this genus. The most commonly isolated, clinically important species are *Enterococcus faecalis* ("pertaining to feces") and *Enterococcus faecium* ("of feces").

Physiology and Structure

The enterococci are gram-positive cocci typically arranged in pairs and short chains (Fig. 24–1). The microscopic morphology of these isolates frequently cannot be differentiated from that of *Streptococcus pneumoniae*. The cocci are facultatively anaerobic and grow optimally at 35°C, although most isolates can grow in the temperature range 10°C to 45°C. They grow readily on blood agar media, with large, white colonies appearing after 24 hours of incubation; the colonies are typically nonhemolytic but can be α-hemolytic or β-hemolytic. The enterococci grow in the presence of 6.5% NaCl, tolerate 40% bile salts, and can hydrolyze esculin. These basic properties can be used to distinguish enterococci from other catalase-negative, gram-positive cocci. Selected phenotypic tests (e.g., fermentation reactions, hydrolysis of pyrrolidonyl-β-naphthylamide [PYR], motility, pigment production) are required to further differentiate the enterococcal species.

Pathogenesis and Immunity

Enterococci are commensal organisms that have a limited potential for causing disease. These bacteria do not possess a potent toxin, and although hydrolytic proteins (e.g., cytolysins, gelatinase) have been identified, their role in disease is undefined. The bacteria generally cannot avoid being engulfed and killed by phagocytic cells.

Despite this lack of significant virulence factors, enterococci cause serious disease. In part, their role in disease is mediated by a combination of virulence factors (Table 24–3). For example, protein and carbohydrate adhesive factors regulate adherence to the cells lining the human intestine and vagina. Enterococci can also produce protein bacteriocins that inhibit competitive bacteria. Perhaps of greater significance is that the enterococci either are inherently resistant to many commonly used antibiotics (e.g., oxacillin, cephalosporins) or have acquired resistance genes (e.g., to aminoglycosides, vancomycin). Thus, in patients who are treated with broad-spectrum antibiotics (and who are typically quite ill), the enterococci that are part of their normal microbial flora are able to proliferate and cause disease.

Epidemiology

As their name implies, enterococci are enteric bacteria, which are commonly recovered in feces collected from humans as well as from a variety of animals. Many *E. faecalis* organisms are found in the large intestine (e.g.,

TABLE 24–1. Human Colonization and Disease Caused by Catalase-Negative, Gram-Positive Cocci

Genus	Human Colonization	Human Disease
Streptococcus	Common	Common
Enterococcus	Common	Common
Abiotrophia	Uncommon	Uncommon
Leuconostoc	Uncommon	Uncommon
Pediococcus	Uncommon	Uncommon
Lactococcus	Uncommon	Uncommon
Aerococcus	Uncommon	Rare
*Alloiococcus**	Rare	Rare
Facklamia	Rare	Rare
Gemella	Rare	Rare
Globicatella	Rare	Rare
Helcococcus	Rare	Rare

*May be catalase-positive (see Chapter 22).

TABLE 24–2. Catalase-Negative, Gram-Positive Cocci and Their Diseases*

Organism	Diseases
Enterococcus	Bacteremia, endocarditis, urinary tract infections, wound infections
Abiotrophia	Bacteremia, endocarditis, eye infections, oral infections
Leuconostoc	Bacteremia, wound infections, central nervous system infections
Pediococcus	Bacteremia, wound infections
Lactococcus	Bacteremia, endocarditis, urinary tract infections, wound infections, eye infections
Aerococcus	Bacteremia, endocarditis, urinary tract infections
Alloiococcus	Chronic middle ear infections
Facklamia	Bacteremia, genitourinary tract infections, wound infections
Gemella	Bacteremia, endocarditis, meningitis, wound infections
Globicatella	Bacteremia, urinary tract infections, meningitis
Helcococcus	Skin infections

Streptococcus is discussed in Chapter 23.

10^7 organisms per gram of feces) and in the genitourinary tract. The distribution of *E. faecium* is similar to that of *E. faecalis*, but the organisms are found less frequently.

The prevalence of the many other enterococcal species is unknown, although they are believed to colonize the intestines in small numbers. Enterococci are not commonly isolated from the respiratory tract or from the skin. Most human infections with enterococci originate from the patient's bowel flora, although the organisms can also be transferred from patient to patient or acquired through the consumption of contaminated food or water.

Clinical Diseases

Despite the paucity of virulence factors, enterococci are well respected for their ability to cause life-threatening infections. Indeed, they have been one of the most feared nosocomial pathogens in the 1990s, because many strains are completely resistant to all conventional antibiotics. Enterococci are one of the leading causes of nosocomial (hospital-acquired) infections, responsible for 10% of all such infections. The urinary tract and blood stream are the most commonly involved sites. Enterococcal infections are particularly common in patients with urinary or intravascular catheters and in patients who have been hospitalized for prolonged periods and have received broad-spectrum antibiotics. A particularly severe complication of enterococcal bacteremia is endocarditis, a disease with a very high mortality rate. Although enterococci are frequently associated with intra-abdominal abscesses (because of their colonization of the intestines) and wound infections, the importance of these isolates is less clear because these infections are generally polymicrobial.

Laboratory Diagnosis

Enterococci grow readily on nonselective media such as blood agar and chocolate agar. Despite the fact that enterococci may resemble *S. pneumoniae* on Gram-stained specimens, the organisms can be readily differentiated on the basis of simple biochemical reactions (e.g., enterococci are resistant to optochin, do not dissolve when exposed to bile, and can hydrolyze PYR).

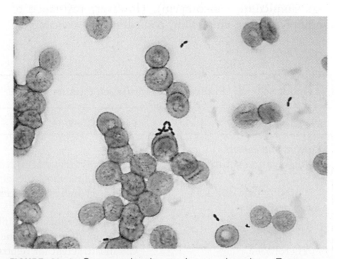

FIGURE 24–1. Gram-stained specimen showing *Enterococcus faecalis.*

BOX 24–1. Summary of *Enterococcus* Infections

Physiology and Structure

Gram-positive cocci arranged in pairs and short chains (similar to *Streptococcus pneumoniae*).

Facultative anaerobe.

Cell wall with group-specific antigen (group D glycerol teichoic acid).

Virulence Factors

Refer to Table 24–3.

Epidemiology

Colonizes the gastrointestinal tracts of humans and animals.

Cell wall structure typical of gram-positive bacteria, so able to survive on environmental surfaces for prolonged periods.

Most infections from patient's bacterial flora; some due to patient-to-patient spread.

Patients at increased risk include those hospitalized for prolonged periods and treated with broad-spectrum antibiotics (particularly cephalosporins, to which enterococci are naturally resistant).

Diseases

Urinary tract infections.

Wound infections (particularly intra-abdominal and usually polymicrobic).

Bacteremia and endocarditis.

Diagnosis

Grows readily on common, nonselective media. Differentiated from related organisms by simple tests (catalase-negative, PYR-positive, resistant to bile and optochin).

Treatment, Prevention, and Control

Therapy for serious infections requires combination of aminoglycosides with a cell wall–active antibiotic (penicillin, ampicillin, or vancomycin). Newer agents include linezolid, quinupristin/dalfopristin, and selected fluoroquinolones.

Antibiotic resistance is becoming increasingly common, and infections with many isolates (particularly *E. faecium*) are not treatable with any antibiotics.

Prevention and control of infections require careful restriction of antibiotic use and implementation of appropriate infection-control practices.

Phenotypic (e.g., pigment production, motility) and biochemical tests are necessary to differentiate among *E. faecalis*, *E. faecium*, and the other *Enterococcus* species, but this topic is beyond the scope of this text.

Treatment, Prevention, and Control

Antimicrobial therapy for enterococcal infections is complicated because most antibiotics are not bactericidal at clinically relevant concentrations. Therapy has traditionally consisted of the synergistic combination of an aminoglycoside and a cell wall–active antibiotic (e.g., ampicillin, vancomycin). However, resistance to aminoglycosides, ampicillin, penicillin, and vancomycin

has become a major problem. Typically, more than 25% of enterococci are resistant to the aminoglycosides; more than 50% of some species (e.g., *E. faecium*) are resistant to ampicillin, and many medical centers report that more than 20% of enterococci are resistant to vancomycin. The resistance in these strains to aminoglycosides and vancomycin is particularly troublesome, because it is mediated by plasmids and can be transferred to other bacteria.

Newer antibiotics have been developed specifically to treat enterococci resistant to ampicillin and vancomycin. They include linezolid, quinupristin/dalfopristin, and selected fluoroquinolones. Although these antibiotics are currently active against many otherwise

---

TABLE 24–3. Enterococcal Virulence Factors

Virulence Factor	Biologic Effect
Colonization Factors	
Aggregation substance	Hairlike protein embedded in cytoplasmic membrane that facilitates plasmid exchange and binding to epithelial cells
Carbohydrate adhesins	Present in individual bacterium in multiple types; mediate binding to host cells
Secreted Factors	
Cytolysin	Protein bacteriocin that inhibits growth of gram-positive bacteria (facilitates colonization); induces local tissue damage
Pheromone	Chemoattractant for neutrophils that may regulate inflammatory reaction
Gelatinase	Hydrolyzes gelatin, collagen, hemoglobin, and other small peptides
Antibiotic resistance	Resistant to aminoglycosides, β-lactams, and vancomycin

resistant isolates, the long-term effectiveness of the drugs remains to be determined.

It is difficult to prevent and control enterococcal infections. Infections typically develop in patients who are hospitalized for a long time and are treated with broad-spectrum antibiotics for other infections. Careful restriction of antibiotic therapy and the implementation of appropriate infection-control practices (e.g., isolation of infected patients, use of gowns and gloves by anyone in contact with patients) can reduce the risk of colonization with these bacteria, but the complete elimination of infections is unlikely.

Other Catalase-Negative, Gram-Positive Cocci

Other catalase-negative, gram-positive cocci or coccobacilli associated with human disease are *Abiotrophia*, *Leuconostoc*, *Pediococcus*, *Lactococcus*, *Aerococcus*, and other less commonly isolated genera. All are relatively avirulent, opportunistic pathogens.

Abiotrophia organisms, formerly called "nutritionally deficient streptococci," are problematic because they will initially grow in blood culture broths or in mixed cultures but do not grow when subcultured (refer to Chapter 23 for additional information).

Leuconostoc and *Pediococcus* can resemble streptococci but are resistant to vancomycin, a trait that has not been seen in streptococci at this time.

Lactococcus can be misidentified as *Enterococcus*, and *Aerococcus* ("air coccus") is typically an airborne organism that can contaminate the patient's skin or the specimen while it is being collected or processed in the laboratory. It is difficult to identify most of these organisms precisely, but a knowledge of their presence and clinical features is useful.

CASE STUDY AND QUESTIONS

■ A 72-year-old man was admitted to the hospital because of a fever that had risen as high as 40°C, myalgias, and respiratory complaints. The clinical diagnosis of influenza was confirmed by the laboratory isolation of influenza virus from respiratory secretions.

This patient's hospitalization was complicated by the development of pneumonia caused by oxacillin-resistant *Staphylococcus aureus* that was treated with a 2-week course of vancomycin. Declining pulmonary function necessitated the use of a ventilator, which led to the development of a secondary infection with *Klebsiella pneumoniae*. Ceftazidime (a cephalosporin) and gentamicin were added to the patient's treatment. After 4 weeks of hospitalization, the patient became septic. *E. faecium* resistant to vancomycin, gentamicin, and ampicillin was cultured from three blood specimens.

1. What predisposing conditions made this patient more susceptible to infection with *E. faecium*?
2. What is the most likely source of this organism?
3. What factors contribute to the virulence of enterococci?

BIBLIOGRAPHY

Edmond MB et al: Vancomycin-resistant *Enterococcus faecium* bacteremia: risk factors for infection, *Clin Infect Dis* 20:1126–1133, 1995.

Elsner HA et al: Virulence factors of *Enterococcus faecalis* and *Enterococcus faecium* blood culture isolates, *Eur J Clin Infect Dis* 19:39–42, 2000.

Facklam R, Elliott JA: Identification, classification, and clinical relevance of catalase-negative, gram-positive cocci, excluding the streptococci and enterococci, *Clin Microbiol Rev* 8:479–495, 1995.

Garbutt JM et al: Association between resistance to vancomycin and death in cases of *Enterococcus faecium* bacteremia, *Clin Infec Dis* 30:466–472, 2000.

Handwerger S et al: Infection due to *Leuconostoc* species: six cases and review, *Rev Infect Dis* 12:602–610, 1990.

Leclercq R, Courvalin P: Resistance to glycopeptides in enterococci, *Clin Infect Dis* 24:545–556, 1997.

Moellering RC: Emergence of *Enterococcus* as a significant pathogen, *Clin Infect Dis* 14:1173–1178, 1992.

Murray BE: β-Lactamase-producing enterococci, *Antimicrob Agents Chemother* 36:2355–2359, 1992.

Murray BE: Vancomycin-resistant enterococci, *Am J Med* 101:284–293, 1997.

Patterson JE, Zervos MJ: High-level gentamicin resistance in *Enterococcus*: microbiology, genetic basis, and epidemiology, *Rev Infect Dis* 12:644–652, 1990.

Ruoff KL: The "new" catalase-negative, gram-positive cocci, *Clin Microbiol Newsletter* 16:153–159, 1994.

Shay DK et al: Epidemiology and mortality risk of vancomycin-resistant enterococcal bloodstream infections, *J Infect Dis* 172:993–1000, 1995.

C H A P T E R   2 5

Bacillus

The family Bacillaceae consists of a diverse collection of bacteria comprising obligate aerobes and strict anaerobes, cocci and bacilli, and gram-positive and gram-negative organisms. The feature they all share is formation of endospores (Fig. 25–1). The two clinically important genera are *Bacillus* (the aerobic and facultative anaerobic spore-formers) and *Clostridium* (the strict anaerobic spore-formers; see Chapter 37). In the past few years, *Bacillus* has been subdivided into six genera, and it is expected that a similar taxonomic reorganization awaits *Clostridium*.

Despite the subdivision of *Bacillus*, more than 50 species remain in the genus. Fortunately, the species that are of medical interest are relatively limited (Table 25–1). *Bacillus anthracis*, the organism responsible for anthrax, is the most important member of this genus. This species is considered one of the most feared agents of biological warfare. The renewed threat of disease due to this organism has refocused interest in *Bacillus*.

Bacillus anthracis

Physiology and Structure

B. anthracis (Greek, *anthrakis*, "coal," describing the coal-like or black lesions of infection) is a large (1 × 3 to 8 μm) organism arranged as single or paired bacilli in clinical specimens and as long, serpentine chains and clumps in culture. Although spores are readily observed in 2- to 3-day-old cultures, they are not seen in clinical specimens.

A prominent polypeptide **capsule** (consisting of poly-D-glutamic acid) is observed in clinical specimens but is not produced in vitro unless special growth conditions are used. Three genes (*cap*A, *cap*B, and *cap*C) are responsible for synthesis of this capsule and are carried on a plasmid. Only one type of capsule has been identified, presumably because it is composed of only glutamic acid.

Virulent *B. anthracis* carry a second plasmid that encodes the following three exotoxins: protective antigen, edema factor, and lethal factor. **Edema toxin** is formed by the combination of protective antigen (responsible for binding to the host cell) and edema factor (adenylate cyclase). A second toxin, **lethal toxin**, is formed when protective antigen combines with lethal factor (a zinc metalloprotease). Both edema toxin and lethal toxin as well as the capsule must be present for disease to occur. Avirulent strains of *B. anthracis* have been made through removal of one or both virulence plasmids.

Pathogenesis and Immunity

The major factors responsible for the virulence of *B. anthracis* are the capsule, edema toxin, and lethal toxin. The capsule inhibits phagocytosis of replicating cells. The adenylate cyclase activity of edema toxin is responsible for the fluid accumulation observed in anthrax. The zinc metalloprotease activity of lethal toxin stimulates macrophages to release tumor necrosis factor-α and interleukin-1β as well as other proinflammatory cytokines.

Epidemiology

Anthrax is primarily a disease of herbivores; humans are infected through exposure to contaminated animals or animal products (Box 25–1). The disease is a serious problem in countries where animal vaccination is not practiced or is impractical (e.g., disease established in African wildlife). In contrast, anthrax is rarely seen in the United States; only five cases were reported between 1981 and 1999.

Although anthrax is rarely encountered in developed countries, the threat of biological warfare has renewed the concern about this disease. At least 17 nations and an unknown number of independent terrorist groups have biological warfare programs. Iran, the former Soviet Union, and the Aum Shinrikyo terrorist group in Japan have experimented with using *B. anthracis* as a weapon. Indeed, much of what we know about anthrax acquired via the inhalation route was learned from the accidental release in 1979 of spores in Sverdlovsk in

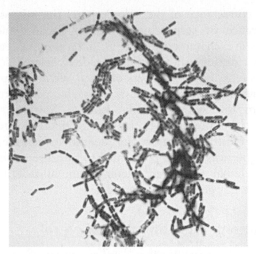

FIGURE 25–1. *Bacillus cereus.* Spores appear as clear areas within the individual bacilli.

TABLE 25–1. *Bacillus* Species and Their Diseases	
Organism	**Diseases**
B. anthracis*	Anthrax (cutaneous, gastrointestinal, inhalation)
B. cereus*	Gastroenteritis (emetic, diarrheal), ocular infections, catheter-related sepsis, opportunistic infections
B. mycoides*	Gastroenteritis, opportunistic infections
B. thuringiensis*	Gastroenteritis, opportunistic infections
Other *Bacillus* species	Opportunistic infections

*Members of the *B. cereus* group.

the former Soviet Union. This accident resulted in at least 79 cases of anthrax with 68 deaths.

Human *B. anthracis* disease is acquired by one of the following three routes: inoculation, ingestion, and inhalation. Approximately 95% of anthrax infections in humans result from the inoculation of *Bacillus* spores through exposed skin, from either contaminated soil or infected animal products such as hides, goat hair, and wool.

Ingestion anthrax is very rare in humans, but ingestion is a common route of infection in herbivores. Because the organism can form resilient spores, contaminated soil or animal products can remain infectious for many years.

Inhalation anthrax, also called **wool-sorters' dis-**

BOX 25–1. **Summary of *Bacillus anthracis* Infections**

Physiology and Structure

Spore-forming gram-positive bacilli.
   Facultative anaerobe.
   Nonfastidious growth of nonhemolytic colonies that are firmly adherent to the agar surface.
   Polypeptide capsule consisting of poly-D-glutamic acid observed in clinical specimens.

Virulence

The capsule is present in virulent stains.
   Virulent strains also produce three exotoxins that combine to form edema toxin (combination of protective antigen and edema factor) and lethal toxin (protective antigen with lethal factor).
   Spores can survive in soil for years.

Epidemiology

B. anthracis primarily infects herbivores with humans as accidental hosts.
   Rarely isolated in developed countries but is prevalent in impoverished areas where vaccination of animals is not practiced.
   Individuals at risk include people in endemic areas in contact with infected animals or contaminated soil, people who work with animal materials imported from endemic areas, and military and nonmilitary people exposed to infectious aerosols.
   There is significant concern that the spores will be used in bioterrorism.

Diseases

Cutaneous anthrax is the most common form.
   Inhalation anthrax is the most deadly form.
   Gastrointestinal anthrax is a rare but commonly fatal disease.

Diagnosis

Isolation of the organism from clinical specimens (e.g., papule or ulcer, blood).

Treatment, Prevention, and Control

Ciprofloxacin is the drug of choice; penicillin, doxycycline, erythromycin, or chloramphenicol can be used (if susceptible), but the bacteria are resistant to sulfonamides and extended-spectrum cephalosporins.
   Vaccination of animal herds and people in endemic areas can control disease, but spores are difficult to eliminate from contaminated soils.
   Animal vaccination is effective, but human vaccines have limited usefulness.

ease, results from the inhalation of *B. anthracis* spores during the processing of goat hair. Although this is currently an uncommon source for human infections, inhalation is the most likely route of infection with biological weapons. The infectious dose of the organism is low (i.e., the LD_{50} [median lethal dose] is estimated to be 2500 to 55,000 spores); however, person-to-person transmission does not occur because bronchopulmonary disease does not develop.

Clinical Diseases

Typically, **cutaneous anthrax** starts with the development of a painless papule at the site of inoculation that rapidly progresses to an ulcer surrounded by vesicles and then to a necrotic eschar. Systemic signs, painful lymphadenopathy, and massive edema can develop. The mortality rate in patients with untreated cutaneous anthrax is 20%.

Clinical symptoms of **gastrointestinal anthrax** are determined by the site of the infection. If organisms invade the upper intestinal tract, ulcers form in the mouth or esophagus, leading to regional lymphadenopathy, edema, and sepsis. If the organism invades the cecum or terminal ileum, the patient presents with nausea, vomiting, and malaise, which rapidly progress to systemic disease. The mortality associated with gastrointestinal anthrax is believed to approach 100%.

Unlike the other two forms of anthrax, **inhalation anthrax** can be associated with a prolonged latent period (2 months or more) during which the infected patient remains asymptomatic. Alveolar macrophages ingest the inhaled spores and transport them to the mediastinal lymph nodes, where the bacteria can remain latent. The initial clinical symptoms of disease are nonspecific—fever, shortness of breath, cough, headache, vomiting, chills, and chest and abdominal pain. The second stage of disease is more dramatic, with a rapidly worsening course of fever, edema, and massive enlargement of the mediastinal lymph nodes (this is responsible for the widened mediastinum observed on chest radiography). Pulmonary disease rarely develops; however, meningeal symptoms are seen in half of patients. Almost all cases progress to shock and death within 3 days of initial symptoms.

Laboratory Diagnosis

B. anthracis can be readily detected by microscopic examination and culture of material from cutaneous papules or ulcers. Large gram-positive bacilli without spores are seen in the tissue (spores form only when nutrients are lacking). *B. anthracis* is not fastidious and can grow on most nonselective laboratory media. The colonies are nonhemolytic, grow rapidly, and are firmly adherent to the agar. The absence of hemolysis, the sticky consistency of the colonies, and the microscopic appearance of serpentine chains of bacilli ("medusa head") are characteristics of *B. anthracis* that can be used to distinguish them from closely related *Bacillus* species (e.g., other members of the *B. cereus* group).

Selected biochemical tests must be conducted to confirm the identity of the isolates; however, most clinical laboratories would need to refer the isolate to a Public Health laboratory for definitive identification. Serologic tests can be performed to measure antibodies to the lethal toxin and edema toxin; however, these tests are not generally performed.

Treatment, Prevention, and Control

In contrast to many other *Bacillus* species, *B. anthracis* is susceptible to penicillin, which has historically been considered the treatment of choice for a suspected infection. Isolates are also susceptible to doxycycline and ciprofloxacin. Because genes encoding resistance to penicillin and doxycycline have been transferred to *B. anthracis*, however, ciprofloxacin is now recommended for empirical therapy. *B. anthracis* strains are resistant to sulfonamides and extended-spectrum cephalosporin.

The control of human disease requires the control of animal disease, which involves the vaccination of animal herds in endemic regions and the burning or burial of animals that die of anthrax. Complete eradication of anthrax is unlikely, because the spores of the organism can exist for many years in soil.

Vaccination of animals is an effective control measure. Vaccination has also been used to protect (1) people who live in areas where the disease is endemic, (2) people who work with animal products imported from countries with endemic anthrax, and (3) military personnel. Although the current vaccine appears to be effective, its widespread use in nonmilitary personnel is unlikely because the vaccine supplies are limited and the risk of infection is currently small.

Bacillus cereus and Other *Bacillus* Species

Bacillus species other than *B. anthracis* are primarily opportunistic pathogens that have relatively low capacities for virulence. Although most of these species have been found to cause disease, *B. cereus* (from the Greek *cereus*, "wax-colored") is clearly the most important pathogen, with gastroenteritis, ocular infections, and intravenous catheter-related sepsis the diseases most commonly observed.

Pathogenesis

Gastroenteritis caused by *B. cereus* is mediated by one of two enterotoxins (Table 25–2). The heat-stable,

TABLE 25–2. *Bacillus cereus* Food Poisoning

	Emetic Form	Diarrheal Form
Implicated food	Rice	Meat, vegetables
Incubation period (hours)	<6 (mean, 2)	>6 (mean, 9)
Symptoms	Vomiting, nausea, abdominal cramps	Diarrhea, nausea, abdominal cramps
Duration (hours)	8–10 (mean, 9)	20–36 (mean, 24)
Enterotoxin	Heat-stable	Heat-labile

proteolysis-resistant enterotoxin causes the **emetic form** of the disease, and the heat-labile enterotoxin causes the **diarrheal form** of the disease. The heat-labile enterotoxin is similar to the enterotoxins produced by *Escherichia coli* and *Vibrio cholerae*; each stimulates the adenylate cyclase–cyclic adenosine monophosphate system in intestinal epithelial cells, leading to profuse watery diarrhea. The mechanism of action of the heat-stable enterotoxin is unknown.

The pathogenesis of *B. cereus* ocular infections is also incompletely defined. At least three toxins have been implicated; they are **necrotic toxin** (a heat-labile enterotoxin), **cereolysin** (a potent hemolysin named after the species), and **phospholipase C** (a potent lecithinase). It is likely that the rapid destruction of the eye that is characteristic of *B. cereus* infections results from the interaction of these toxins and other unidentified factors.

Bacillus species can colonize skin transiently and can be recovered as insignificant contaminants in blood cultures. In the presence of an intravascular foreign body, however, these organisms can be responsible for persistent bacteremia and signs of sepsis (i.e., fever, chills, hypotension, shock).

Epidemiology

B. cereus and other *Bacillus* species are ubiquitous organisms, present in virtually all environments (Box 25–2). Isolation of bacteria from clinical specimens in the absence of characteristic disease usually represents insignificant contamination.

Clinical Diseases

As mentioned previously, *B. cereus* is responsible for two forms of food poisoning, vomiting disease (emetic form) and diarrheal disease (diarrheal form). The emetic form results from the consumption of contaminated rice. Most bacilli are killed during the initial cooking of the rice, but the heat-resistant spores survive. If the cooked rice is not refrigerated, the spores germinate, and the bacilli can multiply rapidly. The heat-stable enterotoxin that is released is not destroyed when the rice is reheated. After ingestion of the enterotoxin and a 1- to 6-hour incubation period, a disease of short duration (less than 24 hours) develops. Symptoms consist of vomiting, nausea, and abdominal cramps. Fever and diarrhea are generally absent. Fulminant liver failure has also been associated with con-

---

BOX 25–2. Summary of *Bacillus cereus* Infections

Physiology and Structure

Spore-forming gram-positive bacilli.
  Facultative anaerobe.
  Nonfastidious growth requirements.

Virulence

Heat-stable enterotoxin.
  Heat-labile enterotoxin.
  Spores can survive in soil.
  Tissue destruction is mediated by cytotoxic enzymes, including cereolysin and phospholipase C.

Epidemiology

Ubiquitous in soils throughout the world.
  People at risk include those who consume food contaminated with the bacterium (e.g., rice, meat, vegetables, sauces), those with penetrating injuries (e.g., to eye), and those who receive intravenous injections.

Diseases

Infections include emetic (vomiting) and diarrheal forms of gastroenteritis; ocular infection following trauma to eye; and other opportunistic infections.

Diagnosis

Isolation of the organism in implicated food product or nonfecal specimens (e.g., eye, wound).

Treatment, Prevention, and Control

Gastrointestinal infections are treated symptomatically.
  Ocular infectious or other invasive diseases require removal of foreign bodies and treatment with vancomycin, clindamycin, ciprofloxacin, or gentamicin.
  Gastrointestinal disease is prevented by proper preparation of food (e.g., foods should be consumed immediately after preparation or refrigerated).

sumption of food contaminated with large amounts of emetic toxin, which impairs mitochondrial fatty acid metabolism. Fortunately, this is a rare complication.

The diarrheal form of *B. cereus* food poisoning results from the consumption of contaminated meat, vegetables, or sauces. There is a longer incubation period, during which the organism multiplies in the patient's intestinal tract and produces the heat-labile enterotoxin. Then the diarrhea, nausea, and abdominal cramps develop. This form of disease generally lasts 1 day or longer.

B. cereus ocular infections usually occur after traumatic, penetrating injuries of the eye with a soil-contaminated object. *Bacillus* panophthalmitis is a rapidly progressive disease that almost universally ends in the complete loss of light perception within 48 hours of the injury. Disseminated infections with ocular manifestations can also develop in intravenous drug abusers.

Other infections with *B. cereus* and other *Bacillus* species are intravenous catheter and central nervous system shunt infections and endocarditis (most common in drug abusers) as well as pneumonitis, bacteremia, and meningitis in severely immunosuppressed patients.

Laboratory Diagnosis

Like *B. anthracis*, other *Bacillus* species can be readily grown in the laboratory. For confirmation of the existence of foodborne disease, the implicated food (e.g., rice, meat, vegetables) should be cultured. Isolation of the organism from the patient should not be attempted, because fecal colonization is common. However, isolation of the organism from the stools of a cluster of epidemiologically related patients is strong evidence implicating *B. cereus* as the causal agent. Tests to detect the heat-stable or heat-labile enterotoxins are not commonly performed. *Bacillus* organisms grow rapidly and are readily detected with Gram stain and culture of specimens collected from infected eyes, intravenous culture sites, and other locations.

Treatment, Prevention, and Control

Because the course of *B. cereus* gastroenteritis is short and uncomplicated, symptomatic treatment is adequate.

The treatment of other *Bacillus* infections is complicated by the fact that they have a rapid and progressive course and a high incidence of multiple-drug resistance (e.g., *B. cereus* carries genes for resistance to penicillins and cephalosporins). Vancomycin, clindamycin, ciprofloxacin, and gentamicin can be used to treat infections. Penicillins and cephalosporins are ineffective. Food poisoning can be prevented by the rapid consumption of foods after cooking and the proper refrigeration of uneaten foods.

QUESTIONS

1. What are three virulence factors found in *B. anthracis* and their modes of action?

2. *B. anthracis* is responsible for what three clinical forms of anthrax? Name the route of acquisition and the prognosis for each.

3. Describe the two forms of *B. cereus* food poisoning. What toxin is responsible for each form? Why is the clinical presentation of these two diseases different?

4. *B. cereus* can cause eye infections. What are two risk factors for this disease?

BIBLIOGRAPHY

Davey RT Jr, Tauber WB: Posttraumatic endophthalmitis: the emerging role of *Bacillus cereus* infection, *Rev Infect Dis* 9:110–123, 1987.

Dixon TC et al: Anthrax, *N Engl J Med* 341:815–826, 1999.

Drobniewski FA: *Bacillus cereus* and related species, *Clin Microbiol Rev* 6:324–338, 1993.

Ihde DC, Armstrong D: Clinical spectrum of infection due to *Bacillus* species, *Am J Med* 55:839–845, 1973.

Ingl TV et al: Anthrax as a biological weapon—medical and public health management, *JAMA* 281:1735–1745, 1999.

Mahler H et al: Fulminant liver failure in association with the emetic toxin of *Bacillus cereus*, *N Engl J Med* 336: 1142–1148, 1997.

Van Ness GB: Ecology of anthrax, *Science* 172:103–109, 1971.

CHAPTER 26

Listeria and Erysipelothrix

The aerobic, non–spore-forming, gram-positive bacilli are a heterogeneous group of bacteria that can be subdivided according to their morphologic appearance. The pathogenic bacilli that are uniform in shape include *Listeria* and *Erysipelothrix*, the subjects of this chapter. A large group of genera constitutes the coryneform bacilli, a group of irregularly shaped bacilli; these bacilli are discussed in Chapter 27. The third group of bacilli are those that have long-chain mycolic acids in their cell walls, rendering the bacilli partially or completely acid-fast. These bacteria, which include *Nocardia*, *Rhodococcus*, and *Mycobacterium*, are discussed in Chapters 39 and 40.

Listeria

The genus *Listeria* consists of seven species, with *Listeria monocytogenes* the only human pathogen. *L. monocytogenes* is a short (0.4 to 0.5 × 0.5 to 2 μm), gram-positive, facultatively anaerobic bacillus (Fig. 26–1). The short bacilli appear singly, in pairs, or in short chains and can be mistaken for *Streptococcus pneumoniae* or *Enterococcus*. The organisms are motile at room temperature but not at 37°C, and they exhibit a characteristic tumbling motion. These differential characteristics are useful for their preliminary identification. Although listeria are widely distributed in nature, human disease due to this organism is uncommon and is restricted to several well-defined populations: neonates, the elderly, pregnant women, and patients with defective cell-mediated immunity.

Pathogenesis and Immunity

L. monocytogenes is a facultative intracellular pathogen that can grow in macrophages, epithelial cells, and cultured fibroblasts. Studies with animal models have shown that infection is initiated in the enterocytes or M cells in Peyer's patches. Entry into nonphagocytic cells is mediated by a family of six or more leucine-rich proteins, **internalins** (e.g., InlA, InlB, InlC), which interact with glycoprotein receptors on the surface of host cells. Following penetration into the cells, the acid pH of the phagolysosome that surrounds the bacteria activates a bacterial exotoxin, **listeriolysin O**, and two different **phospholipase C** enzymes, leading to release of the bacteria into the cell cytosol. The bacteria proceed to replicate and then move through the cell to the cell membrane.

The bacteria's movement is mediated by a bacterial protein, **ActA**. This protein, which is localized on the cell surface at one end of a bacterium, coordinates assembly of actin. The distal ends of the actin tail remain fixed while assembly occurs adjacent to the end of the bacterium. Thus, the bacterium is pushed to the cell membrane, where a protrusion (filopod) is formed, pushing the bacterium into the adjacent cell. Once the bacterium is ingested by the adjacent cell, the process of phagolysosome lysis, bacterial replication, and directional movement repeats. Entry into macrophages following passage through the intestinal lining carries the bacteria to the liver and spleen, leading to disseminated disease.

Humoral immunity is relatively unimportant for management of infections with *L. monocytogenes*. These bacteria can replicate in macrophages and move within cells, thus avoiding antibody-mediated clearance. For this reason, patients with defects in cellular immunity but not in humoral immunity are particularly susceptible to severe infections.

Epidemiology

L. monocytogenes is isolated from soil, water, vegetation, and the intestinal contents of a variety of mammals, birds, fish, insects, and other animals (Box 26–1). Asymptomatic carriage as well as disease is well-documented in humans and other mammals. Although the incidence of human carriage is unknown, fecal carriage is estimated to occur in 1% to 5% of healthy people. Because the organism is ubiquitous, exposure and transient colonization are likely to occur in most individuals. Studies have shown that there are approximately 2500 cases of listeriosis in the United States each year.

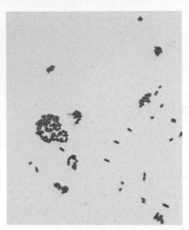

FIGURE 26–1. Gram-stain preparation showing *Listeria monocytogenes.*

This estimate can be misleading, because large outbreaks associated with contaminated food products have been documented. For example, 30 million pounds of contaminated meat were recalled in one outbreak in 1999. Obviously, many people were exposed to the bacteria before the recall could be accomplished. The incidence of disease is also disproportionate in high-risk populations, such as neonates, the elderly, pregnant women, and patients with the acquired immunodeficiency syndrome (AIDS), renal transplants, and solid organ tumors.

Human listeriosis is a sporadic disease seen throughout the year, but the incidence peaks in the warmer months. Focal epidemics and sporadic cases of listeriosis have been associated with consumption of contaminated milk, soft cheese, undercooked meat (e.g., turkey franks, cold cuts), unwashed raw vegetables, and cabbage. Because listeria can grow in a wide pH range as well as in cold temperatures, foods with small numbers of organisms can become grossly contaminated during prolonged refrigeration. If the food is uncooked or inadequately cooked (e.g., microwaving of beef and turkey hot dogs) before consumption, disease can occur. The mortality rate of symptomatic listeria infections (20% to 30%) is higher than that of almost all other foodborne diseases.

Clinical Diseases

Neonatal Disease

Two forms of neonatal disease have been described: **early-onset disease**, acquired transplacentally in utero, and **late-onset disease**, acquired at or soon after birth. Early-onset disease, also called **granulomatosis infantiseptica**, is a devastating disease that has a high mortality rate unless treated promptly. It is characterized

---

BOX 26–1. Summary of *Listeria* Infections

Physiology and Structure

Gram-positive coccobacilli frequently arranged in pairs resembling enterococci.

Facultative anaerobe.

Motile at room temperature, weakly beta-hemolytic, and capable of growth at 4°C (useful identification features).

Virulence

Facultative intracellular pathogen that can avoid antibody-mediated clearance.

Virulent strains produce cell attachment factors (internalins), hemolysins (listeriolysin O, two phospholipase Cs), and a protein that mediates actin-directed motility (ActA).

Growth in refrigerator in contaminated foods can lead to high concentrations of bacteria.

Epidemiology

Isolated in soil, water, and vegetation and from a variety of animals, including humans (low-level gastrointestinal carriage).

Disease associated with consumption of contaminated food products (e.g., soft cheese, milk, turkey, raw vegetables [esp. cabbage]) or transplancental spread from mother to neonate.

Sporadic cases and epidemics occur throughout the year but peak in warmer months.

The young and elderly as well as patients with defects in cellular immunity are at risk for disease.

Diseases

Neonatal infections (e.g., bacteremia, meningitis, meningoencephalitis).

Diseases in adults include a mild influenza-like illness, primary bacteremia, and meningitis.

Diagnosis

Microscopy is insensitive, and culture may require prolonged incubation or enrichment.

Treatment, Prevention, and Control

The treatment of choice for severe disease is penicillin or ampicillin, alone or in combination with gentamicin.

People at high risk should avoid eating raw or partially cooked foods of animal origin, soft cheese, and unwashed raw vegetables.

by the formation of disseminated abscesses and granulomas in multiple organs.

Late-onset disease occurs 2 to 3 weeks after birth in the form of meningitis or meningoencephalitis with septicemia. The clinical signs and symptoms are not unique; thus, other causes of neonatal central nervous system disease, such as group B streptococcal disease, must be excluded.

Disease in Healthy Adults

Most listeria infections in healthy adults are asymptomatic or occur in the form of a mild influenza-like illness. Gastrointestinal symptoms develop in some patients. In contrast, illness in patients with compromised cellular immunity is more severe.

Meningitis in Adults

Meningitis is the most common form of listeria infection in adults. Although the clinical signs and symptoms of meningitis caused by this organism are not specific, listeria should always be suspected in patients with organ transplants or cancer and in pregnant women in whom meningitis develops.

Primary Bacteremia

Patients with bacteremia may have an unremarkable history of chills and fever (commonly observed in pregnant women) or a more acute presentation with high-grade fever and hypotension. Only severely immunocompromised patients and the infants of pregnant women with sepsis appear to be at risk of death.

Laboratory Diagnosis

Microscopy

Gram-stain preparations of cerebrospinal fluid (CSF) typically show no organisms, because the bacteria are generally present in concentrations below the limit of detection (e.g., 10^4 bacteria per mL CSF or less). This is in contrast with most other bacterial pathogens of the central nervous system, which are present in concentrations 100- to 1000-fold higher. If the Gram stain shows organisms, they are intracellular and extracellular gram-positive coccobacilli. Care must be used to distinguish them from other bacteria, such as *S. pneumoniae*, *Enterococcus*, *Corynebacterium*, and, occasionally, *Haemophilus*.

Culture

Listeria grows on most conventional laboratory media, with small, round colonies observed on agar media after incubation for 1 to 2 days. It may be necessary to use selective media and **cold enrichment** (storage of the specimen in the refrigerator for a prolonged period) to detect listeria in specimens contaminated with rapidly growing bacteria. Beta hemolysis on sheep blood agar media can serve to distinguish *Listeria* from morphologically similar bacteria; however, the amount of hemolysis is generally weak and may not be observed initially. The characteristic motility of the organism in a liquid medium or semisolid agar is also helpful for the preliminary identification of listeria. All gram-positive bacilli isolated from blood and CSF should be identified to distinguish between *Corynebacterium* (presumably a contaminant) and *Listeria*.

Identification

Selected biochemical and serologic tests are used to identify the pathogen definitively. A total of 13 serotypes have been described, with 1/2a, 1/2b, and 4b responsible for most infections in neonates and adults. Serotyping is generally not useful in epidemiologic investigations, because relatively few serotypes are isolated from humans with disease. Enzyme profiles (i.e., multilocus enzyme electrophoresis [MLEE]) and genomic analysis (e.g., ribotyping, pulsed-field gel electrophoresis [PFGE], random amplified polymorphic DNA [RAPD] typing) are now used for epidemiologic investigations. Strains of serotype 1/2a are highly heterogeneous and can be typed by any of the methods mentioned. In contrast, serotype 4b is homogeneous, and multiple methods are needed for optimal differentiation.

Treatment, Prevention, and Control

Currently, penicillin or ampicillin, either alone or with gentamicin, is the treatment of choice for infections with *L. monocytogenes*. Listeria are naturally resistant to cephalosporins. Erythromycin can be used in patients allergic to penicillin, but resistance to trimethoprim and the tetracyclines has been observed. Tetracycline resistance was first observed in 1988 and appears to be increasing, in part because of the use of antibiotics in animal herds. Resistance to aminoglycosides has also been reported. Genes for resistance to tetracyclines and aminoglycosides have been found on conjugative plasmids and transposons that originated in enterococci. The rise in antibiotic resistance is of obvious concern and must be monitored closely.

Because listeria are ubiquitous and most infections are sporadic, prevention and control are difficult. People at high risk of infection, however, should avoid eating raw or partially cooked foods of animal origin, soft cheeses, and unwashed raw vegetables. A vaccine is not available, and prophylactic antibiotic therapy for high-risk patients has not been evaluated.

Erysipelothrix

Physiology and Structure

The genus *Erysipelothrix* contains two species, of which *Erysipelothrix rhusiopathiae* (from the Greek words meaning "hair of erysipelas" and "of red disease") is responsible for human disease. *E. rhusiopathiae* is a gram-positive, non–spore-forming, facultatively anaerobic bacillus that is distributed worldwide in wild and domestic animals. The bacilli are slender (0.2 to 0.4 × 0.8 to 2.5 μm) and sometimes pleomorphic, with a tendency to form filaments as long as 60 μm ("hairlike"). They may decolorize readily and appear gram-negative. The organisms are microaerophilic, preferring a reduced oxygen atmosphere and supplemented carbon dioxide. Small, grayish, alpha-hemolytic colonies are observed after 2 to 3 days of incubation. Animal disease—particularly in swine—is widely recognized, but human disease is uncommon.

Pathogenesis

Little is known about specific virulence factors in *Erysipelothrix*. Disease in swine has been associated with production of hyaluronidase and neuraminidase. Because this organism is an uncommon human pathogen, however, similar studies in humans have not been performed.

Epidemiology

Erysipelothrix is a ubiquitous organism that is distributed worldwide. It can be recovered on the tonsils or in the digestive tracts of many wild and domestic animals, including mammals, birds, and fish (Box 26–2). Colonization is particularly high in swine and turkeys. Disease is zoonotic, with butchers, meat processors, farmers, poultry workers, fish handlers, and veterinarians at greatest risk. Cutaneous infections typically develop after the organism is inoculated subcutaneously through an abrasion or puncture wound during the handling of contaminated animal products or soil. The incidence of human disease is unknown, because *Erysipelothrix* infection is not a reportable disease.

Clinical Diseases

The following three forms of human infection with *E. rhusiopathiae* have been described: (1) a localized skin infection (**erysipeloid**), (2) a generalized cutaneous form, and (3) a septicemic form. Erysipeloid is an inflammatory skin lesion that develops at the site of trauma after 1 to 4 days of incubation. The lesion, most commonly present on the fingers or hands, is violaceous and has a raised edge. It slowly spreads peripherally as the discoloration in the central area fades. The painful lesion is pruritic, and the patient experiences a burning or throbbing sensation. Suppuration is uncommon, a feature distinguishing erysipeloid from streptococcal erysipelas. The resolution can be spontaneous but can be hastened with appropriate antibiotic therapy.

The diffuse cutaneous infection is rare. It is often associated with systemic manifestations, but blood culture results are typically negative for the organism.

The septicemic form of *Erysipelothrix* infections is

BOX 26–2. Summary of *Erysipelothrix* Infections

Physiology and Structure

Slender pleomorphic gram-positive bacilli that can form long filaments.

    Microaerophilic, facultative anaerobe.

    Growth is slow, requiring 2 to 3 days of incubation.

    Catalase-positive and nonmotile (useful identification features).

Virulence

Relatively little is known.

    Production of hyaluronidase and neuraminidase is probably important.

Epidemiology

Organism is ubiquitous, but this is an uncommon pathogen in the United States.

    Colonization is high in swine and turkey; found in variety of other animals.

Occupational disease of butchers, meat processors, farmers, poultry workers, fish handlers, and veterinarians.

    Disease is common in swine but rare in humans.

Diseases

Three forms of human infection: localized skin infection, generalized cutaneous infection, and septicemia.

Diagnosis

Organisms typically seen by microscopy and grow readily in culture.

Treatment, Prevention, and Control

Penicillin is drug of choice; organism is susceptible to cephalosporins, erythromycin, and clindamycin; resistant to vancomycin, aminoglycosides, and sulfonamides.

    Workers should cover exposed skin when handling animals and animal products.

    Swine herds should be vaccinated.

also uncommon, but when present, it is frequently associated with endocarditis. *Erysipelothrix* endocarditis may have an acute onset but is usually subacute. Involvement of previously undamaged heart valves (particularly the aortic valve) is common.

Laboratory Diagnosis

The bacilli are located only in the deep tissue of the lesion. Thus, full-thickness biopsy specimens or deep aspirates must be collected from the margin of the lesion. Microscopic studies and the culture of specimens collected from the surface invariably demonstrate the organism. *E. rhusiopathiae* is not fastidious and grows on most conventional laboratory media. The absence of both motility and catalase production distinguishes this organism from *Listeria*. Biochemical testing is used for definitive identification.

Treatment, Prevention, and Control

Erysipelothrix is susceptible to penicillin, which is the antibiotic of choice. Cephalosporins, erythromycin, and clindamycin are also active in vitro, but the organism is resistant to the sulfonamides, aminoglycosides, and vancomycin. Infections in people at a higher occupational risk are prevented by the use of gloves and other appropriate coverings on exposed skin. Vaccination is used to control disease in swine.

CASE STUDY AND QUESTIONS

■ A 35-year-old man was hospitalized because of headache, fever, and confusion. He had received a kidney transplant 7 months before, after which he had been given immunosuppressive drugs to prevent organ rejection. CSF was collected, which revealed a white blood cell count of 36 cells/mm³ with 96% polymorphonuclear leukocytes, a glucose concentration of 40 mg/dL, and a protein concentration of 172 mg/dL. A Gram-stain preparation of CSF was negative for organisms, but gram-positive coccobacilli grew in cultures of the blood and CSF.

1. What is the most likely cause of this patient's meningitis?

2. What are the potential sources of this organism?

3. What virulence factors are associated with this organism?

4. How would this disease be treated? Which antibiotics are effective in vitro? Which antibiotics are ineffective?

BIBLIOGRAPHY

Charpentier E, Courvalin P: Antibiotic resistance in *Listeria* spp., *Antimicrob Agents Chemother* 43:2103–2108, 1999.

Gedde MM et al: Role of listeriolysin O in cell-to-cell spread of *Listeria monocytogenes*, *Infect Immun* 68:999–1003, 2000.

Gorby GL, Peacock JE Jr: *Erysipelothrix rhusiopathiae* endocarditis: microbiologic, epidemiologic, and clinical features of an occupational disease, *Rev Infect Dis* 10:317–325, 1988.

Hof H, Nichterlein T, Kretschmar M: Management of listeriosis, *Clin Microbiol Rev* 10:345–357, 1997.

Ireton K, Cossart P: Host-pathogen interactions during entry and actin-based movement of *Listeria monocytogenes*, *Annu Rev Genet* 31:113–138, 1997.

Jurado RL et al: Increased risk of meningitis and bacteremia due to *Listeria monocytogenes* in patients with human immunodeficiency virus infection, *Clin Infect Dis* 17:224–227, 1993.

Lorber B: Listeriosis, *Clin Infect Dis* 24:1–11, 1997.

Mead P et al: Food-related illness and death in the United States, *Emerg Infect Dis* 5:607–625, 1999.

Moors MA et al: Expression of listeriolysin O and ActA by intracellular and extracellular *Listeria monocytogenes*, *Infect Immun* 67:1331–1339, 1999.

Pinner RW et al: Role of foods in sporadic listeriosis. II. Microbiologic and epidemiologic investigation, *JAMA* 267:2046–2050, 1992.

Schlech W: Foodborne listeriosis, *Clin Infect Dis* 31:770–775, 2000.

Schuchat A et al: Role of foods in sporadic listeriosis. I. Case-control study of dietary risk factors, *JAMA* 267:2041–2045, 1992.

Southwick F, Purich D: Mechanisms of disease: intracellular pathogenesis of listeriosis, *N Engl J Med* 334:770–776, 1996.

Tilney LG, Portnoy DA: Actin filaments and the growth, movement, and spread of the intracellular bacterial parasite, *Listeria monocytogenes*, *J Cell Biol* 109:1597–1608, 1989.

C H A P T E R   2 7

Corynebacterium and Other Gram-Positive Bacilli

The aerobic gram-positive bacilli are a heterogeneous group of bacteria that have been loosely grouped on the basis of their cell morphology, staining properties, and guanine plus cytosine (G + C) content. The **coryneform** group consists of *Corynebacterium* and related genera that are irregularly shaped, non–spore-forming, non–acid-fast, gram-positive bacilli with a high guanine plus cytosine content; these bacteria are the subject of this chapter.

Corynebacterium (Greek, *koryne*, "club"; *bakterion*, "small rod," referring to the fact that an individual organism is a small, club-shaped rod) is a large, heterogeneous collection of species that have a cell wall with arabinose, galactose, meso-diaminopimelic acid, and (in most species) short-chain mycolic acids. Gram stains of these bacteria reveal short chains (V or Y configurations) or clumps resembling Chinese "letters" (Fig. 27–1). Metachromatic granules within the cells may be seen with special stains. Corynebacteria are aerobic or facultatively anaerobic, nonmotile, and catalase-positive. Most species ferment carbohydrates, producing lactic acid as a byproduct. Although many species grow well on common laboratory media, some species require supplementation with lipids for good growth (lipophilic strains). Currently, 46 species have been defined, more than 30 of them associated with human disease.

Corynebacteria are ubiquitous in plants and animals, and they normally colonize the skin, upper respiratory tract, gastrointestinal tract, and urogenital tract in humans. Although all species of corynebacteria can function as opportunistic pathogens, a few are more commonly associated with disease (Table 27–1). The most famous of these is *Corynebacterium diphtheriae*, the etiologic agent of **diphtheria** (Greek, *diphtheria*, "leathery skin," referring to the pseudomembrane that initially forms on the pharynx).

A number of other genera of coryneform bacteria have been characterized. The four genera that have been most commonly associated with human disease are discussed briefly at the end of this chapter (Table 27–2).

Corynebacterium diphtheriae

Physiology and Structure

C. diphtheriae is an irregularly staining, pleomorphic bacillus (0.3 to 0.8 × 1.0 to 8.0 μm). Metachromatic granules have been observed in bacilli stained with methylene blue (Box 27–1). After overnight incubation, 1- to 3-mm colonies are observed on blood agar medium. More selective, differential media can be used to recover this pathogen from specimens in which other organisms are present.

Pathogenesis and Immunity

C. diphtheriae is a classic model of bacterial virulence. The toxicity observed in diphtheria is directly attributed to an exotoxin secreted by the bacteria at the

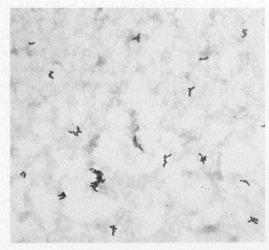

FIGURE 27–1. Gram-stained specimen showing *Corynebacterium* species.

TABLE 27–1. *Corynebacterium* Species Associated with Human Disease

Organism	Diseases
C. diphtheriae	Diphtheria (respiratory, cutaneous); pharyngitis and endocarditis (nontoxigenic strains)
C. jeikeium (group JK)	Septicemia, endocarditis, wound infections, foreign body (catheter, shunt, prosthesis) infections
C. urealyticum (group D2)	Urinary tract infections including pyelonephritis and alkaline-encrusted cystitis, septicemia, endocarditis, wound infections
C. amycolatum	Wound infections, foreign body infections, septicemia, urinary tract infections, respiratory tract infections
C. glucuronolyticum	Genitourinary tract infections (males)
C. riegelii	Genitourinary tract infections (females)
C. macginleyi	Eye infections
C. minutissimum	Wound infections, respiratory tract infections
C. pseudodiphtheriticum	Respiratory tract infections, endocarditis
C. pseudotuberculosis	Lymphadenitis, ulcerative lymphangitis, abscess formation
C. striatum	Wound infections, respiratory tract infections, foreign body infections
C. ulcerans	Respiratory diphtheria

region on the B subunit and a **catalytic region** on the A subunit. The receptor for the toxin is the heparin-binding epidermal growth factor, which is present on the surface of many eukaryotic cells, particularly heart and nerve cells; its presence explains the cardiac and neurologic symptoms observed in patients with severe diphtheria. After the toxin becomes attached to the host cell, the translocation region is inserted into the endosomal membrane, facilitating the movement of the catalytic region into the cytosol. The A subunit then terminates host cell protein synthesis by inactivating **elongation factor 2 (EF-2)**, a factor required for the movement of nascent peptide chains on ribosomes. Because the turnover of EF-2 is very slow and only about one molecule per ribosome is present in a cell, it has been estimated that one exotoxin molecule can inactivate the entire EF-2 content in a cell, completely terminating host cell protein synthesis. Toxin synthesis is regulated by a chromosomally encoded element, **diphtheria toxin repressor (DTxR)**. This protein, activated in the presence of high iron concentrations, can bind to the toxin gene operator and prevent toxin production.

Epidemiology

Diphtheria is a disease found worldwide, particularly in poor urban areas where there is crowding and the protective level of vaccine-induced immunity is low. The largest outbreak in the latter part of the 20th century occurred in the former Soviet Union, where in 1994 almost 48,000 cases were documented, with 1746 deaths. *C. diphtheriae* is maintained in the population by asymptomatic carriage in the oropharynx or on the skin of immune people (after either exposure to *C. diphtheriae* or immunization). It is transmitted from person to person by respiratory droplets or skin con-

focus of infection. The organism does not need to enter the blood stream to produce the systemic signs of disease.

The *tox* gene that codes for the exotoxin is introduced into strains of *C. diphtheriae* by a lysogenic bacteriophage (beta-phage). Two processing steps are necessary for the active gene product to be secreted:

1. Proteolytic cleavage of the leader sequence from the tox protein during secretion from the bacterial cell.
2. Cleavage of the toxin molecule into two polypeptides (A and B) that remain attached by a disulfide bond.

This 58,300-Da protein is an example of the classic **A-B exotoxin.**

Three functional regions exist on the toxin molecule, a **receptor-binding region** and a **translocation**

TABLE 27–2. Less Common Coryneform Gram-Positive Bacilli Associated with Human Disease

Organism	Diseases
Arcanobacterium	Pharyngitis, cellulitis, wound infections, abscess formation, septicemia, endocarditis
Brevibacterium	Septicemia, osteomyelitis, foreign body (catheter, shunt, prosthesis) infections
Oerskovia	Septicemia, endocarditis, meningitis, soft tissue infections, foreign body infections
Turicella	Ear infections

BOX 27–1. Summary of *Corynebacterium diphtheriae*

Physiology and Structure

Gram-positive bacilli with an irregular shape.
Most strains grow well on lipid-free media.
Facultative anaerobe (grows aerobically and anaerobically).

Virulence

A-B exotoxin that inhibits protein synthesis by inactivating elongation factor 2. Additional virulence factors are likely (but unknown), because nontoxigenic strains can cause systemic disease.

Epidemiology

Worldwide distribution maintained in asymptomatic carriers and unvaccinated hosts.
Humans are the only known reservoir, with carriage in oropharynx or on skin surface.
Spread person to person by exposure to respiratory droplets or skin contact.
Disease observed in unvaccinated people living in crowded urban areas and in children or adults with waning immunity.
Disease is uncommon in the United States.

Disease

Respiratory and cutaneous diphtheria.
No seasonal incidence.

Diagnosis

Microscopy is nonspecific. Culture should be performed on nonselective and selective media.
Demonstration of exotoxin is performed by molecular or immunologic methods.

Treatment, Prevention, and Control

Early use of diphtheria antitoxin to neutralize exotoxin.
Use of penicillin or erythromycin to eliminate *C. diphtheriae* and terminate toxin production.
Administration of diphtheria vaccine and booster shots to susceptible population.

tact (see Box 27–1). Humans are the only known reservoir for this organism.

Diphtheria has become uncommon in the United States as the result of an active immunization program, as shown by the fact that more than 200,000 cases were reported in 1921 but fewer than 5 cases per year have been reported since 1980. Diphtheria is primarily a pediatric disease, but the highest incidence has shifted toward older age groups in areas where there are active immunization programs for children. Skin infection with toxigenic *C. diphtheriae* (cutaneous diphtheria) also occurs, but it is not a reportable disease in the United States so its incidence is unknown.

Clinical Diseases

The clinical presentation of diphtheria is determined by (1) the site of infection, (2) the immune status of the patient, and (3) the virulence of the organism. Exposure to *C. diphtheriae* can result in asymptomatic colonization in fully immune people, mild respiratory disease in partially immune patients, or a fulminant, sometimes fatal disease in nonimmune patients.

Respiratory Diphtheria

The symptoms of diphtheria involving the respiratory tract develop after a 2- to 6-day incubation period. Organisms multiply locally on epithelial cells in the pharynx or adjacent surfaces and initially cause localized damage as a result of exotoxin activity. The onset is sudden, with malaise, sore throat, exudative pharyngitis, and a low-grade fever. The exudate evolves into a thick pseudomembrane composed of bacteria, lymphocytes, plasma cells, fibrin, and dead cells that can cover the tonsils, uvula, and palate and can extend up into the nasopharynx or down into the larynx. The pseudomembrane firmly adheres to the respiratory tissue and is difficult to dislodge without making the underlying tissue bleed (unique to diphtheria). As the patient recovers after the approximately 1-week course of the disease, the membrane dislodges and is expectorated. Complications in patients with severe disease include breathing obstruction, cardiac arrhythmia, coma, and, ultimately, death.

Cutaneous Diphtheria

Cutaneous diphtheria is acquired through skin contact with other infected persons. The organism colonizes the skin and gains entry into the subcutaneous tissue through breaks in the skin. A papule develops first and then evolves into a chronic nonhealing ulcer, sometimes covered with a grayish membrane. Systemic signs of disease can occur as a result of the exotoxin effects.

Laboratory Diagnosis

The initial treatment of a patient with diphtheria is instituted on the basis of the clinical diagnosis, not laboratory results, because definitive results are not available for at least a week.

Microscopy

The results of microscopic examination of clinical material are unreliable. Metachromatic granules in bacteria stained with methylene blue have been described, but this appearance is not specific to *C. diphtheriae*, and interpretation of the smear requires technical expertise.

Culture

Specimens for the recovery of *C. diphtheriae* should be collected from both the nasopharynx and the throat and should be inoculated onto nonselective media as well as media developed specifically for this organism (e.g., cysteine-tellurite agar, serum tellurite agar, Löffler's medium). *C. diphtheriae* has a characteristic gray to black color on tellurite agar, and the microscopic morphology is best seen on Löffler's medium.

C. diphtheriae has been described as having the following three colonial morphologies on cysteine-tellurite agar: **gravis, intermedius,** and **mitis.** Gravis colonies are large, irregular, and gray. Intermedius colonies are small, flat, and gray. Mitis colonies are small, round, convex, and black. Although these morphologies were initially correlated with the severity of illness, the distinctions are now not considered valid. They are useful, however, for the epidemiologic classification of isolates. The precise identification of *C. diphtheriae* is determined by the results of specific biochemical tests.

Toxigenicity Testing

All isolates of *C. diphtheriae* should be tested for the production of exotoxin. This has been done historically by an in vitro immunodiffusion assay (**Elek test**), a tissue culture neutralization assay using specific antitoxin, or an in vivo neutralization assay using guinea pigs injected subcutaneously with the isolate from the patient. However, the Centers for Disease Control and Prevention (CDC) has developed an amplification test based on the polymerase chain reaction (PCR) for directly detecting the toxin gene in clinical specimens (e.g., swabs from the diphtheritic membrane or biopsy material). Currently, this test is the diagnostic test of choice. It should be remembered that nontoxigenic strains should not be ignored, because these strains have been associated with significant disease, including septicemia, endocarditis, septic arthritis, osteomyelitis, and abscess formation.

Treatment, Prevention, and Control

The most important aspect of the treatment for diphtheria is the early administration of diphtheria antitoxin to specifically neutralize the exotoxin before it is bound by the host cell. Once the toxin is internalized by the cell, cell death is inevitable. Antibiotic therapy with penicillin or erythromycin is also used to eliminate *C. diphtheriae* and terminate toxin production. Bed rest, isolation to prevent secondary spread, and maintenance of an open airway in patients with respiratory diphtheria are all important.

Symptomatic diphtheria can be prevented by actively immunizing people with diphtheria toxoid during childhood and with booster doses given every 10 years throughout life. The nontoxic, immunogenic toxoid is prepared by formalin treatment of the toxin. Initially, children are given monthly injections of this preparation with pertussis and tetanus antigens (**DPT vaccine**) for 3 months, after which they receive regular booster injections.

Immunity to diphtheria can be determined by measuring the neutralizing antibodies in a person (**Schick test**). This test involves intradermal injection of diphtheria toxin. No skin reaction is observed if neutralizing antibodies are present; localized edema with necrosis occurs if neutralizing antibodies are absent, indicating that the patient is susceptible to diphtheria.

People coming in close contact with patients who have documented diphtheria are at risk for acquiring the disease. Nasopharyngeal specimens for culture should be collected from all close contacts, and antimicrobial prophylaxis with penicillin or erythromycin started immediately. Any contact who has not completed the series of diphtheria immunizations or who has not received a booster dose within the previous 5 years should receive a booster dose of toxoid. People exposed to cutaneous diphtheria should be managed in the same manner as those exposed to respiratory diphtheria. If the respiratory or cutaneous infection is caused by a nontoxigenic strain, it is unnecessary to institute prophylaxis in contacts.

Other *Corynebacterium* Species

A large number of other *Corynebacterium* species have been found as part of the indigenous human flora and are capable of causing disease. The most common species are listed in Table 27–1 and summarized in Box 27–2.

Corynebacterium jeikeium is a well-recognized opportunistic pathogen in immunocompromised patients, particularly those with hematologic disorders or intravascular catheters. Carriage of this organism is uncommon in healthy people, but the skin of as many as 40% of hospitalized patients can be colonized regardless of their immunologic state. Predisposing conditions for disease include prolonged hospitalization, granulocytopenia, prior or concurrent antimicrobial therapy or chemotherapy, as well as a mucocutaneous portal of entry. This organism is very resistant to antibiotics, so antibiotic therapy during hospitalization may foster colonization of the skin. The organism can then gain access through an intravenous catheter and establish disease in the immunologically compromised patient.

Corynebacterium urealyticum is not a common isolate in healthy people; however, the species is an important pathogen of the urinary tract. As the name implies, *C. urealyticum*, which is a strong urease producer, can pro-

---

BOX 27–2. Summary of Other *Corynebacterium* Species

Physiology and Structure

Gram-positive bacilli with an irregular shape.

Some species require lipids for good growth (e.g., *C. jeikeium, C. urealyticum, C. macginleyi*).

Most strains are facultative anaerobes.

Virulence

A-B exotoxin may be carried by *C. ulcerans* and *C. pseudotuberculosis.*

Urinary tract pathogens produce urease (e.g., *C. amycolatum, C. glucuronolyticum, C. riegelii, C urealyticum*).

Many species able to adhere to foreign bodies (e.g., catheters, shunts, prosthetic devices).

Some species resistant to most antibiotics (e.g., *C. amycolatum, C. jeikeium, C. urealyticum*).

Epidemiology

Most infections are endogenous (produced by species that are part of the host's normal bacterial population on the skin surface and mucosal membranes).

Diseases

Septicemia, endocarditis, foreign body infections, wound infections, urinary tract infections, respiratory infections including diphtheria.

Diagnosis

Culture on nonselective media is reliable although growth may be slow and media may require supplementation with lipids.

Treatment, Prevention, and Control

Treatment with effective antibiotics to eliminate the organism.

Removal of foreign body.

---

duce enough urease to make the urine alkaline, possibly leading to the formation of **struvite calculi** or **stones.** Risk factors associated with *C. urealyticum* infections include immunosuppression, underlying genitourinary disorders, an antecedent urologic procedure, and prior antibiotic therapy. Other urease-producing corynebacteria that are associated with urinary tract infections are *Corynebacterium amycolatum, Corynebacterium glucuronolyticum,* and *Corynebacterium riegelii.*

C. amycolatum resides on the skin surface but not in the oropharynx. This species is the most commonly isolated species in clinical specimens, although its importance has been underappreciated because it is frequently misidentified as other corynebacteria species. This species, like *C. jeikeium* and *C. urealyticum,* is resistant to many antibiotics and is an important opportunistic pathogen.

Corynebacterium minutissimum colonizes the skin of healthy people and has been associated with **erythrasma,** a superficial infection of the skin involving the formation of pruritic macular patches. The etiologic role of *C. minutissimum,* however, has been questioned.

Corynebacterium pseudotuberculosis and *Corynebacterium ulcerans* are closely related to *C. diphtheriae* and can carry the diphtheria gene. Although *C. ulcerans* can cause a disease indistinguishable from diphtheria, human infections caused by *C. pseudotuberculosis* are rarely observed.

Numerous other *Corynebacterium* species have been associated with opportunistic infections. These bacteria are commonly present on the skin and mucosal surfaces, so their isolation in a clinical specimen may represent an important finding or may simply represent contamination of the specimen.

Treatment of *Corynebacterium* infections can be problematic. *C. jeikeium, C. urealyticum,* and *C. amycolatum* are typically resistant to most antibiotics, so infected patients usually must be given vancomycin. The other species tend to be more susceptible to antibiotics, but in vitro testing may be required to effect a cure.

Other Coryneform Genera

Other genera of irregularly shaped, gram-positive bacilli have been found to colonize humans and cause disease (see Table 27–2). *Arcanobacterium* can cause pharyngitis with a "scarlet fever–like" rash, polymicrobic wound infections, and, less commonly, systemic infections such as septicemia and endocarditis. Infections can be treated with penicillin or erythromycin.

Brevibacterium colonize the skin surface and, when grown in culture, produce a cheeselike odor. These bacteria have been blamed for malodorous feet in some colonized people. More important diseases attributed to *Brevibacterium* are septicemia, osteomyelitis, and foreign body infections. Treatment is complicated because many strains are resistant to β-lactam antibiotics, erythromycin, clindamycin, and ciprofloxacin. Use of vancomycin, tetracyclines, or gentamicin has proved effective.

Oerskovia is an environmental organism found in the soil and decaying organic matter. This organism has been associated with septicemia, endocarditis, meningitis, soft tissue infections, and infections in the presence of foreign bodies. Effective treatment must be guided by in vitro susceptibility tests, because vancomycin-resistant strains have been reported.

Turicella (Turicella otitidis is the only species) has been isolated in the ears of healthy and infected individuals. The isolates are susceptible to β-lactam antibiotics but may be resistant to clindamycin and erythromycin.

CASE STUDY AND QUESTIONS

■ A 78-year-old man with a history of hypertension was admitted to the hospital because of a severe headache of 4 hours' duration. Evidence of subarachnoid hemorrhage and hydrocephalus was found, and the patient required the placement of a left ventricular-atrial shunt. Fever developed 1 week after the operation. *C. jeikeium* was isolated from blood cultures and a subsequent culture of fluid collected from the shunt.

1. What risk factors are associated with infections with *C. jeikeium?*

2. What antibiotic therapy could be given for infections with this organism?

3. Name two other *Corynebacterium* species that are commonly resistant to multiple antibiotics. What diseases are associated with these organisms?

4. Explain the synthesis and mode of action of the diphtheria exotoxin.

BIBLIOGRAPHY

Esteban J et al: Microbiological characterization and clinical significance of *Corynebacterium amycolatum* strains, *Eur J Clin Microbiol Infect Dis* 18:518–521, 1999.

Funke G et al: Antimicrobial susceptibility patterns of some recently established coryneform bacteria, *Antimicrob Agents Chemother* 40:2874–2878, 1996.

Funke G et al: *Corynebacterium coyleae* sp. nov., isolated from human clinical specimens, *Int Sys Bacteriol* 47:92–96, 1997.

Funke G et al: Clinical microbiology of coryneform bacteria, *Clin Microbiol Rev* 10:125–159, 1997.

Funke G et al: *Corynebacterium macginleyi* has to date been isolated exclusively from conjunctival swabs, *J Clin Microbiol* 36:3670–3673, 1998.

George MJ: Clinical significance and characterization of *Corynebacterium* species, *Clin Microbiol Newsletter* 17:177–180, 1995.

Gutierrez-Rodero F et al: *Corynebacterium pseudodiphtheriticum:* an easily missed respiratory pathogen in HIV-infected patients, *Diagn Microbiol Infect Dis* 33:209–216, 1999.

Lipsky BA et al: Infections caused by nondiphtheria corynebacteria, *Rev Infect Dis* 4:1220–1235, 1982.

Pascual C et al: Phylogenetic analysis of the genus *Corynebacterium* based on 16S rRNA gene sequences, *Int J Syst Bacteriol* 45:724–728, 1995.

Popovic T et al: Molecular epidemiology of diphtheria in Russia, 1985–1994, *J Infect Dis* 174:1064–1072, 1996.

Soriano F et al: Urinary tract infection caused by *Corynebacterium* group D2: report of 82 cases and review, *Rev Infect Dis* 12:1019–1034, 1990.

CHAPTER 28

Neisseria

The genus *Neisseria* (named after German physician A. L. S. Neisser, who originally described the organism responsible for gonorrhea) consists of 10 species. Two species, *Neisseria gonorrhoeae* and *Neisseria meningitidis*, are strictly human pathogens. The remaining species are commonly present on mucosal surfaces of the oropharynx and nasopharynx and occasionally colonize the anogenital mucosal membranes. Members of the genus are aerobic, gram-negative cocci typically arranged in pairs (diplococci) with adjacent sides flattened together (resembling coffee beans) (Fig. 28–1). The bacteria are not motile and do not form endospores. All species are oxidase-positive, and most produce catalase—properties that combined with the Gram-stain morphology allow for a rapid, presumptive identification of a clinical isolate. Acid is produced by oxidation of carbohydrates (not by fermentation). Although diseases caused by *N. gonorrhoeae* and *N. meningitidis* are well known, the other *Neisseria* species have limited virulence and generally produce disease only in compromised patients (Table 28–1).

Neisseria gonorrhoeae

Infection with *N. gonorrhoeae* has been recognized for centuries. Despite effective antibiotic therapy, it is still one of the most common sexually transmitted diseases in the United States.

Physiology and Structure

N. gonorrhoeae is a fastidious organism, requiring complex media for growth and adversely affected by drying and fatty acids. Soluble starch is added to the media to neutralize the toxic effect of the fatty acids. The optimum growth temperature is 35°C to 37°C, with poor survival of the organism at cooler temperatures. A humid atmosphere supplemented with carbon dioxide (CO_2) is either required or enhances growth of *N. gonorrhoeae*. Although the fastidious nature of this organism makes recovery from clinical specimens diffi-

cult, it is nevertheless easy for the organism to be sexually transmitted from person to person.

The structure of *N. gonorrhoeae* is typical of gram-negative bacteria, with the thin peptidoglycan layer sandwiched between the inner cytoplasmic membrane and the outer membrane. The outer surface is not covered with a true carbohydrate capsule, as is found in *N. meningitidis*. The cell surface of *N. gonorrhoeae*, however, has a capsule-like negative charge. Fresh clinical isolates have **pili**, which extend from the cytoplasmic membrane through the outer membrane. The pili are composed of repeating protein subunits (**pilins**), whose expression is controlled by the *pil* gene complex. Pili expression is associated with virulence, in part because the pili mediate attachment to nonciliated epithelial cells as well as provide resistance to killing by neutrophils. Pilin proteins have a conserved region at the amino terminal end and a highly variable region at the exposed carboxyl terminus. The lack of immunity to reinfection with *N. gonorrhoeae* results partially from the antigenic variation among the pilin proteins and partially from the phase variation in pilin expression; these factors complicate attempts to develop effective vaccines.

Other prominent families of proteins are present in the outer membrane. The **Por proteins** (formerly protein I) are porin proteins that form pores or channels in the outer membrane. Two classes of Por proteins (PorA and PorB), each with a variety of antigenic variations, have been identified. Strains expressing PorA are resistant to serum killing and thus are more commonly associated with disseminated disease. The antigenic variation in the Por proteins has been exploited for the serotype classification of *N. gonorrhoeae*.

Opa proteins (opacity proteins; formerly protein II) are a family of membrane proteins that mediate binding to epithelial cells. Multiple alleles of these proteins can be expressed by an individual isolate. Bacteria expressing the Opa proteins appear opaque (versus transparent) when grown in culture. These proteins facilitate bacterial adherence to each other and to eukaryotic cells.

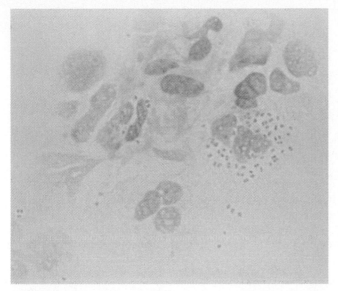

FIGURE 28–1. *Neisseria gonorrhoeae* in urethral exudate. Note the spatial arrangement of the pairs of cocci with sides pressed together, characteristic of this genus.

TABLE 28–1. *Neisseria* Species and Their Diseases

Organism	Diseases
N. gonorrhoeae	Urethritis, cervicitis, salpingitis, pelvic inflammatory disease, proctitis, bacteremia, arthritis, conjunctivitis, pharyngitis
N. meningitidis	Meningitis, meningoencephalitis, bacteremia, pneumonia, arthritis, urethritis
Other *Neisseria* species	Opportunistic infections

tivity. However, LOS does not have the antigenically diverse, strain-specific O polysaccharide antigens found in LPS. Other important gonococcal proteins are an immunoglobulin (Ig) A_1 protease, which degrades secretory IgA, and β-lactamase, which degrades penicillin.

Pathogenesis and Immunity

Gonococci attach to mucosal cells, penetrate into the cells and multiply, and then pass through the cells into the subepithelial space, where infection is established. The presence of pili is important for the initial attachment (Table 28–2). Nonpiliated cells are avirulent.

After the initial attachment, Opa protein directs first a tighter association with the host cell surface and then the migration of bacteria into the epithelial cell. Researchers believe that the Por protein protects the phagocytosed bacteria from intracellular killing by inhibiting phagolysosome fusion. The gonococcal LOS

The third group of proteins in the outer membrane is the highly conserved **Rmp proteins** (reduction-modifiable proteins; formerly protein III). These proteins stimulate antibodies that block serum bactericidal activity against *N. gonorrhoeae*.

Iron is essential for the growth and metabolism of gonococci. Three groups of outer-membrane proteins have been identified that mediate the acquisition of iron by binding transferrin, lactoferrin, and hemoglobin. Another major antigen in the cell wall is lipooligosaccharide (LOS). This antigen is composed of lipid A and a core oligosaccharide, similar to gram-negative lipopolysaccharide (LPS), and possesses endotoxin ac-

TABLE 28–2. Virulence Factors in *Neisseria gonorrhoeae*

Virulence Factor	Biologic Effect
Pilin	Protein that mediates initial attachment to nonciliated human cells (e.g., epithelium of vagina, fallopian tube, and buccal cavity); interferes with neutrophil killing
Por protein (protein I)	Porin protein—promotes intracellular survival by preventing phagolysosome fusion in neutrophils
Opa protein (protein II)	Opacity protein—mediates firm attachment to eukaryotic cells
Rmp protein (protein III)	Reduction-modifiable protein—protects other surface antigens (Por protein, LOS) from bactericidal antibodies
Transferrin-binding proteins	Mediate acquisition of iron for bacterial metabolism
Lactoferrin-binding proteins	Mediate acquisition of iron for bacterial metabolism
Hemoglobin-binding proteins	Mediate acquisition of iron for bacterial metabolism
LOS	Lipooligosaccharide—has endotoxin activity
IgA$_1$ protease	Destroys immunoglobulin A$_1$ (role in virulence is unknown)
β-lactamase	Hydrolyzes β-lactam ring in penicillin

BOX 28–1. Summary of *Neisseria gonorrhoeae*

Physiology and Structure

Gram-negative diplococci with fastidious growth requirements.

Growth best at 35°C to 37°C in a humid atmosphere supplemented with CO_2.

Oxidase- and catalase-positive; acid produced from glucose oxidatively.

Outer surface with multiple antigens: pili protein; Por proteins; Opa proteins; Rmp protein; protein receptors for transferrin, lactoferrin, and hemoglobin; lipooligosaccharide; immunoglobulin protease; β-lactamase.

Virulence

Refer to Table 28–2.

Epidemiology

Humans are the only natural hosts.

Asymptomatic carriage is the major reservoir.

Transmission primarily by sexual contact.

More than 350,000 cases reported in United States in 1998 (underestimates true incidence of disease).

Disease most common in blacks, people aged 15 to 24 years, residents of southeastern states, people who have multiple sexual encounters.

Higher risk of disseminated disease in patients with deficiencies in late components of complement.

Diseases

Refer to Table 28–1.

Diagnosis

Gram stain of urethral specimens is accurate for symptomatic males only.

Culture is sensitive and specific but has been replaced with molecular probe techniques in many laboratories.

Treatment, Prevention, and Control

Ceftriaxone, cefixime, ciprofloxacin, or ofloxacin can be administered in uncomplicated cases.

In vitro susceptibility should be determined in cases unresponsive to therapy, because antibiotic resistance is increasing.

Penicillin should be avoided, because resistance is common.

Doxycycline or azithromycin should be added for infections complicated by *Chlamydia*.

For neonates, prophylaxis with 1% silver nitrate; ophthalmia neonatorum is treated with ceftriaxone.

Prevention consists of patient education, use of condoms or spermicides with nonoxynol 9 (only partially effective), and aggressive follow-up of sexual partners of infected patients.

Effective vaccines are not available.

---

stimulates the inflammatory response and release of tumor necrosis factor-α (TNF-α), which causes most of the symptoms associated with gonococcal disease.

IgG_3 is the predominant IgG antibody formed in response to gonococcal infection. Although the antibody response to Por is minimal, serum antibodies to pilin, Opa protein, and LOS are readily detected. Antibodies to LOS can activate complement, releasing complement component C5a, which has a chemotactic effect on neutrophils. IgG and secretory IgA_1 antibodies directed against Rmp protein can block this bactericidal antibody response, however. People with inherited complement deficiencies are at considerably greater risk for systemic disease.

Epidemiology

Gonorrhea occurs only in humans; it has no other known reservoir (Box 28–1). It is the second most commonly reported sexually transmitted disease in the United States (chlamydia infections are the most common). Infection rates are the same in males and females, are disproportionately higher in blacks than in Hispanic Americans and whites, and are highest in the southeastern United States. The peak incidence of the disease is in the age group 15 to 24 years. Although the incidence of disease has decreased since 1975, this trend was reversed in 1998 and 1999 (Fig. 28–2). More than 360,000 cases were reported in the United States in 1999. Even this large number is an underestimation of the true incidence of disease, however, be-

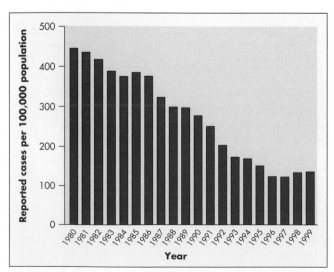

FIGURE 28–2. Gonorrhea in the United States from 1980 to 1999. CDC's morbidity and mortality reports.

cause the diagnosis and reporting of gonococcal infections are incomplete.

N. gonorrhoeae is transmitted primarily by sexual contact. Women have a 50% risk of acquiring the infection as the result of a single exposure to an infected man, whereas men have a risk of approximately 20% as the result of a single exposure to an infected woman. The risk of infection rises as the person has more sexual encounters with infected partners.

The major reservoir for gonococci is the asymptomatically infected person. Asymptomatic carriage is more common in women than in men. As many as half of all infected women have mild or asymptomatic infections, whereas most men are initially symptomatic. The symptoms generally clear within a few weeks in people with untreated disease, and asymptomatic carriage may then become established. The site of infection also determines whether carriage occurs, with rectal and pharyngeal infections more commonly asymptomatic than genital infections.

Clinical Diseases

Genital infection in men is primarily restricted to the urethra. A purulent urethral discharge and dysuria develop after a 2- to 5-day incubation period. Approximately 95% of all infected men have acute symptoms. Although complications are rare, epididymitis, prostatitis, and periurethral abscesses can occur.

The primary site of infection in women is the cervix, because the bacteria infect the endocervical columnar epithelial cells. The organism cannot infect the squamous epithelial cells that line the vagina of postpubescent women. Symptomatic patients commonly experience vaginal discharge, dysuria, and abdominal pain. Ascending genital infection, including salpingitis, tuboovarian abscesses, and pelvic inflammatory disease are observed in 10% to 20% of women.

Disseminated infections with septicemia and infection of skin and joints occur in 1% to 3% of infected women and in a much lower percentage of infected men. The greater proportion of disseminated infections in women is caused by the numerous untreated asymptomatic infections in this population. The clinical manifestations of disseminated disease include fever; migratory arthralgias; suppurative arthritis in the wrists, knees, and ankles; and a pustular rash on an erythematous base over the extremities but not on the head and trunk. *N. gonorrhoeae* is a leading cause of purulent arthritis in adults.

Other diseases associated with *N. gonorrhoeae* are perihepatitis (**Fitz-Hugh–Curtis syndrome**); purulent conjunctivitis, particularly in newborns infected during vaginal delivery (**ophthalmia neonatorum**); anorectal gonorrhea in homosexual men; and pharyngitis.

Laboratory Diagnosis

Microscopy

Gram stain is very sensitive (greater than 90%) and specific (98%) in detecting gonococcal infection in men with purulent urethritis (see Fig. 28–1). However, its sensitivity in detecting infection in asymptomatic men is 60% or less. The test is also relatively insensitive in detecting gonococcal cervicitis in both symptomatic and asymptomatic women, although a positive result is considered reliable when an experienced microscopist sees gram-negative diplococci within polymorphonuclear leukocytes. Thus, the Gram stain can be reliably used to diagnose infections in men with purulent urethritis, but all negative results in women and asymptomatic men must be confirmed by culture.

Gram stain is also useful for the early diagnosis of purulent arthritis but is insensitive for the detection of *N. gonorrhoeae* in patients with skin lesions, anorectal infections, or pharyngitis. Commensal *Neisseria* species in the oropharynx and morphologically similar bacteria in the gastrointestinal tract can be confused with *N. gonorrhoeae*.

Culture

N. gonorrhoeae can be readily isolated from genital specimens if care is taken in collecting and processing the specimens (Fig. 28–3). Because other commensal organisms normally colonize mucosal surfaces, all genital, rectal, and pharyngeal specimens must be inoculated onto both selective media (e.g., modified Thayer-Martin medium) and nonselective media (e.g., chocolate blood agar). Selective media suppress the growth of contaminating organisms. A nonselective medium should also be used, however, because some gonococcal strains are inhibited by the vancomycin present in most selective media. The organisms are also inhibited by the fatty acids and trace metals present in the peptone hydrolysates and agar in other common laboratory media (e.g., blood agar, nutrient agar). The gonococci die rapidly if specimens are allowed to dry. Therefore, drying as well as cold temperatures should be avoided through direct inoculation of the specimen onto prewarmed media at the time of collection.

The endocervix must be properly exposed to ensure that an adequate specimen is collected. Although the endocervix is the most common site of infection in women, the rectal specimen may be the only one positive for gonococci in women who have asymptomatic infections as well as in homosexual and bisexual men. Blood culture results are generally positive for gonococci only during the first week of the infection in patients with disseminated disease. In addition, special handling of blood specimens is required to ensure the

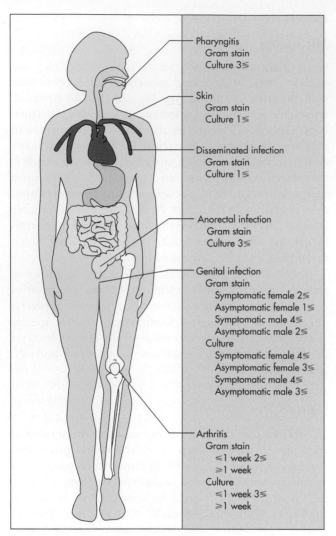

Pharyngitis
Gram stain
Culture 3≤

Skin
Gram stain
Culture 1≤

Disseminated infection
Gram stain
Culture 1≤

Anorectal infection
Gram stain
Culture 3≤

Genital infection
Gram stain
Symptomatic female 2≤
Asymptomatic female 1≤
Symptomatic male 4≤
Asymptomatic male 2≤
Culture
Symptomatic female 4≤
Asymptomatic female 3≤
Symptomatic male 4≤
Asymptomatic male 3≤

Arthritis
Gram stain
≤1 week 2≤
≥1 week
Culture
≤1 week 3≤
≥1 week

FIGURE 28–3. Laboratory detection of *Neisseria gonorrhoeae.*

adequate recovery of gonococci, because supplements present in the blood culture media can be toxic to *Neisseria.* Culture results of specimens from infected joints are positive for the organism if the specimens are collected at the time the arthritis develops, but skin specimen cultures are generally unrewarding.

Identification

N. gonorrhoeae is identified preliminarily on the basis of the isolation of oxidase-positive, gram-negative diplococci that grow on chocolate blood agar or on media that are selective for pathogenic *Neisseria* species. Definitive identification is guided by the detection of acid produced oxidatively from glucose but not from other sugars (Table 28–3).

Genetic Probes

Commercial probes specific for the nucleic acids of *N. gonorrhoeae* have been developed for the direct detection of bacteria in clinical specimens. Tests using these probes are sensitive, specific, and rapid (results are available in 2 to 4 hours). Combination assays for both *N. gonorrhoeae* and *Chlamydia* organisms are also available. In many laboratories, culture for these two pathogens has been replaced with probe assays. The primary problem with this approach is that it cannot be used to monitor antibiotic resistance of the identified pathogens.

Serology

Researchers have developed serologic tests that can detect the gonococcal antigens and antibodies directed against the organism. However, these tests are neither sensitive nor specific, and their use is not recommended.

TABLE 28–3. Differential Characteristics of Commonly Isolated *Neisseria* Species

Characteristic	N. gonorrhoeae	N. meningitidis	N. lactamica	N. sicca	N. mucosa	N. flavescens
Growth on:						
CHOC, BA (22°C)	0	0	V	+	+	+
MTM, ML (35°C)	+	+	+	0	0	0
Nutrient agar (35°C)	0	V	+	+	+	+
Acid from:						
Glucose	+	+	+	+	+	0
Maltose	0	+	+	+	+	0
Lactose	0	0	+	0	0	0
Sucrose	0	0	0	+	+	0
Fructose	0	0	0	+	+	0
Nitrate reduction	0	0	0	0	+	0

BA = blood agar; CHOC = chocolate agar; ML = Martin-Lewis agar; MTM = modified Thayer-Martin agar; V = variable growth.

Treatment, Prevention, and Control

Penicillin is no longer the antibiotic of choice for treatment of gonorrhea, for three reasons. First, the concentration of penicillin required to inhibit growth of *N. gonorrhoeae* has steadily increased, so that doses considerably higher than those used originally are now needed to effect clinical cure. Specifically, the therapeutic dose of penicillin G recommended for the management of uncomplicated gonorrhea has risen from the 200,000 units prescribed in 1945, to the 4.8 million units required currently.

Second, penicillin resistance mediated by enzymatic hydrolysis of the β-lactam ring was initially reported from Southeast Asia and now is seen worldwide. The first case of β-lactamase–producing *N. gonorrhoeae* observed in the United States was reported in 1976. During the next 4 years, relatively few new cases were detected, and most were related to imported cases. Since 1980, however, the number of resistant strains has risen rapidly because the resistance gene is encoded on a transmissible plasmid.

Third, strains of penicillin-resistant *N. gonorrhoeae* that do not produce β-lactamase have also been isolated. This chromosomally mediated resistance is not limited only to penicillin but extends to tetracyclines, erythromycin, and aminoglycosides and results from changes on the cell surface that keep the antibiotic from penetrating into the gonococcal cell. Resistance to fluoroquinolones such as ciprofloxacin has also become prevalent in Africa, Southeast Asia, Australia, and some U.S. cities.

Because the incidence of antibiotic resistance in gonococci is growing, selection of effective empirical therapy is problematic. Currently, the Centers for Disease Control and Prevention (CDC) recommends that ceftriaxone, cefixime, ciprofloxacin, or ofloxacin be used as the initial therapy for cases of uncomplicated gonorrhea and that these agents be given in combination with doxycycline or azithromycin in the management of dual infections with *Chlamydia*. Selection of therapy for cases that do not respond to this empirical treatment should be guided by in vitro susceptibility results.

Although there is tremendous interest in developing a vaccine against *N. gonorrhoeae*, an effective vaccine is not available currently. Immunity to infection with *N. gonorrhoeae* is poorly understood. Antibodies can be detected to pili antigens as well as to the Por proteins and LOS. However, multiple infections are common in sexually promiscuous people. This lack of protective immunity is explained in part by the antigenic diversity of gonococcal strains. The variable region at the carboxyl terminus of the pilin proteins is the immunodominant portion of the molecule. Antibodies developed against this region protect against reinfection with a homologous strain, but cross-protection against heterologous strains is incomplete. This antigenic diversity also explains the ineffectiveness of vaccines developed against pilin proteins.

Chemoprophylaxis is also ineffective, except in the protection of newborns against gonococcal eye infections (ophthalmia neonatorum), in which 1% silver nitrate, 1% tetracycline, or 0.5% erythromycin eye ointments are routinely used. Prophylactic use of penicillin to prevent genital disease is ineffective and may select for resistant strains.

Major efforts to stem the epidemic of gonorrhea encompass education, aggressive detection, and follow-up screening of sexual contacts. It is important to realize that gonorrhea is not an insignificant disease. Chronic infections can lead to sterility, and asymptomatic infections perpetuate the reservoir of disease and lead to a higher incidence of disseminated infections.

Neisseria meningitidis

A paradox surrounds *N. meningitidis*. This encapsulated, gram-negative diplococcus commonly colonizes the nasopharynx of healthy people. It is also the second most common cause of community-acquired meningitis in adults, and the swift progression from good health to life-threatening disease can cause fear and panic in a community unlike the reaction to almost any other disease.

Physiology and Structure

The meningococci form transparent, nonpigmented colonies on chocolate blood agar, and their growth is enhanced in a moist atmosphere with 5% carbon dioxide. Isolates with large polysaccharide capsules appear as mucoid colonies. Meningococci are oxidase-positive and are differentiated from other *Neisseria* species by the production of acid from the oxidation of glucose and maltose but not of sucrose or lactose (see Table 28–3).

N. meningitidis is subdivided into serogroups and serotypes. Thirteen serogroups, with antigenic differences in their polysaccharide capsule, have been described. Serogroups A, B, C, X, Y, and W135 are most commonly associated with meningococcal disease. The serotype classification of isolates is based on differences in the proteins in the outer membrane and in the oligosaccharide component of LOS. Serotype classification has proved useful for epidemiologic classification and for the characterization of virulent strains (certain LOS-based serotypes are more commonly associated with invasive disease); however, molecular analysis (e.g., multilocus enzyme electrophoresis, DNA fingerprinting) has replaced serologic analysis in epidemiologic investigations. All group A meningococci have the same outer-membrane proteins and belong to a single serotype, whereas the meningococci in groups B and C belong to multiple serotypes. The membrane proteins and serotype classification are shared by these two serogroups.

Pathogenesis and Immunity

The outcome in a person exposed to *N. meningitidis* depends on the following four factors:

1. Whether the bacteria are able to colonize the nasopharynx (mediated by pili).
2. Whether specific group- and serotype-specific antibodies are present.
3. Whether systemic spread occurs without antibody-mediated phagocytosis (protection afforded by polysaccharide capsule).
4. Whether toxic effects (mediated by the LOS endotoxin) are expressed.

Experiments with nasopharyngeal tissue organ cultures have shown that meningococci attach selectively to specific receptors for meningococcal pili on nonciliated columnar cells of the nasopharynx. Meningococci without pili are less able to bind to these cells.

Meningococcal disease occurs in the absence of specific antibodies directed against the polysaccharide capsule and other expressed bacterial antigens. Infants are initially afforded protection by the passive transfer of maternal antibodies. By age 6 months, however, this protective immunity has waned, a finding that is consistent with the observation that the incidence of disease is greatest in children younger than 2 years. Immunity can be stimulated by colonization with *N. meningitidis* or other bacteria with cross-reactive antigens (e.g., colonization with nonencapsulated *Neisseria* species; exposure to *E. coli* K1 antigen, which crossreacts with the group B capsular polysaccharide). Bactericidal activity also requires the existence of complement. Patients with deficiencies in C5, C6, C7, or C8 of the complement system are estimated to be at a 6000-fold greater risk for meningococcal disease. Although immunity is mediated primarily by the humoral immune response, lymphocyte responsiveness to meningococcal antigens is markedly depressed in patients with acute disease.

Like *N. gonorrhoeae*, meningococci are internalized into phagocytic vacuoles and are able to avoid intracellular death, replicate, and then migrate to the subepithelial spaces. The antiphagocytic properties of the polysaccharide capsule protect *N. meningitidis* from phagocytic destruction.

The diffuse vascular damage associated with meningococcal infections (e.g., endothelial damage, inflammation of vessel walls, thrombosis, disseminated intravascular coagulation) is largely attributed to the action of the LOS endotoxin present in the outer membrane. *N. meningitidis* produces excess membrane fragments that are released into the extracellular space. This continuous hyperproduction and release of endotoxin may cause the severe endotoxic reaction seen in patients with meningococcal disease.

Epidemiology

Endemic meningococcal disease occurs worldwide, and epidemics are common in developing countries (Box 28–2). Epidemic spread of disease results from the introduction of a new, virulent strain into an immunologically naive population. Pandemics of disease have been uncommon in developed countries since World War II. Approximately 90% of the cases of meningococcal disease in developed countries are caused by serogroup B, C, or Y. Serogroup A strains are associated with disease in underdeveloped countries. Serogroups Y and W135 are most commonly associated with meningococcal pneumonia, whereas serogroups B and C are responsible for meningitis or meningococcemia. *N. meningitidis* is transmitted by respiratory droplets among people in prolonged close contact, such as family members living in the same household and soldiers living together in military barracks. Classmates in schools and hospital employees are not considered close contacts and are not at significantly higher risk of acquiring the disease unless they are in direct contact with the respiratory secretions of an infected person.

Humans are the only natural carriers for *N. meningitidis*. Studies of the asymptomatic carriage of *N. meningitidis* have shown that there is a tremendous variation in its prevalence, from less than 1% to almost 40%. The oral and nasopharyngeal carriage rates are highest for school-aged children and young adults, are higher in lower socioeconomic populations (caused by person-to-person spread in crowded areas), and do not vary with the seasons even though disease is most common during the dry, cold months of the year. Carriage is typically transient, with clearance occurring after specific antibodies develop. Endemic disease is most common in children younger than 5 years, particularly infants (Fig. 28–4). People who are older and who live in closed populations (e.g., military barracks, prisons) are prone to infection during epidemics.

Clinical Diseases

Meningitis

A total of 2725 cases of meningococcal disease (approximately 1 case per 100,000 population) were reported in the United States in 1998. Most of these infections were meningitis. The disease usually begins abruptly

BOX 28–2. Summary of *Neisseria meningitidis*

Physiology and Structure

Gram-negative diplococci with fastidious growth requirements.

Grows best at 35°C to 37°C in a humid atmosphere.

Oxidase- and catalase-positive; acid produced from glucose and maltose oxidatively.

Outer surface antigens include polysaccharide capsule, pili, and lipooligosaccharides (LOS)

Virulence

Capsule protects bacteria from antibody-mediated phagocytosis.

Specific receptors for meningococcal pili allow colonization of nasopharynx.

Bacteria can survive intracellular killing in the absence of humoral immunity.

Endotoxin mediates most clinical manifestations.

Epidemiology

Humans are the only natural hosts.

Person-to-person spread occurs via aerosolization of respiratory tract secretions.

Highest incidence of disease is in children younger than 5 years, institutionalized people, and patients with late complement deficiencies.

Meningitis and meningococcemia most commonly caused by serogroups B and C; pneumonia most commonly caused by serogroups Y and W135; serogroup A associated with disease in underdeveloped countries.

Disease occurs worldwide, most commonly in the dry, cold months of the year.

Diseases

Refer to Table 28–1.

Diagnosis

Gram stain of cerebrospinal fluid is sensitive and specific but is of limited value for blood specimens (too few organisms are generally present except in overwhelming sepsis).

Culture is definitive, but organism is fastidious and dies rapidly when exposed to cold or dry conditions.

Tests to detect meningococcal antigens insensitive and nonspecific.

Treatment, Prevention, and Control

Breast-feeding infants have passive immunity (first 6 months).

Treatment is with penicillin (drug of choice), chloramphenicol, ceftriaxone, and cefotaxime.

Chemoprophylaxis for contacts is with rifampin or sulfadiazine (if isolated organism is susceptible).

For immunoprophylaxis, vaccination is an adjunct to chemoprophylaxis; it is used only for serogroups A, C, Y, and W135; no effective vaccine is available for serogroup B.

Polysaccharide vaccines conjugated with protein carriers offer protection for infants younger than 2 years.

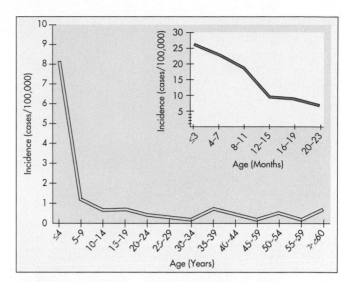

FIGURE 28–4. Incidence of meningococcal disease according to age group in the United States from 1989 to 1991. (From Jackson LA, Wenger JD: *MMWR* 42:21–30, 1993.)

with headache, meningeal signs, and fever. However, very young children may have only nonspecific signs, such as fever and vomiting. Mortality approaches 100% in untreated patients but is less than 10% in patients in whom appropriate antibiotic therapy is instituted promptly. The incidence of neurologic sequelae is low, with hearing deficits and arthritis most commonly reported.

Meningococcemia

Septicemia (meningococcemia) with or without meningitis is a life-threatening disease. Thrombosis of small blood vessels and multiorgan involvement are the characteristic clinical features. Small petechial skin lesions on the trunk and lower extremities are common and may coalesce to form larger hemorrhagic lesions (Fig. 28–5). Overwhelming disseminated intravascular coagulation with shock, together with the bilateral destruction of the adrenal glands (**Waterhouse-Friderichsen syndrome**), may ensue.

A milder, chronic septicemia has also been observed. Bacteremia can persist for days or weeks, and the only signs of infection are a low-grade fever, arthritis, and petechial skin lesions. The response to antibiotic therapy in patients with this form of the disease is generally excellent.

Other Syndromes

Additional infections caused by *N. meningitidis* are pneumonia, arthritis, and urethritis. Meningococcal pneumonia is usually preceded by a respiratory tract infection. Symptoms include cough, chest pain, rales,

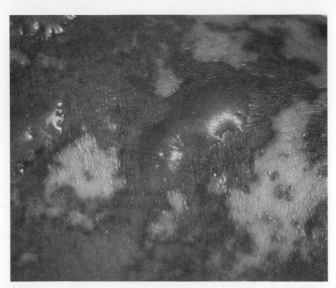

FIGURE 28-5. Skin lesions in a patient with meningococcemia. Note that the petechial lesions have coalesced and formed hemorrhagic bullae.

fever, and chills. Evidence of pharyngitis is observed in most affected patients. The prognosis in patients with meningococcal pneumonia is good.

Laboratory Diagnosis

It is important to identify *N. meningitidis* infection definitively so that specific therapy can be initiated in the patient and prophylaxis can be started for the contacts, when indicated. The most useful specimens for the detection of meningococci are blood and cerebrospinal fluid (CSF). Although the organism is present in the blood of most patients with systemic disease, additives in blood culture broths can be toxic for *Neisseria* and can therefore inhibit or delay bacterial growth. Notification that meningococcal disease is suspected should accompany the specimens sent to the laboratory, so that alternative blood-culturing methods can be used. It is relatively easy to detect and grow the organism from the CSF of untreated patients because of the abundance of organisms in the fluid (i.e., more than 10^7 organisms per mL of fluid are normally found). However, the viability of organisms can be affected adversely in patients previously treated with antibiotics.

Because the bacterial count in CSF is high, the gram-negative diplococci are readily seen within polymorphonuclear leukocytes on Gram stain (Fig. 28-6). Counterimmunoelectrophoresis or the agglutination of latex particles coated with specific antibodies can also be used to detect soluble polysaccharide antigen. The usefulness of these tests is limited, however, because serogroup B *N. meningitidis* is relatively nonimmunogenic and does not react with the test reagents.

Treatment, Prevention, and Control

Antibiotic therapy and supportive management for the complications of meningococcal disease have significantly reduced the mortality associated with the disease. Sulfonamides were the basis for the initial therapeutic successes; however, widespread resistance to the agents has now negated their effectiveness. Penicillin is currently the antibiotic of choice, but resistance to it is also becoming more common. High-level resistance (minimum inhibitory concentration [MIC] of penicillin greater than 2 μg/mL) mediated by β-lactamase is very rare. Moderate resistance (MIC 0.1 to 1.0 μg/mL) caused by the genetic alteration of penicillin-binding proteins is reported with growing frequency; approximately 4% to 5% of isolates in the United States are now resistant via this mechanism. Because penicillin therapy remains effective against most of these isolates, the clinical significance of low-level resistance is unknown. Resistance to chloramphenicol and rifampin has also been observed, so isolates from patients whose disease does not respond to empirical therapy should be evaluated carefully for antibiotic resistance.

Eradication of the pool of healthy carriers of *N. meningitidis* is unlikely. For this reason, efforts have been concentrated on the prophylactic treatment of people exposed to diseased patients and on the enhancement of immunity to the serogroups most commonly associated with disease. As just noted, sulfonamides were used for prophylaxis, but now they are no longer considered reliable. In addition, penicillin is ineffective in eliminating the carrier state. Minocycline and rifampin have been used effectively for antibiotic-mediated chemoprophylaxis because these antibiotics are secreted into the mucus; however, toxic effects have been associated with minocycline, and rifampin-resistant *N. meningitidis* can arise during treatment. At

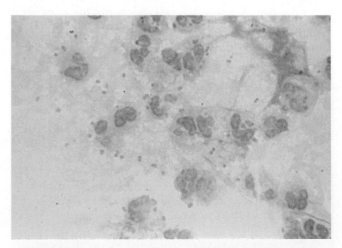

FIGURE 28-6. Gram stain of cerebrospinal fluid showing *Neisseria meningitidis.*

present, prophylaxis with a sulfonamide is recommended for people exposed to susceptible strains, with rifampin used for those with sulfonamide-resistant strains.

Vaccines directed against the group-specific capsular polysaccharides have been developed for antibody-mediated immunoprophylaxis. A polyvalent vaccine effective against serogroups A, C, Y, and W135, which can be administered to children older than 2 years, has been developed. The vaccine cannot be administered to children in younger age groups, however, because they do not respond to polysaccharide antigens. Conjugation of polysaccharide antigens to protein carriers has been used successfully with the *Haemophilus influenzae* vaccine, and a similar conjugated *N. meningitidis* vaccine is under evaluation. Unfortunately, the group B polysaccharide is a weak immunogen and cannot induce a protective antibody response. Thus immunity to group B *N. meningitidis* must develop naturally after exposure to cross-reacting antigens. Vaccination with a suspension containing serogroup A can be used for control of an outbreak of disease, for travelers to hyperendemic areas, or for people at increased risk for disease (e.g., patients with complement deficiency).

Other *Neisseria* Species

Neisseria species such as *Neisseria sicca* and *Neisseria mucosa* are commensal organisms in the oropharynx. These organisms have been implicated in isolated cases of meningitis, osteomyelitis, and endocarditis as well as bronchopulmonary infections, acute otitis media, and acute sinusitis. The true incidence of respiratory tract infections caused by these organisms is not known, because most specimens are contaminated with oral secretions. However, the observation of many gram-negative diplococci associated with inflammatory cells in a well-collected respiratory specimen would support the etiologic role of these organisms. Most isolates of *N. sicca* and *N. mucosa* are susceptible to penicillin, although low-level resistance caused by altered penicillin-binding protein (i.e., PBP$_2$) has been observed.

CASE STUDY AND QUESTIONS

■ A 22-year-old female schoolteacher was brought to the emergency room after a 2-day history of headache and fever. On the day of admission, the patient had failed to come to school or to phone in to explain why. When notified of this fact, the patient's mother had gone to her apartment, where she found the patient in bed, confused and highly agitated.

The patient was comatose when she arrived in the emergency room. Purpuric skin lesions were present on her trunk and arms. Analysis of her CSF revealed the presence of 380 cells/mm^3 (93% polymorphonuclear leukocytes), a protein concentration of 220 mg/dL, and a glucose concentration of 32 mg/dL. Gram stain of CSF showed many gram-negative diplococci, and the same organism was isolated from blood and CSF. The patient died despite prompt initiation of therapy with penicillin.

1. What is the most likely organism responsible for this fulminant disease? What is the most likely source of this organism?
2. Chemoprophylaxis should be administered to which people? What are the criteria for administering chemoprophylaxis?
3. What other diseases are caused by this organism?
4. What virulence factors have been associated with other bacterial species in this genus?

BIBLIOGRAPHY

Campos J et al: Genetic diversity of penicillin-resistant *Neisseria meningitidis*, *J Infect Dis* 166:173–177, 1992.

Van Deuren M et al: Update on meningococcal disease with emphasis on pathogenesis and clinical management, *Clin Microbiol Rev* 13:144–166, 2000.

Feldman HA: The meningococcus: a twenty year perspective, *Rev Infect Dis* 8:288–294, 1986.

Galimand M et al: High-level chloramphenicol resistance in *Neisseria meningitidis*, *N Engl J Med* 339:868–874, 1998.

Hook EW, Holmes KK: Gonococcal infections, *Ann Intern Med* 102:229–243, 1985.

Jackson LA et al: Prevalence of *Neisseria meningitidis* relatively resistant to penicillin in the United States: 1991, *J Infect Dis* 169:438–441, 1994.

Knapp JS: Antimicrobial resistance in *Neisseria gonorrhoeae* in the United States, *Clin Microbiol Newsletter* 21:1–7, 1999.

MacLennan JM et al: Safety, immunogenicity, and induction of immunologic memory by a serogroup C meningococcal conjugate vaccine in infants: a randomized controlled trial, *JAMA* 283:2795–2801, 2000.

Morris SA et al: Perspectives on pathogenic *Neisseria*, *Clin Microbiol Rev* 2(suppl):1–149, 1989.

Rosenstein NE et al: The changing epidemiology of meningococcal disease in the United States, 1992–1996, *J Infect Dis* 180:1894–1901, 1999.

Salyers AA, Whitt DD: *Bacterial pathogenesis: a molecular approach*, Washington, DC, 1994, American Society for Microbiology.

Stephens DS et al: Interaction of *Neisseria meningitidis* with human nasopharyngeal mucosa: attachment and entry into columnar epithelial cells, *J Infect Dis* 148:369–376, 1983.

Winstead JM et al: Meningococcal pneumonia: characterization and review of cases seen over the past 25 years, *Clin Infect Dis* 30:87–94, 2000.

CHAPTER 29

Enterobacteriaceae

The family Enterobacteriaceae is the largest, most heterogeneous collection of medically important gram-negative bacilli. A total of 32 genera and more than 130 species have been described. These genera have been classified based on biochemical properties, antigenic structure, and nucleic acid hybridization and sequencing. Despite the complexity of this family, fewer than 20 species are responsible for more than 95% of the infections (Box 29–1).

Enterobacteriaceae are ubiquitous organisms, being found worldwide in soil, water, and vegetation, and are part of the normal intestinal flora of most animals, including humans. These bacteria cause a variety of human diseases, including 30% to 35% of all septicemias, more than 70% of urinary tract infections (UTIs), and many intestinal infections. Some organisms (e.g., *Salmonella typhi*, *Shigella* species, *Yersinia pestis*) are always associated with disease, whereas others (e.g., *Escherichia coli*, *Klebsiella pneumoniae*, *Proteus mirabilis*) are members of the normal commensal flora that can cause opportunistic infections. A third group of Enterobacteriaceae exists—those normally commensal organisms that become pathogenic when they acquire virulence factor genes on plasmids, bacteriophages, or pathogenicity islands (e.g., *E. coli* associated with gastroenteritis). Infections with the Enterobacteriaceae can originate from an animal reservoir (e.g., most *Salmonella* species, *Yersinia* species), from a human carrier (e.g., *Shigella* species, *S. typhi*), or through the endogenous spread of organisms in a susceptible patient (e.g., *E. coli*) and can involve virtually all body sites (Fig. 29–1).

Physiology and Structure

Members of this family are moderately sized (0.3 to 1.0 × 1.0 to 6.0 μm), gram-negative bacilli (Fig. 29–2). They are either nonmotile or motile with peritrichous flagella and do not form spores. All members can grow rapidly aerobically and anaerobically (facultative anaerobes) on a variety of nonselective (e.g., blood agar) and selective (e.g., MacConkey agar) media. The Enterobacteriaceae have simple nutritional requirements, ferment glucose, reduce nitrate, and are catalase-positive and oxidase-negative. The absence of cytochrome oxidase activity is an important characteristic, because it can be measured rapidly with a simple test and is used to distinguish the Enterobacteriaceae from many other fermentative and nonfermentative gram-negative bacilli.

Characteristics of the organisms' colonies on different media have been used to identify common members of the family Enterobacteriaceae. For example, the ability to ferment lactose has been used to differentiate lactose-fermenting strains (e.g., *Escherichia*, *Klebsiella*, *Enterobacter*, *Citrobacter*, and *Serratia* species) from strains that do not ferment lactose or do so slowly (e.g., *Proteus*, *Salmonella*, *Shigella*, and *Yersinia* species). Resistance to bile salts in some selective media has been used to separate enteric pathogens (e.g., *Shigella*, *Salmonella*) from commensal organisms that are inhibited by bile salts (e.g., gram-positive and some gram-negative bacteria present in the gastrointestinal tract). Some Enterobacteriaceae have prominent capsules (e.g., *Klebsiella*), whereas other strains are surrounded by a loose-fitting, diffusible slime layer.

The heat-stable lipopolysaccharide (LPS) is the major cell wall antigen and consists of three components: the somatic O polysaccharide, a core polysaccharide common to all Enterobacteriaceae (common antigen), and lipid A (Fig. 29–3). The serologic classification of the Enterobacteriaceae is based on three major groups of antigens: somatic O polysaccharides, capsular K antigens (either protein or polysaccharide), and the flagellar H proteins. Specific O antigens are present in each genus, although cross-reactions between closely related genera are common (e.g., *Salmonella* with *Citrobacter*, *Escherichia* with *Shigella*). The antigens are detected by agglutination with specific antibodies. The heat-labile K antigens may interfere with detection of the O antigens. This problem is circumvented by boiling of the organism to remove the K antigens.

Different genera both within and outside the family Enterobacteriaceae possess K antigens; for example, *E.*

BOX 29–1. Common Medically Important Enterobacteriaceae

Citrobacter freundii, Citrobacter koseri
Enterobacter aerogenes, Enterobacter cloacae
Escherichia coli
Klebsiella pneumoniae, Klebsiella oxytoca
Morganella morganii
Proteus mirabilis, Proteus vulgaris
Salmonella enterica
Serratia marcescens
Shigella sonnei, Shigella flexneri
Yersinia pestis, Yersinia enterocolitica, Yersinia pseudo-
    tuberculosis

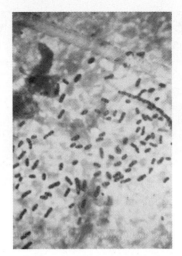

FIGURE 29–2. Gram stain of *Klebsiella pneumoniae.*

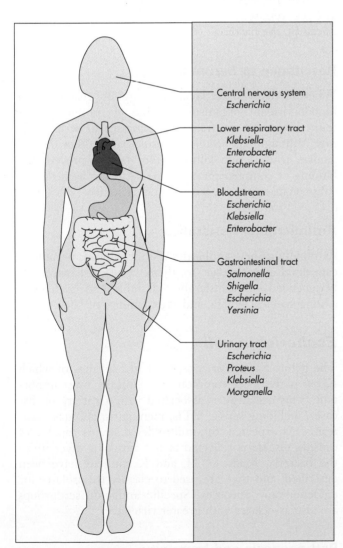

FIGURE 29–1. Sites of infections with common members of the Enterobacteriaceae listed in order of prevalence.

coli K1 cross-reacts with *Neisseria meningitidis* and *Haemophilus influenzae,* and *Klebsiella pneumoniae* cross-reacts with *Streptococcus pneumoniae.* The H antigens are heat-labile, flagellar proteins. They may be absent from a cell, or they may undergo antigenic variation and be present in two phases.

Pathogenesis and Immunity

Numerous virulence factors have been identified in the members of the family Enterobacteriaceae. Some are common to all genera (Box 29–2), and others are unique to specific virulent strains.

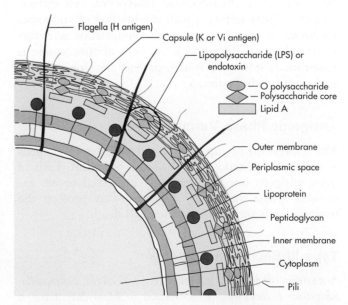

FIGURE 29–3. Antigenic structure of Enterobacteriaceae.

Endotoxin

Endotoxin is a virulence factor shared among all aerobic and some anaerobic gram-negative bacteria. The activity of this toxin depends on the lipid A component of lipopolysaccharide, which is released at cell lysis. Many of the systemic manifestations of gram-negative bacterial infections are initiated by endotoxin, including the following:

1. Activation of complement
2. Release of cytokines
3. Leukocytosis
4. Thrombocytopenia
5. Disseminated intravascular coagulation
6. Fever
7. Decreased peripheral circulation
8. Shock
9. Death

Capsule

Encapsulated Enterobacteriaceae are protected from phagocytosis by the hydrophilic capsular antigens, which repel the hydrophobic phagocytic cell surface. These antigens interfere with the binding of antibodies to the bacteria and are poor immunogens or activators of complement. The protective role of the capsule is diminished, however, if the patient develops specific anti-capsular antibodies.

Antigenic Phase Variation

The expression of capsular K and flagellar H antigens is under the genetic control of the organism. Each of these antigens can be alternately expressed or not expressed (phase variation), a feature that protects the bacteria from antibody-mediated cell death.

Type III Secretion Systems

A variety of distinct bacteria (e.g., *Yersinia*, *Salmonella*, *Shigella*, *Escherichia*, *Pseudomonas*, *Chlamydia*) have a common effector system for delivering their virulence genes into targeted eukaryotic cells. This system, referred to as the **type III secretion system,** consists of approximately 20 proteins that facilitate secretion of bacterial virulence factor into host cells. Although the virulence factors and their effects differ among the various gram-negative bacilli, the general mechanism by which the virulence factors are introduced is the same. In the absence of the type III secretion system, the bacteria lose their virulence.

Sequestration of Growth Factors

Nutrients are provided to the organisms in enriched culture media, but the bacteria must become nutritional scavengers when growing in vivo. Iron is an important growth factor required by bacteria, but it is bound in heme proteins (e.g., hemoglobin, myoglobin) or in iron-chelating proteins (e.g., transferrin, lactoferrin). The bacteria counteract the binding by producing their own competitive iron-chelating compounds (e.g., siderophores **enterobactin** and **aerobactin**). Iron can also be released from host cells by hemolysins produced by the bacteria.

Resistance to Serum Killing

Whereas many bacteria can be rapidly cleared from blood, virulent organisms capable of producing systemic infections are frequently resistant to serum killing. Although the bacterial capsule can protect the organism from serum killing, other factors prevent the binding of complement components to the bacteria and subsequent complement-mediated clearance.

Antimicrobial Resistance

As rapidly as new antibiotics are introduced, organisms can develop resistance to them. This resistance can be encoded on transferable plasmids and exchanged among species, genera, and even families of bacteria.

Escherichia coli

The genus *Escherichia* consists of five species, of which *E. coli* is the most common and clinically most important. This organism is associated with a variety of diseases, including sepsis, UTIs, meningitis, and gastroenteritis. As expected, the multitude of strains capable of causing disease is reflected in the antigenic diversity of the bacteria. Many O, H, and K antigens have been described, and they are used to classify the isolates for epidemiologic purposes. Specific antigenic serogroups are also associated with greater virulence.

Pathogenesis and Immunity

E. coli possesses a broad range of virulence factors (Box 29-3). In addition to the general factors possessed by

BOX 29–3. Specialized Virulence Factors Associated with *Escherichia coli*

Adhesins

Colonization factor antigens CFA/I, CFA/II, and CFA/III.
Aggregative adherence fimbriae AAF/I and AAF/II.
Bundle-forming protein (Bfp).
Intimin.
P pili.
Ipa protein.
Dr fimbriae.

Exotoxins

Heat-stable toxins STa and STb.
Shiga toxins Stx-1 and Stx-2.
Hemolysin HlyA.
Heat-labile toxins LT-I and LT-II.

---

all members of the family Enterobacteriaceae, *Escherichia* strains responsible for diseases such as UTIs and gastroenteritis possess specialized virulence factors. Two general categories are adhesins and exotoxins.

Adhesins

E. coli is able to remain in the urinary tract or gastrointestinal tract because the organisms are able to adhere to the cells at these sites and avoid being eliminated by the flushing action of voided urine or intestinal motility. Strains of *E. coli* possess numerous highly specialized adhesins. They include colonization factor antigens (CFA/I, CFA/II, CFA/III), aggregative adherence fimbriae (AAF/I, AAF/III), bundle-forming pili (Bfp), intimin, P pili (which also binds to P blood group antigens), Ipa (invasion plasmid antigen) protein, and Dr fimbriae (which bind to Dr blood group antigens).

Exotoxins

E. coli also produces a diverse spectrum of exotoxins. These include Shiga toxins (Stx-1, Stx-2), heat-stable toxins (STa and STb), and heat-labile toxins (LT-I and LT-II). Additionally, hemolysins (HlyA) are considered important in the pathogenesis of disease caused by uropathogenic *E. coli*. The precise mechanisms by which these toxins function are described in the following sections.

Epidemiology

Large numbers of *E. coli* are present in the gastrointestinal tract, and the bacteria are common causes of sepsis, neonatal meningitis, infections of the urinary tract, and gastroenteritis (Box 29–4). For example, *E. coli* are (1) the most common gram-negative bacilli isolated from patients with sepsis (Fig. 29–4), (2) responsible for causing more than 80% of all community-acquired UTIs as well as most hospital-acquired infections, and (3) a prominent cause of gastroenteritis in developing countries. Most infections (with the exception of neonatal meningitis and gastroenteritis) are endogenous; that is, the *E. coli* that are part of the patient's normal microbial flora are able to establish infection when the patient's defenses are compromised.

Clinical Diseases

Septicemia

Typically, septicemia caused by gram-negative bacilli such as *E. coli* originates from infections in the urinary or gastrointestinal tract (e.g., an intra-abdominal infection with sepsis following intestinal perforation). The mortality associated with *E. coli* septicemia is high for patients in whom immunity is compromised or the primary infection is in the abdomen or central nervous system.

Urinary Tract Infection

Most gram-negative bacilli that produce UTIs originate in the colon, contaminate the urethra, ascend into the bladder, and may migrate to the kidney or prostate. UTI is an ascending infection, as opposed to an infection caused by the hematogenous spread of the organism to the urinary tract. Although most strains of *E. coli* can produce UTIs, disease is more common with certain specific serogroups. These bacteria are particularly virulent because of their ability to produce adhesins (primarily P pili, AAF/I, AAF/III, and Dr), which bind to cells lining the bladder and upper urinary tract (preventing the elimination of the bacteria in voided urine), and hemolysin HlyA, which lyses erythrocytes and other cell types (leading to cytokine release and stimulation of an inflammatory response).

Neonatal Meningitis

E. coli and group B streptococci cause the majority of central nervous system infections in infants younger than 1 month. Approximately 75% of the *E. coli* strains possess the K1 capsular antigen. This serogroup is also commonly present in the gastrointestinal tracts of pregnant women and newborn infants. However, the reason this serogroup has a predilection for causing disease in newborns is not understood.

Gastroenteritis

The strains of *E. coli* that cause gastroenteritis are subdivided into the following six groups: enterotoxigenic

BOX 29–4. Summary of *Escherichia coli* Infections

Physiology and Structure

Gram-negative bacilli.
    Facultative anaerobe.
    Fermenter.
    Oxidase negative.
    Outer membrane makes the organisms susceptible to drying.
    Lipopolysaccharide consists of outer somatic O polysaccharide, core polysaccharide (common antigen), and lipid A (endotoxin).

Virulence

Refer to Boxes 29–2 and 29–3.
    Endotoxin.
    Permeability barrier of outer membrane.
    Adhesins (e.g., colonization factor antigen, Dr adhesins).
    Exotoxins (e.g., heat-stabile and heat-labile enterotoxins, Shiga toxins).
    Invasive capacity.

Epidemiology

Most common aerobic, gram-negative bacilli in the gastrointestinal tract.
    Most infections are endogenous (patient's normal microbial flora).
    Strains causing gastroenteritis are generally acquired exogenously.

Diseases

Bacteremia (most commonly isolated gram-negative bacillus).

Urinary tract infection (most common cause of bacterial UTIs; limited to bladder (cystitis) or can spread to kidneys (pyelonephritis) or prostate (prostatitis).
    At least six different pathogenic groups cause gastroenteritis (ETEC, EPEC, EIEC, EHEC, EAEC, DAEC); most cause diseases in developing countries, although EHEC is an important cause of hemorrhagic colitis (HC) and hemolytic uremic syndrome (HUS) in the United States.
    Neonatal meningitis (usually with strains carrying the K1 capsular antigen).
    Intra-abdominal infections (associated with intestinal perforation).

Diagnosis

Organisms grow rapidly on most culture media.

Treatment, Prevention, and Control

Treatment guided by in vitro susceptibility tests.
    Infections are controlled by use of appropriate infection-control practices to reduce the risk of nosocomial infections (e.g., restricting use of antibiotics, avoiding unnecessary use of urinary tract catheters).
    Maintenance of high hygienic standards to reduce the risk of exposure to gastroenteritis strains.
    Proper cooking of beef products to reduce risk of EHEC infections.

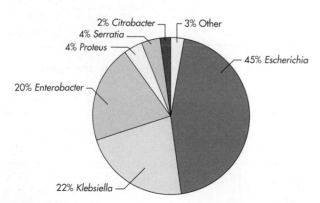

FIGURE 29–4. Incidence of Enterobacteriaceae associated with bacteremia. (Data courtesy Barnes-Jewish Hospital, St. Louis.)

(ETEC), enteropathogenic (EPEC), enteroinvasive (EIEC), enterohemorrhagic (EHEC), enteroaggregative (EAEC), and diffusely adherent *E. coli* (DAEC) (Table 29–1).

ETEC. Disease caused by **enterotoxigenic *E. coli* (ETEC)** is seen most commonly in developing countries, although almost 80,000 cases are estimated to occur annually in the United States. Infections are observed in either young children in developing countries or travelers to these areas. The inoculum for disease is high, so infections are primarily acquired through consumption of fecally contaminated food or water. Person-to-person spread does not occur.

ETEC produce two classes of enterotoxins: heat-labile toxins (LT-I, LT-II) and heat-stabile toxins (STa and STb). Whereas LT-II is not associated with human disease, LT-I is functionally and structurally similar to cholera toxin (see Chapter 30) and is associated with human disease. This toxin consists of one A subunit and five identical B subunits. The B subunits bind to the same receptor as cholera toxin (GM_1 ganglio-

TABLE 29–1. Gastroenteritis Caused by *Escherichia coli*

Organism	Site of Action	Disease	Pathogenesis
Enterotoxigenic *E. coli* (ETEC)	Small intestine	Traveler's diarrhea; infant diarrhea in underdeveloped countries; watery diarrhea, vomiting, cramps, nausea, low-grade fever	Plasmid-mediated heat-stable and/or heat-labile enterotoxins that stimulate hypersecretion of fluids and electrolytes
Enteropathogenic *E. coli* (EPEC)	Small intestine	Infant diarrhea in underdeveloped countries; fever, nausea, vomiting, nonbloody stools	Plasmid-mediated A/E histopathology with disruption of normal microvillus structure resulting in malabsorption and diarrhea
Enteroinvasive *E. coli* (EIEC)	Large intestine	Disease in underdeveloped countries; fever, cramping, watery diarrhea; may progress to dysentery with scant, bloody stools	Plasmid-mediated invasion and destruction of epithelial cells lining colon
Enterohemorrhagic *E. coli* (EHEC)	Large intestine	Hemorrhagic colitis (HC) with severe abdominal cramps, initial watery diarrhea, followed by grossly bloody diarrhea; little or no fever; may progress to hemolytic uremic syndrome (HUS)	Mediation by cytotoxic Shiga toxins (Stx-1, Stx-2), which disrupt protein synthesis; A/E lesions with destruction of intestinal microvillus resulting in decreased absorption
Enteroaggregative *E. coli* (EAEC)	Small intestine	Infant diarrhea in underdeveloped countries; persistent watery diarrhea with vomiting, dehydration, and low-grade fever	Plasmid-mediated aggregative adherence of bacilli ("stacked bricks") with shortening of microvilli, mononuclear infiltration, and hemorrhage; decreased fluid absorption
Diffuse aggregative *E. coli* (DAEC)	Small intestine	Watery diarrhea in infants 1 to 5 years of age	Stimulates elongation of microvilli

sides) as well as other surface glycoproteins on epithelial cells in the small intestine.

Following endocytosis, the A subunit of LT-I translocates across the membrane of the vacuole. The A subunit has ADP (adenosine diphosphate)–ribosyltransferase activity and interacts with a membrane protein (Gs) that regulates adenylate cyclase. The net effect of this interaction is an increase in cyclic adenosine monophosphate (cAMP) levels, with enhanced secretion of chloride and a decreased absorption of sodium and chloride. These changes are manifested in a watery diarrhea. Exposure to the toxin also stimulates prostaglandin secretion and production of inflammatory cytokines, resulting in further fluid loss.

STa but not STb is associated with human disease. STa is a small, monomeric toxin that binds to guanylate cyclase, leading to an increase in the level of cyclic guanosine monophosphate and subsequent hypersecretion of fluids. Genes for LT-I and STa are present on a transferable plasmid, which can also carry the genes for the adhesins (CFA/I, CFA/II, CFA/III). The receptors for these colonization factors are glycoproteins.

Secretory diarrhea caused by ETEC develops after a 1- to 2-day incubation period and persists for an average of 3 to 4 days. The symptoms—cramps, nausea, vomiting (rare), and watery diarrhea—are similar to those of cholera but are milder. Neither histologic changes of the intestinal mucosa nor inflammation is observed. Disease mediated by heat-labile toxin is indistinguishable from that mediated by heat-stable toxin. Toxin production is not associated with specific serogroups, so tissue cultures or animal model assays for toxin activity must be performed if toxigenic strains are to be detected. Nucleic acid probes have also been used to detect the toxin genes.

EPEC. **Enteropathogenic *E. coli*** is the major cause of infant diarrhea in impoverished countries. Disease is rare in older children and adults, presumably because they have developed protective immunity. Although specific O serogroups have been associated with outbreaks of EPEC diarrhea in nurseries, the serotyping of the *E. coli* isolated in random or endemic disease is discouraged except in epidemiologic investigations.

Disease is characterized by bacterial attachment to epithelial cells of the small intestine with subsequent effacement (destruction) of the microvillus (**A/E histopathology**). These strains form microcolonies on the epithelial cell surface with the bacteria attached to the host cells by means of cup-like pedestals. Initially a loose attachment mediated by bundle-forming pili (**Bfp**) occurs, followed by active secretion of proteins by the bacterial type III secretion system into the host epithelial cell. One protein, **translocated intimin receptor** (**Tir**), is inserted into the epithelial cell membrane (this process is mediated by two other secreted proteins) and functions as a receptor for an outer membrane bacterial adhesin, **intimin**. Diarrhea results from malabsorption due to microvilli destruction.

EIEC. **Enteroinvasive *E. coli* (EIEC)** strains are closely related by phenotypic and pathogenic properties to *Shigella*. The bacteria are able to invade and destroy the colonic epithelium, producing a disease characterized initially by watery diarrhea. A minority of patients progress to the dysenteric form of disease, consisting of fever, abdominal cramps, and blood and leukocytes in stool specimens. A series of bacterial genes carried on a plasmid mediate invasion (*pInv* **genes**) into the colonic epithelium. The bacteria then lyse the phagocytic vacuole and replicate in the cell cytoplasm. Movement within the cytoplasm and into adjacent epithelial cells is regulated by formation of actin tails (similar to that observed with *Listeria*). This process of epithelial cell destruction with inflammatory infiltration can progress to colonic ulceration.

EHEC. **Enterohemorrhagic *E. coli* (EHEC)** strains are the most common strains producing disease in developed countries. It is estimated that these bacteria cause more than 100,000 infections and almost 100 deaths each year in the United States. The ingestion of fewer than 100 bacilli can produce disease. The severity of the disease caused by EHEC ranges from mild, uncomplicated diarrhea to **hemorrhagic colitis** with severe abdominal pain, bloody diarrhea, and little or no fever.

Hemolytic uremic syndrome (**HUS**), a disorder characterized by acute renal failure, thrombocytopenia, and microangiopathic hemolytic anemia, is a complication in 10% of infected children younger than 10 years. EHEC disease is most common in the warm months, and the highest incidence is in children younger than 5 years. Most cases of disease have been attributed to the consumption of undercooked ground beef or other meat products, water, unpasteurized milk or fruit juices (e.g., cider made from apples contaminated with feces from cattle), uncooked vegetables, and fruits.

Initially, a nonbloody diarrhea with abdominal pain develops in patients after a 3- to 4-day incubation period. Vomiting is observed in about half the patients.

Within 2 days of onset, disease can progress to a bloody diarrhea with severe abdominal pain. Complete resolution of symptoms typically occurs after 4 to 10 days in most untreated patients; however, HUS is a serious complication, particularly in young children. Death can occur in 3% to 5% of patients with HUS, and severe sequelae (e.g., renal impairment, hypertension, CNS manifestations) can occur in as many as 30% of patients.

EHEC strains express a Shiga toxin (i.e., Stx-1, Stx-2, or both), induce A/E lesions on epithelial cells, and possess a 60-MDa plasmid that carries genes for other virulence factors. Stx-1 is essentially identical to the Shiga toxin produced by *Shigella dysenteriae*; Stx-2 has 60% homology. Both toxins are encoded by lysogenic bacteriophages. Both have one A subunit and five B subunits, with the B subunits binding to a specific glycolipid on the host cell (globotriaosylceramide, Gb_3). A high concentration of Gb_3 receptors are in the intestinal villus and renal endothelial cells. After the A subunit is internalized, it is cleaved into two molecules, and the A_1 fragment binds to 28S ribosomal ribonucleic acid (rRNA) and disrupts protein synthesis. Destruction of the intestinal villus results in decrease absorption with a relative increase in fluid secretion.

HUS has been preferentially associated with the production of Stx-2, which has been shown to destroy glomerular endothelial cells. The destruction results in decreased glomerular filtration and acute renal failure. The Stx toxins also stimulate expression of inflammatory cytokines (e.g., tumor necrosis factor-α [TNF-α], interleukin-6), which among other effects enhance expression of Gb_3. More than 50 serogroups of EHEC have been isolated; however, the majority that cause human disease in the United States are believed to be serotype O157:H7.

EAEC. **Enteroaggregative *E. coli* (EAEC)** strains have been implicated as a cause of persistent, watery diarrhea with dehydration in infants in developing countries. The bacteria are characterized by their autoagglutination in a "stacked brick" arrangement. This process is mediated by bundle-forming fimbriae (aggregative adherence fimbriae I and II [AAF/I and AAF/II]), which are carried on a plasmid. EAEC stimulate secretion of mucus, which traps the bacteria in a biofilm overlying the epithelium of the small intestine. Shortening of the microvilli, mononuclear infiltration, and hemorrhage are then observed. A cytotoxin has not been demonstrated but is likely to be present.

DAEC. **Diffusely adherent *E. coli* (DAEC)** have been recognized from their characteristic adherence to cultured cells. DAEC stimulate elongation of the microvilli with the bacteria embedded in the cell membrane.

The resulting disease is a watery diarrhea found primarily in infants between 1 and 5 years of age.

Salmonella

The taxonomic classification of the genus *Salmonella* is problematic, and 2463 unique serogroups are currently described (Box 29–5). Careful analysis of DNA homology has revealed that the genus consists of two species: *Salmonella enterica* and *Salmonella bongori*. *S. enterica* is further subdivided into six subspecies, with most human pathogens in the first subspecies, *S. enterica* subsp. *enterica*. Unfortunately, the historical approach has been to refer to the numerous serogroups as species (e.g., *S. typhi*, *Salmonella typhimurium*, *Salmonella enteritidis*). In an effort to prevent confusion, this approach is used here.

Pathogenesis and Immunity

After ingestion and passage through the stomach, salmonellae are able to invade and replicate in the **M (microfold) cells** located in Peyer's patches of the terminal portion of the small intestine. These cells typically transport foreign antigens to the underlying macrophages for clearance. Two separate type III secretion systems mediate the initial invasion into the intestinal mucosa (*Salmonella* pathogenicity island 1 [**SPI-1**]) and subsequent systemic disease (**SPI-2**). Binding to M cells is mediated by species-specific fimbriae. The SPI-1 secretion system then introduces salmonella-secreted invasion proteins (**Sips** or **Ssps**) into the M cells, resulting in rearrangement of the host cell actin with subsequent membrane ruffling. The ruffled membranes surround and engulf salmonellae, leading to intracellular replication in the phagosome with subsequent host cell death and spread to adjacent epithelial cells and

---

BOX 29–5. Summary of *Salmonella* Infections

Physiology and Structure

Gram-negative bacilli.
   Facultative anaerobe.
   Fermenter.
   Oxidase-negative.
   Outer membrane makes the organisms susceptible to drying.
   Lipopolysaccharide consists of outer somatic O polysaccharide, core polysaccharide (common antigen), and lipid A (endotoxin).
   More than 2400 O serotypes (commonly referred to as individual *Salmonella* species).

Virulence

Refer to Box 29–2.
   Tolerant to acids in phagocytic vesicles.
   Can survive in macrophages and spread from the intestine to other body sites (particularly true of *S. typhi*).
   Endotoxin.

Epidemiology

Most infections are acquired by eating contaminated food products (poultry, eggs, and dairy products the most common sources of infection).
   Direct fecal-oral spread in children.
   S. typhi and *S. paratyphi* are strict human pathogens (no alternative reservoir); these infections are passed person to person; asymptomatic long-term colonization occurs commonly.
   Individuals at risk for infection include those who eat improperly cooked poultry or eggs, patients with reduced gastric acid levels, and immunocompromised patients (especially patients with acquired immunodeficiency syndrome).

Infections occur worldwide, particularly in the warm months of the year.

Diseases

Asymptomatic colonization (primarily with *S. typhi* and *S. paratyphi*).
   Enteric fever (also called typhoid fever [*S. typhi*] or paratyphoid fever [*S. paratyphi*]).
   Enteritis characterized by fever, nausea, vomiting, bloody or nonbloody diarrhea, and abdominal cramps.
   Bacteremia (most commonly seen with *S. typhi*, *S. paratyphi*, *S. choleraesuis*, and *S. enteritidis*).

Diagnosis

Isolation from stool specimens requires use of selective media.

Treatment, Prevention, and Control

Antibiotic treatment not recommended for enteritis because the duration of disease may be prolonged.
   Infections with *S. typhi* and *S. paratyphi* or disseminated infections with other organisms should be treated with an effective antibiotic (selected by in vitro susceptibility tests); fluoroquinolones (e.g., ciprofloxacin), chloramphenicol, trimethoprim/sulfamethoxazole, or a broad-spectrum cephalosporin can be used.
   Most infections can be controlled by proper preparation of poultry and eggs (completely cooked) and avoidance of contamination of other foods with uncooked poultry products.
   Carriers of *S. typhi* and *S. paratyphi* should be identified and treated.
   Vaccination against *S. typhi* can reduce the risk of disease for travelers into endemic areas.

lymphoid tissue. The inflammatory response confines the infection to the gastrointestinal tract, mediates the release of prostaglandins, and stimulates cAMP and active fluid secretion.

Salmonella species are also protected from stomach acids and the acid pH of the phagosome by an **acid tolerance response (ATR) gene**. Catalase and superoxide dismutase are other factors that protect the bacteria from intracellular killing.

Epidemiology

Salmonella can colonize virtually all animals, including poultry, reptiles, livestock, rodents, domestic animals, birds, and humans. Animal-to-animal spread and the use of *Salmonella*-contaminated animal feeds maintain an animal reservoir. Serogroups such as *S. typhi* and *Salmonella paratyphi* are highly adapted to humans and do not cause disease in nonhuman hosts. Other *Salmonella* strains (e.g., *Salmonella choleraesuis*) are adapted to animals and, when they infect humans, can cause severe disease. Finally, many strains have no host specificity and cause disease in both human and nonhuman hosts.

Most infections result from the ingestion of contaminated food products and, in children, from direct fecal-oral spread. The incidence of disease is greatest in children younger than 5 years and adults older than 60 years, who are infected during the summer and autumn months when contaminated foods are consumed at outdoor social gatherings. The most common sources of human infections are poultry, eggs, dairy products, and foods prepared on contaminated work surfaces (e.g., cutting boards where uncooked poultry was prepared). Approximately 50,000 cases of *Salmonella* infections are reported annually in the United States, although it has been estimated that more than 1.4 million infections occur each year.

S. typhi infections occur when food or water contaminated by infected food handlers is ingested. There is no animal reservoir. A total of 375 *S. typhi* infections was reported in the United States in 1998, most of which were acquired during foreign travel. It is estimated that 16 million cases occur each year worldwide.

The infectious dose for *S. typhi* infections is low, so person-to-person spread is common. In contrast, a large inoculum (e.g., 10^6 to 10^8 bacteria) is required for symptomatic disease to develop with other *Salmonella* species. The organisms can multiply to this high density if contaminated food products are improperly stored (e.g., left at room temperature). The infectious dose is lower for people at high risk for disease because of age, immunosuppression or underlying disease (leukemia, lymphoma, sickle cell disease), or reduced gastric acidity.

Clinical Diseases

The following four forms of *Salmonella* infection exist: enteritis, septicemia, enteric fever, and asymptomatic colonization.

Enteritis

Enteritis is the most common form of salmonellosis. Symptoms generally appear 6 to 48 hours after the consumption of contaminated food or water, with the initial presentation consisting of nausea, vomiting, and nonbloody diarrhea. Fever, abdominal cramps, myalgias, and headache are also common. Colonic involvement can be demonstrated in the acute form of the disease. Symptoms can persist from 2 days to 1 week before spontaneous resolution.

Septicemia

All *Salmonella* species can cause bacteremia, although infections with *S. choleraesuis*, *S. paratyphi*, and *S. typhi* more commonly lead to a bacteremic phase. The risk for *Salmonella* bacteremia is higher in pediatric and geriatric patients as well as in patients with the acquired immunodeficiency syndrome (AIDS). The clinical presentation of *Salmonella* bacteremia is like that of other gram-negative bacteremias; however, localized suppurative infections, such as osteomyelitis, endocarditis, and arthritis, can occur in as many as 10% of patients.

Enteric Fever

S. typhi produce a febrile illness called **typhoid fever**. A mild form of this disease, referred to as **paratyphoid fever**, is produced by *S. paratyphi A*, *Salmonella schottmuelleri* (formerly *S. paratyphi B*), and *Salmonella hirschfeldii* (formerly *S. paratyphi C*). In contrast to other *Salmonella* infections, the bacteria responsible for enteric fever pass through the cells lining the intestines and are engulfed by macrophages. They replicate after being transported to the liver, spleen, and bone marrow. Ten to 14 days after ingestion of the bacilli, patients experience gradually increasing fever with nonspecific complaints of headache, myalgias, malaise, and anorexia. These symptoms persist for a week or longer and are followed by gastrointestinal symptoms. This cycle corresponds to an initial bacteremic phase that is followed by colonization of the gallbladder and then reinfection of the intestines.

Asymptomatic Colonization

The species of *Salmonella* responsible for causing typhoid and paratyphoid fevers are maintained by human colonization. Chronic colonization for more than 1 year after symptomatic disease develops in 1% to 5% of patients, the gallbladder being the reservoir in most patients. Chronic colonization with other species of *Salmonella* occurs in less than 1% of patients and does not represent an important source of human infection.

Shigella

Epidemiology

Unlike the genus *Salmonella*, the taxonomic classification of *Shigella* is quite simple (Box 29–6). Four species consisting of more than 45 O antigen–based serogroups have been described: *S. dysenteriae, Shigella flexneri, Shigella boydii,* and *Shigella sonnei. S. sonnei* is the most common cause of shigellosis in the industrial world, and *S. flexneri* is the most common cause in developing countries. More than 23,600 *Shigella* infections were reported in the United States in 1998; however, it is estimated that almost 450,000 cases occur each year. This figure pales in comparison with the estimated 150 million cases that occur annually worldwide.

Shigellosis is primarily a pediatric disease; 70% of all infections occur in children younger than 15 years. Endemic disease in adults is common in male homosexuals and in household contacts of infected children. Epidemic outbreaks of disease occur in daycare centers, nurseries, and custodial institutions. Shigellosis is transmitted by the fecal-oral route, primarily by people with contaminated hands and less commonly in water or food. Because as few as 200 bacilli can establish disease, shigellosis spreads rapidly in communities where sanitary standards and the level of personal hygiene are low.

Pathogenesis and Immunity

Shigella cause disease by invading and replicating in cells lining the colonic mucosa. Structural gene proteins mediate the adherence of the organisms to the cells as well as their invasion, intracellular replication,

---

BOX 29–6. Summary of *Shigella* Infections

Physiology and Structure

Gram-negative bacilli.
  Facultative anaerobe.
  Fermenter.
  Oxidase-negative.
  Outer membrane makes the organisms susceptible to drying.
  Lipopolysaccharide consists of somatic O polysaccharide, core polysaccharide (common antigen), and lipid A (endotoxin).
  Four species recognized: *S. sonnei* responsible for most infections in developed countries, *S. flexneri* for infections in developing countries, and *S. dysenteriae* for the most severe infections. *S. boydii* is not commonly isolated.

Virulence

Refer to Box 29–2.
  Endotoxin and genes for adherence, invasion, and intracellular replication.
  Permeability barrier of outer membrane.
  Exotoxin (Shiga toxin) is produced by *S. dysenteriae;* disrupts protein synthesis and produces endothelial damage.
  Hemolytic colitis (HC) and hemolytic uremic syndrome (HUS) associated with *Shigella*.

Epidemiology

Humans are only reservoir for these bacteria.
  Disease spread person-to-person by fecal-oral route.
  Patients at highest risk for disease are young children in daycare centers, nurseries, and custodial institutions; siblings and parents of these children; male homosexuals.

  Relatively few organisms can produce disease (highly infectious).
  Disease is worldwide with no seasonal incidence (consistent with person-to-person spread involving a low inoculum).

Diseases

Gastroenteritis (shigellosis).
  Most common form is an initial watery diarrhea progressing within 1 to 2 days to abdominal cramps and tenesmus (with or without bloody stools).
  Asymptomatic carriage develops in a small number of patients (reservoir for future infections).
  A severe form of disease is caused by *S. dysenteriae* (bacterial dysentery).

Diagnosis

Isolation from stool specimens requires use of selective media.

Treatment, Prevention, and Control

Antibiotic therapy shortens the course of symptomatic disease and fecal shedding.
  Treatment should be guided by in vitro susceptibility tests.
  Empiric therapy can be initiated with a fluoroquinolone or trimethoprim/sulfamethoxazole.
  Appropriate infection control measures should be instituted to prevent spread of the organism, including hand washing and proper disposal of soiled linens.

and cell-to-cell spread. These genes are carried on a large virulence plasmid but are regulated by chromosomal genes. Thus, the presence of the plasmid does not ensure functional gene activity.

Shigella species appear unable to attach to differentiated mucosal cells; rather, they first attach to and invade the M cells located in Peyer's patches. The type III secretion system mediates secretion of four proteins (**IpaA, IpaB, IpaC, IpaD**) into epithelial cells and macrophages. These proteins induce membrane ruffling on the target cell, leading to engulfment of the bacteria. Shigella are able to lyse the phagocytic vacuole and replicate in the host cell cytoplasm (unlike *Salmonella*, which replicate in the vacuole). With the rearrangement of actin filaments in the host cells, the bacteria are propelled through the cytoplasm to adjacent cells, where cell-to-cell passage occurs. In this way, *Shigella* organisms are protected from immune-mediated clearance. Shigellae survive phagocytosis by inducing programmed cell death (**apoptosis**). This process also leads to the release of interleukin-1β, resulting in the attraction of polymorphonuclear leukocytes into the infected tissues. This in turn destabilizes the integrity of the intestinal wall and allows the bacteria to reach the deeper epithelial cells.

S. dysenteriae produce an exotoxin, **Shiga toxin**. Like the toxin produced by EHEC, the Shiga toxin has one A subunit and five B subunits. The B subunits bind to a host cell glycolipid (Gb$_3$) and facilitate transfer of the A subunit into the cell. The A subunit cleaves the 28S rRNA in the 60S ribosomal subunit, thereby preventing the binding of aminoacyl-transfer RNA and disrupting protein synthesis. The primary manifestation of toxin activity is damage to the intestinal epithelium; however, in a small subset of patients, the Shiga toxin can mediate damage to the glomerular endothelial cells, resulting in renal failure (HUS).

Clinical Diseases

Shigellosis is characterized by abdominal cramps, diarrhea, fever, and bloody stools. The clinical signs and symptoms of the disease appear 1 to 3 days after bacilli are ingested. The bacilli initially colonize the small intestine and begin to multiply within the first 12 hours. The first sign of infection, profuse watery diarrhea without histologic evidence of mucosal invasion, is mediated by an enterotoxin. However, the cardinal feature of shigellosis is lower abdominal cramps and tenesmus, with abundant pus and blood in the stool. It results from invasion of the colonic mucosa by the bacilli. Abundant neutrophils, erythrocytes, and mucus are found in the stool. Infection is generally self-limited, although antibiotic treatment is recommended to reduce the risk of secondary spread to family members and other contacts. Asymptomatic colonization of the

organism in the colon develops in a small number of patients and represents a persistent reservoir for infection.

Yersinia

The genus *Yersinia* consists of 10 species, with *Y. pestis*, *Yersinia enterocolitica*, and *Yersinia pseudotuberculosis* the well-known human pathogens (Box 29–7). *Y. enterocolitica* can be subdivided into six biogroups (1A, 1B, 2, 3, 4, and 5). 1A strains are not associated with human disease, but the other biogroups are all capable of causing human disease.

Pathogenesis and Immunity

Y. pestis is a highly virulent pathogen that causes systemic disease with a high mortality rate; *Y. enterocolitica* and *Y. pseudotuberculosis* are primarily enteric pathogens that are rarely isolated from the blood stream. All three species of *Yersinia* carry plasmids with virulence genes.

A common characteristic of the pathogenic *Yersinia* species is their ability to resist phagocytic killing. This property is mediated by the type III secretion system. On contact with phagocytic cells, the bacteria secrete proteins into the phagocyte that dephosphorylate several proteins required for phagocytosis (YopH gene product), induce cytotoxicity by disrupting actin filaments (YopE gene product), and initiate apoptosis in macrophages (YopJ/P gene product). The type III secretion system also suppresses cytokine production, in turn diminishing the inflammatory immune response to infection.

Y. pestis has the following two additional plasmids that encode virulence genes: (1) fraction 1 (F1) gene, which codes for an antiphagocytic protein capsule, and (2) plasminogen activator (Pla) protease gene, which degrades complement components C3b and C5a, preventing opsonization and phagocytic migration, respectively. The Pla gene also degrades fibrin clots, permitting *Y. pestis* to spread rapidly. Other virulence factors specifically associated with *Y. pestis* are serum resistance and the ability of the organism to absorb organic iron as a result of a siderophore-independent mechanism.

Epidemiology

All *Yersinia* infections are zoonotic, with humans the accidental hosts. There are two forms of *Y. pestis* infection, **urban plague**, for which rats are the natural reservoirs, and **sylvatic plague**, which causes infections in squirrels, rabbits, field rats, and domestic cats. Pigs, rodents, livestock, and rabbits are the natural reservoirs for *Y. enterocolitica*, whereas rodents, wild animals, and

BOX 29–7. Summary of *Yersinia* Infections

Physiology and Structure

Gram-negative bacilli.
  Facultative anaerobe.
  Fermenter.
  Oxidase-negative.
  Outer membrane makes the organisms susceptible to drying.
  Lipopolysaccharide consists of somatic O polysaccharide, core polysaccharide (common antigen), and lipid A (endotoxin).
  Y. pestis is covered with a protein capsule.
  Some species (e.g., *Y. enterocolitica*) can grow at cold temperatures (e.g., can grow to high numbers in contaminated, refrigerated food or blood products).

Virulence

Refer to Box 29–2.
  Capsule on *Y. pestis* is antiphagocytic.
  Y. pestis is also resistant to serum killing.
  Yersinia with genes for adherence, cytotoxic activity, inhibition of phagocytic migration and engulfment, and inhibition of platelet aggregation.

Epidemiology

Y. pestis is a zoonotic infection with humans the accidental host. Natural reservoirs include rats, squirrels, rabbits, and domestic animals. Disease is spread by flea bites or direct contact with infected tissues or person-to-person by inhalation of infectious aerosols from a patient with pulmonary disease.

Other *Yersinia* infections are spread through exposure to contaminated food products or blood products (*Y. enterocolitica*).
  Colonization with other *Yersinia* species can occur.

Diseases

Y. pestis causes bubonic plague (most common) and pulmonary plague, both having a high mortality rate.
  Other *Yersinia* species cause gastroenteritis (acute watery diarrhea or chronic diarrhea) and transfusion-related sepsis.
  Enteric disease in children may manifest as enlarge mesenteric lymph nodes and mimic acute appendicitis.

Diagnosis

Organisms grow on most culture media; prolonged storage at 4°C can selectively enhance isolation.

Treatment, Prevention, and Control

Y. pestis infections are treated with streptomycin; tetracyclines, chloramphenicol, or trimethoprim/sulfamethoxazole can be administered as alternative therapy.
  Enteric infections with other *Yersinia* species are usually self-limited. If antibiotic therapy is indicated, most organisms are susceptible to broad-spectrum cephalosporins, aminoglycosides, chloramphenicol, tetracyclines, and trimethoprim/sulfamethoxazole.
  Plague is controlled by reduction of the rodent population and vaccination of individuals at risk.
  Other *Yersinia* infections are controlled by the proper preparation of food products.

---

game birds are the natural reservoirs for *Y. pseudotuberculosis*.

Plague, caused by *Y. pestis*, was one of the most devastating diseases in history. Epidemics of the plague were recorded in the Old Testament. The first of three major pandemics (urban plague) started in Egypt in 541 AD and spread throughout North Africa, Europe, central and southern Asia, and Arabia. By the time this pandemic ended in the mid-700s, a major proportion of the population in these countries had died from plague. The second pandemic, which started in the 1320s, resulted over a 5-year period in more than 25 million deaths in Europe alone (30% to 40% of the population). The third pandemic began in China in the 1860s and spread to Africa, Europe, and the Americas. Epidemic and sporadic cases of the disease continue to this day. In the last decade, an average of 10 cases annually were reported in the United States, with disease (sylvatic plague) primarily in the western United States.

Urban plague is maintained in rat populations and is spread among rats or between rats and humans by infected fleas. Fleas become infected during a blood meal from a bacteremic rat. After the bacteria replicate in the flea gut, the organisms can be transferred to another rodent or to humans. Urban plague has been eliminated from most communities by the effective control of rats and better hygiene. In contrast, sylvatic plague is difficult or impossible to eliminate, because the mammalian reservoirs and flea vectors are widespread. *Y. pestis* produces a fatal infection in the animal reservoir. Thus, cyclic patterns of human disease occur as the opportunity for contact with the reservoir population increases or decreases. Infections can also be acquired through the ingestion of contaminated animals or the handling of contaminated animal tissues. Although the organism is highly infectious, human-to-human spread is uncommon unless the patient has pulmonary involvement.

Y. enterocolitica is a common cause of enterocolitis in Scandinavian and other European countries as well as in the colder areas of North America. It is estimated that more than 96,000 cases occur annually in the United States, 90% of the infections being associated with consumption of contaminated meat, milk, and water. Most studies show that infections are more common during the cold months. Virulence with this organism is associated with specific serogroups. The most common serogroups found in Europe, Africa, Japan, and Canada are O3 and O9. Serogroup O8 has been identified in the United States. *Y. pseudotuberculosis* is a relatively uncommon cause of human disease.

Clinical Diseases

The two clinical manifestations of *Y. pestis* infection are bubonic plague and pneumonic plague. **Bubonic plague** is characterized by an incubation period of no more than 7 days after a person has been bitten by an infected flea. Patients have a high fever and a painful bubo (inflammatory swelling of the lymph nodes) in the groin or axilla. Bacteremia develops rapidly if patients are not treated, and as many as 75% die. The incubation period (2 to 3 days) is shorter in patients with **pneumonic plague**. Initially, these patients experience fever and malaise, and pulmonary signs develop within 1 day. The patients are highly infectious; person-to-person spread occurs by aerosols. The mortality rate in untreated patients with pneumonic plague exceeds 90%.

Approximately two thirds of all *Y. enterocolitica* infections are enterocolitis, as the name implies. The gastroenteritis is typically associated with ingestion of contaminated food products or water. After an incubation period of 1 to 10 days (average, 4 to 6 days), the patient experiences disease characterized by diarrhea, fever, and abdominal pain that last for as long as 1 to 2 weeks. A chronic form of the disease can also develop and persist for months. Disease involves the terminal ileum and, if the mesenteric lymph nodes become enlarged, can mimic acute appendicitis. *Y. enterocolitica* infection is most common in children, with pseudoappendicitis posing a particular problem in this age group. *Y. pseudotuberculosis* can also produce an enteric disease with the same clinical features. Other manifestations seen in adults are septicemia, arthritis, intra-abdominal abscess, hepatitis, and osteomyelitis.

In 1987, *Y. enterocolitica* was first reported to cause blood transfusion–related bacteremia and endotoxic shock. Because *Yersinia* organisms can grow at 4°C, this organism can multiply to toxic concentrations in nutritionally rich blood products that are contaminated and refrigerated for at least 3 weeks. There is no reliable method for detecting contaminated blood products. Use of products stored for a shorter time would probably eliminate the problem, because the organisms would not be able to multiply to toxic levels. However, this method is not practical given the current shortage of blood products.

Other Enterobacteriaceae

Klebsiella

Members of the genus *Klebsiella* have a prominent capsule that is responsible for the mucoid appearance of isolated colonies and the enhanced virulence of the organisms in vivo. The most commonly isolated member of this genus is *K. pneumoniae*, which can cause community-acquired primary lobar pneumonia. Alcoholics and people with compromised pulmonary function are at increased risk for pneumonia because of their inability to clear aspirated oral secretions from the lower respiratory tract. Pneumonia due to *Klebsiella* species frequently involves the necrotic destruction of alveolar spaces, formation of cavities, and the production of blood-tinged sputum. These bacteria also cause wound, soft tissue, and UTIs.

Proteus

Infection of the urinary tract with *P. mirabilis* is the most common disease produced by this genus. *P. mirabilis* produces large quantities of urease, which splits urea into carbon dioxide and ammonia. This process raises the urine pH and facilitates the formation of renal stones. The increased alkalinity of the urine is also toxic to the uroepithelium. Despite the serologic diversity of these organisms, infection has not been associated with any specific serogroup. Furthermore, in contrast to *E. coli*, the pili on *P. mirabilis* may decrease its virulence by enhancing phagocytosis of the bacilli.

Enterobacter, Citrobacter, Morganella, Serratia

Primary infections caused by *Enterobacter*, *Citrobacter*, *Morganella*, or *Serratia* are rare in immunocompetent patients. They are more common causes of hospital-acquired infections in neonates and immunocompromised patients. For example, *Citrobacter koseri* has been recognized to have a predilection for causing meningitis and brain abscesses in neonates. Antibiotic therapy for these genera can be ineffective, because the organisms are frequently resistant to multiple antibiotics. Resistance is a particularly serious problem with *Enterobacter* species.

Laboratory Diagnosis

Culture

Members of the family Enterobacteriaceae grow readily on culture media. Specimens of normally sterile material, such as spinal fluid and tissue collected at surgery, can be inoculated onto nonselective blood agar media. Selective media (e.g., MacConkey agar, eosin–methylene blue [EMB] agar) are used for the culture of specimens normally contaminated with other organisms (e.g., sputum, feces). Use of these selective differential agars enables the separation of lactose-fermenting Enterobacteriaceae from nonfermentative strains, thereby providing information that can be used to guide empirical antimicrobial therapy. Highly selective or organism-specific media are useful for the recovery of organisms such as *Salmonella* and *Shigella* in stool specimens, where an abundance of normal flora can obscure the presence of these important pathogens.

It is difficult to recover *Y. enterocolitica*, because this organism grows slowly at traditional incubation temperatures and prefers cooler temperatures, at which it is more active metabolically. Clinical laboratories have exploited this property, however, by mixing the fecal specimen with saline and then storing the specimen at 4°C for 2 weeks or more before subculturing it to agar media. This **cold enrichment** permits the growth of *Yersinia* but inhibits or kills other organisms in the specimen. Although use of the cold enrichment method does not aid in the initial management of a patient with *Yersinia* gastroenteritis, it has helped elucidate the role of this organism in chronic intestinal disease.

Biochemical Identification

There are many diverse species in the family Enterobacteriaceae. The citations listed in the Bibliography of this chapter provide additional information about their biochemical identification. Biochemical test systems have become increasingly sophisticated, and now virtually all members of the family can be identified accurately in less than 24 hours with one of several commercially available identification systems.

Serologic Classification

Serologic testing is very useful for determining the clinical significance of an isolate (e.g., serotyping specific pathogenic strains, such as *E. coli* O157:H7 or *Y. enterocolitica* O8) and for classifying isolates for epidemiologic purposes. The usefulness of this procedure is limited, however, by cross-reactions with antigenically related Enterobacteriaceae as well as with organisms from other bacterial families.

Treatment, Prevention, and Control

Antibiotic therapy for infections with Enterobacteriaceae must be guided by in vitro susceptibility test results and clinical experience. Whereas some organisms such as *E. coli* and *P. mirabilis* are susceptible to many antibiotics, others can be highly resistant. Furthermore,

susceptible organisms exposed to subtherapeutic concentrations of antibiotics in a hospital setting can rapidly develop resistance. In general, antibiotic resistance is more common in hospital-acquired infections than in community-acquired infections. Antibiotic therapy is not recommended for some infections. For example, symptomatic relief, but not antibiotic treatment, is usually recommended for patients with *E. coli* or *Salmonella* gastroenteritis, because antibiotics can prolong the fecal carriage of these organisms or increase the risk of secondary complications (e.g., HUS with EHEC infections in children).

It is difficult to prevent infections with Enterobacteriaceae because these organisms are a major part of the endogenous microbial population. However, some risk factors for the infections should be avoided; they are as follows:

1. The unrestricted use of antibiotics that can select for resistant bacteria.
2. The performance of procedures that traumatize mucosal barriers without prophylactic antibiotic coverage.
3. The use of urinary catheters.

Unfortunately, many of these factors are present in patients at greatest risk for infection (e.g., immunocompromised patients confined to the hospital for extended periods).

Exogenous infection with Enterobacteriaceae is theoretically easier to control. For example, the source of infections with organisms such as *Salmonella* is well-defined. However, these bacteria are ubiquitous in poultry and eggs. Unless care is taken in the preparation and refrigeration of such foods, little can be done to control these infections. *Shigella* organisms are predominantly transmitted in young children, but it is difficult to interrupt the fecal-hand-mouth transmission responsible for spreading the infection in this population. Outbreaks of these infections can be effectively prevented and controlled only through education and the introduction of appropriate infection-control procedures (e.g., hand washing, proper disposal of soiled diapers and linens) in the settings where these infections typically occur.

Vaccination with formalin-killed *Y. pestis* has proved effective for people at high risk. Chemoprophylaxis with tetracycline has also proved useful for people in close contact with a patient with pneumonic plague. Improvements in the live, attenuated *S. typhi* vaccines have led to development of significant protection in populations in which the incidence of endemic disease is high. This protection can persist for up to 5 years. Inactivated whole-cell vaccines, as well as vaccination with purified Vi antigen (the polysaccharide capsular antigen of *S. typhi* associated with virulence), are also protective.

CASE STUDY AND QUESTIONS

■ A 25-year-old, previously healthy woman came to the emergency room for the evaluation of bloody diarrhea and diffuse abdominal pain of 24 hours' duration. She complained of nausea and had vomited twice. She reported no history of inflammatory bowel disease, previous diarrhea, or contact with other people with diarrhea. The symptoms began 24 hours after she had eaten an undercooked hamburger at a local fast food restaurant. Rectal examination revealed watery stool with gross blood. Sigmoidoscopy showed diffuse mucosal erythema and petechiae with a modest exudation but no ulceration or pseudomembranes.

1. Name four genera of Enterobacteriaceae that can cause gastrointestinal disease. Name two genera that can cause hemorrhagic colitis.

2. What virulence factor mediates this disease?

3. Name the six groups of *E. coli* that can cause gastroenteritis. What is characteristic of each group of organisms?

4. What are the four forms of *Salmonella* infection?

5. Differentiate between disease caused by *S. typhi* and that caused by *S. sonnei*.

6. Describe the epidemiology of the two forms of disease caused by *Y. pestis*.

BIBLIOGRAPHY

Abbott S: *Klebsiella, Enterobacter, Citrobacter,* and *Serratia.* In Murray PR et al, editors: *Manual of clinical microbiology,* ed 7, Washington, DC, 1999, American Society of Microbiology.

Ackers ML et al: Laboratory-based surveillance of *Salmonella* serotype *typhi* infections in the United States: antimicrobial resistance on the rise, *JAMA* 283:2668–2673, 2000.

Bopp CA et al: *Escherichia, Salmonella,* and *Shigella.* In Murray PR et al, editors: *Manual of clinical microbiology,* ed 7, Washington, DC, 1999, American Society of Microbiology

Bottone EJ: *Yersinia enterocolitica:* the charisma continues, *Clin Microbiol Rev* 10:257–276, 1997.

Brenner F et al: *Salmonella* nomenclature, *J Clin Microbiol* 38:2465–2467, 2000.

Butler T: *Yersinia* infections: centennial of the discovery of the plague bacillus, *Clin Infect Dis* 19:655–663, 1994.

Darwin KH, Miller VL: Molecular basis of the interaction of *Salmonella* with the intestinal mucosa, *Clin Microbiol Rev* 12:405–428, 1999.

Doran TI: The role of *Citrobacter* in clinical disease of children: review, *Clin Infect Dis* 28:384–394, 1999.

Farmer JJ: Enterobacteriaceae: introduction and identification. In Murray PR et al, editors: *Manual of clinical microbiology,* ed 7, Washington, DC, 1999, American Society of Microbiology.

Glandt M et al: Enteroaggregative *Escherichia coli* as a cause of traveler's diarrhea: clinical response to ciprofloxacin, *Clin Infect Dis* 29:335–338, 1999.

Glynn MK et al: Emergence of multidrug-resistant *Salmonella enterica* serotype *typhimurium* DT104 infections in the United States, *N Engl J Med* 338:1333–1338, 1998.

Holt JG et al: *Bergey's manual of determinative bacteriology,* ed 9, Baltimore, 1994, Williams & Wilkins.

Hueck C: Type III protein secretion systems in bacterial pathogens of animals and plants, *Microbiol Mol Biol Rev* 62:379–433, 1998.

Johnson JR: Virulence factors in *Escherichia coli* urinary tract infection, *Clin Microbiol Rev* 4:80–128, 1991.

Koornhof HJ et al: Yersiniosis II: the pathogenesis of *Yersinia* infections, *Eur J Clin Microbiol Infect Dis* 18:87–112, 1999.

Mead P et al: Food-related illness and death in the United States, *Emerging Infect Dis* 5:607–625, 1999.

Miller VL et al, editors: *Molecular genetics of bacterial pathogenesis,* Washington, DC, 1994, American Society of Microbiology.

Nataro JP, Kaper JB: Diarrheagenic *Escherichia coli, Clin Microbiol Rev* 11:142–201, 1998.

Paton JC, Paton AW: Pathogenesis and diagnosis of Shiga toxin-producing *Escherichia coli* infections, *Clin Microbiol Rev* 11:450–479, 1998.

Perry RD, Fetherston JD: *Yersinia pestis*—etiologic agent of plague, *Clin Microbiol Rev* 10:35–66, 1997.

Podschun R, Ullmann U: *Klebsiella* spp. as nosocomial pathogens: epidemiology, taxonomy, typing methods, and pathogenicity factors, *Clin Microbiol Rev* 11:589–603, 1998.

Reisner BS: Plague—past and present, *Clin Microbiol Newsletter* 18:153–160, 1996.

Salyers AA, Whitt DD: *Bacterial pathogenesis: a molecular approach,* Washington, DC, 1994, American Society of Microbiology.

Sanders WE, Sanders CC: *Enterobacter* spp: pathogens poised to flourish at the turn of the century, *Clin Microbiol Rev* 10:220–241, 1997.

Sansonetti PJ: Molecular and cellular biology of *Shigella flexneri* invasiveness: from cell assay systems to shigellosis, *Curr Topics Microbiol Immunol* 180:1–19, 1992.

Slutsker L et al: *Escherichia coli* O157:H7 diarrhea in the United States: clinical and epidemiologic features, *Ann Intern Med* 126:505–513, 1997.

Smego RA et al: Yersiniosis I: microbiological and clinicoepidemiological aspects of plague and non-plague *Yersinia* infections, *Eur J Clin Microbiol Infect Dis* 18:1–15, 1999.

Su C, Brandt LJ: *Escherichia coli* O157:H7 infection in humans, *Ann Intern Med* 123:698–714, 1995.

Wong CS et al: The risk of the hemolytic-uremic syndrome after antibiotic treatment of *Escherichia coli* O157:H7 infections, *N Engl J Med* 342:1930–1936, 2000.

C H A P T E R 3 0

Vibrio, Aeromonas, and Plesiomonas

The second major group of gram-negative, facultatively anaerobic (i.e., growing aerobically and anaerobically), fermentative bacilli are the genera *Vibrio*, *Aeromonas*, and *Plesiomonas*. These organisms were at one time classified together in the family Vibrionaceae and were separated from the Enterobacteriaceae on the basis of a positive oxidase reaction and the presence of polar flagella. These organisms were also classified together because they are primarily found in water and are able to cause gastrointestinal disease. Molecular biology techniques have established, however, that these genera are only distantly related and belong in three separate families: *Vibrio* and *Aeromonas* are now classified in the families Vibrionaceae and Aeromonadaceae, respectively. It is interesting (at least to taxonomists) that *Plesiomonas* are closely related to *Proteus* and have now been placed in the Enterobacteriaceae family, notwithstanding the differences noted previously. Despite this taxonomic reorganization, it is appropriate to consider these bacteria together because their epidemiology and range of diseases are similar.

Vibrio

The genus *Vibrio* is composed of many species of curved bacilli, and 12 species have been implicated in human infections (Table 30–1). *Vibrio cholerae*, *Vibrio parahaemolyticus*, and *Vibrio vulnificus* are the most prominent.

Physiology and Structure

Vibrio species can grow on a variety of simple media within a broad temperature range (from 18°C to 37°C). *V. cholerae* (Box 30–1) can grow in the absence of salt; most other species that are pathogenic in humans require salt (halophilic). *V. cholerae*, the etiologic agent of cholera, is the best-known member of the genus. Members of the species are subdivided on the basis of their somatic O antigens, with more than 200 serogroups described to date. *V. cholerae* O1 and O139 are responsible for causing classic cholera, which can occur in epidemics or worldwide pandemics. Other strains of *V. cholerae* can also cause human disease but not in epidemics.

V. cholerae O1 can be subdivided into the following two biotypes: El Tor and classical. These groups are important for the epidemiologic classification of isolates. *V. parahaemolyticus* can also be subdivided on the basis of differences in the somatic O and capsular K antigens.

Pathogenesis and Immunity

Multiple chromosomal genes involved in the virulence of *V. cholerae* O1 have been characterized (Table 30–2). These include genes for the two subunits of **cholera toxin** (*ctx*A and *ctx*B), the toxin coregulated pilus (*tcp*) gene complex, accessory colonization factor (*acf*) genes, the hemagglutination-protease (*hap*) gene, and neuraminidase. Regulatory genes (e.g., *ToxR* regulator) control the expression of these genes.

Clearly, the best-studied and most important of these virulence factors is cholera toxin. This toxin is a complex A-B toxin that is structurally and functionally similar to the heat-labile enterotoxin of *Escherichia coli*. The B subunit of cholera toxin binds to the ganglioside GM_1 receptors on the intestinal epithelial cells. The A subunit is internalized and activates adenylate cyclase, resulting in a hypersecretion of water and electrolytes (Fig. 30–1). Severely infected patients can lose as much as 1 L of fluid per hour during the height of the disease. Such a tremendous loss of fluid would normally flush the organisms out of the gastrointestinal tract; however, *V. cholerae* are able to adhere to the mucosal cell layer by means of (1) the pili encoded by the *tcp* gene complex and (2) chemotaxis proteins encoded by the *acf* genes. Nonadherent strains are unable to establish infection.

The *hap* gene is largely responsible for the mild to moderate diarrhea seen with *ctx*-negative *V. cholerae* vaccine strains. Stimulation of interleukin-8 production by the *hap* gene product and degradation of the tight junctions in the intestinal mucosa result in intestinal

TABLE 30-1. *Vibrio* **Species Associated with Human Disease**

Species	Source of Infection	Clinical Disease
V. cholerae	Water, food	Gastroenteritis
V. parahaemolyticus	Shellfish, seawater	Gastroenteritis, wound infection, bacteremia
V. vulnificus	Shellfish, seawater	Bacteremia, wound infection, cellulitis
V. alginolyticus	Seawater	Wound infection, external otitis
V. hollisae	Shellfish	Gastroenteritis, wound infection, bacteremia
V. fluvialis	Seafood	Gastroenteritis, wound infection, bacteremia
V. damsela	Seawater	Wound infection
V. metschnikovii	Unknown	Bacteremia
V. mimicus	Fresh water	Gastroenteritis, wound infection, bacteremia
*V. furnissii**	Seawater	Gastroenteritis
*V. cincinnatiensis**	Unknown	Bacteremia, meningitis
*V. carchariae**	Seawater	Wound (shark bite)

* Isolates rarely associated with human infection.

BOX 30-1. **Summary of** *Vibrio cholerae* **Infections**

Physiology and Structure

Curved gram-negative bacilli.
   Facultative anaerobe.
   Fermenter.
   Simple nutritional requirements; do not require salt for growth but can tolerate it.
   Strains subdivided by their O cell wall antigens.
   Two biotypes of *V. cholerae* O1 strains—El tor and classical (this is important for epidemiologic classification of isolates).

Virulence

Refer to Table 30-2 for complete listing.
   Cholera toxin is primarily responsible for the watery diarrhea characteristic of this species.
   Adherence factors are important for establishing the initial colonization in the intestines, permitting the toxin to function.

Epidemiology

Organism responsible for major pandemics (worldwide epidemics), with significant mortality in underdeveloped countries.
   All pandemics of cholera caused by serotype O1, although O139 can cause similar diseases and may cause a pandemic.
   Organism found in estuarine and marine environments worldwide (including along the coast of the United States) associated with chitinous shellfish.
   Organism can multiply freely in water.

Bacterial levels increase in contaminated waters during the warm months.
   Spread by consumption of contaminated food or water.
   Direct person-to-person spread is rare because the infectious dose is high.
   The infectious dose is high because most organisms are killed by stomach acids.

Disease

Cholera.
   Presentation can range from mild disease to severe life-threatening disease.
   Disease is characterized by profuse watery diarrhea.
   Death is caused by electrolyte abnormalities and massive fluid loss.

Diagnosis

Culture should be performed early in course of disease with fresh stool specimens.

Treatment, Prevention, and Control

Fluid and electrolyte replacement are crucial.
   Antibiotic therapy reduces the bacterial burden and exotoxin production, as well as duration of diarrhea.
   Doxycycline (adults), trimethoprim-sulfamethoxazole (children), or furazolidone (pregnant women) is administered.
   Improved hygiene is critical for control.
   The killed parenteral vaccine is of no value, but the newer oral vaccine has some protective value.

TABLE 30–2. Virulence Factors of *Vibrio cholerae* O1 and O139

Virulence Factor	Biologic Effect
Cholera toxin	Hypersecretion of electrolytes and water
Coregulated pilus	Adherence to mucosal cells
Accessory colonization	Adhesin factor
Hemagglutination-protease (mucinase)	Induces intestinal inflammation and degradation of tight junctions
Siderophores	Iron sequestration
Neuraminidase	Increase toxin receptors

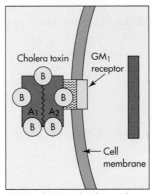

The complete toxin binding to the GM₁-ganglioside receptor on the cell membrane via the binding subunits (B).

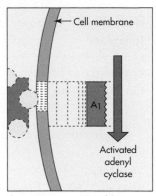

The active portion (A₁) of the A subunit enters the cell and activates adenyl cyclase.

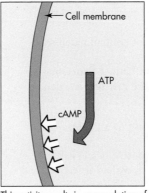

This activity results in accumulation of cyclic adenosine 3′, 5′–monophosphate (cAMP) along the cell membrane.

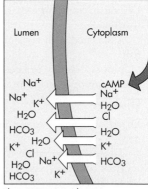

The cAMP causes the active secretion of sodium (Na⁺), chloride (Cl⁻), potassium (K⁺), bicarbonate (HCO₃), and water (H₂O) out of the cell into the intestinal lumen.

FIGURE 30–1. Mechanism of action of cholera toxin.

inflammation and diarrhea. Unlike other, non-O1 serotypes, *V. cholerae* O139 possesses the same virulence complex as that of the O1 strains. Thus, the ability of the O139 strains to adhere to the intestinal mucosa and produce cholera toxin is the reason these strains can produce a watery diarrhea similar to cholera.

The means by which other *Vibrio* species cause disease is less clearly understood, although a variety of potential virulence factors have been identified (Table 30–3). Most virulent strains of *V. parahaemolyticus* (Box 30–2) produce thermostable direct hemolysin (TDH). TDH is an enterotoxin that induces chloride ion secretion in epithelial cells by increasing intracellular calcium.

Epidemiology

Vibrio species, including *V. cholerae,* grow naturally in estuarine and marine environments worldwide. All *Vibrio* species are able to survive and replicate in contaminated waters with increased salinity and at temperatures of 10°C to 30°C. Pathogenic vibrios can also flourish in waters with chitinous shellfish—hence the association between *Vibrio* infections and the consumption of shellfish. Asymptomatically infected humans can also be an important reservoir for this organism in areas where *V. cholerae* disease is endemic.

Seven major pandemics of cholera have occurred since 1817, resulting in thousands of deaths and major socioeconomic changes. Sporadic disease and epidemics occurred before this time, but worldwide spread of the disease became possible only with intercontinental travel resulting from increased commerce as well as wars.

The seventh pandemic, which was caused by *V. cholerae* O1 biotype El Tor, began in Asia in 1961 and spread to Africa, Europe, and Oceania in the 1970s and 1980s. In 1991, the pandemic strain spread to Peru

TABLE 30–3. Virulence Factors of Other *Vibrio* Species

Organism	Virulence Factors
V. parahaemolyticus	Thermostable direct hemolysin
V. vulnificus	Serum resistance, antiphagocytic polysaccharides, cytolysins, collagenase, protease, siderophore
V. alginolyticus	Collagenase
V. hollisae	Heat-stable and heat-labile enterotoxin, hemolysin
V. damsela	Cytolysin

BOX 30–2. Summary of *Vibrio parahaemolyticus* Infections

Physiology and Structure

Curved gram-negative bacilli.
    Facultative anaerobe.
    Fermenter.
    Simple nutritional requirements but requires salt for growth.

Virulence

Refer to Table 30–3 for complete listing.
    Hemolysin.
    Adhesin.

Epidemiology

Organism found in estuarine and marine environments worldwide.
    Associated with consumption of contaminated shellfish.
    Not commonly isolated in the United States but is a major pathogen in countries where raw fish is eaten.

Diseases

Diarrhea ranging from mild disease to a cholera-like illness.
    Typical presentation is an explosive, watery diarrhea.
    Less commonly associated with wound infections and bacteremia.

Diagnosis

Culture should be performed as with *V. cholerae*.

Treatment, Prevention, and Control

Self-limited disease, although antibiotics can shorten symptoms and fluid loss.
    Disease prevented by proper cooking of shellfish.
    No vaccines are available.

---

and subsequently has caused disease in most countries in South and Central America as well as in the United States and Canada. By June 1995, more than 1 million cases and 10,000 deaths resulting from the disease had been reported in the Americas. A new epidemic strain emerged in 1992 in India and rapidly spread across Asia into Europe and the United States. This strain, *V. cholerae* O139 Bengal, produces the cholera toxin and shares other traits with *V. cholerae* O1. This is the first non-O1 strain capable of causing epidemic disease and is capable of producing disease in adults who were previously infected with the O1 strain (showing that no protective immunity is conferred).

Cholera is spread by contaminated water and food. Direct person-to-person spread is unusual, because a high inoculum (e.g., more than 10^8 organisms) is required to establish infection in a person with normal gastric acidity. In a person with achlorhydria or hypo-

chlorhydria, the infectious dose can be as low as 10^3 to 10^5 organisms. Cholera is usually seen in communities with poor sanitation. Indeed, one benefit from the cholera pandemics was recognition of the role of contaminated water in the spread of disease and the need to improve community sanitation systems so that the disease could be controlled.

Infections caused by *V. parahaemolyticus*, *V. vulnificus*, and other pathogenic vibrios result from the consumption of improperly cooked seafood, particularly oysters, or exposure to contaminated seawater. Gastroenteritis caused by vibrios occurs throughout the year, because oysters are typically contaminated with abundant organisms year-round. In contrast, septicemia and wound infections with *Vibrio* occur during the warm months, when the organisms in seawater can multiply to high numbers.

Clinical Diseases

Vibrio cholerae

Infection with *V. cholerae* O1 can range from asymptomatic colonization or a mild diarrheal disease to severe, rapidly fatal diarrhea. The clinical manifestations of cholera begin an average of 2 to 3 days after ingestion of the bacilli, with the abrupt onset of watery diarrhea and vomiting. As more fluid is lost, the feces-streaked stool specimens become colorless and odorless, free of protein, and speckled with mucus (rice-water stools). The resulting severe fluid and electrolyte loss can lead to dehydration, metabolic acidosis (bicarbonate loss), and hypokalemia and hypovolemic shock (potassium loss), with cardiac arrhythmia and renal failure. The mortality rate is 60% in untreated patients but less than 1% in patients who are promptly treated with replacement of lost fluids and electrolytes. Cholera can resolve spontaneously after a few days of symptoms. Disease caused by *V. cholerae* O139 can be as severe as disease caused by *V. cholerae* O1. Gastroenteritis caused by other serotypes of *V. cholerae* is milder and is not associated with epidemics.

Vibrio parahaemolyticus

The severity of gastroenteritis caused by *V. parahaemolyticus* can range from a self-limited diarrhea to a mild cholera-like illness. In general, the disease develops after a 5- to 72-hour incubation period (mean, 24 hours) with an explosive, watery diarrhea. No grossly evident blood or mucus is found in stool specimens except in very severe cases. Headache, abdominal cramps, nausea, vomiting, and low-grade fever may persist for 72 hours or more. The patient usually experiences an uneventful recovery. Wound infections with this organism can occur in people exposed to contaminated seawater.

Vibrio vulnificus

V. vulnificus (Box 30–3) is a particularly virulent species of *Vibrio* responsible for rapidly progressive wound infections after exposure to contaminated seawater and for septicemia after consumption of contaminated raw oysters. The wound infections are characterized by initial swelling, erythema, and pain followed by the development of vesicles or bullae and eventual tissue necrosis. Patients usually experience systemic signs of fever and chills. The mortality in patients with *V. vulnificus* septicemia can be as high as 50% unless antimicrobial therapy is started rapidly. Infections are most severe in patients with hepatic disease, hematopoietic disease, or chronic renal failure and in those receiving immunosuppressive drugs.

Other *Vibrio* Species

V. alginolyticus can cause infection in superficial wounds exposed to contaminated seawater. Infections of the ear, eye, and gastrointestinal tract have also been reported rarely. *V. hollisae, V. mimicus, V. fluvialis, V. furnissii,* and *V. damsela* are responsible for causing gastroenteritis, wound infections, and bacteremia. Single cases of infections with *V. metschnikovii* (bacteremia), *V. cincinnatiensis* (meningitis), and *V. carchariae* (wound infection) have been documented.

Laboratory Diagnosis

Microscopy

Vibrio species are small (0.5×1.5 to 3 μm), curved, gram-negative bacilli. The organisms are rarely seen in Gram-stained stool or wound specimens; however, an experienced observer using darkfield microscopy may be able to detect the characteristic motile bacilli in stool specimens.

Culture

Vibrio organisms survive poorly in an acidic or dry environment. Specimens must be collected early in the disease and inoculated promptly onto culture media. If culture will be delayed, the specimen should be mixed in a Cary-Blair transport medium and refrigerated. Vibrios survive poorly in buffered glycerol-saline, the transport medium used for most enteric pathogens.

Vibrios grow on most media used in clinical laboratories for stool cultures, including blood agar and MacConkey agar. Special selective agar for vibrios (e.g., thiosulfate citrate bile salts sucrose agar), as well as an enrichment broth (e.g., alkaline peptone broth; pH 8.6), can also be used. Isolates are identified with selective biochemical tests and serotyped using polyvalent antisera. In tests performed to identify halophilic

---

BOX 30–3. Summary of *Vibrio vulnificus* Infections

Physiology and Structure

Curved gram-negative bacilli.
    Facultative anaerobe.
    Fermenter.
    Simple nutritional requirements but requires salt for growth.

Virulence

Refer to Table 30–3 for complete listing.
    Resistant to complement- and antibody-mediated serum killing (thus, systemic infections).
    Antiphagocytic capsule.
    Production of hydrolytic enzymes (cytolysins, collagenase, proteases).

Epidemiology

Infection associated with exposure of a wound to contaminated salt water or ingestion of improperly prepared shellfish.

Diseases

Wound infections that can progress rapidly to formation of bullae and tissue necrosis.
    Septicemia following ingestion of contaminated shellfish.
    High mortality rate in immunocompromised patients.

Diagnosis

Culture wounds and blood.

Treatment, Prevention, and Control

Life-threatening illnesses that must be promptly treated with antibiotics.
    Tetracyclines or aminoglycosides treatment of choice.
    No vaccine is available.

---

vibrios, the media must be supplemented with 1% sodium chloride.

Treatment, Prevention, and Control

Patients with cholera must be promptly treated with fluid and electrolyte replacement before the resultant massive fluid loss leads to hypovolemic shock. Antibiotic therapy, although of secondary value, can reduce exotoxin production and more rapidly eliminate the organism. Doxycycline or tetracycline is the drug of choice for adults, furazolidone is used for pregnant women, and trimethoprim-sulfamethoxazole is used for children. *V. cholerae* has been reported to be resistant to tetracycline and trimethoprim-sulfamethoxazole.

V. parahaemolyticus gastroenteritis is usually a self-limited disease, although antibiotic therapy can be used in addition to fluid and electrolyte therapy in patients with severe infections. *V. vulnificus* wound infections

TABLE 30–4. Characteristics of *Aeromonas* and *Plesiomonas* Gastroenteritis

Epidemiologic and Clinical Features	*Aeromonas*	*Plesiomonas*
Natural habitat	Fresh or brackish water	Fresh or brackish water
Source of infection	Contaminated food or water	Contaminated food or water; contact with amphibians or reptiles
Clinical presentation:		
Diarrhea	Present	Present
Vomiting	Present	Present
Abdominal cramps	Present	Present
Fever	Absent	Absent
Blood/leukocytes in stool	Absent	Present
Pathogenesis	Enterotoxin (?)	Invasive

and septicemia must be promptly treated with antibiotic therapy. Tetracycline is the most effective drug in vivo, although some success has been reported for the aminoglycosides.

People infected with *V. cholerae* can shed bacteria for the first few days of acute illness and so represent important sources of new infections. Although long-term carriage of *V. cholerae* does not occur, vibrios are free-living in estuarine and marine reservoirs. Only improvements in sanitation can lead to effective control of the disease. They involve adequate sewage management, the use of purification systems to eliminate contamination of the water supply, and the implementation of appropriate steps to prevent contamination of food.

Although there is a killed parenteral cholera vaccine for O1 strains, the protection it confers is short-lived. Currently, this vaccine is not recommended for people traveling to areas with endemic disease. Two new oral vaccines have been developed and are licensed in various industrialized countries for travelers to cholera-endemic countries. One is a killed whole cell, *ctxs*B subunit toxoid combination vaccine, and the other is a genetically engineered attenuated *V. cholerae* vaccine. There is no vaccine for the O139 strains. Tetracycline prophylaxis has also been used to reduce the risk of infection in people traveling to areas where the disease is endemic but has not prevented the spread of cholera. Because the infectious dose of *V. cholerae* is high, antibiotic prophylaxis is generally unnecessary in people who use appropriate hygiene.

Aeromonas

Aeromonas is a gram-negative, facultative anaerobic bacillus that morphologically resembles members of the Enterobacteriaceae. A total of 16 species of *Aeromonas* has been described, including 11 associated with human disease. The most important pathogens are *Aeromonas hydrophila*, *Aeromonas caviae*, and *Aeromonas ve-*

ronii biovar *sobria*. The organisms are ubiquitous in fresh and brackish water.

The two major diseases associated with *Aeromonas* are gastroenteritis and wound infections (with or without bacteremia). Gastrointestinal carriage has been observed in approximately 3% of individuals, with the highest carriage in the warm months. Therefore, the isolation of this organism in enteric specimens does not indicate disease, which is determined by the clinical presentation of the patient. Gastroenteritis typically occurs after the ingestion of contaminated water or food, whereas wound infections result from exposure to contaminated water.

Although numerous potential virulence factors (e.g., endotoxin, hemolysins, enterotoxin, proteases, siderophores, adherence factors) have been identified for *Aeromonas*, their precise role is unknown. *Aeromonas* species cause (1) opportunistic systemic disease in immunocompromised patients (particularly those with hepatobiliary disease or an underlying malignancy), (2) diarrheal disease in otherwise healthy people, and (3) wound infections (Table 30–4).

Gastrointestinal disease in children is usually an acute, severe illness, whereas that in adults tends to be chronic diarrhea. Severe *Aeromonas* gastroenteritis resembles shigellosis, in that blood and leukocytes are present in the stool of affected patients. Acute diarrheal disease is self-limited, and only supportive care is indicated in affected patients.

Antimicrobial therapy is necessary in patients with chronic diarrheal disease or systemic infection. *Aeromonas* are resistant to penicillins, most cephalosporins, and erythromycin; only gentamicin, trimethoprim-sulfamethoxazole, and chloramphenicol are consistently active.

Plesiomonas

The genus *Plesiomonas* consists of facultative anaerobic, gram-negative bacilli that are oxidase-positive, have multiple polar flagella, and are differentiated from *Aeromonas* by selected biochemical reactions. Only one species has been described, *Plesiomonas shigelloides*, which is taxonomically related to *Proteus* species and serologically related to *Shigella sonnei*. The organism is found in fresh water and estuarine waters and is acquired through contact with fresh water, the consumption of seafood, or exposure to amphibians or reptiles.

As with *Aeromonas*, the absence of an animal model has prevented researchers from defining the pathogenic mechanisms of *Plesiomonas* disease. The primary disease caused by *P. shigelloides* is a self-limited gastroenteritis with onset 48 hours after exposure to the organism. A variety of uncommon extraintestinal infections has also been described. Asymptomatic carriage is rare, so isolation of this organism in a clinical specimen is generally significant. The organism is susceptible to chloramphenicol, cephalosporins, imipenem, trimethoprim-sulfamethoxazole, and fluoroquinolones and is resistant to ampicillin, carbenicillin, erythromycin, and many aminoglycosides.

CASE STUDY AND QUESTIONS

■ A 57-year-old man was hospitalized in New York City with a 2-day history of severe, watery diarrhea. The illness had begun 1 day after his return from Ecuador. The patient was dehydrated and suffering from an electrolyte imbalance (acidosis, hypokalemia). The patient made an uneventful recovery after fluid and electrolyte replacement was instituted to compensate for the losses resulting from the watery diarrhea. Stool cultures were positive for *V. cholerae*.

1. What are the characteristic clinical symptoms of cholera?

2. What is the most important virulence factor in this disease? What other virulence factors have been described? What are the modes of their action?

3. How did this patient acquire this infection? How does this situation differ from the acquisition of infections caused by *V. parahaemolyticus* or *V. vulnificus*?

4. How can cholera be controlled in areas where infection is endemic?

BIBLIOGRAPHY

Albert MJ: *Vibrio cholerae* O139 Bengal, *J Clin Microbiol* 32: 2345–2349, 1994.

Besser RE et al: Diagnosis and treatment of cholera in the United States: are we prepared? *JAMA* 272:1203–1205, 1994.

Calia KE: *Vibrio cholerae* O139: an emerging pathogen, *Clin Microbiol Newsletter* 18:17–22, 1996.

Clark RB, Janda JM: *Plesiomonas* and human disease, *Clin Microbiol Newsletter* 13:49–52, 1991.

Hlady WG, Klontz KC: The epidemiology of *Vibrio* infections in Florida, 1981–1993, *J Infect Dis* 173:1176–1183, 1996.

Holmberg SD, Farmer JJ III: *Aeromonas hydrophila* and *Plesiomonas shigelloides* as causes of intestinal infections, *Rev Infect Dis* 6:633–639, 1984.

Janda JM et al: *Aeromonas* species in septicemia: laboratory characteristics and clinical observations, *Clin Infect Dis* 19: 77–83, 1994.

Ko W-C, Chuang Y-C: *Aeromonas* bacteremia: review of 59 episodes, *Clin Infect Dis* 20:1298–1304, 1995.

Lacey SW: Cholera: calamitous past, ominous future, *Clin Infect Dis* 20:1409–1419, 1995.

Lang DR, Guerrant RL: Summary of the 29th United States–Japan Joint Conference on Cholera and Related Diarrheal Diseases, *J Infect Dis* 171:8–12, 1995.

Mahon BE et al: Reported cholera in the United States, 1992–1994: a reflection of global changes in cholera epidemiology, *JAMA* 276:307–312, 1996.

Tauxe RV et al: Epidemic cholera in the new world: translating field epidemiology into new prevention strategies, *Emerging Infect Dis* 1:141–146, 1995.

Waldor MK, Mekalanos JJ: Emergence of a new cholera pandemic: molecular analysis of virulence determinants in *Vibrio cholerae* O139 and development of a live vaccine prototype, *J Infect Dis* 170:278–283, 1994.

C H A P T E R 3 1

Campylobacter and *Helicobacter*

The classification of *Campylobacter* and *Helicobacter* has undergone many changes since the bacteria were first isolated at the beginning of this century. However, molecular biology techniques (e.g., sequence analysis of 16S rRNA genes), characterization of cell wall proteins and lipids, serologic characterization, and analysis of biochemical properties have been used to resolve much of the taxonomic confusion. These genera, along with *Arcobacter*, *Wolinella*, and *Flexispira*, belong to the same rRNA superfamily, which consists of spiral, gram-negative bacilli with (1) a low DNA guanosine plus cytosine base ratio, (2) an inability to ferment or oxidize carbohydrates (in contrast with the bacteria discussed in Chapters 29 and 30), and (3) microaerophilic growth requirements (i.e., growth only in the presence of a reduced oxygen level). *Campylobacter* and *Arcobacter* are grouped into the family Campylobacteriaceae; *Helicobacter*, *Wolinella*, and *Flexispira* are grouped into an unnamed family. Because *Campylobacter* and *Helicobacter* species are the most commonly isolated and clinically most important members of this superfamily, they are the only genera discussed in this chapter.

Campylobacter

The genus *Campylobacter* (from the Greek word *kampylos* for "curved") consists of small, comma-shaped, gram-negative bacilli (Fig. 31–1) that are motile by means of a polar flagellum. Most species are microaerobic, requiring an atmosphere with decreased oxygen and increased hydrogen and carbon dioxide levels for aerobic growth. A total of 18 species and subspecies are now recognized; 13 have been associated with human disease (Table 31–1).

Diseases caused by campylobacters are primarily gastroenteritis and septicemia. *Campylobacter jejuni* is the most common cause of bacterial gastroenteritis in the United States, and *Campylobacter coli* is responsible for 2% to 5% of the cases of campylobacter gastroenteritis. The latter is a more common cause of gastroenteritis in underdeveloped countries.

Campylobacter upsaliensis is most likely an important cause of gastroenteritis in humans; however, the true incidence of disease caused by this organism is underestimated by conventional culture methods (*C. upsaliensis* is inhibited by the antibiotics used in isolation media for other campylobacters). A variety of other species are rare causes of gastroenteritis or systemic infections. Unlike other species, *Campylobacter fetus* is most commonly responsible for causing systemic infections such as bacteremia, septic thrombophlebitis, arthritis, septic abortion, and meningitis.

Physiology and Structure

Campylobacters have a typical gram-negative cell wall structure (Box 31–1). The major antigen of the genus is the lipopolysaccharide of the outer membrane. In addition, the different somatic O polysaccharide antigens and the heat-labile capsular and flagellar antigens have been used for the epidemiologic classification of clinical isolates.

Recognition of the role of campylobacters in gastrointestinal disease was delayed, because the organisms grow best in an atmosphere of reduced oxygen (5% to 7%, microaerophilic) and increased carbon dioxide (5% to 10%). In addition, *C. jejuni* grow better at 42°C than at 37°C. These properties have now been exploited for the selective isolation of pathogenic campylobacters in stool specimens. The small size of the organisms (0.3 to 0.6 μm in diameter) has also been used to recover the bacteria by filtration of stool specimens. Campylobacters pass through 0.45-μm filters, whereas other bacteria are retained. This method was also used to demonstrate that *C. upsaliensis* caused human gastroenteritis as well as disease in domestic dogs and cats. Unfortunately, filtration of stool specimens is a cumbersome procedure and is not used in most clinical laboratories.

Pathogenesis and Immunity

Efforts to define the role of specific virulence factors in *Campylobacter* disease have been thwarted by a lack of

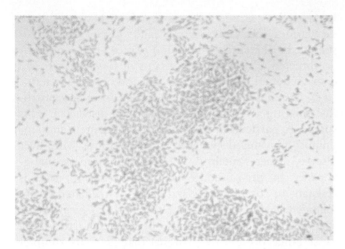

FIGURE 31–1. Gram stain showing *Campylobacter jejuni.* Note the small, curved bacilli.

an animal model to study the disease. *C. jejuni* is the best-studied species. Although adhesins, cytotoxic enzymes, and enterotoxins have been detected in this species, their specific role in disease remains poorly defined. It is clear that the probability of disease is influenced by the infectious dose. The organisms are killed when exposed to gastric acids, so conditions that decrease or neutralize gastric acid secretion favor disease. The patient's immune status also affects the se-

verity of disease. People in a population of high endemic disease develop measurable levels of specific serum and secretory antibodies and have less severe disease. Patients with hypogammaglobulinemia have prolonged, severe disease with *C. jejuni.*

C. jejuni gastrointestinal disease characteristically produces histologic damage to the mucosal surfaces of the jejunum (as implied by the species name), ileum, and colon. The mucosal surface appears ulcerated, edematous, and bloody, with crypt abscesses in the epithelial glands and infiltration of the lamina propria with neutrophils, mononuclear cells, and eosinophils. This inflammatory process is consistent with invasion of the organisms into the intestinal tissue. However, the precise roles of cytopathic toxins, enterotoxins, and endotoxic activity that have been detected in *C. jejuni* isolates have not been defined. For example, strains lacking enterotoxin activity are still fully virulent. An adhesin that mediates the attachment of the organisms to the mucosal layer has been described; however, strains without the adhesin as well as nonmotile strains are avirulent.

C. jejuni and *C. upsaliensis* have been associated with Guillain-Barré syndrome, an autoimmune disorder of the peripheral nervous system characterized by development of symmetrical weakness over a period of several days and recovery requiring weeks to months. As many as 20% of patients have residual neurologic de-

TABLE 31–1. *Campylobacter* Species Associated with Human Disease

Species	Reservoir Host	Human Disease	Frequency
C. jejuni	Poultry, pigs, bulls, dogs, cats, birds, minks, rabbits, insects	Gastroenteritis, septicemia, meningitis, spontaneous abortion, proctitis, Guillain-Barré syndrome	Common
C. jejuni subsp. *doylei*	Humans	Gastroenteritis, gastritis, septicemia	Uncommon
C. coli	Pigs, poultry, bulls, sheep, birds	Gastroenteritis, septicemia, gastroenteritis, spontaneous abortion, meningitis	Uncommon
C. upsaliensis	Dogs, cats	Gastroenteritis, septicemia, abscesses	Uncommon
C. fetus	Cattle, sheep	Septicemia, gastroenteritis, spontaneous abortion, meningitis	Uncommon
C. fetus subsp. *venerealis*	Cattle	Septicemia	Uncommon
C. hyointestinalis	Pigs, cattle, hamsters, deer	Gastroenteritis	Rare
C. concisus	Humans	Periodontal disease, gastroenteritis	Rare
C. sputorum subsp. *sputorum*	Humans, cattle, pigs	Abscesses, gastroenteritis	Rare
C. curvus	Humans	Periodontal disease, gastroenteritis	Rare
C. rectus	Humans	Periodontal disease	Rare
C. showae	Humans	Periodontal disease	Rare
C. lari	Poultry, birds, dogs, cats, monkeys, horses, seals	Gastroenteritis, septicemia	Rare

---

BOX 31–1. Summary of *Campylobacter* Infections

Physiology and Structure

Thin, curved gram-negative bacilli; too thin to be seen in most clinical specimens by brightfield microscopy.

Virulence

Factors that regulate adhesion, motility, and invasion into intestinal mucosa are poorly defined for *C. jejuni*, *C. upsaliensis*, and *C. coli*.

S protein in *C. fetus* inhibits C3b binding and subsequent complement-mediated phagocytosis and killing (i.e., resistant to serum killing).

Guillain-Barré syndrome believed to be an autoimmune disease due to antigenic cross-reactivity between oligosaccharides in bacterial capsule and glycosphingolipids on surface of neural tissues.

Epidemiology

Zoonotic infection; improperly prepared poultry is a common source of human infections.

Infections acquired by ingestion of contaminated food, unpasteurized milk, or contaminated water.

Person-to-person spread is unusual.

Infectious dose is high unless the gastric acids are neutralized or absent.

Worldwide distribution, with enteric infections most commonly seen in warm months.

Diseases

Refer to Table 31–1.

Acute enteritis with diarrhea, malaise, fever, and abdominal pain. Most infections are self-limited but can persist for a week or more.

C. fetus is associated with septicemia and is disseminated to multiple organs.

Diagnosis

Microscopy is insensitive.

Culture requires use of specialized media incubated with reduced oxygen, increased carbon dioxide, and (for thermophilic species) elevated temperatures; slow grower requiring incubation for 2 days or more.

Nonfermenter.

Treatment, Prevention, and Control

For gastroenteritis, infection is self-limited and is managed by fluid and electrolyte replacement.

Severe gastroenteritis and septicemia are treated with erythromycin (drug of choice), tetracyclines, quinolones.

Gastroenteritis is prevented by proper preparation of food and consumption of pasteurized milk; prevention of contaminated water supplies also controls infection.

---

fects. Although this is an uncommon complication of *Campylobacter* disease, the syndrome has been associated with specific serotypes (primarily *C. jejuni* serotype O:19). The pathogenesis of this disease is believed to be related to antigenic cross-reactivity between oligosaccharides of *Campylobacter* and glycosphingolipids present on the surface of neural tissues. Thus, antibodies directed against specific strains of *Campylobacter* can damage neural tissue in the peripheral nervous system.

C. fetus has a propensity to spread from the gastrointestinal tract to the blood stream and distal foci. This spread is particularly common in debilitated and immunocompromised patients, such as those with liver disease, diabetes mellitus, chronic alcoholism, or malignancies. In vitro studies have shown that *C. fetus* is resistant to complement- and antibody-mediated serum killing, whereas *C. jejuni* and most other *Campylobacter* species are killed rapidly. *C. fetus* is covered with a capsule-like protein (**S protein**) that prevents complement-mediated killing in serum (inhibition of C3b binding to the bacteria). *C. fetus* loses its virulence if this protein layer is removed.

Epidemiology

Campylobacter infections are zoonotic, with a variety of animals serving as reservoirs (see Table 31–1). Humans acquire the infections with *C. jejuni* and *C. coli* after consumption of contaminated food, milk, or water; contaminated poultry are responsible for more than half of the *Campylobacter* infections in developed countries. In contrast, *C. upsaliensis* infections are acquired primarily after contact with domestic dogs (either healthy carriers or pets with diarrheal disease). Food products that neutralize gastric acids (e.g., milk) effectively reduce the infectious dose. Fecal-oral transmission from person to person may also occur, but it is uncommon for the disease to be transmitted by food handlers.

The actual incidence of *Campylobacter* infections is unknown, because disease is not reported to public health officials. It has been estimated, however, that more than 2.5 million infections occur annually in the United States, and these infections are more common than *Salmonella* and *Shigella* infections combined (Fig. 31–2). The number of *Campylobacter* infections may be even higher, because *C. upsaliensis* is believed to be responsible for approximately 10% of the *Campylobacter* infections, and this species would not be isolated by commonly used techniques. Disease is most common in the warm months but occurs throughout the year. The peak incidence of disease is in young adults. In underdeveloped countries, symptomatic disease occurs in young children, and persistent, asymptomatic carriage is observed in adults.

C. fetus infections are relatively uncommon, with fewer than 250 cases reported annually. Unlike *C. jejuni*, *C. fetus* primarily infects immunocompromised elderly people.

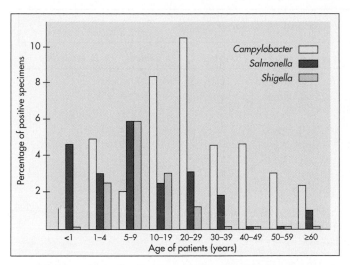

FIGURE 31–2. Age distribution of diarrheal disease caused by *Campylobacter*, *Salmonella*, and *Shigella* organisms.

Clinical Diseases

Gastrointestinal infections with *C. jejuni, C. coli, C. upsaliensis,* and other enteric pathogens are seen most commonly as acute enteritis with diarrhea, malaise, fever, and abdominal pain. Affected patients can have 10 or more bowel movements per day during the peak of disease, and stools may be bloody on gross examination. The disease is generally self-limited, although symptoms may last for a week or longer. The range of clinical manifestations includes colitis, acute abdominal pain, and bacteremia, and chronic infections can develop. In the most common presentation of *C. fetus* infection, the patient experiences initial gastroenteritis, followed by septicemia with dissemination to multiple organs.

Laboratory Diagnosis

Microscopy

Campylobacters are thin (0.3 μm) and cannot be easily seen when specimens are stained. The organism, with its characteristic darting motility, can be detected on darkfield or phase-contrast microscopy in freshly collected stool specimens; however, these examinations are rarely performed. The organisms in cultured specimens appear as small, curved bacilli, arranged either singly or in end-to-end pairs (either resembling the curved wings of a seagull or in an S shape).

Culture

C. jejuni, C. coli, and *C. upsaliensis* went unrecognized for many years, because their isolation requires growth in a microaerophilic atmosphere (i.e., 5% to 7% oxy-gen, 5% to 10% carbon dioxide, and the balance nitrogen), at an elevated incubation temperature (i.e., 42°C), and on selective media. The selective media must contain blood or charcoal to remove toxic oxygen radicals, and antibiotics are added to inhibit the growth of contaminating organisms. Campylobacters are slow-growing organisms, usually requiring incubation for 48 to 72 hours or longer. *C. fetus* is not thermophilic and cannot grow at 42°C; however, its isolation still requires a microaerophilic atmosphere.

Identification

Preliminary identification of isolates is based on growth under selective conditions and typical microscopic morphology. Definitive identification of all isolates is determined from the reactions summarized in Table 31–2.

Treatment, Prevention, and Control

Campylobacter gastroenteritis is typically a self-limited infection managed by the replacement of lost fluids and electrolytes. Antibiotic therapy may be used in patients with severe infections or septicemia. Campylobacters are susceptible to a wide variety of antibiotics, including macrolides (i.e., erythromycin, azithromycin, clarithromycin), tetracyclines, aminoglycosides, chloramphenicol, quinolones, clindamycin, amoxicillin/clavulanic acid, and imipenem. Most isolates are resistant to penicillins, cephalosporins, and sulfonamide antibiotics. Erythromycin is the antibiotic of choice for the treatment of enteritis, with tetracycline or quinolones used as secondary antibiotics. Resistance to quinolones has increased, so these drugs may be less effective. Amoxicillin/clavulanic acid can be used in place of tetracycline, which is contraindicated in young children. Systemic infections are treated with an aminoglycoside, chloramphenicol, or imipenem.

Exposure to enteric campylobacters is prevented by the proper preparation of food (particularly poultry), avoidance of unpasteurized dairy products, and the implementation of safeguards to prevent the contamination of water supplies. It is unlikely that *Campylobacter* carriage in animal reservoirs such as chickens and turkeys will be eliminated, so the risk of infections from these sources will remain.

Helicobacter

In 1983, spiral, gram-negative bacilli resembling campylobacters were found in patients with type B gastritis. The organisms were originally classified as *Campylobacter* but were subsequently reclassified as a new genus, *Helicobacter*. The bacteria, *Helicobacter pylori*, have now been associated with gastritis, peptic ulcers,

TABLE 31–2. Phenotypic Properties of Selected *Campylobacter* and *Helicobacter* Species

Characteristics	C. jejuni	C. coli	C. upsaliensis	C. fetus	H. pylori	H. cinaedi	H. fennelliae
Oxidase	+	+	+	+	+	+	+
Catalase	+	+	−/W	+	+	+	+
Nitrate reduction	+	+	+	+	−	+	−
Urease	−	−	−	−	+	−	−
Hydrolysis of:							
Hippurate	+	−	−	−	−	−	−
Indoxyl acetate	+	+	+	−	−	−	+
Growth at:							
25°C	−	−	−	+	−	−	−
37°C	+	+	+	+	+	+	+
42°C	+	+	+	−	−	−	−
Growth in 1% glycine	+	+	V	+	−	+	+
Susceptibility to:							
Nalidixic acid	S	S	S	V	R	S	S
Cephalothin	R	R	S	S	S	I	S

+ = Positive reaction; − = negative reaction; I = intermediate; R = resistant; S = susceptible; V = variable reaction; W = weak reaction.
Modified from Murray PR et al, editors: *Manual of clinical microbiology*, ed 7, Washington, DC, 1999, American Society for Microbiology.

gastric adenocarcinoma, and gastric mucosa–associated lymphoid type (MALT) B-cell lymphomas (Table 31–3; Box 31–2). Helicobacters have been isolated from the stomachs of many other mammals (e.g., monkeys, dogs, cats, cheetahs, ferrets, mice, rats). The intestinal tract is also colonized by helicobacters including *Helicobacter cinaedi* and *Helicobacter fennelliae* that have been isolated from homosexual men with proctitis, proctocolitis, or enteritis.

Physiology and Structure

Helicobacter species are characterized according to sequence analysis of their 16S rRNA genes, their cellular fatty acids, and the presence of polar flagella. Cur-rently, 23 species have been characterized, but this taxonomy is changing rapidly. Helicobacters have a spiral shape in young cultures but can assume coccoid forms in older cultures (Fig. 31–3).

H. pylori is highly motile (corkscrew motility) and produces an abundance of urease. Urease production is a consistent finding in *Helicobacter* species of humans that colonize the stomach but is uncommon in species found in the intestines. Helicobacters do not ferment or oxidize carbohydrates, although they can metabolize amino acids by fermentative pathways. Growth of *H. pylori* and other helicobacters requires a complex medium supplemented with blood, serum, charcoal, starch, or egg yolk, in microaerophilic conditions (decreased oxygen and increased carbon dioxide), and in a temperature range between 30°C and 37°C.

TABLE 31–3. *Helicobacter* Species Associated with Human Disease*

Species	Reservoir Host	Human Disease	Frequency
H. pylori	Humans, primates, pigs	Gastritis, peptic ulcers, gastric adenocarcinoma	Common
H. cinaedi	Humans, hamsters	Gastroenteritis, septicemia, proctocolitis, cellulitis	Uncommon
H. fennelliae	Humans	Gastroenteritis, septicemia, proctocolitis	Uncommon
H. canis	Dogs	Gastroenteritis	Rare
H. pullorum	Poultry	Gastroenteritis	Rare
H. rappini	Humans, sheep, mice	Gastroenteritis	Rare
H. canadensis	Humans	Gastroenteritis	Rare

*Species associated with only one or two reported infections are not included in this table.
Modified from On SLW: Identification methods for compylobacters, helicobacters, and related organisms, *Clin Microbiol Rev* 9:405–422, 1996.

Physiology and Structure

Curved gram-negative bacilli.

Urease production at very high levels is typical of gastric helicobacters (e.g., *H. pylori*) and uncommon in intestinal helicobacters (important diagnostic test for *H. pylori*).

Virulence

Refer to Table 31–4.

Epidemiology

Infections are common, particularly in people in a low socioeconomic class or in developing nations.

Humans are the primary reservoir.

Person-to-person spread is important (typically fecal-oral).

An animal reservoir has not been identified.

Ubiquitous and worldwide with no seasonal incidence of disease.

Diseases

Refer to Table 31–3.

Diagnosis

Microscopy—histologic examination of biopsy specimens is sensitive and specific.

Culture requires incubation in microaerophilic conditions; growth is slow.

Serology useful for demonstrating exposure to *H. pylori*.

Treatment, Prevention, and Control

Multiple regimens have been evaluated for treatment of *H. pylori* infections. Therapy with tetracycline, metronidazole, bismuth, and omeprazole for 2 weeks has had a high success rate.

Prophylactic treatment of colonized individuals has not been useful and potentially has adverse effects, such as predisposing patients to adenocarcinomas of the lower esophagus.

Human vaccines are not currently available.

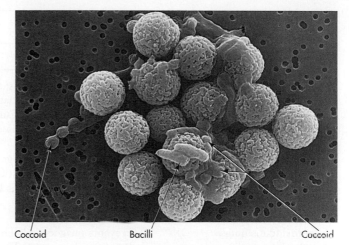

Coccoid   Bacilli   Coccoid

FIGURE 31–3. Scanning electron micrograph of *Helicobacter pylori* in a 7-day culture. Bacilli and coccoid forms (*arrows*) are bound to paramagnetic beads used in immunomagnetic separation. (Courtesy Dr. L. Engstrand, Uppsala.)

Pathogenesis and Immunity

Most of the research into virulence factors in helicobacters has focused on *H. pylori*. Multiple factors contribute to the gastric inflammation, alteration of gastric acid production, and tissue destruction that are characteristic of *H. pylori* disease (Table 31–4). Initial colonization is facilitated by (1) blockage of acid production by a bacterial acid–inhibitory protein and (2) neutralization of gastric acids by the ammonia produced by bacterial urease activity. The activity of bacterial urease is enhanced by a **heat shock protein (HspB)** that is coexpressed with **urease** on the bacterial surface. The actively motile helicobacters can then pass through the gastric mucus and adhere to the epithelial cells. Localized tissue damage is mediated by urease byproducts, **mucinase, phospholipases,** and the activity of the **vacuolating cytotoxin** that induces epithelial cell damage and, together with urease and bacterial lipopolysaccharide, stimulates the inflammatory response. *H. pylori* is protected from phagocytosis and intracellular killing by production of **superoxide dismutase** and **catalase**. *H. pylori* also produces factors that stimulate (1) secretion of interleukin-8 (IL-8), (2) production of platelet-activating factor that causes hypersecretion of gastric acid, and (3) programmed death of gastric epithelial cells.

Epidemiology

An enormous amount of information about the prevalence of *H. pylori* has been collected since 1984, when the organism was first isolated in culture. The highest incidence of carriage is found in developing countries, where 70% to 90% of the population is colonized, most before the age of 10 years. In contrast, developed countries such as the United States have documented that the incidence of *H. pylori* colonization in healthy people is relatively low during childhood but increases to approximately 45% in older adults (see Box 31–2). These studies have also demonstrated that 70% to 100% of patients with gastritis, gastric ulcers, or duodenal ulcers are infected with *H. pylori*. The differences in colonization rates between developing and developed countries is believed to be due to improved hygienic standards in the latter. Humans are the primary reser-

TABLE 31–4. Virulence Factors of *Helicobacter pylori*

Virulence Factors	Function
Urease	Neutralizes gastric acids; stimulates monocytes and neutrophil chemotaxis; stimulates production of inflammatory cytokines
Heat shock protein (HspB)	Enhances expression of urease
Acid-inhibitory protein	Induces hypochlorhydria during acute infection by blocking acid secretion from parietal cells
Flagella	Allow penetration into gastric mucous layer and protection from acid environment
Adhesins	Mediate binding to host cells; examples of adhesins are hemagglutinins, sialic acid–binding adhesin, Lewis blood group adhesin
Mucinase	Disrupts gastric mucus
Phospholipases	Disrupt gastric mucus
Superoxide dismutase	Prevents phagocytic killing by neutralizing oxygen metabolites
Catalase	Prevents phagocytic killing by neutralizing peroxides
Vacuolating cytotoxin	Induces vacuolation in epithelial cells; stimulates neutrophil migration into mucosa
Poorly defined factors	*H. pylori:*
	Stimulates interleukin-8 secretion by gastric epithelial cells, which recruits and activates neutrophils
	Stimulates gastric mucosal cells to produce platelet-activating factor (PAF), which stimulates gastric acid secretion
	Induces nitric oxide synthase in gastric epithelial cells, which mediates tissue injury
	Induces death of gastric epithelial cells

voir for *H. pylori*, and transmission is most likely by the fecal-oral route. Thus, it is expected that the risk of colonization will decrease with improved hygienic standards.

An interesting observation about *H. pylori* colonization has been made. This organism is clearly associated with diseases such as gastritis, gastric ulcers, gastric adenocarcinoma, and gastric MALT lymphomas. It is anticipated that treatment of colonized or infected individuals will lead to a reduction of these diseases. However, colonization with *H. pylori* appears to offer protection from gastroesophageal reflux disease and adenocarcinomas of the lower esophagus and gastric cardia. Thus, it may be unwise to eliminate *H. pylori* in patients without symptomatic disease. Certainly, the complex relationship between *H. pylori* and its host remains to be defined.

Clinical Diseases

Clinical evidence is now overwhelming that *H. pylori* is the etiologic agent in virtually all cases of type B gastritis. This evidence includes (1) virtually a 100% association between gastritis and infection with the bacterium, (2) production of experimental infection in both animals and humans, and (3) histologic resolution of the pathologic changes when specific therapy is used to eradicate the organism. *H. pylori* is now generally ac-

cepted to be the cause of most gastric and duodenal ulcers, with elimination of the organism leading to healing of the ulcers and a significant reduction in the rate of recurrence.

Chronic gastritis is a risk factor for gastric carcinoma, so it is not surprising that there is a relationship between infection with *H. pylori* and adenocarcinoma of the body and antrum of the stomach but not the cardia (an area of the stomach that is not infected by *H. pylori*). *H. pylori* colonization is also associated with gastric MALT B-cell lymphomas. Supporting the role of *H. pylori* in these malignancies is the observation that therapy directed against the bacteria is associated with regression of the lymphoma.

H. cinaedi and *H. fennelliae* can cause gastroenteritis and proctocolitis with septicemia in homosexual men. *H. cinaedi* also causes recurrent cellulitis with fever and bacteremia in immunocompromised patients.

Laboratory Diagnosis

Microscopy

H. pylori is detected by histologic examination of gastric biopsy specimens. Although the organism can be seen in specimens stained with hematoxylin-eosin or Gram stain, the Warthin-Starry silver stain is the most sensitive. The sensitivity and specificity of histologic analysis approach 100%.

Urease Test

The **urease test** is the most rapid way to detect *H. pylori*. Urease activity can be measured directly in the clinical specimen or after an organism has been isolated. The abundance of urease produced by the organism permits detection of the alkaline byproduct in less than 2 hours. The sensitivity of the direct test with biopsy specimens varies from 75% to 95%; however, the specificity approaches 100%, so a positive reaction is compelling evidence of an active infection.

Culture

H. pylori can grow only in a microaerophilic atmosphere on enriched medium supplemented with blood, hemin, or charcoal. The supplementation of the medium protects the bacteria from oxygen free radicals, hydrogen peroxide, and fatty acids. Specimens should not be inoculated onto media used for the recovery of *Campylobacter*, because these media are too inhibitory. Culture is insensitive unless multiple biopsy specimens from the gastric mucosa are processed. Additionally, the success of culture is influenced by the experience of the microbiologist.

Identification

Preliminary identification of isolates is based on their growth characteristics under selective conditions, typical microscopic morphologic findings, and detection of oxidase, catalase, and urease activity. Definitive identification of *H. pylori* and related bacteria is guided by the reactions summarized in Table 31–2.

Serology

Infection with *H. pylori* stimulates a humoral immune reaction that persists as the result of continuous exposure to the bacteria. Because the antibody titers persist for many years, the test cannot be used to discriminate between past and current infection. Furthermore, the titer of antibodies measured does not correlate with the severity of the disease or the response to therapy. The tests are useful, however, for documenting exposure to the bacteria, either for epidemiologic studies or for the initial evaluation of a symptomatic patient.

Treatment, Prevention, and Control

Numerous antibiotic regimens have been evaluated for treating *H. pylori* infections. Use of a single antibiotic or an antibiotic combined with bismuth is ineffective. The greatest success in curing gastritis or peptic ulcer disease has been accomplished with the combination of a proton pump inhibitor (e.g., omeprazole) and one or more antibiotics (e.g., tetracycline, clarithromycin, amoxicillin, metronidazole). Bismuth can also be added. At this time, multiple treatment regimens are in use; however, therapy with the combination of tetracycline, metronidazole, bismuth, and omeprazole for 2 weeks has an eradication rate greater than 90%. Growing resistance to metronidazole may necessitate use of an alternative antibiotic mixture. Infections caused by *H. cinaedi* and *H. fennelliae* can generally be treated with ampicillin or gentamicin.

Efforts are under way to develop a vaccine against *H. pylori*. Urease and the heat shock protein HspB are expressed uniquely on the surface of the bacteria. The success of using these antigens in a vaccine remains to be demonstrated.

CASE STUDY AND QUESTIONS

■ A mother and her 4-year-old son came to the local emergency room with a 1-day history of diarrhea and abdominal cramping. Both patients had low-grade fevers, and blood was grossly evident in the child's stool specimen. The symptoms had developed 18 hours after the patients had consumed a dinner consisting of mixed green salad, chicken, corn, bread, and apple pie. Culture of blood samples was negative for organisms, but *C. jejuni* was isolated from stool specimens of both the mother and the child.

1. What is the most likely food responsible for these infections? What measures should be used to prevent these infections?
2. Name three *Campylobacter* species that have been associated with gastroenteritis. Name the species of *Campylobacter* that is most commonly associated with septicemia.
3. What diseases have been associated with *H. pylori*? *H. cinaedi*? *H. fennelliae*?
4. *H. pylori* has multiple virulence factors. Which factors are responsible for interfering with gastric acid secretion? For adhering to the gastric epithelium? For disrupting the gastric mucus? For interfering with phagocytic killing?

BIBLIOGRAPHY

Blaser MJ: In a world of black and white, *Helicobacter pylori* is gray, *Ann Intern Med* 130:695–697, 1999.

Bourke B et al: *Campylobacter upsaliensis*: waiting in the wings, *Clin Microbiol Rev* 1:440–449, 1998.

Cover TL, Blaser MJ: *Helicobacter pylori* infection: a paradigm for chronic mucosal inflammation: pathogenesis and implications for eradication and prevention, *Adv Intern Med* 41:85–117, 1996.

Dunn B et al: *Helicobacter pylori, Clin Microbiol Rev* 10:720–741, 1997.

Friedman L: *Helicobacter pylori* and nonulcer dyspepsia, *N Engl J Med* 339:1928–1930, 1998 (editorial).

Hunt R, editor: Proceedings of a symposium: *Helicobacter pylori*: from theory to practice, *Am J Med* 100:1–64, 1996.

Nachamkin I et al: *Campylobacter* species and Guillain-Barré syndrome, *Clin Microbiol Rev* 11:555–567, 1998.

NIH Consensus Development Panel: *Helicobacter pylori* in peptic ulcer disease, *JAMA* 272:65–69, 1994.

On SLW: Identification methods for campylobacters, helicobacters, and related organisms, *Clin Microbiol Rev* 9:405–422, 1996.

Parsonnet J et al: Fecal and oral shedding of *Helicobacter pylori* from healthy infected adults, *JAMA* 282:2240–2245, 1999.

Soll A: Medical treatment of peptic ulcer disease: practice guidelines, *JAMA* 275:622–629, 1996.

Staat MA et al: A population-based serologic survey of *Helicobacter pylori* infection in children and adolescents in the United States, *J Infect Dis* 174:1120–1123, 1996.

Van Enk R: Serologic diagnosis of *Helicobacter pylori* infection, *Clin Microbiol Newsletter* 18:89–92, 1996.

Wassenaar T. Toxin production by *Campylobacter* spp., *Clin Microbiol Rev* 10:466–476, 1997.

CHAPTER 32

Pseudomonas and Related Organisms

Clinically important aerobic, gram-negative bacilli can be artificially classified into the following four general groups:

1. Facultatively anaerobic and microaerophilic fermenters (i.e., bacilli discussed in Chapters 29 to 31).
2. Aerobic nonfermenters (i.e., Pseudomonadaceae).
3. *Haemophilus* and related genera.
4. Uncommon or fastidious bacilli.

Of the bacilli isolated in clinical specimens, 70% to 80% are members of the first group, 10% to 15% are in the second group, 10% to 15% are in the third group, and fewer than 5% are classified into the uncommon or fastidious bacilli group. The focus of this chapter is *Pseudomonas* and related nonfermentative, gram-negative bacilli, whereas *Haemophilus* and the other bacilli are discussed in Chapters 33 to 35.

Pseudomonas and related bacilli are a complex mixture of opportunistic pathogens of plants, animals, and humans. To complicate the understanding of these organisms, the taxonomic classification has undergone numerous changes in recent years. A partial listing of clinically important nonfermentative organisms is summarized in Box 32–1. Despite the many genera, only a few are isolated commonly and are of interest to us here. *Pseudomonas aeruginosa*, *Burkholderia cepacia*, *Stenotrophomonas maltophilia*, *Acinetobacter baumannii*, and *Moraxella catarrhalis* constitute more than 75% of all isolates.

Pseudomonas

Pseudomonads are ubiquitous organisms found in soil, decaying organic matter, vegetation, and water. They are also found throughout the hospital environment in moist reservoirs, such as food, cut flowers, sinks, toilets, floor mops, respiratory therapy and dialysis equipment, and even disinfectant solutions. It is uncommon for carriage to persist in humans as part of the normal microbial flora, except in hospitalized patients and ambulatory, immunocompromised hosts.

The broad environmental distribution of pseudomonads is made possible by their simple growth requirements. They are capable of using many organic compounds as sources of carbon and nitrogen, and some strains can even grow in distilled water by using trace nutrients. *Pseudomonas* species also possess many structural factors, enzymes, and toxins that enhance their virulence as well as render them resistant to most commonly used antibiotics. Indeed, it is surprising that these organisms are not more common pathogens, considering their ubiquitous presence, ability to grow in virtually any environment, virulence properties, and resistance to many antibiotics. Instead, *Pseudomonas* infections are primarily opportunistic (i.e., restricted to patients with compromised host defenses). This feature illustrates the importance of the host's ability to prevent colonization and subsequent invasion with pseudomonads.

Physiology and Structure

Pseudomonads are straight or slightly curved gram-negative bacilli (0.5 to 1.0 × 1.5 to 5.0 μm) with polar flagella that render them motile. The organisms are nonfermentative, utilizing carbohydrates through respiratory metabolism with oxygen the terminal electron acceptor. Although pseudomonads are defined as obligate aerobes, they can grow anaerobically using nitrate or arginine as an alternate electron acceptor. The presence of cytochrome oxidase in *Pseudomonas* species is used to differentiate them from the Enterobacteriaceae. Some strains appear mucoid because of the abundance of a polysaccharide capsule; these strains are particularly common in patients with cystic fibrosis. Some pseudomonads produce diffusible pigments (e.g., pyocyanin [blue], fluorescein [yellow], pyorubin [red-brown]).

Although the genus consisted of a large number of species at one time, most of the species have been reclassified in other genera (e.g. *Acidovorax*, *Brevundimonas*, *Burkholderia*, *Comamonas*, *Ralstonia*, *Stenotrophomonas*). The genus now consists of approximately 10 species that have been isolated in clinical specimens,

BOX 32–1. **Clinically Important Nonfermentative Gram-Negative Bacilli**

Achromobacter	Burkholderia	Pseudomonas
Acinetobacter	Chryseobacterium	Psychrobacter
Agrobacterium	Flavobacterium	Ralstonia
Alcaligenes	Methylobacterium	Roseomonas
Balneatrix	Moraxella	Shewanella
Bordetella	Ochrobactrum	Sphingomonas
Brevundimonas	Oligella	Stenotrophomonas

with *P. aeruginosa* the most common pseudomonad and the species that is emphasized in this chapter.

Pathogenesis and Immunity

P. aeruginosa has many virulence factors, including structural components, toxins, and enzymes (Table 32–1); however, defining the role that each factor plays in disease is difficult, and most experts in this field believe that its virulence is multifactorial.

Adhesins

Adherence of *P. aeruginosa* to host cells is mediated by pili and nonpilus adhesins. Pili are important for bind-ing to epithelial cells and are similar in structure to the pili found in *Neisseria gonorrhoeae*. *P. aeruginosa* also produces neuraminidase, which removes sialic acid resi-dues from the pili receptor, thereby enhancing adher-ence of the bacteria to the epithelial cells.

Polysaccharide Capsule

P. aeruginosa produces a polysaccharide capsule (also known as mucoid exopolysaccharide, alginate coat, or glycocalyx) that has multiple functions. The polysac-charide layer anchors the bacteria to epithelial cells and tracheobronchial mucin. The capsule also protects the organism from phagocytosis and activity of antibiotics such as aminoglycosides. The production of this mu-coid polysaccharide is under complex regulation. The genes controlling production of the polysaccharide can be activated in patients, such as those with cystic fibro-sis or other chronic respiratory diseases, who are pre-disposed to long-term colonization with these mucoid strains of *P. aeruginosa*. The mucoid strains can revert to a nonmucoid phenotype when cultured in vitro.

Endotoxin

Lipopolysaccharide endotoxin is a major cell wall anti-gen in *P. aeruginosa*, as it is in other gram-negative bacilli. The lipid A component of endotoxin mediates the various biologic effects of the sepsis syndrome.

TABLE 32–1. Virulence Factors Associated with *Pseudomonas aeruginosa*

Virulence Factors	Biologic Effects
Structural Components	
Capsule	Mucoid exopolysaccharide; adhesin; inhibits antibiotic (e.g., aminoglycoside) killing; suppresses neutrophil and lymphocyte activity
Pili	Adhesin
Lipopolysaccharide (LPS)	Endotoxin activity
Pyocyanin	Impairs ciliary function; stimulates inflammatory response; mediates tissue damage through production of toxic oxygen radicals (i.e., hydrogen peroxide, superoxide, hydroxyl radicals)
Toxins and Enzymes	
Exotoxin A	Inhibitor of protein synthesis; produces tissue damage (e.g., skin, cornea); immunosuppressive
Exotoxin S	Inhibits protein synthesis; immunosuppressive
Cytotoxin (leukocidin)	Cytotoxic for eukaryotic membranes (e.g., disrupts leukocyte function, produces pulmonary microvascular injury)
Elastase	Destruction of elastin-containing tissues (e.g., blood vessels, lung tissue, skin), collagen, immunoglobulins, and complement factors
Alkaline protease	Tissue destruction; inactivation of interferon and tumor necrosis factor-α
Phospholipase C	Heat-labile hemolysin; mediates tissue damage; stimulates inflammatory response
Rhamnolipid	Heat-stable hemolysin; disrupts lecithin-containing tissues; inhibits pulmonary ciliary activity
Antibiotic resistance	Complicates antimicrobial therapy

Pyocyanin

A blue pigment produced by *P. aeruginosa*, pyocyanin, catalyzes the production of superoxide and hydrogen peroxide, toxic forms of oxygen. In the presence of pyochelin (an iron-binding siderophore), the more toxic hydroxyl radical is produced, which can mediate tissue damage. This pigment also stimulates the inflammatory response.

Exotoxin A

Exotoxin A is believed to be one of the most important virulence factors produced by pathogenic strains of *P. aeruginosa*. This toxin blocks protein synthesis in eukaryotic cells much like the diphtheria toxin, which is produced by *Corynebacterium diphtheriae*. However, the toxins produced by these two organisms are structurally and immunologically different, and exotoxin A is less potent than diphtheria toxin. Exotoxin A most likely contributes to the dermatonecrosis that occurs in burn wounds, corneal damage in ocular infections, and tissue damage in chronic pulmonary infections. The toxin is also immunosuppressive.

Exoenzymes S and T

Exoenzymes S and T are extracellular toxins produced by *P. aeruginosa*. They possess adenosine diphosphate–ribosyltransferase activity, the function of which is unclear. When the proteins are introduced into their target eukaryotic cells by the type III secretion system, however, epithelial cell damage occurs, facilitating bacterial spread, tissue invasion, and necrosis. This cytotoxicity is mediated by actin rearrangement.

Elastases

Two enzymes, LasA (serine protease) and LasB (zinc metalloprotease), act synergistically to degrade elastin, resulting in damage to elastin-containing tissues and producing the lung parenchymal damage and hemorrhagic lesions (**ecthyma gangrenosum**) associated with disseminated *P. aeruginosa* infections. These enzymes can also degrade complement components and inhibit neutrophil chemotaxis and function, leading to further spread and tissue damage in acute infections. Chronic *Pseudomonas* infections are characterized by the formation of antibodies to LasA and LasB, with the deposition of immune complexes in the infected tissues.

Alkaline Protease

Like the elastases, alkaline protease contributes to tissue destruction and spread of *P. aeruginosa*. It also interferes with the host immune response.

Phospholipase C

Phospholipase C is a heat-labile hemolysin that breaks down lipids and lecithin, facilitating tissue destruction. The exact role of this enzyme in respiratory and urinary tract infections is unclear, although an important association between hemolysin production and disease has been recognized.

Rhamnolipid

Rhamnolipid is a heat-stable hemolysin that disrupts lecithin-containing tissues. This hemolysin is also associated with inhibition of ciliary activity of the respiratory tract.

Antibiotic Resistance

P. aeruginosa is inherently resistant to many antibiotics and can mutate to even more resistant strains during therapy. Although numerous resistance mechanisms have been identified, the mutation of porin proteins constitutes the major mechanism of resistance. Penetration of antibiotics into the pseudomonad cell is primarily through pores in the outer membrane. If the proteins forming the walls of these pores are altered to restrict flow through the channels, resistance to many classes of antibiotics can develop. *P. aeruginosa* also produces a number of different β-lactamases that can inactivate many β-lactam antibiotics (e.g., penicillins, cephalosporins, carbapenems).

Epidemiology

Pseudomonads are opportunistic pathogens present in a variety of environments (Box 32–2). The ability to isolate these organisms from moist surfaces may be limited only by the efforts to look for the organism. Pseudomonads have minimal nutritional requirements, can tolerate a wide range of temperatures (4°C to 42°C), and are resistant to many antibiotics and disinfectants. Indeed, the recovery of *Pseudomonas* from an environmental source (e.g., hospital sink or floor) means very little unless there is epidemiologic evidence that the contaminated site is a reservoir for infection.

Furthermore, isolation of pseudomonads from a hospitalized patient is worrisome but does not normally justify therapeutic intervention unless there is evidence of disease. The recovery of *Pseudomonas*, particularly species other than *P. aeruginosa*, from a clinical specimen may represent simple colonization of the patient or environmental contamination of the specimen during collection or laboratory processing.

BOX 32-2. Summary of *Pseudomonas aeruginosa* Infections

Physiology and Structure

Small gram-negative bacilli.
> Strict aerobe.
> Nonfermenter.
> Simple nutritional requirements.
> Mucoid exopolysaccharide capsule.

Virulence

Refer to Table 32-1 for complete listing.

Epidemiology

Ubiquitous in moist environmental sites in the hospital (e.g., flowers, sinks, toilets, respiratory and dialysis equipment) as well as in nature.
> No seasonal incidence of disease.
> Can transiently colonize the respiratory and gastrointestinal tracts of hospitalized patients, particularly those treated with broad-spectrum antibiotics, exposed to respiratory therapy equipment, or hospitalized for extended periods.

Diseases

Pulmonary infections (common in patients with cystic fibrosis).
> Burn wound infections and other skin and soft tissue infections (can be life-threatening).
> Urinary tract infections (primarily in catheterized patients).
> External otitis (varying from mild "swimmer's ear" to malignant otitis externa).
> Eye infections (commonly associated with contaminated contact lens cleaning fluids).

Diagnosis

Readily grow on common laboratory media. *P. aeruginosa* is identified by colonial characteristics (e.g., hemolytic, green pigment, grapelike odor) and simple biochemical tests (e.g., positive oxidase reaction).

Treatment, Prevention, and Control

Combined use of effective antibiotics (e.g., aminoglycoside and β-lactam antibiotics) frequently required. Monotherapy is generally ineffective and can select for resistant strains.
> Hyperimmune globulin and granulocyte transfusions may be beneficial in selected infections in immunocompromised patients.
> Hospital infection control efforts should concentrate on preventing contamination of sterile medical equipment and nosocomial infections.
> Unnecessary use of broad-spectrum antibiotics can select for resistant organisms such as *P. aeruginosa*.

Clinical Diseases

Pulmonary Infections

P. aeruginosa infections of the lower respiratory tract can range in severity from asymptomatic colonization or benign tracheobronchitis to severe necrotizing bronchopneumonia. Colonization is seen in patients with cystic fibrosis, other chronic lung diseases, and neutropenia. Infections in patients with cystic fibrosis have been associated with exacerbation of the underlying disease as well as invasive pulmonary disease. Mucoid strains are commonly isolated from specimens from such patients and are difficult to eradicate with antibiotic therapy.

Conditions that predispose immunocompromised patients to infections with *Pseudomonas* include (1) previous therapy with broad-spectrum antibiotics that disrupt the normal, protective bacterial population and (2) use of respiratory therapy equipment, which may introduce the organism to the lower airways. Invasive disease in this population is characterized by a diffuse, typically bilateral bronchopneumonia with microabscess formation and tissue necrosis. The mortality rate is as high as 70%.

Primary Skin Infections

P. aeruginosa can cause a variety of skin infections. The most recognized are infections of burn wounds. Colonization of a burn wound, followed by localized vascular damage, tissue necrosis, and, ultimately bacteremia, is common in patients with severe burns. The moist surface of the burn and the lack of a neutrophilic response to tissue invasion predispose patients to such infections. Wound management with topical antibiotic creams has had only limited success in controlling these infections.

Folliculitis is another common infection caused by *Pseudomonas*, resulting from immersion in contaminated water (e.g., hot tubs, whirlpools, swimming pools). Secondary infections with *Pseudomonas* also occur in people who have acne or who depilate their legs. Finally *P. aeruginosa* can cause nail infections in people whose hands are frequently exposed to water.

Urinary Tract Infections

Infection of the urinary tract is seen primarily in patients with long-term indwelling urinary catheters. Typically such patients are treated with multiple courses of antibiotics, which tend to select for the more resistant strains of bacteria such as *Pseudomonas*.

Ear Infections

External otitis is frequently caused by *P. aeruginosa*, with swimming ("**swimmer's ear**") an important risk factor. This localized infection can be managed with topical antibiotics and drying agents. **Malignant external otitis** is a virulent form of disease seen primarily in diabetics and elderly patients. It can invade the underlying tissues, can damage the cranial nerves and bones, and can be life-threatening. Aggressive antimicrobial and surgical intervention is required for patients with the latter disease. *P. aeruginosa* is also associated with **chronic otitis media**.

Eye Infections

Infections of the eye occur after initial trauma to the cornea (e.g., abrasion from contact lens, scratch on the eye surface) and then exposure to *P. aeruginosa* in contaminated water. **Corneal ulcers** develop and can progress to eye-threatening disease unless prompt treatment is instituted.

Bacteremia and Endocarditis

Bacteremia due to *P. aeruginosa* is clinically indistinguishable from that due to other gram-negative bacteria. The mortality rate in affected patients is higher with *P. aeruginosa* bacteremia, however, because of (1) the predilection of the organism for immunocompromised patients and (2) the inherent virulence of *Pseudomonas*. Bacteremia occurs most often in patients with neutropenia, diabetes mellitus, extensive burns, and hematologic malignancies. Most bacteremias originate from infections of the lower respiratory tract, urinary tract, and skin and soft tissue (particularly burn wound infections). Although seen in a minority of bacteremic patients, characteristic skin lesions (**ecthyma gangrenosum**) may develop. The lesions manifest as erythematous vesicles that become hemorrhagic, necrotic, and ulcerated. Microscopic examination of the lesion shows abundant organisms, vascular destruction (which explains the hemorrhagic nature of the lesions), and an absence of neutrophils, as would be expected in neutropenic patients.

Pseudomonas **endocarditis** is most commonly observed in intravenous drug abusers. These patients acquire the infection from the use of drug paraphernalia contaminated with the waterborne organisms. The tricuspid valve is often involved, and the infection is associated with a chronic course but with a more favorable prognosis than that in patients who have infections of the aortic or mitral valve.

Other Infections

P. aeruginosa is also the cause of a variety of other infections, including those localized in the gastrointestinal tract, central nervous system, and musculoskeletal system. The underlying conditions required for most infections are (1) the presence of the organism in a moist reservoir and (2) the circumvention or elimination of host defenses (e.g., cutaneous trauma, elimination of normal microbial flora as a result of antibiotic usage, neutropenia).

All *Pseudomonas* species can cause opportunistic infections in immunocompromised patients. Most true infections with these organisms have been localized to the respiratory tract in patients with underlying pulmonary disease or to the urinary tract in patients who have instrumentation of the tract or catheterization. The clinical significance of an isolate is often difficult to assess, because specific signs and symptoms of disease may be absent and the organism may be an insignificant waterborne contaminant.

Laboratory Diagnosis

Culture

Because pseudomonads have simple nutritional requirements, they grow easily on common isolation media such as blood agar and MacConkey agar. They do require aerobic incubation (unless nitrate is available), so their growth in broth is generally confined to the broth-air interface.

Identification

The colonial morphology (e.g., colony size, hemolytic activity, pigmentation, odor) combined with the results of selected rapid biochemical tests (e.g., positive oxidase reaction) is sufficient for the preliminary identification of these isolates. For example, *P. aeruginosa* grows rapidly and has flat colonies with a spreading border, β-hemolysis, a green pigmentation caused by the production of the blue pyocyanin and the yellow fluorescein, and a characteristic sweet, grapelike odor.

Although definitive identification of *P. aeruginosa* is relatively easy, an extensive battery of physiologic tests may be required to identify other pseudomonads. Biochemical profiles, antibiotic susceptibility patterns, susceptibility to bacteriophages (phage typing), production of pyocins, serologic typing, and the molecular characterization of DNA or ribosomal RNA are used for the specific classification of isolates for epidemiologic purposes.

Treatment, Prevention, and Control

The antimicrobial therapy for *Pseudomonas* infections is frustrating, because (1) the bacteria are typically resistant to most antibiotics and (2) the infected patient with compromised host defenses cannot augment the antibiotic activity (Table 32–2). Even susceptible organisms can become resistant during therapy by inducing the formation of antibiotic-inactivating enzymes (e.g., β-lactamases) or the mutation of the genes coding the

TABLE 32–2. Mechanisms of Antibiotic Resistance in *Pseudomonas aeruginosa*

Antibiotic	Resistance Mechanisms
β-lactams	β-lactamase hydrolysis, decreased permeability, altered binding proteins
Aminoglycosides	Enzymatic hydrolysis by acetylation, adenylation, or phosphorylation; decreased permeability; altered ribosomal target
Chloramphenicol	Enzymatic hydrolysis by acetyltransferase; decreased permeability
Fluoroquinolones	Altered target (DNA gyrase); decreased permeability

outer membrane pore proteins or through the transfer of plasmid-mediated resistance from a resistant organism to a susceptible one. Furthermore, some groups of antibiotics, such as the aminoglycosides, are ineffective at certain sites of infection (e.g., poor activity in the acidic environment of an abscess). A combination of active antibiotics is generally required for therapy to be successful in patients with serious infections. The administration of hyperimmune globulin and granulocyte transfusions to augment compromised immune function may be beneficial in selected patients who have infections.

Attempts to eliminate *Pseudomonas* from the hospital are practically useless, given the ubiquitous presence of the organism in water supplies. Effective infection-control practices should concentrate on preventing the contamination of sterile equipment, such as respiratory therapy and dialysis machines, and the cross-contamination of patients by medical personnel. The inappropriate use of broad-spectrum antibiotics should also be avoided because such use can suppress the normal microbial flora and permit the overgrowth of resistant pseudomonads.

Burkholderia

Four species formerly classified as *Pseudomonas* have been reclassified as members of the genus *Burkholderia* (Table 32–3). *B. cepacia* and *Burkholderia pseudomallei* are important human pathogens; *Burkholderia gladioli* and *Burkholderia mallei* do not cause human disease.

Like *P. aeruginosa*, *B. cepacia* can colonize a variety of moist environmental surfaces and is commonly associated with nosocomial infections. Infections caused by this organism include the following:

1. Respiratory tract infections in patients with cystic fibrosis or chronic granulomatous disease.

2. Urinary tract infections in catheterized patients.
3. Septicemia, particularly in patients with contaminated intravascular catheters.
4. Other opportunistic infections.

With the exception of pulmonary infections, *B. cepacia* has a relatively low level of virulence, and infections with the organism do not commonly result in death. *B. cepacia* is susceptible to trimethoprim-sulfamethoxazole. Although the organism appears to be susceptible in vitro to piperacillin, to broad-spectrum cephalosporins, and to ciprofloxacin, the clinical response is generally poor.

B. pseudomallei is a saprophyte found in soil, water, and vegetation. It is endemic in Southeast Asia, India, Africa, and Australia. The organism causes opportunistic infections; however, such an infection (**melioidosis**) can occur in a previously healthy person as an acute suppurative infection or a chronic pulmonary infection. The disease can occur from a few days to many years after exposure. Thus, although *B. pseudomallei* is not found in the United States, latent disease can occur in people who have traveled in endemic areas.

Melioidosis has protean manifestations. Most people exposed to *B. pseudomallei* remain **asymptomatic**. However, a localized suppurative **cutaneous infection** accompanied by regional lymphadenitis, fever, and malaise can develop in some patients. This form of disease can resolve without incident or can rapidly progress to overwhelming sepsis. The third form of infection is **pulmonary disease**, which may range in severity from a mild bronchitis to necrotizing pneumonia. Cavitation can develop if appropriate antimicrobial therapy is not instituted. Isolation of *B. pseudomallei* for diagnostic purposes should be approached carefully because the organism is highly infectious. The combina-

TABLE 32–3. *Burkholderia* Species and Associated Diseases

Species	Diseases
B. cepacia	Respiratory tract infections, particularly in patients with cystic fibrosis; urinary tract infections; septic arthritis; peritonitis; septicemia; opportunistic infections
B. pseudomallei	Asymptomatic colonization; cutaneous infection with regional lymphadenitis, fever, and malaise; pulmonary disease ranging from bronchitis to necrotizing pneumonia
B. gladioli	Colonization of respiratory tracts of patients with cystic fibrosis
B. mallei	Glanders in livestock

tion of trimethoprim-sulfamethoxazole and a broad-spectrum cephalosporin is recommended for the treatment of systemic infections.

Stenotrophomonas maltophilia

S. maltophilia is one of the most commonly isolated nonfermentative, gram-negative bacilli. This organism was originally classified in the genus *Pseudomonas* and then more recently in the genus *Xanthomonas*. Despite the confusion created by these taxonomic changes, the clinical importance of this opportunistic pathogen is well-known. It is responsible for infections in debilitated patients with impaired host defense mechanisms. Also, because *S. maltophilia* is resistant to most commonly used β-lactam and aminoglycoside antibiotics, patients receiving long-term antibiotic therapy are particularly at risk for acquiring infections with this organism.

The spectrum of nosocomial infections with *S. maltophilia* includes bacteremia, pneumonia, meningitis, wound infections, and urinary tract infections. Hospital epidemics with this organism have been traced to contaminated disinfectant solutions, respiratory therapy or monitoring equipment, and ice machines.

Antimicrobial therapy is complicated because the organism is resistant to many commonly used drugs. Trimethoprim-sulfamethoxazole is the agent most active against the organism; good activity is also seen with chloramphenicol and ceftazidime.

Acinetobacter

The genus *Acinetobacter* has also undergone taxonomic reorganization. At the present time, 7 species are recognized, but 21 DNA groups ("genomospecies") have been recognized. Whether or not all these groups will achieve species status is probably of little clinical significance. The most important species currently are *A. baumannii*, *Acinetobacter lwoffii*, and *Acinetobacter haemolyticus*.

Acinetobacters are recovered in nature and in the hospital. They survive on moist surfaces, including respiratory therapy equipment, and on dry surfaces such as the human skin (the latter feature is unusual for gram-negative bacilli). These bacteria are also part of the normal oropharyngeal flora of a small number of healthy people and can proliferate to large numbers during hospitalization.

Acinetobacters are opportunistic pathogens that cause infections in the respiratory tract, urinary tract, and wounds; they also cause septicemia. Treatment of *Acinetobacter* infections is problematic because these organisms, particularly *A. baumannii*, are often resistant to antibiotics. Specific therapy must be guided by in vitro susceptibility tests, but empirical therapy for serious infections should consist of a β-lactam antibiotic (e.g., ceftazidime, imipenem) and an aminoglycoside.

Moraxella

Like other genera discussed in this chapter, the genus *Moraxella* has been reorganized on the basis of nucleic acid analysis. Although the species classified in the genus continue to change, *M. catarrhalis* is the most important pathogen. *M. catarrhalis* is a common cause of bronchitis and bronchopneumonia (in elderly patients with chronic pulmonary disease), sinusitis, and otitis. The latter two infections occur most commonly in previously healthy people. Most isolates produce β-lactamases and are resistant to penicillin; however, these bacteria are uniformly susceptible to most other antibiotics, including cephalosporins, erythromycin, tetracycline, trimethoprim-sulfamethoxazole, and the combination of penicillins with a β-lactamase inhibitor (e.g., clavulanic acid).

CASE STUDY AND QUESTIONS

■ A 63-year-old man has been hospitalized for 21 days for the management of newly diagnosed leukemia. Three days after the patient entered the hospital, a urinary tract infection with *Escherichia coli* developed. He was treated for 14 days with broad-spectrum antibiotics. On hospital day 21, the patient experienced fever and shaking chills. Within 24 hours, he became hypotensive, and ecthymic skin lesions appeared. Despite aggressive therapy with antibiotics, the patient died. Multiple blood cultures were positive for *P. aeruginosa*.

1. What factors put this man at increased risk for infection with *P. aeruginosa*?
2. What virulence factors possessed by the organism make it a particularly serious pathogen? What are the biologic effects of these factors?
3. What three mechanisms are responsible for the antibiotic resistance found in *P. aeruginosa*?
4. What diseases are caused by *B. cepacia*? *S. maltophilia*? *A. baumannii*? *M. catarrhalis*? What antibiotics can be used to treat these infections?

BIBLIOGRAPHY

Bergogne-Berezin E, Towner K: *Acinetobacter* spp. as nosocomial pathogens: microbiological, clinical, and epidemiological features, *Clin Microbiol Rev* 9:148–165, 1996.

Berlau J et al: Distribution of *Acinetobacter* species on skin of healthy humans, *Eur J Clin Microbiol Infect Dis* 18:179–183, 1999.

Dance DAB: Melioidosis: the tip of the iceberg, *Clin Microbiol Rev* 4:52–60, 1991.

Denton M, Kerr K: Microbiological and clinical aspects of infection associated with *Stenotrophomonas maltophilia*, *Clin Microbiol Rev* 11:57–80, 1998.

Forster D, Dashner F: *Acinetobacter* species as nosocomial pathogens, *Eur J Clin Microbiol Infect Dis* 17:73–77, 1998.

Govan J, Deretic V: Microbial pathogenesis in cystic fibrosis: mucoid *Pseudomonas aeruginosa* and *Burkholderia cepacia*. *Microbiol Rev* 60:539–574, 1996.

Krueger K, Barbieri J: The family of bacterial ADP-ribosylating exotoxins, *Clin Microbiol Rev* 8:34–47, 1995.

Mendelson M et al: *Pseudomonas aeruginosa* bacteremia in patients with AIDS, *Clin Infect Dis* 18:886–895, 1994.

McGregor K et al: *Moraxella catarrhalis*: clinical significance, antimicrobial susceptibility and BRO beta-lactamases, *Eur J Clin Microbiol Infect Dis* 17:219–234, 1998.

Muder R et al: Bacteremia due to *Stenotrophomonas (Xanthomonas) maltophilia*: a prospective, multicenter study of 91 episodes, *Clin Infect Dis* 22:508–512, 1996.

Pier G: *Pseudomonas aeruginosa*: a key problem in cystic fibrosis. *ASM News* 64:339–347, 1998.

Robin T, Janda JM: Pseudo-, Xantho-, *Stenotrophomonas maltophilia*: an emerging pathogen in search of a genus, *Clin Microbiol Newsletter* 18:9–13, 1996.

Sadoff JC, Sanford JP: Symposium on *Pseudomonas aeruginosa* infections, *Rev Infect Dis* 5(suppl):833–1004, 1983.

Salyers AA, Whitt DD: *Bacterial pathogenesis: a molecular approach*, Washington, DC, 1994, American Society of Microbiology.

Wick MJ et al: Structure, function, and regulation of *Pseudomonas aeruginosa* exotoxin A, *Annu Rev Microbiol* 44:335–363, 1990.

CHAPTER 33

Bordetella, Francisella, and *Brucella*

Whereas most of the gram-negative bacilli discussed in the previous chapters are commonly found in the environment or as normal members of the human microbial flora, some bacteria are always clinically significant when isolated from clinical specimens. The three genera discussed in this chapter, *Bordetella, Francisella,* and *Brucella,* are small, aerobic, nonfermentative gram-negative coccobacilli whose isolation is always associated with disease.

Bordetella

Bordetella organisms are extremely small (0.2 to 0.5 $\times$ 1 μm), strictly aerobic, nonfermentative, gram-negative coccobacilli (Box 33–1). Seven species are currently recognized, with three species responsible for human disease: *Bordetella pertussis* (Latin for "severe cough"), the agent responsible for pertussis or whooping cough; *Bordetella parapertussis* (Latin for "like pertussis"), responsible for a milder form of pertussis; and *Bordetella bronchiseptica,* responsible for respiratory disease in dogs, swine, laboratory animals, and occasionally pertussis-like symptoms in humans.

Physiology and Structure

Bordetella species are differentiated on the basis of their growth characteristics, biochemical reactivity, and antigenic properties (Table 33–1). Despite phenotypic differences, genetic studies have shown that the three species pathogenic for humans are closely related or identical species, differing only in the expression of virulence genes. At this time, however, the species have not been reclassified and should be considered as distinct.

B. *pertussis* organisms do not grow on common laboratory media; they require media supplemented with charcoal, starch, blood, or albumin to absorb the toxic substances present in agar. Nicotinamide is also required for growth. The organisms are nonmotile and oxidize amino acids but do not ferment carbohydrates. The other *Bordetella* species are less fastidious and can grow on blood and MacConkey agars. *Bordetella* species possess a genus-specific O antigen and strain-specific, heat-labile K antigens. The K antigens are used for differentiating isolates in epidemiologic investigations.

Pathogenesis and Immunity

Infection with *B. pertussis* and the development of whooping cough require exposure to the organism, bacterial attachment to the ciliated epithelial cells of the respiratory tract, proliferation of the bacteria, and production of localized tissue damage and systemic toxicity. Attachment of the organisms to ciliated epithelial cells is mediated primarily by two bacterial adhesins: filamentous hemagglutinin and pertussis toxin (Table 33–2). The filamentous hemagglutinin binds to sulfated glycolipids on the membranes of ciliated respiratory cells. This adhesin also binds to CR3, a glycoprotein receptor on the surface of polymorphonuclear leukocytes. This interaction initiates the phagocytic uptake of the bacteria. The intracellular survival of *B. pertussis* protects the bacteria from humoral antibodies and may permit persistent carriage. Pertussis toxin is a classic A-B toxin consisting of a toxic subunit (S1) and five binding subunits (S2 to S5; two S4 subunits are present in each toxin molecule). The S2 subunit binds to lactosylceramide, a glycolipid present on ciliated respiratory cells. The S3 subunit binds to receptors on phagocytic cells, leading to an increase in CR3 on the cell surface, further bacterial attachment mediated by the filamentous hemagglutinin, and subsequent bacterial phagocytosis. Two other adhesins have been identified in *B. pertussis:* pili and pertactin, the latter a protein on the surface of the bacteria. Although both proteins mediate the binding to cultured mammalian cells, their role in the attachment to ciliated cells in vivo is unknown.

B. *pertussis* produces several toxins that mediate the localized and systemic manifestations of disease. The S1 portion of pertussis toxin has adenosine diphosphate–ribosylating activity for the membrane surface G protein (a guanosine triphosphate–hydrolyzing pro-

---

BOX 33–1. Summary of *Bordetella pertussis* Infections

Physiology and Structure

Very small gram-negative coccobacilli.

Nonfermentative.

Strict aerobe.

Requires specialized media and prolonged incubation for growth in culture.

Virulence

Refer to Table 33–2.

Epidemiology

Human reservoir host.

Worldwide distribution.

Children younger than 1 year at greatest risk for infection, but prevalence of disease is increasing in older children and adults.

Nonvaccinated individuals at greatest risk for disease.

Disease spread person to person by infectious aerosols.

Diseases

Pertussis characterized by three stages: catarrhal, paroxysmal, and convalescent stages.

Most severe disease is in nonvaccinated individuals.

Diagnosis

Microscopy is insensitive and nonspecific.

Culture is specific but insensitive.

Nucleic acid amplification tests, although not readily available, are the most sensitive and specific tests.

Detection of IgG or IgA can confirm the clinical diagnosis.

Treatment, Prevention, and Control

Treatment with macrolide (i.e., erythromycin, azithromycin) is effective in eradicating organisms and reducing length of infectious stage. Treatment does not alleviate symptoms.

Erythromycin has been used for prophylaxis. Effectiveness is unknown.

Vaccination with whole-cell vaccines is effective but associated with side effects. Acellular vaccines are effective and associated with fewer adverse effects.

---

tein), which regulates adenylate cyclase activity. This causes the cyclic adenosine monophosphate levels to be unregulated, resulting in increased respiratory secretions and mucus production characteristic of the paroxysmal stage of pertussis.

Adenylate cyclase/hemolysin is a bifunctional toxin (also called *cyclolysin*) that is activated by intracellular calmodulin and catalyzes the conversion of endogenous adenosine triphosphate to cyclic adenine monophosphate in eukaryotic cells (as pertussis toxin does). Adenylate cyclase toxin also inhibits leukocyte chemotaxis, phagocytosis, and killing. This toxin may be im-

portant for the initial protection of the bacteria during the early stages of disease.

Dermonecrotic toxin is a heat-labile toxin that at low doses causes vasoconstriction of peripheral blood vessels in mice; this is accompanied by localized ischemia, the movement of leukocytes to extravascular spaces, and hemorrhage. At high doses, this toxin causes fatal reactions in mice. The toxin probably is responsible for the localized tissue destruction in human infections, although further work is necessary to confirm this.

Tracheal cytotoxin is a low-molecular-weight cell wall peptidoglycan monomer that has a specific affinity for ciliated epithelial cells. At low concentrations, it causes ciliostasis (inhibition of cilia movement), and at the higher concentrations produced later in the infection, it causes extrusion of ciliated cells. Tracheal cytotoxin specifically interferes with DNA synthesis, thereby impairing the regeneration of damaged cells. This process disrupts the normal clearance mechanisms in the respiratory tree and leads to the characteristic cough associated with pertussis. The toxin also stimulates the release of the cytokine interleukin-1, which leads to fever.

B. pertussis produces two distinct lipopolysaccharides, one with lipid A and the other with lipid X. Both lipopolysaccharide molecules can activate the alternate complement pathway and stimulate cytokine release. Their role in the disease process is unknown.

Epidemiology

B. pertussis is a human disease with no other recognized animal or environmental reservoir. Although the incidence of pertussis, with its associated morbidity and mortality, was reduced considerably after the introduction of effective vaccines in 1949, the disease is still endemic worldwide and affects more than 60 million people annually. Between 4000 and 8000 new cases are reported each year in the United States (Fig. 33–1), but this is certainly an underestimation of the true incidence of disease. Historically, pertussis has been considered a pediatric disease, and certainly the majority of infections are found in children younger than 1 year (Fig. 33–2). In recent years, however, there has been a dramatic increase in disease in older children and adults. This is attributed to waning immunity over time (even in vaccinated individuals).

Clinical Diseases

Infection is initiated when infectious aerosols are inhaled and the bacteria become attached to and proliferate on ciliated epithelial cells. After a 7- to 10-day incubation, the typical patient experiences the first of three stages (Fig. 33–3). The first stage, the **catarrhal stage,** resembles a common cold, with serous rhinor-

TABLE 33–1. Differential Characteristics of *Bordetella* Species

Characteristics	*B. pertussis*	*B. parapertussis*	*B. bronchiseptica*
Oxidase	+	–	+
Urease	–	+	+
Motility	–	–	+
Growth on			
Sheep blood agar	–	+	+
MacConkey agar	–	+/–	+

Modified from Murray P et al: *Manual of clinical microbiology,* ed 7, Washington, DC, 1999, American Society for Microbiology.

rhea, sneezing, malaise, anorexia, and low-grade fever. Because the peak number of bacteria is produced during this stage and the cause of the disease is not yet recognized, patients in the catarrhal stage pose the highest risk to their contacts. After 1 to 2 weeks, the **paroxysmal stage** begins. During this time, ciliated epithelial cells are extruded from the respiratory tract and the clearance of mucus is impaired. This stage is characterized by the classic whooping cough paroxysms (i.e., a series of repetitive coughs followed by an inspiratory whoop). Mucus production in the respiratory tract is common and is partially responsible for causing airway restriction. The paroxysms are frequently terminated with vomiting and exhaustion. A marked lymphocytosis is also prominent during this stage. Affected patients may experience as many as 40 to 50 paroxysms daily during the height of the illness. After 2 to 4 weeks, the disease enters the **convalescent stage;** at this time, the paroxysms diminish in number and severity but secondary complications can occur. This classic presentation of pertussis may not be seen in patients with partial immunity. Such patients may have a history of a chronic persistent cough with or without vomiting.

Laboratory Diagnosis

Specimen Collection and Transport

B. pertussis organisms are extremely sensitive to drying and do not survive unless care is taken during the collection and transport of the specimen to the labora-

TABLE 33–2. Virulence Factors Associated with *Bordetella pertussis*

Virulence Factor	Biologic Effect
Adhesins	
Filamentous hemagglutinin	Binds to sulfated glycolipids on ciliated cell membranes; binds to CR3 on surface of polymorphonuclear leukocytes and initiates phagocytosis.
Pertussis toxin	S2 subunit binds to glycolipid on surface of ciliated respiratory cells; S3 subunit binds to ganglioside on surface of phagocytic cells.
Pili	Binds to mammalian cells. Role in disease is unknown.
Pertactin	Binds to mammalian cells. Role in disease is unknown.
Toxins	
Pertussis toxin	S1 subunit adenosine diphosphate–ribosylates host cell G protein, causing deregulation of host cell adenylate cyclase; toxin inhibits phagocytic killing and monocyte migration.
Adenylate cyclase/hemolysin toxin	Increases intracellular level of adenylate cyclase and inhibits phagocytic killing and monocyte migration.
Dermonecrotic toxin	Causes dose-dependent skin lesions or fatal reactions in experimental animal model. Role in disease is unknown.
Tracheal cytotoxin	A peptidoglycan fragment that kills ciliated respiratory cells and stimulates the release of interleukin-1 (fever).
Lipopolysaccharide	Two distinct lipopolysaccharide molecules with either lipid A or lipid X; activates alternate complement pathway and stimulates cytokine release. Role in disease is unknown.

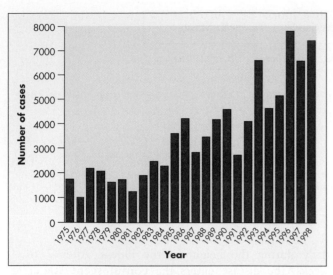

FIGURE 33–1. Incidence of pertussis in the United States from 1975 to 1998.

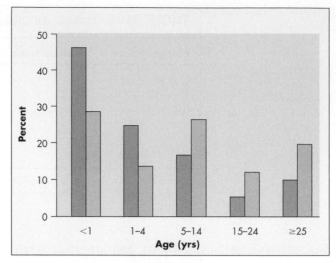

FIGURE 33–2. Age distribution for pertussis infections reported in 1988 (*blue bars*) and 1998 (*orange bars*).

tory. The optimal diagnostic specimen is a nasopharyngeal aspirate. The yield from specimens obtained by oropharyngeal swabs is lower than that from nasopharyngeal aspirates, and synthetic fiber swabs (e.g., calcium alginate or Dacron) must be used. Cotton swabs should not be used because they contain fatty acids that are toxic to *B. pertussis*.

The most important factors affecting the recovery of *Bordetella* are the speed with which the specimen is cultured and the quality of the culture media. The specimen must be either directly inoculated onto freshly prepared isolation media (e.g., charcoal-horse blood agar, Bordet-Gengou medium) at the patient's bedside or placed in a suitable transport medium (e.g., Regan-Lowe transport medium). Specimens cannot be delivered to the laboratory in traditional transport media, because the organisms will not survive. Inoculated culture media must be kept moist because drying kills the organisms. A portion of the specimen can also be used for microscopic examination.

Microscopy

A direct fluorescent antibody procedure can be used to examine the specimens. In this method, the aspirated specimen is smeared onto a microscopic slide, air dried and heat fixed, and then stained with fluorescein-labeled antibodies directed against *B. pertussis*. Antibodies against *B. parapertussis* should also be used to detect mild forms of pertussis caused by this organism. The direct fluorescent antibody test results are positive in slightly more than half of the patients with pertussis, but false-positive results can occur as a result of cross-reactions with other bacteria.

Culture

After the inoculated media are received in the laboratory, they are incubated in air at 35°C and in a humidified chamber. Prolonged incubation (e.g., 7 days) is necessary because the tiny colonies can be observed only after 3 or more days of incubation. Because the quality of the media dramatically affects the success of culture, laboratories that infrequently culture specimens for *Bordetella* should arrange for the state public health department to process these specimens. Despite use of optimized culture conditions, fewer than half the infected patients have positive cultures.

	Incubation	Catarrhal	Paroxysmal	Convalescent
Duration	7–10 days	1–2 weeks	2–4 weeks	3–4 weeks (or longer)
Symptoms	None	Rhinorrhea, malaise, fever, sneezing, anorexia	Repetitive cough with whoops, vomiting, leukocytosis	Diminished paroxysmal cough, development of secondary complications (pneumonia, seizures, encephalopathy)
Bacterial culture				

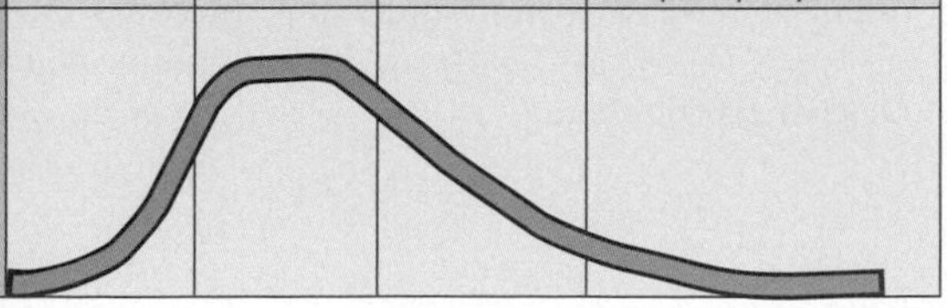

FIGURE 33–3. Clinical presentation of *Bordetella pertussis* disease.

Nucleic Acid Amplification

The most promising diagnostic technique appears to be nucleic acid amplification by methods such as polymerase chain reaction. Several studies have demonstrated a sensitivity of 80% to 100%. Although these tests have been restricted to "home-brew" procedures, it is anticipated that commercial tests (either for *Bordetella* only or for a panel of respiratory pathogens) will be offered soon.

Identification

B. pertussis organisms are identified by their characteristic microscopic and colonial morphology on selective media and their reactivity with a specific antiserum (either in an agglutination reaction or with the reagents used in the direct fluorescent antibody test). The reactions summarized in Table 33–1 can be used to differentiate *B. pertussis* and *B. parapertussis*.

Serology

It is difficult to interpret the results of serologic tests because microscopy and culture techniques are relatively insensitive standards by which to evaluate these results. Most investigators recommend using several tests (e.g., measure immunoglobulin [Ig] G and IgA antibodies against filamentous hemagglutinin and IgG antibodies against pertussis toxin). A significant rise in antibody titer between acute and convalescent serum or an initially high titer is consistent with a recent infection.

Treatment, Prevention, and Control

The treatment for pertussis is primarily supportive, with nursing supervision during the paroxysmal and convalescent stages of the illness. Antibiotics do not ameliorate the clinical course; in fact, convalescence depends on the rapidity and degree to which the layer of ciliated epithelial cells regenerates. Erythromycin is effective in eradicating the organisms and can reduce the duration of infectivity; however, this effect has limited value because the illness is usually unrecognized during the peak of contagiousness.

Whole-cell, inactivated vaccines have been available for almost 50 years. In the United States, they are commonly administered with vaccines for diphtheria and tetanus (DPT vaccine) and are considered 80% to 85% effective in eliminating symptomatic pertussis. However, concern about the associated complications has limited the acceptance of the current whole-cell vaccine in some countries. Multivalent cellular pertussis vaccines have been developed; these vaccines use components believed to evoke protective immunity, such as

filamentous hemagglutinin, pertussis toxin, fimbriae agglutinins, and pertactin. Numerous clinical trials have shown that these vaccines confer a protective immunity at least equivalent to that conferred by whole-cell vaccines, and these vaccines are associated with a lower incidence of side effects. On the basis of these results, it has been recommended that multivalent acellular vaccines should replace the older vaccines.

Because pertussis is highly contagious in a susceptible population and unrecognized infections in family members of a symptomatic patient can maintain disease in a community, erythromycin has been used for prophylaxis in select instances.

Other *Bordetella* Species

B. parapertussis is responsible for causing 10% to 20% of the cases of mild pertussis occurring annually in the United States. *B. bronchiseptica* causes respiratory disease primarily in animals but has been associated with human respiratory tract colonization and bronchopulmonary disease. Both organisms can be readily isolated on conventional laboratory media, and unlike *B. pertussis*, both have easily recognizable metabolic properties.

Francisella Tularensis

F. tularensis is the causative agent of **tularemia** (also called **glandular fever, rabbit fever, tick fever,** and **deer fly fever**) in animals and humans. The organism was originally named *Bacterium tularensis* because it was discovered to be a pathogen of rodents in Tulare County, California. It was later discovered to be an important human pathogen, and, because Edward Francis spent his professional life studying this organism and the pathology of human disease, the organism was renamed *Francisella tularensis*.

Physiology and Structure

F. tularensis is a very small (0.2 × 0.2 to 0.7 μm), faintly staining, gram-negative coccobacillus (Fig. 33–4). The organism is nonmotile, has a thin lipid capsule, and has fastidious growth requirements (i.e., most strains require cysteine for growth). Like *Bordetella*, this organism is strictly aerobic and requires enriched media and incubation for a minimum of 3 days.

Pathogenesis and Immunity

F. tularensis is an intracellular parasite that can survive for prolonged periods in macrophages of the reticuloendothelial system because the organism inhibits phagosome-lysosome fusion. Pathogenic strains possess an antiphagocytic capsule, and loss of the capsule is associated with decreased virulence (Box 33–2). Like all

FIGURE 33-4. Gram stain of *Francisella tularensis* isolated in culture.

gram-negative bacilli, this organism has endotoxin, but it is considerably less active than the endotoxin found in other gram-negative bacilli (e.g., *Escherichia coli*).

Epidemiology

Although *F. tularensis* has a worldwide distribution, reports of disease are somewhat restricted. For example, in the United States, disease primarily occurs in the states of Missouri, Oklahoma, and Arkansas. The organism is found in many wild mammals, domestic animals, birds, fish, and blood-sucking arthropods, as well as in contaminated water. The most common reservoirs of *F. tularensis* in the United States are rabbits, ticks, and muskrats. Human tularemia is acquired most often from the bite of an infected tick or from contact with an infected animal or domestic pet (e.g., cat) that has caught an infected animal (e.g., rabbit). However, disease can also be acquired from the consumption of contaminated meat or water or from the inhalation of an infectious aerosol (most commonly in a laboratory or while dressing an infected animal). Infection with *F. tularensis* requires as few as 10 organisms when exposure is by an arthropod bite or contamination of unbroken skin, 50 organisms when inhaled, and 10^8 organisms when ingested.

The reported incidence of disease is low. Approximately 100 cases are recognized in the United States each year; however, the actual number of infections is likely to be much higher because tularemia is frequently unsuspected and is difficult to confirm by laboratory tests. In addition, the Centers for Disease Control and Prevention has not required reporting tularemia since 1994. Thus, awareness of the disease has waned for many physicians.

Most of the infections occur during the summer (when exposure to infected ticks is greatest) and the winter (when hunters are exposed to infected rabbits). The incidence of disease increases dramatically when a relatively warm winter is followed by a wet summer and the tick population proliferates. People at greatest risk for infection are hunters, those exposed to ticks, and laboratory personnel. In areas where the organism is endemic, it is said that if a rabbit is moving so slowly that it can be shot by a hunter or caught by a pet, the rabbit could be infected.

BOX 33-2. Summary of *Francisella tularensis* Infections

Physiology and Structure

Very small gram-negative coccobacilli.
Strict aerobe.
Nonfermenter.
Requires specialized media and prolonged incubation for growth in culture.

Virulence

Antiphagocytic capsule.
Intracellular pathogen resistant to killing in serum and by phagocytes.

Epidemiology

Wild mammals, domestic animals, birds, fish, and blood-sucking arthropods are reservoirs; rabbits and ticks most common hosts; humans are accidental hosts.
Worldwide distribution.
Approximately 100 cases seen in United States, although the actual number is not known because this is not a reportable disease.
The infectious dose is small when exposure is by arthropod, through skin, or by inhalation; large numbers of organisms must be ingested for infection by this route.

Disease

Clinical symptoms and prognosis determined by route of infection: ulceroglandular, oculoglandular, glandular, typhoidal, oropharyngeal, gastrointestinal, and pneumonic.

Diagnosis

Microscopy is insensitive.
Culture on cysteine-supplemented media is sensitive and specific if prolonged incubation is used.
Serology can be used to confirm the clinical diagnosis.

Treatment, Prevention, and Control

Streptomycin is the antibiotic of choice, with gentamicin an acceptable alternative. Penicillins and some cephalosporins are ineffective.
Disease prevented by avoiding reservoirs and vectors of infection. Clothing and gloves are protective.
Live-attenuated vaccine available but rarely used in human disease.

Clinical Diseases

The symptoms of tularemia develop abruptly after a 3- to 5-day incubation period and include fever, chills, malaise, and fatigue. *F. tularensis* disease is subdivided into several different forms based on the clinical presentation: ulceroglandular, oculoglandular, glandular, typhoidal, oropharyngeal, pneumonic, and gastrointestinal.

Ulceroglandular tularemia is the most common manifestation. A skin lesion, which starts as a painful papule in the area of the enlarged lymph node, develops at the site of the tick bite. The papule then ulcerates and has a necrotic center and raised border. Localized lymphadenopathy and bacteremia are also typically present.

Oculoglandular tularemia is a specialized form of the disease and results from direct contamination of the eye. The organism can be introduced into the eyes, for example, by contaminated fingers or through exposure to water or aerosols. Affected patients have a painful conjunctivitis and regional lymphadenopathy.

Patients with **glandular tularemia** initially have a painful adenopathy without the overlying ulcer. **Typhoidal tularemia** is a systemic illness characterized by sepsis with multiorgan involvement. This is the most difficult form to recognize and is associated with the highest mortality. **Oropharyngeal tularemia** and **gastrointestinal tularemia** result from the ingestion of contaminated meat or water. **Pneumonic tularemia** results from inhalation of infectious aerosols and is also associated with high morbidity and mortality unless the organism is recovered rapidly in blood cultures (it is generally not recovered in respiratory cultures).

Laboratory Diagnosis

Specimen Collection

The collection and processing of specimens for the isolation of *F. tularensis* are extremely hazardous for both the physician and the laboratory worker. The organism, by virtue of its small size, can penetrate through unbroken skin and the mucous membranes during collection of the sample, or it can be inhaled if aerosols are produced (a particular concern during processing of specimens in the laboratory). Even though tularemia is rare, it is commonly reported as a laboratory-acquired infection. Gloves should be worn during collection of the specimen (e.g., aspiration of an ulcer or lymph node), and all processing should be performed in a biohazard hood.

Microscopy

Detection of *F. tularensis* in Gram-stained aspirates from infected nodes or ulcers is almost always unsuc-

cessful because the organism is extremely small and stains faintly (see Fig. 33–4). A more sensitive and specific approach is direct staining of the clinical specimen with fluorescein-labeled antibodies directed against the organism; however, most clinical laboratories do not perform this test.

Culture

It is stated that *F. tularensis* cannot be isolated on common laboratory media because the organism requires sulfhydryl-containing substances (e.g., cysteine) for it to grow. However, *F. tularensis* can grow on the chocolate agar plates used in most laboratories (medium is supplemented with cysteine) and occasionally will grow on blood agar media. Thus, it is usually not necessary for a laboratory to use specialized media such as cysteine blood agar or glucose cysteine agar. If infection with *F. tularensis* is suspected, the laboratory should be notified. *F. tularensis* grows slowly and may be overlooked if the cultures are not incubated for a prolonged period. Blood cultures are generally negative for the organism unless the cultures are incubated for a week or longer. Cultures of respiratory specimens will be positive if appropriate selective media are used to suppress the more rapidly growing bacteria from the upper respiratory tract. *F. tularensis* also grows on the selective media used for *Legionella* because the media are supplemented with cysteine. Aspirates of lymph nodes or draining sinuses are usually positive if the cultures are incubated for 3 days or longer.

Identification

Preliminary identification of *F. tularensis* is based on the slow growth of very small gram-negative coccobacilli. Growth on chocolate agar but not blood agar is also helpful. The identification is confirmed by demonstrating the reactivity of the bacteria with specific antiserum (i.e., agglutination of the organism with antibodies against *Francisella*). Further biochemical testing is not helpful and can be hazardous.

Serology

Tularemia is diagnosed in most patients by finding of a fourfold or greater increase in the titer of antibodies during the illness or a single titer of 1:160 or greater. However, antibodies (including IgG, IgM, and IgA) can persist for many years, making it difficult to differentiate between past and current disease. Antibodies directed against *Brucella* can also cross react with *Francisella*. Therefore, the diagnosis of tularemia should not be based solely on serologic tests.

Treatment, Prevention, and Control

Streptomycin is the antibiotic of choice for the treatment of all forms of tularemia. Gentamicin is an acceptable alternative, but there has been less clinical experience with this drug. *F. tularensis* strains produce β-lactamase, which renders penicillins and some cephalosporins ineffective. The use of ciprofloxacin or imipenem has proved useful for a limited number of patients, but additional studies are needed before these antibiotics can be recommended. Tetracycline and chloramphenicol have been used to treat infections; however, these bacteriostatic antibiotics are associated with an unacceptably high rate of relapse. The mortality rate is less than 1% if patients are treated promptly.

To prevent infection, people should avoid the reservoirs and vectors of infection (e.g., rabbits, ticks, biting insects), but this is often difficult. At a minimum, people should not handle ill-appearing rabbits and should wear gloves when skinning and eviscerating animals. Because the organism is present in the arthropod's feces and not saliva, the tick must feed for a prolonged time before the infection is transmitted. Prompt removal of the tick can therefore prevent infection. Wearing protective clothing and using insect repellents reduce the risk of exposure.

Live-attenuated vaccines are not completely effective in preventing disease but can lessen the severity of the disease. These are recommended for people at a significantly increased risk of exposure to the organism. Inactivated vaccines do not elicit protective cellular immunity.

Brucella

The genus *Brucella* consists of seven species, four of which cause human brucellosis: *Brucella abortus*, *Brucella melitensis*, *Brucella suis*, and *Brucella canis*. The diseases caused by members of this genus are characterized by a number of names based on the original microbiologists who isolated and described the organisms (Sir David Bruce [**brucellosis**], Bernhard Bang [**Bang's disease**]),

its clinical presentation (**undulant fever**), and the sites of recognized outbreaks (e.g., Malta fever, Mediterranean remittent fever, rock fever of Gibraltar, county fever of Constantinople, fever of Crete). However, the most commonly used term is *brucellosis*, and that will be used in this text.

Physiology and Structure

The individual species are distinguished by their reservoir host, growth properties, and biochemical reactivities, as well as by the fatty acid composition of their cell walls. Brucellae are small (0.5×0.6 to 1.5 μm), nonmotile, nonencapsulated, gram-negative coccobacilli. The organism grows slowly on culture (taking a week or more); is strictly aerobic, with some strains requiring supplemental carbon dioxide for growth; and does not ferment carbohydrates. Human isolates are catalase- and oxidase-positive, are able to reduce nitrate, and have variable urease activity. *B. abortus*, *B. melitensis*, and *B. suis* have two surface antigens in common: **A and M antigens**. *B. abortus* has the highest concentration of A antigen, and *B. melitensis* has the highest concentration of M antigen. *B. canis* is antigenically distinct and thus is not detected by the serologic assays that are used to recognize the other pathogenic species. Some characteristics of the four species that cause human disease are summarized in Table 33–3.

Pathogenesis and Immunity

Like *Francisella*, *Brucella* is an intracellular parasite of the reticuloendothelial system. After the initial exposure, the organisms are phagocytosed by macrophages and monocytes and then are carried to the spleen, liver, bone marrow, lymph nodes, and kidneys. Granulomas form in these organs, and destructive changes in these and other tissues occur in patients with advanced disease. These organisms are able to survive intracellularly because they can inhibit polymorphonuclear leukocyte degranulation, and their survival in cells can be prolonged unless specific cellular immunity develops.

TABLE 33–3. **Characteristics of Human Brucellosis**

Species	Animal Reservoir	Clinical Disease
Brucella melitensis	Goats, sheep	Severe acute disease with complications (common)
Brucella abortus	Cattle	Mild disease with suppurative complications (uncommon)
Brucella suis	Swine	Chronic, suppurative, destructive disease
Brucella canis	Dogs	Mild disease with suppurative complications (uncommon)

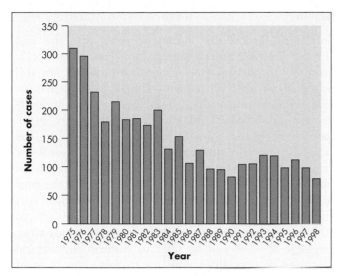

FIGURE 33–5. Incidence of brucellosis in the United States from 1975 to 1998.

B. melitensis is the species most able to resist the bactericidal effect of serum and phagocytic killing, consistent with the increased virulence of this species.

Epidemiology

Brucella infections have a worldwide distribution, with more than 500,000 documented cases reported annually. However, the incidence of disease in the United States is much lower (79 reported infections in 1998 [Fig. 33–5]), with approximately 1 reported case per 3 million people. The disease is rare in the United States because disease in the animal reservoir is well controlled.

Brucella causes mild or asymptomatic disease in the natural host: *B. abortus* infects cattle; *B. melitensis*, goats and sheep; *B. suis*, swine; and *B. canis*, dogs, foxes, and coyotes (Box 33–3). The organism has a predilection for infecting organs rich in erythritol, a sugar metabolized by many *Brucella* strains in preference to glucose. Animal (but not human) tissues, including breast, uterus, placenta, and epididymis, are rich in erythritol. The organisms thus localize in these tissues in nonhuman reservoirs and can cause sterility, abortions, or asymptomatic carriage. Human disease in the United States results primarily from consumption of contaminated unpasteurized milk and other dairy products. California and Texas are the areas in the United States where the highest number of cases is reported, and most of these infections occur in residents from Mexico or visitors to that country. Laboratory personnel are also at significant risk for infection through direct contact or inhalation of the organism. Disease in the animal population in the United States has been effectively eliminated through the destruction of infected animals and the vaccination of disease-free animals;

thus, infections in veterinarians, slaughterhouse workers, and farmers is now much less common than before 1980.

Clinical Diseases

The disease spectrum of brucellosis depends on the infecting organism. *B. abortus* and *B. canis* tend to produce mild disease with rare suppurative complications. In contrast, *B. suis* causes the formation of destructive lesions and has a prolonged course. *B. melitensis*, the

---

BOX 33–3. Summary of *Brucella* Infections

Physiology and Structure

Very small gram-negative coccobacilli.
Nonfermentative.
Strict aerobe.
Requires specialized media and prolonged incubation for growth in culture.

Virulence

Intracellular pathogen that is resistant to killing in serum and by phagocytes.

Epidemiology

Animal reservoirs are goats and sheep (*Brucella melitensis*), cattle (*Brucella abortus*), swine (*Brucella suis*), and dogs (*Brucella canis*).
Worldwide distribution, although vaccination of herds has controlled disease in the United States.
Most disease in the United States is reported in the Hispanic population in California and Texas.
No seasonal incidence.
Individuals at greatest risk for disease are people who consume unpasteurized dairy products, people in direct contact with infected animals, and laboratory workers.

Disease

Brucellosis

Diagnosis

Microscopy is insensitive.
Culture is sensitive and specific if prolonged incubation is used.
Serology can be used to confirm the clinical diagnosis.

Treatment, Prevention, and Control

Treatment for 3 to 6 weeks with doxycycline either alone or with rifampin or gentamicin for patients older than 8 years; doxycycline is replaced with trimethoprim-sulfamethoxazole for children younger than 8 years or for pregnant women.
Human disease is controlled by eradication of the disease in the animal reservoir through vaccination and serologic monitoring of the animals for evidence of disease; pasteurization of dairy products; and use of proper safety techniques in clinical laboratories working with this organism.

most common cause of brucellosis, also causes severe disease with a high incidence of serious complications because the organisms can survive in phagocytic cells and multiply to high concentrations.

Acute disease develops in approximately half of the patients infected with *Brucella*, with symptoms first appearing up to 2 months after exposure. Initial symptoms are nonspecific and consist of malaise, chills, sweats, fatigue, weakness, myalgias, weight loss, arthralgias, and nonproductive cough. Almost all patients have fever, and this can be intermittent in untreated patients, hence the name **undulant fever.** Patients with advanced disease can have gastrointestinal tract symptoms (70% of patients), osteolytic lesions or joint effusions (20% to 60%), respiratory tract symptoms (25%), and less commonly, cutaneous, neurologic, or cardiovascular manifestations. Chronic infections can also develop in inadequately treated patients.

Laboratory Diagnosis

Specimen Collection

Several blood samples should be collected for culture and serologic testing. Bone marrow cultures, as well as cultures of infected tissues, may also be useful. To ensure safe handling of the specimen, the laboratory should be notified if brucellosis is suspected.

Microscopy

Brucella organisms are readily stained using conventional techniques, but their intracellular location and small size make them difficult to detect in clinical specimens.

Culture

Brucella organisms are slow-growing during primary isolation. The organisms can grow on most enriched blood agars and occasionally on MacConkey agar; however, incubation for 3 or more days may be required. Blood cultures should be incubated for 2 weeks before they are considered negative.

Identification

Preliminary identification of *Brucella* is based on the isolate's microscopic and colonial morphology, a positive oxidase reaction, and reactivity with antibodies directed against *Brucella*. Because isolates are uncommon in the United States, most laboratories refer the organism to a state public health laboratory for definitive identification.

Serology

Subclinical brucellosis and many cases of acute and chronic diseases are identified by a specific antibody response in the infected patient. Antibodies are detected in virtually all patients. Initially observed is an IgM response, after which both IgG and IgA antibodies are produced. Antibodies can persist for many months or years; thus, a significant increase in the antibody titer is required to provide definitive serologic evidence of current disease. A presumptive diagnosis can be made if there is a fourfold increase in the titer or a single titer is greater than or equal to 1:80. High antibody titers (1:160 or more) are noted in 5% to 10% of the population living in endemic areas; thus, serologic tests should be used to confirm the clinical diagnosis of brucellosis and not to form the basis of the diagnosis. The antigen used in the *Brucella* agglutination test is from *B. abortus.* Antibodies directed against *B. melitensis* or *B. suis* cross react with this antigen; however, there is no cross-reactivity with *B. canis.* The specific *B. canis* antigen must be used to diagnose infections with this organism. Antibodies directed against other genera of bacteria are also reported to cross react with the *B. abortus* antigen.

Treatment, Prevention, and Control

Tetracyclines, with doxycycline the preferred agent, are generally active against most strains of *Brucella*; however, because this is a bacteriostatic drug, relapse is common after an initially successful response. The combination of doxycycline with rifampin or gentamicin has proved effective and yields a low incidence of relapse. Because the tetracyclines are toxic to young children and fetuses, doxycycline should be replaced with trimethoprim-sulfamethoxazole for pregnant women and children younger than 8 years. Treatment must be continued for 6 weeks or longer for it to be successful. Relapse of disease is due to inadequate therapy and not the development of antibiotic resistance.

Control of human brucellosis is accomplished through control of the disease in livestock, as demonstrated in the United States. This requires systematic identification (by serologic testing) and elimination of infected herds and animal vaccination. The avoidance of unpasteurized dairy products, the observance of appropriate safety procedures in the clinical laboratory, and the wearing of protective clothing by abattoir workers, are further ways to prevent brucellosis. The live-attenuated *B. abortus* and *B. melitensis* vaccines have been used successfully to prevent infection in animal herds. Vaccines have not been developed against *B. suis* or *B. canis*, and the existing vaccines cannot be used in humans because they produce symptomatic disease. The lack of an effective human vaccine is of concern because *Brucella* (as well as *Bordetella* and *Francisella*) could be used as an agent of bioterrorism.

CASE STUDY AND QUESTIONS

■ A 5-year-old girl was brought to the local public health clinic because of a severe, intractable cough. During the previous 10 days she had a persistent cold that had become worse. The cough developed the previous day and was so severe that it was frequently followed by vomiting. The child appeared exhausted from the coughing episodes. A blood cell count showed a marked leukocytosis with a predominance of lymphocytes. The examining physician suspected that the child had pertussis.

1. What laboratory tests can be performed to confirm the physician's clinical diagnosis? What specimens should be collected, and how should they be submitted to the laboratory?
2. What virulence factors are produced by *B. pertussis*, and what are their biologic effects?
3. What is the natural progression and prognosis for this disease? How can it be prevented? What are the differences between whole-cell and acellular vaccines?
4. Describe the epidemiology and clinical manifestations of *F. tularensis* infections.
5. Describe the epidemiology and clinical manifestations of infection with *Brucella*.

BIBLIOGRAPHY

Capellan J, Fong I: Tularemia from a cat bite: case report and review of feline-associated tularemia, *Clin Infect Dis* 16:472–475, 1993.

Centers for Disease Control and Prevention: Pertussis: United States, *MMWR* 47:1–92, 1999.

Cherry J, Robbins J: Pertussis in adults: epidemiology, signs, symptoms, and implications for vaccination, *Clin Infect Dis* 28 (suppl 2), 1999.

Chomel B et al: Changing trends in the epidemiology of human brucellosis in California from 1973 to 1992: a shift toward foodborne transmission, *J Infect Dis* 170:1216–1223, 1994.

Edwards K, Decker M: Acellular pertussis vaccines for infants, *N Engl J Med* 334:391–392, 1996 (editorial).

Guris D et al: Changing epidemiology of pertussis in the United States: increasing reported incidence among adolescents and adults, 1990–1996, *Clin Infect Dis* 28:1230–1237, 1999.

He Q et al: Whooping cough caused by *Bordetella pertussis* and *Bordetella parapertussis* in an immunized population, *JAMA* 280:635–637, 1998.

Hoppe J: Update on epidemiology, diagnosis, and treatment of pertussis, *Eur J Clin Microbiol Infect Dis* 15:189–193, 1996.

Kerr J, Matthews R: *Bordetella pertussis* infection: pathogenesis, diagnosis, management, and the role of protective immunity, *Eur J Clin Microbiol Infect Dis* 19:77–88, 2000.

Loeffelholz M et al: Comparison of PCR, culture, and direct fluorescent-antibody testing for detection of *Bordetella pertussis*, *J Clin Microbiol* 37:2872–2876, 1999.

Muller F et al: Laboratory diagnosis of pertussis: state of the art in 1997, *J Clin Microbiol* 35:2435–2443, 1997.

Nennig M et al: Prevalence and incidence of adult pertussis in an urban population, *JAMA* 275:1672–1674, 1996.

Tilley P et al: Detection of *Bordetella pertussis* in a clinical laboratory by culture, polymerase chain reaction, and direct fluorescent antibody staining: accuracy and cost. *Diagn Microbial Infect Dis* 37:17–23, 2000.

Vancanney M et al: Differentiation of *Bordetella pertussis*, *B. parapertussis*, and *B. bronchiseptica* by whole-cell protein electrophoresis and fatty acid analysis, *Int J Syst Bacteriol* 45:843–847, 1995.

Woolfrey BF, Moody JA: Human infections associated with *Bordetella bronchiseptica*, *Clin Microbiol Rev* 4:243–255, 1991.

Wright S et al: Pertussis infection in adults with persistent cough, *JAMA* 273:1044–1046, 1996.

Yagupsky P: Detection of Brucellae in blood cultures, *J Clin Microbiol* 37:3437–3442, 1999.

CHAPTER 34

Pasteurellaceae

The family Pasteurellaceae consists of three genera, *Haemophilus*, *Pasteurella*, and *Actinobacillus*. *Haemophilus* is the most common human pathogen (Table 34–1). Although these genera are clearly related to one other, the taxonomic classification of the individual species is controversial. Because the classification is unsettled, the traditional nomenclature has been maintained in this chapter.

The members of the family Pasteurellaceae are small (0.2 × 0.3 to 1.0 × 2.0 μm), gram-negative, non–spore-forming, nonmotile, and aerobic or facultative anaerobic bacilli. Most have fastidious growth needs, requiring enriched media for isolation.

Haemophilus

Haemophilus organisms are small, sometimes pleomorphic, gram-negative bacilli (Fig. 34–1; Box 34–1). They are obligate parasites present on the mucous membranes of humans and certain species of animals. *Haemophilus influenzae* is the species most commonly associated with disease. Although less frequently isolated, *Haemophilus ducreyi* is well-recognized as the etiologic agent of the sexually transmitted disease **soft chancre**, or **chancroid**. *Haemophilus aphrophilus* is an uncommon but important cause of endocarditis. The other members of the genus are commonly isolated in clinical specimens but are rarely pathogenic, being responsible primarily for opportunistic infections.

Physiology and Structure

Most species of *Haemophilus* (from the Greek words for "blood-loving") require media supplemented with the following growth-stimulating factors: (1) **X factor** (hematin), (2) **V factor** (nicotinamide adenine dinucleotide [NAD]), or (3) both. Although both factors are present in blood-enriched media, sheep blood agar must be gently heated to destroy the inhibitors of V factor. For this reason, heated-blood ("chocolate") agar is used for the in vitro isolation of *Haemophilus*.

The cell wall structure of *Haemophilus* is typical of other gram-negative bacilli. Lipopolysaccharide with endotoxin activity is present in the cell wall, and strain-specific and species-specific proteins are found in the outer membrane. Analysis of these strain-specific proteins is valuable in epidemiologic investigations. The surface of many but not all strains of *H. influenzae* is covered with a **polysaccharide capsule**, and six antigenic serotypes (**a** through **f**) have been identified. Before the introduction of haemophilus vaccines, *H. influenzae* serotype b was responsible for more than 95% of all invasive *Haemophilus* infections. After the introduction of vaccines directed against the type b capsular antigen, most disease caused by this serotype disappeared. Currently, serotypes c and f as well as nonencapsulated *H. influenzae* are responsible for most *H. influenzae* disease.

In addition to the serologic differentiation of *H. influenzae*, the species is subdivided into eight biotypes (I through VIII) on the basis of the following three biochemical reactions: indole production, urease activity, and ornithine decarboxylase activity. The separation of these biotypes is useful for epidemiologic purposes. Finally, *H. influenzae* has been subdivided into biogroups. This subdivision is useful for clinical purposes. *H. influenzae* biogroup *aegypticus* is important because it causes purulent conjunctivitis and a systemic disease called Brazilian purpuric fever. Although biogroup *aegyptius* and *H. influenzae* biotype III have identical biochemical profiles, they can be distinguished on the basis of (1) the nature of the clinical disease, (2) their in vitro growth properties, and (3) the outer membrane protein profiles.

In summary, *H. influenzae* is subdivided as follows:

1. Serotypes a through f (determined by the presence of capsular antigens; type b the most important).
2. Biotypes I through VIII (determined by biochemical properties).
3. Biogroups (with biogroup *aegypticus* the most important clinically).

TABLE 34–1. *Haemophilus* Species Associated with Human Disease

Species	Primary Diseases	Frequency
H. influenzae	Pneumonia, sinusitis, otitis, conjunctivitis, meningitis, epiglottitis, cellulitis, bacteremia	Common
H. ducreyi	Chancroid	Uncommon (in U.S.)
H. aphrophilus	Endocarditis, opportunistic infections	Uncommon
H. parainfluenzae	Bacteremia, endocarditis, opportunistic infections	Rare
H. haemolyticus	Opportunistic infections	Rare
H. parahaemolyticus	Opportunistic infections	Rare
H. paraphrophilus	Opportunistic infections	Rare
H. segnis	Opportunistic infections	Rare

Pathogenesis and Immunity

Haemophilus species, particularly *Haemophilus parainfluenzae* and nonencapsulated *H. influenzae*, colonize the upper respiratory tract in virtually all people within the first few months of life. These organisms can spread locally and cause disease in the ears (otitis media), sinuses (sinusitis), and lower respiratory tract (bronchitis, pneumonia). Disseminated disease, however, is relatively uncommon. In contrast, encapsulated *H. influenzae* (particularly serotype b) is uncommon in the upper respiratory tract or is present in only very small numbers but has been a common cause of disease in children (i.e., meningitis, epiglottitis, cellulitis). Pili and nonpilus adhesins mediate colonization of the oropharynx with *H. influenzae*. Cell wall components of the bacteria (e.g., lipopolysaccharide and a low-molecular-weight glycopeptide) impair ciliary function, leading to damage of the respiratory epithelium. The bacteria can then be translocated across both epithelial and endothelial cells and can enter the blood stream. In the absence of specific opsonic antibodies directed against the polysaccharide capsule, high-grade bacteremia can develop, with dissemination to the meninges or other distal foci.

The major virulence factor in *H. influenzae* type b is the antiphagocytic polysaccharide capsule, which contains ribose, ribitol, and phosphate (commonly referred to as **polyribitol phosphate [PRP]**). Antibodies directed against the capsule greatly stimulate bacterial phagocytosis and complement-mediated bactericidal activity. These antibodies develop as a result of natural infection, vaccination with purified PRP, or the passive transfer of maternal antibodies. The severity of systemic disease is inversely related to the rate of clearance of bacteria from the blood stream. The risk of meningitis and epiglottitis is significantly greater in patients with no anti-PRP antibodies, those with depletion of complement, and those who have undergone splenectomy. The lipopolysaccharide lipid A component induces meningeal inflammation in an animal model and may be responsible for initiating this response in humans. Immunoglobulin (Ig) A1 proteases are produced by *H. influenzae* (both encapsulated and nonencapsulated strains) and may facilitate colonization of the organisms on mucosal surfaces by interfering with humoral immunity.

Epidemiology

Haemophilus species are present in almost all individuals. Most of the isolates are nonencapsulated *H. influenzae*, with encapsulated strains detectable in small numbers and only when highly selective culture methods are used. *H. influenzae* type b is the most common serotype that causes systemic disease; however, it is rarely isolated in healthy children (a fact that emphasizes the virulence of this bacterium). In contrast, *H. parainfluenzae* constitutes 10% of the bacterial flora in saliva, and the other species are associated with dental plaque and periodontal disease. *Haemophilus* species can also be isolated in the gastrointestinal and genitourinary tracts but typically in relatively low numbers.

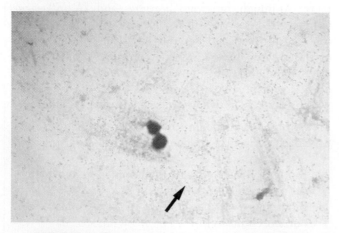

FIGURE 34–1. Gram stain of *Haemophilus influenzae*.

BOX 34–1. Summary of *Haemophilus* Infections

Physiology and Structure

Small, pleomorphic, gram-negative bacilli or coccobacilli. Facultative anaerobes, fermentative.

Most species require X and/or V factor for growth.

H. influenzae subdivided serologically (types a to f), biochemically (biotypes I to VIII), and clinically (biogroup *aegypticus*).

Virulence

H. influenzae type b is clinically most virulent (with PRP, [polyribitol phosphate] in capsule).

Haemophilus adhere to host cells via pili and nonpilus structures.

Epidemiology

Noncapsular *Haemophilus* commonly colonized humans; encapsulated *Haemophilus* species, particularly *H. influenzae* type b, are uncommon members of normal flora.

Disease caused by *H. influenzae* type b was primarily a pediatric problem; eliminated in immunized populations.

H. ducreyi disease is uncommon in the United States.

With the exception of *H. ducreyi*, which is spread by sexual contract, most *Haemophilus* infections are caused by the patient's bacterial flora (endogenous infections).

Patients at greatest risk for disease are those with inadequate levels of protective antibodies, those with depleted complement, and those who have undergone splenectomy.

Diseases

H. influenzae is responsible for meningitis, epiglottitis, cellulitis, arthritis, otitis, sinusitis, lower respiratory tract disease, conjunctivitis, and Brazilian purpuric fever.

H. ducreyi is responsible of the ulcerative genital infection chancroid.

Diagnosis

Microscopy is a sensitive test for detecting *H. influenzae* in CSF, synovial fluid, and lower respiratory specimens.

Culture is performed using chocolate agar.

Antigen tests for *H. influenzae* type b are less useful following the introduction of vaccination for this organism.

Treatment, Prevention, and Control

Haemophilus infections are treated with broad-spectrum cephalosporins, azithromycin, or fluoroquinolones; many strains are resistant to ampicillin.

Active immunization with conjugated PRP vaccines prevents most *H. influenzae* type b infections.

Rifampin prophylaxis is used to eliminate carriage of *H. influenzae* in children at high risk for disease.

The epidemiology of *Haemophilus* disease has changed dramatically. Before the introduction of conjugated *H. influenzae* type b vaccines, an estimated 20,000 cases of invasive *H. influenzae* type b disease occurred annually in children younger than 5 years. The first polysaccharide vaccines for *H. influenzae* type b were not protective for children younger than 18 months (the population at greatest risk for disease), because there is a natural delay in the maturation of the immune response to polysaccharide antigens. Vaccines containing purified PRP antigens conjugated to protein carriers (i.e., diphtheria toxoid, tetanus toxoid, meningococcal outer membrane protein), however, were found to elicit a protective antibody response in infants 2 months and older. Since the introduction of conjugated vaccines in December 1987, there has been a 95% reduction in the incidence of systemic disease in children younger than 5 years, with only approximately 250 cases reported in 1999. Most of the *H. influenzae* type b infections now occur in children who are not immune (because of incomplete vaccination or a poor response to the vaccine) and in elderly adults with waning immunity. In addition, invasive *H. influenzae* disease due to other serotypes of encapsulated bacteria and by nonencapsulated strains has now become proportionally more common than that due to serotype b. It should be noted that the successful elimination of *H. influenzae* type b disease in the United States has not been seen in many developing countries where vaccination programs have not been implemented successfully. Thus, *H. influenzae* type b remains the most significant pediatric pathogen in many countries of the world.

The epidemiology of disease caused by nonencapsulated *H. influenzae* and other *Haemophilus* species is distinct. Because it is common for people to be colonized with these species, invasive disease is relatively uncommon. Ear and sinus infections caused by these organisms are primarily pediatric diseases but can occur in adults. Pulmonary disease most commonly affects elderly people, particularly those with a history of underlying obstructive pulmonary disease or conditions predisposing to aspiration (e.g., alcoholism, altered mental state).

H. ducreyi is an important cause of genital ulcers (chancroid) in Africa and Asia but is less common in Europe and North America. The incidence of disease in the United States is cyclic. A peak incidence of more than 5000 cases was reported in 1988, which decreased to fewer than 250 cases in 1999. Despite this favorable trend, the Centers for Disease Control and Prevention have documented that the disease is significantly underreported, so the true incidence is unknown.

Clinical Diseases

The clinical syndromes seen in patients with *H. influenzae* infections are represented in Figure 34–2. The

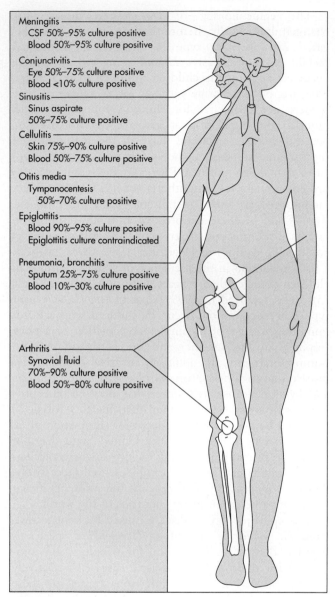

Meningitis
  CSF 50%–95% culture positive
  Blood 50%–95% culture positive

Conjunctivitis
  Eye 50%–75% culture positive
  Blood <10% culture positive

Sinusitis
  Sinus aspirate
  50%–75% culture positive

Cellulitis
  Skin 75%–90% culture positive
  Blood 50%–75% culture positive

Otitis media
  Tympanocentesis
  50%–70% culture positive

Epiglottitis
  Blood 90%–95% culture positive
  Epiglottitis culture contraindicated

Pneumonia, bronchitis
  Sputum 25%–75% culture positive
  Blood 10%–30% culture positive

Arthritis
  Synovial fluid
  70%–90% culture positive
  Blood 50%–80% culture positive

FIGURE 34–2. Infections caused by *Haemophilus influenzae*. With the advent of the conjugated vaccine, most infections in adults involve areas contiguous with the oropharynx (i.e., lower respiratory tract, sinuses, ears). Serious systemic infections (e.g., meningitis, epiglottitis) can occur in nonimmune patients. CSF = Cerebrospinal fluid.

diseases caused by all *Haemophilus* species are described in the following sections.

Meningitis

H. influenzae type b was the most common cause of pediatric meningitis, but this situation changed rapidly once the conjugated vaccines became widely used. Disease in nonimmune patients results from the bacteremic spread of the organisms from the nasopharynx and cannot be differentiated clinically from other causes of bacterial meningitis. The initial presentation is a 1- to 3-day history of mild upper respiratory disease, after which the typical signs and symptoms of meningitis appear. Mortality is less than 10% in patients who receive prompt therapy, and carefully designed studies have documented a low incidence of serious neurologic sequelae (in contrast with the 50% incidence of severe residual damage in nonimmune children seen in initial studies).

Epiglottitis

Epiglottitis, characterized by cellulitis and the swelling of the supraglottic tissues, represents a life-threatening emergency. Although epiglottitis is a pediatric disease, the peak incidence of this disease during the prevaccine era occurred in children 2 to 4 years of age; in contrast, the peak incidence of meningitis was seen in children 3 to 18 months of age. Children with epiglottitis have pharyngitis, fever, and difficulty breathing, which can progress rapidly to complete obstruction of the airway and death. Since the introduction of the vaccine, the incidence of this disease has also decreased dramatically in children and remains relatively rare in adults.

Cellulitis

Like meningitis and epiglottitis, cellulitis is a pediatric disease due to *H. influenzae* that has largely been eliminated by vaccination. When it is observed, patients have fever and cellulitis characterized by the development of reddish blue patches on the cheeks or periorbital areas. The diagnosis is strongly suggested by the typical clinical presentation, cellulitis proximal to the oral mucosa, and lack of documented vaccination in the child.

Arthritis

Before the advent of conjugated vaccines, the most common form of arthritis in children younger than 2 years was an infection of a single large joint secondary to the bacteremic spread of *H. influenzae* type b. Disease does occur in older children and adults, but it is very uncommon and generally affects immunocompromised patients and patients with previously damaged joints.

Otitis, Sinusitis, and Lower Respiratory Tract Disease

Nonencapsulated strains of *H. influenzae* are opportunistic pathogens that can cause infections of the upper and lower airways. Most studies have shown that *H. influenzae* and *Streptococcus pneumoniae* are the two most common causes of acute and chronic otitis and sinusitis. Primary pneumonia is uncommon in children and adults who have normal pulmonary function. These organisms commonly colonize patients who have chronic pulmonary disease (including cystic fibrosis), and frequently are associated with exacerbation of bronchitis as well as frank pneumonia.

Conjunctivitis and Brazilian Purpuric Fever

Both epidemic conjunctivitis and endemic conjunctivitis can be caused by *H. influenzae* biogroup *aegyptius*. A specific strain of this organism has also been found to cause Brazilian purpuric fever, a fulminant pediatric disease characterized by an initial conjunctivitis followed a few days later by the acute onset of fever, vomiting, and abdominal pain. In untreated patients, petechiae, purpura, and shock culminating in death rapidly ensue. The pathogenesis of Brazilian purpuric fever and the specific virulence characteristics of the pathogen are poorly understood.

Chancroid

Chancroid is a sexually transmitted disease that is most commonly diagnosed in men, presumably because women can have asymptomatic or inapparent disease. Approximately 5 to 7 days after exposure, a tender papule with an erythematous base develops on the genitalia or perianal area. The lesion then ulcerates and becomes painful, and inguinal lymphadenopathy is frequently present. Other causes of genital ulcers, such as syphilis and herpes simplex disease, must be excluded.

Other Infections

Other species of *Haemophilus* can cause opportunistic infections, such as otitis media, conjunctivitis, sinusitis, meningitis, and dental abscesses. Some species, such as *H. aphrophilus*, can spread from the mouth to the blood stream and then infect a previously damaged heart valve, leading to subacute endocarditis. Subacute endocarditis is particularly difficult to diagnose with laboratory testing because organisms cultured from blood grow slowly.

Laboratory Diagnosis

Specimen Collection and Transport

It is necessary to obtain samples of cerebrospinal fluid (CSF) and blood to diagnose *Haemophilus* meningitis. Because there are approximately 10^7 bacteria per mL of CSF in patients with untreated meningitis, 1 to 2 mL of fluid is generally adequate for microscopy, culture, and antigen-detection tests. Blood cultures should also be performed for the diagnosis of epiglottitis, cellulitis, arthritis, or pneumonia. These cultures are less useful, however, for the diagnosis of localized upper respiratory tract diseases (e.g., sinusitis, otitis). Culture of ma-

terial obtained by direct needle aspiration is necessary for definitive microbiologic confirmation of these diseases. Specimens should not be collected from the posterior pharynx in patients with suspected epiglottitis, because the procedure may stimulate coughing and completely obstruct the airway. Specimens for the detection of *H. ducreyi* should be collected with a moistened swab from the base or margin of the ulcer. The laboratory should be notified that this organism is suspected, because special culture techniques must be used for its isolation.

Microscopy

If microscopy is performed carefully, the detection of *Haemophilus* species in clinical specimens is both sensitive and specific. Small gram-negative coccobacilli can be detected in more than 80% of CSF specimens from patients with untreated *Haemophilus* meningitis. The microscopic examination of Gram-stain specimens is also useful for the rapid diagnosis of the organism in arthritis and lower respiratory tract disease.

Culture

It is relatively easy to isolate *H. influenzae* from clinical specimens inoculated onto media supplemented with growth factors. Chocolate agar or Levinthal's agar is used in most laboratories. If chocolate agar is overheated during preparation, however, V factor is destroyed, and *Haemophilus* species requiring this growth factor will not grow; thus, each preparation of medium must be tested before use. The bacteria appear as 1- to 2-mm, smooth, opaque colonies after 24 hours of incubation. They can also be detected growing around colonies of *Staphylococcus aureus* on unheated blood agar (**satellite phenomenon**). The staphylococci provide the requisite growth factors by lysing the erythrocytes in the medium and releasing intracellular V factor. The colonies of *H. influenzae* in these cultures are much smaller than they are on chocolate agar, however, because the V factor inhibitors are not inactivated.

The growth of *Haemophilus* in blood cultures is generally delayed, because most commercially prepared blood culture broths are not supplemented with optimum concentrations of X and V factors. Furthermore, the growth factors are released only when the blood cells lyse, but inhibitors of V factor present in the medium can delay recovery of the bacteria. Isolates of *H. influenzae* frequently grow better in anaerobically incubated blood cultures because under these conditions the organisms do not require X factor for growth.

H. influenzae biogroup *aegyptius* and *H. ducreyi* are fastidious and require specialized growth conditions. Biotype *aegyptius* grows best on chocolate agar supplemented with 1% IsoVitaleX (BBL Microbiology Systems, Cockeysville, Md), with growth detected after incubation in a carbon dioxide atmosphere for 2 to 4 days. The recovery of *H. ducreyi* in culture is relatively insensitive (less than 85% of cultures yield organisms under optimal conditions) but reportedly is best on GC agar supplemented with 1% to 2% hemoglobin, 5% fetal bovine serum, 10% CVA enrichment, and vancomycin (3 μg/mL). Cultures should be incubated at 33°C in 5% to 10% carbon dioxide for 7 days or more.

Antigen Detection

The immunologic detection of *H. influenzae* antigen, specifically the PRP capsular antigen, is a rapid and sensitive way to diagnose *H. influenzae* type b disease. PRP can be detected with particle agglutination, which can detect less than 1 ng/mL of PRP. In this test, antibody-coated latex particles are mixed with the clinical specimen; agglutination occurs if PRP is present. Antigen can be detected in CSF and urine (in which the antigen is eliminated intact). This test has limited utility, however, because it can detect only *H. influenzae* type b, which is uncommon in the United States. Other capsular serotypes and nonencapsulated strains do not give a positive reaction.

Identification

H. influenzae is readily identified by the demonstration of a requirement for both X and V factors and the specific biochemical properties summarized in Table 34-2. Further subgrouping of *H. influenzae* can be done with biotyping, electrophoretic characterization of the membrane protein antigens, and analysis of the strain-specific nucleic acid sequences.

Treatment, Prevention, and Control

Patients with systemic *H. influenzae* infections require prompt antimicrobial therapy, because the mortality rate in patients with meningitis or epiglottitis approaches 100%. Serious infections are treated with broad-spectrum cephalosporins. Less severe infections, such as sinusitis and otitis, can be treated with ampicillin (if susceptible—approximately 35% of strains are resistant), an active cephalosporin, azithromycin, or a fluoroquinolone.

The primary approach to preventing *H. influenzae* type b disease is through active immunization with purified capsular PRP. As discussed previously, the use of conjugated vaccines has been remarkably successful in reducing the incidences of *H. influenzae* type b disease and colonization. Currently, it is recommended that children receive three doses of vaccine against *H. influenzae* type b disease before the age of 6 months, followed by booster doses.

Antibiotic chemoprophylaxis is used to eliminate the carriage of *H. influenzae* type b in children at high risk for disease (e.g., children younger than 2 years in a family or daycare center where systemic disease is documented). Rifampin prophylaxis has been used in these settings.

Pasteurella

Pasteurella are small facultatively anaerobic, fermentative coccobacilli (Fig. 34-3) commonly found as commensals in the oropharynx of healthy animals. Most human infections result from animal contact (e.g., animal bites, scratches, shared food). *Pasteurella multocida* and, less commonly, *Pasteurella canis* are human pathogens; the other *Pasteurella* species are rarely responsible for human infections (Table 34-3). The following three general forms of disease are reported:

TABLE 34-2. Differential Characteristics of Common Members of the Family Pasteurellaceae

Organism	Catalase	Growth Factor Requirement X	V	Enhanced Growth with CO$_2$	Fermentation of Glucose	Sucrose	Lactose	Mannose
Haemophilus:								
H. influenzae	+	+	+	−	+	−	−	−
H. parainfluenzae	+/−	−	+	−	+	+	−	+
H. aphrophilus	−	−	−	+	+	+	+	+
H. ducreyi	−	+	−	−	−	−	−	−
Pasteurella:								
P. multocida	+	−	−	−	+	+	−	+
P. canis	+	−	−	−	+	+/−	−	−
Actinobacillus actinomycetemcomitans	+	−	−	+	+	−	−	+

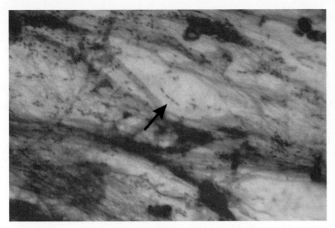

FIGURE 34–3. *Pasteurella multocida* in respiratory specimen from patient with pneumonia.

TABLE 34–3. *Pasteurella* Species Associated with Human Disease

Species	Primary Disease	Frequency
P. multocida	Bite wound infections, chronic pulmonary disease, bacteremia, meningitis	Common
P. canis	Bite wound infections	Uncommon
P. bettyae	Opportunistic infections (abscesses, bite wound infections, urogenital infections, bacteremia)	Rare
P. dagmatis	Bite wound infections	Rare
P. stomatis	Bite wound infections	Rare

1. A localized cellulitis and lymphadenitis that occur after an animal bite or scratch (*P. multocida* from contact with cats or dogs; *P. canis* from dogs).
2. An exacerbation of chronic respiratory tract disease in patients with underlying pulmonary dysfunction (presumably related to colonization of the patient's oropharynx followed by the aspiration of oral secretions).
3. A systemic infection in immunocompromised patients, particularly those with underlying hepatic disease.

P. multocida grows well on blood and chocolate agars but poorly on MacConkey agar and other media typically selective for gram-negative bacilli. After overnight incubation on blood agar, large buttery colonies with a characteristic musty odor caused by the production of indole are present. They can be readily differentiated from other Pasteurellaceae, as indicated in Table 34–2. *P. multocida* is susceptible to a variety of antibiotics. Penicillin is the antibiotic of choice, and tetracycline, cephalosporins, or fluoroquinolones are acceptable alternatives.

Actinobacillus

Actinobacillus species are small, facultatively anaerobic, gram-negative bacilli that grow slowly (generally requiring 2 to 3 days of incubation). *Actinobacillus actinomycetemcomitans* is the most important human pathogen, and the other species are rarely encountered (Table 34–4). The cumbersome name is derived from the fact that this organism is frequently associated with (*comitans*, from the Latin word for "accompanying") *Actinomyces*.

Members of the genus *Actinobacillus* colonize the oropharynx of humans and animals and are responsible for periodontitis, endocarditis, bite wound infections, and opportunistic infections. *A. actinomycetemcomitans* is a relatively uncommon cause of subacute bacterial endocarditis. In patients in whom this disease occurs, however, typically there is preexisting valvular heart disease and evidence of oral disease (e.g., periodontitis, oral abscess, poor oral hygiene). The organism spreads from the oropharynx through the blood stream and adheres to the damaged heart valve. An interesting characteristic of *Actinobacillus* noted in vitro is that the

TABLE 34–4. *Actinobacillus* Species Associated with Human Disease

Species	Primary Diseases	Frequency
A. actinomycetemcomitans	Periodontitis, endocarditis, bite wound infections	Common
A. equuli	Bite wound infections	Rare
A. hominis	Opportunistic infections (bacteremia, pneumonia)	Rare
A. lignieresii	Bite wound infections	Rare
A. ureae	Opportunistic infections (bacteremia, meningitis, pneumonia)	Rare

bacteria are sticky, adhering to the surfaces of blood culture bottles and agar plates in much the same way as they adhere to damaged heart valves.

Serious infections with *Actinobacillus* species are treated with ampicillin, either alone or in combination with an aminoglycoside. Strains resistant to ampicillin can be treated with cephalosporins or fluoroquinolones.

CASE STUDY AND QUESTIONS

■ A 78-year-old man confined to a nursing home awoke with a severe headache and stiff neck. Because he had a high fever and signs of meningitis, the nursing home staff took him to a local emergency department. The CSF specimen was cloudy. Analysis revealed 400 white blood cells per mm³ (95% polymorphonuclear neutrophils), a protein concentration of 75 mg/dL, and a glucose concentration of 20 mg/dL. Small gram-negative bacilli were seen on Gram stain of the CSF, and cultures of CSF and blood were positive for *Haemophilus influenzae*.

1. Discuss the epidemiology of *H. influenzae* meningitis, and compare it with the epidemiology of meningitis caused by *Streptococcus pneumoniae* and by *Neisseria meningitidis*.

2. Compare the biology of the *H. influenzae* strain that is likely to be the cause of this patient's disease with that of the strains that historically caused pediatric diseases (prior to vaccination).

3. What other diseases are caused by this organism? What other *Haemophilus* species cause disease and what are the diseases?

4. Why is chocolate agar needed for the isolation of *Haemophilus* organisms?

5. What diseases are caused by *Pasteurella multocida*? What is the source of this organism?

6. What diseases are caused by *Actinobacillus actinomycetemcomitans*? What is the source of this organism?

BIBLIOGRAPHY

Albritton WL: Infections due to *Haemophilus* species other than *H. influenzae*, *Ann Rev Microbiol* 36:199–216, 1982.

Campos J: *Haemophilus*. In Murray P et al, editors: *Manual of clinical microbiology*, Washington, DC, 1999, American Society of Microbiology.

Daum R et al: Epidemiology, pathogenesis, and prevention of *Haemophilus influenzae* disease, *J Infect Dis* 165(suppl):1–206, 1992.

Doern G et al: *Haemophilus influenzae* and *Moraxella catarrhalis* from patients with community-acquired respiratory tract infections: antimicrobial susceptibility patterns from the SENTRY antimicrobial surveillance program (United States and Canada, 1997), *Antimicrob Agents Chemother* 43:385–389, 1999.

Holst E et al: Characterization and distribution of *Pasteurella* species recovered from infected humans, *J Clin Microbiol* 30:2984–2987, 1992.

Kaplan AH et al: Infection due to *Actinobacillus actinomycetemcomitans*: 15 cases and review, *Rev Infect Dis* 11:46–63, 1989.

Mortensen J, Giger O, Rodgers G: In vitro activity of oral antimicrobial agents against clinical isolates of *Pasteurella multocida*, *Diagn Microbiol Infect Dis* 30:99–102, 1998.

Peltola H: Worldwide *Haemophilus influenzae* type b disease at the beginning of the 21st century: global analysis of the disease burden 25 years after the use of the polysaccharide vaccine and a decade after the advent of conjugates, *Clin Microbiol Rev* 13:302–317, 2000.

Talan D et al: Bacteriologic analysis of infected dog and cat bites, *N Engl J Med* 340:85–92, 1999.

Trees D, Morse S: Chancroid and *Haemophilus ducreyi*: an update, *Clin Microbiol Rev* 8:357–375, 1995.

Urwin G et al: Invasive disease due to *Haemophilus influenzae* serotype f: clinical and epidemiologic characteristics in the *H. influenzae* serotype b vaccine era, *Clin Infect Dis* 22:1069–1076, 1996.

CHAPTER 35

Miscellaneous Gram-Negative Bacilli

Gram-negative bacilli are an extremely diverse group of organisms. A variety of miscellaneous gram-negative organisms that cause human disease are discussed in this chapter (Table 35–1).

Legionella

In the summer of 1976, public attention was focused on an outbreak of severe pneumonia that caused many deaths in members of the American Legion convention in Philadelphia. After months of intensive investigations, a previously unknown gram-negative bacillus was isolated. Subsequent studies found this organism, named *Legionella pneumophila*, to be the cause of multiple epidemic and sporadic infections. The organism was previously not known to exist, because it stains poorly with conventional dyes and does not grow on common laboratory media. Despite the initial problems with the isolation of *Legionella* organisms, it is now recognized to be a ubiquitous aquatic saprophyte.

Taxonomic studies have shown that the family Legionellaceae consists of one genus, *Legionella*, with 39 species and more than 60 serogroups. Approximately half of these species and serogroups have been implicated in human disease, with the others found in environmental sources. *L. pneumophila* is the cause of almost 85% of all infections; serotypes 1 and 6 are most commonly isolated (Fig. 35–1).

Physiology and Structure

Members of the genus *Legionella* are slender, pleomorphic, gram-negative bacilli measuring 0.3 to 0.9 × 2 to 5 μm (Box 35–1). The organisms characteristically appear as short coccobacilli in tissue but are very pleomorphic on artificial media (Fig. 35–2). Legionellae in clinical specimens do not stain with common reagents but can be seen in tissues stained with Dieterle's silver stain. One species, *Legionella micdadei*, can also be stained with weak acid-fast stains, but the organism loses this property when it grows in culture.

Legionellae are nutritionally fastidious; their growth is enhanced with iron salts and depends on the supplementation of media with L-cysteine. Growth of these bacteria on supplemented media but not on conventional blood agar media has been used as the basis for the preliminary identification of clinical isolates. The organisms are nonfermentative and derive energy from the metabolism of amino acids. Most species are motile and catalase-positive, liquefy gelatin, and do not reduce nitrate or hydrolyze urea.

Pathogenesis and Immunity

Respiratory tract disease caused by *Legionella* species develops in susceptible people who inhale infectious aerosols. Legionellae are facultative intracellular parasites that can multiply in alveolar macrophages and monocytes. The replicative cycle is initiated by binding complement to an outer membrane porin protein and deposition of complement component C3b on the bacterial surface. This permits the bacteria to bind to CR3 complement receptors on mononuclear phagocytes, after which the organisms penetrate into the cell through endocytosis. The bacteria are not killed in the cells through exposure to toxic superoxide, hydrogen peroxide, and hydroxyl radicals, because phagolysosome fusion is inhibited. The bacilli proliferate in their intracellular vacuole and produce proteolytic enzymes, phosphatase, lipase, and nuclease, which eventually kill the host cell when the vacuole is lysed. Immunity to disease is primarily cell-mediated, with humoral immunity playing a minor role. The bacteria are not killed until sensitized T cells activate the parasitized macrophages.

Epidemiology

Sporadic and epidemic legionellosis has a worldwide distribution. The bacteria are commonly present in natural bodies of water, such as lakes and streams, as well as in air conditioning cooling towers and condensers and in water systems (e.g., showers, hot tubs). The organisms can survive in moist environments for a long

TABLE 35–1. Miscellaneous Gram-Negative Bacilli and Their Diseases

Organism	Disease
Legionella	Legionnaires' disease, Pontiac fever
Bartonella	Cat-scratch disease, Oroya fever, bacteremia, endocarditis, bacillary angiomatosis
Eikenella	Human bite wound infections, head and neck infections, respiratory tract infections, bacteremia, endocarditis
Cardiobacterium	Endocarditis
Kingella	Endocarditis
Capnocytophaga	Periodontitis, septicemia, endocarditis, bite wound infections
Streptobacillus	Rat-bite fever
Spirillum	Rat-bite fever
Calymmatobacterium	Granuloma inguinale (donovanosis) granulomatis

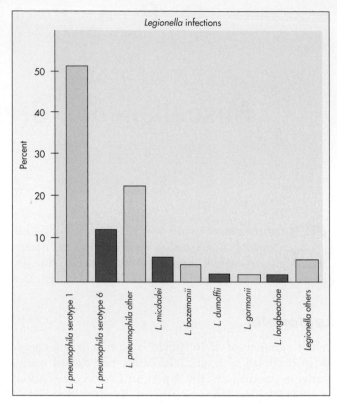

FIGURE 35–1. *Legionella* species associated with human disease.

time, at relatively high temperatures, and in the presence of disinfectants such as chlorine. One reason for this is that the bacteria can parasitize amebae in the water and replicate in this protected environment (like their replication in human macrophages).

The incidence of infections caused by *Legionella* species is unknown because it is difficult to document disease. The number of reported cases has steadily risen during the past decade, with 1500 to 1800 cases reported annually. However, the Centers for Disease Control and Prevention (CDC) estimate that between 10,000 and 20,000 cases of Legionnaire's disease occur

---

BOX 35–1. Summary of *Legionella* Infections

Physiology and Structure

Slender, pleomorphic, gram-negative bacilli.
    Stains poorly with common reagents.
    Nutritionally fastidious with requirement for L-cysteine and enhanced growth with iron salts.
    Nonfermentative.

Virulence

Capable of replication in alveolar macrophages (and amoeba in nature).
    Prevents phagolysosome fusion.

Epidemiology

Capable of sporadic and epidemic disease.
    Commonly found in natural bodies of water, cooling towers, condensers, and water systems (including hospital systems).
    Estimated to be between 10,000 and 20,000 cases in United States annually.
    Patients at high risk for symptomatic disease include patients with compromised pulmonary function and patients with decreased cellular immunity (particularly transplant patients).

Diseases

Legionnaires' disease.
    Pontiac fever.

Diagnosis

Culture on BCYE agar is the diagnostic test of choice. Antigen tests are species-specific and serology is sensitive, but positive titers develop late in the course of disease.

Treatment, Control, and Prevention

Severe disease treated with azithromycin or levofloxacin; less severe disease can be treated with erythromycin or tetracycline.
    Decrease environmental exposure to reduce risk of disease.
    For environmental sources associated with disease, treat with hyperchlorination, superheating, or copper-silver ionization.

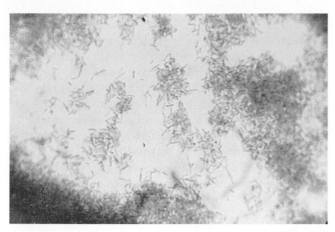

FIGURE 35–2. Gram stain of *Legionella pneumophila* grown on buffered charcoal–yeast extract agar. Note the pleomorphic forms characteristic of *Legionella*. (Courtesy, Dr. Janet Stout.)

each year in the United States. Serologic studies have also shown that a significant proportion of the population has acquired immunity to this group of organisms. On the basis of these studies and the knowledge that legionellae are ubiquitous aquatic saprophytes, it is reasonable to conclude that contact with the organism and acquisition of immunity after an asymptomatic infection are common.

Although sporadic outbreaks of the disease occur throughout the year, most epidemics of the infection occur in the late summer and autumn, presumably because the organism proliferates in water reservoirs during the warm months. The elderly are at greatest risk for disease because of their decreased cellular immunity and compromised pulmonary function. Almost 25% of reported cases are acquired in hospitals, presumably because of the predominance of high-risk patients

there. Person-to-person spread or an animal reservoir has not been demonstrated.

Clinical Diseases

Asymptomatic *Legionella* infections are relatively common. Symptomatic infections primarily affect the lungs and present in one of two forms (Table 35–2): (1) an influenza-like illness (referred to as Pontiac fever) and (2) a severe form of pneumonia (i.e., legionnaires' disease).

Pontiac Fever

L. pneumophila was responsible for causing a self-limited, febrile illness in people working in the Pontiac, Michigan, Public Health Department in 1968. The disease was characterized by fever, chills, myalgia, malaise, and headache but no clinical evidence of pneumonia. The symptoms developed over a 12-hour period, persisted for 2 to 5 days, and then resolved spontaneously, with minimal morbidity and no deaths. Additional epidemics of **Pontiac fever** have been documented, and the incidence of disease has been high in the people exposed.

Legionnaires' Disease

Legionnaires' disease (legionellosis) is characteristically more severe and causes considerable morbidity, leading to death unless therapy is initiated promptly. After an incubation period of 2 to 10 days, systemic signs of an acute illness appear abruptly (e.g., fever and chills, a dry nonproductive cough, headache). Multiorgan disease involving the gastrointestinal tract, central nervous system, liver, and kidneys is common. The primary manifestation is pneumonia, with multilobar

TABLE 35–2. Comparison of Diseases Caused by *Legionella*

	Legionnaires' Disease	Pontiac Fever
Epidemiology		
Presentation	Epidemic, sporadic	Epidemic
Attack rate (%)	<5	>90
Person-to-person spread	No	No
Underlying pulmonary disease	Yes	No
Time of onset	Epidemic disease in late summer or autumn; endemic disease throughout year	Throughout year
Clinical Manifestations		
Incubation period (days)	2–10	1–2
Pneumonia	Yes	No
Course	Requires antibiotic therapy	Self-limited
Mortality (%)	15–20; higher if diagnosis is delayed	<1

consolidation and inflammation and microabscesses in lung tissue observed on histopathologic studies. Pulmonary function steadily deteriorates in susceptible patients with untreated disease. The overall mortality rate is 15% to 20% but can be much higher in patients with severely depressed cell-mediated immunity (e.g., recipients of renal or cardiac transplants).

Laboratory Diagnosis

Microscopy

Legionellae in clinical specimens stain poorly with Gram stain. Nonspecific staining methods, such as those using Dieterle's silver or Gimenez's stain, can be used to visualize the organisms but are of little value if the specimens are contaminated with normal oral bacteria. The most sensitive way of detecting legionellae microscopically in clinical specimens is to use the direct fluorescent antibody (DFA) test, in which fluorescein-labeled monoclonal or polyclonal antibodies directed against *Legionella* species are used (Fig. 35–3). The test is specific, with false-positive reactions observed only rarely if monoclonal antibody preparations are used. However, the sensitivity of the DFA test is low because (1) the antibody preparations are serotype- or species-specific and (2) many organisms must be present for detection. The latter problem is due to the relatively small size and predominantly intracellular location of the bacteria. Positive test results revert to negative after about 4 days of treatment. The primary advantage of microscopy over other diagnostic tests is that a positive result can be obtained rapidly.

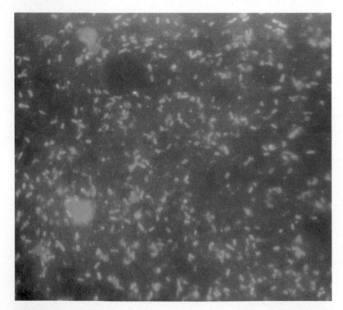

FIGURE 35–3. Direct fluorescent antibody stain of *Legionella micdadei.*

Culture

Although legionellae were difficult to grow initially, commercially available media now make growth easy. As mentioned earlier, legionellae require L-cysteine, and their growth is enhanced with iron (supplied in hemoglobin or ferric pyrophosphate). The medium most commonly used for the isolation of legionellae is buffered charcoal–yeast extract (BCYE) agar, although other supplemented media have also been used. Antibiotics can be added to suppress the growth of rapidly growing contaminating bacteria. Legionellae grow in air or 3% to 5% carbon dioxide at 35°C after 3 to 5 days. Their small (1- to 3-mm) colonies have a ground-glass appearance.

Antigen Detection

Enzyme-linked immunoassays, radioimmunoassays, the agglutination of antibody-coated latex particles, and nucleic acid analysis studies have all been used to detect legionellae in respiratory specimens and urine. Although the immunologic assays are relatively sensitive, the serotype-specific reagents limit the clinical usefulness of the tests. In addition, antigen may be excreted in urine for as long as 1 year after the infection has resolved. Currently, commercial tests have been developed only for *L. pneumophila* serogroup 1. Thus, if another serogroup is responsible for disease (e.g., serogroup 5 has been responsible for an outbreak of infections in Baltimore), a negative antigen test result can be misleading. If an antigen test is used, culture should always be performed. Nucleic acid analyses have been disappointing to date. The presence of inhibitors in clinical specimens has compromised the test sensitivity, and reliable commercial tests are not available currently.

Serology

Legionellosis is commonly diagnosed with the use of the indirect fluorescent antibody test to measure a serologic response to infection. A fourfold or greater increase in the antibody titer (to a level of 1:128 or greater) is considered diagnostic. The response may be delayed, however, with a significant increase in the titer typically not seen until after 3 weeks of illness. High titers can persist occasionally for prolonged periods.

Identification

It is easy to identify an isolate as *Legionella* from the findings of typical morphology and specific growth requirements. Legionellae appear as weakly staining, pleomorphic, thin, gram-negative bacilli. Their growth on BCYE but not on media without L-cysteine is presumptive evidence that the organism is *Legionella*. Specific staining with fluorescein-labeled antibodies can confirm the identity of the organisms. In contrast to the identification of the genus, species classification is problematic and is generally relegated to reference laboratories. Although biochemical tests and the ability of bacilli to fluoresce under long-wave ultraviolet light are useful for differentiating species, the species can be identified definitively only through analysis of the major branched-chain fatty acids in the cell wall and DNA homology.

Treatment, Prevention, and Control

In vitro susceptibility tests are not performed routinely with legionellae, because the organisms grow poorly on the media commonly used for these tests. However, in vitro testing and accumulated clinical experience indicate that azithromycin or levofloxacin should be used to treat disease in hospitalized or immunocompromised patients. Erythromycin or tetracycline can be used to treat community-acquired disease. β-lactam antibiotics are ineffective, because most isolates produce β-lactamases. Specific therapy for Pontiac fever is generally unnecessary because it is a self-limited disease.

Prevention of legionellosis requires identification of the environmental source of the organism and reduction of the microbial burden. Hyperchlorination of the water supply and the maintenance of elevated water temperatures have proved moderately successful. However, complete elimination of *Legionella* organisms from a water supply is often difficult or impossible. Because the organism has a low potential for causing disease, reducing the number of organisms in the water supply is frequently an adequate control measure. Hospitals with patients at high risk for disease should monitor their water supply on a regular basis for the presence of *Legionella* and their hospital population for disease. If hyperchlorination or superheating of the water does not eliminate disease (complete elimination of the organisms in the water supply is probably not possible), continuous copper-silver ionization of the water supply may be necessary.

Bartonella

As with many groups of bacteria studied in the past 10 years, analysis of the 16S ribosomal RNA has led to the reorganization of the genus *Bartonella*. The genus *Rochalimaea* was transferred into the genus *Bartonella*, which now consists of 11 species, including 5 that cause human disease (Table 35–3). The bacteria are short (0.3 to 0.5 × 1.0 to 1.7 μm), gram-negative, aerobic bacilli with fastidious growth requirements. Although the organisms can grow on enriched blood agar, prolonged incubation (1 to 6 weeks) in a humid,

TABLE 35–3. *Bartonella* Species Associated with Human Infections

Species	Diseases
B. bacilliformis	Oroya fever (bartonellosis, Carrión's disease)
B. quintana	Trench fever; cutaneous, subcutaneous, and osseous manifestations of bacillary angiomatosis; endocarditis
B. henselae	Cat-scratch disease; bacteremia; cutaneous, lymphatic, and hepatosplenic (peliosis hepatis) manifestions of bacillary angiomatosis; endocarditis
B. clarridgeiae	Endocarditis, cat scratch disease (rare)
B. elizabethae	Endocarditis (rare)

37°C atmosphere supplemented with carbon dioxide is required for their initial recovery.

Members of the genus are found in a variety of animal reservoirs and are typically present without evidence of disease. Insect vectors have also been shown or implicated in human infections. Because *Bartonella* organisms do not cause disease in other hosts, an animal model is not available for studying the pathogenesis of these infections.

Bartonella bacilliformis, the original member of the genus, is responsible for bartonellosis, an acute febrile illness consisting of severe anemia (**Oroya fever**) followed by a chronic cutaneous form (**verruga**). Bartonellosis is restricted to Peru, Ecuador, and Colombia, the endemic regions of the sandfly vector *Phlebotomus*. After the bite of an infected sandfly, the bacteria enter the blood stream, multiply, and penetrate into erythrocytes. This process increases the fragility of the infected cells and facilitates their clearance by the reticuloendothelial system, leading to acute anemia. Myalgias, arthralgias, and headaches are also common. This stage of illness ends with the development of humoral immunity. In the chronic stage of bartonellosis, 1- to 2-cm cutaneous nodules appear over the course of 1 to 2 months and may persist for months to years.

Bartonella quintana was originally described as the causative organism of **trench fever** ("5-day" fever), a disease prevalent during World War I. Infection can vary from asymptomatic to a severe, debilitating illness. Typically, patients have severe headaches, fever, weakness, and pain in the long bones (particularly the tibia). The fever can recur at 5-day intervals; hence the name of the disease. Although trench fever does not cause death, the illness can be very severe. No animal reservoir for this disease has been identified. Rather, disease is spread person-to-person by the human body louse.

More recently, *B. quintana* has been associated with **bacillary angiomatosis,** a vascular proliferative disorder seen primarily in immunocompromised patients (e.g., patients with the human immunodeficiency virus [HIV]) as well as with endocarditis in immunocompetent patients. Bacillary angiomatosis due to *B. quintana* primarily involves the skin, subcutaneous tissues, and bones (in contrast with disease due to *Bartonella henselae*). As with trench fever, the vector of these diseases appears to be the human body louse, and disease is primarily restricted to the homeless population, in whom personal hygiene is substandard. The etiologic role of *B. quintana* and other *Bartonella* species in "culture-negative" endocarditis is supported by serologic studies.

B. henselae is also responsible for bacillary angiomatosis, but primarily involving the skin, lymph nodes, or liver and spleen (**peliosis hepatis**). The reasons for this differential tissue affinity are not known. *B. henselae* can cause subacute bacterial endocarditis, like *B. quintana*. Finally, *B. henselae* is responsible for **cat-scratch disease.** The disease is acquired after exposure to cats (e.g., scratches, bites, contact with cat fleas). Typically, cat-scratch disease is a benign infection in children, characterized by chronic regional adenopathy of the lymph nodes draining the site of contact. Although bacilli can be seen in the lymph node tissues, culture is usually negative for organisms. A definitive diagnosis is based on the characteristic presentation and serologic evidence of a recent infection. In contrast, *B. henselae* can be isolated from blood collected from patients with chronic bacteremia if the cultures are incubated for 3 weeks or more. The reason this organism can be isolated in one disease but not the other is not understood.

Treatment of *Bartonella* infections is complicated, because minimal information is available about the in vitro susceptibility of the organisms. Cat-scratch disease does not appear to respond to antimicrobial therapy. Trench fever, bacillary angiomatosis and peliosis hepatis, and endocarditis can be treated with gentamicin, either alone or with erythromycin. Broad-spectrum cephalosporins appear to be effective, and erythromycin or doxycycline has been used with initial success, but the bacteriostatic antibiotics are associated with a high rate of relapse. Penicillinase-resistant penicillins, first-generation cephalosporins, and clindamycin do not appear active in vitro.

Eikenella

In the early 1960s, a collection of small, fastidious, gram-negative bacilli were classified by workers at the CDC as members of the HB group (named after the patient infected with the original isolate). The organisms were subsequently subdivided into subgroup HB-1 (now known as *Eikenella corrodens*), subgroup HB-2 (*Haemophilus aphrophilus*; see Chapter 34), and subgroups HB-3 and HB-4 (*Actinobacillus actinomycetemcomitans*; see Chapter 34). In addition to being morphologically similar, these organisms colonize the human oropharynx and, in the setting of preexisting heart disease, can cause subacute bacterial endocarditis. In fact, the group of fastidious gram-negative bacilli associated with subacute endocarditis is known by the acronym HACEK (*H. aphrophilus*, *A. actinomycetemcomitans*, *Cardiobacterium hominis*, *E. corrodens*, and *Kingella kingae*).

E. corrodens is a moderate-sized (0.2 × 2 μm), non-motile, non–spore-forming, facultatively anaerobic gram-negative bacillus. The organism is named after Eiken, who characterized the bacterium and observed the ability of the organism to pit or "corrode" agar (from its ability to split polygalacturonic acid). *E. corrodens* is a normal inhabitant of the human upper respiratory tract, but because of its fastidious growth requirements, it is difficult to detect unless specific selective culture media are used. It is an opportunistic pathogen that causes infections in patients who are immunocompromised or have diseases or trauma of the oral cavity. *E. corrodens* is most commonly isolated in the settings of a human bite wound or fistfight injury. Other infections are endocarditis, sinusitis, meningitis, brain abscesses, pneumonia, and lung abscesses. Because most infections originate from the oropharynx, polymicrobial mixtures of aerobic and anaerobic bacteria are frequently present in cultures.

A slow-growing, fastidious organism, *E. corrodens* requires 5% to 10% carbon dioxide to grow. Small (0. 5- to 1-mm) colonies are observed after 48 hours of incubation on blood or chocolate agar, but the organism grows poorly or not at all on selective media for gram-negative bacilli. Pitting in agar is a useful differential characteristic, but fewer than half of all isolates exhibit pitting. The organism also produces a characteristic bleachlike odor. Thus, a preliminary identification of the organism can be made if a slow-growing gram-negative bacilli is found to pit blood agar and produce a bleachlike odor.

E. corrodens is susceptible to penicillin, ampicillin, extended-spectrum cephalosporins, tetracyclines, and fluoroquinolone, but is resistant to oxacillin, first-generation cephalosporins, clindamycin, erythromycin, and the aminoglycosides. Thus, *E. corrodens* is resistant to many antibiotics that are selected empirically to treat bite wound infections.

Cardiobacterium

Cardiobacterium hominis, named for the predilection of this bacterium to cause endocarditis in humans, is the only member of the genus. The bacteria are nonmotile, characteristically small (1×1 to 2 μm) but sometimes pleomorphic, gram-negative bacilli. The bacteria are fermentative, indole- and oxidase-positive, and catalase-negative. *C. hominis* is present in the upper respiratory tract of almost 70% of healthy people.

Endocarditis is the primary human disease caused by *C. hominis*. Although endocarditis due to *C. hominis* is uncommon, many infections are likely to be unreported or undiagnosed because of the low virulence of this organism and its slow growth in vitro. Most patients with *C. hominis* endocarditis have preexisting heart disease and either have a history of oral disease or underwent dental procedures before the clinical symptoms developed. The organisms are able to enter the blood stream from the oropharynx, adhere to the damaged heart tissue, and then slowly multiply. The course of disease is insidious and subacute; patients typically have symptoms (fatigue, malaise, and low-grade fever) for months before seeking medical care. Complications are rare, and complete recovery after appropriate antibiotic therapy is common.

The isolation of *C. hominis* from blood cultures confirms the diagnosis of endocarditis. The organism grows slowly in culture. It takes 1 to 2 weeks for growth to be detected, which is the reason that infections with these organisms are not confirmed in some patients. *C. hominis* appears in broth cultures as discrete clumps that can be easily overlooked. The organism requires enhanced carbon dioxide and humidity levels to grow on agar media, with pinpoint (1-mm) colonies seen on blood or chocolate agar plates after 3 days of incubation. The organism does not grow on MacConkey agar or other selective media commonly used for gram-negative bacilli. *C. hominis* can be readily identified from its growth properties, microscopic morphology, and reactivity in biochemical tests.

C. hominis is susceptible to multiple antibiotics, and most infections are successfully treated with penicillin or ampicillin for 2 to 6 weeks. *C. hominis* endocarditis in people with preexisting heart disease is prevented by the maintenance of good oral hygiene and the use of antibiotic prophylaxis at the time of dental procedures. A long-acting penicillin is effective prophylaxis, but erythromycin should not be used, because *C. hominis* is commonly resistant to it.

Kingella

Kingella species are small, gram-negative coccobacilli that morphologically resemble *Neisseria* species and reside in the human oropharynx. The bacteria are facultatively anaerobic, ferment carbohydrates, and have fastidious growth requirements. *K. kingae*, the most commonly isolated species, has been primarily responsible for septic arthritis in children and endocarditis in patients of all ages. Because the organism grows slowly,

it may take 3 or more days of incubation for the organism to be detected in clinical specimens. Most strains are susceptible to β-lactam antibiotics, including penicillin, tetracyclines, erythromycin, fluoroquinolones, and aminoglycosides.

Capnocytophaga

Members of the genus *Capnocytophaga* are filamentous gram-negative bacilli capable of aerobic and anaerobic growth in the presence of carbon dioxide. The genus is subdivided into two groups, (1) dysgonic fermenter 1 (DF-1), with three species, and (2) dysgonic fermenter 2 (DF-2), with two species. DF-1 strains colonize the human oropharynx and are associated with periodontitis, bacteremia, and, rarely, endocarditis. DF-2 strains colonize the dog oropharynx and are associated with bite wounds.

Overwhelming sepsis due to *Capnocytophaga* can occur in patients who have undergone splenectomy or who have compromised hepatic function (e.g., cirrhosis). Most *Capnocytophaga* infections can be treated with broad-spectrum cephalosporins, fluoroquinolones, or penicillin; strains are typically resistant to the aminoglycosides.

Streptobacillus and Spirillum

Streptobacillus moniliformis and *Spirillum minus* are the causative agents of two distinct diseases referred to collectively as **rat-bite fever** (Table 35–4). *S. moniliformis* is a long, thin (0.1 to 0.5×1 to 5 μm), gram-negative bacillus that tends to stain poorly and to be more pleomorphic in older cultures. Granules and bulbous swellings resembling a string of beads may be seen (Fig. 35–4). *S. minus* is a spiral, gram-negative bacillus (0.2 to 0.5×3 to 5 μm).

Both *Streptobacillus* and *Spirillum* organisms are found in the nasopharynx of rats and other small rodents as well as transiently in animals that feed on rodents (e.g., dogs, cats). Turkeys exposed to rats and mice, as well as contaminated water and milk, have also been implicated in *Streptobacillus* infections.

Although the infections caused by the two organisms are similar in epidemiology and the clinical presentation of recurrent fevers, distinct differences have been observed. For example, the incubation period for *Streptobacillus* infections is shorter than that for *Spirillum* infections, and the clinical course in patients with *Spirillum* infections does not usually include the myalgias, arthralgias, and frank arthritis seen in *Streptobacillus* infections. Patients with one form of *S. moniliformis* infection, **Haverhill's fever** or **erythema arthriticum epidemicum,** typically have fever, rash, arthralgia, chills, vomiting, and gastrointestinal and respiratory symptoms. Ulceration at the bite site with lymphade-

TABLE 35–4. Comparison of *Streptobacillus* and *Spirillum* Species

	Streptobacillus moniliformis	*Spirillum minus*
Distribution	Worldwide	Worldwide, primarily Asia
Reservoir	Rats and other small rodents	Rats and other small rodents
Transmission	Bite of rat or another rodent, contact with animals that feed on rodents, consumption of water or other contaminated food or fluid	Bite of rat or another rodent, contact with animals that feed on rodents
Disease	Rat-bite fever (Haverhill's fever)	Rat-bite fever
Incubation period	<10 days	2 weeks
Clinical presentation	Abrupt onset; high fever; chills, headache, myalgias, rash, arthritis or arthralgia; recurrent fevers if untreated	Abrupt onset; fever, chills, rash, lymphagitis, lymphadenopathy; recurrent fevers if untreated
Mortality	10% if untreated	6% if untreated
Treatment	Penicillin	Penicillin
Diagnosis	Culture, serologic tests	Darkfield microscopy examination, Wright- or Giemsa-stained blood smears, animal inoculation

nopathy and lymphangitis is observed in patients with *Spirillum* rat-bite infections. Recurrent febrile episodes are observed in patients with untreated disease due to either organism.

S. moniliformis, but not *S. minus*, can be cultured in vitro. Blood and joint fluid should be collected for this purpose and mixed with citrate to prevent clotting during transport to the laboratory. The organism can grow on enriched media supplemented with 15% blood, 20% horse or calf serum, or 5% ascitic fluid. S. moniliformis is slow growing, taking at least 3 days to be isolated. When grown in broth, it has the appearance of "puffballs"; small round colonies are seen on agar, as are cell wall–defective forms, with their typical fried-egg appearance. It is difficult to identify the organisms because they are relatively inactive, although acid

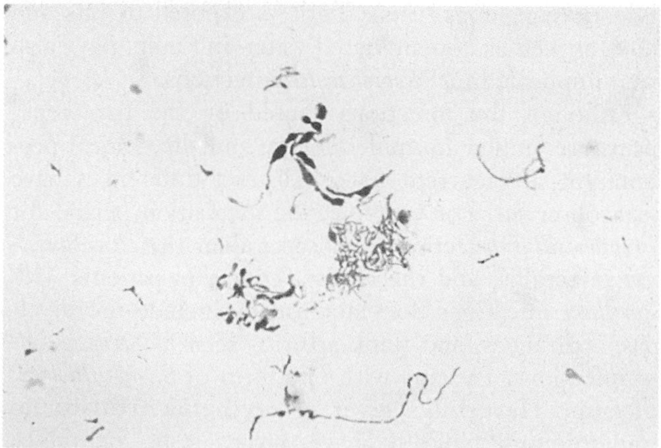

is produced from glucose and other selected carbohydrates. The serologic tests that can detect antibodies against *Streptobacillus* antigens are available in reference laboratories. A titer greater than or equal to 1:80 or a fourfold rise in the titer is considered diagnostic, although this test has not been standardized or carefully evaluated for cross-reactivity.

S. minus, which is more common in countries outside the United States, has not been cultured in vitro. Darkfield microscopy examination of blood, ulcer exudates, or lymph node aspirates is used to detect *S. minus*. Blood smears can be stained with Giemsa's or Wright's stain. *S. minus* can also be detected in the blood of rodents 1 to 3 weeks after the intraperitoneal inoculation of the clinical specimen.

Penicillin is the antibiotic of choice for treating rat-bite fever. Tetracycline can be used in penicillin-allergic patients.

FIGURE 35–4. Gram stain of *Streptobacillus moniliformis*. Note the pleomorphic forms and bulbous swellings.

Calymmatobacterium

The etiologic agent of **granuloma inguinale,** a granulomatous disease affecting the genitalia and inguinal area, has been called historically *Calymmatobacterium (Donovania) granulomatis*. The organism was discovered by Donovan and subsequently renamed to reflect its encapsulated appearance in tissues (*kalymma* is Greek for "hood" or "veil"). Recently, this organism was transferred into the genus Klebsiella based on genomic criteria and the fact this organism produces clinical and pathologic changes similar to two other species of *Klebsiella*—*K. rhinoscleromatis* (causes a granulomatous disease of the nose) and *K. ozaenae* (causes chronic atrophic rhinitis). Because the literature still refers to this organism in the genus *Calymmatobacterium*, that name will be used in this text.

C. granulomatis has been isolated in a monocyte culture system but does not appear to grow in cell-free systems. The laboratory diagnosis is made through staining of infected tissues with Wright's or Giemsa's stain. The organisms appear as small (0.5 to 1.0 × 1.5 μm) bacilli in the cytoplasm of histiocytes, polymorphonuclear leukocytes, and plasma cells. From 1 to 25 bacteria per phagocytic cell can be seen; a prominent capsule surrounds the organisms.

Granuloma inguinale is a rare disease in the United States but is encountered in tropical areas such as the Caribbean and New Guinea. It can be transmitted after repeated exposure through sexual intercourse or nonsexual trauma to the genitalia. After a prolonged incubation of weeks to months, subcutaneous nodules appear on the genitalia or in the inguinal area. The nodules subsequently break down, revealing one or more painless granulomatous lesions that can extend and coalesce.

Laboratory confirmation of granuloma inguinale is made by scraping the border of the lesion, by spreading the collected tissue on a slide, and by staining it with Giemsa or Wright's stain. Pathognomonic **Donovan bodies** are observed within mononuclear phagocytes. Tetracyclines, erythromycin, and trimethoprim-sulfamethoxazole have been used successfully for treatment, although relapses have occurred with use of these agents. Antibiotic prophylaxis has not proved effective in preventing and controlling infection.

CASE STUDY AND QUESTIONS

■ A 73-year-old man was admitted to the hospital because of breathing difficulties, chest pain, chills, and fever of several days' duration. He had been well until 1 week before admission, when he noted the onset of a persistent headache and a productive cough. The patient smoked 2 packs of cigarettes a day for more than 50 years and drank a 6-pack of beer daily; he also had a history of bronchitis. Physical examination revealed an elderly man in severe respiratory distress with a temperature of 39.0°C, pulse of 120 beats/min, respiratory rate of 36 breaths/min, and blood pressure of 145/95 mm Hg. Chest radiograph revealed an infiltrate in the middle and lower lobes of the right lung. The white blood cell count was 14,000 cells/mm³ (80% polymorphonuclear neutrophils). Gram stain of the sputum showed neutrophils but no bacteria, and routine bacterial cultures of sputum and blood were negative for organisms. Infection with *Legionella pneumophila* was suspected.

1. What laboratory tests can be used to confirm this diagnosis? Why were the routine culture and Gram-stained specimen negative for *Legionella* organisms?

2. How are *Legionella* species able to survive phagocytosis by the alveolar macrophages?

3. What environmental factors are implicated in the spread of *Legionella* infections? How can this risk be eliminated or minimized?

4. What infections are caused by *Bartonella quintana* and *Bartonella henselae*? How does the epidemiology of these infections differ?

5. What infection is common to *Eikenella*, *Kingella*, and *Cardiobacterium*? What is the common reservoir of these organisms? What other infections are caused by *Eikenella*?

6. What infection is caused by *Spirillum* and *Streptobacillus*?

BIBLIOGRAPHY

Anderson B, Neuman M: *Bartonella* spp. as emerging human pathogens, *Clin Microbiol Rev* 10:203–219, 1997.

Carter J et al: Phylogenetic evidence for reclassification of *Calymmatobacterium granulomatis* as *Klebsiella granulomatis* Combr, *Nov Internatl J: System Bacteriol* 49:1695–1700, 1999.

Decker M: *Eikenella corrodens*, *Infect Control* 7:36–41, 1986.

Edelstein P: Antimicrobial chemotherapy for Legionnaires disease: time for a change, *Ann Intern Med* 129:328–330, 1998.

Kharsany A et al: Culture of *Calymmatobacterium granulomatis*, *Clin Infect Dis* 22:391, 1996.

Koehler J et al: Molecular epidemiology of *Bartonella* infections in patients with bacillary angiomatosis-peliosis, *N Engl J Med* 337:1876–1883, 1997.

La Scola B, Raoult D: Culture of *Bartonella quintana* and *Bartonella henselae* from human samples: a 5-year experience (1993 to 1998), *J Clin Microbiol* 37:1899–1905, 1999.

Maurin M, Raoult D: *Bartonella* (*Rochalimaea*) *quintana* infections, *Clin Microbiol Rev* 9:273–292, 1996.

Maurin M, Birtles R, Raoult D: Current knowledge of *Bartonella* species, *Eur J Clin Microbiol Infect Dis* 16:487–506, 1997.

Schulin T et al: Susceptibilities of *Legionella* spp. to newer antimicrobials in vitro, *Antimicrob Agents Chemother* 42:1520–1523, 1998.

Schwartzman W: *Bartonella* infections: beyond cat scratch, *Annu Rev Med* 47:355–364, 1996.

Spach D et al: *Bartonella* (*Rochalimaea*) species as a cause of apparent "culture-negative" endocarditis, *Clin Infect Dis* 20:1044–1047, 1995.

Stoloff AL, Gillies ML: Infections with *Eikenella corrodens* in a general hospital: a report of 33 cases, *Rev Infect Dis* 8:50–53, 1986.

Stout J, Yu V: Legionellosis, *N Engl J Med* 337:681–687, 1997.

Wormser GP, Bottone EJ: *Cardiobacterium hominis*: review of microbiologic and clinical features, *Rev Infect Dis* 5:680–691, 1983.

CHAPTER 36

Anaerobic Gram-Positive Cocci and Non–Spore-Forming Bacilli

The anaerobic gram-positive cocci and non–spore-forming bacilli are a heterogeneous group of bacteria that characteristically colonize the skin and mucosal surfaces. These organisms are opportunistic pathogens, typically responsible for endogenous infections and usually recovered in mixtures of aerobic and anaerobic bacteria. Additionally, most of these anaerobes have fastidious nutritional requirements and grow slowly on laboratory media. Thus, the isolation and identification of individual strains are difficult and frequently time-consuming. Fortunately, the appropriate management and treatment of most infections with these organisms can be based on the knowledge that a mixture of aerobic and anaerobic organisms is present in the clinical specimen and does not require the isolation and identification of the individual organisms.

Anaerobic Gram-Positive Cocci

The taxonomic classifications of most bacteria have become more complex; however, classification of the clinically significant anaerobic cocci has been simplified. Virtually all important anaerobic cocci belong to the genus *Peptostreptococcus*. Unfortunately, this simplified classification is destined to be revised, because it is now recognized that the 13 species in the genus *Peptostreptococcus* are not closely related and should be subdivided into at least seven genera. Until the taxonomists have completed their exercises and the microbiologists and clinicians have accepted the new nomenclature, however, the genus *Peptostreptococcus* is adequate for our purposes.

These gram-positive cocci normally colonize the oral cavity, gastrointestinal tract, genitourinary tract, and skin. They produce infections when they spread from these sites to normally sterile sites. For example, bacteria colonizing the upper airways can cause sinusitis and pleuropulmonary infections; bacteria in the intestines can cause intra-abdominal infections; bacteria in the genitourinary tract can cause endometritis, pelvic abscesses, and salpingitis; bacteria on the skin can cause cellulitis and soft tissue infections; and bacteria that invade the blood stream can produce infections in bones and solid organs (Fig. 36–1).

Laboratory confirmation of infections with peptostreptococci is complicated by the following three factors:

1. Care must be taken to prevent contamination of the clinical specimen with peptostreptococci that normally colonize the mucosal surface.
2. The collected specimen must be transported in an oxygen-free container to prevent loss of the organisms.
3. Specimens should be cultured on nutritionally enriched media for a prolonged period (i.e., 5 to 7 days); this practice is in contrast with that for other anaerobic bacteria that typically grow in 1 to 2 days.

Additionally, some species of staphylococci and streptococci grow initially only in an anaerobic atmosphere. These organisms eventually grow well in air supplemented with 10% CO_2, however, so they cannot be classified as anaerobes. The problem that occurs with these organisms is that they tend to be more resistant to antibiotics than the peptostreptococci.

Members of the genus *Peptostreptococcus* are usually susceptible to penicillin, metronidazole, imipenem, and chloramphenicol. They have intermediate susceptibility to broad-spectrum cephalosporins, clindamycin, erythromycin, and the tetracyclines and are resistant to the aminoglycosides (as are all anaerobes). Specific therapy is generally indicated in monomicrobic infections. Because most infections with these organisms are polymicrobic, however, broad-spectrum therapy against aerobic and anaerobic bacteria is usually selected.

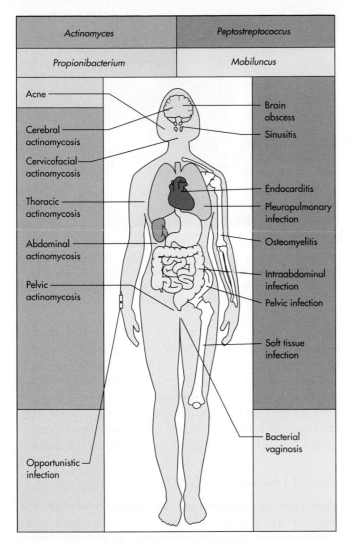

FIGURE 36–1. Diseases associated with *Peptostreptococcus, Actinomyces, Propionibacterium,* and *Mobiluncus,* which are all anaerobic, non–spore-forming, gram-positive bacilli.

TABLE 36–1. Anaerobic, Non–Spore-Forming, Gram-Positive Bacilli

Anaerobic Bacilli	Human Disease
Actinomyces spp.	Actinomycosis (cervicofacial, thoracic, abdominal, pelvic, central nervous system)
Propionibacterium spp.	Acne, lacrimal canaliculitis, opportunistic infections
Mobiluncus spp.	Bacterial vaginosis, opportunistic infections
Lactobacillus spp.	Endocarditis, opportunistic infections
Eubacterium spp.	Opportunistic infections
Bifidobacterium spp.	Opportunistic infections

acid-fast (in contrast to the morphologically similar *Nocardia* species), they grow slowly in culture, and they tend to produce chronic, slowly developing infections. They typically form delicate filamentous forms or hyphae, similar to those of fungi, when detected in clinical specimens or isolated in culture (Fig. 36–2). In fact, the name *Actinomyces* is derived from the Greek words for "ray fungus." However, these organisms are true bacteria in that they lack mitochondria and a nuclear membrane, reproduce by fission, and are inhibited by penicillin but not by antifungal antibiotics. Numerous species have been described; *Actinomyces israelii, Actinomyces meyeri, Actinomyces naeslundii, Actinomyces odontolyticus,* and *Actinomyces viscosus* are responsible for most human infections. Only *A. meyeri* is a strict anaerobe. The other species grow best in anaerobic conditions but can grow aerobically.

Anaerobic, Non–Spore-Forming, Gram-Positive Bacilli

The non–spore-forming, gram-positive bacilli are a diverse collection of facultatively anaerobic or strictly anaerobic bacteria that colonize the skin and mucosal surfaces (Table 36–1). *Actinomyces, Mobiluncus, Lactobacillus,* and *Propionibacterium* are well-recognized opportunistic pathogens, whereas members of the genera *Bifidobacterium* and *Eubacterium* can be isolated in clinical specimens but rarely cause human disease.

Actinomyces

Physiology and Structure

Actinomyces organisms are facultatively anaerobic or strictly anaerobic, gram-positive bacilli. They are not

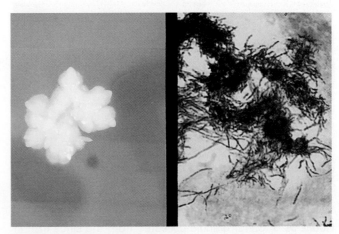

FIGURE 36–2. Macroscopic colony *(left)* and gram stain *(right)* of *Actinomyces.*

Pathogenesis and Immunity

Actinomyces colonize the upper respiratory tract, gastrointestinal tract, and female genital tract. These bacteria are not normally present on the skin surface. The organisms have a low virulence potential and cause disease only when the normal mucosal barriers are disrupted by trauma, surgery, or infection.

Disease caused by actinomyces is termed **actinomycosis** (in keeping with the original idea that these organisms were fungi or "mycoses"). Actinomycosis is characterized by the development of chronic granulomatous lesions that become suppurative and form abscesses connected by sinus tracts. Macroscopic colonies of organisms resembling grains of sand can frequently be seen in the abscesses and sinus tracts. These colonies, called **sulfur granules** because they appear yellow or orange, are masses of filamentous organisms bound together by calcium phosphate (Fig. 36–3). The areas of suppuration are surrounded by fibrosing granulation tissue, which gives the surface overlying the involved tissues a hard or woody consistency.

Epidemiology

Actinomycosis is an endogenous infection with no evidence of person-to-person spread or disease originating from an external source such as soil or water. Disease is classified according to the organ systems involved. Cervicofacial infections are seen in patients who have poor oral hygiene or who have undergone an invasive dental procedure or oral trauma. In these patients, the actinomyces that are present in the mouth invade into the diseased tissue and initiate the infectious process.

Patients with thoracic infections generally have a history of aspiration, with the disease becoming established in the lungs and then spreading to adjoining tissues. Abdominal infections most commonly occur in

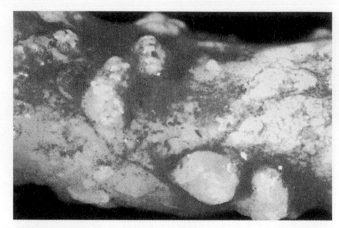

FIGURE 36–4. *Actinomyces* species can colonize the surface of foreign bodies, such as this intrauterine device, leading to the development of pelvic actinomycosis. (From Smith E: In Lambert H, Farrar W, editors: *Infectious diseases illustrated*, London, 1982, Gower.)

patients who have undergone gastrointestinal surgery or have suffered trauma to the bowel. Pelvic infection can be a secondary manifestation of abdominal actinomycosis or may be a primary infection in a woman with an intrauterine device (Fig. 36–4). Central nervous system infections usually represent hematogenous spread from another infected tissue, such as the lungs.

Clinical Diseases

Most cases of actinomycosis are the **cervicofacial** type (Fig. 36–5). The disease may occur as an acute pyogenic infection or, more commonly, as a slowly evolving, relatively painless process. The finding of tissue swelling with fibrosis and scarring as well as draining sinus tracts along the angle of the jaw and neck should alert the physician to the possibility of actinomycosis.

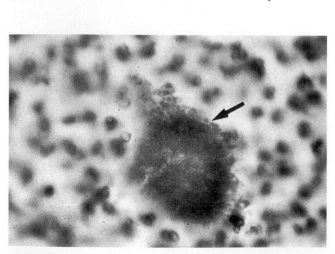

FIGURE 36–3. Sulfur granule collected from the sinus tract in a patient with actinomycosis. Note the delicate filamentous bacilli (*arrow*) at the periphery of the crushed granule.

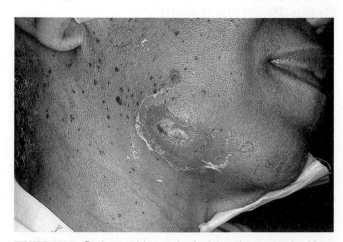

FIGURE 36–5. Patient with cervicofacial actinomycosis. Note the draining sinus tract.

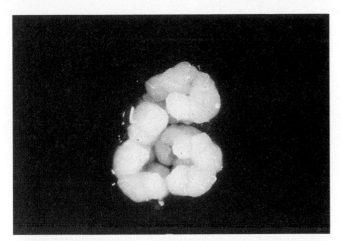

FIGURE 36–6. Molar tooth appearance of *Actinomyces israelii* after incubation for 1 week. This colonial morphology serves as a reminder that the bacteria are normally found in the mouth.

Symptoms of **thoracic actinomycosis** are nonspecific. Abscesses may form in the lung tissue early in the disease and then spread into adjoining tissues as the disease progresses. **Abdominal actinomycosis** can spread throughout the abdomen, potentially involving virtually every organ system. **Pelvic actinomycosis** can occur as a relatively benign form of vaginitis, or more commonly, there can be extensive tissue destruction, including the development of tuboovarian abscesses or ureteral obstruction. The most common manifestation of **central nervous system actinomycosis** is a solitary brain abscess, but meningitis, subdural empyema, and epidural abscess are also seen.

Laboratory Diagnosis

Laboratory confirmation of actinomycosis is frequently difficult. Care must be used during collection of clinical specimens that they not become contaminated with actinomyces that are part of the normal bacterial population on mucosal surfaces. The significance of actinomyces isolated from contaminated specimens cannot be determined. Because the organisms are concentrated in sulfur granules and are sparse in involved tissues, a large amount of tissue or pus should be collected. If sulfur granules are detected in a sinus tract or in tissue, the granule should be crushed between two glass slides, stained, and examined microscopically. Thin, gram-positive, branching bacilli can be seen along the periphery of the granules.

Actinomyces are fastidious and grow slowly under anaerobic conditions; it can take 2 weeks or more for the organisms to be isolated. Colonies appear white and have a domed surface that can become irregular after incubation for a week or more, resembling the top of a molar (Fig. 36–6). The individual species of actinomyces can be differentiated by biochemical tests; however, this process can be time-consuming. Generally, it is necessary only to determine that the isolate is a member of the genus *Actinomyces*.

Treatment, Prevention, and Control

Treatment for actinomycosis involves the combination of surgical débridement of the involved tissues and the prolonged administration of antibiotics. Actinomyces are uniformly susceptible to penicillin (considered the antibiotic of choice) as well as to erythromycin and clindamycin. Most species are resistant to metronidazole, and the tetracyclines have variable activity. An undrained focus should be suspected in patients with infections that do not appear to respond to prolonged therapy (e.g., 4 to 12 months). The clinical response is generally good even in patients who have suffered extensive tissue destruction. Maintenance of good oral hygiene and the use of appropriate antibiotic prophylaxis when the mouth or gastrointestinal tract is penetrated can lower the risk of these infections.

Propionibacterium

Propionibacteria are small gram-positive bacilli that are frequently arranged in short chains or clumps (Fig. 36–7). They are commonly found on the skin (in contrast with the actinomyces), conjunctiva, and external ear and in the oropharynx and female genital tract. The organisms are anaerobic or aerotolerant, nonmotile, catalase-positive, and capable of fermenting carbohydrates, producing propionic acid as their major byproduct (hence the name). The two most commonly isolated species are *Propionibacterium acnes* and *Propionibacterium propionicus*.

P. acnes is responsible for two types of infections, acne (as the name implies) in teenagers and young

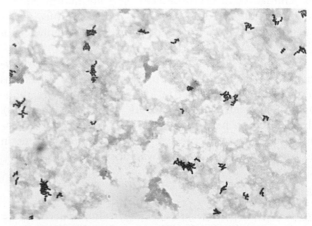

FIGURE 36–7. Gram stain of *Propionibacterium*.

adults and opportunistic infections in patients with prosthetic devices (e.g., artificial heart valves or joints) or intravascular lines (e.g., catheters, cerebrospinal fluid shunts). Propionibacteria are also commonly isolated in blood cultures, but this finding usually represents contamination with bacteria on the skin at the phlebotomy site.

The central role of *P. acnes* in acne is to stimulate an inflammatory response. Production of a low-molecular-weight peptide by the bacilli residing in sebaceous follicles attracts leukocytes. The bacilli are then phagocytosed, followed by the release of hydrolytic enzymes that, together with bacterial lipases, proteases, neuraminidase, and hyaluronidase, precipitate the inflammatory response, leading to rupture of the follicle. When injected into experimental animals, *P. propionicus* causes lacrimal canaliculitis (inflammation of the tear duct) and abscesses.

Propionibacteria can grow on most common media, although it may take 2 to 5 days for growth to appear. Care must be taken to avoid contamination of the specimen with the organisms normally found on the skin. The significance of the recovery of an isolate must also be interpreted in light of the clinical presentation (e.g., a catheter or other foreign body can serve as a focus for these opportunistic pathogens).

Acne is unrelated to the effectiveness of skin cleansing, because the lesion develops within the sebaceous follicles. For this reason, acne is managed primarily through the topical application of benzoyl peroxide and antibiotics. Antibiotics such as erythromycin and clindamycin have proved effective.

Mobiluncus

Members of the genus *Mobiluncus* are obligate anaerobic, gram-variable or gram-negative, curved bacilli with tapered ends. Despite their appearance in Gram-stained specimens, they are classified as gram-positive bacilli because they (1) have a gram-positive cell wall, (2) lack endotoxin, and (3) are susceptible to vancomycin, clindamycin, erythromycin, and ampicillin but resistant to colistin. The organisms are fastidious, growing slowly even on enriched media supplemented with rabbit or horse serum.

Two species, *Mobiluncus curtisii* and *Mobiluncus mulieris*, have been identified in humans. The organisms colonize the genital tract in low numbers but are abundant in women with **bacterial vaginosis** (vaginitis). Their microscopic appearance is a useful marker for this disease, but the precise role of these organisms in the pathogenesis of bacterial vaginosis is unclear.

Lactobacillus

Lactobacillus species are facultatively anaerobic or strictly anaerobic bacilli. They are found as part of the normal flora of the mouth, stomach, intestines, and genitourinary tract. The organisms are most commonly isolated in urine specimens and blood cultures. Because lactobacilli are the most common organism in the urethra, their recovery in urine cultures invariably stems from contamination of the specimen, even when large numbers of the organisms are present. The reason lactobacilli rarely cause infections of the urinary tract is their inability to grow in urine. Invasion into the blood stream occurs in one of the following three settings: (1) transient bacteremia from a genitourinary source (e.g., after childbirth or a gynecologic procedure), (2) endocarditis, and (3) opportunistic septicemia in an immunocompromised patient.

Treatment of endocarditis and opportunistic infections is difficult, because lactobacilli are resistant to vancomycin (an antibiotic commonly active against gram-positive bacteria) and are inhibited but not killed by other antibiotics. A combination of penicillin with an aminoglycoside is required for bactericidal activity.

Bifidobacterium and Eubacterium

Bifidobacterium and *Eubacterium* species are commonly found in the oropharynx, large intestine, and vagina. These bacteria can be isolated in clinical specimens but have a very low virulence potential and usually represent clinically insignificant contaminants. Confirmation of their etiologic role in an infection requires their repeated isolation in large numbers from multiple specimens and the absence of other pathogenic organisms.

CASE STUDY AND QUESTIONS

■ A 42-year-old man entered the university hospital for the treatment of a chronically draining wound in the jaw. The patient had undergone extraction of many teeth 3 months before admission and had poor oral hygiene and fetid breath at the time of admission. Multiple pustular nodules were observed overlying the carious teeth, and some nodules had ruptured. The drainage material consisted of serosanguineous fluid containing small, hard granules.

1. The diagnosis of actinomycosis is considered. How would you collect and transport specimens for confirmation of this diagnosis? What diagnostic tests can be performed?

2. Describe the epidemiology of actinomycosis. What is the risk factor for this patient?

3. What diseases are caused by *Propionibacterium*? What is the source of this organism?

BIBLIOGRAPHY

Antonio M, Hawes S, Hillier S: The identification of vaginal *Lactobacillus* species and the demographic and microbiologic characteristics of women colonized by these species, *J Infect Dis* 180:1950–1956, 1999.

Antony S, Stratton C, Dummer S: *Lactobacillus* bacteremia: description of the clinical course in adult patients without endocarditis, *Clin Infect Dis* 23:773–778, 1996.

Brook I, Frazier EH: Infections caused by *Propionibacterium* species, *Rev Infect Dis* 3:819–822, 1991.

Fruchart C et al: *Lactobacillus* species as emerging pathogens in neutropenic patients, *Eur J Clin Microbiol Infect Dis* 16: 681–684, 1997.

Hofstad T: Current taxonomy of medically important nonsporing anaerobes, *Rev Infect Dis* 12(suppl):122–126, 1990.

Hollick G: Isolation and identification of aerobic actinomycetes, *Clin Microbiol Newsletter* 17:25–29, 1995.

Murdoch D: Gram-positive anaerobic cocci, *Clin Microbiol Rev* 11:81–120, 1998.

Smego RA: Actinomycosis of the central nervous system, *Rev Infect Dis* 9:855–865, 1987.

Spiegel CA: Bacterial vaginosis, *Clin Microbiol Rev* 4:485–502, 1991.

Stackebrandt E, Rainey F, Ward-Rainey N: Proposal for a new hierarchic classification system, *Actinobacteria classis* nov., *Int J Syst Bacteriol* 47:479–491, 1997.

Tiveljung A, Forsum U, Monstein H-J: Classification of the genus *Mobiluncus* based on comparative partial 16S rRNA gene analysis, *Int J Syst Bacteriol* 46:332–336, 1996.

CHAPTER 37

Clostridium

The genus *Clostridium* includes all anaerobic, gram-positive bacilli capable of forming endospores. Although most members of the genus are strict anaerobes, some are aerotolerant (e.g., *Clostridium tertium*, *Clostridium histolyticum*) and can grow on agar media exposed to air. Some clostridia appear to be gram-negative (e.g., *Clostridium ramosum*, *Clostridium clostridiiforme*), and spores may not be observed in some species (*Clostridium perfringens*, *C. ramosum*). The traditional method for classifying an isolate in the genus *Clostridium* was based on a combination of diagnostic tests, including the demonstration of spores, optimal growth in anaerobic conditions, a complex pattern of biochemical reactivity, and the findings yielded by gas chromatography analysis of the metabolic byproducts. With these methods, more than 130 species have been defined. Fortunately, most of the clinically important isolates fall within a few species (Table 37–1). It should not be surprising that the use of gene sequencing techniques has enabled the subdivision of this heterogeneous collection of organisms into 16 groups. Because the reclassification of these spore-forming anaerobes has not been resolved at this time, the conventional organization of these bacteria in the genus *Clostridium* is used in the present discussion.

The organisms are ubiquitous, being present in soil, water, and sewage and as part of the normal microbial flora in the gastrointestinal tracts of animals and humans. Most clostridia are harmless saprophytes, but some are well-recognized human pathogens with a clearly documented history of causing diseases, such as tetanus (*Clostridium tetani*), botulism (*Clostridium botulinum*, *Clostridium barati*, *Clostridium butyricum*), and myonecrosis or **gas gangrene** (*C. perfringens*, *Clostridium novyi*, *Clostridium septicum*, *C. histolyticum*, *Clostridium sordellii*). Despite the notoriety of these diseases, we now know that clostridia are more commonly associated with skin and soft tissue infections, food poisoning, and antibiotic-associated diarrhea and colitis. The remarkable capacity of clostridia to cause diseases is attributed to the following features:

1. Ability to survive adverse environmental conditions through spore formation.

2. Rapid growth in a nutritionally enriched, oxygen-deprived environment.
3. Production of numerous histolytic toxins, enterotoxins, and neurotoxins.

The most important human pathogens in the genus are discussed in this chapter.

Clostridium perfringens

Physiology and Structure

C. perfringens, the clostridial species most commonly isolated in clinical specimens, can be associated with simple colonization or can cause severe, life-threatening disease. *C. perfringens* is a large, rectangular, gram-positive bacillus, with spores rarely observed either in vivo or after in vitro cultivation (Fig. 37–1). This organism is one of the few nonmotile clostridia, but rapidly spreading growth on laboratory media (resembling the growth of motile organisms) is characteristic (Fig. 37–2). The organism grows rapidly in tissues and in culture, is hemolytic, and is metabolically active, features that make possible its rapid identification in the laboratory. The production of one or more lethal toxins of *C. perfringens* (α, β, ϵ, and ι toxins) is used to subdivide isolates into five types (A through E; Table 37–2). Type A *C. perfringens* causes most of the human infections in the United States.

Pathogenesis and Immunity

C. perfringens can cause a spectrum of diseases, from a self-limited gastroenteritis to an overwhelming destruction of tissue (e.g., clostridial myonecrosis) associated with a very high mortality, even in patients who receive early medical intervention. This pathogenic potential is attributed primarily to the 12 toxins and enzymes produced by this organism (Table 37–3). α **Toxin**, the most important toxin and the one produced by all types of *C. perfringens*, is a lecithinase (phospholipase C) that lyses erythrocytes, platelets, leukocytes, and endothelial cells (Fig. 37–3). This toxin increases

TABLE 37–1. Pathogenic Clostridia and Their Associated Human Diseases*

Species	Human Disease	Frequency
C. difficile	Antibiotic-associated diarrhea, pseudomembranous colitis	Common
C. perfringens	Soft tissue infections (i.e., cellulitis, suppurative myositis, myonecrosis or gas gangrene), food poisoning, enteritis necroticans, septicemia	Common
C. septicum	Gas gangrene, septicemia	Uncommon
C. tertium	Opportunistic infections	Uncommon
C. botulinum	Botulism	Uncommon
C. tetani	Tetanus	Uncommon
C. barati	Botulism	Rare
C. butyricum	Botulism	Rare
C. histolyticum	Gas gangrene	Rare
C. novyi	Gas gangrene	Rare
C. sordellii	Gas gangrene	Rare

*Other clostridial species have been associated with human disease but primarily as opportunistic pathogens. Additionally, some species (e.g., *C. clostridioforme*, *C. innocuum*, *C. ramosum*) are commonly isolated but are rarely associated with disease.

vascular permeability, resulting in massive hemolysis and bleeding, tissue destruction (as found in myonecrosis), hepatic toxicity, and myocardial dysfunction (bradycardia, hypotension). The largest quantities of α-toxin are produced by *C. perfringens* type A. **β Toxin** is responsible for the necrotic lesions in necrotizing enteritis (**enteritis necroticans, pig-bel**). **ε Toxin**, a protoxin, is activated by trypsin and increases the vascular permeability of the gastrointestinal wall. **ι Toxin**, the fourth major lethal toxin produced by *C. perfringens*, has necrotic activity and increases vascular permeability.

The *C. perfringens* **enterotoxin** is produced primarily by type A strains. The toxin is heat-labile and is susceptible to pronase but not to trypsin or other proteases. The enterotoxin is produced during the phase transition from vegetative cells to spores and is released when the bacterial cells undergo lysis, releasing the formed spores. The alkaline conditions in the small intestine stimulate sporulation. The released entero-

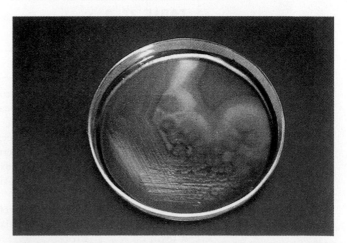

FIGURE 37–2. Growth of *Clostridium perfringens* on sheep blood agar. Note the flat, rapidly spreading colonies and the hemolytic activity of the organism. *C. perfringes* can be identified preliminarily from the finding of a zone of complete hemolysis (caused by the θ toxin) and a wider zone of partial hemolysis (caused by the α toxin), combined with the characteristic microscopic morphology.

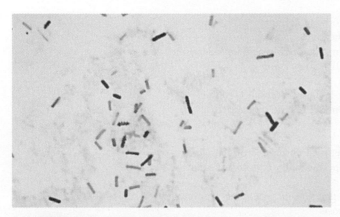

FIGURE 37–1. Gram stain of *Clostridium perfringens*.

TABLE 37-2. Distribution of Lethal Toxins in *Clostridium perfringens* Types A-E

Type of Isolate	Lethal Toxins			
	α	β	ϵ	ι
A	+	−	−	−
B	+	+	+	−
C	+	+	−	−
D	+	−	+	−
E	+	−	−	+

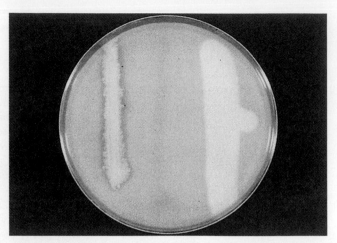

FIGURE 37-3. Growth of *Clostridum perfringens* on egg-yolk agar. The α toxin (lecithinase) hydrolyzes phospholipids in serum and egg yolk, producing an opaque precipitate *(right)*. This precipitate is not observed when the organism is grown in the presence of antibodies against the toxin *(left)*. This reaction (Nagler's reaction) is characteristic of *C. perfringens.*

toxin binds to receptors on the brush border membrane of the small intestine epithelium. This disrupts ion transport in the ileum (primarily) and jejunum and alters membrane permeability. Antibodies to enterotoxin, indicating previous exposure, are commonly found in adults but are not protective. The activities of the other toxins and enzymes of *C. perfringens* are summarized in Table 37-3.

Epidemiology

C. perfringens type A commonly inhabits the intestinal tract of humans and animals and is widely distributed in nature, particularly in soil and water contaminated with feces (Box 37-1). Spores are formed under adverse environmental conditions and can survive for prolonged periods. Strains of types B through E do not survive in soil but rather colonize the intestinal tracts of animals and occasionally humans. *C. perfringens* type A is responsible for most human infections, including soft tissue infections, food poisoning, and primary septicemia. *C. perfringens* type C is responsible for one other important infection in humans—enteritis necroticans.

TABLE 37-3. Virulence Factors Associated with *Clostridium perfringens*

Virulence Factors	Biologic Activity
α toxin	Lethal toxin; phospholipase C (lecithinase); increases vascular permeability; hemolysin; produces necrotizing activity
β toxin	Lethal toxin; necrotizing activity
ϵ toxin	Lethal toxin; permease
ι toxin	Lethal binary toxin; necrotizing activity; adenosine diphosphate (ADP) ribosylating
δ toxin	Hemolysin
θ toxin	Heat- and oxygen-labile hemolysin; cytolytic
κ toxin	Collagenase; gelatinase; necrotizing activity
λ toxin	Protease
μ toxin	Hyaluronidase
ν toxin	Deoxyribonuclease; hemolysin; necrotizing activity
Enterotoxin	Alters membrane permeability (cytotoxic, enterotoxic)
Neuraminidase	Alters cell surface ganglioside receptors; promotes capillary thrombosis

---

BOX 37–1. Summary of *Clostridium perfringens* Infections

Physiology and Structure

Large, rectangular, gram-positive bacillus.

Forms spores but they are rarely seen in clinical specimens or culture.

Replicates rapidly, so large spreading colonies are seen within first day of culture; "double zone" of hemolysis on blood agar (due to α and δ toxins).

Produces many toxins and hemolytic enzymes, so white blood cells are not seen in Gram-stained clinical specimens.

Produces lecithinase (phospholipase C).

Subdivided into 5 types (A–E) on the basis of toxin production (refer to Table 37–2).

Virulence

Refer to Table 37–3.

Epidemiology

Ubiquitous; present in soil, water, and intestinal tract of humans and animals.

Type A is responsible for most human infections (also only type capable of surviving in soil).

Disease follows exogenous or endogenous exposure.

Diseases

Soft tissue infections (cellulitis, suppurative myositis, myonecrosis).

Food poisoning.

Septicemia.

Diagnosis

Characteristic forms seen on Gram stain.

Grows rapidly in culture.

Treatment, Prevention, and Control

Rapid treatment is essential for serious infections.

Systemic infections require surgical débridement and high-dose penicillin therapy; antiserum against α toxin not used now, and the value of hyperbaric oxygen treatment is unproven.

Treat with débridement and penicillin for localized infections.

Symptomatic treatment for food poisoning.

Proper wound care and judicious use of prophylactic antibiotics will prevent most infections.

Clinical Diseases

Soft Tissue Infections

Soft tissue infections caused by *C. perfringens* are subdivided into (1) cellulitis, (2) fasciitis or suppurative myositis, and (3) myonecrosis or gas gangrene. Clostridial species can colonize wounds and skin with no clinical consequences. Indeed, most isolates of *C. per-* *fringens* and other clostridial species from wound cultures are insignificant. However, these organisms can also initiate **cellulitis** (Fig. 37–4) with gas formation in the soft tissue. This process can progress to **suppurative myositis** characterized by an accumulation of pus in the muscle planes, but muscle necrosis and systemic symptoms are absent.

Clostridial myonecrosis is a life-threatening disease that illustrates the full virulence potential of histotoxic clostridia. The onset of disease, characterized by intense pain, generally develops within a week after clostridia are introduced into tissue by trauma or surgery. The onset is followed rapidly by extensive muscle necrosis, shock, renal failure, and death, frequently within 2 days of initial onset. Macroscopic examination of muscle reveals devitalized necrotic tissue. Gas found in the tissue is caused by the metabolic activity of the rapidly dividing bacteria (hence the name **gas gangrene**). Microscopic examination reveals abundant rectangular, gram-positive bacilli in the absence of inflammatory cells (resulting from lysis by clostridial toxins). The clostridial toxins characteristically cause extensive hemolysis and bleeding. Clostridial myonecrosis is most commonly caused by *C. perfringens*, although other species can also produce this disease (e.g., *C. septicum*, *C. histolyticum*, *C. sordellii*, and *C. novyi*).

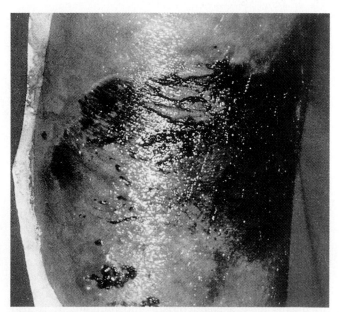

FIGURE 37–4. Clostridial cellulitis. Clostridia can be introduced into tissue during surgery or by a traumatic injury. The patient suffered a compound fracture of the tibia. Five days after the injury, the skin became discolored, and bullae and necrosis developed. A serosanguineous exudate and subcutaneous gas were present, but there was no evidence of muscle necrosis. The patient had an uneventful recovery. (From Lambert H, Farrar W, editors: *Infectious diseases illustrated*, London, 1982, Gower.)

Food Poisoning

Clostridial food poisoning, a relatively common but underappreciated bacterial disease, is characterized by (1) a short incubation period (8 to 24 hours), (2) a clinical presentation that includes abdominal cramps and watery diarrhea but no fever, nausea, or vomiting, and (3) a clinical course lasting less than 24 hours. Disease results from the ingestion of meat products contaminated with large numbers (10^8 to 10^9 organisms) of type A *C. perfringens*. The refrigeration of food after preparation prevents the production of enterotoxin. Alternatively, reheating of the food can destroy the heat-labile enterotoxin.

Necrotizing Enteritis

Necrotizing enteritis, or **enteritis necroticans**, is a rare, acute necrotizing process in the jejunum characterized by abdominal pain, bloody diarrhea, shock, and peritonitis. The mortality in patients with the infection approaches 50%. β-Toxin–producing *C. perfringens* type C is responsible for this disease. Necrotizing enteritis is most common in Papua New Guinea, with sporadic cases reported from other countries. Risk factors for the disease are exposure to large numbers of organisms and malnutrition (with loss of the proteolytic activity that inactivates the enterotoxin).

Septicemia

The isolation of *C. perfringens* or other clostridial species in blood cultures can be alarming. More than half of the isolates are clinically insignificant, however, representing a transient bacteremia or, more likely, contamination of the culture with clostridia colonizing the skin. The significance of an isolate must be viewed in light of other clinical findings.

Laboratory Diagnosis

The laboratory performs only a confirmatory role in the diagnosis of clostridial soft tissue diseases, because therapy must be initiated immediately in affected patients. The microscopic detection of gram-positive bacilli in clinical specimens, usually in the absence of leukocytes, can be a very useful finding, because these organisms have a characteristic morphology. It is also relatively simple to culture these anaerobes; *C. perfringens* can be detected on simple media after incubation for 1 day or less. Under appropriate conditions, *C. perfringens* can divide every 8 to 10 minutes, so growth on agar media or in blood culture broths can be detected after incubation for only a few hours. The role of *C. perfringens* in food poisoning is documented by recovery of more than 10^5 organisms per gram of food

or more than 10^6 bacteria per gram of feces collected within 1 day of the onset of disease. Immunoassays have also been developed for detection of the enterotoxin in fecal specimens.

Treatment, Prevention, and Control

C. perfringens infections such as suppurative myositis and myonecrosis must be treated aggressively with surgical débridement and high-dose penicillin therapy. Hyperbaric oxygen treatment has been used to manage these infections; however, the results are inconclusive. Antiserum against α-toxin also has not been successful and is no longer available.

Despite all therapeutic efforts, the prognosis in patients with these diseases is poor, reported mortality ranging from 40% to almost 100%. Less serious, localized clostridial diseases can be successfully treated with penicillin, with resistance only rarely reported for species other than *C. perfringens*. Antibiotic therapy for clostridial food poisoning is unnecessary.

Prevention and control of *C. perfringens* infections are difficult because of the ubiquitous distribution of the organisms. Disease requires introduction of the organism into devitalized tissues and maintenance of an anaerobic environment favorable for bacterial growth. Thus, proper wound care and the judicious use of prophylactic antibiotics can do much to prevent most infections.

Clostridium tetani

Physiology and Structure

C. tetani is a small, motile, spore-forming bacillus that commonly gram stains weakly. The organism produces round, terminal spores that give it the appearance of a drumstick (Fig. 37–5). Unlike *C. perfringens*, *C. tetani* is difficult to grow and identify, because it is extremely sensitive to oxygen toxicity and is relatively inactive metabolically.

Pathogenesis and Immunity

Although the vegetative cells of *C. tetani* die rapidly when exposed to oxygen, spore formation allows the organism to survive in the most adverse conditions. Of greater significance is the fact *C. tetani* produces two toxins, an oxygen-labile hemolysin (**tetanolysin**) and a plasmid-encoded, heat-labile neurotoxin (**tetanospasmin**). Tetanolysin is serologically related to other clostridial hemolysins and streptolysin O. The clinical significance of this enzyme is unknown, however, because it is inhibited by oxygen and serum cholesterol.

Tetanospasmin is produced during the stationary phase of growth, is released when the cell is lysed, and

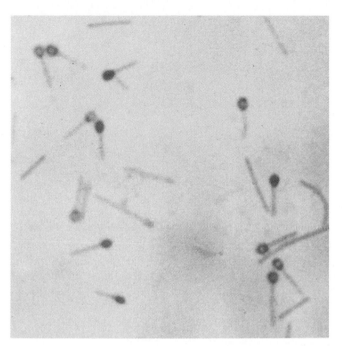

FIGURE 37–5. Gram stain of *Clostridium tetani.* Note the terminal spores.

is responsible for the clinical manifestations of tetanus. Tetanospasmin (an A-B toxin) is synthesized as a single 151,000-Da peptide that is cleaved into a light (A-chain) subunit and a heavy (B-chain) subunit by an endogenous protease when the cell releases the neurotoxin. The two chains are held together by a disulfide bond and noncovalent forces. The carboxyl-terminal portion of the heavy (100,000-Da) chain binds to a surface receptor on neuronal membranes. The light chain of the toxin, a zinc endopeptidase, is then internalized and moves from the peripheral nerve terminals to the central nervous system by retrograde axonal transport. It is released from the postsynaptic dendrites, crosses the synaptic cleft, and is localized within vesicles in the presynaptic nerve terminals.

Tetanospasmin acts by blocking the release of neurotransmitters (e.g., gamma-aminobutyric acid [GABA], glycine) for inhibitory synapses, thus causing excitatory synaptic activity to be unregulated (**spastic paralysis**). It does not affect acetylcholine transmission (in contrast to *C. botulinum*). The toxin binding is irreversible, so recovery depends on whether new axonal terminals form.

Epidemiology

C. tetani is ubiquitous. It is found in fertile soil and colonizes the gastrointestinal tracts of many animals, including humans (Box 37–2). The vegetative forms of *C. tetani* are extremely susceptible to oxygen toxicity, but the organisms sporulate readily and can survive in nature for a long time. Disease is relatively rare in the

---

BOX 37–2. Summary of *Clostridium tetani* Infections

Physiology and Structure

Gram-positive bacilli with prominent terminal spores (drumstick appearance).

Strict anaerobe (vegetative cells are extremely oxygen sensitive).

Difficult to isolate from clinical specimens.

Virulence

Spore formation.

Tetanospasmin (heat-labile neurotoxin; blocks release of neurotransmitters [i.e., gamma-aminobutyric acid, glycine] for inhibitory synapses).

Tetanolysin (heat-stable hemolysin of unknown significance).

Epidemiology

Ubiquitous; spores are found in most soils and can colonize gastrointestinal tract of humans and animals.

Exposure to spores is common, but disease is uncommon except in underdeveloped countries, where there is poor vaccination compliance and medical care is inadequate.

Risk is greatest for people with inadequate vaccine-induced immunity; disease does not induce immunity.

Diseases

Generalized tetanus (most common form).
  Cephalic tetanus (high mortality).
  Localized or wound tetanus (good prognosis).
  Neonatal tetanus (high mortality).

Diagnosis

Diagnosis is based on clinical presentation.
  Microscopy and culture with poor sensitivity.
  Neither tetanus toxin nor antibodies are typically detected.

Treatment, Prevention, and Control

Treatment requires débridement, antibiotic therapy (metronidazole), passive immunization with antitoxin globulin, and vaccination with tetanus toxoid.

Prevention through use of vaccination, consisting of three doses of tetanus toxoid followed by boosters every 10 years.

United States because of the high incidence of immunity brought about by vaccination. Fewer than 50 cases are reported annually, and the disease occurs primarily in elderly patients with waning immunity. However, tetanus is still responsible for causing many deaths in people living in underdeveloped areas where vaccination is unavailable or medical practices are lax. It is estimated that more than 1 million cases occur worldwide, with a mortality rate ranging from 20% to 50%. At least half the deaths occur in neonates.

TABLE 37–4. Clinical Manifestations of Tetanus	
Disease	**Clinical Manifestations**
Generalized	Involvement of bulbar and paraspinal muscles (trismus or lockjaw, risus sardonicus, difficulty swallowing, irritability, opisthotonos); involvement of autonomic nervous system (sweating, hyperthermia, cardiac arrhythmias, fluctuations in blood pressure)
Cephalic	Primary infection in head, particularly ear; isolated or combined involvement of cranial nerves, particularly seventh cranial nerve; very poor prognosis
Localized	Involvement of muscles in area of primary injury; infection may precede generalized disease; favorable prognosis
Neonatal	Generalized disease in neonates; infection typically originates from umbilical stump; very poor prognosis in infants whose mothers are nonimmune

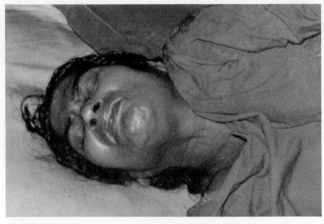

FIGURE 37–6. Risus sardonicus in tetanus caused by sustained spasms of the masseter muscles. (From Emond RT, Rowland HAK, Welsby P: *Colour atlas of infectious diseases,* ed 3, London, 1995, Wolfe.)

Clinical Diseases

The clinical symptoms of tetanus are summarized in Table 37–4. The incubation period for tetanus varies from a few days to weeks. The duration of the incubation period is directly related to the distance of the primary wound infection from the central nervous system.

Generalized tetanus is the most common form.

Involvement of the masseter muscles (trismus or lockjaw) is the presenting sign in most patients. The characteristic sardonic smile that results from the sustained contraction of the facial muscles is known as *risus sardonicus* (Fig. 37–6). Other early signs are drooling, sweating, irritability, and persistent back spasms (*opisthotonos*) (Fig. 37–7). The autonomic nervous system is involved in patients with more severe disease; the signs and symptoms include cardiac arrhythmias, fluctuations in blood pressure, profound sweating, and dehydration.

Another form of *C. tetani* disease is **localized tetanus**, in which the disease remains confined to the musculature at the site of primary infection. A variant is **cephalic tetanus**, in which the primary site of infection is the head. In contrast to the prognosis for pa-

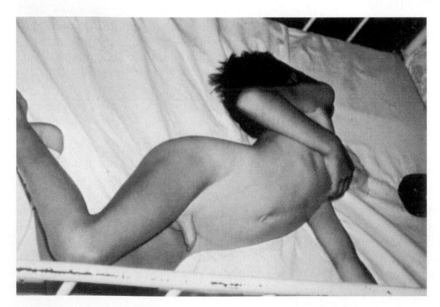

FIGURE 37–7. A child with tetanus and opisthotonos resulting from persistent spasms of the back muscles. (From Emond RT, Rowland HAK, Welsby P: *Colour atlas of infectious diseases,* ed 3, London, 1995, Wolfe.)

tients with localized tetanus, the prognosis for patients with cephalic tetanus is very poor.

Neonatal tetanus (tetanus neonatorum) is typically associated with an initial infection of the umbilical stump that progresses to become generalized. The mortality in infants exceeds 90%, and developmental defects are present in survivors.

Laboratory Diagnosis

The diagnosis of tetanus, as with that of most other clostridial diseases, is made on the basis of the clinical presentation. The microscopic detection or isolation of *C. tetani* is useful but frequently unsuccessful. Culture results are positive in only about 30% of patients with tetanus, because disease can be caused by relatively few organisms and the slow-growing bacteria are killed rapidly when exposed to air. Neither tetanus toxin nor antibodies to the toxin are detectable in the patient. If the organism is recovered in culture, production of toxin by the isolate can be confirmed with the tetanus antitoxin neutralization test in mice (a procedure performed only in Public Health reference laboratories).

Treatment, Prevention, and Control

The mortality associated with tetanus has steadily decreased during the past century, resulting in large part from the decreased incidence of tetanus in the United States. The highest mortality is in newborns and in patients in whom the incubation period is shorter than 1 week.

Treatment of tetanus requires débridement of the primary wound (which may appear innocuous), use of metronidazole, passive immunization with human tetanus immunoglobulin, and vaccination with tetanus toxoid. Wound care and metronidazole therapy eliminate the vegetative bacteria that produce toxin, and the antitoxin antibodies work by binding free tetanospasmin molecules. Metronidazole and penicillin have equivalent activity against *C. tetani*; however, penicillin, like tetanospasmin, inhibits GABA activity and hence should not be used. Toxin bound to nerve endings is protected from antibodies. Thus, the toxic effects must be controlled symptomatically until the normal regulation of synaptic transmission is restored. Vaccination with a series of three doses of tetanus toxoid followed by booster doses every 10 years is highly effective in preventing tetanus.

Clostridium botulinum

Physiology and Structure

C. botulinum (from the Latin *botulus*, "sausage"), the etiologic agent of botulism, is a heterogeneous group of fastidious, spore-forming, anaerobic bacilli. Seven antigenically distinct botulinum toxins (A to G) have been described; human disease is associated with types A, B, E, and F. Only one toxin is produced by most individual isolates. Like tetanus toxin, *C. botulinum* toxin is a 150,000- to 165,000-Da progenitor protein (A-B toxin) consisting of the neurotoxin subunit (light or A chain) and one or more nontoxic subunits (B or heavy chain). Each nontoxic subunit protects the neurotoxin from being inactivated by stomach acids.

Pathogenesis and Immunity

Botulinum toxin is similar in structure and function to tetanus toxin, differing only in the target neural cell. This toxin is very specific for cholinergic nerves. It blocks neurotransmission at peripheral cholinergic synapses by preventing release of the neurotransmitter acetylcholine. As with tetanus, recovery of function after botulism requires regeneration of the nerve endings. *C. botulinum* also produces a binary toxin consisting of two components that combine to disrupt vascular permeability.

Epidemiology

C. botulinum is commonly isolated in soil and water samples throughout the world (Box 37–3). In the United States, type A strains are found mainly in neutral or alkaline soil west of the Mississippi River; type B strains are found primarily in the eastern part of the country in rich, organic soil; and type E strains are found only in wet soil. Even though *C. botulinum* is commonly found in soil, disease is uncommon in the United States.

The following three forms of botulism have been identified: (1) classic or foodborne botulism, (2) infant botulism, and (3) wound botulism. Fewer than 50 cases of **foodborne botulism** are seen annually; most are associated with the consumption of home-canned foods (types A and B toxins) and occasionally with the consumption of preserved fish (type E toxin). The food may not appear spoiled, but even a small taste can cause full-blown clinical disease. **Infant botulism** is more common (although fewer than 100 cases are reported annually) and has been associated with the consumption of foods (particularly honey) contaminated with botulinum spores. The incidence of **wound botulism** is unknown, but the disease is very rare.

Clinical Diseases

Foodborne Botulism

Patients with foodborne botulism typically become weak and dizzy 1 to 2 days after consuming the con-

BOX 37–3. Summary of *Clostridium botulinum* Infections

Physiology and Structure

Gram-positive, spore-forming bacillus.

Strict anaerobe (vegetative cells extremely oxygen-sensitive).

Fastidious growth requirements.

Can produce one of seven distinct botulinum toxins (A–G).

Strains associated with human disease produce lipase, digest milk proteins, hydrolyze gelatin, and ferment glucose.

Virulence

Spore formation.

Botulinum toxin (prevents release of neurotransmitter acetylcholine).

Binary toxin.

Epidemiology

Ubiquitous; *C. botulinum* spores are found in soil worldwide

Human diseases associated with toxins A, B, E, and F.

Relatively few cases of botulism in the United States.

Infant botulism more common than other forms.

Diseases

Foodborne botulism.

Infant botulism.

Wound botulism.

Diagnosis

Botulism confirmed by isolating the organism or detecting the toxin in food products or the patient's feces or serum.

Treatment, Prevention, and Control

Treatment involves administration of metronidazole or penicillin, trivalent botulinum antitoxin, and ventilatory support.

Spore germination in foods prevented by maintaining food in an acid pH, by high sugar content (e.g., fruit preserves), or by storing the foods at 4°C or colder.

Toxin is heat-labile so can be destroyed by heating of food for 20 minutes at 80°C.

Infant botulism is associated with consumption of contaminated foods (particularly honey). Infants younger than 1 year should not be given honey or foods containing it.

---

taminated food. The initial signs include blurred vision with fixed dilated pupils, dry mouth (indicative of the anticholinergic effects of the toxin), constipation, and abdominal pain. Fever is absent. Bilateral descending weakness of the peripheral muscles develops in patients with progressive disease (flaccid paralysis), and death is most commonly attributed to respiratory paralysis. Pa-

tients maintain a clear sensorium throughout the disease. Despite aggressive management of the patient's condition, the disease may continue to progress, because the neurotoxin is irreversibly bound and inhibits the release of excitatory neurotransmitters for a prolonged period. Complete recovery in patients frequently requires many months to years, or until the affected nerve endings regrow. Mortality in patients with foodborne botulism, which once approached 70%, has been reduced to 10% through the use of better supportive care, particularly in the management of respiratory complications.

Infant Botulism

Infant botulism was first recognized in 1976 and is now the most common form of botulism in the United States. In contrast with foodborne botulism, this disease is caused by neurotoxin produced in vivo by *C. botulinum* colonizing the gastrointestinal tracts of infants. Although adults certainly are exposed to the organism in their diet, *C. botulinum* cannot survive and proliferate in their intestines. In the absence of competitive bowel microbes, however, the organism can become established in the gastrointestinal tracts of infants. The disease typically affects infants younger than 1 year (most between 1 and 6 months), and the symptoms are initially nonspecific (e.g., constipation, weak cry, or "failure to thrive"). Progressive disease with flaccid paralysis and respiratory arrest can develop; however, mortality in documented cases of infant botulism is very low (1% to 2%). Some infant deaths attributed to other conditions (e.g., sudden infant death syndrome) may actually be caused by botulism.

Wound Botulism

As the name implies, wound botulism develops from toxin production by *C. botulinum* in contaminated wounds. Although the symptoms of disease are identical to those of foodborne disease, the incubation period is generally longer (4 days or more), and the gastrointestinal tract symptoms are less prominent.

Laboratory Diagnosis

The clinical diagnosis of botulism is confirmed if the organism is isolated or toxin activity is demonstrated. Toxin activity is most likely to be found early in the disease. An attempt should be made to culture *C. botulinum* from the feces of patients with foodborne disease and from the implicated food if it is available (Fig. 37–8).

Isolation of *C. botulinum* from specimens contaminated with other organisms can be improved by heating the specimen for 10 minutes at 80°C to kill all

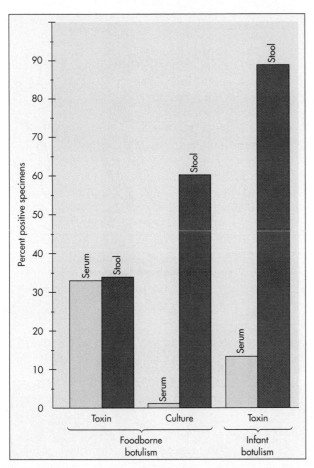

FIGURE 37-8. Rates of detection of *Clostridium botulinum* and botulinal toxin in serum and stool specimens collected from patients with foodborne botulism and infant botulism. Confirmation of foodborne disease requires testing of the implicated food and the patient's serum and stool specimen for botulinal toxin activity and culture of the food and stool specimen for the organism. No single test for foodborne botulism has a sensitivity greater than 60%. Serum and stool specimens from an infant with botulism should be tested for toxin activity, and the stool specimen cultured. (Data from Dowell V et al: Coproexamination for botulinum toxin and *Clostridium botulinum*: a new procedure for laboratory diagnosis of botulism, *JAMA* 238:1829–1832, 1977; and Hatheway C, McCroskey L: Examination of feces and serum for diagnosis of infant botulism in 336 patients. *J Clin Microbiol* 25:2334–2338, 1987.)

vegetative cells. Culture of the heated specimen on nutritionally enriched anaerobic media allows the heat-resistant *C. botulinum* spores to germinate. The strains of *C. botulinum* associated with human botulism are characterized by lipase production (appears as an iridescent film on colonies grown on egg-yolk agar) as well as the ability to digest milk proteins, hydrolyze gelatin, and ferment glucose.

Demonstration of toxin production (typically performed at Public Health laboratories) must be done with a mouse bioassay. This procedure consists of the preparation of two aliquots of the isolate, mixing of one aliquot with antitoxin, and intraperitoneal inoculation of each aliquot into mice. If the antitoxin treatment protects the mice, toxin activity is confirmed. Samples of the implicated food, stool specimen, and patient's serum should also be tested for toxin activity.

The diagnosis of infant botulism is supported if (1) *C. botulinum* is isolated from feces or (2) toxin activity is detected in feces or serum. The organism can be isolated from stool cultures in virtually all patients, because carriage of the organism may persist for many months even after a baby has recovered. Wound botulism is confirmed by isolation of the organism from the wound or by detection of toxin activity in wound exudate or serum.

Treatment, Prevention, and Control

Patients with botulism require the following treatment measures:

1. Adequate ventilatory support.
2. Elimination of the organism from the gastrointestinal tract through the judicious use of gastric lavage and metronidazole or penicillin therapy.
3. The use of trivalent botulinum antitoxin versus toxins A, B, and E to bind toxin circulating in the blood stream.

Ventilatory support is extremely important in reducing mortality. Protective levels of antibodies do not develop after disease, so patients are susceptible to secondary infections.

Disease is prevented by destroying the spores in food (virtually impossible for practical reasons), preventing spore germination (by maintaining the food in an acid pH or storage at 4°C or colder), or destroying the preformed toxin (by heating the food for 20 minutes at 80°C). Infant botulism has been associated with the consumption of honey contaminated with *C. botulinum* spores, so children younger than 1 year should not eat honey.

Clostridium difficile

Until the mid-1970s, the clinical importance of *C. difficile* was not appreciated. This organism was infrequently isolated in fecal cultures and rarely associated with human disease. Systematic studies now clearly show, however, that toxin-producing *C. difficile* is responsible for antibiotic-associated gastrointestinal diseases ranging from a relatively benign, self-limited diarrhea to severe, life-threatening pseudomembranous colitis (Figs. 37–9 and 37–10).

C. difficile produces two toxins (Table 37–5), an **enterotoxin** (toxin A) and a **cytotoxin** (toxin B). Al-

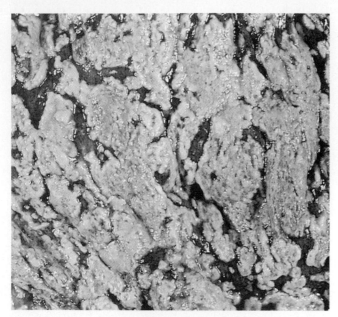

FIGURE 37–9. Antibiotic-associated colitis: gross section of the lumen of the colon. Note the white plaques of fibrin, mucus, and inflammatory cells overlying the normal intestinal mucosa *(red).*

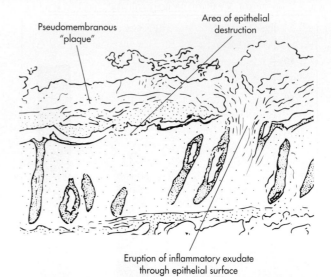

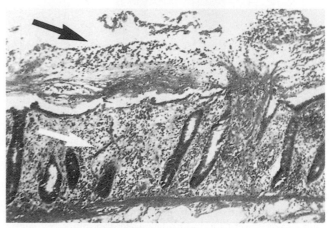

FIGURE 37–10. Antibiotic-associated colitis caused by *Clostridium difficile.* Histologic section of colon showing an intense inflammatory response, with the characteristic "plaque" *(black arrow)* overlying the intact intestinal mucosa *(white arrow).* (Hematoxylin & eosin.) (From Lambert HP, Farrar WE, editors: *Infectious diseases illustrated,* London, 1982, Gower.)

though these toxins are immunologically distinct, their purification has proved difficult. The enterotoxin is chemotactic for neutrophils, with infiltration of polymorphonuclear neutrophil leukocytes into the ileum, resulting in the release of cytokines, hypersecretion of fluid, and development of hemorrhagic necrosis. The cytotoxin causes actin to depolymerize, with the resultant destruction of the cellular cytoskeleton both in vivo and in vitro. The precise role that each toxin plays in the pathogenesis of disease is still unclear, because both toxins are produced in clostridia associated with disease (Box 37–4). Other *C. difficile* virulence factors are summarized in Table 37–5.

C. difficile is part of the normal intestinal flora in a small number of healthy people and hospitalized patients. The disease develops in people taking antibiotics because the agents alter the normal enteric flora, either permitting the overgrowth of these relatively resistant organisms or making the patient more susceptible to the exogenous acquisition of *C. difficile.* The disease occurs if the organisms proliferate in the colon and produce their toxins there.

The diagnosis of *C. difficile* infection is confirmed if (1) the organisms are isolated from cultures of feces on highly selective media, (2) the cytotoxin is detected by an in vitro cytotoxicity assay with tissue culture cells, or (3) enterotoxin is detected by immunoassays. The most specific test for *C. difficile* disease is the cytotoxicity assay. To detect colonization, a combination of diagnostic tests is performed to maximize sensitivity.

Discontinuation of the implicated antibiotic (e.g., ampicillin, clindamycin) is generally sufficient to alleviate mild disease. However, specific therapy with metronidazole or vancomycin is necessary for the management of serious disease. Relapses may occur in as many as 20% to 30% of patients after the completion of therapy, because only the vegetative forms of *C. difficile* are killed by the antibiotics; the spores are resistant. A second course of treatment with the same antibiotic is frequently successful. It is difficult to prevent the disease, because the organism commonly exists in hospitals, particularly in areas adjacent to infected patients. The spores of *C. difficile* are difficult to destroy; thus, the organism can contaminate an environment for

TABLE 37–5. Virulence Factors Associated with *Clostridium difficile*

Virulence Factor	Biologic Activity
Enterotoxin (toxin A)	Produces chemotaxis; induces cytokine production with hypersecretion of fluid; produces hemorrhagic necrosis
Cytotoxin (toxin B)	Induces depolymerization of actin with loss of cellular cytoskeleton
Adhesin factor	Mediates binding to human colonic cells
Hyaluronidase	Produces hydrolytic activity
Spore formation	Permits organism's survival for months in hospital environment

many months and can be a major source of nosocomial outbreaks of *C. difficile* disease.

Other Clostridial Species

Many other clostridia have been associated with clinically significant disease. Their virulence is due to their ability to survive exposure to oxygen by forming spores and producing many diverse toxins and enzymes. The virulence factors produced by some of the more important clostridia are summarized in Table 37–6. *C. septicum* is a particularly important pathogen because it is a cause of nontraumatic myonecrosis and frequently exists in patients with occult colon cancer, acute leukemia, and diabetes (Fig. 37–11). If the integrity of the bowel mucosa is compromised and the patient's body is less able to mount an effective response to the organism, *C. septicum* can spread into tissue and rapidly proliferate there. Most patients have a fulminant course, dying within 1 to 2 days after initial presentation.

CASE STUDY AND QUESTIONS

■ A 61-year-old woman with left-sided face pain came to the emergency department of a local hospital.

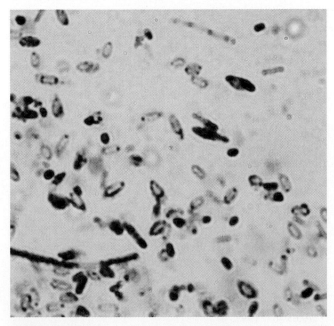

FIGURE 37–11. *Clostridium septicum:* Note the spores within the bacilli.

BOX 37–4. Summary of *Clostridium difficile* Infections

Physiology and Structure

Gram-positive, spore-forming bacillus.
  Strict anaerobe (vegetative cells are extremely oxygen-sensitive).

Virulence

Refer to Table 37–5.

Epidemiology

The organism is ubiquitous.
  Colonizes the intestines of a small proportion of healthy individuals (<5%).
  Exposure to antibiotics is associated with overgrowth of *C. difficile* and subsequent disease (endogenous infection).
  Spores can be detected in hospital rooms of infected patients (particularly around beds and in the bathrooms); these can be an exogenous source of infection.

Diseases

Asymptomatic colonization.
  Antibiotic-associated diarrhea.
  Pseudomembranous colitis.

Diagnosis

C. difficile disease is confirmed by isolating the organism or detecting the cytotoxin or enterotoxin in the patient's feces.

Treatment, Prevention, and Control

The implicated antibiotic should be discontinued.
  Treatment with metronidazole or vancomycin should be used in severe disease.
  Relapse is common, because the spores are not affected by antibiotics; a second course of therapy with the same antibiotic is usually successful.
  The hospital room should be carefully cleaned after the infected patient is discharged.

TABLE 37–6. Virulence Factors Associated with Other Clostridial Species

Species and Their Virulence Factors	Biologic Activity
C. septicum	
α toxin	Necrotizing, hemolytic toxin
β toxin	Heat-stable deoxyribonuclease
γ toxin	Hyaluronidase
δ toxin	Oxygen-labile hemolysin
Neuraminidase	Alters cell membrane glycoproteins
C. sordellii	
Lecithinase	Phospholipase C
Hemolysin	Oxygen-labile hemolytic activity
Fibrinolysin	Tissue destruction
Lethal β toxin	Necrotic enterotoxin activity
Hemorrhagic toxin	Hemorrhagic cytotoxin activity
C. histolyticum	
α toxin	Necrotizing (not hemolytic) toxin
β toxin	Collagenase
γ toxin	Protease
δ toxin	Elastase
ε toxin	Oxygen-labile hemolysin
C. novyi	
α toxin	Necrotizing toxin
β toxin	Lecithinase; necrotizing, hemolytic toxin
γ toxin	Lecithinase; necrotizing, hemolytic toxin
δ toxin	Oxygen-labile hemolysin
ε toxin	Lipase
ζ toxin	Hemolysin
η toxin	Tropomyosinase
θ toxin	Lecithinase
C. barati	
Botulinum toxin	Neurotoxin
C. butyricum	
Botulinum toxin	Neurotoxin

She was unable to open her mouth because of facial muscle spasms and had been unable to eat for 4 days because of severe pain in her jaw. Her attending physician had noted trismus and risus sardonicus.

The patient reported that 1 week before presentation, she had incurred a puncture wound to her toe while walking in her garden. She had cleaned the wound and removed small pieces of wood from it but she had not sought medical attention. Although she had received tetanus immunizations as a child, she had not had a booster vaccination since she was 15 years old. The presumptive diagnosis of tetanus was made.

1. How should this diagnosis be confirmed?
2. What is the recommended procedure for treating this patient? Should management wait until the laboratory results are available? What is the long-term prognosis for this patient?

3. Compare the mode of action of the toxins produced by *C. tetani* and *C. botulinum*.
4. What virulence factors are produced by *C. perfringens*? What diseases are caused by this organism?
5. What disease is caused by *C. difficile*? Why are infections caused by this organism difficult to manage?

BIBLIOGRAPHY

Bongaerts G, Lyerly D: Role of toxins A and B in the pathogenesis of *Clostridium difficile* disease, *Microb Pathog* 17:1–12, 1994.

Boone J, Carman R: *Clostridium perfringens*: food poisoning and antibiotic-associated diarrhea, *Clin Microbiol Newsletter* 19:65–67, 1997.

Bryant A et al: Clostridial gas gangrene. I and II, *J Infect Dis* 182:799–807, 808–815, 2000.

Domachowske J: Infant botulism, *Clin Microbiol Newsletter* 20: 189–191, 1998.

Gergen P et al: A population-based serologic survey of immunity to tetanus in the United States, *N Engl J Med* 332: 761–766, 1995.

Kelly C, LaMont JT: *Clostridium difficile* infection, *Annu Rev Med* 49:375–390, 1998.

Kornbluth AA, Danzid JB, Bernstein LH: *Clostridium septicum* infection and associated malignancy, *Medicine* 68:30–37, 1989.

Lyerly DM: *Clostridium difficile* testing, *Clin Microbiol Newsletter* 17:17–22, 1995.

Midura T: Update: infant botulism, *Clin Microbiol Rev* 9:119–125, 1996.

Montecucco C, Schiavo G: Mechanism of action of tetanus and botulinum neurotoxins, *Mol Microbiol* 13:1–8, 1994.

Riley T: *Clostridium difficile*: a pathogen of the nineties, *Eur J Clin Microbiol Infect Dis* 17:137–141, 1998 (editorial).

Samore M et al: Clinical and molecular epidemiology of sporadic and clustered cases of nosocomial *Clostridium difficile* diarrhea, *Am J Med* 100:32–40, 1996.

Sanford J: Tetanus: forgotten but not gone, *N Engl J Med* 332:812–813, 1995 (editorial).

Schiavo G et al: Tetanus and botulinum neurotoxins are zinc proteases specific for components of the neuroexocytosis apparatus, *Ann N Y Acad Sci* 710:65–75, 1994.

Shapiro R, Hatheway C, Swerdlow D: Botulism in the United States: a clinical and epidemiologic review, *Ann Intern Med* 129:221–228, 1998.

Simpson L: Botulinum toxin: a deadly poison sheds its negative image, *Ann Intern Med* 125:616–617, 1996 (editorial).

Stevens DL et al: Spontaneous, nontraumatic gangrene due to *Clostridium septicum*, *Rev Infect Dis* 12:286–296, 1990.

Woodruff B et al: Clinical and laboratory comparison of botulism from toxin types A, B, and E in the United States, 1975–1988, *J Infect Dis* 166:1281–1286, 1992.

CHAPTER 38

Anaerobic Gram-Negative Bacilli

With each edition of this text, the number of genera of anaerobic gram-negative bacilli and gram-negative cocci has expanded. Many new genera represent reclassification of well-known organisms, and some represent newly discovered bacteria. The most important gram-negative anaerobes that colonize the human upper respiratory tract, gastrointestinal tract, and genitourinary tract are the bacilli in the genera *Bacteroides*, *Fusobacterium*, *Porphyromonas*, and *Prevotella*, and the cocci in the genus *Veillonella*. Anaerobes are the predominant bacteria at each of these sites, outnumbering aerobic bacteria by 10- to 1000-fold. The anaerobic species are also numerous, with as many as 50 different species of gram-negative anaerobes present in these anatomic locations. Despite the abundance and diversity of these bacteria, most infections are caused by relatively few species (Table 38–1). Among these pathogens, the most important is *Bacteroides fragilis*, the prototypical endogenous anaerobic pathogen.

Physiology and Structure

At one time, the genus *Bacteroides* consisted of almost 50 species, but many of these species have now been transferred to new genera. Species of pigmented, asaccharolytic bacilli were reclassified as *Porphyromonas* (from the Greek word for "purple"), and saccharolytic, bile-sensitive bacilli were transferred into the genus *Prevotella*. The genus *Bacteroides* now consists of the anaerobes previously categorized into the *B. fragilis* group and some closely related species. *B. fragilis*, the most important member of this genus, is pleomorphic in size and shape, resembling a mixed population of organisms in a casually examined Gram stain (Fig. 38–1). Other gram-negative bacilli can be very small (e.g., *Prevotella* species) or elongated (e.g., *Fusobacterium*, so-named because the type species, *Fusobacterium nucleatum*, is long and thin—"fusiform") (Fig. 38–2). Most gram-negative anaerobes respond weakly to Gram stain, so stained specimens must be carefully examined. Although *Bacteroides* species grow rapidly in culture,

the other anaerobic, gram-negative bacilli are fastidious, and cultures may have to be incubated for 3 days or longer before the bacteria can be detected.

Bacteroides have a typical gram-negative cell wall structure, which can be surrounded by a polysaccharide capsule. A major component of the cell wall is a surface lipopolysaccharide (LPS). In contrast to the LPS molecules in *Fusobacterium* and the aerobic gram-negative bacilli, however, the *Bacteroides* glycolipid has little or no endotoxin activity. This is because the lipid A component of LPS lacks phosphate groups on the glucosamine residues and the number of fatty acids linked to the amino sugars is reduced; both factors are correlated with the loss of pyrogenic activity.

The anaerobic cocci are rarely isolated in clinical specimens, except when present as contaminants. Members of the genus *Veillonella* are the predominant anaerobes in the oropharynx, but they represent less than 1% of all anaerobes isolated in clinical specimens. The other cocci are rarely isolated.

Pathogenesis and Immunity

Despite the variety of anaerobic species that colonize the human body, relatively few are responsible for causing disease. For example, *Bacteroides distasonis* and *Bacteroides thetaiotaomicron* are the predominant species of *Bacteroides* found in the gastrointestinal tract; however, more than 80% of intra-abdominal infections are associated with *B. fragilis*, an organism that is a minor member of the gastrointestinal flora. The enhanced virulence of this and other pathogenic anaerobes is attributed to a variety of virulence factors that facilitate adherence of the organisms to host tissues, protection from the host immune response, and tissue destruction (Table 38–2).

Adhesins

B. fragilis and *Prevotella melaninogenica* strains can adhere to peritoneal surfaces more effectively than other anaerobes because their surface is covered with a poly-

TABLE 38–1. Predominant Anaerobic Gram-Negative Bacteria Responsible for Human Disease

Infection	Bacteria
Head and neck	*Bacteroides ureolyticus*
	Fusobacterium nucleatum
	Fusobacterium necrophorum
	Porphyromonas asaccharolytica
	Porphyromonas gingivalis
	Prevotella intermedia
	Prevotella melaninogenica
	Veillonella parvula
Intra-abdominal	*Bacteroides fragilis*
	Bacteroides thetaiotaomicron
	P. melaninogenica
Gynecologic	*B. fragilis*
	Prevotella bivia
	Prevotella disiens
Skin and soft tissue	*B. fragilis*
Bacteremia	*B. fragilis*
	B. thetaiotaomicron
	Fusobacterium spp.

FIGURE 38–2. *Fusobacterium nucleatum.* Organisms are elongated with tapered ends (e.g., fusiform).

saccharide capsule. *B. fragilis* and other *Bacteroides* species as well as *Porphyromonas gingivalis* can adhere to epithelial cells by means of pili and fimbriae.

Protection Against Phagocytosis

The capsular polysaccharide of these organisms is antiphagocytic like other bacterial capsules. In addition, the short-chain fatty acids (e.g., succinic acid) produced during anaerobic metabolism inhibit phagocytosis and intracellular killing. Finally, proteases are produced by

TABLE 38–2. Virulence Factors in Anaerobic Gram-Negative Bacilli

Virulence Factor	Bacteria
Adhesins	
Capsule	*Bacteroides fragilis, Prevotella melaninogenica*
Fimbriae	*B. fragilis, Porphyromonas gingivalis*
Hemagglutinin	*P. gingivalis*
Lectin	*Fusobacterium nucleatum*
Resist Oxygen Toxicity	
Superoxide dismutase	Many species
Catalase	Many species
Antiphagocytic	
Capsule	*B. fragilis, P. melaninogenica*
Immunoglobulin (Ig)A, IgM, IgG proteases	*Porphyromonas* spp., *Prevotella* spp.
Lipopolysaccharide	*Fusobacterium* species
Succinic acid	Many species
Tissue Destruction	
Phospholipase C	*Fusobacterium necrophorum*
Hemolysins	Many species
Proteases	Many species
Collagenase	Many species
Fibrinolysin	Many species
Neuraminidase	Many species
Heparinase	Many species
Chondroitin sulfatase	Many species
Glucuronidases	Many species
N-Acetylglucosaminidase	Many species
Volatile fatty acids	Many species

Modified from Duerden B: Virulence factors in anaerobes. *Clin Infect Dis* 18(suppl 4):S253–259, 1994; and Lorber B: *Bacteroides, Prevotella, Porphyromonas,* and *Fusobacterium* species. In *Mandell, Douglas and Bennett's Principles and practice of infectious diseases,* ed 5, New York, 2000, Churchill Livingstone.

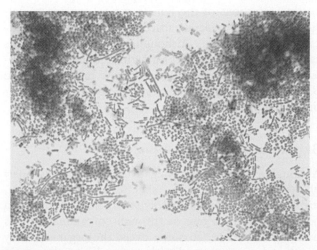

FIGURE 38–1. *Bacteroides fragilis.* Organisms appear as faintly staining, pleomorphic, gram-negative bacilli.

some *Porphyromonas* and *Prevotella* species that degrade immunoglobulins.

Protection Against Oxygen Toxicity

Anaerobes capable of causing disease can generally tolerate exposure to oxygen. Catalase and superoxide dismutase, which inactivate hydrogen peroxide and the superoxide free radicals (O_2^-), respectively, are present in many pathogenic strains.

Tissue Destruction

A variety of enzymes have been associated with gram-negative anaerobes. Many of these enzymes are found in both virulent and avirulent isolates. Nonetheless, the ability of these organisms to cause tissue destruction and inactivate immunoglobulins as well as to resist oxygen toxicity (superoxide dismutase) most likely plays an important role in the pathogenesis of anaerobic infections.

Epidemiology

As already stated, anaerobic gram-negative cocci and bacilli colonize the human body in large numbers. Their numerous important functions at these sites include stabilizing the resident bacterial flora, preventing colonization by pathogenic organisms from exogenous sources, and aiding in the digestion of food. These normal protective organisms produce serious disease when they move from their endogenous homes to normally sterile sites (i.e., the same as is described for gram-positive, non–spore-forming anaerobes in Chapter 36). Thus, the organisms in the resident flora are able to spread by trauma or disease from the normally colonized mucosal surfaces to sterile tissues or fluids.

As expected, these endogenous infections are characterized by the presence of a polymicrobial mixture of organisms. It is important to realize, however, that the mixture of organisms present on healthy mucosal surfaces differs from that in diseased tissues. The difference relates to the virulence potential of pathogenic organisms and their ability to increase from existing in relatively small numbers on mucosal surfaces to being the predominant organisms at the site of infection. For example, *B. fragilis* is commonly associated with pleuropulmonary, intra-abdominal, and genital infections. The organism constitutes less than 1% of the colonic flora, however, and is rarely isolated from the oropharynx or genital tract of healthy people unless highly selective techniques are used.

Clinical Diseases

Respiratory Tract Infections

Up to half of the chronic infections of the sinuses and ears and virtually all periodontal infections involve mixtures of gram-negative anaerobes, with *Prevotella*, *Porphyromonas*, *Fusobacterium*, and non-*fragilis Bacteroides* most commonly isolated. Anaerobes are less commonly associated with infections of the lower respiratory tract unless there is a history of aspiration of oral secretions.

Brain Abscess

Anaerobic infections of the brain are typically associated with a history of chronic sinusitis or otitis. Such history is confirmed by radiologic evidence of direct extension into the brain. A less common cause of such infections is bacteremic spread from a pulmonary source. In this case, multiple abscesses are present. The most common anaerobes in these polymicrobial infections are species of *Prevotella*, *Porphyromonas*, and *Fusobacterium* (as well as *Peptostreptococcus* and aerobic cocci).

Intra-Abdominal Infections

Despite the diverse population of bacteria that colonize the gastrointestinal tract, relatively few species are associated with intra-abdominal infections. Anaerobes are recovered in virtually all of these infections, with *B. fragilis* the most common organism. Other important anaerobes are *B. thetaiotaomicron* and *P. melaninogenica* as well as the peptostreptococci and aerobic bacteria.

Gynecologic Infections

Mixtures of anaerobes are frequently responsible for causing infections of the female genital tract (e.g., pelvic inflammatory disease, abscesses, endometritis, surgical wound infections). Although a variety of anaerobes can be isolated in patients with these infections, *Prevotella bivia* and *Prevotella disiens* are the most important; *B. fragilis* is commonly responsible for abscess formation.

Skin and Soft Tissue Infections

Although anaerobic gram-negative bacteria are not part of the normal flora of the skin (in contrast to *Peptostreptococcus* and *Propionibacterium* organisms), they can be introduced by a bite or through contamination of a traumatized surface. In some cases, the organisms may simply colonize a wound without producing disease; in other cases, colonization may quickly progress to life-threatening disease such as myonecrosis. *B. fragilis* is the organism most commonly associated with significant disease.

Bacteremia

Anaerobes were at one time responsible for more than 20% of all clinically significant cases of bacteremia; however, these organisms now cause less than 5% of such infections. The reduced incidence of disease is not completely understood but probably can be attributed to the widespread use of broad-spectrum antibiotics. The anaerobes most commonly isolated in blood cultures are *B. fragilis*, *B. thetaiotaomicron*, and *Fusobacterium* species.

Laboratory Diagnosis

Microscopy

Microscopic examination of specimens from patients with suspected anaerobic infections can be useful. Although the bacteria may stain faintly and irregularly, the finding of pleomorphic, gram-negative bacilli can be useful preliminary information.

Culture

Specimens should be collected and transported to the laboratory in an oxygen-free system, promptly inoculated onto specific media for the recovery of anaerobes, and incubated in an anaerobic environment. Because most anaerobic infections are endogenous, it is important to collect specimens so that they are not contaminated with the normal bacterial population present on the adjacent mucosal surface. Specimens should also be kept in a moist environment, because drying causes significant bacterial loss.

Most *Bacteroides* grow rapidly and should be detected within 2 days; however, other gram-negative anaerobes may have to be incubated longer. In addition, it is sometimes difficult to recover all clinically significant bacteria because of the different organisms present in polymicrobial infections. The use of selective media has facilitated the recovery of most important anaerobes (Fig. 38–3).

Biochemical Identification

The preliminary identification of the *B. fragilis* group can be made from (1) Gram stain and colonial morphology, (2) resistance to kanamycin, vancomycin, and colistin, and (3) stimulated growth in 20% bile. The definitive identification of this group and other gram-negative anaerobes is made with the use of commercially prepared biochemical systems that measure the

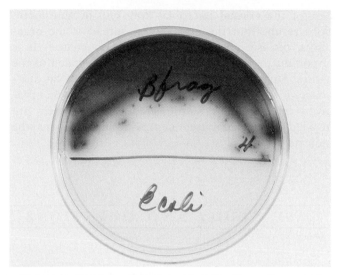

FIGURE 38–3. Growth of *Bacteroides fragilis* on *Bacteroides* bile-esculin agar. Most aerobic and anaerobic bacteria are inhibited by bile and gentamicin in this medium, whereas the *B. fragilis* group of organisms is stimulated by bile, resistant to gentamicin, and able to hydrolyze esculin, producing a black precipitate.

activity of preformed enzymes. Gas chromatography has occasionally proved to be a useful, simple technique for detecting metabolic byproducts (short-chain fatty acids) and can be used to supplement biochemical testing.

Treatment, Prevention, and Control

Antibiotic therapy combined with surgical intervention is the main approach for managing serious anaerobic infections. β-Lactamase is produced by virtually all members of the *B. fragilis* group, many *Prevotella* and *Porphyromonas* species, and some *Fusobacterium* isolates. This enzyme renders the bacteria resistant to penicillin and to many cephalosporins. Nevertheless, high concentrations of some penicillins (e.g., carbenicillin, piperacillin), cefoxitin, imipenem, or β-lactams combined with β-lactamase inhibitors can be used to treat these infections.

Clindamycin resistance in *Bacteroides*, which is plasmid-mediated, has become more prevalent; an average of 7% to 10% of the isolates in the United States are now resistant. Metronidazole is active against *Bacteroides* species and other gram-negative bacilli and is the antibiotic of choice for treating infections caused by these organisms. The anaerobic gram-negative cocci are usually susceptible to penicillin, cephalosporins, clindamycin, chloramphenicol, and metronidazole. However, it is often unnecessary to use specific therapy against them.

Because *Bacteroides* species constitute an important

part of the normal microbial flora and because infections result from the endogenous spread of the organisms, disease is virtually impossible to control. It is important to recognize, however, that disruption of the natural barriers around the mucosal surfaces by diagnostic or surgical procedures can introduce these organisms into normally sterile sites. If the barriers are invaded, prophylactic treatment with antibiotics may be indicated.

CASE STUDY AND QUESTIONS

■ A 65-year-old man entered the emergency department of a local hospital. He appeared to be acutely ill, with abdominal tenderness and a temperature of 40.0°C. The patient was taken to surgery because appendicitis was suspected. A ruptured appendix surrounded by approximately 20 mL of foul-smelling pus was found at laparotomy. The pus was drained and submitted for aerobic and anaerobic bacterial culture analysis. Postoperatively, the patient was started on antibiotic therapy. Gram stain of the specimen revealed a polymicrobial mixture of organisms, and culture was positive for *B. fragilis*, *Escherichia coli*, and *Enterococcus faecalis*.

1. Which organism or organisms are responsible for causing the abscess formation? What virulence factors are responsible for causing abscess formation?

2. *B. fragilis* causes infections at what other body sites?

3. What antibiotics should be selected to manage this polymicrobial infection?

4. What other anaerobic gram-negative bacilli are important causes of human disease?

BIBLIOGRAPHY

Bjornson AB: Role of humoral factors in host resistance to the *Bacteroides fragilis* group, *Rev Infect Dis* 12:S161–S168, 1990.

Cuchural GJ et al: Susceptibility of the *Bacteroides fragilis* group in the United States: analysis by site of isolation, *Antimicrob Agents Chemother* 32:717–722, 1988.

Duerden B: Virulence factors in anaerobes, *Clin Infect Dis* 18(suppl 4):S253–S259, 1994.

Finegold SM, Baron EJ, Wexler HM: *A clinical guide to anaerobic infections*, Belmont, Calif, 1992, Star.

Jousimies-Somer H, Summanen P, Finegold S: *Bacteroides, Porphyromonas, Prevotella, Fusobacterium*, and other anaerobic gram-negative bacteria. In Murray P et al, editors: *Manual of clinical microbiology*, ed 7, Washington, DC, 1999, American Society for Microbiology.

Lindberg AA et al: Structure-activity relationships in lipopolysaccharides of *Bacteroides fragilis*, *Rev Infect Dis* 12:S133–S140, 1990.

Tessier F et al: Antigenic relationships among *Bacteroides* species studied by rocket-line immunoelectrophoresis, *Int J Syst Bacteriol* 43:191–195, 1993.

CHAPTER 39

Nocardia, Rhodococcus, and Related Actinomycetes

The aerobic actinomycetes are gram-positive, catalase-positive bacilli. These bacteria, which can colonize animals and humans, are found in soil and decaying vegetation. Some actinomycetes have delicate filamentous forms (also called **hyphae**), similar to fungal hyphal forms, in clinical specimens and in culture (hence the fungal reference in the name). However, the cell wall structure and antimicrobial susceptibility patterns are typical of bacteria.

The **mycolic acid**–containing members of this group consist of three families: Corynebacteriaceae (see Chapter 26), Nocardiaceae, and Mycobacteriaceae (see Chapter 40). Four genera are currently placed in the family Nocardiaceae: *Nocardia*, *Rhodococcus*, *Tsukamurella*, and *Gordona*. Organisms from all four genera stain irregularly with Gram stain and are **partially acid-fast** (resistant to decolorization with weak acid solutions). This property of acid-fastness is an extremely useful clinical tool for identifying members of the families Nocardiaceae and Mycobacteriaceae. Numerous other genera of actinomycetes have been described, but the genera most commonly isolated in clinical specimens or associated with human disease are listed in Box 39–1.

The spectrum of the diseases associated with the aerobic actinomycetes is extensive and includes insignificant colonization (many genera), pulmonary disease (*Nocardia*, *Rhodococcus*), systemic infections (*Nocardia*, *Rhodococcus*), mycetoma (*Actinomadura*, *Nocardiopsis*, *Streptomyces*, and *Nocardia*), other opportunistic cutaneous infections (most genera), Whipple's disease (*Tropheryma*), and allergic pneumonitis (thermophilic actinomycetes) (Table 39–1).

Nocardia

Physiology and Structure

The genus *Nocardia* was named after French veterinarian Edmond Nocard, who was the first to describe the involvement of these bacteria in a bovine disease characterized by pyogenic pulmonary and cutaneous lesions. The organisms are strict aerobic bacilli that form branched hyphae in tissues and culture (Box 39–2). The organisms are gram-positive, although many stain poorly and appear to be gram-negative with intracellular gram-positive beads (Fig. 39–1). Nocardia have a cell wall structure similar to that of mycobacteria, with mycolic acids present, and like mycobacteria, these organisms are acid-fast (Fig. 39–2). This acid-fastness is a helpful characteristic for distinguishing *Nocardia* organisms from morphologically similar organisms, such as *Actinomyces*. *Nocardia* species are catalase-positive, use carbohydrates oxidatively, and can grow on most nonselective laboratory media; however, their isolation can require at least a week of incubation. The appearance of colonies varies from dry to waxy and from white to orange.

Phylogenetic analysis of 16S rDNA has identified 10 species of *Nocardia*. Unfortunately, it is difficult to distinguish many of these species on the basis of their phenotypic properties (e.g., reactivity in biochemical tests). The species most commonly associated with human disease are *Nocardia farcinica*, *Nocardia asteroides*, *Nocardia brasiliensis*, and *Nocardia otitidiscaviarum*. However, the role that *N. farcinica* plays in the pathogenesis of human disease is certainly underestimated, because most laboratories classify this species within the *N. asteroides* complex.

Pathogenesis and Immunity

Organisms in the *N. asteroides* complex cause approximately 90% of human *Nocardia* infections. They cause bronchopulmonary disease in immunocompromised patients, with a high predilection for hematogenous spread to the central nervous system (CNS) or skin. Patients at greatest risk for disease are those with T-cell deficiencies produced by disease (e.g., leukemia,

---

BOX 39-1. Pathogenic Aerobic Actinomycetes

Actinomycetes with Mycolic Acids

Corynebacteriaceae
Nocardiaceae
   Nocardia
   Rhodococcus
   Gordona
   Tsukamurella
Mycobacteriaceae

Actinomycetes with No Mycolic Acids

Actinomadura
Nocardiopsis
Streptomyces
Dermatophilus
Oerskovia
Rothia
Tropheryma
Thermophilic actinomycetes
   Saccharopolyspora
   Saccharomonospora
   Thermoactinomyces

---

the acquired immunodeficiency syndrome [AIDS]) or immunosuppressive therapy (e.g., corticosteroids for renal or cardiac transplantation). Disease can also occur in patients with chronic pulmonary diseases such as bronchitis, emphysema, asthma, bronchiectasis, and alveolar proteinosis. *N. brasiliensis* and *N. otitidiscaviarum* most commonly cause primary cutaneous infections (e.g., mycetoma, lymphocutaneous infections, superficial abscesses, cellulitis) in immunocompetent patients, with infrequent hematogenous dissemination.

Bronchopulmonary infections develop after the initial colonization of the oropharynx by inhalation and then aspiration of oral secretions into the lower airways. Primary cutaneous nocardiosis develops after traumatic introduction of organisms into subcutaneous tissues. Disease is characterized by necrosis and abscess formation similar to those caused by other pyogenic bacteria. Chronic infections with sinus tract formation can occur, particularly with primary cutaneous infections. Although sulfur granules are observed with *Actinomyces* species, they are uncommon with *Nocardia*, being seen only with cutaneous involvement. Colonization of the oropharynx or wounds can occur, so the significance of isolating *Nocardia* organisms in clinical specimens must be judged in light of the clinical presentation.

TABLE 39-1. Diseases of Selected Pathogenic Actinomycetes

Organism	Diseases	Frequency
Nocardia	Pulmonary diseases (bronchitis, pneumonia, lung abscesses); primary or secondary cutaneous infections (e.g., mycetoma, lymphocutaneous infections, cellulitis, subcutaneous abscesses); secondary CNS infections (e.g., meningitis, brain abscesses)	Common
Rhodococcus	Pulmonary diseases (pneumonia, lung abscesses); disseminated diseases (e.g., meningitis, pericarditis); opportunistic infections (e.g., wound infections, peritonitis, traumatic endophthalmitis)	Uncommon
Gordona	Opportunistic infections	Rare
Tsukamurella	Opportunistic infections	Rare
Actinomadura	Mycetoma	Rare (in U.S.)
Nocardiopsis	Mycetoma	Rare (in U.S.)
Streptomyces	Mycetoma	Rare (in U.S.)
Dermatophilus	Exudative dermatitis	Rare (in U.S.)
Oerskovia	Opportunistic infections (e.g., peritonitis, traumatic endophthalmitis, CNS shunt infections, catheter-associated bacteremia, endocarditis)	Rare
Rothia	Dental plaque	Rare
Tropheryma	Whipple's disease	Common
Thermoactinomyces	Allergic pneumonitis	Common
Saccharopolyspora	Allergic pneumonitis	Common
Saccharomonospora	Allergic pneumonitis	Common

CNS = central nervous system.

BOX 39–2. Summary of *Nocardia* Infections

Physiology and Structure

Gram-positive, partially acid-fast, filamentous bacilli; cell wall with mycolic acid.

Strict aerobe capable of growth on most nonselective bacterial media; however, prolonged incubation (7 days or more) required for recovery of most isolates.

Virulence

Specific factors not well-characterized.
Opportunistic pathogen.

Epidemiology

Worldwide distribution in soil rich with organic matter.

Exogenous infections acquired by inhalation (pulmonary) or traumatic introduction (cutaneous).

Disease most common in immunocompetent patients with chronic pulmonary disease (bronchitis, emphysema, bronchiectasis, alveolar proteinosis), immunocompromised patients with T-cell deficiencies (transplant recipients, patients with malignancies, patients infected with the human immunodeficiency virus, patients receiving corticosteroids), and people who have suffered skin wounds through which the organisms could be introduced into subcutaneous tissues.

Diseases

Bronchopulmonary disease.

Primary or secondary cutaneous infections (e.g., mycetoma, lymphocutaneous infection, cellulitis, subcutaneous abscesses).

Secondary central nervous system infections (e.g., brain abscesses).

Diagnosis

Microscopy is sensitive and relatively specific when branching, partially acid-fast organisms are seen.

Culture is slow, requiring incubation for up to 1 week. Selective media (e.g., BCYE agar) may be required for isolating *Nocardia* in mixed cultures.

Treatment, Prevention, and Control

Infections are treated with antibiotic therapy with sulfonamides or antibiotics with proven in vivo activity, and proper wound care.

Exposure cannot be avoided because nocardia are ubiquitous.

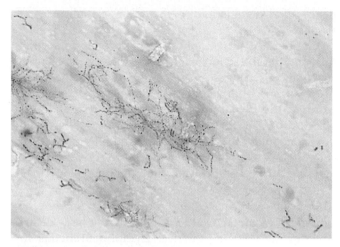

FIGURE 39–1. Gram stain of *Nocardia asteroides* in expectorated sputum. Note that the delicate beaded filaments cannot be distinguished from those of *Actinomyces* organisms (see Chapter 36).

noticeable in high-risk populations, such as patients who are infected with human immunodeficiency virus (HIV) or who have received solid organ transplants.

Clinical Diseases

Bronchopulmonary infections caused by *Nocardia* species cannot be distinguished from infections caused by other pyogenic organisms, although *Nocardia* infections tend to develop more slowly. Signs such as cough, dyspnea, and fever are usually present but are not diagnostic. Cavitation and spread into the pleura are common. Even though the clinical picture is not specific for *Nocardia*, these organisms should be considered when immunocompromised patients experience pneumonia with cavitation, particularly if there is evi-

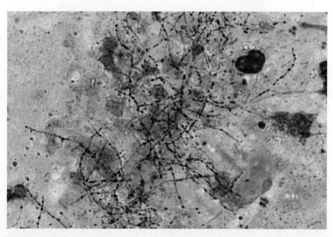

FIGURE 39–2. Acid-fast stain of *Nocardia asteroides* in expectorated sputum. In contrast with the family Mycobacteriaceae, genera in the family Nocardiaceae do not uniformly retain the stain ("partially acid-fast").

Epidemiology

Nocardia infections are exogenous (i.e., caused by organisms not normally part of the normal human flora but rather transient inhabitants). The ubiquitous presence of the organism in soil rich with organic matter and the abundance of immunocompromised patients in hospitals have led to dramatic increases in disease caused by this organism. The increase is particularly

dence of dissemination to the CNS or subcutaneous tissues.

Cutaneous infections may be primary infections (e.g., mycetoma, lymphocutaneous infections, cellulitis, subcutaneous abscesses) or may result from the spread of organisms from a primary pulmonary infection. **Actinomycotic mycetoma** is a painless, chronic infection characterized by localized subcutaneous swelling, suppuration, and the formation of multiple sinus tracts (Fig. 39–3). The underlying connective tissues, muscle, and bone can be involved, and draining sinus tracts usually open on the skin surface. A variety of organisms can cause mycetoma, although *N. brasiliensis* is the most common cause in North America, Central America, and South America. **Lymphocutaneous infections** can manifest as cutaneous nodules and ulcerations along the lymphatics and regional lymph node involvement. These infections resemble cutaneous infections caused by species of mycobacteria and by the fungus *Sporothrix schenckii*. *Nocardia* can also cause

chronic ulcerative lesions, subcutaneous abscesses, and cellulitis.

As many as a third of all patients with *Nocardia* infections have CNS involvement, most commonly involving the formation of single or multiple brain abscesses. The disease can manifest initially as chronic meningitis.

Laboratory Diagnosis

Which specimens are collected for the isolation of *Nocardia* is dictated by the clinical presentation. Multiple sputum specimens should be collected from patients with pulmonary disease. Because *Nocardia* are usually distributed throughout the tissue and abscess material, it is relatively easy to detect them with microscopy and to recover them in culture of specimens from patients with cutaneous or CNS disease. The delicate hyphae of *Nocardia* in tissues cause them to resemble *Actinomyces* organisms; however, *Nocardia* stain poorly with Gram stain and are typically partially acid-fast (see Figs. 39–1 and 39–2).

The organisms grow on most laboratory media incubated in an atmosphere of 5% to 10% carbon dioxide, but the presence of these slow-growing organisms may be obscured by that of more rapidly growing commensal bacteria. If a specimen sent for analysis for *Nocardia* is potentially contaminated with other bacteria (e.g., oral bacteria in sputum), selective media should be inoculated. Success has been achieved with the medium used for the isolation of *Legionella* species (buffered charcoal–yeast extract [BCYE] agar). Indeed, this medium can be used to recover both organisms from pulmonary specimens. *Nocardia* occasionally grows on media used for the isolation of mycobacteria and fungi; however, this method is less reliable than the use of special bacterial media. It is important to notify the laboratory that nocardiosis is suspected, because most laboratories do not routinely incubate clinical specimens for more than 1 to 3 days. It takes more time (i.e., as long as a week) for *Nocardia* species to be isolated.

The preliminary identification of *Nocardia* is uncomplicated. Members of the genus can be classified initially on the basis of the presence of filamentous, partially acid-fast bacilli. Definitive identification is frequently delayed, however, because *N. asteroides* complex, the species group most commonly isolated, is nonreactive with most differential tests used for biochemical classification (Table 39–2).

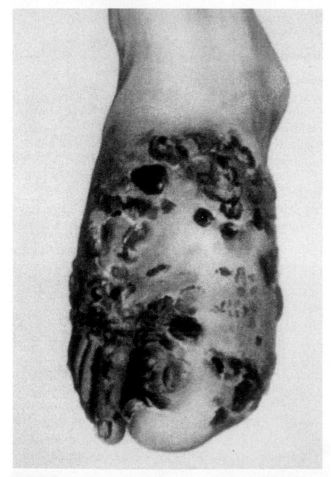

FIGURE 39–3. Mycetoma caused by *Nocardia brasiliensis*. The foot is grossly enlarged and covered with multiple draining sinus tracts. (From Binford CH, Connor DH, editors: *Pathology of tropical and extraordinary diseases*, vol 2, Washington, DC, 1976, Armed Forces Institute of Pathology.)

Treatment, Prevention, and Control

Nocardia infections are treated with the combination of antibiotics and appropriate surgical intervention. Sulfonamides are the antibiotics of choice for treating nocardiosis. Amikacin, imipenem, and broad-spectrum

TABLE 39–2. Identification Tests for Common *Nocardia* Species

Tests	N. asteroides complex*	N. brasiliensis	N. otitidis-caviarum
Decomposition of:			
Casein	−	+	−
Tyrosine	−	+	−
Xanthine	−	−	+
Gelatin	−	+	−
Starch	−	−	−
Urea	+		+
Acid from:			
Glucose	+	+	+
Rhamnose	+/−	−	−

* *Nocardia asteroides* complex includes *Nocardia asteroides, Nocardia farcinica,* and *Nocardia nova.*

cephalosporins also have good in vitro activity, but their in vivo effectiveness is unproved.

Of the clinically important *Nocardia* species, *N. farcinica* is the most resistant to antibiotics, including sulfa drugs. Because *Nocardia* can disseminate and produce significant disease, in vitro susceptibility testing should be used to guide the selection of antibiotic therapy. Therapy should be extended for 6 weeks or more. Whereas the clinical response is favorable in patients with localized infections, the prognosis is poor for immunocompromised patients with disseminated disease.

Because *Nocardia* are ubiquitous, it is impossible to avoid exposure to them. However, bronchopulmonary disease caused by *Nocardia* is uncommon in immunocompetent persons, and primary cutaneous infections can be prevented with proper wound care. The complications associated with disseminated disease can be minimized if nocardiosis is considered in the differential diagnosis for immunocompromised patients with cavitary pulmonary disease and promptly treated.

Rhodococcus

The genus *Rhodococcus* ("red-pigmented coccus") consists of more than 20 species of gram-positive, obligate aerobic actinomycetes. The cell wall of these catalase-positive coccobacilli is similar to that of *Nocardia* and *Mycobacterium*: It contains mycolic acid and tuberculostearic acid, rendering the organisms acid-fast. At least seven species have been associated with human disease; however, *Rhodococcus equi* is the most important human pathogen. Originally, *R. equi* (formerly *Corynebacterium equi*) was considered a well-recognized veterinary pathogen, particularly in herbivores, that rarely caused occupational disease in farmers and veterinarians. This organism, however, has become an increasingly more common pathogen of immunocompromised patients

(e.g., patients with malignancies or transplants, those receiving corticosteroids, those infected with the human immunodeficiency virus). Interestingly, most infected patients do not have a history of contact with grazing animals or of exposure to soil contaminated with herbivore manure. The rise in the incidence of human infection is most likely related to the increase in the number of patients with immunosuppressive diseases, particularly AIDS, and to the enhanced awareness of the organism. It is likely that many isolates were ignored previously and considered insignificant coryneform bacteria.

R. equi is a facultative, intracellular organism that survives in macrophages and causes granulomatous inflammation, which leads to abscess formation. Although numerous putative virulence factors have been identified, the precise pathophysiology of the infections is incompletely understood. Immunocompromised patients most typically present with invasive pulmonary disease (e.g., pneumonia, lung abscesses), and evidence of dissemination to distal sites (lymph nodes, meninges, pericardium, and skin) is commonly observed. Rhodococci usually cause opportunistic infections in immunocompetent patients (e.g., post-traumatic cutaneous infections, peritonitis in patients undergoing long-term dialysis, traumatic endophthalmitis).

Rhodococcus grows readily on nonselective media incubated aerobically, although the characteristic pigment may not be obvious for 4 days or longer. The organisms can be identified initially from their slow growth, microscopic morphology (pleomorphic, gram-positive coccobacilli), and ability to weakly retain the acid-fast stain. Definitive identification is problematic, because the organisms are relatively inert.

Rhodococcus infections have proved difficult to treat. Although in vitro tests and tests in animal models have identified specific combinations of drugs as effective, only limited success has been realized in the treatment of human infections using these agents, particularly in immunocompromised patients. Currently, treatment with vancomycin or the combination of erythromycin and rifampin is recommended, but relapses are frequently observed. Penicillins and cephalosporins should not be used because resistance to these agents is common in *Rhodococcus*.

Gordona and Tsukamurella

Gordona and *Tsukamurella* were previously classified with *Rhodococcus* because they are morphologically similar, contain mycolic acids, and are partially acid-fast. The organisms are present in soil and are rare opportunistic pathogens in humans. *Gordona* has been associated with pulmonary and cutaneous infections as well as nosocomial infections such as those resulting from contaminated intravascular catheters. *Tsukamurella* has been associated with catheter infections. The significance of isolating either organism in clinical specimens must be evaluated carefully.

Actinomadura, Nocardiopsis, and *Streptomyces*

Mycetoma can be caused by fungi as well as by bacteria in the genera *Actinomadura, Nocardiopsis, Streptomyces,* and *Nocardia.* The precise etiology of this disease can be determined only by isolation of the pathogen in culture, because (1) many of these organisms resemble fungi when seen in tissue and (2) the diseases they cause are clinically indistinguishable. Infection usually results from the traumatic introduction of the bacteria or fungi into tissue, most commonly in an extremity. Chronic cutaneous and subcutaneous infections with abscess and sinus tract formation then develop.

These pathogens can be isolated on Sabouraud's dextrose agar (typically considered a fungal medium) or on nonselective bacterial media. It may take as long as 3 weeks of incubation for growth to be apparent. The isolates are identified on the basis of morphologic criteria and the results of selected biochemical tests.

Effective therapy includes both surgical débridement and an appropriate antibiotic, such as trimethoprim-sulfamethoxazole, streptomycin, rifampin, dapsone, or a combination of these agents. Because the clinical diagnosis is noncontributory and culture results may be delayed for 3 weeks or longer, empirical therapy for bacterial and fungal infection must be initiated. Broad-spectrum antibiotics that are effective against all potential pathogens should be chosen.

Other Actinomycetes

Dermatophilus, an actinomycete found in the soil, causes infections in humans who are exposed to infected animals or contaminated animal products (e.g., slaughterhouse workers, butchers, hunters, dairy farmers, veterinarians). The disease is an exudative dermatitis with encrustations that typically involve the hands or feet. This organism is susceptible to many antibiotics, and most infections are treated with the combination of penicillin and an aminoglycoside.

Oerskovia is an opportunistic human pathogen associated with peritonitis in patients who are undergoing long-term peritoneal dialysis as well as with traumatic endophthalmitis, CNS shunt infections, catheter-associated bacteremia, and endocarditis occurring after the placement of a homograft. Most infections do not respond to antibiotics unless the foreign body is removed.

Rothia, part of the normal bacterial flora of the oropharynx, is associated with dental plaque. Invasive disease has been rarely reported.

Tropheryma whippelii is a newly classified bacterium responsible for **Whipple's disease,** a disorder charac-

terized by arthralgia, diarrhea, abdominal pain, weight loss, lymphadenopathy, fever, and increased skin pigmentation. Historically, the disease was diagnosed on the basis of the clinical presentation and the finding of periodic acid–Schiff positive inclusions in foamy macrophages that infiltrated the lamina propria of the small intestine. Through the use of molecular diagnostic techniques, the bacterial etiology of this infection was confirmed. Analysis of the ribosomal DNA of these bacteria revealed that they are members of the actinomycetes. Although techniques to culture these organisms have not been developed, nucleic acid–based diagnostic tests are now available.

Allergic pneumonitis ("farmer's lung") is a hypersensitivity reaction to repeated exposure to **thermophilic actinomycetes** commonly found in decaying vegetation. The clinically significant genera are *Thermoactinomyces* (three species), *Saccharopolyspora* (one species), and *Saccharomonospora* (one species). Patients with the disease have granulomatous changes in the lung, with pulmonary edema, eosinophilia, and elevations of immunoglobulin E. Clinical diagnosis is confirmed by detection of specific precipitin antibodies to these agents in serum.

CASE STUDY AND QUESTIONS

■ A 47-year-old renal transplant recipient who had been receiving prednisone and azathioprine for 2 years was admitted to the university medical center. Two weeks before, the patient had noticed the development of a dry, persistent cough. Five days before admission, the cough became productive, and pleuritic chest pain developed. On the day of admission, the patient was in mild respiratory arrest, and chest radiographs revealed a patchy right upper lobe infiltrate. Sputum specimens were initially sent for bacterial culture; results were reported as negative for organisms after 2 days of incubation. Antibiotic therapy with cephalothin was ineffective, so additional specimens were collected for the culture of bacteria, mycobacteria, *Legionella* species, and fungi. After 4 days of incubation, *Nocardia* was isolated on the media inoculated for mycobacteria, *Legionella* species, and fungi.

1. Why did the organism fail to grow initially? What can be done to correct this problem?

2. If this organism disseminates, what two target tissues are most likely to be involved?

3. What diseases are caused by *N. asteroides* complex? *N. brasiliensis*? *N. otitidiscaviarum*?

4. What disease is caused by *Rhodococcus* in immunocompromised patients? What diagnostic property does this organism share with *Nocardia*? Which two

other genera discussed in this chapter have the same property?

    5. Which bacteria cause mycetoma?

BIBLIOGRAPHY

Baba T, Nishiuchi Y, Yano I: Composition of mycolic acid molecular species as a criterion in nocardial classification, *Int J Syst Bacteriol* 47:795–801, 1997.

Beaman B, Beaman L: Nocardia species: host-parasite relationships, *Clin Microbiol Rev* 7:213–264, 1994.

Chun J, Goodfellow M: A phylogenetic analysis of the genus *Nocardia* with 16S rRNA gene sequences, *Int J Syst Bacteriol* 45:240–245, 1995.

Dobbins W: The diagnosis of Whipple's diseases, *N Engl J Med* 332:390–392, 1995 (editorial).

Harvey RL, Sunstrum JC: *Rhodococcus equi* infection in patients with and without human immunodeficiency virus infection, *Rev Infect Dis* 13:139–145, 1991.

Johnson D, Burke C: *Rhodococcus equi* pneumonia, *Semin Respir Infect* 12:57–60, 1997.

Lerner P: Nocardiosis, *Clin Infect Dis* 22:891–905, 1996.

Maiwald M et al: Reassessment of the phylogenetic position of the bacterium associated with Whipple's disease and determination of the 16S–23S ribosomal intergenic spacer sequence, *Int J Syst Bacteriol* 46:1078–1082, 1996.

McNeil M, Brown J: The medically important aerobic actinomycetes: epidemiology and microbiology, *Clin Microbiol Rev* 7:357–417, 1994.

Prescott JF: *Rhodococcus equi*: an animal and human pathogen, *Clin Microbiol Rev* 4:20–34, 1991.

Relman D et al: Identification of the uncultured bacillus of Whipple's disease, *N Engl J Med* 327:293–301, 1992.

Smego RA, Gallis HA: The clinical spectrum of *Nocardia brasiliensis* infection in the United States, *Rev Infect Dis* 6: 164–180, 1984.

Steingrube V et al: Rapid identification of clinically significant species and taxa of aerobic actinomycetes, including *Actinomadura, Gordona, Nocardia, Rhodococcus, Streptomyces,* and *Tsukamurella* isolates, by DNA amplification and restriction endonuclease analysis, *J Clin Microbiol* 35:817–822, 1997.

Torres O et al: Infection caused by *Nocardia farcinica*: case report and review, *Eur J Clin Microbiol Infect Dis* 19:205–212, 2000.

C H A P T E R 4 0

Mycobacterium

The genus *Mycobacterium* consists of nonmotile, non–spore-forming, aerobic bacilli that are 0.2 to 0.6 × 1 to 10 μm in size. The bacilli occasionally form branched filaments, but these can be readily disrupted. The cell wall is rich in lipids, making the surface hydrophobic and the mycobacteria resistant to many disinfectants as well as to common laboratory stains. Once stained, the bacilli also cannot be decolorized with acid solutions; hence the name **acid-fast bacilli**. Because the mycobacterial cell wall is complex and this group of organisms is fastidious, most mycobacteria grow slowly, dividing every 12 to 24 hours. Isolation of the slow-growing organisms (e.g., *Mycobacterium tuberculosis*, *Mycobacterium avium-intracellulare* [*Mycobacterium avium* complex], *Mycobacterium kansasii*) can require 3 to 8 weeks of incubation whereas the more "rapidly growing" mycobacteria (e.g., *Mycobacterium fortuitum*, *Mycobacterium chelonae*, *Mycobacterium abscessus*) require incubation for 3 days or more. *Mycobacterium leprae*, the etiologic agent of leprosy, cannot be grown in cell-free cultures.

Mycobacteria are still a significant cause of morbidity and mortality, particularly in countries with limited medical resources. Currently, more than 70 species of mycobacteria have been identified, many of which are associated with human disease (Table 40–1). Despite the abundance of mycobacterial species, the following few species or groups cause most human infections: *M. tuberculosis*, *M. leprae*, *M. avium* complex, *M. kansasii*, *M. fortuitum*, *M. chelonae*, and *M. abscessus*.

Physiology and Structure

Bacteria are classified in the genus *Mycobacterium* on the basis of (1) their acid-fastness, (2) the presence of mycolic acids containing 60 to 90 carbons that are cleaved by pyrolysis to C22 to C26 fatty acid methyl esters, and (3) a high (61% to 71%) guanosine plus cytosine (G + C) content in their DNA. Although other species of bacteria can be acid-fast (i.e., *Nocardia*, *Rhodococcus*, *Tsukamurella*, *Gordona*), they stain less intensely (are partially acid-fast), their mycolic acids chains are shorter, and their G + C content is lower.

Mycobacteria possess a complex, lipid-rich cell wall. This cell wall is responsible for many of the characteristic properties of the bacteria (e.g., acid-fastness, slow growth, resistance to detergents, resistance to common antibacterial antibiotics, antigenicity, clumping or **cord formation**). The basic structure of the cell wall is typical of gram-positive bacteria: an inner cytoplasmic membrane overlaid with a thick peptidoglycan layer and no outer membrane. The peptidoglycan skeleton is covalently linked with polysaccharides (arabinogalactan) whose terminal ends are esterified to high-molecular-weight mycolic acids. This layer is overlaid with polypeptides and a hydrophobic layer of highly antigenic mycolic acids consisting of free lipids, glycolipids, and peptidoglycolipids (Fig. 40–1). These lipids constitute 60% of the dry weight of the cell wall. The peptide chains in the outer layer constitute 15% of the cell wall weight and are biologically important antigens, stimulating the patient's cellular immune response to infection. Extracted and partially purified preparations of these protein derivatives (**purified protein derivatives, or PPDs**) are used as skin test reagents to measure exposure to *M. tuberculosis*. Similar preparations from other mycobacteria have been used as species-specific skin test reagents.

Growth properties and colonial morphology are used for the preliminary identification of mycobacteria. As noted earlier, *M. tuberculosis* and closely related species are slow-growing bacteria. The colonies of these mycobacteria are either nonpigmented or buff-colored (Fig. 40–2). Runyon classified the other mycobacteria ("nontuberculous mycobacteria") into four groups on the basis of their rate of growth and their ability to produce pigments in the presence or absence of light. The pigmented mycobacteria produce intensely **yellow carotenoids**. Photochromogenic organisms (Runyon group I) produce these pigments only after exposure to light (Fig. 40–3), whereas scotochromogenic organisms (Runyon group II) produce the pigments in the dark and the light. The slow-growing, nonpigmented myco-

TABLE 40-1. Classification of Selected Mycobacteria Pathogenic for Humans

Organism	Pathogenicity	Frequency in United States
M. tuberculosis *Complex*		
M. tuberculosis	Strictly pathogenic	Common
M. leprae	Strictly pathogenic	Uncommon
M. africanum	Strictly pathogenic	Rare
M. bovis	Strictly pathogenic	Rare
M. ulcerans	Strictly pathogenic	Rare
Runyon Group I (Slow-Growing Photochromogens)		
M. kansasii	Usually pathogenic	Common
M. marinum	Usually pathogenic	Uncommon
M. simiae	Usually pathogenic	Uncommon
Runyon Group II (Slow-Growing Scotochromogens)		
M. szulgai	Usually pathogenic	Uncommon
M. scrofulaceum	Sometimes pathogenic	Uncommon
M. xenopi	Sometimes pathogenic	Uncommon
Runyon Group III (Slow-Growing Nonchromogens)		
M. avium complex	Strictly pathogenic	Common
M. genavense	Strictly pathogenic	Uncommon
M. haemophilum	Usually pathogenic	Uncommon
M. malmoense	Usually pathogenic	Uncommon
Runyon Group IV (Rapid Growers)		
M. fortuitum	Sometimes pathogenic	Common
M. chelonae	Sometimes pathogenic	Common
M. abscessus	Sometimes pathogenic	Uncommon
M. mucogenicum	Sometimes pathogenic	Uncommon

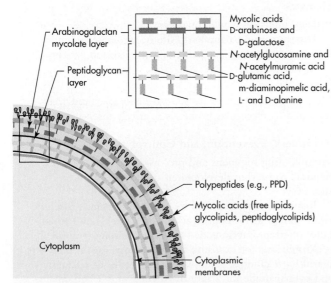

FIGURE 40-1. Mycobacterial cell wall structure. Mycolic acids are attached to the arabinose-galactose layer at the arabinose side chain. Phosphodiester linkage binds the arabinogalactan layer to the underlying peptidoglycan layer at the muramic acid subunit. *PPD,* Purified protein derivative. (Redrawn and modified from Kubica GP, Wayne LG, editors: *The mycobacteria: a sourcebook.* New York, 1984, Marcel Dekker.)

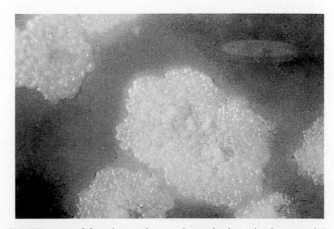

FIGURE 40-2. *Mycobacterium tuberculosis* colonies on Löwenstein-Jensen agar after 8 weeks of incubation. (From Baron EJ, Peterson LR, Finegold SM: *Bailey and Scott's diagnostic microbiology,* ed 9, St Louis, 1994, Mosby.)

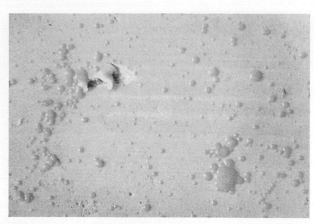

FIGURE 40–3. *Mycobacterium kansasii* colonies on Middle-brook agar 1 day after exposure to light. (From Baron EJ, Peterson LR, Finegold SM: *Bailey and Scott's diagnostic microbiology,* ed 9, St Louis, 1994, Mosby.)

bacteria are classified as Runyon group III, whereas the relatively rapidly growing mycobacteria are classified as Runyon group IV. The **Runyon classification** is a useful differentiation scheme for organizing this diverse collection of clinically important species (see Table 40–1).

Mycobacterium tuberculosis

Pathogenesis and Immunity

Tuberculosis is the classic human mycobacterial disease (Box 40–1). The infection is acquired through the inhalation of aerosolized infectious particles, which then travel to the terminal airways. At these sites, the bacteria penetrate into unactivated alveolar macrophages. The phagocytized bacilli inhibit acidification of the phagosome and subsequent phagosome-lysosome fusion, and proceed to replicate freely (it is unclear whether the bacilli replicate in the phagosome or in the cytoplasm). The infected phagocytic cells are eventually destroyed, after which there are further cycles of phagocytosis by macrophages, mycobacterial replication, and cell lysis.

Although phagocytosis is initiated by alveolar macrophages, circulating macrophages and lymphocytes are attracted to the infectious focus by the bacilli, cellular

---

BOX 40–1. Summary of *Mycobacterium tuberculosis* Infections

Physiology and Structure

Weakly gram-positive, strongly acid-fast, aerobic bacilli.

Lipid-rich cell wall, making the organism resistant to disinfectants, detergents, common antibacterial antibiotic, and traditional stains.

Virulence

Capable of intracellular growth in unactivated alveolar macrophages.

Disease primarily from host response to infection.

Epidemiology

Worldwide; one third of the world population is infected with this organism.

Sixteen million existing cases of disease and 8 million new cases each year.

Disease most common in Southeast Asia, sub-Saharan Africa, and Eastern Europe.

Approximately 20,000 new cases in United States annually.

Populations at greatest risk for disease are immunocompromised patients (particularly those with HIV infection), drug or alcohol abusers, homeless, and individuals exposed to diseased patients.

Humans are the only natural reservoir.

Person-to-person spread by infectious aerosols.

Diseases

Primary infection is pulmonary.

Dissemination to any body site occurs most commonly in immunocompromised patients and untreated patients.

Diagnosis

Microscopy and culture are sensitive and specific. Direct detection by molecular probes is relatively insensitive.

Treatment, Prevention, and Control

Multiple-drug regimens and prolonged treatment are required to prevent development of drug-resistant strains.

Regimens recommended for treatment include isoniazid and rifampin for 9 months, with pyrazinamide and ethambutol or streptomycin added for drug-resistant strains.

Prophylaxis for exposure to tuberculosis can include isoniazid for 9 months, rifampin for 4 months, or rifampin and pyrazinamide for 2 months. Pyrazinamide and ethambutol or levofloxacin are used for 6 to 12 months following exposure to drug-resistant *M. tuberculosis*.

Immunoprophylaxis with BCG in endemic countries.

Control of disease through active surveillance, prophylactic and therapeutic intervention, and careful case monitoring.

debris, and host chemotactic factors (e.g., complement component C5a). The histologic characteristic of this focus is formation of **multinucleated giant cells** of fused macrophages, also called **Langhans' cells**. Infected macrophages can also spread during the initial phase of disease to the local lymph nodes as well as into the blood stream and other tissues (e.g., bone marrow, spleen, kidneys, central nervous system).

The histologic signs of mycobacterial infection are primarily the components of the host response to the infection rather than specific virulence factors elaborated by the mycobacteria. The intracellular replication of mycobacteria stimulates both helper (CD4+) T cells and cytotoxic (CD8+) T cells. Activation of CD4+ cells leads to antibody production, but this response is ineffective in controlling mycobacterial disease because the bacteria are protected in their intracellular location. T cells also release interferon-γ and other cytokines that activate macrophages. Activated macrophages can engulf and kill mycobacteria. The cytotoxic T cells can also lyse phagocytic cells with replicating mycobacteria, thus permitting phagocytosis and bacterial killing by activated phagocytic cells.

If a small antigenic burden is present at the time that the macrophages are stimulated, the bacilli are destroyed with minimal tissue damage. If many bacilli are present, however, the cellular immune response results in tissue necrosis. Multiple host factors are involved in this process, including cytokine toxicity, local activation of the complement cascade, ischemia, and exposure to macrophage-derived hydrolytic enzymes and reactive oxygen intermediates. No known mycobacterial toxin or enzyme has been associated with tissue destruction.

The effectiveness of bacillary elimination is in part related to the size of the focus of infection. Localized collections of activated macrophages (**granulomas**) prevent further spread of the bacilli. These macrophages can penetrate into small granulomas (less than 3 mm) and kill all the bacilli contained in them. However, larger necrotic or caseous granulomas become encapsulated with fibrin that effectively protects the bacilli from macrophage killing. The bacilli can remain dormant in this stage or can be reactivated years later, when the patient's immunologic responsiveness wanes as the result of old age or immunosuppressive disease or therapy. This process is the reason that disease may not develop until late in life in patients exposed to *M. tuberculosis*.

Epidemiology

Although tuberculosis can be established in primates and laboratory animals such as guinea pigs, humans are the only natural reservoir. The disease is spread by close person-to-person contact through the inhalation of infectious aerosols. Large particles are trapped on mucosal surfaces and removed by the ciliary action of the respiratory tree. However, small particles containing one to three tubercle bacilli can reach the alveolar spaces and establish infection.

It was estimated that in 2000, one third of the world's population (1.9 billion people) were infected with *M. tuberculosis*. There were 8 million new cases and 16 million preexisting cases of disease, with 1.9 millions deaths that year. Countries with the highest incidence of disease were Southeast Asia, sub-Saharan Africa, and Eastern Europe. These data are relevant for the United States, because with the decrease in domestically acquired disease in the last decade, most new cases in the United States are found in immigrant populations or contacts with immigrants.

Other populations at greater risk for *M. tuberculosis* disease are the homeless, drug and alcohol abusers, prisoners, and people infected with the human immunodeficiency virus (HIV). Because it is difficult to eradicate disease in these patients, spread of the infection to other populations, including health care workers, poses a significant public health problem. This statement is particularly true for drug-resistant *M. tuberculosis*, because patients who receive inadequate treatment may remain infectious for a long time.

Clinical Diseases

Although tuberculosis can involve any organ, most infections in immunocompetent patients are restricted to the lungs. The initial pulmonary focus is the middle or lower lung fields, where the tubercle bacilli can multiply freely. The patient's cellular immunity is activated, and mycobacterial replication ceases in most patients within 3 to 6 weeks after exposure to the organism. Approximately 5% of patients exposed to *M. tuberculosis* progress to having active disease within 2 years, and another 5% to 10% experience disease sometime later in life.

The likelihood that infection will progress to active disease is a function of both the infectious dose and the patient's immune competence. For example, active disease develops in approximately 10% of patients who are infected with HIV within 1 year of exposure, compared with a 10% risk of disease during the lifetime of patients without HIV infection. In patients with HIV infection, disease usually appears before the onset of other opportunistic infections, is twice as likely to spread to extrapulmonary sites, and can progress rapidly to death.

The clinical signs and symptoms of tuberculosis reflect the site of infection, with primary disease usually restricted to the lower respiratory tract. The disease is insidious in onset. Patients typically have nonspecific complaints of malaise, weight loss, cough, and night sweats. Sputum may be scant or bloody and purulent. Sputum production with hemoptysis is associated with tissue destruction (e.g., cavitary disease). The clinical diagnosis is supported by (1) radiographic evidence of pulmonary disease (Fig. 40–4), (2) positive skin test reactivity, and (3) the laboratory detection of mycobacteria either with microscopy or in cultures. One or both upper lobes of the lungs are usually involved in patients with active disease that includes pneumonitis or abscess formation and cavitation.

As noted earlier, extrapulmonary tuberculosis can occur as the result of the hematogenous spread of the bacilli during the initial phase of multiplication. There may be no evidence of pulmonary disease in patients with disseminated or miliary tuberculosis.

Mycobacterium leprae

Pathogenesis and Immunity

Leprosy (also called **Hansen's disease**) is caused by *M. leprae* (Box 40–2). Like the manifestations of infection with *M. tuberculosis*, the clinical manifestations of leprosy depend on the patient's immune reaction to the bacilli. Leprosy manifests as tuberculoid leprosy or lepromatous leprosy, with intermediate forms also recognized. Patients with **tuberculoid leprosy** have a strong cellular immune reaction but a weak humoral antibody response. Infected tissues typically have many lymphocytes and granulomas but relatively few bacilli (Table 40–2). As in *M. tuberculosis* infections in immunocompetent patients, the bacteria produce cytokines (e.g., interferon-γ, interleukin-2) that mediate macrophage activation, phagocytosis, and bacillary clearance.

Patients with **lepromatous leprosy**, however, have a strong antibody response but a specific defect in the cellular response to *M. leprae* antigens. Thus, an abundance of bacilli are typically observed in dermal macrophages and the Schwann cells of the peripheral nerves.

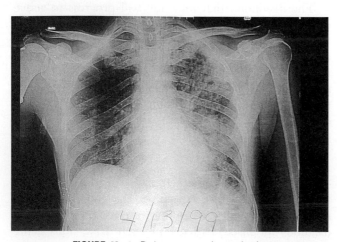

FIGURE 40–4. Pulmonary tuberculosis.

BOX 40–2. Summary of *Mycobacterium leprae* Infections

Physiology and Structure

Weakly gram-positive, strongly acid-fast bacilli.
Lipid-rich cell wall.
Unable to be cultured on artificial media.
Diagnosis made with specific skin test (tuberculoid form of disease) or acid-fast stain (lepromatous form).

Virulence

Capable of intracellular growth.
Disease primarily from host response to infection.

Epidemiology

Rare in United States but common in other countries (e.g., Asia, Africa).
Armadillos are naturally infected and represent an indigenous reservoir.
Lepromatous form of disease, but not the tuberculoid form, is highly infectious.
Person-to-person spread by direct contact or inhalation of infectious aerosols.
People in close contact with patients who have lepromatous disease are at greatest risk.

Diseases

Tuberculoid form of leprosy.
Lepromatous form of leprosy.
Intermediate forms of leprosy.

Diagnosis

Microscopy is sensitive for the lepromatous form but not the tuberculoid form.
Skin testing required to confirm tuberculoid leprosy. Culture cannot be used.

Treatment, Prevention, and Control

Dapsone with or without rifampin is used to treat the tuberculoid form of disease; clofazimine is added for the treatment of the lepromatous form. Therapy is prolonged.
Dapsone is recommended for long-term prophylaxis in treated patients.
Disease is controlled through the prompt recognition and treatment of infected people.

As would be expected, this is the most infectious form of leprosy.

Epidemiology

More than 6 million cases of leprosy are recognized worldwide, particularly in Asia and Africa. In the United States, leprosy is much less common, with only about 125 new cases reported each year. Most cases occur in California, Texas, and Hawaii and primarily in

TABLE 40-2. Clinical and Immunologic Manifestations of Leprosy

Features	Tuberculoid Leprosy	Lepromatous Leprosy
Skin lesions	Few erythematous or hypopigmented plaques with flat centers and raised, demarcated borders; peripheral nerve damage with complete sensory loss; visible enlargement of nerves	Many erythematous macules, papules, or nodules; extensive tissue destruction (e.g., nasal cartilage, bones, ears); diffuse nerve involvement with patchy sensory loss; lack of nerve enlargement
Histopathology	Infiltration of lymphocytes around center of epithelial cells; presence of Langhans' cells; few or no acid-fast bacilli observed	Predominantly "foamy" macrophages with few lymphocytes; lack of Langhans' cells; numerous acid-fast bacilli in skin lesions and internal organs
Infectivity	Low	High
Immune response		
Delayed hypersensitivity	Reactivity to lepromin	Nonreactivity to lepromin
Immunoglobulin levels	Normal	Hypergammaglobulinemia
Erythema nodosum leprosum	Absent	Usually present

immigrants from Mexico, Asia, Africa, and the Pacific Islands. Interestingly, leprosy is endemic in armadillos found in Texas and Louisiana, producing a disease similar to the highly infectious lepromatous form of leprosy in humans. Thus, these armadillos represent a potential endemic focus in this country.

Disease is spread by person-to-person contact. Although the most important route of infection is unknown, it is believed that *M. leprae* is spread either through the inhalation of infectious aerosols or through skin contact with respiratory secretions and wound exudates. Numerous *M. leprae* are found in the nasal secretions from patients with lepromatous leprosy.

M. leprae cannot grow in cell-free cultures. Thus, laboratory confirmation of leprosy requires histopathologic findings consistent with the clinical disease and either skin test reactivity to lepromin or the presence acid-fast bacilli in the lesions.

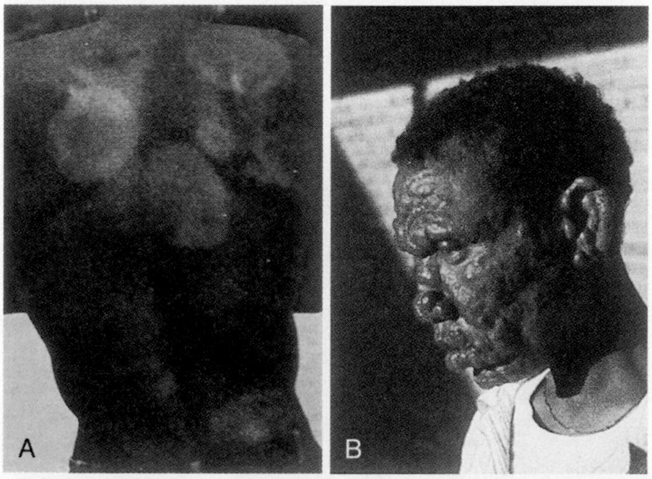

Clinical Diseases

As noted earlier, leprosy presents clinically as tuberculoid or lepromatous disease; each manifests typical clinical and immunologic characteristics (Fig. 40-5; see Table 40-2). Lepromatous leprosy is the form characteristically associated with disfiguring skin lesions.

Mycobacterium avium Complex

M. avium complex consists of common environmental isolates present in water (fresh, brackish, ocean, drinking water) and soil (Box 40-3). Before the acquired immunodeficiency syndrome (AIDS) epidemic, recovery of the organism in clinical specimens typically represented a transient colonization in asymptomatic patients. When disease was observed, it was generally restricted to patients with compromised pulmonary function (e.g., patients with chronic bronchitis or obstructive pulmonary disease, previous pulmonary damage as the result of infection, or other disease) and was

FIGURE 40-5. *A,* Tuberculoid leprosy. Early tuberculoid lesions are characterized by anesthetic macules with hypopigmentation. *B,* Lepromatous leprosy with extensive infiltration, edema, and corrugation of the face. (From Peters W, Gilles HM: *Color atlas of tropical medicine and parasitology,* ed 4, London, 1995, Wolfe.)

stages of their immune disorder, when their CD4+ cell counts fall below 10 cells/mm³.

Although some patients with AIDS develop *M. avium* complex disease following pulmonary exposure (e.g., infectious aerosols of contaminated water), many infections are believed to develop after ingestion of the bacilli. After exposure to the mycobacteria, replication is initiated in localized lymph nodes, followed by systemic spread. The clinical manifestations of disease are not observed until the mass of replicating bacilli impairs normal organ function. Person-to-person transmission has not been demonstrated.

Other Slow-Growing Mycobacteria

Many other slow-growing mycobacteria can cause human disease, and new species continue to be reported as better diagnostic test methods are developed. The spectrum of diseases produced by these mycobacteria also continues to expand, in large part because diseases such as AIDS, malignancies, and organ transplantation

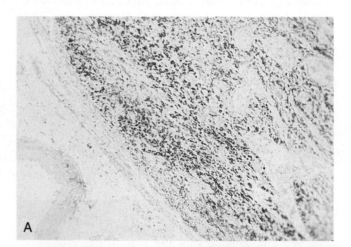

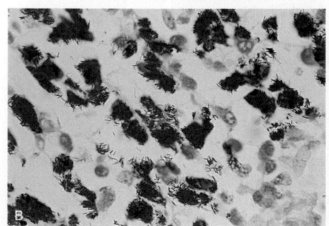

FIGURE 40–6. Tissue from a patient with AIDS who is infected with *Mycobacterium avium* complex photographed under low *(top)* and high *(bottom)* magnification.

clinically identical to pulmonary tuberculosis. However, a new spectrum of disease has arisen in patients with AIDS, making infection with *M. avium* complex the most common mycobacterial disease in these patients in the United States. (*M. tuberculosis* infections are more common than *M. avium* complex in countries such as Africa, where tuberculosis is highly endemic.)

In contrast to disease in other groups of patients, *M. avium* complex infection in patients with AIDS is typically disseminated, with virtually no organ spared. The magnitude of these infections is remarkable; the tissues of some patients are literally filled with the mycobacteria (Fig. 40–6), and there are hundreds to thousands of bacilli per milliliter of blood. Overwhelming disseminated infections with *M. avium* complex are particularly common in patients who are in the terminal

with concomitant use of immunosuppressive drugs have created a population of patients who are highly susceptible to organisms with relatively low virulence potentials. Some mycobacteria produce disease identical to pulmonary tuberculosis (e.g., *Mycobacterium bovis*, *M. kansasii*), other species commonly cause infections localized to lymphatic tissue (*Mycobacterium scrofulaceum*), and others that grow optimally at cool temperatures primarily produce cutaneous infections (*Mycobacterium ulcerans*, *Mycobacterium marinum*, *Mycobacterium haemophilum*). However, disseminated disease can be observed in patients with AIDS who are infected with these same species as well as with relatively uncommon mycobacteria (e.g., *Mycobacterium genavense*, *Mycobacterium simiae*).

Most of these mycobacteria have been isolated in water and soil and occasionally from infected animals (e.g., *M. bovis* causes bovine tuberculosis). Frequently, the isolation of these mycobacteria in clinical specimens simply represents a transient colonization with organisms that the patient ingested. With the exception of *M. bovis* and other mycobacteria closely related to *M. tuberculosis*, person-to-person spread of these mycobacteria does not occur.

Rapid-Growing Mycobacteria

The many mycobacteria have been subdivided into slow-growing species and rapid-growing species (growth in less than 7 days). Five members of the latter group are recognized as important opportunistic pathogens of humans. The most common isolates are *M. fortuitum*, *M. chelonae*, and *M. abscessus*. It is important to distinguish between the rapid-growing and slow-growing mycobacteria, because the rapid-growing species have a relatively low virulence potential, stain irregularly with traditional mycobacterial stains, and are more susceptible to "conventional" antibacterial antibiotics than to drugs used to treat mycobacterial infections.

The rapid-growing mycobacteria rarely cause disseminated infections. Rather, they are most commonly associated with disease occurring after bacteria are introduced into the deep subcutaneous tissues by trauma or iatrogenic infections (e.g., infections associated with an intravenous catheter, contaminated wound dressing, prosthetic device such as a heart valve, peritoneal dialysis, or bronchoscopy). Unfortunately, the incidence of infections with these organisms is increasing as more invasive procedures are performed in hospitalized patients and advanced medical care lengthens the life expectancy of immunocompromised patients.

Laboratory Diagnosis

The various laboratory tests used in the diagnosis of infections caused by mycobacteria are listed in Box 40-4.

Skin Test

Reactivity to an intradermal injection of mycobacterial antigens can differentiate between infected and noninfected people. The only evidence of infection with mycobacteria in most patients is a lifelong positive skin test reaction and radiographic evidence of calcification of the initial active foci in the lungs or other organs. Tests with protein antigens extracted from *M. tuberculosis* have been used most commonly and are the best-standardized ones, although skin tests with other species-specific mycobacterial antigens have also been developed.

The methods of antigen preparation and skin inoculation have been changed many times since the tests were first developed. The currently recommended tuberculin antigen is the PPD of the cell wall. In this test, a specific amount of the antigen (0.1 μg [5 tuberculin units] of PPD) is inoculated into the intradermal layer of the patient's skin. Skin test reactivity is measured 48 hours later. Positive reactivity is defined differently, depending on the population (Table 40-3). A positive PPD reaction usually develops 3 to 4 weeks after exposure to *M. tuberculosis*. Exposure to other mycobacteria may cause a patient to show cross-reactivity with tuberculin, but the reaction is generally less than a 10-mm induration. Patients infected with *M. tuberculosis* may not show a response to the tuberculin skin test if they are anergic (particularly true of HIV-infected patients); thus, control antigens should always be used with tuberculin tests.

TABLE 40–3. Criteria Defining Positive Purified Protein Derivative Reactivity in Patients Exposed to *Mycobacterium tuberculosis*

Reactivity to PPD	Populations
≥5 mm of induration	HIV-positive patients; patients receiving immunosuppressive therapy; recent contacts of patients with tuberculosis; patients with abnormal chest radiographs consistent with prior tuberculosis
≥10 mm of induration	Recent immigrants from high-prevalence countries; injection drug users; residents and employees of high-risk settings (e.g., prisons; residential facilities for the elderly, patients with AIDS, and the homeless; health care facilities; mycobacteriology laboratory); persons with conditions of high risk (e.g., silicosis, diabetes, chronic renal failure, hematologic disorders, significant weight loss, gastrectomy, jejunoileal bypass); children younger than 4 years or exposed to adults at high risk
≥15 mm of induration	Persons at low risk for tuberculosis

Reactivity to lepromin, which is prepared from inactivated *M. leprae*, is valuable for confirming the clinical diagnosis of tuberculoid leprosy. Papular induration develops 3 to 4 weeks after the intradermal injection of the antigen. This test is not useful for identifying patients with lepromatous leprosy, because such patients are anergic to the antigen.

Microscopy

The microscopic detection of acid-fast bacilli in clinical specimens is the most rapid way to confirm mycobacterial disease. The clinical specimen is stained with carbolfuchsin (Ziehl-Neelsen or Kinyoun methods) or fluorescent auramine-rhodamine dyes (Truant fluorochrome method), decolorized with an acid-alcohol solution, and then counterstained. The specimens are examined with a light microscope or, if fluorescent dyes are used, a fluorescent microscope (Fig. 40–7). The Truant fluorochrome method is more sensitive, because the specimen can be scanned rapidly under low magnification for fluorescent areas, and then the presence of acid-fact bacilli can be confirmed with higher magnification.

In approximately a third to half of all culture-positive specimens, the bacilli are detected by acid-fast microscopy. The sensitivity of this test is high for (1) respiratory specimens (particularly from patients with radiographic evidence of cavitation) and (2) specimens for which many mycobacteria are isolated in culture. Thus, a positive acid-fast stain reaction corresponds to higher infectivity. The specificity of the test is greater than 95%.

Nucleic Acid Probes

Although microscopy provides useful information regarding the presence of mycobacterial disease, it can-

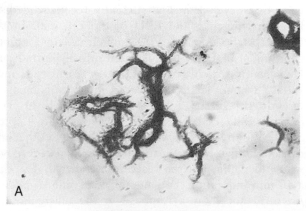 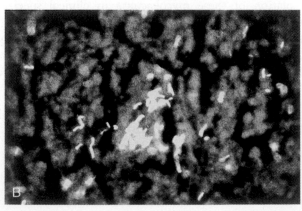

FIGURE 40–7. Acid-fast stains of *Mycobacterium tuberculosis*. *A,* Stained with carbolfuchsin using the Kinyoun method. *B,* Stained with the fluorescent dyes auramine and rhodamine using the Truant fluorochrome method.

not identify the particular mycobacterial species involved. For this reason, techniques have been developed to detect specific mycobacterial nucleic acid sequences present in clinical specimens. Because only a few bacteria may be present, a variety of amplification techniques are used (e.g., polymerase chain reaction, ligase chain reaction, transcription-mediated amplification). The procedures currently used are specific for *M. tuberculosis* but relatively insensitive. With further refinements, however, these procedures will most likely prove to be useful diagnostic tools.

Culture

Mycobacteria that cause pulmonary disease, particularly in patients with evidence of cavitation, are abundant in the respiratory secretions (e.g., 10^8 bacilli per mL or more). Recovery of the organisms is virtually assured in patients from whom early morning respiratory specimens are collected for 3 consecutive days. It is more difficult, however, to isolate *M. tuberculosis* and other mycobacteria from other sites in patients with disseminated disease (e.g., genitourinary tract, tissues, cerebrospinal fluid). In such cases, additional specimens must be collected for cultures, and a large volume of fluid must be processed.

The in vitro growth of mycobacteria is complicated by the fact that most isolates grow slowly and can be obscured by the rapid-growing bacteria that normally colonize people. Thus, specimens such as sputum are initially treated with a decontaminating reagent (e.g., 2% sodium hydroxide) to remove organisms that could confound results. Mycobacteria can tolerate brief alkali treatment, which kills the rapid-growing bacteria and permits the selective isolation of mycobacteria. Extended decontamination of the specimen kills mycobacteria, so the procedure is not performed when normally sterile specimens are being tested or when few mycobacteria are expected.

In former times, when specimens were inoculated onto egg-based (e.g., Löwenstein-Jensen) and agar-based (e.g., Middlebrook) media, it generally took a long time for *M. tuberculosis*, *M. avium* complex, and other important slow-growing mycobacteria to be detected. However, this time has been shortened through the use of specially formulated broth cultures that support the rapid growth of most mycobacteria. Thus, the average time to grow mycobacteria has been decreased from 3 to 4 weeks to 10 to 14 days.

Preliminary Identification

Growth properties and colonial morphology can be used for the preliminary identification of the most common species of mycobacteria. This step is important, because only mycobacteria in the *M. tuberculosis* complex are transmitted from person to person. Thus, only patients infected with these organisms must be isolated and their close contacts given prophylactic antibiotics. The preliminary identification of an isolate can also be used to guide empirical antimicrobial therapy.

Definitive Identification

The mycobacteria can be identified definitively through the use of a variety of techniques. Biochemical tests are a standard way to identify mycobacteria (Table 40–4), but results are not available for at least 3 weeks or more. Mycobacterial species can also be identified through chromatographic analysis of their characteristic cell wall lipids. However, species-specific molecular probes are the most useful means of identifying commonly isolated mycobacteria (e.g., *M. tuberculosis*, *M. avium* complex, *M. kansasii*). Because many organisms are present after in vitro cultivation, it is not necessary to amplify the target genomic sequence. The commercially prepared probe identification systems currently used are rapid (test time, 2 hours), sensitive, and specific.

An additional way to identify mycobacterial species for which probes are not available involves the amplifi-

---

TABLE 40–4. Selected Biochemical Reactions for Five Commonly Isolated Mycobacteria

Organism	Niacin	Nitrate Reductase	Heat-Stable Catalase	Tween-80 Hydrolysis	Iron Uptake	Arylsulfatase	Urease
M. tuberculosis	+	+	−	−		−	+
M. kansasii	−	+	+	+		−	+
M. avium complex	−	−	+/−	−		−	−
M. fortuitum	−	+	+	V	+	+	+
M. chelonae	V	−	V	V	−	+	+

V = Variable.

Modified from Murray PR et al, editors: *Manual of clinical microbiology*, ed. 7, Washington, DC, 1999, American Society for Microbiology.

cation of the species-specific, hypervariable regions of the 16S ribosomal RNA genes followed by sequence analysis to identify the species. This method is rapid (2 days) and is not limited by the availability of specific probes. It is likely that this method will eventually replace biochemical methods of identifying many mycobacterial species.

Treatment, Prevention, and Control

Treatment

The treatment and prophylaxis of mycobacterial infections, unlike those for most other bacterial infections, are complex and controversial. Slow-growing mycobacteria are resistant to most antibiotics used to treat other bacterial infections. In general, patients must take multiple antibiotics for an extended period (e.g., a minimum of 6 to 9 months), or antibiotic-resistant strains will develop. In 1990, the first outbreaks of multiple-drug–resistant *M. tuberculosis* were observed in patients with AIDS and in the homeless in New York City and Miami. Although there has been a dramatic reduction in resistant *M. tuberculosis* strains in such populations, all therapy must be directed against these organisms until antimicrobial susceptibility results are available for the individual patient.

The number of treatment regimens that have been developed for drug-susceptible and drug-resistant tuberculosis is too complex to review here comprehensively. A traditional regimen that has been used successfully is to treat the patient with the combination of isoniazid and rifampin for 9 months. This combination of drugs can be administered either daily or (with a higher dosage of isoniazid) twice weekly. Pyrazinamide and either ethambutol or streptomycin should be given with this regimen until susceptibility results are available.

M. avium complex and many other slow-growing mycobacteria are resistant to common antimycobacterial agents. One regimen recommended currently for *M. avium* complex infections is clarithromycin or azithromycin combined with ethambutol and rifabutin. The American Thoracic Society has recommended that *M. kansasii* infections be treated with isoniazid, rifampin, and ethambutol with or without streptomycin. The duration of treatment and final selection of drugs are determined by (1) the response to therapy and (2) interactions among these drugs and other drugs the patient is receiving (e.g., toxic and pharmacokinetic interactions of these drugs with protease inhibitors used to treat HIV infection).

Unlike the slow-growing mycobacteria, the rapid-growing species are resistant to most commonly used antimycobacterial agents but are susceptible to antibiotics such as clarithromycin, imipenem, amikacin, ce-

foxitin, and the sulfonamides. The specific activity of these agents must be determined with in vitro tests. Because infections with these mycobacteria are generally confined to the skin or are associated with prosthetic devices, surgical débridement or removal of the prosthesis is also necessary.

Treatment of patients with *M. leprae* infections is based on clinical experience, because in vitro testing is not possible and in vivo testing with animal models (e.g., mouse footpad inoculations) is not practical. Treatment regimens, particularly those advanced by the World Health Organization, have been controversial and are not universally accepted. It has been recommended that the tuberculoid form of leprosy (few bacilli present, so less infectious) should be treated with dapsone alone or in combination with rifampin. The more infectious lepromatous form should be treated with dapsone, clofazimine, and rifampin. The duration of treatment is not well-defined, but many believe that lifelong dapsone therapy is necessary to prevent relapses.

Chemoprophylaxis

The American Thoracic Society and the Centers for Disease Control and Prevention have examined a number of prophylactic regimens for use in patients (HIV-positive and HIV-negative) exposed to *M. tuberculosis*. The three regimens that have been recommended are as follows: (1) daily or twice weekly isoniazid for 9 months, (2) daily rifampin for 4 months, and (3) daily rifampin and pyrazinamide for 2 months. Patients who have been exposed to drug-resistant *M. tuberculosis* should receive prophylaxis with pyrazinamide and either ethambutol or levofloxacin for 6 to 12 months. Because *M. avium* complex intracellulare infections are common in patients with AIDS, chemoprophylaxis is recommended for patients whose CD4+ T cell counts fall to less than 75 cells/mm^3. Prophylaxis with clarithromycin, azithromycin, or rifabutin is recommended. Combinations of these drugs have been used, but they are generally more toxic and no more effective than the single agent. Chemoprophylaxis is unnecessary for patients with other mycobacterial infections.

Immunoprophylaxis

Vaccination with attenuated *M. bovis* (bacille Calmette-Guérin [**BCG**]) is commonly used in countries where tuberculosis is endemic and is responsible for significant morbidity and mortality. This practice can lead to a significant reduction in the incidence of tuberculosis if BCG is administered to people when they are young (it is less effective in adults). Unfortunately, BCG immunization cannot be used in immunocompromised patients (e.g., those with HIV infection). Thus, it is unlikely to be useful in countries with a high prevalence of HIV infections (e.g., Africa) or to control the spread of drug-resistant tuberculosis. An additional problem with BCG immunization is that positive skin test reactivity develops in all patients and may persist for a prolonged time. However, skin test reactivity is generally low, so a strongly reactive skin test result (e.g., >20 mm of induration) is generally significant. BCG immunization is not widely used in the United States or in other countries where the incidence of tuberculosis is low.

Control

Because one third of the world population is infected with *M. tuberculosis*, the elimination of this disease is highly unlikely. Disease can be controlled, however, with a combination of active surveillance, prophylactic and therapeutic intervention, and careful case monitoring. The success of this approach was demonstrated in the 44% reduction of drug-resistant tuberculosis in the New York City area from 1991 to 1996.

CASE STUDY AND QUESTIONS

■ A 35-year-old man with a history of intravenous drug use entered the local health clinic with complaints of a dry, persistent cough; fever; malaise; and anorexia. Over the preceding 4 weeks, he had lost 15 pounds and experienced chills and sweats. A chest radiograph revealed patchy infiltrates throughout the lung fields. Because the patient had a nonproductive cough, sputum was induced and submitted for bacterial, fungal, and mycobacterial cultures as well as examination for *Pneumocystis* organisms. Blood cultures and serologic tests for HIV infection were performed. The patient was found to be HIV-positive. The results of all cultures were negative after 2 days of incubation; however, cultures were positive for *M. tuberculosis* after an additional week of incubation.

1. What is unique about the cell wall of mycobacteria and what biologic effects can be attributed to the cell wall structure?
2. Why is *M. tuberculosis* more virulent in patients with HIV infection than in patients without it?
3. What is the definition of a positive skin test (PPD) result for *M. tuberculosis*?
4. What are the two clinical presentations of *M. leprae* infections? How do the diagnostic tests differ for these two presentations?
5. Why do mycobacterial infections have to be treated for 6 months or more? What is the recommended therapy for *M. tuberculosis*? *M. avium* complex? *M. kansasii*? *M. fortuitum*?

BIBLIOGRAPHY

Cantwell MF et al: Epidemiology of tuberculosis in the United States, 1985–1992, *JAMA* 272:535–539, 1994.

Centers for Disease Control and Prevention: Targeted tuberculin testing and treatment of latent tuberculosis infection. *MMWR* 49:1–51, 2000.

Cohn ZA, Kaplan G: Hansen's disease, cell-mediated immunity, and recombinant lymphokines, *J Infect Dis* 163:1195–1200, 1991.

Dye C et al: Global burden of tuberculosis: estimated incidence, prevalence, and mortality by country, *JAMA* 282:677–686, 1999.

Falkinham J: Epidemiology of infection by nontuberculous mycobacteria, *Clin Microbiol Rev* 9:177–215, 1996.

Hastings RC et al: Leprosy, *Clin Microbiol Rev* 1:330–348, 1988.

Horsburgh C: Epidemiology of *Mycobacterium avium* complex disease, *Am J Med* 102:11–15, 1997.

Huebner RE, Castro KG: The changing face of tuberculosis, *Annu Rev Med* 46:47–55, 1995.

Jacobson K et al: Clinical and radiological features of pulmonary disease caused by rapidly growing mycobacteria in cancer patients, *Eur J Clin Microbiol Infect Dis* 17:615–621, 1998.

Jacobson K et al: *Mycobacterium kansasii* infections in patients with cancer, *Clin Infect Dis* 30:965–969, 2000.

Kiehn TE, Armstrong D: Current topic: mycobacteriology, *Eur J Clin Microbiol Infect Dis* 13:881–1006, 1994.

Kubica GP, Wayne LG: *The mycobacteria: a sourcebook*, New York, 1984, Marcel Dekker.

Moore M et al: Trends in drug-resistant tuberculosis in the United States, 1993–1996, *JAMA* 278:833–837, 1997.

Pierce M et al: A randomized trial of clarithromycin as prophylaxis against disseminated *Mycobacterium avium* complex infection in patients with advanced acquired immunodeficiency syndrome, *N Engl J Med* 335:384–391, 1996.

Raviglione MC, Snider DE, Kochi A: Global epidemiology of tuberculosis: morbidity and mortality of a worldwide epidemic, *JAMA* 273:220–226, 1995.

Salyers AA, Whitt DD: *Bacterial pathogenesis: a molecular approach*, Washington, DC, 1994, American Society for Microbiology.

Saubolle MA et al: *Mycobacterium haemophilum*: microbiology and expanding clinical and geographic spectra of disease in humans, *Clin Microbiol Rev* 9:435–447, 1996.

Sepkowitz KA et al: Tuberculosis in the AIDS era, *Clin Microbiol Rev* 8:180–199, 1995.

Shafran S et al: A comparison of two regimens for the treatment of *Mycobacterium avium* complex bacteremia in AIDS: rifabutin, ethambutol, and clarithromycin versus rifampin, ethambutol, clofazimine, and ciprofloxacin, *N Engl J Med* 335:377–383, 1996.

Verdon R et al: Tuberculous meningitis in adults: review of 48 cases, *Clin Infect Dis* 22:982–988, 1996.

CHAPTER 41

Treponema, Borrelia, and *Leptospira*

The bacteria in the order Spirochaetales have been grouped together on the basis of their common morphologic properties. These spirochetes are thin, helical (0.1 to 0.5 × 5 to 20 μm), gram-negative bacteria. The order Spirochaetales is subdivided into two families and eight genera, of which three (*Treponema, Borrelia,* and *Leptospira*) are responsible for human disease (Table 41–1).

Treponema

The two treponemal species that cause human disease are *Treponema pallidum* (with three subspecies) and *Treponema carateum*. All are morphologically identical, produce the same serologic response in humans (e.g., positive reactivity in the Venereal Disease Research Laboratory [VDRL] test, fluorescent treponemal antibody absorption [FTA-ABS] test, and microhemagglutination test for *T. pallidum* [MHA-TP]), and are susceptible to penicillin. The organisms are distinguished by their epidemiologic characteristics and clinical presentation. *T. pallidum* subspecies *pallidum* (referred to as *T. pallidum* in this chapter) is the etiologic agent of the venereal disease **syphilis**; *T. pallidum* subspecies *endemicum* causes endemic syphilis, or **bejel**; *T. pallidum* subspecies *pertenue* causes **yaws**; and *T. carateum* causes **pinta**. Bejel, yaws, and pinta are nonvenereal diseases. Syphilis is discussed initially; the other treponemal diseases are discussed at the end of the section.

Physiology and Structure

Syphilis is a sexually transmitted disease that has plagued humans for centuries. The spirochete that causes this disease is a strict human pathogen. Natural syphilis is not found in any other species, and experimental syphilis has been established only in rabbits. *T. pallidum* is a thin, coiled spirochete (0.1 × 5 to 15 μm) that cannot be grown in cell-free cultures. Limited growth of the organisms has been achieved in cultured rabbit epithelial cells, but replication is slow (doubling time is 30 hours) and can be maintained for only a few generations. The spirochetes were once considered strict anaerobes; however, it is now known that they can use glucose oxidatively.

The spirochetes are too thin to be seen with light microscopy in specimens stained with Gram or Giemsa stain. However, motile forms can be visualized by darkfield illumination or by staining with specific antitreponemal antibodies labeled with fluorescent dyes.

Pathogenesis and Immunity

The inability to grow *T. pallidum* to high concentrations in vitro has limited detection of specific virulence factors in this organism. However, several investigators have now cloned *T. pallidum* genes in *Escherichia coli* and isolated the protein products. Several gene products have been associated specifically with virulent strains, although their role in pathogenesis remains to be delineated. The outer membrane proteins are associated with adherence to the surface of host cells, and virulent spirochetes produce hyaluronidase, which may facilitate perivascular infiltration. Virulent spirochetes are also coated with host cell fibronectin, which can protect against phagocytosis.

The tissue destruction and lesions observed in syphilis are primarily the consequence of the patient's immune response to infection. The clinical course of syphilis evolves through three phases. The initial or **primary phase** is characterized by one or more skin lesions (**chancres**) at the site where the spirochete penetrated. Although spirochetes are disseminated in the blood stream soon after infection, the chancre represents the primary site of initial replication. Histologic examination of the lesion reveals endarteritis and periarteritis (characteristic of syphilitic lesions at all stages) and infiltration of the ulcer with polymorphonuclear leukocytes and macrophages. Spirochetes are ingested by the phagocytic cells, but the organisms frequently survive. In the **secondary phase,** the clinical signs of disseminated disease appear, with prominent skin lesions dispersed over the entire body surface (Fig. 41–1). Spontaneous remission may occur after the primary

TABLE 41–1. Order Spirochaetales

Spirochaetales	Human Disease	Etiologic Agent
Family Spirochaetaceae		
Genus *Borrelia*	Epidemic relapsing fever	*Borrelia recurrentis*
	Endemic relapsing fever	Many *Borrelia* species
	Lyme borreliosis	*Borrelia burgdorferi, Borrelia garinii, Borrelia afzelii*
Genus *Cristispira*	None	—
Genus *Serpulina*	None	—
Genus *Spirochaeta*	None	—
Genus *Treponema*	Syphilis	*Treponema pallidum* subspecies *pallidum*
	Bejel	*T. pallidum* subspecies *endemicum*
	Yaws	*T. pallidum* subspecies *pertenue*
	Pinta	*Treponema carateum*
Family Leptospiraceae		
Genus *Leptonema*	None	—
Genus *Leptospira*	Leptospirosis	*Leptospira interrogans*
Genus *Turneria*	None	—

or secondary stages, or the disease may progress to the **late phase** of disease, in which virtually all tissues may be involved. Each stage represents localized multiplication of the spirochete and tissue destruction. Although replication is slow, numerous organisms are present in the initial chancre as well as in the secondary lesions, making the patient highly infectious at these stages.

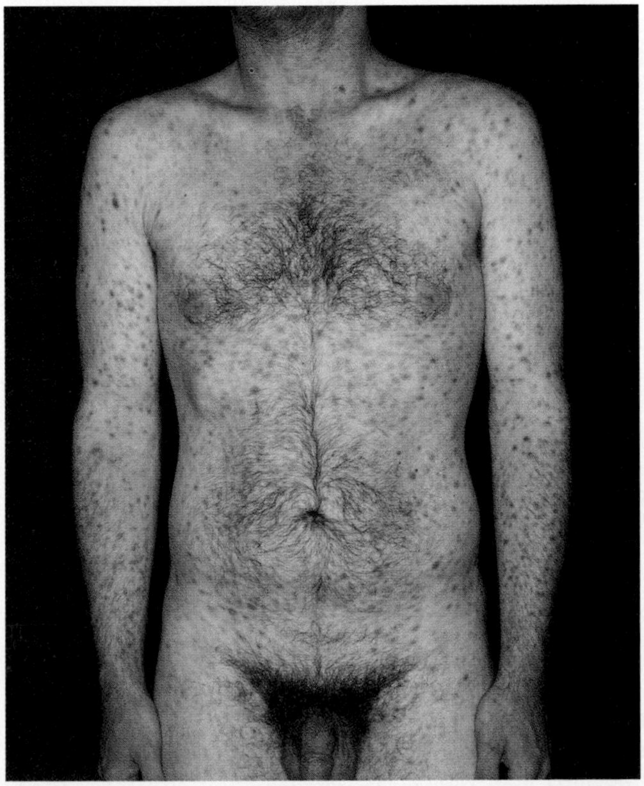

Epidemiology

Syphilis is found worldwide and is the third most common sexually transmitted bacterial disease in the United States (after *Neisseria gonorrhoeae* and *Chlamydia* infections) (Box 41–1). The incidence of disease has steadily decreased since the advent of penicillin therapy in the early 1940s. However, almost 50,000 new cases in the United States were reported in 1999. Numerous infections remain unreported, thus contributing to a gross underestimation of the true incidence of this disease.

Natural syphilis is exclusive to humans and has no other known natural hosts. *T. pallidum* is extremely labile, unable to survive exposure to drying or disinfectants. Thus, syphilis cannot be spread through contact with inanimate objects such as toilet seats. The most common route of spread is by direct sexual contact. The disease can also be acquired congenitally or by transfusion with contaminated blood. Syphilis is not highly contagious; the risk of a person's contracting the disease after a single sexual contact is estimated to be 30%. However, contagiousness is influenced by the stage of disease in the infectious person. As mentioned previously, the spirochetes cannot survive on dry skin surfaces. Thus, *T. pallidum* is transferred primarily during the early stages of disease, when many organisms are present in moist cutaneous or mucosal lesions. During the early stages of disease, the patient becomes bacteremic, and if the disease is untreated, bacteremia can persist for as long as 8 years. Congenital transmis-

FIGURE 41–1. Disseminated rash in secondary syphilis. (From Habif TP: *Clinical dermatology: a color guide to diagnosis and therapy,* St Louis, 1996, Mosby.)

BOX 41–1. Summary of *Treponema* Infections

Physiology and Structure

Thin, coiled spirochete, 0.1 × 5 to 15 μm.

Cannot be seen with Gram or Giemsa stains; observed by darkfield microscopy.

Cannot be grown in vitro except in selected cultured cells.

Virulence Factors

Outer membrane proteins promote adherence to host cells.

Hyaluronidase may facilitate perivascular infiltration.

Coating of fibronectin protects against phagocytosis.

Tissue destruction primarily results from host's immune response to infection.

Epidemiology

Humans are the only natural host.

Venereal syphilis transmitted by sexual contact or congenitally; patients at risk include sexually active adolescents and adults, and children born of mothers with active disease.

Other *Treponema* infections transmitted by contact of mucous membranes with infectious lesions; congenital infections rare; patients at risk are children or adults in contact with infectious lesions.

Venereal syphilis occurs worldwide; endemic syphilis (bejel) occurs in desert and temperate regions of North Africa, Middle East, and northern Australia; yaws occurs in tropical or desert regions of Africa, South America, and Indonesia; pinta occurs in tropical areas of Central and South America.

No seasonal incidence.

Diseases

Venereal syphilis (*Treponema pallidum* subspecies *pallidum*).

Endemic syphilis or bejel (*T. pallidum* subspecies *endemicum*).

Yaws (*T. pallidum* subspecies *pertenue*).

Pinta (*Treponema carateum*).

Diagnosis

Refer to Table 41–2.

Treatment, Prevention, and Control

Penicillin is drug of choice; tetracycline, erythromycin, or chloramphenicol is administered if the patient is allergic to penicillin.

Safe sex practices should be emphasized, and sexual partners of infected patients should be treated.

Endemic syphilis, yaws, and pinta can be eliminated through organized public health measures (treatment, education); however, these efforts have been inconsistently applied.

---

sion from mother to fetus can occur at any time during this period. After 8 years, the disease can remain active, but bacteremia is not believed to occur.

With the advent of effective antimicrobial therapy, the incidence of late (tertiary) syphilis has markedly decreased. Although antibiotic therapy has led to a decrease in the length of infectivity in infected persons, the incidence of primary and secondary syphilis has remained high because of sexual practices, particularly prostitution to support drug habits. The incidence of congenital syphilis corresponds to the pattern of syphilis in women of childbearing age. It should be noted that when active genital lesions are present, the patient is at greater risk for transmitting and acquiring human immunodeficiency virus.

Clinical Diseases

The natural history of untreated acquired syphilis is illustrated in Figure 41–2.

Primary Syphilis

As noted earlier, the initial syphilitic chancre develops at the site where the spirochete is inoculated. Many chancres can be observed in immunocompromised pa-

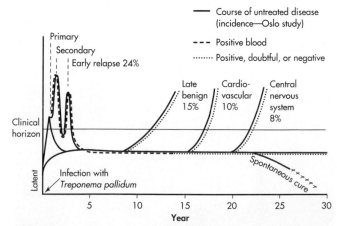

FIGURE 41–2. The natural history of untreated acquired syphilis was carefully chronicled at the University of Oslo. (Modified from Morgan H: *South Med J* 26:18–22, 1933; incidence data from Clark E, Danbolt N: The Oslo study of the natural history of untreated syphilis, *J Chron Dis* 2: 311–344, 1955.)

tients such as those infected with the human immunodeficiency virus. The lesion starts as a papule but then erodes to become a **painlesss ulcer** with raised borders. In most patients, a painless regional lymphadenopathy develops 1 to 2 weeks after the appearance of the chancre, which represents a local focus for the proliferation of spirochetes. Abundant spirochetes are present in the chancre and can be disseminated throughout the patient by way of the lymphatic system and blood stream. The fact that this ulcer heals spontaneously within 2 months gives the patient a false sense of relief.

Secondary Syphilis

The clinical evidence of disseminated disease marks the second stage of syphilis. In this stage, patients typically experience a "flu-like" syndrome with sore throat, headache, fever, myalgias, anorexia, lymphadenopathy, and a **generalized mucocutaneous rash.** The "flu-like" syndrome and lymphadenopathy generally appear first and then are followed a few days later by the disseminated skin rash. The rash can be variable (macular, papular, pustular), can cover the entire skin surface (including the palms and soles), and may resolve slowly over a period of weeks to months. As with the primary chancre, the rash in secondary syphilis is highly infectious. The rash and symptoms gradually resolve spontaneously, and the patient enters the latent or clinically inactive stage of disease.

Late Syphilis

A small proportion of cases can progress to the tertiary stage of syphilis. The diffuse, chronic inflammation characteristic of late syphilis can cause a devastating destruction of virtually any organ or tissue (e.g., arteritis, dementia, blindness). Granulomatous lesions (**gum-** mas) may be found in bone, skin, and other tissues. The nomenclature of late syphilis reflects the organs of primary involvement (e.g., neurosyphilis, cardiovascular syphilis). An increased incidence of neurosyphilis despite adequate therapy for early syphilis has been documented in patients with the acquired immunodeficiency syndrome.

Congenital Syphilis

In utero infections can lead to serious fetal disease, resulting in latent infections, multiorgan malformations, or death of the fetus. Most infected infants are born without clinical evidence of the disease, but rhinitis then develops and is followed by a widespread desquamating maculopapular rash. Late bony destruction and cardiovascular syphilis are common in untreated infants who survive the initial course of disease.

Laboratory Diagnosis

Microscopy

The diagnosis of primary, secondary, or congenital syphilis can be made rapidly by darkfield examination of the exudate from skin lesions (Table 41–2 and Fig. 41–3). However, the test is reliable only when clinical material with actively motile spirochetes is examined immediately by an experienced microscopist. The spirochetes do not survive transport to the laboratory, and tissue debris can be mistaken for spirochetes. Material collected from oral lesions should not be examined because nonpathogenic oral spirochetes can contaminate the specimen. *T. pallidum* can be identified specifically using fluorescein-labeled antitreponemal antibodies. Histologic staining of tissue lesions may be beneficial in showing the organisms; silver stains are used most commonly.

TABLE 41–2. Diagnostic Tests for Syphilis

Diagnostic Test	Method or Examination
Microscopy	Darkfield
	Direct fluorescent antibody staining
Culture	Not available
Serology	Nontreponemal tests
	Venereal Disease Research Laboratory (VDRL)
	Rapid plasma reagin (RPR)
	Treponemal tests
	Fluorescent treponemal antibody absorption (FTA-ABS)
	Microhemagglutination test for *Treponema pallidum* (MHA-TP)

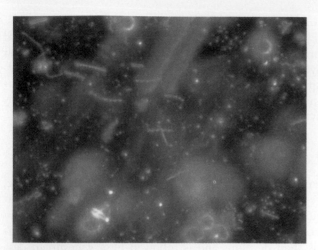

FIGURE 41–3. *T. pallidum* in a darkfield microscopy study. (From Peters W, Gilles HM: *A color atlas of tropical medicine and parasitology,* ed 4, London, 1995, Wolfe.)

Culture

Efforts to culture *T. pallidum* in vitro should not be attempted because the organism does not grow in artificial cultures.

Serology

Syphilis is diagnosed in most patients on the basis of serologic tests. The two general types of tests used are biologically nonspecific (**nontreponemal**) tests and the specific **treponemal** tests (Table 41–3). Nontreponemal tests measure immunoglobulin (Ig) G and IgM antibodies (also called **reagin antibodies**) developed against lipids released from damaged cells during the early stage of disease and present on the cell surface of treponemes. The antigen used for the nontreponemal tests is **cardiolipin,** which is derived from beef heart.

The two tests used most commonly are the **VDRL test** and the **rapid plasma reagin (RPR) test.** Both tests measure the flocculation of cardiolipin antigen by the patient's serum. Both tests can be performed rapidly, although complement in serum must be inactivated for 30 minutes before the VDRL test can be performed. Only the VDRL test should be used to test cerebrospinal fluid from patients with suspected neurosyphilis.

Treponemal tests are specific antibody tests used to confirm positive reactions with the VDRL or RPR tests. The treponemal test results can also be positive before the nontreponemal test results become positive in early syphilis, or they can remain positive when the nonspecific test results revert to negative in some patients who have late syphilis. The tests most commonly used are the **FTA-ABS** and **MHA-TP.** The MHA-TP test is technically easier to perform and the results easier to interpret than the FTA-ABS test. The Western blot assay with whole-cell *T. pallidum* as the antigen has been used successfully as a confirmatory treponeme-specific test.

Because positive reactions with the nontreponemal tests develop late during the first phase of disease, the serologic findings are negative in many patients who initially have chancres. However, serologic results are positive within 3 months in all patients and remain positive in untreated patients with secondary syphilis. The antibody titers decrease slowly in patients with untreated syphilis, and serologic results are negative in approximately 25% to 30% of patients with late syphilis. Although the results of treponemal tests generally remain positive for the life of the person who has syphilis, a negative test is unreliable in patients with the acquired immunodeficiency syndrome.

Successful treatment of primary or secondary syphilis and, to a lesser extent, late syphilis leads to reduced titers measured in the VDRL and RPR tests (Fig. 41–

TABLE 41–3. Sensitivity and Specificity of Serologic Tests for Syphilis

Test	Sensitivity (%)				Specificity (%)
	Primary	*Secondary*	*Latent*	*Late*	
Nontreponemal					
VDRL	78 (74–87)	100	95 (88–100)	71 (37–94)	98 (96–99)
RPR	86 (77–100)	100	98 (95–100)	73	98 (93–99)
Treponemal					
FTA-ABS	84 (70–100)	100	100	96	97 (94–100)
MHA-TP	76 (69–90)	100	97 (97–100)	94	99 (98–100)

FTA-ABS = fluorescent treponemal antibody absorption test; MHA-TP = microhemagglutination test for *Treponema pallidum*; RPR = rapid plasma reagin; VDRL = Venereal Disease Research Laboratory.

Based on data from Larsen S, Steiner B, Rudolph A: Laboratory diagnosis and interpretation of tests for syphilis, *Clin Microbiol Rev* 8:1–21, 1995.

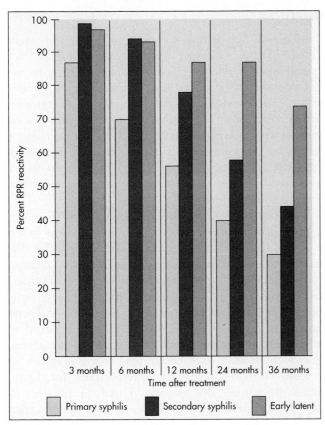

FIGURE 41–4. Effect of treatment for syphilis on rapid plasma reagin reactivity. (Data from Romanowski B et al: Serologic response to treatment of infectious syphilis, *Ann Intern Med* 114: 1005–1009, 1991.)

4). Thus, these tests can be used to monitor the effectiveness of therapy, although seroreversion is slowed in patients in an advanced stage of disease, those with high initial titers, and those who have previously had syphilis. The treponemal tests are influenced less by therapy than the VDRL and RPR tests are, with seroconversion observed in less than 25% of patients successfully treated during the primary stage of the disease.

The specificity of the nontreponemal tests is at least 98%. However, transient false-positive reactions are seen in patients with acute febrile diseases, after immunizations, and in pregnant women. Long-term false-positive reactions occur most often in patients with chronic autoimmune diseases or infections that involve the liver or that cause extensive tissue destruction. The specificity of the treponemal tests is 97% to 99%, with most false-positive reactions observed in patients with elevated immune globulin levels and autoimmune diseases (Box 41–2). Many of the false-positive reactions can be resolved using the Western blot assay, which may become the preferred confirmatory test.

Positive serologic test results in infants of infected

BOX 41–2. Conditions Associated with False-Positive Serologic Test Results

Nontreponemal Tests	Treponemal Tests
Viral infection	Pyoderma
Rheumatoid arthritis	Skin neoplasm
Systemic lupus erythematosus	Acne vulgaris
Acute or chronic illness	Mycoses
Pregnancy	Crural ulceration
Recent immunization	Rheumatoid arthritis
Drug addiction	Psoriasis
Leprosy	Systemic lupus erythematosus
Malaria	Pregnancy
	Drug addiction
	Herpes genitalis

mothers can represent a passive transfer of antibodies or a specific immunologic response to infection. These two possibilities are distinguished by measuring the antibody titers in the sera of the infant during a 6-month period. The antibody titers in noninfected infants decrease to undetectable levels within 3 months of birth but remain elevated in infants who have congenital syphilis.

Treatment, Prevention, and Control

Penicillin is the drug of choice for treating infections with *T. pallidum.* Long-acting benzathine penicillin is used for the early stages of syphilis, and penicillin G is recommended for congenital and late syphilis. Tetracycline and doxycycline can be used as alternative antibiotics for patients allergic to penicillin. Only penicillin can be used for the treatment of neurosyphilis; thus, penicillin-allergic patients must undergo desensitization. This is also true for pregnant women, who should not be treated with the tetracyclines.

Because protective vaccines are not available, syphilis can be controlled only through the practice of safe sex techniques and adequate contact and treatment of the sex partners of patients who have documented infections. The control of syphilis and other venereal diseases has been complicated by an increase in prostitution among drug abusers.

Other Treponemes

Three other nonvenereal treponemal diseases are important: bejel, yaws, and pinta. These diseases are primarily observed in impoverished children. *T. pallidum* subspecies *endemicum* is responsible for **bejel,** also called **endemic syphilis.** Disease is spread person to person by the use of contaminated eating utensils. The initial oral lesions are rarely observed, but secondary lesions include oral papules and mucosal patches. Gummas of the skin, bones, and nasopharynx are late manifestations. The disease is present in Africa, Asia, and Australia.

T. pertenue is the etiologic agent of **yaws,** a granulomatous disease in which patients have skin lesions early in the disease (Fig. 41–5) and then late destructive lesions of the skin, lymph nodes, and bones. The disease is present in primitive tropical areas of South America, Central Africa, and Southeast Asia and is spread by direct contact with infected skin lesions.

T. carateum is responsible for causing **pinta,** a disease that primarily affects the skin. Small pruritic papules develop on the skin surface after a 1- to 3-week incubation period. These lesions enlarge and persist for months to years before resolving. Disseminated, recurrent, hypopigmented lesions can develop over years, resulting in scarring and disfigurement. Pinta is present in Central and South America and is also spread by direct contact with infected lesions.

Bejel, yaws, and pinta are diagnosed by their typical clinical manifestation in an endemic area. The diagnoses of yaws and pinta are confirmed by the detection of spirochetes in skin lesions by darkfield microscopy, but this test cannot be used to detect spirochetes in patients with the oral lesions of bejel. The results of serologic tests for syphilis are also positive.

Penicillin, tetracycline, and chloramphenicol have been used to treat these diseases. The diseases are controlled through the treatment of infected people and the elimination of person-to-person spread.

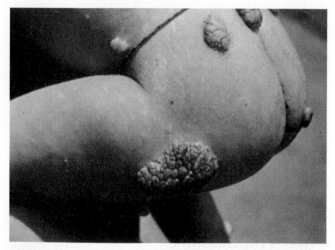

FIGURE 41–5. The elevated papillomatous nodules characteristic of early yaws are widely distributed and painless. They contain numerous spirochetes, which are easily seen on darkfield microscopy studies. (From Peters W, Gilles HM: *A color atlas of tropical medicine and parasitology,* ed 4, London, 1995, Wolfe.)

Borrelia

Members of the genus *Borrelia* cause two important human diseases: relapsing fever and Lyme disease. Relapsing fever is a febrile illness characterized by recurrent episodes of fever and septicemia separated by afebrile periods. Two forms of the disease are recognized. *Borrelia recurrentis* is the etiologic agent of **epidemic** or **louse-borne relapsing fever** and is spread person to person by the human body **louse** (*Pediculus humanus*). **Endemic relapsing fever** is caused by as many as 15 species of borreliae and is spread by infected **soft ticks** of the genus *Ornithodoros*.

The history of **Lyme disease** begins in 1977, when an unusual cluster of children with arthritis was noted in Lyme, Connecticut. Five years later, Burgdorfer discovered the spirochete responsible for this disease. Lyme disease is a tick-borne disease with protean manifestations, including dermatologic, rheumatologic, neurologic, and cardiac abnormalities. All cases of Lyme disease (or Lyme borreliosis) were initially believed to be caused by one organism, *B. burgdorferi*. However, subsequent studies have determined that a complex of at least 10 *Borrelia* species is responsible for Lyme disease in animals and humans. Three species (i.e., *B. burgdorferi, Borrelia garinii, Borrelia afzelii*) cause human disease, with *B. burgdorferi* found in the United States and Europe and *B. garinii* and *B. afzelii* found in Europe and Japan. For the purposes of this chapter, the discussion focuses on *B. burgdorferi* infections.

Physiology and Structure

Members of the genus *Borrelia* are weakly staining, gram-negative bacilli that resemble other spirochetes. They tend to be larger than other spirochetes (0.2 to 0.5 × 3 to 30 μm), stain well with aniline dyes (e.g., Giemsa or Wright stain), and can be easily seen in smears of peripheral blood from patients with relapsing fever (Fig. 41–6) but not those with Lyme disease. From 7 to 20 periplasmic flagella (depending on the species) are present between the periplasmic cylinder and the outer envelope and are responsible for the organism's twisting motility (Fig. 41–7). Borreliae are microaerophilic and have complex nutritional requirements, making it difficult to recover them in culture. The species that have been successfully cultured have generation times of 18 hours or longer. Because culture is generally unsuccessful, diagnosis of diseases caused by borreliae is by microscopy (relapsing fever) or serology (Lyme disease).

Pathogenesis and Immunity

After a person is exposed to infected arthropods, borreliae spread in the blood stream to many organs. Mem-

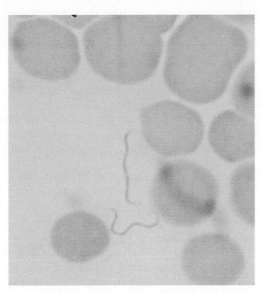

FIGURE 41–6. *Borrelia* organisms present in the blood of a patient with endemic relapsing fever (Giemsa stain).

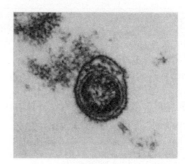

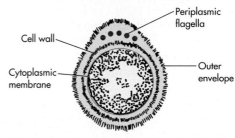

FIGURE 41–7. Electron micrograph and drawing of a cross section through *Borrelia burgdorferi,* the agent that causes Lyme borreliosis. The protoplasmic core of the bacterium is enclosed in a cytoplasmic membrane and conventional cell wall. This in turn is surrounded by an outer envelope, or sheath. Between the protoplasmic core and outer sheath are periplasmic flagella (also called *axial fibrils*), which are anchored at either end of the bacterium and wrap around the protoplasmic core. (From Steere AC et al: The spirochetal etiology of Lyme disease, *N Engl J Med* 308:733–740, 1983.)

bers of the genus do not produce recognized toxins and are removed rapidly when a specific antibody response is mounted. The periodic febrile and afebrile cycles of relapsing fever stem from the ability of the borreliae to undergo antigenic variation. When specific IgM antibodies are formed, agglutination with complement-mediated lysis occurs, and the borreliae are cleared rapidly from the blood stream. However, organisms residing in internal tissues can alter their serotype-specific outer envelope proteins through gene rearrangement and emerge as antigenically novel organisms. The clinical manifestations of relapsing fever are in part a response to the release of endotoxin by the organism.

B. burgdorferi organisms are present in low numbers in the skin when erythema migrans develops. This has been shown by culture of the organism from skin lesions or detection of bacterial nucleic acids by polymerase chain reaction amplification. Spirochetes are infrequently isolated from clinical material late in the disease. It is not known whether the viable organisms cause these late manifestations of disease or whether they represent immunologic cross-reactivity to *Borrelia* antigens. Although the immune response to the organism is depressed at the time that skin lesions initially develop, antibodies develop over months to years and are responsible for producing the complement-mediated clearance of the borreliae.

Epidemiology

The etiologic agent of louse-borne epidemic relapsing fever is *B. recurrentis,* the vector is the human body louse, and humans are the only reservoir (Box 41–3 and Fig. 41–8). Lice become infected after feeding on an infected person. The organisms are ingested, pass through the wall of the gut, and multiply in hemolymph. Disseminated disease is not believed to occur in lice; thus, human infection occurs when the lice are crushed during feeding. Because infected lice do not

Infection	Reservoir	Vector
Relapsing fever Epidemic (louse-borne)	Humans	Body louse
Relapsing fever Endemic (tick-borne)	Rodents, soft-shelled ticks	Soft-shelled tick
Lyme disease	Rodents, deer, domestic pets, hard-shelled ticks	Hard-shelled tick

FIGURE 41–8. Epidemiology of *Borrelia* infections.

BOX 41–3. Summary of *Borrelia* Infections

Physiology and Structure

Epidemic relapsing fever—etiologic agent is *Borrelia recurrentis*.

Endemic relapsing fever—many *Borrelia* species are responsible.

Lyme disease—*Borrelia burgdorferi* causes disease in the United States and Europe; *Borrelia garinii* and *Borrelia afzelii* cause disease in Europe and Asia.

Spirochetes measure 0.2×0.5 to $30 \ \mu m$.

Can be seen when stained with aniline dyes (e.g., Giemsa, Wright stains).

Can grow in culture, but bacteria are microaerophilic and have complex nutritional requirements.

Virulence Factors

Borrelia responsible for relapsing fever are able to undergo antigenic shift and escape immune clearance; periodic febrile and afebrile periods result from antigenic variation.

Immune reactivity against the Lyme disease agents may be responsible for the clinical disease.

Epidemiology

Epidemic relapsing fever: transmitted person to person; reservoir—humans; vector—human body louse.

Endemic relapsing fever: transmitted rodents to humans; reservoirs—rodents, small mammals, and soft ticks; vector—soft ticks.

Individuals at risk for relapsing fever include people exposed to lice (epidemic disease) in crowded or unsanitary conditions and people exposed to ticks (endemic disease) in rural areas.

Epidemic relapsing fever is endemic in Ethiopia, Rwanda, and the Andean foothills.

Endemic relapsing fever has worldwide distribution and is in the western states of the United States.

Lyme disease: transmitted by hard ticks from mice to humans; reservoir—mice, deer, ticks; vectors include *Ixodes scapularis* in eastern and midwestern United States, *Ixodes pacificus* in the western United States, *Ixodes ricinus* in Europe, and *Ixodes persulcatus* in Eastern Europe and Asia.

Individuals at risk for Lyme disease include people exposed to ticks in areas of high endemicity.

Lyme disease has worldwide distribution.

Seasonal incidence corresponds to feeding patterns of vectors; most cases of Lyme disease in the United States occur in late spring and early summer (feeding pattern of nymphs).

Diseases

Epidemic relapsing fever.

Endemic relapsin fever.

Lyme disease.

Diagnosis

Refer to Box 41–4.

Treatment, Prevention, and Control

For relapsing fever, treatment is with tetracycline or erythromycin.

For Lyme disease, treatment is with amoxicillin, tetracycline, cefuroxime, or ceftriaxone.

Exposure to the insect vector can be decreased by using insecticides and applying insect repellents to clothing and by wearing protective clothing that reduces exposure of skin to insects.

Recombinant ospA vaccine is available for Lyme disease.

---

survive for more than a few months, maintenance of the disease requires crowded, unsanitary conditions (e.g., wars, natural disasters) that permit frequent human contact with infected lice. Although epidemics of louse-borne relapsing fever swept from Eastern to Western Europe in the past century, disease now appears to be restricted to Ethiopia, Rwanda, and the Andean foothills.

Several features distinguish endemic relapsing fever from epidemic disease. Tick-borne endemic relapsing fever is a zoonotic disease, with rodents, small mammals, and soft ticks (*Ornithodoros* species) the main reservoirs and many species of *Borrelia* responsible for the disease. Unlike the louse-borne infections, the borreliae that cause endemic disease produce a disseminated infection in ticks. However, the arthropods can survive and maintain an endemic reservoir of infection by transsovarian transmission. Furthermore, ticks can survive for months between feedings. A history of a tick

bite may also not be elicited because soft ticks are primarily nocturnal feeders and remain attached for only a few minutes. The ticks contaminate the bite wound with borreliae present in saliva or feces. Tick-borne disease is found worldwide, corresponding to the distribution of the *Ornithodoros* tick. In the United States, disease is primarily found in the western states.

Despite the relatively recent recognition of Lyme disease in the United States, retrospective studies have shown that the disease was present for many years in this and other countries. Lyme disease has now been described on 6 continents, in at least 20 countries, and in 49 states of the United States. The incidence of disease has risen dramatically since 1982, when 497 cases were reported, to 1998, when more than 16,802 cases were reported (Fig. 41–9). Lyme disease is the leading vector-borne disease in the United States. The three principal foci of infection in the United States are the Northeast (Massachusetts to Maryland), the up-

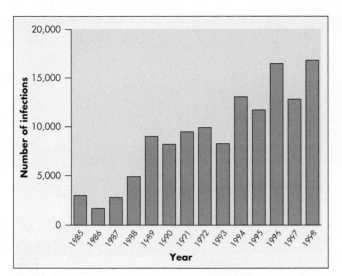

FIGURE 41-9. Lyme disease in the United States, 1985 to 1998.

per Midwest (Minnesota and Wisconsin), and the Pacific West (California and Oregon). Hard ticks are the major vectors of Lyme disease: *Ixodes scapularis* in the Northeast and Midwest and *Ixodes pacificus* on the West Coast. *Ixodes ricinus* is the major tick vector in Europe, and *Ixodes persulcatus* in Eastern Europe and Asia. The major reservoir hosts in the United States are the white-footed mouse and white-tailed deer. The white-footed mouse is the primary host of larval and nymph forms of *Ixodes* species, and the adult *Ixodes* species infest the white-tailed deer. Because the nymph stage causes more than 90% of the cases of documented disease, the mouse host is more relevant for human disease.

Ixodes larvae become infected when they feed on the mouse reservoir. The larva molts to a nymph in late spring and takes a second blood meal; in this case, humans can be accidental hosts. Although the borreliae are transmitted in the tick's saliva during a prolonged period of feeding (48 hours or more), most patients do not remember having had a specific tick bite because the nymph is the size of a poppy seed. The nymphs mature into adults in the late summer and take a third feeding. Although the white-tailed deer is the natural host, humans can also be infected at this stage. Most infected patients are identified in May to August, although disease can be encountered throughout the year.

Clinical Diseases

Relapsing Fever

The clinical presentations of epidemic louse-borne and endemic tick-borne relapsing fever are essentially the same, although a small pruritic eschar may develop at

the site of the tick bite (Fig. 41–10). After a 1-week incubation period, the disease is heralded by the abrupt onset of shaking chills, fever, muscle aches, and headache. Splenomegaly and hepatomegaly are common. These symptoms correspond to the bacteremic phase of the disease and resolve after 3 to 7 days, when the borreliae are cleared from the blood. Bacteremia and fever return after a 1-week afebrile period. The clinical symptoms are generally milder and last a shorter time during this and subsequent febrile episodes. A single relapse is characteristic of epidemic louse-borne disease, and repeated relapses are common in endemic tick-borne disease. The clinical course and outcome of epidemic relapsing fever tend to be more severe than they are in those with endemic disease, but this may be related to the patients' underlying poor state of health. Mortality with endemic disease is less than 5% but can be 4% to 40% in epidemic disease.

Lyme Disease

Clinical diagnosis of Lyme disease is complicated by the varied manifestations of disease caused by *B. burg-*

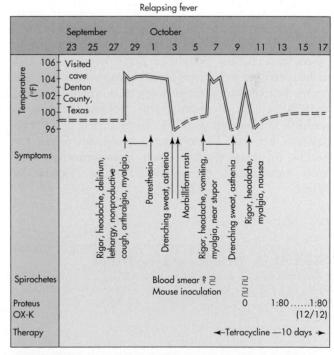

FIGURE 41–10. The clinical evolution of tick-borne relapsing fever in a 14-year-old boy. The initial febrile episode is typically the most severe. Subsequent episodes tend to be shorter and less intense. Although nonspecific reactivity with *Proteus* Ox-K antigens is frequently observed, the specific diagnosis is made on the basis of the observation of borreliae in peripheral blood smears. These are positive for organisms only during the febrile periods. (Modified from Southern P, Sanford J: Relapsing fever: a clinical and microbiological review, *Medicine* 48:129–149, 1969.)

dorferi and other *Borrelia* species, as well as the lack of reliable diagnostic tests. The clinical and laboratory definitions of Lyme disease that are recommended by the Centers for Disease Control and Prevention are summarized in Box 41–4. The following is a description of Lyme disease in the United States. The frequency of the skin lesions and late manifestations differ in disease observed in other countries.

After an incubation period of 3 to 30 days, one or more skin lesions typically develop at the site of the tick bite. The lesion (**erythema migrans**) begins as a small macule or papule and then enlarges over the next few weeks, ultimately covering an area ranging from 5 cm to more than 50 cm in diameter (Fig. 41–11). The lesion typically has a flat red border and central clearing as it develops; however, erythema, vesicle formation, and central necrosis can also be seen. The lesion fades and disappears within weeks, although new transient lesions may subsequently appear. Other early signs and symptoms of Lyme disease include malaise, severe fatigue, headache, fever, chills, musculoskeletal pains, myalgias, and lymphadenopathy. These last for an average of 4 weeks.

Late manifestations develop in almost 80% of patients with untreated Lyme disease. These can develop from within a week of the onset of disease to more than 2 years later. The late stage consists of two phases. The first involves neurologic symptoms (meningitis, encephalitis, peripheral nerve neuropathy) and cardiac dysfunction (heart block, myopericarditis, congestive heart failure). These symptoms are encountered in 10% to 15% of patients and can last for days to months. The second phase is characterized by arthralgias and arthritis. These complications can persist for months to years, during which spirochetes are only rarely visualized in the involved tissue or isolated in culture.

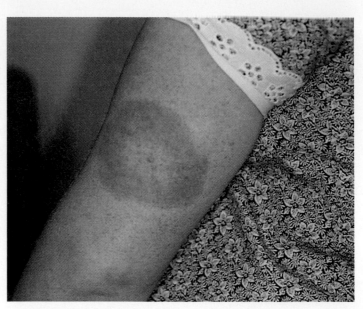

FIGURE 41–11. Erythema migrans rash on the arm of a patient with Lyme borreliosis.

Laboratory Diagnosis

Microscopy

Because of their relatively large size, borreliae that cause relapsing fever can be seen during the febrile period on Giemsa- or Wright-stained preparation of blood. This is the most sensitive method for diagnosing relapsing fever, with smears positive for organisms in more than 70% of patients. The sensitivity of the test can be improved by inoculating a mouse with blood from infected patients and then after 1 to 10 days examining the mouse's blood for the presence of borreliae. Microscopic examination of blood or tissues from patients with Lyme disease is not recommended because *B. burgdorferi* is rarely seen in clinical specimens.

Culture

Some borreliae, including *B. recurrentis* and *Borrelia hermsii* (a common cause of endemic relapsing fever in the United States), can be cultured in vitro on specialized media. The cultures are rarely performed in most clinical laboratories, however, because the media are not readily available and the organisms grow slowly on them. There has been limited success with the culture of *B. burgdorferi*, although isolation of the organism has been improved through the use of specialized media. However, the sensitivity of culture is low for all specimens except the initial skin lesion, which is pathognomonic, thus making culture rarely necessary.

BOX 41–4. Definition of Lyme Disease

Clinical Case Definition

Either of the following:
  Erythema migrans (≥5 cm in diameter)
  At least one late manifestation (i.e., musculoskeletal, nervous system, or cardiovascular involvement) and laboratory confirmation of infection

Laboratory Criteria for Diagnosis

At least one of the following:
  Isolation of *Borrelia burgdorferi*
  Demonstration of diagnostic levels of IgM or IgG antibodies to the spirochetes
  Significant increase in antibody titer between acute and convalescent serum samples

Serology

Serologic tests are not useful in the diagnosis of relapsing fever because the borreliae that cause this condition undergo antigenic phase variation. In contrast, serologic testing is an important confirmatory test for patients with suspected Lyme disease. The tests most commonly used are the immunofluorescence assay and enzyme-linked immunosorbent assay (ELISA). ELISA is preferred because it is more sensitive and specific for all stages of Lyme disease. Unfortunately, all serologic tests are relatively insensitive during the early acute stage of disease. IgM antibodies appear 2 to 4 weeks after the onset of erythema migrans in untreated patients; the levels peak after 6 to 8 weeks of illness and then decline to a normal range after 4 to 6 months. The IgM level may remain elevated in some patients with a persistent infection. The IgG antibodies appear later. Their levels peak after 4 to 6 months of illness and persist during the late manifestations of the disease. Thus, most patients with late complications of Lyme disease have detectable antibodies to *B. burgdorferi*, although the antibody level may be ablated in patients treated with antibiotics. Detection of antibodies in cerebrospinal fluid is strong evidence for neuroborreliosis.

Although cross-reactions are uncommon, positive serologic results must be interpreted carefully, particularly if the titers are low (Box 41–5). Most false-positive reactions occur in patients with syphilis. These can be excluded by performing a nontreponemal test for syphilis; the result is negative in patients with Lyme disease.

Western blot analysis has been used to confirm the specificity of a positive ELISA reaction. The 41-kDa flagellar antigen (common to many spirochetes) is the major target of IgM antibodies. IgG antibodies against other antigens (e.g., 31-kDa outer surface protein A [ospA], 34-kDa ospB, 21-kDa ospC, 60-kDa common heat shock protein) develop late in disease. However, specific reactions with antigens unique to *B. burgdorferi*

BOX 41–5. **Bacteria and Diseases Associated with Cross-Reactions in Serologic Tests for Lyme Borreliosis**

Treponema pallidum
Oral spirochetes
Other *Borrelia* species
Juvenile rheumatoid arthritis
Rheumatoid arthritis
Systemic lupus erythematosus
Infectious mononucleosis
Subacute bacterial endocarditis

---

need to be detected for this test to be considered useful.

Antigenic heterogeneity in *B. burgdorferi* and other *Borrelia* species that cause Lyme disease affects the test sensitivity. The magnitude of this problem in the United States is unknown, but it should be significant in Europe and Asia, where many *Borrelia* species are found to cause Lyme disease. At present, serologic tests should be considered confirmatory and should not be performed in the absence of an appropriate history and clinical symptoms of Lyme disease. Preliminary studies have shown that the detection of *Borrelia*-specific DNA amplified by polymerase chain reaction may be an effective diagnostic test for Lyme disease. However, this test is not yet commercially available.

Treatment, Prevention, and Control

Relapsing fever has been treated most effectively with tetracycline or erythromycin. Tetracycline is the drug of choice but is contraindicated for pregnant women and young children. A Jarisch-Herxheimer reaction (shocklike profile with rigors, leukopenia, an increase in temperature, and a decrease in blood pressure) can occur in patients within a few hours after therapy is started and must be carefully managed. This reaction corresponds to the rapid killing of borreliae and the possible release of toxic products such as endotoxin.

The early manifestations of Lyme disease are effectively managed with orally administered doxycycline or amoxicillin. Cefuroxime can be used as alternative therapy. Antibiotic treatment lessens the likelihood and the severity of late complications. Despite this intervention, Lyme arthritis and other complications occur in a small number of patients. Ceftriaxone, doxycycline, or amoxicillin has been used for the treatment of these manifestations. Patients with neurologic and musculoskeletal disease typically require prolonged treatment, and relapses may necessitate re-treatment.

Prevention of tick-borne *Borrelia* diseases includes avoiding ticks and their natural habitats, wearing protective clothing such as long pants tucked into socks, and applying insect repellents. Rodent control is also important in the prevention of endemic relapsing fever. Epidemic louse-borne disease is controlled through the use of delousing sprays and improvements in hygienic conditions.

Vaccines are not available for relapsing fever. A recombinant vaccine directed against the ospA antigen of *B. burgdorferi* elicits protective antibodies in experimental animals and humans. In two human trials, efficacy was demonstrated in 76% to 92% of the vaccinees who received the primary dose and two booster doses. The mode of action of the vaccine is unique. Antibodies develop against the ospA antigen. However, this antigen is not expressed in infected individuals. Thus, circulating antibodies must be present at the time the tick feeds. The antibodies are transferred to the tick and in turn inactivate the borreliae in the tick gut. This approach to vaccine protection is problematic because ospA heterogeneity among *Borrelia* species is well-known. Circulating antibodies reactive with the specific ospA antigen must be maintained for the vaccine to be effective. Thus, there is considerable interest in replacing these first-generation vaccines with more broadly reactive products.

Leptospira

Physiology and Structure

The taxonomy of the genus *Leptospira* is the source of great confusion. Traditionally, the genus has been grouped by serologic relationships and pathogenicity. Pathogenic strains were placed in the species *Leptospira interrogans*, which currently contains 218 serovars. Nonpathogenic strains were placed in the species *Leptospira biflexa*, with 63 serovars. However, this classification is not consistent with nucleic acid analysis, which supports subdividing the genus into three genera with 17 species. Maybe it is fortunate that this nomenclature has not yet been adopted universally; the more traditional subdivision into two species is used here. The species names are derived from the fact that *Leptospira* organisms are thin, coiled bacilli (0.1 × 6 to 12 μm) with a hook at one or both ends (*interrogans*, meaning "shaped like a question mark"; *biflexa*, for "twice bent") (Fig. 41–12). *L. biflexa* is a free-living saprophyte found in moist environmental sites and is not associated with disease in humans or animals. *L. interrogans* is pathogenic for many wild and domestic animals, as well as humans. About 22 serotypes of *L. interrogans* cause human disease in the United States, with serotypes *icterohaemorrhagiae, canicola, pomona,* and *autumnalis* the most common. Some serotypes have been historically associated with specific clinical presentations (*icterohaemorrhagiae,* **Weil's disease;** *pomona,* **swineherd's disease;** *autumnalis,* **Fort Bragg fever** or pretibial eruptions), but it is now recognized that the illnesses are not specific to individual serotypes.

The pathogenic leptospires are obligatively aerobic and motile by means of two periplasmic flagella, each anchored at opposite ends of the bacterium. They use fatty acids and alcohols as sources of carbon and energy. The leptospires can be grown on specially formulated media enriched with rabbit serum or bovine serum albumin.

Pathogenesis and Immunity

L. interrogans can cause subclinical infection, a mild influenza-like febrile illness, or severe systemic disease

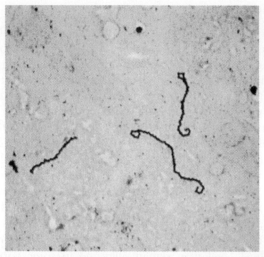

FIGURE 41–12. *Leptospira interrogans* serotype *icterohaemorrhagiae.* Silver staining of organisms grown in culture. Notice the tightly coiled body with hooked ends (more typically a characteristic of *Leptospira biflexa*). (From Emond R, Rowland H: *Color atlas of infectious diseases,* ed 3, London, 1995, Wolfe.)

(Weil's disease), with renal and hepatic failure, extensive vasculitis, myocarditis, and death. The severity of the disease is influenced by the number of infecting organisms, the host's immunologic defenses, and the virulence of the infecting strain.

Because leptospires are thin and highly motile, they can penetrate intact mucous membranes or skin through small cuts or abrasions. They can then spread in the blood stream into all tissues, including the central nervous system. *L. interrogans* multiplies rapidly and damages the endothelium of small blood vessels, resulting in the major clinical manifestations of disease (e.g., meningitis, hepatic and renal dysfunction, hemorrhage). Organisms can be found in blood and cerebrospinal fluid early in the disease and in urine during the later stages. Clearance of leptospires occurs when humoral immunity develops. However, some clinical manifestations may stem from immunologic reactions with the organisms. For example, meningitis develops after the organisms have been removed from the cerebrospinal fluid and immune complexes have been detected in renal lesions.

Epidemiology

Leptospirosis has a worldwide distribution (Box 41–6). Fewer than 100 human infections are normally documented in the United States each year; most cases are reported from Hawaii. However, the incidence of disease is significantly underestimated because most infec-

---

BOX 41–6. Summary of *Leptospira* Infections

Physiology and Structure

Complex taxonomy with many species and many serovars; traditional classification subdivides genus into saprophytic strains (*Leptospira biflexa*) and pathogenic strains (*Leptospira interrogans*).

Thin, coiled spirochetes (0.1×6 to $12 \ \mu m$). One or both ends hook-shaped.

Obligate aerobe; slow growing in culture.

Virulence Factors

Direct invasion and replication in tissues.
Immune complex glomerulonephritis.

Epidemiology

U.S. reservoirs: rodents (particularly rats), dogs, farm animals, and wild animals.

Humans: accidental end-stage host.

Organism can penetrate the skin through minor breaks in the epidermis.

People are infected with leptospires through exposure to water contaminated with urine from an infected animal or handling of tissues from an infected animal.

People at risk are those exposed to urine-contaminated streams, rivers, and standing water; occupational exposure to infected animals for farmers, meat handlers, veterinarians.

Infection is rare in the United States but has worldwide distribution.

Disease is more common during warm months (recreational exposure).

Diseases

Mild virus-like syndrome.

Systemic leptospirosis with aseptic meningitis.

Overwhelming disease (Weil's disease) with vascular collapse, thrombocytopenia, hemorrhage, and hepatic and renal dysfunction.

Diagnosis

Refer to Table 41–4.

Treatment, Prevention, and Control

Treatment of severe infections involves intravenous penicillin or ampicillin; mild infections treated with oral ampicillin, amoxicillin, or doxycycline.

Doxycycline, but not the penicillins, is used for prophylaxis.

Herds and domestic pets should be vaccinated.

Rats should be controlled.

---

tions are mild and misdiagnosed as a "viral syndrome" or viral aseptic meningitis. Because many states failed to report this disease to the public health service, mandatory reporting was discontinued in 1995. Thus, it will be impossible to determine the true prevalence of this disease in the future.

Many wild and domestic animals are colonized with leptospires. Rodents (particularly rats), dogs, and farm animals are the most common sources of human disease in the United States. Serologic studies have shown a high incidence of exposure to leptospires in urban youths. This is attributed to their contact with the urine of infected rats. Chronic carriage in humans has not been demonstrated.

Leptospires usually cause asymptomatic infections in their reservoir host, in which the spirochetes colonize the renal tubules and are shed in urine in large numbers. Streams, rivers, standing water, and moist soil can be contaminated with urine from infected animals and can serve as a source for human infection, with organisms surviving for as long as 6 weeks in such sites. Leptospires require a moist, alkaline environment to survive. Most human infections result from recreational exposure to contaminated water or occupational exposure to infected animals (farmers, slaughterhouse workers, and veterinarians). Most human infections occur during the warm months, when recreational exposure is greatest. Person-to-person spread has not been documented.

Clinical Diseases

Most infections with *L. interrogans* are clinically inapparent and detected only through the demonstration of specific antibodies. Symptomatic infections develop after a 1- to 2-week incubation period. The initial presentation is similar to an influenza-like illness, with fever and myalgias. During this phase, the patient is bacteremic with the leptospires, and the organisms can frequently be isolated in cerebrospinal fluid, even though no meningeal symptoms are present. The fever and myalgias may remit after 1 week, or the patient may develop a more advanced disease—including aseptic meningitis—or a generalized illness with headache, rash, vascular collapse, thrombocytopenia, hemorrhage, and hepatic and renal dysfunction (Weil's disease).

Leptospirosis confined to the central nervous system can be mistaken for viral meningitis because the course of the disease is generally uncomplicated and has a very low mortality rate. Culture of cerebrospinal fluid is usually negative at this stage. In contrast, the icteric form of generalized disease (approximately 10% of all symptomatic infections) is more severe and is associated with a mortality approaching 10%. Although hepatic involvement with jaundice is striking in patients with severe leptospirosis, hepatic necrosis is not seen, and surviving patients do not suffer permanent hepatic damage. Similarly, most patients recover full renal function.

Congenital leptospirosis can also occur. This disease is characterized by the sudden onset of headache, fever, myalgias, and a diffuse rash.

Laboratory Diagnosis

The tests used to diagnose leptospirosis are summarized in Table 41–4.

Microscopy

Because leptospires are thin, they are at the limit of the resolving power of a light microscope and thus cannot be seen easily by conventional light microscopy. Neither Gram stain nor silver stain is reliable in the detection of leptospires. Darkfield microscopy is also relatively insensitive and can yield nonspecific findings. Although leptospires can be seen in blood specimens early in the disease, protein filaments from erythrocytes can be easily mistaken for organisms. Fluorescein-labeled antibody preparations have been used to stain leptospires but are not available in most clinical laboratories.

Culture

Leptospires can be cultured on specially formulated media (Fletcher, EMJH, or Tween 80–albumin). They grow slowly (generation time, 6 to 16 hours), requiring incubation at 28°C to 30°C for as long as 4 months; however, most cultures are positive within 2 weeks.

L. interrogans can be recovered in blood or cerebrospinal fluid during the first 10 days of infection and in urine after the first week and for as long as 3 months. Because the concentration of organisms in blood, cerebrospinal fluid, and urine may be low, several specimens should be collected if leptospirosis is suspected. In addition, inhibitors present in blood and urine may delay or prevent recovery of leptospires.

Nucleic Acid Probes

Preliminary work with the detection of leptospires using nucleic acid probes has had limited success. Techniques using nucleic acid amplification (e.g., polymerase chain reaction) are more sensitive than direct hybridization methods. Unfortunately, commercial molecular diagnostic systems are not currently available.

Serology

Because of the need for specialized media and prolonged incubation, most laboratories do not attempt to culture leptospires and thus rely on serologic techniques. The reference method for all serologic tests is the **microscopic agglutination test.** This test measures the ability of the patient's serum to agglutinate live leptospires. Because the test is directed against specific serotypes, it is necessary to use pools of leptospiral antigens. In this test, serial dilutions of the patient's serum are mixed with the test antigens and then examined microscopically for agglutination. Agglutinins appear in the blood of untreated patients during the second week of illness, although this response may be delayed for as long as several months. Infected patients have a titer of at least 1:100, and it may be 1:25,000 or higher. Patients treated with antibiotics may have a

TABLE 41–4. Diagnostic Tests for Leptospirosis		
Diagnostic Test	**Method**	**Test Accuracy**
Microscopy	Gram stain	Organisms too thin to be detected
	Darkfield examination	Insensitive, nonspecific
	Silver stain	Insensitive, nonspecific
	Direct fluorescent antibody	Insensitive, specific
Culture	Blood	Positive during first 10 days
	Cerebrospinal fluid	Positive during first 10 days
	Urine	Positive after first week
Nucleic acid probes	Direct hybridization	Insensitive, specific
	Amplification (e.g., polymerase chain reaction)	Sensitive, specific
Serology	Indirect hemagglutination, slide agglutination, enzyme-linked immunosorbent assay	Insensitive, nonspecific
	Microscopic agglutination test	Sensitive, specific, reference laboratory test, serovar specific

diminished antibody response or nondiagnostic titers. Agglutinating antibodies are detectable for many years after the acute illness; thus, their presence may represent either a blunted antibody response in a treated patient with acute disease or residual antibodies in a person with a distant, unrecognized infection with leptospires. Because the microscopic agglutination test uses live organisms, it is performed only in reference laboratories. Alternative tests such as indirect hemagglutination, slide agglutination, and ELISA are less sensitive and specific and are not recommended.

Treatment, Prevention, and Control

Leptospirosis is usually not fatal, particularly in the absence of icteric disease. Patients with severe disease should be treated with intravenously administered penicillin or ampicillin, and patients with less severe disease can be treated with orally administered doxycycline, ampicillin, or amoxicillin. Doxycycline, but not the penicillins, can be used to prevent disease in persons exposed to infected animals or water contaminated with urine. It is difficult to eradicate leptospirosis because the disease is widespread in wild and domestic animals. However, vaccination of livestock and pets has proved successful in reducing the incidence of disease in these populations and therefore subsequent human exposure. Rodent control is also effective in eliminating leptospirosis in communities.

CASE STUDY AND QUESTIONS

■ An 18-year-old woman seen by her physician complained of knee pain that started 2 weeks previously. Three months earlier, soon after vacationing in Connecticut, she noticed a circular area of redness on her lower leg; it was approximately 10 cm in diameter. During the next 2 weeks, the area enlarged and the border became more clearly demarcated; however, the rash gradually disappeared. A few days after the rash disappeared, she experienced the onset of headaches, an inability to concentrate, and nausea. These symptoms also gradually abated. The pain in her knee developed approximately 1 month after these symptoms disappeared. On examination of the knee, mild tenderness and pain were elicited. A small amount of serous fluid was aspirated from the joint, and it had an elevated white blood cell count. Antibodies to *B. burgdorferi* were present in the patient's serum (titers of 1:32 and 1:1024 for IgM and IgG, respectively), confirming the clinical diagnosis of Lyme arthritis.

1. What are the initial and late manifestations of Lyme disease?
2. What are the limitations of the following diagnostic tests for Lyme disease: microscopy, culture, and serology? How does this compare with the diagnostic tests for other relapsing fevers?
3. Name two examples each of nontreponemal and treponemal tests for syphilis. What reactions to those tests would you expect in patients with primary, secondary, and late syphilis?
4. What are the reservoir and vectors for syphilis, epidemic and endemic relapsing fever, Lyme disease, and leptospirosis?
5. What diagnostic tests can be used for the diagnosis of leptospirosis?

BIBLIOGRAPHY

Balmelli T, Piffaretti J: Analysis of the genetic polymorphism of *Borrelia burgdorferi sensu lato* by multilocus enzyme electrophoresis, *Int J Syst Bacteriol* 46:167–172, 1996.

Barbour AG, Hayes SF: Biology of *Borrelia* species, *Microbiol Rev* 50:381–400, 1986.

Butler T et al: Infection with *Borrelia recurrentis:* pathogenesis of fever and petechiae, *J Infect Dis* 140:665–672, 1979.

Centers for Disease Control and Prevention: Surveillance for Lyme Disease — United States, 1992–1998, *MMWR* 49:1–12, 2000.

Cutler S et al: *Borrelia recurrentis* characterization and comparison with relapsing fever, Lyme-associated, and other *Borrelia* spp., *Int J Syst Bacteriol* 47:958–968, 1997.

Gardner P: Lyme disease vaccines, *Ann Intern Med* 129:583–585, 1998 (editorial).

Heath CW, Alexander AD, Galton MM: Leptospirosis in the United States: analysis of 483 cases in man, 1949–1961, *N Engl J Med* 273:857–864, 915–922, 1965.

Johnson B et al: Serodiagnosis of Lyme disease: accuracy of a two-step approach using a flagella-based ELISA and immunoblotting, *J Infect Dis* 174:346–353, 1996.

Larsen S, Steiner B, Rudolph A: Laboratory diagnosis and interpretation of tests for syphilis, *Clin Microbiol Rev* 8:1–21, 1995.

Mouritsen C et al: Polymerase chain reaction detection of Lyme disease: correlation with clinical manifestations and serologic responses, *Am J Clin Pathol* 105:647–654, 1996.

Ras N et al: Phylogenesis of relapsing fever *Borrelia* spp., *Int J Syst Bacteriol* 46:859–865, 1996.

Rolfs R: Treatment of syphilis, 1993, *Clin Infect Dis* 20(suppl 1):S23–S38, 1995.

Romanowski B et al: Serologic response to treatment of infectious syphilis, *Ann Intern Med* 114:1005–1009, 1991.

Southern PM, Sanford JP: Relapsing fever: a clinical and microbiological review, *Medicine* 48:129–149, 1969.

Spach D et al: Tick-borne diseases in the United States, *N Engl J Med* 329:936–947, 1993.

Steigbigel R, Benach J: Immunization against Lyme Disease — an important first step, *N Engl J Med* 339:263–264, 1998.

Tugwell P et al: Guidelines for laboratory evaluation in the diagnosis of Lyme disease, I and II, *Ann Intern Med* 127: 1106–1123, 1997.

Van Dam A et al: Different genospecies of *Borrelia burgdorferi* are associated with distinct clinical manifestations of Lyme borreliosis, *Clin Infect Dis* 17:708–717, 1993.

Vinetz J et al: Sporadic urban leptospirosis, *Ann Intern Med* 125:794–798, 1996.

Wang G et al: Molecular typing of *Borrelia burgdorferi sensu lata:* taxonomic, epidemiological, and clinical implications, *Clin Microbiol Rev* 12:633–653, 1999.

Wormser G et al: Practice guidelines for the treatment of Lyme disease, *Clin Infect Dis* 31 (S1):1–14, 2000.

CHAPTER 42

Mycoplasma and *Ureaplasma*

The class of organisms Mollicutes is subdivided into four families, with the human pathogens placed in the family Mycoplasmataceae. This family contains two genera, *Mycoplasma* and *Ureaplasma*, 13 species of which colonize or cause disease in humans (Table 42–1). The most important species is *Mycoplasma pneumoniae* (also called **Eaton's agent** after the investigator who originally isolated it). *M. pneumoniae* causes respiratory tract diseases, such as tracheobronchitis and pneumonia (Box 42–1). Other pathogens that are commonly isolated are *Mycoplasma hominis*, *Mycoplasma genitalium*, and *Ureaplasma urealyticum*, which cause genitourinary tract diseases. These and other mycoplasmas that colonize humans have been associated with a variety of maladies (e.g., infertility, spontaneous abortion, vaginitis, cervicitis, epididymitis, prostatitis). However, their etiologic role in these diseases remains incompletely defined.

Physiology and Structure

Mycoplasma and *Ureaplasma* organisms are the smallest free-living bacteria (Table 42–2). They are unique among bacteria because they do not have a cell wall and their cell membrane contains **sterols**. In contrast, other cell wall–deficient bacteria (also called **L forms**) do not have sterols in their cell membrane and can form cell walls under the appropriate growth conditions. The absence of the cell wall renders the mycoplasmas resistant to penicillins, cephalosporins, vancomycin, and other antibiotics that interfere with synthesis of the cell wall.

The mycoplasmas form pleomorphic filaments with an average diameter of 0.1 to 0.3 μm, and many can pass through the 0.45-μm filters used to remove bacteria from solutions. For these reasons, the mycoplasmas were originally thought to be viruses. However, the organisms divide by binary fission (typical of all bacteria), grow on artificial cell-free media, and contain both RNA and DNA. Mycoplasmas are facultatively anaerobic (except *M. pneumoniae*, which is a strict aerobe) and require exogenous sterols supplied by animal serum added to the growth medium. The mycoplasmas grow slowly, with a generation time of 1 to 6 hours, and most form small colonies that have a fried-egg appearance (Fig. 42–1). *M. pneumoniae* is an exception in this respect as well, because its colonies do not have a thin halo and have been described as "mulberry-shaped." Colonies of *Ureaplasma* (formerly called "T strains" for tiny strains) are extremely small, measuring 10 to 50 μm in diameter.

Because the Mycoplasmataceae do not have a cell wall, the major antigenic determinants are membrane glycolipids and proteins. These antigens cross-react with human tissues and other bacteria.

Pathogenesis and Immunity

M. pneumoniae is an extracellular pathogen that adheres to the respiratory epithelium by means of a specialized terminal protein attachment factor. This adhesin protein, called **P1**, interacts specifically with sialated glycoprotein receptors at the base of cilia on the epithelial cell surface (as well as on the surface of erythrocytes). Ciliostasis then occurs, after which first the cilia then the ciliated epithelial cells are destroyed. The loss of these cells interferes with the normal clearance of the upper airways and permits the lower respiratory tract to become contaminated with microbes and mechanically irritated. This process is responsible for the persistent cough present in patients with symptomatic disease. *M. pneumoniae* functions as a superantigen, stimulating inflammatory cells to migrate to the site of infection and release cytokines, initially tumor necrosis factor-α (TNF-α) and interleukin-1 (IL-1) and later IL-6. This process contributes to both the clearance of the bacteria and the observed disease.

Epidemiology

Pneumonia caused by *M. pneumoniae* occurs worldwide throughout the year, with no consistent increase in seasonal activity. However, because pneumonia caused by other infectious agents (e.g., *Streptococcus pneumoniae*,

TABLE 42–1. Mycoplasmataceae Isolated in Humans

Organism	Site	Disease
Mycoplasma pneumoniae	Respiratory tract	Upper respiratory tract disease, atypical pneumonia, tracheobronchitis
Mycoplasma hominis	Genitourinary tract	Pyelonephritis, pelvic inflammatory disease, postpartum fever
Mycoplasma genitalium	Genitourinary tract	Urethritis
Mycoplasma orale	Respiratory tract	Unknown
Mycoplasma salivarium	Respiratory tract	Unknown
Mycoplasma buccale	Respiratory tract	Unknown
Mycoplasma faucium	Respiratory tract	Unknown
Mycoplasma lipophilum	Respiratory tract	Unknown
Mycoplasma primatum	Respiratory and genitourinary tracts	Unknown
Mycoplasma fermentans	Genitourinary tract	Unknown
Mycoplasma fermentans var. *incognitus*	Blood	Fulminant disseminated disease in patients with acquired immunodeficiency syndrome (AIDS)
Mycoplasma pirum	Blood	Septicemia in patients with AIDS
Ureaplasma urealyticum	Genitourinary tract	Urethritis

viruses) is more common during the cold months, *M. pneumoniae* disease is proportionally more common during the summer and fall. Epidemic disease occurs every 4 to 8 years. Disease is most common in school-aged children and young adults (5 to 15 years). Disease was once believed to be uncommon in older adults; however, studies have now demonstrated that all age groups are susceptible to infections with this organism.

It has been estimated that 2 million cases of *M. pneumoniae* pneumonia and more than 20 million cases of other respiratory diseases caused by this organism occur annually in the United States. *M. pneumoniae* disease is not reportable, and reliable diagnostic tests are not readily available, so the true incidence is not known.

Infection is spread by nasal secretions. Close contact is necessary for transmission, and the infection usually occurs among classmates or family members. The attack rate is higher in children than in adults (overall average, approximately 60%), presumably because most adults are partially immune from previous exposure. The incubation period and time of infectivity are pro-

BOX 42–1. Summary of *Mycoplasma pneumoniae* Infections

Physiology and Structure

The smallest free-living bacterium; able to pass through 0.45-μm pore filters.

Absence of cell wall and a cell membrane containing sterols are unique among bacteria.

Slow rate of growth (generation time, 1 to 6 hours); strict aerobe.

Virulence

P1 adhesin binds to base of cilia on epithelial cells, leading to eventual loss of ciliated epithelial cells.

Acts as superantigen, stimulating migration of inflammatory cells and release of cytokines.

Epidemiology

Worldwide disease with no seasonal incidence (in contrast to disease caused by most respiratory pathogens).

Primarily infects children aged 5 to 15 years, but all populations susceptible to disease.

Transmitted by inhalation of aerosolized droplet.

Strict human pathogen.

Diseases

Upper respiratory infections.

Lower respiratory infections, including tracheobronchitis and bronchopneumonia.

Diagnosis

(Refer to Table 42–3.)

Treatment, Control, and Prevention

Drug of choice is erythromycin or tetracycline (not used in young children).

Immunity to reinfection is not lifelong, and vaccines have proved ineffective.

longed; thus, disease can persist for months among classmates or family members.

Infants, particularly girls, are colonized with *M. hominis*, *M. genitalium*, and *Ureaplasma* species at birth, with *Ureaplasma* organisms being isolated most frequently. Although carriage of these mycoplasmas usually does not persist, a small proportion of prepubertal children remains colonized. The incidence of genital mycoplasmas rises after puberty, corresponding to sexual activity. Approximately 15% of sexually active men and women are colonized with *M. hominis*, and 45% to 75% are colonized with *Ureaplasma*. The incidence of carriage in adults who are sexually inactive is no greater than that in prepubertal children.

Clinical Diseases

Infection with *M. pneumoniae* typically produces mild **upper respiratory tract disease**. Low-grade fever, malaise, headache, and a dry, nonproductive cough develop 2 to 3 weeks after exposure. Symptoms gradually worsen over the next few days and can persist for 2 weeks or longer. More severe disease with lower respiratory tract symptoms occurs in less than 10% of patients. **Tracheobronchitis**, in which the bronchial passages primarily become infiltrated with lymphocytes and plasma cells, can occur. Pneumonia (referred to as primary **atypical pneumonia** or walking pneumonia) can also develop, with a patchy bronchopneumonia seen on chest radiographs that is typically more impressive than the physical findings. Myalgias and gas-

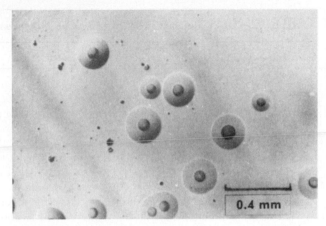

FIGURE 42–1. Fried-egg appearance of colonies of mycoplasmas. All mycoplasmas except *Mycoplasma pneumoniae* typically show this morphology. *M. pneumoniae* has a strict aerobic atmosphere requirement. It is one of the slowest growing mycoplasmas, and it appears as homogeneous granular colonies after incubation for 1 week or longer. The other mycoplasmas generally grow within 1 to 4 days. (From Razin S, Oliver O: Morphogenesis of *Mycoplasma* and bacterial L-form colonies, *J Gen Microbiol* 24: 225–237, 1961.)

trointestinal tract symptoms are uncommon. Secondary complications include otitis media, erythema multiforme (**Stevens-Johnson syndrome**), hemolytic anemia, myocarditis, pericarditis, and neurologic abnormalities. The disease resolves slowly. Secondary infections can occur because immunity is incomplete.

The role of other mycoplasmas in human disease is less clearly defined. *M. genitalium* and *U. urealyticum* can cause **nongonococcal urethritis**, and *M. hominis* has been implicated as a cause of **pyelonephritis**, **pelvic inflammatory disease**, and **postpartum fever**. The evidence implicating the organisms in these diseases is based on (1) recovery of the bacteria from specimens from infected patients, (2) a serologic response to the organism, (3) clinical improvement after treatment with specific antibiotics, (4) demonstration of disease in animal models, or (5) a combination of these findings. It is common, however, for the genitourinary tract to be colonized with these organisms, and their presence can mask a more important pathogen.

Laboratory Diagnosis

The diagnostic tests for *M. pneumoniae* infections are summarized in Table 42–3 and Figure 42–2.

Microscopy

Microscopy is of no diagnostic value. Mycoplasmas stain poorly because they have no cell wall.

TABLE 42–2. Properties of *Mycoplasma* and *Ureaplasma*

Properties	Characteristics
Size	0.1–0.3 μm
Cell wall	Absent
Growth:	
Atmosphere	Facultatively anaerobic*
Nutritional requirement	Sterols
Nutritional supplements	Vitamins, amino acids, nucleic acid precursors
Other	Cell-free growth
Replication	Binary fission
Generation time	1–6 hr
Antibiotic susceptibility:	
Penicillins	Resistant
Cephalosporins	Resistant
Tetracycline	Susceptible
Erythromycin	Susceptible†

* *Mycoplasma pneumoniae* is an obligate aerobe.
† *Mycoplasma hominis* is resistant.

TABLE 42–3. Diagnostic Tests for *Mycoplasma pneumoniae* Infections

Test	Assessment
Microscopy	Test is not useful because organisms do not have a cell wall and do not stain with conventional reagents
Culture	Test is slow (2–6 weeks before positive) and insensitive; it is not available in most laboratories
Serology	
Complement fixation	Titers peak in 4 weeks and persist for 6–12 months; diagnostic titer is $\geq 1:32$, or a fourfold increase; has good sensitivity but can be non-specific
Enzyme-linked immunosorbent assay (ELISA) or immunofluorescence	Test is sensitive and easier to perform than complement fixation; nonspecific reactions can occur
Cold agglutinins	Diagnostic titer is $>1:128$, or a fourfold increase; seroconversion occurs in 34% to 68% (insensitive); test is nonspecific

Culture

Unlike other mycoplasmas, *M. pneumoniae* is a strict aerobe. This mycoplasma can be isolated from throat washings, bronchial washings, or expectorated sputum. Washings are more reliable than sputum specimens, because most infected patients have a dry, nonproductive cough and do not produce sputum. The specimen should be inoculated into special media supplemented with serum (provides sterols), yeast extract (for nucleic acid precursors), glucose, a pH indicator, and penicillin (to inhibit other bacteria). The organisms grow slowly in culture, with a generation time of 6 hours.

Although a positive culture result is definitive evidence of disease, it is relatively insensitive. In one well-designed study, 36% of the isolates were detected within 2 weeks, whereas detection of the remaining isolates required prolonged incubation (as long as 6 weeks). In another study, only 64% of cultures from patients with serologic evidence of an acute mycoplasma infection had positive results. Growth of the organisms in culture is indicated by the metabolism of glucose with a corresponding pH change.

Colonies of *M. pneumoniae* are small and have a homogeneous granular appearance ("mulberry-shaped"), unlike the fried-egg morphology of other mycoplasmas. Identification of isolates can be confirmed by inhibition of their growth with specific antisera. Because this organism is difficult to grow and results are typically not available for many weeks, however, most laboratories do not perform cultures.

M. hominis is a facultative anaerobe that grows within 1 to 4 days and metabolizes arginine but not glucose. The colonies have a typical large fried-egg appearance (see Fig. 42–1). Inhibition of their growth with specific antisera is used to differentiate them from other genital mycoplasmas. *Ureaplasma* requires urea for growth but is inhibited by the higher alkalinity resulting from the metabolism of urea. Thus, the growth medium must be supplemented with urea and be highly buffered. Even if these steps are taken, ureaplasmas die rapidly after initial isolation.

Serology

Serologic tests are available only for *M. pneumoniae*. Detection of antibodies directed against *M. pneumoniae* by complement fixation is a useful but technically cumbersome test. The antibody is initially detected soon

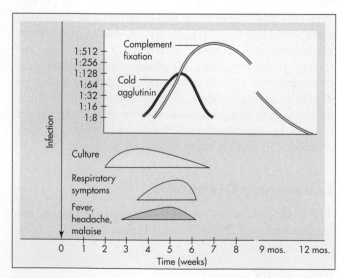

FIGURE 42–2. Correlation between clinical course of *Mycoplasma pneumoniae* infection and results of diagnostic tests.

after the onset of infection. The titer peaks within 4 weeks and persists for 6 to 12 months. As many as 90% of patients with a positive culture result have diagnostic antibody titers, although these results may not be observed until 1 month after the onset of disease. Because the antibodies are directed against outer membrane glycolipids common to other organisms and tissues, false-positive reactions are observed; these occur (1) in patients with infections caused by other mycoplasmas, (2) in the presence of some plant antigens, and (3) in patients with bacterial meningitis, syphilis, or pancreatitis. Thus, the high sensitivity of this serologic test is offset by the delay in obtaining a diagnostic titer, its low specificity, and the technical complexity of the test. Alternative antibody-directed tests, such as enzyme-linked immunosorbent assays and immunofluorescence, have been developed and are now used more commonly than the complement fixation test. The tests are easier to perform and are highly sensitive if both immunoglobulin M (IgM) and IgG are measured. Nevertheless, problems with test specificity persist.

It is also possible to measure nonspecific reactions to the outer membrane glycolipids of *M. pneumoniae*. The most useful of these reactions is the production of cold agglutinins (e.g., IgM antibodies that bind the I antigen on the surface of human erythrocytes at 4°C). The cold agglutinin assay is positive in approximately 65% of patients with *M. pneumoniae* infections, particularly those who are symptomatic, and is frequently positive at the time the patient presents with symptoms. Because this test is not specific for *M. pneumoniae*, cross-reactions are observed in patients with respiratory tract diseases caused by other organisms (e.g., Epstein-Barr virus, cytomegalovirus, adenovirus). A strongly reactive cold agglutinin titer, of at least 1:128, or a significant increase in the titer constitutes presumptive evidence of *Mycoplasma* disease.

Treatment, Prevention, and Control

Erythromycin and tetracycline (or doxycycline) are equally effective in treating *M. pneumoniae* infections, although the tetracyclines are reserved for use in adults. Tetracyclines have the advantage of also being active against most other mycoplasmas and chlamydia, a common cause of nongonococcal urethritis. Erythromycin is used to treat *Ureaplasma* infections, because these organisms are resistant to tetracycline. Unlike the other mycoplasmas, *M. hominis* is resistant to erythromycin and occasionally to the tetracyclines. Clindamycin has been used to treat infections caused by these resistant strains.

The prevention of *Mycoplasma* disease is problematic. *M. pneumoniae* infections are spread by close contact; thus, the isolation of infected people could theoretically reduce the risk of infection. Isolation is impractical, however, because patients are typically infectious for a prolonged period, even while receiving appropriate antibiotics. Inactivated vaccines as well as attenuated live vaccines have also proved disappointing. The protective immunity conferred by infection has been low. Infections with *M. hominis*, *M. genitalium*, and *Ureaplasma* are transmitted by sexual contact. Therefore, these diseases can be prevented by avoidance of sexual activity or the use of proper barrier precautions.

CASE STUDY AND QUESTIONS

■ Increased lethargy, headache, cough, a low-grade fever, and chills and sweats at night developed in a 21-year-old university student. When she was seen at the student health center, she had a nonproductive cough and shortness of breath on exertion. Her pulse rate was 95 beats/min, and her respiratory rate was 28 breaths/min. Her pharynx was erythematous; scattered rhonchi and rales but no consolidation were noted on auscultation. A chest radiograph showed patchy infiltrates. A Gram stain of sputum revealed many white blood cells but no organisms. The antibody titer for a *Mycoplasma* complement fixation test performed on a specimen collected at admission was 1:8; the titer for a specimen collected a week later was 1:32. The patient was treated with erythromycin, to which her disease responded slowly during the next 2 weeks.

1. If cultures were performed, what would be the best specimen? When would the results be available? What are the sensitivity and specificity of culture in a patient infected with *M. pneumoniae*?

2. How do *Mycoplasma* species differ from other bacteria?

3. Describe the epidemiology of *M. pneumoniae* infections. What aspects of this case are characteristic of such infections?

4. What other mycoplasmas cause human disease? What diseases?

BIBLIOGRAPHY

Barile MF et al: Current topics in mycoplasmology, *Rev Infect Dis* 4:1–277, 1982.

Cassell GH, Cole BC: Mycoplasmas as agents of human disease, *N Engl J Med* 304:80–89, 1981.

Cole B, Sawitzke A: Mycoplasmas, superantigens and autoimmune arthritis. In Henderson B et al, editors: *Mechanisms and models in rheumatoid arthritis*, San Diego, 1996, Academic.

Foy HM et al: Long-term epidemiology of infections with *Mycoplasma pneumoniae*, *J Infect Dis* 139:681–687, 1979.

Kenny GE et al: Diagnosis of *Mycoplasma pneumoniae* pneumonia: sensitivities and specificities of serology with lipid antigen and isolation of the organism on soy peptone medium for identification of infections, *J Clin Microbiol* 28:2087–2093, 1990.

Lo S: New understandings of mycoplasmal infections and diseases, *Clin Microbiol Newsletter* 17:169–173, 1995.

Luby JP: Pneumonia caused by *Mycoplasma pneumoniae* infection, *Clin Chest Med* 12:237–244, 1991.

Maniloff J et al, editors: *Mycoplasmas: molecular biology and pathogenesis*, Washington, DC, 1992, American Society of Microbiology.

McMahon DK et al: Extragenital *Mycoplasma hominis* infections in adults, *Am J Med* 89:275–281, 1990.

Waites K et al: Laboratory diagnosis of mycoplasmal and ureaplasmal infections, *Clin Microbiol Newsletter* 18:105–112, 1996.

CHAPTER 43

Rickettsia, Orientia, Ehrlichia, and *Coxiella*

Rickettsia, Orientia, Ehrlichia, and *Coxiella* are aerobic, gram-negative bacilli that are obligate intracellular parasites. Although they were classified originally in a single family, analysis of their DNA sequences revealed that this classification was invalid. They are therefore discussed as distinct, unrelated genera in this chapter.

These bacteria were originally thought to be viruses because they are small (0.3×1 to 2 μm), stain poorly with the Gram stain, and grow only in the cytoplasm of eukaryotic cells. Nevertheless, these organisms have the following characteristics of bacteria:

1. Are structurally similar to gram-negative bacilli.
2. Contain DNA, RNA, and enzymes for the Krebs cycle and ribosomes for protein synthesis.
3. Multiply by binary fission.
4. Are inhibited by antibiotics (e.g., tetracycline, chloramphenicol).

The pathogenic species of these four genera are maintained in animal and arthropod reservoirs and are transmitted by arthropod vectors (e.g., ticks, mites, lice, fleas). Humans are accidental hosts. The most common species that cause human disease are summarized in Table 43–1 and Figure 43–1.

Physiology and Structure

The structure of the cell wall in the bacteria of all four genera is typical of gram-negative bacilli, with a peptidoglycan layer and lipopolysaccharide (LPS). The peptidoglycan layer is minimal in some bacteria, however, and the LPS has only weak endotoxin activity (or is absent, as in *Ehrlichia* species). The bacteria do not have flagella and are surrounded by a loosely adherent slime layer. All organisms are seen best with Giemsa or Gimenez stains and stain weakly with the Gram stain. All the bacteria are strict intracellular parasites, but their intracellular locations vary: *Rickettsia* and *Orientia* are found free in the cytoplasm, whereas *Coxiella* and *Ehrlichia* multiply in cytoplasmic vacuoles.

The bacteria enter eukaryotic cells by stimulating phagocytosis. After engulfment, *Rickettsia* and *Orientia* must degrade the phagosome membrane by producing phospholipase A and must be released into the cytoplasm, or the organisms will not survive. Multiplication by binary fission is slow (generation time, 9 to 12 hours). *Rickettsia prowazekii* accumulates in the cell until it lyses; in contrast, *Rickettsia rickettsii* and *Orientia tsutsugamushi* are continually released from cells through long cytoplasmic projections.

After *Coxiella* enters the cell, it remains in the phagolysosome, where the organism has become adapted to growing in the acidic environment. In contrast, *Ehrlichia* species are killed if lysosomes fuse with their cytoplasmic vacuoles. Figure 43–2 illustrates the growth cycle of *Ehrlichia* species, which comprises the following three stages of growth: elementary body, initial body, and morula.

The reason that these bacteria must grow inside eukaryotic cells is not understood. The bacteria are capable of protein synthesis and can produce adenosine triphosphate (ATP) by means of the tricarboxylic acid cycle. It appears that the bacteria are energy parasites that use the host cell ATP as long as it is available. They also use host cell coenzyme A, nicotinamide adenine dinucleotide, and available amino acids.

Once these bacteria are released from the host cell, they are unstable and die quickly. The exception is *Coxiella* species, which is highly resistant to desiccation and remains viable in the environment for months to years. This characteristic is extremely important in the epidemiology of *Coxiella* infections.

Rickettsia rickettsii

Pathogenesis and Immunity

Rickettsiae are subdivided into the spotted fever group and the typhus group. At least 12 species of rickettsiae in the spotted fever group have been associated with

TABLE 43–1. Distribution of *Rickettsia, Orientia, Ehrlichia,* and *Coxiella* Species Associated with Human Disease

Organism	Human Disease	Distribution
Spotted fever group:		
R. rickettsii	Rocky Mountain spotted fever	Western hemisphere
R. akari	Rickettsialpox	United States, former Soviet Union, Korea
R. conorii	Boutonneuse fever	Mediterranean countries, Africa, India, Southwest Asia
R. africae	African tick bite fever	Eastern and southern Africa
R. sibirica	Siberian tick typhus	Siberia, Mongolia, northern China
R. japonica	Oriental spotted fever	Japan
R. australis	Australian tick typhus	Australia
Typhus group:		
R. prowazekii	Epidemic typhus	South America and Africa
	Recrudescent typhus	Worldwide
	Sporadic typhus	United States
R. typhi	Murine typhus	Worldwide
Scrub typhus group:		
O. tsutsugamushi	Scrub typhus	Asia, northern Australia, Japan, Pacific Islands
Ehrlichia organisms:		
E. canis group		
E. ewingii	Human granulocytic ehrlichiosis	United States: southeast and south central states
E. chaffeensis	Human monocytic ehrlichiosis	United States: southeast and south central states
E. phagocytophila-equi group		
E. phagocytophila	Human granulocytic ehrlichiosis	United States: northern and central midwest states, northeastern and central Atlantic states, northern California
E. risticii-sennetsu group		
E. sennetsu	Sennetsu fever	Japan
Coxiella burnetii	Q fever	Worldwide

human disease, and 7 more species have been isolated in arthropod vectors. The most common human pathogen in the United States is *R. rickettsii,* the agent responsible for **Rocky Mountain spotted fever**.

There is no evidence that *R. rickettsii* produces toxins or that the host's immune response is responsible for the pathologic manifestations of Rocky Mountain spotted fever. The primary clinical manifestations appear to result from the replication of bacteria in endothelial cells, with subsequent damage to the cells and leakage of the blood vessels. Hypovolemia and hypoproteinemia caused by the loss of plasma into tissues can lead to reduced perfusion of various organs and organ failure.

Epidemiology

Approximately 400 to 800 documented cases of Rocky Mountain spotted fever are reported annually in the United States (Box 43–1). Although the disease was first described in Idaho and later in Montana, most cases are now seen in the southeastern Atlantic and south central states. The reason for this shift is un-known, but it could result from changes in the tick population or changes in the proportion of infected ticks in the specific areas. The principal reservoir and vector for *R. rickettsii* are infected **hard ticks**: the wood tick (*Dermacentor andersoni*) in Rocky Mountain states and the dog tick (*Dermacentor variabilis*) in the southeastern states and the West Coast. Other tick reservoirs are *Rhipicephalus sanguineus* in Mexico, and *Amblyomma cajennense* in Central and South America. It is not clear whether the Lone Star tick (*Amblyomma americanum*) in the south central states is a reservoir. The rickettsiae are maintained in the tick population by transovarian transmission. Mammals such as wild rodents can also serve as reservoirs, but this source is considered uncommon for tick-to-human infections.

Rickettsial infections are spread to humans by the adult ticks when they feed. More than 90% of all infections occur from April through October, corresponding to the period of greatest tick activity. To become infected, a person must be exposed to the tick for a lengthy period (e.g., 24 to 48 hours). The dormant avirulent rickettsiae are activated by the warm blood meal, then must be released from the tick sali-

Disease	Organism	Vector	Reservoir
Rocky Mountain spotted fever	R. rickettsii	Tick-borne 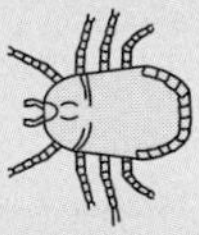	Ticks, wild rodents
Ehrlichiosis	E. chaffeensis E. phagocytophila E. ewingii		Ticks
Rickettsialpox	R. akari	Mite-borne 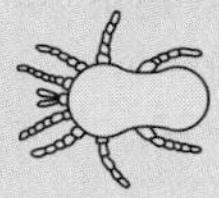	Mites, wild rodents
Scrub typhus	O. tsutsugamushi		Mites (chiggers), wild rodents
Epidemic typhus	R. prowazekii	Louse-borne 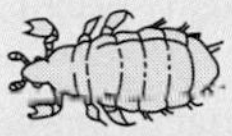	Humans, squirrel fleas, flying squirrels
Trench fever	R. quintana		Humans
Murine typhus	R. typhi	Flea-borne 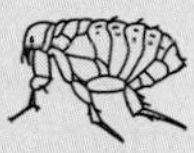	Wild rodents
Q fever	C. burnetii	None*	Cattle, sheep, goats, cats

* Tick vectors may be responsible for animal-to-animal transmission.

FIGURE 43–1. Epidemiology of common *Rickettsia, Ehrlichia, Orientia,* and *Coxiella* infections.

vary glands to penetrate the blood stream of the human host.

Clinical Diseases

Clinically symptomatic disease develops 2 to 14 days (average, 7 days) after the tick bite (Table 43–2). The patient may not recall the painless tick bite. The onset

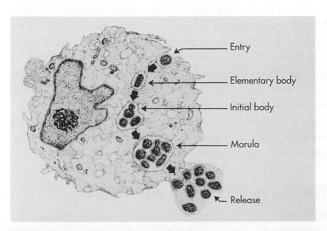

FIGURE 43–2. The growth of *Ehrlichia* in an infected cell. (From McDade JE: Ehrlichiosis—a disease of animals and humans. *J Infect Dis* 161:609–617, 1990 © 1990, the University of Chicago Press.)

Labels: Entry · Elementary body · Initial body · Morula · Release

of disease is heralded by fever, chills, headache, and myalgias. A rash may develop after 3 or more days and can evolve from a macular to petechial form. It initially involves the extremities and then spreads to the trunk. The palms and soles can be involved. Complications of Rocky Mountain spotted fever include gastrointestinal symptoms, respiratory failure, encephalitis, and renal failure. Complications increase and the prognosis is worse when the characteristic rash does not develop or develops late in the disease, because the diagnosis is delayed.

Laboratory Diagnosis

Although the rickettsiae stain poorly with the Gram stain, they can be stained with Giemsa or Gimenez stains. Specific fluorescein-labeled antibodies can also

TABLE 43–2. Clinical Course of Human Diseases Caused by *Rickettsia, Orientia, Ehrlichia,* and *Coxiella* Species

Disease	Average Incubation Period (days)	Clinical Presentation	Rash	Eschar	Mortality (%)
Rocky Mountain spotted fever	7	Abrupt onset; fever, chills, headache, myalgia	>90%; macular; centripetal spread	No	20
Rickettsialpox	9–14	Abrupt onset; fever, headache, chills, myalgia, photophobia	100%; papulovesicular; generalized	Yes	<1
Typhus:					
Epidemic	8	Abrupt onset; fever, headache, chills, myalgia, arthralgia	40–80%; macular; centrifugal spread	No	Variable
Endemic	7–14	Gradual onset; fever, headache, myalgia, cough	>55%; maculopapular rash on trunk	No	1–2
Scrub	10–12	Abrupt onset; fever, headache, myalgia	<50%; maculopapular rash; centrifugal	No	7
Ehrlichiosis	12	Abrupt onset; fever, headache, myalgia, malaise, leukopenia, thrombocytopenia	10–80%; nonspecific	No	<5
Q fever					
Acute	20	Abrupt onset; fever, headache, chills, myalgia; granulomatous hepatitis	No	No	1
Chronic	Months to years	Chronic disease with subacute onset; endocarditis, hepatic dysfunction	No	No	High

be used to stain biopsy tissue specimens; however, this procedure is less sensitive in patients who have received effective antibiotics.

The rickettsiae can be isolated in tissue culture or embryonated eggs. Bacterial isolation is performed mainly in reference laboratories because the bacteria grow slowly and their recovery is traditionally considered a hazardous procedure.

The primary diagnostic procedure for Rocky Mountain spotted fever is serologic. Although the **Weil-Felix test** (which involves the differential agglutination of *Proteus* antigens) has been used historically for the diagnosis of rickettsial infections, it is not recommended now because it is insensitive and nonspecific.

The test most commonly used for detecting *Rickettsia*-specific antibodies is the indirect fluorescent antibody (IFA) test. The test is reactive with heat-labile proteins and the LPS antigen is shared among the *Rickettsia* and so is not species-specific. However, commercially prepared reagents are available that differentiate between the spotted fever group and the typhus group. The IFA test is both sensitive (94% to 100%) and specific (100%); the finding of a fourfold rise in

the antibody titers or an initial titer of 1:64 or more is considered a positive result. The initial antibody response is detected 2 to 3 weeks after the onset of disease, and antibodies remain detectable for a long time.

The direct detection of rickettsial antigens in skin biopsy specimens is a rapid, specific method for confirming the clinical diagnosis of Rocky Mountain spotted fever. This can be accomplished with the use of specific antibodies labeled with fluorescent dyes that can stain the intracellular bacteria. Alternatively, nucleic acid probes are an accurate method for detecting rickettsiae. Unfortunately, both tests are offered only in reference laboratories, so there is some delay before test results are available.

Treatment, Prevention, and Control

Rickettsiae are susceptible to the tetracyclines (i.e., doxycycline), chloramphenicol, and fluoroquinolones (e.g., ciprofloxacin). The prompt diagnosis and institution of appropriate therapy usually result in a satisfactory prognosis; unfortunately, this scenario may not occur if key clinical signs (such as the rash) develop late or not at all. In addition, the serologic findings frequently are not available until 2 to 4 weeks after the onset of disease, also delaying the start of treatment. The morbidity and mortality are high if the diagnosis or specific therapy is delayed.

There is no vaccine for Rocky Mountain spotted fever. Thus, avoidance of tick-infested areas, the use of protective clothing and insect repellents, and the prompt removal of attached ticks are the best preventive measures. It is virtually impossible to eliminate the tick reservoir, because the ticks can survive for as long as 4 years without feeding.

Other Spotted Fever Rickettsiae

At least six other rickettsial species in the spotted fever group cause human disease (see Table 43–1). *Rickettsia akari*, the agent responsible for causing **rickettsialpox**, is occasionally isolated in the United States. Infections with *R. akari* are maintained in the rodent population through the bite of mouse ectoparasites (e.g., mites) and in mites by transovarian transmission. Humans become accidental hosts when bitten by infected mites. The other rickettsiae in the spotted fever group are transmitted by ticks.

Clinical infection with *R. akari* is biphasic. First, a papule develops at the site where the mite has bitten the host. The papule appears approximately 1 week after the bite and quickly progresses to ulceration and then eschar formation. During this period, the rickettsiae spread systemically. After an incubation period of 7 to 24 days (average, 9 to 14 days), the second phase of the disease develops abruptly, with high fever, severe headache, chills, sweats, myalgias, and photophobia. A generalized papulovesicular rash forms within 2 to 3 days. A poxlike progression of the rash is then seen, in which vesicles form and then crust over. Despite the appearance of the disseminated rash, rickettsialpox is usually mild and uncomplicated, and complete healing is seen within 2 to 3 weeks without treatment. Specific therapy with doxycycline or chloramphenicol speeds the process.

Rickettsia prowazekii

Epidemiology

R. prowazekii is the etiologic agent of **epidemic typhus**, also called **louse-borne typhus**, and the principal vector is the human body louse, Pediculus humanus (Box 43–2). Unlike with most other rickettsial diseases, humans are the primary reservoir of typhus. Epidemic typhus occurs among people living in crowded, unsanitary conditions that favor the spread of body lice — conditions such as those that arise during wars, fam-

---

> **BOX 43–2.** **Summary of *Rickettsia prowazekii* Infections**
>
> **Physiology and Structure**
>
> Small, intracellular bacteria.
>   Stain poorly with Gram stain; best with Giemsa or Gimenez stains.
>   Replicate in cytoplasm of infected cells.
>
> **Virulence**
>
> Intracellular growth protects the bacteria from immune clearance.
>   Replicates in endothelial cells with resulting vasculitis.
>
> **Epidemiology**
>
> Humans are the primary reservoir, with person-to-person transmission by louse vector.
>   Sporadic disease is believed to be spread from squirrels to humans by squirrel fleas.
>   Recrudescent disease can develop years after initial infection.
>   People at greatest risk are those in crowded unsanitary conditions.
>   Infection occurs most commonly in Central and South America and Africa; less commonly in the United States.
>   Sporadic disease is seen in the eastern United States.
>
> **Diseases**
>
> Epidemic typhus (louse-borne typhus).
>   Recrudescent typhus (Brill-Zinsser disease).
>   Sporadic typhus.
>
> **Diagnosis**
>
> The IFA test is the diagnostic test of choice.
>
> **Treatment, Prevention, and Control**
>
> The tetracyclines are the drugs of choice; alternative antibiotics include chloramphenicol.
>   Control through improvements in living conditions and reduction of the lice population through use of insecticides.
>   Inactivated vaccine is available for high-risk populations.

---

ines, and natural disasters. Lice die from their infection within 2 to 3 weeks, preventing the transovarian transmission of *R. prowazekii*. The disease is present in Central and South America, Africa, and less commonly in the United States.

The incidence of the disease in the United States is unknown, because it is not classified as a disease reportable to public health departments. Sporadic disease in the United States is primarily restricted to rural areas of the eastern states. It occurs in this area because flying squirrels as well as squirrel fleas and lice are infected with *R. prowazekii*. Squirrel lice do not feed on humans, but the fleas are less discriminating and may be responsible for transmitting the *Rickettsia* from squirrels to humans. Epidemiologic and serologic evidence supports this hypothesis, but such transmission has not been documented.

Recrudescent disease with *R. prowazekii* (**Brill-Zinsser disease**) can occur in people years after their initial infection. Such people in the United States are primarily Eastern European immigrants who were exposed to epidemic typhus during World War II.

Clinical Diseases

In one study of epidemic typhus in Africa, clinical disease was found to develop after a 2- to 30-day incubation period (average, 8 days). Most of the patients initially had nonspecific symptoms; then within 1 to 3 days, high fever, severe headache, and other symptoms such as chills, myalgias, arthralgia, and anorexia developed. Less than 40% of the patients had a petechial or macular rash, but darkly pigmented skin can obscure the rash. Complications of epidemic typhus include myocarditis and central nervous system dysfunction; a mortality rate as high as 66% has been reported in some epidemics. This high mortality rate undoubtedly stems from the poor general health, nutrition, and hygiene of the population together with the lack of antibiotic therapy and proper supportive medical care. In patients with uncomplicated disease, the body temperature returns to normal within 2 weeks, but complete convalescence may take 3 months or longer.

As noted earlier, reactivation or recrudescent epidemic typhus (Brill-Zinsser disease) can occur years after the initial disease. However, the course is generally milder than that of epidemic typhus, and the convalescence is shorter.

Laboratory Diagnosis

The IFA test is the diagnostic method of choice for documenting disease with *R. prowazekii*.

Treatment, Prevention, and Control

The tetracyclines and chloramphenicol are highly effective in the treatment of epidemic typhus. However, antibiotic treatment must be combined with effective louse-control measures for the management of an epidemic. A formaldehyde-inactivated typhus vaccine is available, and its use is recommended in high-risk populations.

Rickettsia typhi

Epidemiology

Endemic or murine typhus is caused by *Rickettsia typhi*. Until 1994, this was a reportable disease in the United States. However, mandatory reporting was discontinued because of the relatively small number of cases observed (i.e., less than 30 annually). In the United States, most reported cases were from the Gulf states (especially Texas) and southern California. Endemic disease continues to be reported in people living in the temperate and subtropical coastal areas of Africa, Asia, Australia, Europe, and South America. Rodents are the primary reservoir, and the rat flea (*Xenopsylla cheopis*) is the principal vector. However, the cat flea (*Ctenocephalides felis*), which infests cats, opossums, raccoons, and skunks, is considered an important vector for disease in the United States. Most cases occur during the warm months.

Clinical Disease

The incubation period for *R. typhi* disease is 7 to 14 days. The symptoms appear abruptly, with fever, severe headache, chills, myalgia, and nausea most common. A rash develops in approximately half of infected patients, most commonly late in the illness. It is typically restricted to the chest and abdomen but may extend to the palms and soles. The course of disease is generally uncomplicated, lasting less than 3 weeks even in untreated patients.

Laboratory Diagnosis

A *R. typhi*–specific IFA test is used to confirm the diagnosis of murine typhus. A fourfold increase in the titer or a single titer of at least 1:128 is diagnostic. Significant titers are usually detectable within 1 to 2 weeks of the onset of disease.

Treatment, Prevention, and Control

Tetracycline, doxycycline, or chloramphenicol is effective in the treatment of murine typhus, and patients respond promptly to these agents. It is difficult to control or prevent endemic typhus, because the reservoir and vector are widely distributed. Any such efforts should be directed at controlling the rodent reservoir. An effective vaccine is not available.

Orientia tsutsugamushi

O. tsutsugamushi, formerly classified with the *Rickettsia*, is the etiologic agent for **scrub typhus**, a disease transmitted to humans by mites (chiggers, red mites). The reservoir is the mite population, in which the bacteria are transmitted by transovarian means. Infection is also present in the rodent population, which can serve as a reservoir for mite infections. Because mites feed only once during their life span, rodents are not believed to be an important reservoir for human disease. Scrub typhus is present in people living in eastern Asia, Aus-

TABLE 43–3. Epidemiology of *Ehrlichia* Species Responsible for Human Disease

Species	Reservoir	Vector or Source	Disease
E. chaffeensis	White-tailed deer, domestic dogs	*Amblyomma americanum* (Lone Star tick)	Monocytic ehrlichiosis
E. ewingii	Canines	*Amblyomma americanum*	Granulocytic ehrlichiosis
E. phagocytophila	Small mammals (e.g., white-footed mouse, chipmunks, voles)	*Ixodes* (including *I. scapularis*, *I. pacificus*, *I. ricinus*)	Granulocytic ehrlichiosis
E. sennetsu	Unknown	Ingestion of raw fish infested with infected flukes	Sennetsu fever

BOX 43–3. Summary of Human *Ehrlichia* Infections

Physiology and Structure

Small, intracellular bacteria.
Stain poorly with Gram stain; best with Giemsa or Gimenez stains.
Replicates in phagosome of infected cells.

Virulence

Intracellular growth protects bacteria from immune clearance.
Able to prevent fusion of phagosome with lysosome of monocytes or granulocytes.

Epidemiology

Depending on the species of *Ehrlichia*, important reservoirs are white-tailed deer, white-footed mouse, chipmunks, voles, and canines.
Ticks are important vectors.
Disease in United States is most common in the Atlantic states; northern, central, and southern midwestern states; and northern California.
People at greatest risk are those exposed to ticks in the endemic areas.
Disease is most common from April to October.

Diseases

Human granulocytic ehrlichiosis.
Human monocytic ehrlichiosis.
Sennetsu fever.

Diagnosis

Microscopy of limited value.
Serology and DNA probe tests methods of choice.

Treatment, Prevention, and Control

Doxycycline is the drug of choice; fluoroquinolones are an acceptable alternative.
Prevention involves avoidance of tick-infested areas, use of protective clothing and insect repellents, and prompt removal of embedded ticks.
Vaccines are not available.

tralia, and Japan and other western Pacific islands. It can also be imported into the United States.

O. tsutsugamushi disease develops suddenly after a 6- to 18-day incubation period (average, 10 to 12 days), with severe headache, fever, and myalgias. A macular to papular rash develops on the trunk in less than half of patients and spreads centrifugally to the extremities. Generalized lymphadenopathy, splenomegaly, central nervous system complications, and heart failure can occur. Fever in untreated patients disappears after 2 to 3 weeks, whereas fever in patients who receive appropriate treatment with tetracycline, doxycycline, or chloramphenicol responds promptly. No vaccine is available, so the disease is prevented by avoidance of exposure to chiggers (i.e., the wearing of protective clothing, the use of insect repellents).

Ehrlichia

Pathogenesis and Immunity

The genus *Ehrlichia* (organisms named after Paul Ehrlich, one of the fathers of microbiology) consists of intracellular bacteria that parasitize mononuclear and granulocytic phagocytes, but not erythrocytes. The intracellular location of the organisms protects them from the host's antibody response.

Epidemiology

The genus *Ehrlichia* is subdivided into three groups, with species that cause human disease found in each group (Tables 43–1 and 43–3; Box 43–3). *Ehrlichia sennetsu*, which is primarily restricted to Japan, causes **Sennetsu fever** and was the first species found to cause human disease. Disease produced by this species differs from that caused by the other *Ehrlichia* because it is associated with ingestion of raw fish infested with ehrlichia-infected flukes. Ticks are the vectors of ehrlichiosis caused by all other species associated with human and animal disease.

Tick-borne ehrlichiosis was first recognized in the

United States in 1986. The disease, **human monocytic ehrlichiosis**, was believed initially to be caused by *Ehrlichia canis*; however, a serologically distinct species, *Ehrlichia chaffeensis*, within the *E. canis* group was recognized to be the etiologic agent. This organism was first isolated from an Army reservist at Fort Chaffee, Arkansas (hence the species name). Disease is found predominantly in the southeastern, mid-Atlantic, and south central areas of the United States (e.g., Oklahoma, Texas, Arkansas, Missouri, Georgia, South Carolina). This area corresponds to the geographic distribution of *A. americanum* (Lone Star tick), the primary vector responsible for transmitting the organism, and of white-tailed deer, the reservoir for *E. chaffeensis*. Domestic dogs have also been identified as a reservoir for human infections. The prevalence of this disease has been underestimated (fewer than 1000 infections have been identified), because serologic studies have shown that antibodies to *E. chaffeensis* are at least as common as antibodies to *R. rickettsii*, which has a similar geographic distribution.

Human granulocytic ehrlichiosis is caused by two species of *Ehrlichia*—*Ehrlichia ewingii* and *Ehrlichia phagocytophila*. *E. ewingii* is a newly identified species in the *E. canis* group that has a geographic distribution similar to *E. chaffeensis*. The frequency with which it is associated with human disease and the geographic distribution is unknown, because serologic response to this organism cross-reacts with antibodies against *E. chaffeensis*. Disease caused by *E. phagocytophila* is found primarily in the northern and central Midwestern states and northeast and central Atlantic states. The reservoirs are small mammals (e.g., white-footed mouse, chipmunks, voles), and the vectors are *Ixodes* ticks. More than 90% of all disease caused by *Ehrlichia* in the United States occurs between mid-April and late October.

Clinical Diseases

Patients with Sennetsu fever typically have an acute febrile illness similar to infectious mononucleosis, consisting of lethargy, cervical lymphadenopathy, and rises in numbers of peripheral mononuclear cells and atypical lymphocytes.

Human monocytic ehrlichiosis and granulocytic ehrlichiosis have similar manifestations and resemble Rocky Mountain spotted fever. Approximately 12 days after the tick bite (range, 1 to 3 weeks), a high fever, headache, malaise, and myalgia develop. Leukopenia caused by the destruction of leukocytes and thrombocytopenia are also observed. A rash develops in only 20% of patients, more commonly in children than adults and in monocytic ehrlichiosis than granulocytic ehrlichiosis. The absence of a rash has been partly responsible for the difficulty in diagnosing these diseases. Mortality is less than 5% in patients with ehrlichiosis, and death is primarily seen in the elderly, in patients with delays in treatment, and in patients with immunocompromising diseases (e.g., acquired immunodeficiency syndrome [AIDS]).

Laboratory Diagnosis

Microscopy is of limited value for diagnosing human ehrlichiosis. Giemsa stain preparations of peripheral blood should be performed, because detection of intracellular organisms (called **morulae**) is diagnostic. However, morulae are detected in less than 10% of patients with human monocytic ehrlichiosis and in 20% to 80% of patients with human granulocytic ehrlichiosis. Likewise, although *Ehrlichia* have been cultured in vitro, this procedure is difficult and would not be performed in a clinical laboratory. The most common methods used for confirming the clinical diagnosis of ehrlichiosis are serologic and DNA probe tests. An increase in the antibody titer is typically observed 2 weeks or longer after the initial presentation. *E. chaffeensis* and *E. ewingii* are closely related and are not distinguished serologically. Species-specific DNA probes are available and can distinguish among the strains pathogenic for humans.

Treatment, Prevention, and Control

Patients with suspected ehrlichiosis should be treated with doxycycline. Therapy should not be delayed to wait for laboratory confirmation of the disease. Although chloramphenicol has been used, it is not believed to be effective. The fluoroquinolones are effective in vitro, but the clinical experience with these drugs is limited. Infection is prevented by avoidance of tick-infested areas, wearing of protective clothing, and use of insect repellents. Embedded ticks should be removed promptly. Vaccines are not available.

Coxiella burnetii

Pathogenesis and Immunity

Coxiella were originally classified with *Rickettsia* because they stain weakly with the Gram stain, grow intracellularly in eukaryotic cells, and are associated with arthropods (i.e., ticks). However, it is now recognized that these bacteria are more closely related to *Legionella* and *Francisella*. The disease caused by *Coxiella* is **Q fever**, which may be asymptomatic in humans and may either manifest acutely or develop as a chronic infection.

Understanding of the pathogenesis of Q fever is limited, because most infections are self-limited and there is no animal model for the chronic disease. Human infection usually occurs after the inhalation of airborne particles from a contaminated environmental source rather than from the bite of an arthropod vector, as occurs in *Rickettsia, Orientia,* and *Ehrlichia* infections. *Coxiella* proliferate in the respiratory tract and then disseminate to other organs. Pneumonia and granulomatous hepatitis develop in patients with severe, acute infections, whereas most chronic infections manifest as endocarditis.

An important characteristic of *Coxiella* infections is the ability to undergo **antigenic variation** in expression of the cell wall LPS antigen. The highly infectious form of the bacterium possesses LPS with a complex carbohydrate (**phase I antigen**) that blocks antibody interaction with surface proteins. After cultivation of the bacterium, the LPS is modified (**phase II antigen**), exposing the surface proteins to antibodies and producing a less infectious form. Antibody response to these antigens in disease is a useful marker for acute and chronic diseases. Acute disease is characterized by antibodies against the exposed phase II antigen, whereas high antibody titers against the phase I and II antigens are detected in patients with chronic infections. The high antibody titers observed in patients with chronic disease lead to the formation of immune complexes and are responsible for producing some of the signs and symptoms of this disease. Thus, humoral immunity contributes to the pathologic manifestations of the disease and clinical improvement is associated with cellular immunity.

Epidemiology

Coxiella burnetii is extremely stable in harsh environmental conditions and can survive in soil for months to years. The range of hosts for *C. burnetii* is wide, infections being found in mammals, birds, and numerous different genera of ticks (Box 43–4). Farm animals such as sheep, cattle, and goats as well as recently infected cats, dogs, and rabbits are the primary reservoirs for human disease. Ticks are an important vector for disease in animals but not in humans. The bacteria can reach high concentrations in the placenta of infected livestock. Dried placentas left on the ground after parturition as well as feces, urine, and tick feces can contaminate soil, which in turn can serve as a focus for infection if these bacteria become airborne and are inhaled. *C. burnetii* is also excreted in milk, so people who consume contaminated unpasteurized milk can become infected.

Q fever has a worldwide distribution. Although only 20 to 30 cases are reported annually in the United States, this figure is certainly an underestimation of the actual prevalence of the disease. Infection is common in livestock in the United States; however, actual disease in livestock is rare. Human exposure, particularly for ranchers, veterinarians, and food handlers, is fre-

---

> **BOX 43–4.** **Summary of *Coxiella* Infections**
>
> **Physiology and Structure**
>
> Small, intracellular bacteria.
>
> Stain poorly with Gram stain; best with Giemsa or Gimenez stains.
>
> Replicate in phagolysosome of infected cells.
>
> Capable of phase transition with phase I (infectious) and phase II lipopolysaccharide antigens.
>
> **Virulence**
>
> Intracellular growth protects the bacteria from immune clearance.
>
> Able to replicate in acidic environment of fused phagosomes and lysosomes.
>
> Phase I forms are protected from antibody interaction with bacterial surface proteins.
>
> Extracellular form extremely stable so can survive in nature for a prolonged period.
>
> **Epidemiology**
>
> Many reservoirs, including mammals, birds, and ticks.
>
> Most human infections associated with contact with infected cattle, sheep, goats, dogs, and cats.
>
> Most disease acquired through inhalation; possible disease from consumption of contaminated milk; ticks are not an important vector for human disease.
>
> Worldwide distribution, although disease in the United States is relatively uncommon.
>
> No seasonal incidence.
>
> **Diseases**
>
> Acute diseases include influenza-like syndrome, atypical pneumonia, hepatitis, pericarditis, myocarditis, meningoencephalitis.
>
> Chronic diseases include endocarditis, hepatitis, pulmonary disease, and infection of pregnant women.
>
> **Diagnosis**
>
> Detection of antibody response to phase I and phase II antigens test of choice.
>
> **Treatment, Prevention, and Control**
>
> Tetracyclines are the drugs of choice for acute infections; rifampin combined with either doxycycline or trimethoprim-sulfamethoxazole is used to treat chronic infections.
>
> Phase I antigen vaccines are protective and safe if administered in a single dose before the animal or human has been exposed to *Coxiella*.

---

quent, and experimental studies have shown that the infectious dose of *C. burnetii* is small. Thus, most human infections are mild or asymptomatic. This finding is confirmed by serologic studies, which have shown that more than half of all patients with detectable antibodies do not have a history of disease. Infections also go undiagnosed because *C. burnetii* is frequently not considered in patients who have symptomatic disease.

Clinical Diseases

C. burnetii infection can present in an acute or a chronic fashion. Acute disease is characterized by a long incubation period (average, 20 days), followed by the sudden onset of severe headache, high fever, chills, and myalgias. Respiratory symptoms are generally mild, mimicking the **"atypical pneumonia"** caused by *Mycoplasma* species (see Chapter 42) and *Chlamydia* organisms (see Chapter 44) but can be severe. Hepatosplenomegaly is present in approximately half of patients. Histologically diffuse granulomas are seen in the livers of most patients who have acute Q fever.

The most common presentation of chronic Q fever is **subacute endocarditis**, generally on a prosthetic or previously damaged heart valve. The incubation period for chronic Q fever can be months to years, and the presentation is insidious. Unfortunately, chronic disease frequently progresses in an unrelenting fashion, and the prognosis is poor.

Laboratory Diagnosis

At present, Q fever can be diagnosed by culture (not commonly performed) or by specific serologic tests. *C. burnetii* undergoes phase variation, characterized by the development of phase I and II antigens. The phase I antigens are only weakly antigenic. In acute Q fever, immunoglobulin (Ig) M and IgG antibodies are developed primarily against phase II antigens. Acute Q fever is diagnosed on the basis of (1) a fourfold increase in antibody titers, (2) an IgM titer of at least 1:50, or (3) an IgG titer of at least 1:200. The IgM complement fixation titer in untreated patients is first positive after 2 weeks and then reverts to negative after 12 weeks. The IgG titer is positive after 12 weeks and persists for more than 1 year in 90% of patients. A diagnosis of chronic Q fever is confirmed by the demonstration of antibodies against both phase I and II antigens, with the titers to the phase I antigen typically higher. Nucleic acid amplification techniques have been used to detect *Coxiella* and are as sensitive as culture techniques; however, these newer techniques are currently available only in research laboratories.

Treatment, Prevention, and Control

In vitro susceptibility tests have not proved useful for predicting clinical efficacy. For this reason, treatment of acute and chronic *C. burnetii* infections is guided by clinical experience. Currently, it is recommended that acute infections be treated with a tetracycline (e.g., doxycycline). Chronic disease should be treated for a prolonged period with a bactericidal combination of drugs, such as rifampin and either doxycycline or trimethoprim-sulfamethoxazole. The difficulty in the treatment of patients with these infections is that antibiotic activity is suboptimal against the bacteria replicating in intracellular, acidic vacuoles.

Inactivated whole cell vaccines and partially purified antigen vaccines for Q fever have been developed, and the vaccines prepared from phase I organisms have been shown to provide the best protection. Vaccination of animal herds appears efficacious unless the animals have been previously infected naturally. Vaccination does not eradicate *Coxiella* in infected animals or decrease asymptomatic shedding. Likewise, vaccination of humans with phase I vaccines is protective if the vaccinees are uninfected. Vaccination of previously infected individuals is contraindicated, because immune stimulation can lead to an increase in adverse reactions. For this reason, a single-dose vaccine with no booster immunizations is recommended.

CASE STUDY AND QUESTIONS

■ A 37-year-old man came to the local emergency department because of fever, arthralgias, myalgias, and malaise. He was well until 4 days before admission, when he developed a fever reaching 40°C, a diffuse headache, photophobia, nausea, and vomiting. His family physician prescribed a cephalosporin antibiotic at the time of his initial illness, but the patient did not experience any relief of symptoms. Physical examination in the emergency room revealed a critically ill man with a temperature of 39.7°C, pulse of 110 beats/min, respiratory rate of 28 breaths/min, and blood pressure of 100/60 mm Hg. Leukopenia, thrombocytopenia, and elevated serum transaminase levels were noted. A dermatologic evaluation revealed no ulcerations, rashes, or petechiae. The patient recalled having had numerous tick bites 2 weeks before the onset of symptoms. Serologic tests for *Rickettsia* species yielded negative findings; however, tests for *E. chaffeensis* were positive.

1. Name one rickettsial infection and three ehrlichial infections that are observed in the United States. What are the organisms responsible, the reservoirs, and the vectors for each disease?
2. How are *Rickettsia*, *Orientia*, *Ehrlichia*, and *Coxiella* able to survive phagocytosis?
3. What are the major differences in clinical diseases caused by *R. rickettsii* and *E. chaffeensis*?
4. Describe the epidemiology of Q fever. How does the etiologic agent for it differ from that for rickettsial infection?
5. What serologic results would be diagnostic for acute and chronic *Coxiella* infections?

BIBLIOGRAPHY

Archibald L, Sexton D: Long-term sequelae of Rocky Mountain spotted fever, *Clin Infect Dis* 20:1122–1125, 1995.

Bakken J et al: Human granulocytic ehrlichiosis in the upper Midwest United States: a new species emerging? *JAMA* 272:212–218, 1994.

Dumler JS: Laboratory diagnosis of human rickettsial and ehrlichial infections, *Clin Microbiol Newsletter* 18:57–61, 1996.

Dumler JS, Bakken JS: Human ehrlichiosis: newly recognized infections transmitted by ticks, *Annu Rev Med* 49:201–213, 1998.

Fournier P, Marrie T, Raoult D: Minireview: diagnosis of Q fever, *J Clin Microbiol* 36:1823–1834, 1998.

La Scola B, Raoult D: Minireview: laboratory diagnosis of rickettsioses: current approaches to diagnosis of old and new rickettsial diseases, *J Clin Microbiol* 35:2715–2727, 1997.

Magnarelli L, Dumler J: Ehrlichioses: emerging infectious diseases in tick-infected areas, *Clin Microbiol Newsletter* 18: 81–83, 1996.

Maurin M, Raoult D: Q fever, *Clin Microbiol Rev* 12:518–553, 1999.

Raoult D, Roux V: Rickettsioses as paradigms of new or emerging infectious diseases, *Clin Microbiol Rev* 10:694–719, 1997.

Rolain J et al: In vitro susceptibilities of 27 rickettsiae to 13 antimicrobials, *Antimicrob Agents Chemother* 42:1537–1541, 1998.

Schaffner W, Standaert S: Ehrlichiosis—in pursuit of an emerging infection, *N Engl J Med* 334:262–263, 1996 (editorial).

Spach D et al: Tick-borne diseases in the United States, *N Engl J Med* 329:936–947, 1993.

Walker DH: *Biology of rickettsial diseases*, Boca Raton, Fla, 1988, CRC.

C H A P T E R 4 4

Chlamydiaceae

In 1999, the taxonomy of the family Chlamydiaceae was revised extensively on the basis of genomic studies of these organisms (Box 44–1). Previously, the family consisted of one genus, *Chlamydia*, with four species. Now the family has been divided into two genera, *Chlamydia* and *Chlamydophila*. *Chlamydia trachomatis* was retained in the genus *Chlamydia*, but *Chlamydia psittaci* and *Chlamydia pneumoniae* were transferred into the new genus, *Chlamydophila*. Other species have been placed into the two genera, but they are uncommon human pathogens and are not discussed in this chapter.

The Chlamydiaceae were once considered viruses because they are small enough to pass through 0.45-μm filters and are obligate intracellular parasites. However, the organisms have the following properties of bacteria:

1. Possess inner and outer membranes similar to those of gram-negative bacteria.
2. Contain both DNA and RNA.
3. Possess prokaryotic ribosomes.
4. Synthesize their own proteins, nucleic acids, and lipids.
5. Are susceptible to numerous antibacterial antibiotics.

Unlike other bacteria, however, the Chlamydiaceae lack a peptidoglycan layer. Properties that differentiate the three important human pathogens in this family are summarized in Table 44–1.

Physiology and Structure

The Chlamydiaceae exist in two morphologically distinct forms, the small (300- to 400-nm) infectious **elementary body** (EB) and the larger (800- to 1000-nm) noninfectious **reticulate body** (RB).

Much like a spore, the EB is resistant to many harsh environmental factors. Even though these bacteria lack the rigid peptidoglycan layer found in most other bacteria, their outer membrane proteins are extensively cross-linked by disulfide bonds between cysteine resi-

dues. The bacteria do not replicate in the EB form, but they are infectious in this form; that is, they can bind to receptors on host cells and stimulate uptake by the infected cell. The RB is the metabolically active, replicating chlamydial form. Because the extensive cross-linked proteins are absent in RBs, this form is osmotically fragile; however, RBs are protected by their intracellular location.

Other important structural components of Chlamydiaceae are a genus-specific lipopolysaccharide (LPS) that can be detected in a complement fixation (CF) test and species- and strain-specific outer membrane proteins.

The Chlamydiaceae replicate by means of a unique growth cycle that occurs within susceptible host cells (Fig. 44–1). The cycle is initiated when the infectious EBs become attached to the microvilli of susceptible cells, followed by active penetration into the host cell. After they are internalized, the bacteria remain within cytoplasmic phagosomes, where the replicative cycle proceeds. The fusion of cellular lysosomes with the EB-containing phagosome and subsequent intracellular killing is inhibited. Phagolysosomal fusion is prevented if the outer membrane is intact. If the outer membrane is damaged or the bacteria are inactivated by heat or coated with antibodies, phagolysosomal fusion occurs with subsequent bacterial killing.

Within 6 to 8 hours after entering the cell, the EBs reorganize into the metabolically active RBs. RBs are able to synthesize their own DNA, RNA, and protein but lack the necessary metabolic pathways to produce their own high-energy phosphate compounds. The Chlamydiaceae have been termed **energy parasites** because of this defect. Some strains may also depend on the host to provide specific amino acids. The RBs replicate by binary fission, which continues for the next 18 to 24 hours. The phagosome with accumulated RBs, called an **inclusion**, can be readily detected by histologic stains. Approximately 18 to 24 hours after infection, the RBs begin reorganizing into the smaller EBs, and between 48 and 72 hours, the cell ruptures and then releases the infective EBs.

BOX 44–1. Revised Classification of the Family Chlamydiaceae

Genus *Chlamydia*	Genus *Chlamydophila*
C. trachomatis	*C. pneumoniae*
C. muridarum	*C. psittaci*
C. suis	*C. pecorum*
	C. abortus
	C. caviae
	C. felis

Chlamydia trachomatis

C. trachomatis has a very limited host range with infections restricted to humans (Box 44–2). The species has been subdivided into two biovars, **trachoma** and **LGV (lymphogranuloma venereum)**. The biovars (Table 44–2) have been further divided into 19 serotypes (commonly called serologic variants, or **serovars**) on the basis of antigenic differences in the major outer membrane protein (MOMP). The LGV biovar consists of 4 serovars (L_1, L_2, L_{2a}, and L_3); the remaining 15 serovars (**A, B, Ba, C, D, Da, E, F, G, Ga, H, I, Ia, J,** and **K**) are in the trachoma biovar.

Pathogenesis and Immunity

The range of cells that *C. trachomatis* can infect is limited. Receptors for EBs are primarily restricted to nonciliated columnar, cuboidal, or transitional epithelial cells, which are found on the mucous membranes of the urethra, endocervix, endometrium, fallopian tubes, anorectum, respiratory tract, and conjunctivae. The LGV biovar replicates in mononuclear phagocytes present in the lymphatic system. The clinical manifestations of chlamydial infections are due to (1) the direct destruction of cells during replication and (2) the host inflammatory response.

Chlamydiae gain access through minute abrasions or lacerations. In lymphogranuloma venereum, the lesions form in the lymph nodes, draining the site of primary infection (Fig. 44–2). Granuloma formation is characteristic. The lesions may become necrotic, attract polymorphonuclear leukocytes, and cause the inflammatory process to spread to surrounding tissues. Subsequent rupture of the lymph node leads to formation of abscesses or sinus tracts. Infection with non-LGV serotypes of *C. trachomatis* stimulates a severe inflammatory response consisting of neutrophils, lymphocytes, and plasma cells. True lymphoid follicles with germinal centers eventually are induced.

Infection does not confer long-lasting immunity. Rather, reinfection characteristically induces a vigorous inflammatory response with subsequent tissue damage. This response produces the vision loss in patients with chronic ocular infections, and scarring with sterility and sexual dysfunction in patients with genital infections.

Epidemiology

C. trachomatis is found worldwide and causes trachoma (chronic keratoconjunctivitis), oculogenital disease,

TABLE 44–1. Differentiation of Chlamydiaceae That Cause Human Disease

Property	Chlamydia trachomatis	Chlamydophila pneumoniae	Chlamydophila psittaci
Host range	Primarily human pathogen	Primarily human pathogen	Primarily animal pathogen; occasionally infects humans
Biovars	LGV and trachoma	TWAR	Many
Diseases	LGV: lymphogranuloma venereum	Bronchitis, pneumonia, sinusitis, pharyngitis, coronary artery disease (?)	Pneumonia (psittacosis)
	Trachoma: ocular trachoma, oculogenital disease, infant pneumonia		
Elementary body (EB) morphology	Round, narrow periplasmic space	Pear-shaped, large periplasmic space	Round, narrow periplasmic space
Inclusion body morphology	Single, round inclusion per cell	Multiple, uniform inclusions per cell	Multiple, variably sized inclusions per cell
Plasmid DNA	Yes	No	Yes
Iodine-staining glycogen in inclusions	Yes	No	No
Susceptibility to sulfonamides	Yes	No	No

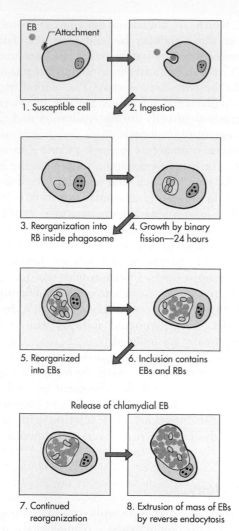

1. Susceptible cell
2. Ingestion
3. Reorganization into RB inside phagosome
4. Growth by binary fission—24 hours
5. Reorganized into EBs
6. Inclusion contains EBs and RBs

Release of chlamydial EB

7. Continued reorganization
8. Extrusion of mass of EBs by reverse endocytosis

FIGURE 44–1. The growth cycle of *Chlamydia trachomatis.* (Redrawn from Batteiger B, Jones R: Chlamydial infections, *Infect Dis Clin North Am* 1:55–81, 1987.)

pneumonia, and LGV (Table 44–2). An estimated 500 million people worldwide are infected with the serovar trachoma, 7 to 9 million of whom are blinded as a result.

Trachoma is endemic in the Middle East, North Africa, and India. Infections occur predominantly in children, who are the chief reservoir of *C. trachomatis* in endemic areas. The incidence of infection is lower in older children and adolescents; however, the incidence of blindness continues to rise through adulthood as the disease progresses. Trachoma is transmitted eye-to-eye by droplet, hands, contaminated clothing, and eye-seeking flies, which transmit ocular discharges from the eyes of infected children to the eyes of uninfected children. Because a high percentage of children in endemic areas harbor *C. trachomatis* in their respiratory and gastrointestinal tracts, the pathogen may also be transmitted by respiratory droplet or through fecal

---

BOX 44–2. Summary of *Chlamydia trachomatis* Infections

Physiology and Structure

Small, gram-negative bacilli with no peptidoglycan layer in cell wall.

Strict intracellular parasite of humans.

Two distinct forms: infectious elementary bodies and noninfectious reticulate bodies.

Lipopolysaccharide (LPS) antigen shared by *Chlamydia* and *Chlamydophila* species.

Major outer membrane proteins (MOMPs) are species-specific.

Two human biovars: trachoma (with 15 serovars) and lymphogranuloma venereum (LGV; 4 serovars).

Infects nonciliated columnar, cuboidal, or transitional epithelial cells.

Virulence

Intracellular replication.

Prevents fusion of phagosome with cellular lysosomes.

Pathologic effects of trachoma due to repeated infections.

Epidemiology

Most common sexually transmitted bacteria in United States.

Ocular trachoma worldwide (most common in Middle East, North Africa, India), with blindness developing in 7 to 9 million patients.

LGV highly prevalent in Africa, Asia, and South America.

Diseases

Trachoma biovar responsible for ocular trachoma, adult inclusion conjunctivitis, neonatal conjunctivitis, infant pneumonia, and urogenital infections.

LGV biovar responsible for LGV and ocular LGV.

Diagnosis

Culture is highly specific but is relatively insensitive. Antigen tests (DFA, ELISA) are relatively insensitive. The molecular amplification tests are the most sensitive and specific tests currently available.

Treatment, Prevention, and Control

Treat LGV with tetracyclines, macrolides, or sulfisoxazole.

Treat ocular or genital infections with azithromycin, doxycycline, or ofloxacin.

Treat newborn conjunctivitis or pneumonia with erythromycin.

Safe sex practices and prompt treatment of patient and sexual partners help control infections.

TABLE 44–2. Clinical Spectrum of *Chlamydia trachomatis* Infections

Serovars	Site of Infection
A, B, Ba, C	Primarily conjunctiva
D through K	Primarily urogenital tract
L_1, L_2, L_{2a}, L_3	Inguinal lymph nodes

contamination. Trachoma generally is endemic in communities where the living conditions are crowded, sanitation is poor, and the personal hygiene of the people is poor—all risk factors that promote the transmission of infections.

Most cases of *C. trachomatis* **adult inclusion conjunctivitis** occur in people who are 18 to 30 years of age, and genital infection probably precedes eye involvement. Autoinoculation and oral-genital contact are believed to be the routes of transmission. A third form of *C. trachomatis* eye infections is **inclusion conjunctivitis in the newborn**, an infection acquired during passage of the infant through an infected birth canal. *C. trachomatis* conjunctivitis develops in approximately 25% of infants whose mothers have active genital infections.

Pulmonary infection with *C. trachomatis* also occurs in newborns. A diffuse interstitial pneumonia develops

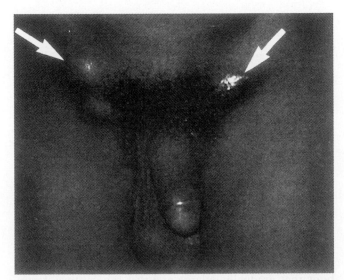

FIGURE 44–2. Patient with lymphogranuloma venereum, showing bilateral inguinal buboes (*arrows*) with adenopathy above and below the inguinal ligament on one side (the groove sign) and thinning of the skin over the adenopathy on the opposite side, where the node is about to rupture. (Reproduced, with permission, from Holmes KK et al, editors: *Sexually transmitted diseases*, ed 3, New York, 1997, the McGraw-Hill Companies.)

in 10% to 20% of infants exposed to the pathogen at birth.

C. trachomatis is thought to be the most common **sexually transmitted bacterial disease** in the United States, with an estimated 4 million new cases per year. It is estimated that 50 million new infections occur each year worldwide. Most genital tract infections are caused by serotypes D through K. *Neisseria gonorrhoeae* and chlamydiae are the most common causes of epididymitis in sexually active men. As much as 15% of the cases of proctitis in homosexual men are caused by *C. trachomatis*.

Lymphogranulosum venereum (LGV) is a chronic sexually transmitted disease caused by *C. trachomatis* serotypes L_1, L_2, L_{2a}, and L_3. It occurs sporadically in North America, Australia, and Europe but is highly prevalent in Africa, Asia, and South America. In the United States, 200 to 500 cases have been reported annually during the past decade, with male homosexuals being the major reservoir of disease. Acute LGV is seen more frequently in men, primarily because symptomatic infection is less common in women.

Clinical Diseases

Trachoma

Trachoma is a chronic disease caused by serovars A, B, Ba, and C. Initially, patients have a follicular conjunctivitis with diffuse inflammation that involves the entire conjunctiva. The conjunctivae become scarred as the disease progresses, causing the patient's eyelids to turn inward. The in-turned eyelashes abrade the cornea, eventually resulting in corneal ulceration, scarring, pannus formation (invasion of vessels into the cornea), and loss of vision. It is common for trachoma to recur after apparent healing, most likely as a result of subclinical infections that have been documented in children in endemic areas and in immigrants to the United States who acquired trachoma during childhood in their native countries.

Adult Inclusion Conjunctivitis

An acute follicular conjunctivitis caused by the *C. trachomatis* strains associated with genital infections (A, B, Ba, D to K) has been documented in sexually active adults. The infection is characterized by mucopurulent discharge, keratitis, corneal infiltrates, and, occasionally, some corneal vascularization. Corneal scarring has been observed in patients with chronic infection.

Neonatal Conjunctivitis

Eye infections can also develop in infants exposed to *C. trachomatis* at birth. After an incubation of 5 to 12 days, the infant's eyelids swell, hyperemia occurs, and copious purulent discharge appears. Untreated infections may run a course as long as 12 months, during which time conjunctival scarring and corneal vascularization occur. Infants who are untreated or are treated with topical therapy only are at risk for *C. trachomatis* pneumonia.

Infant Pneumonia

The incubation period for infant pneumonia is variable, but the onset generally occurs 2 to 3 weeks after birth. Rhinitis is initially observed in such infants, after which a distinctive staccato cough develops. The child remains afebrile throughout the clinical illness, which can last for several weeks. Radiographic signs of infection can persist for months.

Ocular Lymphogranuloma Venereum

The LGV serotypes of *C. trachomatis* have been implicated in Parinaud's oculoglandular conjunctivitis, a conjunctival inflammation associated with preauricular, submandibular, and cervical lymphadenopathy.

Urogenital Infections

Most genital tract infections in women are asymptomatic (as many as 80%) but can nevertheless become symptomatic; the clinical manifestations include cervicitis, endometritis, urethritis, salpingitis, bartholinitis, and perihepatitis. Chlamydial infection may be overlooked in asymptomatic patients. A mucopurulent discharge and hypertrophic ectopy are seen in patients with symptomatic infection, whose specimens generally yield more organisms on cultures than specimens from patients with asymptomatic infections. Urethritis due to *C. trachomatis* may occur with or without a concurrent cervical infection.

As noted earlier, most genital infections in men caused by *C. trachomatis* are symptomatic; however, as many as 25% of chlamydial infections in men may be asymptomatic (Fig. 44–3). Approximately 35% to 50% of cases of nongonococcal urethritis are caused by *C. trachomatis*; dual infections with both sexually transmitted pathogens, *C. trachomatis* and *Neisseria gonorrhoeae*, are not uncommon. The symptoms of the chlamydial infection develop after successful treatment of the gonorrhea, because the incubation period is longer and the use of β-lactam antibiotics to treat gonorrhea would be ineffective against *C. trachomatis*. Although there is less purulent exudate in patients with chlamydial urethral infections, such infections cannot be differentiated reliably from gonorrhea, so specific diagnostic tests for both organisms should be performed.

Reiter's syndrome (urethritis, conjunctivitis, poly-

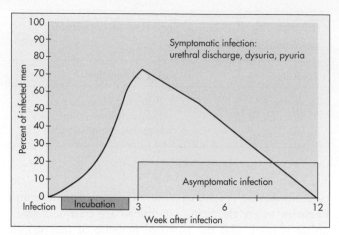

FIGURE 44–3. Time course of untreated chlamydial urethritis in men.

arthritis, and mucocutaneous lesions) is believed to be initiated by genital infection with *C. trachomatis*. Although chlamydiae have not been isolated from the synovial fluid of such patients, EBs have been observed in synovial fluid or tissue specimens from men with sexually acquired reactive arthritis. The disease usually occurs in young white men. Approximately 50% to 65% of patients with Reiter's syndrome have a chlamydial genital infection at the onset of arthritis, and serologic studies indicate that more than 80% of men with Reiter's syndrome have evidence of a preceding or concurrent infection with *C. trachomatis*.

Lymphogranuloma Venereum

After an incubation of 1 to 4 weeks, a primary lesion appears at the site of infection (e.g., penis, urethra, glans, scrotum, vaginal wall, cervix, vulva) in patients with LGV. The lesion (either a papule or an ulcer) is often overlooked, however, because it is small, painless, and inconspicuous and heals rapidly. The absence of pain differentiates these ulcers from those observed in syphilis and herpes simplex virus infections. The patient may experience fever, headache, and myalgia at the time of the lesion.

The second stage of infection is marked by inflammation and swelling of the lymph nodes draining the site of initial infection. The inguinal nodes are most commonly involved, becoming painful, fluctuant **buboes** that gradually enlarge and that can rupture, forming draining fistulas. Systemic manifestations include fever, chills, anorexia, headache, meningismus, myalgias, and arthralgias.

Proctitis is common in women with LGV, resulting from lymphatic spread from the cervix or the vagina. Proctitis develops in men after anal intercourse or as the result of lymphatic spread from the urethra. Untreated LGV may resolve at this stage or it may progress to a chronic ulcerative phase, in which genital ulcers, fistulas, strictures, or genital elephantiasis develops.

Laboratory Diagnosis

C. trachomatis infection can be diagnosed (1) on the basis of cytologic, serologic, or culture findings, (2) through the direct detection of antigen in clinical specimens, and (3) through the use of molecular probes. The sensitivity of each method depends on the patient population examined, the site where the specimen is obtained, and the nature of the disease. For example, symptomatic infections are generally easier to diagnose than asymptomatic infections, because more chlamydiae are present in the specimen from a patient with symptoms. The quality of the specimen is also important. Because chlamydiae are obligate intracellular bacteria, specimens must be obtained from the involved site (e.g., urethra, cervix, rectum, oropharynx, conjunctiva). A specimen of pus or a urethral exudate is inadequate. It has been estimated that 30% of the specimens submitted for study in patients with suspected *Chlamydia* infection are inappropriate.

Cytology

Examination of Giemsa-stained cell scrapings for the presence of inclusions was the first method used for the diagnosis of *C. trachomatis* infection. However, this method is insensitive compared with culture and direct immunofluorescence. Likewise, Papanicolaou's staining of cervical material has been found to be an insensitive and nonspecific method.

Culture

The isolation of *C. trachomatis* in cell culture remains the most specific method of diagnosing *C. trachomatis* infections. The bacteria infect a restricted range of cell lines in vitro (e.g., HeLa-229, McCoy, BHK-21, Buffalo green monkey kidney cells), similar to the narrow range of cells they infect in vivo. The test sensitivity has been improved as the result of modifications in the culture procedures. Some of these modifications are as follows:

1. Pretreatment of the specimen with chemical inhibitors of host cell metabolism (e.g., cycloheximide).
2. Centrifugation of the specimen onto the cell monolayers (modifies the host cell).
3. Use of the shell vial technique (growth of the host cell monolayer on glass coverslips rather than in small microtiter wells).
4. Multiple passages or subcultures of infected cells.
5. The use of iodine stains or fluorescein-conjugated

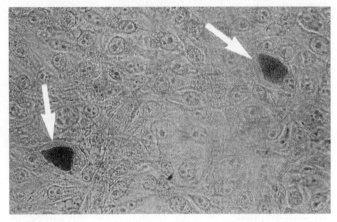

FIGURE 44–4. Iodine-stained *Chlamydia trachomatis* inclusion bodies (*arrows*).

antibodies to detect intracellular inclusions (iodine stains glycogen-containing *C. trachomatis* inclusions; Fig. 44–4).

Despite these improvements, the sensitivity of culture is compromised if inadequate specimens are used and if chlamydial viability has been lost during transport of the specimen. It has been estimated that the sensitivity of the findings yielded by a single endocervical specimen may be only 70% to 85%.

Antigen Detection

Two general approaches have been used to detect chlamydial antigens in clinical specimens, direct immunofluorescence staining (DFA) with fluorescein-conjugated monoclonal antibodies (Fig. 44–5) and enzyme-linked immunoassays (ELISAs). In both assays, antibodies are used that have been prepared against either the chlamydial MOMP or the cell wall LPS. Because antigenic determinants on LPS may be shared

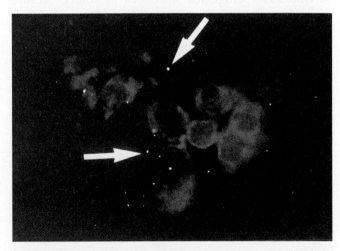

FIGURE 44–5. Fluorescent-stained elementary bodies (*arrows*) in a clinical sample.

with other bacteria, particularly those in fecal specimens, antibody tests that target the LPS antigen are considered less specific. The sensitivity of each assay method has been reported to vary enormously, but neither is considered as sensitive as culture, particularly if male urethral specimens or specimens from asymptomatic patients are used. The latter pose a problem because they may contain relatively few chlamydiae.

Nucleic Acid Probes

Different nucleic acid probe tests are currently available. The tests measure for the presence of a species-specific sequence of 16S rRNA. The advantage of these tests is that the nucleic acid does not have to be amplified so the tests are rapid and relatively inexpensive. However, these tests are relatively insensitive for the detection of small numbers of chlamydiae. For this reason, a number of molecular diagnostic tests have been developed that first amplify a specific sequence of genetic information and then detect it with species-specific probes.

The amplification procedures that are now commercially available for chlamydia testing are (1) the polymerase chain reaction (PCR), (2) ligase chain reaction (LCR), (3) transcription-mediated amplification (TMA), and (4) strand displacement amplification (SDA). These amplification techniques are highly sensitive (generally reported to be 90% to 98% sensitive) and, if properly monitored, are very specific. With further refinements in the technical manipulations used in nucleic acid probe tests, it is expected that they will become the tests of choice for the laboratory diagnosis of *C. trachomatis* infection.

Serology

Serologic testing is of limited value in the diagnosis of *C. trachomatis* urogenital infections in adults, because antibody titers can persist for a prolonged period. Thus, the test cannot differentiate between current and past infections. Demonstration of a significant increase in antibody levels can be useful; however, this increase may not be demonstrated for a month or longer, particularly in patients who receive antibiotic treatment. Testing for immunoglobulin (Ig) M antibodies is also usually not helpful, because adolescents and adults frequently do not produce these antibodies. An exception is the detection of IgM antibodies in infants with chlamydial pneumonitis.

Additionally, antibody tests for the diagnosis of LGV can be helpful. Infected patients produce a vigorous antibody response that can be detected by complement fixation (CF), microimmunofluorescence (MIF), or enzyme immunoassay (EIA). The CF test is directed against the genus-specific LPS antigen. Thus, a posi-tive result (i.e., four-fold increase in titer or a single titer ≥ 1:256) is highly suggestive of LGV. Confirmation is determined by the MIF test, which is directed against species- and serovar-specific antigens (the chlamydial MOMPs). Like the CF test, EIAs are genus-specific. The advantage of these tests is they are less technically cumbersome. However, the results must be confirmed by MIF.

Treatment, Prevention, and Control

It is recommended that patients with LGV be treated with a tetracycline (e.g., doxycycline) for 21 days. Treatment with a macrolide (e.g., erythromycin, azithromycin) or sulfisoxazole is recommended for children younger than 9 years, pregnant women, and patients unable to tolerate tetracyclines. Ocular and genital infections in adults should be treated with one dose of azithromycin, doxycycline for 7 days, or a fluoroquinolone (e.g., ofloxacin) for 7 days. Newborn conjunctivitis and pneumonia should be treated with erythromycin for 10 to 14 days. The effectiveness of tetracyclines, macrolides, and fluoroquinolones is unknown because resistance to all of these antibiotics has now been observed.

It is difficult to prevent *C. trachomatis* infections, because the population with endemic disease commonly has limited access to medical care. The blindness associated with advanced stages of trachoma can be prevented only by prompt treatment of early disease and the prevention of reexposure. Although treatment can be successful in individuals living in areas where the disease is endemic, it is difficult to eradicate the disease within a population and to prevent reinfections unless sanitary conditions are improved. *Chlamydia* conjunctivitis and genital infections are prevented through the use of safe sexual practices and the prompt treatment of symptomatic patients and their sexual partners.

Chlamydophila pneumoniae

C. pneumoniae was first isolated from the conjunctiva of a child in Taiwan. It was initially considered a psittacosis strain, because the morphology of the inclusions produced in cell culture was similar. However, it was shown subsequently that the Taiwan isolate (TW-183) was related serologically to a pharyngeal isolate designated AR-39 and was unrelated to psittacosis strains. This new organism was initially called TWAR, then classified as *Chlamydia pneumoniae*, and finally placed in the new genus *Chlamydophila*. Only a single serotype (TWAR) has been identified. Infection is transmitted by respiratory secretions; no animal reservoir has been identified.

C. pneumoniae is a human pathogen. It is an important cause of bronchitis, pneumonia, and sinusitis, infections being transmitted person-to-person by respiratory secretions. Infection is believed to be common (estimated 200,000 to 300,000 cases of *C. pneumoniae* pneumonia occur annually), and most common in adults. More than 50% of people have serologic evidence of past infections. Most *C. pneumoniae* infections are asymptomatic or mild, causing a persistent cough and malaise; most patients do not require hospitalization. More severe respiratory tract infections typically involve a single lobe of the lungs. These infections cannot be differentiated from other atypical pneumonias, such as those caused by *Mycoplasma pneumoniae*, *Legionella pneumoniae*, and respiratory viruses.

The role of *C. pneumoniae* in the pathogenesis of atherosclerosis remains to be defined. It is known that *C. pneumoniae* can infect and grow in smooth muscle cells, endothelial cells of the coronary artery, and macrophages. The organism has also been demonstrated in biopsy specimens of atherosclerotic lesions by means of culture, PCR amplification, immunohistologic staining, electron microscopy, and in situ hybridization. Thus, the association of *C. pneumoniae* with atherosclerotic lesions is clear. What is not clear is the role of the organism in the development of atherosclerosis. The disease is believed to result from an inflammatory response to chronic infection; however, this remains to be proven.

Diagnosis of *C. pneumoniae* infections is difficult. The organisms do not grow in the cell lines used for the isolation of *C. trachomatis*, and although *C. pneumoniae* will grow in the HEp-2 cell line, this cell line is not used in most clinical laboratories. Detection of *C. pneumoniae* by nucleic acid amplification techniques has been successful, and these may be the most sensitive diagnostic methods available. However, these tests are primarily research tools and are not currently available commercially. CF or MIF tests can be used to make a serologic diagnosis. Because the CF test reacts with *Chlamydia* and *Chlamydophila*, it is not specific for *C. pneumoniae* infection. The MIF test uses *C. pneumoniae* EBs as antigen, so it is specific.

Macrolides (erythromycin, azithromycin, clarithromycin), tetracyclines (tetracycline, doxycycline), or levofloxacin administered for 10 to 14 days has been used to treat infections. Control of exposure to *C. pneumoniae* is likely to be difficult because the bacterium is ubiquitous.

Chlamydophila psittaci

C. psittaci is the cause of psittacosis (parrot fever), which can be transmitted to humans. The disease was first observed in parrots, thus the name **psittacosis** (*psittakos* is the Greek word for "parrot"). In reality, however, the natural reservoir of *C. psittaci* is virtually any species of bird, and the disease has been referred to more appropriately as **ornithosis** (derived from the Greek word *ornithos* for "bird"). Other animals, such as sheep, cows, and goats, as well as humans can become infected. The organism is present in the blood, tissues, feces, and feathers of infected birds that may appear either ill or healthy.

Infection occurs by means of the respiratory tract, after which the bacteria spread to the reticuloendothelial cells of the liver and spleen. The organisms multiply in these sites, producing focal necrosis. The lung and other organs are then seeded as the result of hematogenous spread, which causes a predominantly lymphocytic inflammatory response in the alveolar and interstitial spaces. Edema, thickening of the alveolar wall, infiltration of macrophages, necrosis, and occasionally hemorrhage occur at these sites. Mucous plugs develop in the bronchioles, causing cyanosis and anoxia.

Fewer than 50 cases of the disease are reported annually in the United States, with most infections in adults. This number certainly is an underestimation of the true prevalence of disease, however, because (1) human infections may be asymptomatic or mild, (2) exposure to an infected bird may not be suspected, (3) convalescent serum may not be collected so that the clinical diagnosis can be confirmed, and (4) antibiotic therapy may blunt the antibody response. Furthermore, because of the serologic cross-reactions with *C. pneumoniae*, specific estimates of the prevalence of disease will remain unreliable until a definitive diagnostic test is developed.

The bacterium is usually transmitted to humans through the inhalation of dried bird excrement, urine, or respiratory secretions. Most infections result from exposure to psittacine birds (e.g., parrots, parakeets, macaws, cockatiels). Person-to-person transmission is rare. Veterinarians, zookeepers, pet shop workers, and employees of poultry-processing plants are at increased risk for this infection.

The illness develops after an incubation of 5 to 14 days and usually manifested as headache, high fever, chills, malaise, and myalgia (Fig. 44–6). Pulmonary signs include a nonproductive cough, rales, and consolidation. Central nervous system involvement is common, usually consisting of headache, but encephalitis, convulsions, coma, and death may occur in severe, untreated cases. Patients may suffer gastrointestinal tract symptoms such as nausea, vomiting, and diarrhea. Other systemic symptoms are carditis, hepatomegaly, splenomegaly, and follicular keratoconjunctivitis.

Psittacosis is usually diagnosed on the basis of serologic findings. A fourfold increase in titer, shown by the CF testing of paired acute and convalescent phase sera, is suggestive of *C. psittaci* infection, but the species-specific MIF test must be performed to confirm the diagnosis. *C. psittaci* can be isolated in cell culture

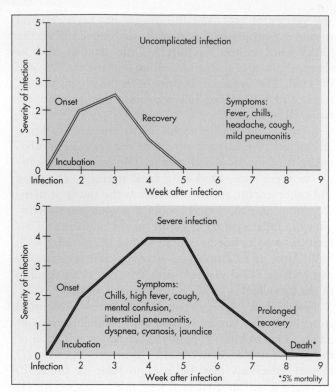

FIGURE 44-6. Time course of *Chlamydophila psittaci* infection.

(e.g., with L cells) after 5 to 10 days of incubation, although this procedure is rarely performed in clinical laboratories.

Infections can be treated successfully with tetracyclines or macrolides. Person-to-person transmission occurs rarely, so isolation of the patient and prophylactic treatment of contacts are not necessary. Psittacosis can be prevented only through the control of infections in domestic and imported pet birds. Such control can be achieved by treating birds with chlortetracycline hydrochloride for 45 days. No vaccine currently exists for this disease.

CASE STUDY AND QUESTIONS

■ A 22-year-old man came to the emergency department with a history of urethral pain and purulent discharge that developed after he had sexual contact with a prostitute. Gram stain of the discharge revealed abundant gram-negative diplococci resembling *Neisseria gonorrhoeae*. The patient was treated with penicillin and sent home. Two days later, the patient returned to the emergency room with a complaint of persistent, watery urethral discharge. Abundant white blood cells but no organisms were observed on Gram stain of the discharge. Culture of the discharge was negative for *N. gonorrhoeae* but positive for *C. trachomatis*.

1. Why is penicillin ineffective against *Chlamydia*? What antibiotic can be used to treat this patient?

2. Describe the growth cycle of *Chlamydia*. What structural features make the EBs and RBs well suited for their environment?

3. Describe the differences among the three species in the family Chlamydiaceae that cause human disease.

4. *C. trachomatis*, *C. pneumoniae*, and *C. psittaci* each cause respiratory tract infections. Describe the patient population most commonly infected and the epidemiology of these infections.

BIBLIOGRAPHY

Black C: Current methods of laboratory diagnosis of *Chlamydia trachomatis* infections, *Clin Microbiol Rev* 10:160–184, 1997.

Boman J, Gaydos C, Quinn T: Minireview: molecular diagnosis of *Chlamydia pneumoniae* infection, *J Clin Microbiol* 37:3791–3799, 1999.

Centers for Disease Control and Prevention: Compendium of psittacosis (chlamydiosis) control, *MMWR* 46 (RR-13): 1–13, 1997.

Everett K, Bush R, Andersen A: Emended description of the order Chlamydiales, proposal of Parachlamydiaceae fam. nov. and Simkaniaceae fam. nov., each containing one monotypic genus, revised taxonomy of the family Chlamydiaceae, including a new genus and five new species, and standards for the identification of organisms, *Int J System Bacteriol* 49:415–440, 1999.

Gibbs R, Carrey N, Davies A: Review: *Chlamydia pneumoniae* and vascular disease, *Br J Surg* 85:1191–1197, 1998.

Grayston J et al: Evidence that *Chlamydia pneumoniae* causes pneumonia and bronchitis, *J Infect Dis* 168:1231–1235, 1993.

Hammerschlag M: Current knowledge of *Chlamydia pneumoniae* and atherosclerosis, *Eur J Clin Microbiol* Infect Dis 17:305–308, 1998 (editorial).

Morre S et al: Urogenital *Chlamydia trachomatis* serovars in men and women with a symptomatic or asymptomatic infection: an association with clinical manifestations? *J Clin Microbiol* 38:2292–2296, 2000.

Ramirez J and the *Chlamydia pneumoniae* Atherosclerosis Study Group: Isolation of *Chlamydia pneumoniae* from the coronary artery of a patient with coronary atherosclerosis, *Ann Intern Med* 125:979–982, 1996.

Schacter J: Biology of *Chlamydia trachomatis*. In Holmes KK et al, editors: *Sexually transmitted diseases*, New York, 1984, McGraw-Hill.

Welsh L, Gaydos C, Quinn T: In vitro activities of azithromycin, clarithromycin, erythromycin, and tetracycline against 13 strains of *Chlamydia pneumoniae*, *Antimicrob Agents Chemother* 40:212–214, 1996.

CHAPTER 45

Role of Bacteria in Disease

A summary of the bacteria most commonly associated with human disease is presented in this chapter. Human diseases develop as pathogenic processes in one or more organ systems. The etiology in some diseases can be attributed to a single organism (e.g., tetanus—*Clostridium tetani*). More commonly, however, multiple organisms can produce a disease syndrome. The clinical management of infections is therefore predicated on the ability to develop a differential diagnosis; that is, it is critical to know which organisms are most commonly associated with a particular infectious process (e.g., bacteremia, pneumonia, gastroenteritis) or an epidemiologic situation (e.g., foodborne or waterborne diseases, arthropod-associated infections).

The development of an infection depends on the complex interactions of (1) the host's susceptibility to infection, (2) the organism's virulence potential, and (3) the opportunity for interaction between host and organism. It is impossible to summarize in a single chapter the complex interactions that lead to the development of disease in each organ system. That is the domain of texts in infectious disease. Rather, this chapter is intended to serve as a very broad overview of the bacteria commonly associated with infections at specific body sites and with specific clinical manifestations (Tables 45–1 to 45–4). Because many factors influence the relative frequency with which specific organisms cause disease (e.g., age, underlying disease, epidemiologic factors, host immunity), no attempt is made to define all the factors associated with disease caused by specific organisms. That material is provided, in part, in the preceding chapters as well in comprehensive infectious disease texts cited in this chapter and in the preceding chapters. Furthermore, the roles of fungi, viruses, and parasites are not considered here but rather in the subsequent sections of this book.

TABLE 45–1. Summary of Bacteria Associated with Human Disease

System Affected	Pathogens
Upper Respiratory Infections	
Pharyngitis	Groups A and C *Streptococcus, Arcanobacterium haemolyticum, Chlamydophila pneumoniae, Neisseria gonorrhoeae, Corynebacterium diphtheriae, Corynebacterium ulcerans, Mycoplasma pneumoniae*
Sinusitis	*Streptococcus pneumoniae, Haemophilus influenzae,* mixed anaerobes, *Staphylococcus aureus, Moraxella catarrhalis,* group A *Streptococcus, Chlamydophila pneumoniae, Pseudomonas aeruginosa* and other gram-negative bacilli
Epiglottitis	*Haemophilus influenzae, Streptococcus pneumoniae, Staphylococcus aureus*
Ear Infections	
Otitis externa	*Pseudomonas aeruginosa, Staphylococcus aureus,* group A *Streptococcus*
Otitis media	*Streptococcus pneumoniae, Haemophilus influenzae, Moraxella catarrhalis, Staphylococcus aureus,* group A *Streptococcus,* mixed anaerobes
Eye Infections	
Conjunctivitis	*Streptococcus pneumoniae,* group B *Streptococcus,* viridans *Streptococcus, Staphylococcus aureus, Moraxella catarrhalis, Haemophilus aegyptius, Neisseria gonorrhoeae, Pseudomonas aeruginosa, Corynebacterium* species, *Francisella tularensis, Chlamydia trachomatis*
Keratitis	*Staphylococcus aureus,* coagulase-negative *Staphylococcus, Streptococcus pneumoniae,* viridans *Streptococcus,* group A *Streptococcus, Pseudomonas aeruginosa, Proteus mirabilis* and other Enterobacteriaceae, *Bacillus* species, *Clostridium perfringens, Neisseria gonorrhoeae*
Endophthalmitis	*Staphylococcus aureus,* coagulase-negative *Staphylococcus, Pseudomonas aeruginosa, Bacillus* species, *Propionibacterium* species, *Corynebacterium* species
Pleuropulmonary and Bronchial Infections	
Bronchitis	*Bordetella pertussis, Mycoplasma pneumoniae, Chlamydophila pneumoniae, Moraxella catarrhalis, Haemophilus influenzae, Streptococcus pneumoniae*
Empyema	*Staphylococcus aureus, Streptococcus pneumoniae,* group A *Streptococcus, Bacteroides fragilis, Klebsiella pneumoniae* and other Enterobacteriaceae, *Actinomyces* species, *Nocardia* species, *Mycobacterium tuberculosis* and other species
Pneumonia	*Streptococcus pneumoniae, Staphylococcus aureus, Haemophilus influenzae, Neisseria meningitidis, Mycoplasma pneumoniae, Chlamydia trachomatis, Chlamydophila pneumoniae, Chlamydophila psittaci, Klebsiella pneumoniae* and other Enterobacteriaceae, *Pseudomonas aeruginosa, Burkholderia* species, *Legionella* species, *Francisella tularensis, Bacteroides fragilis, Nocardia* species, *Rhodococcus equi, Mycobacterium tuberculosis* and other species, *Coxiella burnetii, Rickettsia rickettsii,* and many other species
Urinary Tract Infections	
Cystitis and pyelonephritis	*Escherichia coli, Proteus mirabilis,* other Enterobacteriaceae, *Pseudomonas aeruginosa, Staphylococcus aureus, Staphylococcus epidermidis, Staphylococcus saprophyticus,* group B *Streptococcus, Enterococcus* species, *Aerococcus urinae, Mycobacterium tuberculosis*
Renal calculi	*Proteus* species, *Morganella morganii, Klebsiella pneumoniae, Corynebacterium urealyticum, Staphylococcus saprophyticus, Ureaplasma urealyticum*
Renal abscess	*Staphylococcus aureus,* mixed anaerobes
Prostatitis	*Escherichia coli, Klebsiella pneumoniae,* other Enterobacteriaceae, *Enterococcus* species, *Neisseria gonorrhoeae, Mycobacterium tuberculosis* and other species
Intra-abdominal Infections	
Peritonitis	*Escherichia coli, Klebsiella pneumoniae,* other Enterobacteriaceae, *Pseudomonas aeruginosa, Streptococcus pneumoniae, Staphylococcus aureus, Enterococcus* species, *Bacteroides fragilis* and other species, *Fusobacterium* species, *Clostridium* species, *Peptostreptococcus* species, *Neisseria gonorrhoeae, Chlamydia trachomatis, Mycobacterium tuberculosis*

(continued)

System Affected	Pathogens
Dialysis-associated peritonitis	Coagulase-negative *Staphylococcus, Staphylococcus aureus, Streptococcus* species, *Corynebacterium* species, *Propionibacterium* species, *Escherichia coli* and other Enterobacteriaceae, *Pseudomonas aeruginosa, Acinetobacter* species
Visceral abscesses	*Escherichia coli* and other Enterobacteriaceae, *Enterococcus* species, *Staphylococcus aureus, Bacteroides fragilis, Fusobacterium* species, *Actinomyces* species, mixed anaerobic infections, *Yersinia enterocolitica, Mycobacterium tuberculosis* and other species
Cardiovascular Infections	
Endocarditis	Viridans *Streptococcus, Streptococcus pneumoniae, Abiotrophia* species, *Staphylococcus aureus,* coagulase-negative *Staphylococcus, Stomatococcus mucilaginosus, Enterococcus* species, HACEK organisms, *Bartonella* species, *Coxiella burnetii, Brucella* species, *Erysipelothrix rhusiopathiae,* Enterobacteriaceae, *Pseudomonas aeruginosa, Corynebacterium* species, *Propionibacterium* species
Myocarditis	*Corynebacterium diphtheriae, Clostridium perfringens,* group A *Streptococcus, Borrelia burgdorferi, Neisseria meningitidis, Staphylococcus aureus, Mycoplasma pneumoniae, Chlamydophila pneumoniae, Chlamydophila psittaci, Rickettsia rickettsii, Orientia tsutsugamushi*
Pericarditis	*Streptococcus pneumoniae, Staphylococcus aureus, Neisseria gonorrhoeae, Neisseria meningitidis, Mycoplasma pneumoniae, Mycobacterium tuberculosis* and other species
Sepsis	
General sepsis	*Staphylococcus aureus,* coagulase-negative *Staphylococcus, Streptococcus pneumoniae* and other species, *Enterococcus* species, *Escherichia coli, Klebsiella* species, *Enterobacter* species, *Proteus mirabilis,* other Enterobacteriaceae, *Pseudomonas aeruginosa,* many other bacteria
Transfusion-associated sepsis	*Yersinia enterocolitica,* coagulase-negative *Staphylococcus, Staphylococcus aureus, Pseudomonas fluorescens* group, *Salmonella* species, other Enterobacteriaceae, *Campylobacter jejuni* and other species, *Treponema pallidum, Bacillus cereus* and other species, *Borrelia* species
Septic thrombophlebitis	*Staphylococcus aureus, Klebsiella* species, *Enterobacter* species, *Pseudomonas aeruginosa, Bacteroides* species, *Fusobacterium* species
Central Nervous System Infections	
Meningitis	Group B *Streptococcus, Streptococcus pneumoniae, Neisseria meningitidis, Listeria monocytogenes, Haemophilus influenzae, Escherichia coli,* other Enterobacteriaceae, *Staphylococcus aureus,* coagulase-negative *Staphylococcus, Propionibacterium* species, *Nocardia* species, *Mycobacterium tuberculosis* and other species, *Borrelia burgdorferi, Leptospira* species, *Treponema pallidum, Brucella* species
Encephalitis	*Listeria monocytogenes, Treponema pallidum, Leptospira* species, *Actinomyces* species, *Nocardia* species, *Borrelia* species, *Rickettsia rickettsii, Coxiella burnetii, Mycoplasma pneumoniae, Mycobacterium tuberculosis* and other species
Brain abscess	*Staphylococcus aureus,* Enterobacteriaceae, *Pseudomonas aeruginosa,* viridans *Streptococcus, Bacteroides* species, *Prevotella* species, *Porphyromonas* species, *Fusobacterium* species, *Peptostreptococcus* species, *Actinomyces* species, *Clostridium perfringens, Listeria monocytogenes, Nocardia* species, *Rhodococcus equi, Mycobacterium tuberculosis* and other species
Subdural empyema	*Staphylococcus aureus, Streptococcus pneumoniae,* group B *Streptococcus, Neisseria meningitidis,* mixed anaerobes
Skin and Soft Tissue Infections	
Impetigo	Group A *Streptococcus, Staphylococcus aureus*
Folliculitis	*Staphylococcus aureus, Pseudomonas aeruginosa*
Furuncles and carbuncles	*Staphylococcus aureus*
Paronychia	*Staphylococcus aureus,* group A *Streptococcus, Pseudomonas aeruginosa*
Erysipelas	Group A *Streptococcus*

(continued)

TABLE 45–1. *continued*

System Affected	Pathogens
Skin and Soft Tissue Infections (*continued*)	
Cellulitis	Group A *Streptococcus, Staphylococcus aureus, Haemophilus influenzae,* many other bacteria
Necrotizing cellulitis and fasciitis	Group A *Streptococcus, Clostridium perfringens* and other species, *Bacteroides fragilis,* other anaerobes, Enterobacteriaceae, *Pseudomonas aeruginosa*
Bacillary angiomatosis	*Bartonella henselae, Bartonella quintana*
Infections of burns	*Pseudomonas aeruginosa, Enterobacter* species, *Enterococcus* species, *Staphylococcus aureus,* group A *Streptococcus,* many other bacteria
Bite wounds	*Eikenella corrodens, Pasteurella multocida, Pasteurella canis, Staphylococcus aureus,* group A *Streptococcus,* mixed anaerobes, many gram-negative bacilli
Surgical wounds	*Staphylococcus aureus,* coagulase-negative *Staphylococcus,* groups A and B *Streptococcus, Clostridium perfringens, Corynebacterium* species, many other bacteria
Traumatic wounds	*Bacillus* species, *Staphylococcus aureus,* group A *Streptococcus,* many gram-negative bacilli
Gastrointestinal Infections	
Gastritis	*Helicobacter pylori*
Gastroenteritis	*Campylobacter jejuni* and other species, *Salmonella* species, *Shigella* species, *Vibrio cholerae, Vibrio parahaemolyticus,* other *Vibrio* species, *Yersinia enterocolitica, Escherichia coli* (ETEC, EIEC, EHEC, EPEC, others), *Edwardsiella tarda, Bacillus cereus, Pseudomonas aeruginosa, Aeromonas* species, *Plesiomonas shigelloides, Bacteroides fragilis, Clostridium botulinum, Clostridium perfringens, Clostridium difficile*
Food intoxication	*Staphylococcus aureus, Bacillus cereus, Clostridium botulinum, Clostridium perfringens*
Proctitis	*Neisseria gonorrhoeae, Chlamydia trachomatis, Treponema pallidum*
Bone and Joint Infections	
Osteomyelitis	*Staphylococcus aureus,* coagulase-negative *Staphylococcus,* β-hemolytic *Streptococcus, Streptococcus pneumoniae, Escherichia coli, Salmonella* species and other Enterobacteriaceae, *Pseudomonas aeruginosa, Mycobacterium tuberculosis* and other species, many less common bacteria
Arthritis	*Staphylococcus aureus, Neisseria gonorrhoeae, Streptococcus pneumoniae, Salmonella* species, *Pasteurella multocida, Mycobacterium* species
Prosthetic-associated infections	*Staphylococcus aureus,* coagulase-negative *Staphylococcus,* group A *Streptococcus,* viridans *Streptococcus, Corynebacterium* species, *Propionibacterium* species, *Peptostreptococcus* species
Genital Infections	
Genital ulcers	*Treponema pallidum, Haemophilus ducreyi, Chlamydia trachomatis, Francisella tularensis, Calymmatobacterium* (*Klebsiella*) *granulomatis, Mycobacterium tuberculosis*
Urethritis	*Neisseria gonorrhoeae, Chlamydia trachomatis, Ureaplasma urealyticum*
Vaginitis	*Mobiluncus* species, *Gardnerella vaginalis, Mycoplasma hominis*
Cervicitis	*Neisseria gonorrhoeae, Neisseria meningitidis, Chlamydia trachomatis,* group B *Streptococcus, Mycobacterium tuberculosis, Actinomyces* species
Granulomatous Infections	
General	*Mycobacterium tuberculosis* and other species, *Nocardia* species, *Brucella* species, *Francisella tularensis, Listeria monocytogenes, Burkholderia pseudomallei, Actinomyces* species, *Bartonella henselae, Tropheryma whippelii, Chlamydia trachomatis, Coxiella burnetii, Treponema pallidum, Treponema carateum*

EHEC = Enterohemorrhagic *E. coli;* EIEC = enteroinvasive *E. coli;* EPEC = enteropathogenic *E. coli;* ETEC = enterotoxic *E. coli;* HACEK organisms = *Haemophilus influenzae, Actinobacillus actinomycetemcomitans, Cardiobacterium hominis, Eikenella corrodens,* and *Kingella kingae.*

TABLE 45-2. Selected Bacteria Associated with Foodborne Diseases

Organism	Implicated Food(s)
Aeromonas species	Meats, produce, dairy products
Bacillus cereus	Fried rice, meats, vegetables
Brucella species	Unpasteurized dairy products, meat
Campylobacter species	Poultry, unpasteurized dairy products
Clostridium botulinum	Vegetables, fruits, fish, honey
Clostridium perfringens	Beef, poultry, pork, gravy
Escherichia coli	
Enterohemorrhagic	Beef, unpasteurized milk, fruit juices
Enterotoxigenic	Lettuce, fruits, vegetables
Enteroinvasive	Lettuce, fruit, vegetables
Francisella tularensis	Rabbit meat
Listeria monocytogenes	Unpasteurized dairy products, coleslaw, poultry
Plesiomonas shigelloides	Seafood
Salmonella species	Poultry, unpasteurized dairy products
Shigella species	Eggs, lettuce
Staphylococcus aureus	Ham, poultry, egg dishes, pastries
Streptococcus, group A	Egg dishes
Vibrio cholerae	Shellfish
Vibrio parahaemolyticus	Shellfish
Yersinia enterocolitica	Unpasteurized dairy products, pork

TABLE 45-3. Selected Bacteria Associated with Waterborne Diseases

Organism	Disease
Aeromonas species	Gastroenteritis, wound infections, septicemia
Campylobacter species	Gastroenteritis
Francisella tularensis	Tularemia
Legionella species	Respiratory disease
Leptospira species	Systemic disease
Mycobacterium marinum	Cutaneous infection
Plesiomonas shigelloides	Gastroenteritis
Pseudomonas species	Dermatitis
Salmonella species	Gastroenteritis
Shigella species	Gastroenteritis
Vibrio species	Gastroenteritis, wound infection, septicemia
Yersinia enterocolitica	Gastroenteritis

TABLE 45–4. Arthropod-Associated Diseases

Arthropod	Organism	Disease
Tick	*Borrelia burgdorferi*	Lyme disease
	Borrelia garinii	Lyme disease
	Borrelia afzelii	Lyme disease
	Borrelia, other species	Endemic relapsing fever
	Coxiella burnetii	Q fever
	Ehrlichia chaffeensis	Human monocytic ehrlichiosis
	Ehrlichia phagocytophila	Human granulocytic ehrlichiosis
	Ehrlichia ewingii	Human granulocytic ehrlichiosis
	Francisella tularensis	Tularemia
	Rickettsia rickettsii	Rocky Mountain spotted fever
	Rickettsia conorii	Mediterranean spotted fever
	Rickettsia sibirica	Siberian tick typhus
	Rickettsia australis	Australian tick typhus
	Rickettsia japonica	Oriental spotted fever
Flea	*Rickettsia conorii*	Mediterranean spotted fever
	Rickettsia prowazekii	Sporadic typhus
	Rickettsia typhi	Murine typhus
	Yersinia pestis	Plague
Lice	*Bartonella quintana*	Trench fever
	Borrelia recurrentis	Epidemic relapsing fever
	Rickettsia prowazekii	Epidemic typhus
Mite	*Rickettsia akari*	Rickettsialpox
	Orientia tsutsugamushi	Scrub typhus
Sandfly	*Bartonella bacilliformis*	Bartonellosis (Carrión's disease)

BIBLIOGRAPHY

Balows A, Truper HG, editors: *The prokaryotes*, ed 2, New York, 1992, Springer-Verlag.

Finegold SM, George WL: *Anaerobic infections in humans*, San Diego, 1989, Academic.

Kelley WN et al: *Textbook of internal medicine*, Philadelphia, 1989, JB Lippincott.

Mandell GL, Bennett JE, Dolin R, editors: *Principles and practice of infectious diseases*, ed 5, New York, 2000, Churchill Livingstone.

Murray P: *Pocket guide to clinical microbiology*, ed 2, Washington, DC, 1998, American Society for Microbiology.

Murray PR et al, editors: *Manual of clinical microbiology*, ed 7, Washington, DC, 1999, American Society for Microbiology.

Virology

CHAPTER 46

Mechanisms of Viral Pathogenesis

Viruses cause disease after they break through the natural protective barriers of the body, evade immune control, and either kill cells of an important tissue (e.g., brain) or trigger a destructive immune and inflammatory response. The outcome of a viral infection is determined by the nature of the virus-host interaction and the host's response to the infection (Box 46–1). The immune response is the best treatment, but it often contributes to the pathogenesis of a viral infection. The tissue targeted by the virus affects the nature of the disease and its symptoms. Viral and host factors govern the severity of the disease; they include the strain of virus, the inoculum size, and the general health of the infected person. The ability of the infected person's immune response to control the infection determines the severity and duration of the disease.

A particular disease may be caused by several viruses that have a common tissue **tropism** (preference) (e.g., hepatitis, liver; common cold, upper respiratory tract; encephalitis, central nervous system). On the other hand, a particular virus may cause several different diseases or no observable symptoms. For example, herpes simplex virus (HSV) type 1 (HSV-1) can cause gingivostomatitis, pharyngitis, herpes labialis (cold sores), genital herpes, encephalitis, or keratoconjunctivitis, depending on the affected tissue, or it can cause no disease at all. Although normally benign, this virus can be life-threatening in a newborn or an immunocompromised person.

Many viruses encode activities (**virulence factors**) that promote the efficiency of viral replication, viral transmission, the access and binding of the virus to target tissue, or the escape of the virus from host defenses and immune resolution (see Chapter 14). These activities may not be essential for viral growth in tissue culture but are necessary for the pathogenicity or the survival of the virus in the host. Loss of these virulence factors results in **attenuation** of the virus. Many live-virus vaccines are attenuated virus strains.

The discussion in this chapter focuses on viral disease at the cellular level (cytopathogenesis), the host level (mechanisms of disease), and the population level (epidemiology and control). The antiviral immune response is discussed here and in Chapter 14.

Basic Steps in Viral Disease

Viral disease in the body progresses through defined steps, just like viral replication in the cell (Fig. 46–1*A*). The early steps are as follows:

1. **Acquisition** (entry into the body).
2. **Initiation of infection** at a primary site.
3. An **incubation period,** when the virus is amplified and may spread to a secondary site.

The incubation period may proceed without symptoms (**asymptomatic**) or may produce nonspecific early symptoms, termed the **prodrome.** The **symptoms of the disease** are caused by tissue damage and systemic effects caused by the virus and possibly the immune system. These symptoms may continue through the **convalescence**, while the body repairs the damage. The individual usually develops a memory immune response for future protection against a similar challenge with this virus.

Infection of the Target Tissue

The virus gains **entry into the body** through breaks in the skin or through the mucoepithelial membranes that line the orifices of the body (eyes, respiratory tract, mouth, genitalia, and gastrointestinal tract). The skin is an otherwise excellent barrier to infection, and the orifices are protected by tears, mucus, ciliated epithelium, stomach acid, bile, and immunoglobulin A. *Inhalation is probably the most common route of viral infection.*

On entry into the body, the virus replicates in cells that express viral receptors and that have the appropriate biosynthetic machinery. Many viruses initiate infection in the oral mucosa or upper respiratory tract. Symptoms may accompany viral replication at the primary site. The virus may replicate and remain at the primary site, may disseminate to other tissues via the blood stream or the mononuclear phagocyte and lym-

BOX 46-1. Determinants of Viral Disease

Nature of the Disease

Target tissue
 Portal of entry of virus
 Access of virus to target tissue
 Tissue tropism of virus
 Permissiveness of cells for viral replication
Viral pathogen (strain)

Severity of Disease

Cytopathic ability of virus
Immune status
 Competence of the immune system
 Prior immunity to the virus
Immunopathology
Virus inoculum size
Length of time before resolution of infection
General health of the person
 Nutrition
 Other diseases influencing immune status
Genetic makeup of the person
Age

phatic system, or may disseminate through neurons (Fig. 46–1*B*).

The blood stream and the lymphatic system are the predominant means of viral transfer in the body. The virus may gain access to them after tissue damage, by means of phagocytosis, or upon transport past the mucoepithelial cells of the oropharynx, gastrointestinal tract, vagina, or anus. Several enteric viruses (picornaviruses and reoviruses) bind to receptors on M cells, which translocate the virus to the underlying Peyer's patches of the lymphatic system.

The transport of virus in the blood is termed **viremia.** The virus may be either free in the plasma or may be cell-associated in lymphocytes or macrophages. Viruses taken up by phagocytic macrophages may be inactivated, may replicate, or may be delivered to other tissues by way of the mononuclear phagocyte system. Replication of a virus in macrophages, the endothelial lining of blood vessels, or the liver can cause the infection to be amplified and initiate the development of a **secondary viremia.** In many cases, a secondary viremia precedes delivery of the virus to the **target tissue** (e.g., liver, brain, skin) and the manifestation of symptoms.

Viruses can gain access to the central nervous system or brain (1) from the blood stream (e.g., arboencephalitis viruses), (2) from infected meninges or cerebrospinal fluid, or (3) by means of the migration of infected macrophages or the infection of peripheral and sensory (olfactory) neurons. Viruses in the blood may infect and disrupt the endothelial cell lining and exit the blood vessels or traverse the blood-brain bar-

rier to infect the central nervous system. The meninges are accessible to many of the viruses spread by viremia, which may also provide access to neurons. Herpes simplex, varicella-zoster, and rabies viruses initially infect mucoepithelium, skin, or muscle and then the peripheral innervating neuron, which transports the virus to the central nervous system or brain.

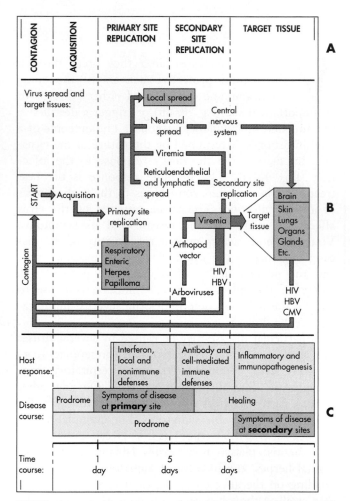

FIGURE 46-1. *A,* The stages of viral infection. The virus is released from one person, is acquired by another, replicates, and initiates a primary infection at the site of acquisition. Depending on the virus, it may then spread to other body sites and finally to a target tissue characteristic of the disease. *B,* The cycle starts with acquisition, as indicated, and proceeds until the release of new virus. The thickness of the *arrow* denotes the degree to which the original virus inoculum is amplified on replication. The *boxes* indicate a site or cause of symptoms. *C,* Time course of viral infection. The time course of symptoms and the immune response correlate with the stage of viral infection and depend on whether the virus causes symptoms at the primary site or only after dissemination to another (secondary) site. HIV = human immunodeficiency virus; HBV = hepatitis B virus; CMV = cytomegalovirus.

BOX 46–2. Determinants of Viral Pathogenesis

Interaction of Virus with Target Tissue

Access of virus to target tissue
   Stability of virus in the body
     Temperature
     Acid and bile of the gastrointestinal tract
   Ability to cross skin or mucous epithelial cells (e.g., cross the gastrointestinal tract into the blood stream)
   Ability to establish viremia
   Ability to spread through the reticuloendothelial system
Target tissue
   Specificity of viral attachment proteins
   Tissue-specific expression of receptors

Cytopathologic Activity of the Virus

Efficiency of viral replication in the cell
   Optimum temperature for replication
   Permissiveness of cell for replication
Cytotoxic viral proteins
Inhibition of cell's macromolecular synthesis
Accumulation of viral proteins and structures (inclusion bodies
Altered cell metabolism (e.g., cell immortalization)

Host Protective Responses

Antigen-nonspecific antiviral responses
   Interferon
   Natural killer cells and macrophages
Antigen-specific immune responses
   T-cell responses
   Antibody responses
Viral mechanisms of escape of immune responses

Immunopathology

Interferon: flu-like systemic symptoms
T-cell responses: delayed-type hypersensitivity
Antibody: complement, antibody-dependent cellular cyto toxicity, immune complexes
Other inflammatory responses

Viral Pathogenesis

Cytopathogenesis

The three potential outcomes of a viral infection of a cell are as follows (Box 46–2 and Table 46–1):

1. Failed infection (**abortive infection**).
2. Cell death (**lytic infection**).
3. Infection without cell death (**persistent infection**).

Viral mutants, which cause abortive infections, do not multiply and therefore disappear. Persistent infections may be (1) **chronic** (nonlytic, productive), (2) **latent** (limited viral macromolecular but no virus synthesis), (3) **recurrent**, or (4) **transforming (immortalizing)**.

TABLE 46–1. Types of Viral Infections at the Cellular Level

Type	Virus Production	Fate of Cell
Abortive	−	No effect
Cytolytic	+	Death
Persistent		
Productive	+	Senescence
Latent	−	No effect
Transforming		
DNA viruses	−	Immortalization
RNA viruses	+	Immortalization

The nature of the infection is determined by the characteristics of both the viruses and the cell. A **nonpermissive cell** does not allow replication of a particular type or strain of virus. A **permissive cell** provides the biosynthetic machinery (e.g., transcription factors, post-translational processing enzymes) to support the complete replicative cycle of the virus. A **semipermissive cell** may be very inefficient or may support some but not all the steps in viral replication.

Replication of the virus can initiate changes in cells that lead to cytolysis or to alterations in the cell's appearance, functional properties, or antigenicity. The effects on the cell may result from viral takeover of macromolecular synthesis, the accumulation of viral proteins or particles, or a modification or disruption of cellular structures (Table 46–2).

Lytic Infections

Lytic infection results when virus replication kills the target cell. Some viruses prevent cellular growth and repair by inhibiting the synthesis of cellular macromolecules or by producing degradative enzymes and toxic proteins. For example, herpes simplex and other viruses produce proteins that inhibit the synthesis of cellular DNA and messenger RNA (mRNA) and synthesize other proteins that degrade host DNA to provide substrates for viral genome replication. Cellular protein synthesis may be actively blocked (e.g., poliovirus inhibits translation of 5'-capped cellular mRNA) or pas-

TABLE 46–2. Mechanisms of Viral Cytopathogenesis

Mechanism	Examples
Inhibition of cellular protein synthesis	Polioviruses, herpes simplex virus, togaviruses, poxviruses
Inhibition and degradation of cellular DNA	Herpesviruses
Alteration of cell membrane structure	Enveloped viruses
Glycoprotein insertion	All enveloped viruses
Syncytia formation	Herpes simplex virus, varicella-zoster virus, paramyxoviruses, human immunodeficiency virus
Disruption of cytoskeleton	Nonenveloped viruses (accumulation), herpes simplex virus
Permeability	Togaviruses, herpesviruses
Inclusion bodies	
Negri bodies (intracytoplasmic)	Rabies
Owl's eye (intranuclear)	Cytomegalovirus
Cowdry type A (intranuclear)	Herpes simplex virus, subacute sclerosing panencephalitis (measles) virus
Intranuclear basophilic	Adenoviruses
Intracytoplasmic acidophilic	Poxviruses
Perinuclear cytoplasmic acidophilic	Reoviruses
Toxicity of virion components	Adenovirus fibers

sively blocked (e.g., through the production of much viral mRNA that successfully competes for ribosomes) (see Chapter 6).

Replication of the virus and the accumulation of viral components and progeny within the cell can disrupt the structure and function of the cell or disrupt lysosomes, causing autolysis. The expression of viral antigens on the cell surface and disruption of the cytoskeleton can cause the cell-to-cell interactions and cellular appearance to change, making the cell a target for immune cytolysis.

Cell surface expression of the glycoproteins of some paramyxoviruses, herpesviruses, and retroviruses triggers the fusion of neighboring cells into multinucleated giant cells called **syncytia**. Cell-to-cell fusion may occur in the absence of new protein synthesis (fusion from without), as occurs in infections with Sendai virus and other paramyxoviruses, or may require new protein synthesis (fusion from within), as occurs in infection with the HSV. Syncytia formation allows the virus to spread from cell to cell and escape antibody detection. The syncytia formation that occurs in infection with the human immunodeficiency virus (HIV) also causes death of the cells.

Virus infection or cytolytic immune responses may induce **apoptosis** in the infected cell. Apoptosis is a preset cascade of events that, when triggered, leads to cellular suicide. This process may facilitate release of the virus from the cell but it also limits the amount of virus that is produced by destroying the viral "factory." As a result, *many viruses (e.g., herpesviruses, adenovirus, hepatitis C virus) encode methods for inhibiting apoptosis.*

Some viral infections cause characteristic changes in the appearance and properties of the target cells. For example, chromosomal aberrations and degradation may occur and can be detected with histologic staining (e.g., marginated chromatin ringing the nuclear membrane in HSV-infected and adenovirus-infected cells). In addition, new, stainable structures called **inclusion bodies** may appear within the nucleus or cytoplasm. These structures may result from virus-induced changes in the membrane or chromosomal structure or may represent the sites of viral replication or accumulations of viral capsids. Because the nature and location of these inclusion bodies are characteristic of particular viral infections, the presence of such bodies facilitates laboratory diagnosis (see Table 46–2). Viral infection may also cause vacuolization, or rounding of the cells, and other nonspecific histologic changes indicative of sick cells.

Nonlytic Infections

A **persistent infection** occurs in an infected cell that is not killed by the virus. Some viruses cause a persistent productive infection because the virus is released gently from the cell through exocytosis or through budding (enveloped viruses) from the plasma membrane.

A **latent** or **immortalizing infection** may result from DNA virus infection of a cell that restricts or lacks the machinery for transcribing all the viral genes. The specific transcription factors required by such a virus may be expressed only in specific tissues, in growing but not resting cells, or after hormone or cytokine induction. For example, HSV establishes a latent infection in neurons that lack the nuclear factors required to transcribe the immediate early viral genes, but stress and other stimuli can activate viral replication.

Oncogenic Viruses

Some DNA viruses and retroviruses establish persistent infections that can also stimulate uncontrolled cell growth, causing the **transformation** or **immortalization** of the cell (Fig. 46–2). Characteristics of transformed cells include continued growth without senescence, alterations in cell morphology and metabolism, increased cell growth rate and sugar transport, loss of cell-contact-inhibition of growth, and ability to grow in a suspension or a semisolid agar.

Different **oncogenic** viruses have different mechanisms for immortalizing cells. Viruses immortalize cells by (1) promoting or providing growth-stimulating genes, (2) removing the inherent braking mechanisms that limit DNA synthesis and cell growth, or (3) preventing apoptosis. Immortalization by DNA viruses occurs in semipermissive cells, which express only select viral genes but do not produce virus. The synthesis of viral DNA, late mRNA, late proteins, or virus leads to cell death, which precludes immortalization. Most oncogenic DNA viruses integrate into the host cell chromosome. Papillomavirus, SV40 virus, and adenovirus encode proteins that bind and inactivate cell growth-regulatory proteins, such as p53 and the retinoblastoma gene product. Loss of p53 also makes the cell more susceptible to mutation, thus releasing the brakes on cell growth. Epstein-Barr virus immortalizes B cells by stimulating cell growth (as a B-cell mitogen) and by inducing expression of the cell's *bcl-2* oncogene, which prevents programmed cell death (apoptosis).

Retroviruses (RNA viruses) use two approaches to oncogenesis. Some oncoviruses encode **oncogene** proteins (e.g., *sis, ras, src, mos, myc, jun, fos*), which are almost identical to the cellular proteins involved in

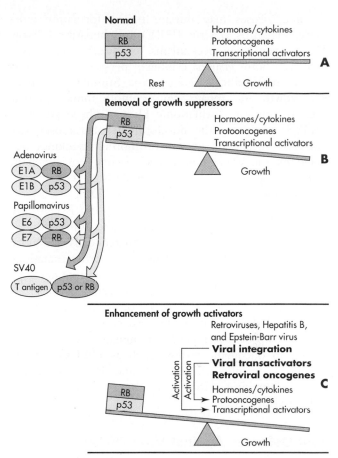

FIGURE 46–2. Mechanisms of viral transformation and immortalization. Cell growth is controlled (*A*) by the maintenance of a balance in the external and internal growth activators (accelerators) and by growth suppressors such as p53 and the retinoblastoma gene product (RB) (brakes). Oncogenic viruses alter the balance by removing the brakes (*B*) or enhancing the effects of the accelerators (*C*).

cellular growth control (e.g., components of a growth factor signal cascade or growth-regulating transcription factors). The overproduction or altered function of these oncogene products stimulates cell growth. These oncogenic viruses *rapidly* cause tumors to form. *However, no human retrovirus of this type has been identified.*

Human T-cell lymphotropic virus (HTLV-1), the only human oncogenic retrovirus identified, uses more subtle mechanisms of leukemogenesis. It encodes a protein (**tax**) that **transactivates** gene expression, including genes for growth-stimulating lymphokines (e.g., interleukin-2). This constitutes the second approach to oncogenesis. The integration of HTLV-1 near a cellular growth-stimulating gene can also cause the gene to be activated by the strong viral enhancer and promoter sequences encoded at each end of the viral genome (LTR sequences). *HTLV-1–associated leukemias* **develop slowly**, *occurring 20 to 30 years after infection.* Retroviruses continue to produce virus in immortalized or transformed cells.

Some viruses may initiate tumor formation indirectly. Hepatitis B virus (HBV) and hepatitis C virus (HCV) may have mechanisms for direct oncogenesis; however, both viruses establish persistent infections and initiate significant tissue repair. Stimulation of liver cell growth and repair may promote mutations that lead to tumor formation. Human herpesvirus 8 (HHV8) promotes the development of Kaposi's sarcoma by means of growth-promoting cytokines encoded by the virus; this disease occurs most often in immunosuppressed patients, such as those with the acquired immunodeficiency syndrome (AIDS).

Viral transformation is the first step but is generally not sufficient to cause oncogenesis and tumor formation. Instead, over time, immortalized cells are more likely than normal cells to accumulate other mutations or chromosomal rearrangements that promote development of tumor cells. Immortalized cells may also be more susceptible to cofactors and tumor promoters (e.g., phorbol esters, butyrate) that enhance tumor formation. Approximately 15% of human cancers can be related to oncogenic viruses such as HTLV-1, HBV and HCV, papillomaviruses 16 and 18, HHV8, and Epstein-Barr virus. HSV-2 may be a co-factor for human cervical cancer.

Host Defenses Against Viral Infection

The skin is the best barrier to infection, but openings in the skin, whether natural orifices (e.g., mouth, eyes, nose, ears, anus) or due to trauma such as abrasion or puncture, provide pathogens with access to the body. The natural openings have basic protections that, in addition to skin, are part of **the natural barriers of the body** (e.g., mucus, ciliated epithelium, gastric acid, tears, bile). After the virus penetrates the natural barriers, it activates the **antigen-nonspecific (innate) immune defenses** (e.g., fever, interferon, macrophages, natural killer cells), which attempt to limit and control local viral replication and spread. **Antigen-specific immune responses** (e.g., antibodies, helper T [TH] cells) are the last to be activated and can be divided into (1) early-local responses (**TH1**), (2) later-systemic-antibody responses (**TH2**), and (3) **immune memory**. Interferon and cytotoxic T-cell responses may have evolved primarily as antiviral defense mechanisms.

*The ultimate goal of the host response is to eliminate the virus and the cells harboring or replicating the virus (**resolution**). The immune response is the best and in most cases the only means of controlling a viral infection. Both humoral and cellular immune responses are important for antiviral immunity.* A detailed description of the antiviral immune response is presented in Chapter 14.

A viral infection resolves when all infectious virus and virus-infected cells are cleared from the body. The nonspecific responses produced by interferon and local antigen are often sufficient to limit infection and promote resolution. **Antibody** *is effective against extracellular virus, especially* **viremias**, and may be sufficient to *control cytolytic viruses* because the virion factory within the infected cell is eliminated by viral replication. **Cell-mediated immunity** *is required for lysis of the target cell in the setting of* **noncytolytic infections** (*e.g., hepatitis A virus*) *and infections caused by* **enveloped viruses.** Failure to resolve the infection may lead to persistent infection, chronic disease or death of the patient.

Prior immunity, due to memory B and T cells, may not prevent the initial stages of infection but in most cases does prevent disease progression. Upon rechallenge, serum antibody can prevent viremic spread of the virus, and secondary responses develop much more rapidly and are more effective than primary responses; this is the basis for the development of vaccine programs.

Immunopathology

The hypersensitivity and inflammatory reactions initiated by antiviral immunity can be the major cause of the pathologic manifestations and symptoms of viral disease (Table 46–3). Early responses to the virus and viral infection, such as interferon and lymphokines, and activation of the C3 component of complement by the alternative pathway can initiate local inflammatory as well as systemic responses. For example, interferon and lymphokines stimulate the **flu-like systemic symptoms** that are usually associated with *respiratory viral infections and viremias* (e.g., fever, runny nose, malaise, headache). These symptoms often precede (**prodrome**) the characteristic symptoms of the viral infection, during the viremic stage. Later, immune complexes and complement activation (classic pathway), CD4 T-cell–induced delayed-type hypersensitivity, and CD8 cytolytic T cell action may induce tissue damage. These actions often promote neutrophil infiltration and more cell damage.

The inflammatory response initiated by cell-mediated immunity is difficult to control and damages tissue. *Infections by enveloped viruses in particular induce cell-mediated immune responses that usually produce more extensive immunopathologic conditions.* For example, the classic symptoms of measles and mumps result from the T-cell–induced inflammatory and hypersensitivity responses rather than from cytopathologic effects of the virus. The presence of large amounts of antigen in blood during viremias or chronic infections (e.g., hepatitis B virus infection) can initiate the **classic type III immune complex hypersensitivity reactions. Immune complexes** containing virus or viral antigen can activate the complement system, triggering inflammatory responses and tissue destruction. These immune complexes often accumulate in the kidney and cause renal problems.

In the case of dengue and measles viruses, partial

TABLE 46–3. Viral Immunopathogenesis

Immunopathogenesis	Immune Mediators	Examples
Flu-like symptoms	Interferon, lymphokines	Respiratory viruses, arboviruses (viremia-inducing viruses)
Delayed type hypersensitivity and inflammation	T cells, macrophages, and polymorphonuclear leukocytes	Enveloped viruses
Immune complex disease	Antibody, complement	Hepatitis B virus, rubella
Hemorrhagic disease	T cell, antibody, complement	Dengue virus
Postinfection cytolysis	T cells	Enveloped viruses (e.g., postmeasles encephalitis)
Immunosuppression	—	Human immunodeficiency virus, cytomegalovirus, measles virus, influenza virus

immunity to a related or inactivated virus can result in a more severe host response and disease upon subsequent challenge with a related or virulent virus. This is because antigen-specific T-cell and antibody responses are enhanced and induce significant inflammatory and hypersensitivity damage to infected endothelial cells (*dengue hemorrhagic fever*) or skin and the lung (*atypical measles*). In addition, a non-neutralizing antibody can facilitate the uptake of dengue and yellow fever viruses into macrophages through Fc receptors, where they can replicate.

Children generally have a less active cell-mediated immune response than adults and therefore usually have milder symptoms during infections by some viruses (e.g., measles, mumps, Epstein-Barr, and varicella-zoster viruses). However, in the case of hepatitis B virus, mild or no symptoms correlate with an inability to resolve the infection, resulting in chronic disease.

Viral Disease

The relative **susceptibility** of a person and the **severity** of the disease depend on the following factors:

1. The nature of the exposure.
2. The immune status, age, and general health of the person.
3. The viral dose.
4. The genetics of the virus and the host.

Once the host is infected, however, the host's immune status and competence are probably the major factors that determine whether a viral infection causes a life-threatening disease, a benign lesion, or no symptoms at all.

The stages of viral disease are shown in Figure 46–1C. The initial period before the characteristic symptoms of a disease are detected is termed the **incubation period**. During this period, the virus is replicating but has not reached the target tissue or induced sufficient damage to cause the disease. *The incubation period*

is relatively short if infection of the primary site produces the characteristic symptoms of the disease. During the **prodrome**, nonspecific or flu-like symptoms may precede the characteristic symptoms of the disease. The incubation periods for many common viral infections are listed in Table 46–4. Specific viral diseases are dis-

TABLE 46–4. Incubation Periods of Common Viral Infections

Disease	Incubation Period (days)*
Influenza	1–2
Common cold	1–3
Bronchiolitis, croup	3–5
Acute respiratory disease (adenoviruses)	5–7
Dengue	5–8
Herpes simplex	5–8
Enteroviruses	6–12
Poliomyelitis	5–20
Measles	9–12
Smallpox	12–14
Chickenpox	13–17
Mumps	16–20
Rubella	17–20
Mononucleosis	30–50
Hepatitis A	15–40
Hepatitis B	50–150
Rabies	30–100
Papilloma (warts)	50–150
Human immunodeficiency virus (acquired immunodeficiency syndrome)	1–10 years

*Until first appearance of prodromal symptoms. Diagnostic signs (e.g., rash, paralysis) may not appear until 2 to 4 days later.

Modified from White DO, Fenner F: *Medical virology*, ed 3, New York, 1986, Academic.

cussed in subsequent chapters and reviewed in Chapter 65.

The nature and severity of the symptoms of a viral disease are related to the function of the infected target tissue (e.g., liver, hepatitis; brain, encephalitis) and the extent of the immunopathologic responses triggered by the infection. **Inapparent infections** result if (1) the infected tissue is undamaged, (2) the infection is controlled before the virus reaches its target tissue, (3) the target tissue is expendable, (4) the damaged tissue is rapidly repaired, or (5) the extent of damage is below a functional threshold for that particular tissue. For example, many infections of the brain are inapparent or are below the threshold of severe loss of function, but encephalitis results if the loss of function becomes significant. However, *asymptomatic infections are major sources of contagion.* Inapparent infections are frequently detected in people as the finding of virus-specific antibody. For example, although 97% of adults have antibody (seropositive) to varicella-zoster virus, less than half remember having had chickenpox.

Viral infections may cause **acute** or **chronic disease (persistent infection)**. The ability and speed with which a person's immune system controls and resolves a viral infection usually determine whether acute or chronic disease ensues as well as the severity of the symptoms (Fig. 46–3). The acute episode of a persistent infection may be asymptomatic (JC papovavirus) or may, later in life, cause symptoms that are similar to (varicella and zoster) or different from (HIV) those of the acute disease. **Slow viruses** have long incubation periods during which sufficient virus or tissue destruction accumulates prior to a rapid progression of symptoms.

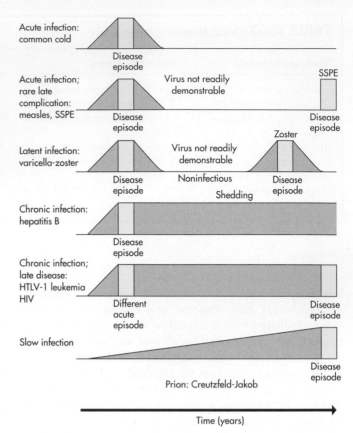

FIGURE 46–3. Acute infection and various types of persistent infection, as illustrated by the diseases indicated in the column at the *left. Blue* represents presence of virus; *green* indicates episode of disease. SSPE = subacute sclerosing panencephalitis. (Modified from White DO, Fenner F: *Medical virology,* ed 3, New York, 1986, Academic.)

Epidemiology

Epidemiology studies the spread of disease through a population. Infection of a population is similar to infection of a person, in that the virus must spread through the population and is controlled by immunization of the population (Box 46–3). To endure, viruses must continue to infect new, immunologically naive, susceptible hosts.

Exposure

People are exposed to viruses throughout their lives. However, some situations, vocations, lifestyles, and living arrangements increase the likelihood that a person will come in contact with certain viruses. In addition, many viruses are **ubiquitous**, as borne out by the fact that evidence of exposure (antibodies to the virus) can be detected in most young children (HSV-1, HHV6, varicella-zoster virus, parvovirus B19) or by early adulthood (Epstein-Barr virus and many respiratory and enteric viruses).

Poor hygiene and crowded living, school, and job conditions promote exposure to respiratory and enteric viruses. Daycare centers are consistent sources of viral infections, especially viruses spread by the respiratory and fecal-oral routes. Travel, summer camp, and vocations that bring people in contact with a virus vector, such as mosquitos, put them at particular risk for infection by arboviruses and other zoonoses. Sexual promiscuity also promotes the spread and acquisition of several viruses. Health care workers, such as physicians, dentists, nurses, and technicians, are frequently exposed to respiratory and other viruses but are uniquely at risk for acquiring viruses from contaminated blood (HBV, HIV) or vesicle fluid (HSV).

Transmission of Viruses

Viruses are transmitted by direct contact (including sexual contact), injection with contaminated fluids or blood, the transplantation of organs, and the respiratory and fecal-oral routes (Table 46–5). *The route of transmission depends on the source of the virus (the tissue*

BOX 46-3. Viral Epidemiology*

Mechanisms of Viral Transmission†

Aerosols
Food, water
Fomites (e.g., tissues, clothes)
Direct contact with secretions (e.g., saliva, semen)
Sexual contact, birth
Blood transfusion or organ transplant
Zoonoses (animals, insects [arboviruses])

Disease and Viral Factors that Promote Transmission

Stability of virion in response to the environment (e.g., drying, detergents, temperature)
Replication and secretion of virus into transmissible aerosols and secretions (e.g., saliva, semen)
Asymptomatic transmission
Transience or ineffectiveness of immune response to control reinfection or recurrence

Risk Factors

Age
Health
Immune status
Occupation: contact with agent or vector
Travel history

Risk Factors—cont'd

Lifestyle
Children in daycare centers
Sexual activity

Critical Community Size

Seronegative, susceptible people

Geography and Season

Presence of co-factors or vectors in the environment
Habitat and season for arthropod vectors (mosquitos)
School session: close proximity and crowding
Home-heating season

Modes of Control

Quarantine
Elimination of the vector
Immunization
    Natural infection
    Vaccination
Treatment

*Infection of a population instead of a person.
†See also Table 46–5.

---

site of viral replication and secretion) and the ability of the virus to endure the hazards and barriers of the environment and the body en route to the target tissue. For example, viruses that replicate in the respiratory tract (e.g., influenza A virus) are released in aerosol droplets, whereas enteric viruses (e.g., picornaviruses and reoviruses) are passed by the fecal-oral route. Cytomegalovirus is transmitted in most bodily secretions because it infects mucoepithelial, secretory, and other cells found in the skin, secretory glands, lungs, liver, and other organs. Togaviruses and rhabdoviruses can be introduced into human hosts by means of arthropod or animal bites.

The presence or absence of an envelope is the major structural determinant of the mode of viral transmission. **Nonenveloped viruses** (naked capsid viruses) can withstand drying, the effects of detergents, and extremes of pH and temperature, whereas enveloped viruses generally cannot. Specifically, most nonenveloped viruses can withstand the acidic environment of the stomach and the detergent-like bile of the intestines as well as mild disinfection and insufficient sewage treatment. These viruses are generally transmitted by the respiratory and fecal-oral routes and can often be acquired from contaminated objects, termed **fomites**. For example, hepatitis A virus, a picornavirus, is a nonen-

veloped virus that is transmitted by the fecal-oral route and acquired from contaminated water, shellfish, and food. Rhinoviruses and many other nonenveloped viruses can be spread by contact with fomites such as handkerchiefs and toys.

Unlike the sturdy nonenveloped viruses, **enveloped viruses** are comparatively fragile. They require an intact envelope for infectivity. These viruses must remain wet and are spread (1) in respiratory droplets, blood, mucus, saliva, or semen, (2) by injection, or (3) in organ transplants. Most enveloped viruses are also labile in response to acid and detergents, a feature that precludes their being transmitted by the fecal-oral route. Exceptions are HBV and coronaviruses.

Animals can also act as **vectors** that spread viral disease to other animals and humans and even to other locales. They can also be **reservoirs** for the virus, which maintain and amplify the virus in the environment. Viral diseases that are shared by animals or insects and humans are called **zoonoses**. For example, raccoons, foxes, bats, dogs, and cats are vectors for the rabies virus. Arthropods, including mosquitos, ticks, and sandflies, can act as vectors for togaviruses, flaviviruses, bunyaviruses, and reoviruses. These viruses are often referred to as **arboviruses** because they are *ar-*

TABLE 46–5. Viral Transmission

Mode	Examples
Respiratory transmission	Paramyxoviruses, influenza viruses, picornaviruses, rhinoviruses, enteroviruses, varicella-zoster virus, B19 virus
Fecal-oral transmission	Picornaviruses, rotavirus, reovirus, caliciviruses, Norwalk virus, adenovirus
Contact (lesions, saliva, fomites)	Herpes simplex virus, rhinoviruses, poxviruses, adenovirus
Zoonoses (animals, insects)	Togaviruses (alpha), flaviviruses, bunyaviruses, orbiviruses, arenaviruses, rabies virus, orf (pox)
Transmission via blood	Human immunodeficiency virus, human T-cell lymphotropic virus-1, hepatitis B virus, hepatitis C virus, hepatitis delta virus, cytomegalovirus
Sexual contact	Blood-borne viruses, herpes simplex virus, human papillomavirus
Maternal-neonatal transmission	Rubella virus, cytomegalovirus, B19 virus, echovirus, herpes simplex virus, varicella-zoster virus
Genetic	Prions, retroviruses

thropod *bo*rne. Most arboviruses have a very broad host range, capable of replicating in specific insects, birds, amphibians, and mammals in addition to humans. Also, the arboviruses must establish a viremia in the animal reservoir so that the insect can acquire the virus during its blood meal.

Other factors that can promote the transmission of viruses are the potential for asymptomatic infection, crowded living conditions, certain occupations, certain lifestyles, daycare centers, and travel. With regard to the first of these conditions, many viruses (e.g., HIV, varicella-zoster virus) are released before symptoms appear, making it difficult to restrict transmission. Viruses that cause persistent productive infections (e.g., cytomegalovirus, HIV) are a particular problem because the infected person is a continual source of virus that can be spread to immunologically naive people. Viruses with many different serotypes (rhinoviruses) or viruses capable of changing their antigenicity (influenza and HIV) also readily find immunologically naive populations.

Maintenance of a Virus in the Population

The persistence of a virus in a community depends on the availability of a critical number of immunologically naive (seronegative), susceptible people. The efficiency of virus transmission determines the size of the susceptible population necessary for maintenance of the virus in the population. Immunization, produced by natural means or by vaccination, is the best way of reducing the number of such susceptible people.

Age

The age of the person is an important factor in determining his or her susceptibility to viral infections. Infants, children, adults, and the elderly are susceptible to different viruses and have different symptomatic responses to the infection. These differences may result from variations in body size, tissue characteristics, recuperative abilities, and, most important, immune status in people in these age groups. Differences in lifestyles, habits, school environments, and job settings at different ages also determine when people are exposed to viruses.

Infants and children acquire a series of respiratory and exanthematous viral diseases at first exposure because they are immunologically naive. Infants are especially prone to more serious presentations of paramyxovirus respiratory infections and gastroenteritis because of their small size and physiologic requirements (e.g., nutrients, water, electrolytes). However, children generally do not mount as severe an immunopathologic response as adults, and some diseases (herpesviruses) are more benign in children.

The elderly are especially susceptible to new viral infections and the reactivation of latent viruses. Because they are less able to initiate a new immune response, repair damaged tissue, and recover, they are therefore more susceptible to outbreaks of the new strains of the influenza A and B viruses. The elderly are also more prone to zoster (shingles), a recurrence of varicella-zoster virus, as a result of the decline in this specific immune response with age.

Immune Status

The competence of a person's immune response and his or her immune history determine how quickly and efficiently the infection is resolved and can also determine the severity of the symptoms. The rechallenge of a person with prior immunity usually results in asymptomatic or mild disease without transmission. People who are in an immunosuppressed state as a result of AIDS, cancer, or immunosuppressive therapy are at greater risk of suffering more serious disease upon primary infection (measles, vaccinia) and more prone to suffer recurrences of infections with latent viruses (e.g., herpesviruses, papovaviruses).

Other Host Factors

The general health of a person plays an important role in determining the competence and nature of his or her immune response and ability to repair diseased tissue. Poor nutrition can compromise a person's immune system and decrease his or her tissue regenerative capacity. Immunosuppressive diseases and therapies may allow viral replication or recurrence to proceed unchecked. A person's genetic makeup also plays an important role in determining the response of his or her immune system to viral infection. Specifically, genetic differences in immune response genes, genes for viral receptors, and other genetic loci affect the person's susceptibility to a viral infection as well as the severity of infection.

Geographic and Seasonal Considerations

The geographic distribution of a virus is usually determined by whether the requisite cofactors or vectors are present or whether there is an immunologically naive, susceptible population. For example, many of the arboviruses are limited to the ecologic niche of their arthropod vectors. Extensive global transportation is eliminating many of the geographically determined restrictions to virus distribution.

Seasonal differences in the occurrence of viral disease correspond with behaviors that promote the spread of the virus. For example, respiratory viruses are more prevalent in the winter because crowding facilitates the spread of such viruses and the temperature and humidity conditions stabilize them. Enteric viruses, on the other hand, are more prevalent during the summer, possibly because hygiene is more lax during this season. The seasonal differences in arboviral diseases reflect the life cycle of the arthropod vector or its reservoir (e.g., birds).

Outbreaks, Epidemics, and Pandemics

Outbreaks of a viral infection often result from the introduction of a virus (such as hepatitis A) into a new location. The outbreak originates from a **common source** (e.g., food preparation) and often can be stopped once the source is identified. **Epidemics** occur over a larger geographic area and generally result from the introduction of a new strain of virus into an immunologically naive population. **Pandemics** are worldwide epidemics, usually resulting from the introduction of a new virus (e.g., HIV). Pandemics of influenza A used to occur approximately every 10 years as the result of the introduction of new strains of the virus.

Control of Viral Spread

The spread of a virus can be controlled by quarantine, good hygiene, changes in lifestyle, elimination of the vector, or immunization of the population. **Quarantine** was once the only means of limiting epidemics of viral infections and is most effective for limiting the spread of viruses that always cause symptomatic disease (e.g., smallpox). It is now used especially in hospitals to limit the **nosocomial spread** of viruses, especially to high-risk patients (e.g., immunosuppressed people). The proper sanitation of contaminated items and disinfection of the water supply are means of limiting the spread of enteric viruses. Changes in lifestyle have made a difference in the spread of sexually transmitted viruses such as HIV, HBV, and HSV. Elimination of an arthropod or its ecologic niche (e.g., drainage of the swamps it inhabits) has proved effective for controlling arboviruses.

The best way to limit viral spread, however, is to immunize the population. Immunization, whether produced by natural infection or by vaccination, protects the person and reduces the size of the immunologically naive, susceptible population necessary to promote the spread and maintenance of the virus.

QUESTIONS

1. What are the routes by which viruses gain entry into the body? For each route, list the barriers to infection and a virus that infects by it.

2. Describe or draw the disease path of a virus that is transmitted by an aerosol and causes lesions on the skin (similar to varicella).

3. Identify the structures that elicit a protective antibody response to adenovirus, influenza A virus, poliovirus, and rabies virus.

4. Describe the major roles of each of the following in promoting resolution of a viral infection: interferon, macrophage, natural killer cells, CD4 T cells, CD8 T cells, and antibody.

5. Why are α- and β-interferons produced before γ-interferon?

6. How does the nucleoprotein of influenza virus become an antigen for cytolytic CD8 T cells?

7. What events occur during the prodromal periods of a respiratory virus disease (e.g., parainfluenza virus) and encephalitis (e.g., St. Louis encephalitis virus)?

8. List the viral characteristics (structure, replication, target tissue) that would promote transmission by the fecal-oral route, by arthropods, by fomites, by mother's milk, and by sexual activity.

9. What are the different mechanisms by which oncogenic viruses immortalize cells? Describe them.

BIBLIOGRAPHY

Armstrong D, Cohen J: *Infectious diseases*, St. Louis, 1999, Mosby.

Belshe RB: *Textbook of human virology*, ed 2, St. Louis, 1991, Mosby.

Ellner PD, Neu HC: *Understanding infectious disease*, St. Louis, 1992, Mosby.

Emond RT et al: *Color atlas of infectious diseases*, ed 3, St. Louis, 1995, Mosby.

Evans AS, Kaslow RA: *Viral infections of humans. Epidemiology and control*, 4th ed, New York, 1997, Plenum.

Fields BN et al, editors: *Virology*, ed 3, New York, 1996, Lippincott-Raven.

Gorbach SL et al: *Infectious diseases*, Philadelphia, 1992, WB Saunders.

Hart CA, Broadhead RL: *Color atlas of pediatric infectious diseases*, St. Louis, 1992, Mosby.

Hart CA, Broadhead RL: *Color atlas of medical microbiology*, London, 1996, Mosby-Wolfe.

Katz SL, Gershon AA, Hotez PJ: *Krugman's infectious diseases of children*, ed 10, St. Louis, 1998, Mosby.

Mandell GL et al: *Principles and practice of infectious disease*, ed 5, New York, 2000, Churchill Livingstone.

Mims CA, White DO: *Viral pathogenesis and immunology*, Oxford, 1984, Blackwell.

Richman DD et al: *Clinical virology*, New York, 1997, Churchill Livingstone.

Shulman ST et al: *The biologic and clinical basis of infectious diseases*, ed 4, Philadelphia, 1992, WB Saunders.

Stark GR et al: How cells respond to interferons, *Ann Rev Biochem* 67:227–264, 1998.

White DO, Fenner FJ: *Medical virology*, ed 4, San Diego, 1994, Academic.

Zuckerman AJ, Banatvala JE, Pattison JR: *Principles and practice of clinical virology*, Chichester, New York, 2000, Wiley.

INTERNET RESOURCES

All the virology on the Internet and specific viruses: Available at http://www.virology.net/garryfavwebindex.html

Centers for Disease Control Health Topics A to Z: Available at http://www.cdc.gov/health/diseases.htm

http://www.virology.net/

National Center for Infectious Disease: Disease Information: Available at http://www.cdc.gov/ncidod/diseases/index.htm

National Center for Infectious Disease: Traveler's Health: Available at http://www.cdc.gov/travel/diseases.html

National Foundation for Infectious Diseases Fact Sheets on Diseases: Available at http://www.nfid.org/factsheets/Default.html

Power Point slide sets for different viral diseases: Available at http://sites.netscape.net/derekwongkk/slidesets

World Health Organization: Diseases and Vaccines: Available at http://www.who.int/vaccines-diseases/index.html

World Health Organization: Infectious Diseases: Available at http://www.who.int/health-topics/idindex.htm

CHAPTER 47

Antiviral Agents

The development of antiviral chemotherapy has lagged significantly behind that of antibacterial drugs. Antibacterial drugs, such as the β-lactam and aminoglycoside antibiotics, are targeted at enzymes and structures unique to the prokaryote and essential to their viability. Unlike most bacteria, however, viruses are obligate intracellular parasites that use the host cell's biosynthetic machinery and enzymes for replication (see Chapter 6). Hence, it is more difficult to inhibit viral replication without also being toxic to the host.

Early antiviral drugs were selective poisons, similar to cancer chemotherapies and targeted cells with extensive DNA and RNA synthesis. Newer antiviral drugs are targeted toward viral-encoded enzymes or structures of the virus that are important for replication. Most of these compounds are classic biochemical inhibitors of viral-encoded enzymes. Unlike the activity of antibacterial drugs, the activity of antiviral drugs is generally limited to specific families of viruses. Antiviral drugs have been developed against viruses that cause significant morbidity and mortality and also provide reasonable targets for drug action (Box 47–1). As has occurred with antibacterial drugs, however, resistance to antiviral drugs is becoming more of a problem because of the higher rate of long-term treatment of some patients, especially immunocompromised people (e.g., patients with the acquired immunodeficiency syndrome [AIDS]).

Targets for Antiviral Drugs

The steps of the viral replication cycle provide potential targets for antiviral drugs (e.g., structures, enzymes, or processes important or essential for virus production). These targets are described in this chapter, and examples of antiviral drugs developed to target these sites are also given. These targets and their respective antiviral agents are listed in Table 47–1 and shown in Figure 6–10.

Attachment, the first step in viral replication, is mediated by the interaction of a viral attachment protein with its cell surface receptor. This interaction can be blocked by **neutralizing antibodies**, which bind and coat the virion, or by **receptor antagonists**. The administration of specific antibodies (**passive immunization**) is the oldest form of antiviral therapy. Receptor antagonists include peptide or sugar analogues of the cell receptor or the viral attachment protein that competitively block the interaction of the virus with the cell. Specific peptides of the human immunodeficiency virus (HIV) glycoprotein gp120 or its receptor, the CD4 molecule of T cells, block infection and are being investigated for their clinical potential. Acidic polysaccharides, such as heparan and dextran sulfate, interfere with viral binding and have been suggested for the treatment of infection with herpes simplex virus (HSV), HIV, and other viruses.

Penetration and uncoating of the virus are required to deliver the viral genome into the cytoplasm of the host cell. After uptake of many viruses, the acidic environment of the endocytic vesicle is used to initiate uncoating. Specifically, the acidic pH promotes conformational changes in attachment proteins that promote fusion or membrane disruption. **Amantadine**, **rimantadine**, and other hydrophobic amines (weak organic bases) are antiviral agents that can neutralize the pH of these compartments and inhibit virion uncoating. **Tromantadine**, a derivative of amantadine, inhibits penetration of HSV. Arildone, disoxaril, **pleconaril**, and other **methylisoxazole** compounds block uncoating by fitting into a cleft in the receptor-binding canyon of the picornavirus capsid.

Amantadine and rimantadine have a more specific activity against influenza A. These compounds bind to and block the H^+ channel formed by the M_2 protein. Without the influx of H^+, the M_1 matrix proteins do not dissociate from the nucleocapsid (uncoating), so movement of the nucleocapsid to the nucleus, transcription, and replication are prevented. Blockage of this proton pore also disrupts the proper processing of the hemagglutinin protein late in the replication cycle. In the absence of a functional M_2 proton pore, the hemagglutinin inopportunely changes its conformation

BOX 47–1. Viruses Treatable with Antiviral Drugs

Herpes simplex virus
Varicella-zoster virus
Cytomegalovirus
Human immunodeficiency virus
Influenza A virus
Respiratory syncytial virus
Hepatitis A, B, and C viruses*
Papillomavirus*
Picornavirus

* Experimental protocols are available.

into its "fusion form" and is inactivated as it traverses the normally acidic Golgi environment.

Although messenger RNA (mRNA) synthesis is essential for the production of virus, it is not a good target for antiviral drugs. It would be difficult to inhibit viral mRNA synthesis without affecting cellular mRNA synthesis. DNA viruses use the host cell's transcriptases for mRNA synthesis. The RNA polymerases encoded by RNA viruses may not be sufficiently different from host cell transcriptases to selectively inhibit this activity. Alternatively, the high rate at which RNA viruses mutate may result in the generation of many drug-resistant strains. **Guanidine** and 2-hydroxybenzyl-benzimidine are two compounds that can block picor-

navirus RNA synthesis by binding to the 2C picornavirus protein, which is essential for RNA synthesis. Inhibition of RNA synthesis and induction of hypermutation are activities attributed to **ribavirin.**

The proper processing (splicing) and translation of viral mRNA can be inhibited by interferon, antisense oligonucleotides, and other agents. Viral infection of an **interferon**-treated cell triggers a cascade of biochemical events that block viral replication. Specifically, the degradation of viral and cellular mRNA is enhanced, and mRNA binding to the ribosome is blocked, preventing protein synthesis and viral replication. Interferon is described further in Chapter 14. Interferon and artificial interferon inducers (Ampligen, poly rI:rC) have been approved for clinical use (papilloma, hepatitis B and C) or are in clinical trials.

Antisense oligonucleotides are short, oligomeric sequences (20 nucleotides) that are complementary to specific sequences of the viral genome. These oligomers are chemically synthesized from nucleotide analogues and are resistant to nuclease digestion. The binding of antisense oligonucleotides to newly transcribed viral RNA prevents its being processed (spliced) into mRNA in the nucleus, its delivery to the cytoplasm, and its binding to the ribosome. RO 24-7429 is an antisense oligonucleotide that inhibits the tat trans-activation function and prevents activation of the transcription of HIV mRNA and HIV replication. **Isatin-β-thiosemicarbazone** induces mRNA degradation in

TABLE 47–1. Examples of Targets for Antiviral Drugs

Replication Step or Target	Agent	Targeted Virus*
Attachment	Peptide analogues of attachment protein	Human immunodeficiency virus (gp 120/CD4 receptor)
	Neutralizing antibodies	Most viruses
	Dextran sulfate, heparin	Human immunodeficiency virus; herpes simplex virus
Penetration and uncoating	Amantadine, rimantadine	Influenza A virus
	Tromantadine	Herpes simplex virus
	Arildone, disoxaril, pleconaril	Picornaviruses
Transcription	Interferon	Hepatitis A, B, and C viruses; papillomavirus
	Antisense oligonucleotides	Papillomavirus
Protein synthesis	Interferon	Hepatitis A, B, and C viruses; papillomavirus
DNA replication (polymerase)	Nucleoside analogues	Herpesviruses; human immunodeficiency virus; hepatitis B virus
	Phosphonoformate, phosphonoacetic acid	Herpesviruses
Nucleoside biosynthesis	Ribavirin	Respiratory syncytial virus; Lassa fever virus
Nucleoside scavenging (thymidine kinase)	Nucleoside analogues	Herpes simplex virus; varicella-zoster virus
Glycoprotein processing	—	Human immunodeficiency virus
Assembly (protease)	Hydrophobic substrate analogues	Human immunodeficiency virus
Virion integrity	Nonoxynol-9	Human immunodeficiency virus; herpes simplex virus

*Therapies may not have received approval for human use.

poxvirus-infected cells and was used as a treatment for smallpox.

Viral **DNA polymerases** (including **reverse transcriptases**) are the prime target for most antiviral drugs, because they are *essential* for virus replication and different from host enzymes. Most antiviral drugs are **nucleoside analogues,** which are nucleosides with modifications of the base, sugar, or both (Fig. 47–1). Before being used by the polymerase, the nucleoside analogues must be phosphorylated to the triphosphate form by viral enzymes (e.g., HSV thymidine kinase), cellular enzymes, or both. For example, the thymidine kinase of HSV and varicella-zoster virus (VZV) applies the first phosphate to **acyclovir (ACV)**, and the cellular enzymes apply the rest. HSV mutants lacking thymidine kinase activity are resistant to ACV. **Azidothymidine (AZT)** and many other nucleoside analogues are phosphorylated by cellular enzymes.

Nucleoside analogues selectively inhibit viral polymerases because these enzymes are less accurate than host cell enzymes. The binding of a nucleoside analogue with modifications of the base, sugar, or both is several 100-fold better than the host cell enzyme. These drugs either **prevent chain elongation**, as a result of the absence of a 3′-hydroxyl on the sugar, or **alter recognition and base pairing**, as a result of a base modification (see Fig. 47–1). Antiviral drugs that cause termination of the DNA chain by means of modified nucleoside sugar residues include **ACV, ganciclovir (GCV), valacyclovir, famciclovir, adenosine arabinoside (vidarabine, ara-A), zidovudine (AZT), dideoxycytidine,** and **dideoxyinosine.** Antiviral drugs that become incorporated into the viral genome and cause errors in replication (mutation) and transcription (inactive mRNA and proteins) because of modified nucleoside bases include **5-iododeoxyuridine (idoxuridine)** and **trifluorothymidine (trifluridine).** The rapid rate and large extent of nucleotide incorporation during viral replication make DNA viral replication especially susceptible to these drugs. A variety of other nucleoside analogues are also being developed as antiviral drugs.

Pyrophosphate analogues resembling the byproduct of the polymerase reaction, such as **phosphohacetic acid (foscarnet, PFA)** and **phosphonacetic acid,** are classic inhibitors of the herpesvirus polymerases. **Nevirapine, delavirdine,** and other non–nucleoside reverse transcriptase inhibitors do not bind to the substrate site and are noncompetitive inhibitors of the enzyme.

Deoxyribonucleotide scavenging enzymes (e.g., the thymidine kinase and ribonucleoside reductase of the herpesviruses) are also enzyme targets of antiviral drugs. These enzymes generate nucleoside substrates, which are necessary for the replication of the DNA virus genome.

Some antiviral drugs target cellular enzymes or pathways that are important to viral replication but not

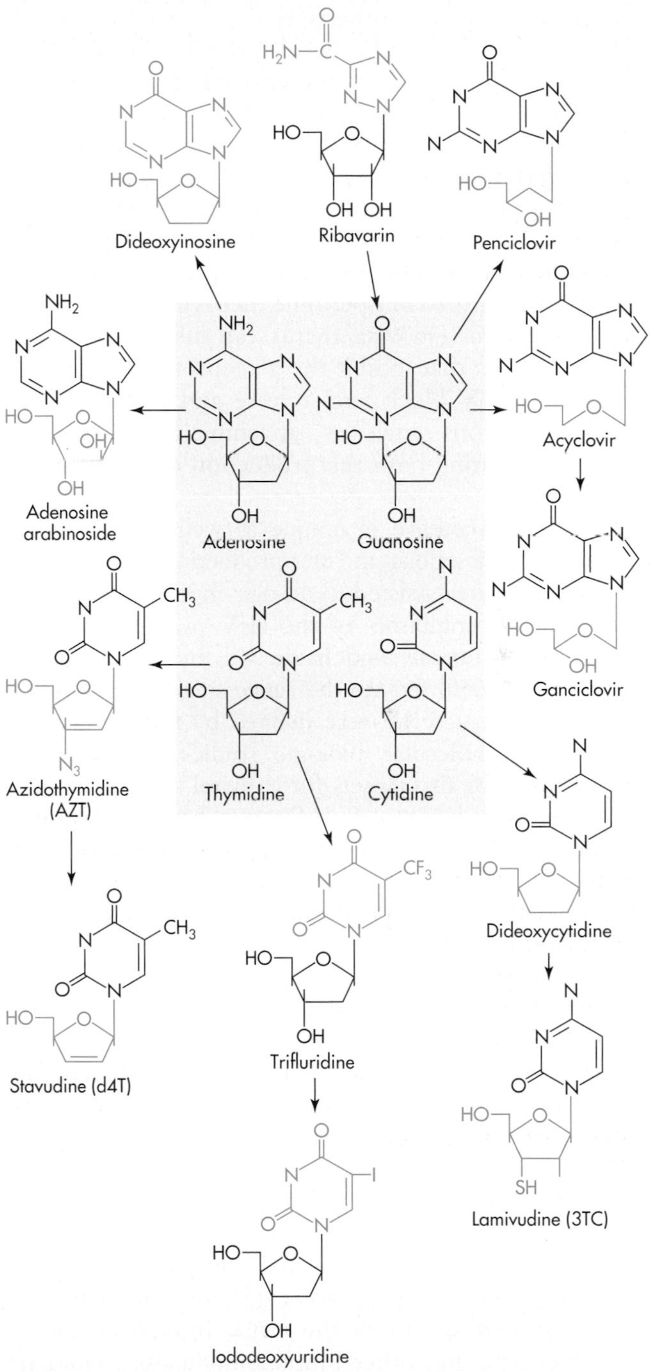

FIGURE 47–1. Structure of nucleoside analogues that are antiviral drugs. The chemical distinctions between the natural deoxynucleoside and the antiviral drug analogues are highlighted. *Arrows* indicate related drugs. Valacyclovir (not shown) is the L-valylester of acyclovir. Famciclovir (not shown) is the diacetyl 6-deoxyanalogue of penciclovir. Both of these drugs are metabolized to the active drug in the liver or intestinal wall.

to cell viability. **Ribavirin** is such an agent. It resembles guanosine monophosphate and inhibits nucleoside biosynthesis, mRNA capping, and other processes important to the replication of many viruses.

Bacterial protein synthesis is the target for several antibacterial compounds. Viral protein synthesis, in contrast, is a poor target for antiviral drugs, because the virus uses host cell ribosomes and synthetic mechanisms for replication, so selective inhibition is not possible. Interferons α and β stop a virus by inhibiting total cell protein synthesis of the infected cell. Inhibition of the post-translational modification of proteins, such as the proteolysis of a viral polyprotein, glycoprotein processing (castanospermine, deoxynojirimycin), or phosphorylation (D609:xanthate), can inhibit virus replication. Agents that inhibit the glycoprotein processing of HIV or HSV block viral release and inhibit glycoprotein functions such as attachment and fusion, thereby preventing both the production and the spread of the virus.

The **HIV protease** is unique as well as *essential* to the assembly of virions and the production of infectious virions. Computer-assisted molecular modeling has been used to design inhibitors of the HIV protease, such as **saquinavir**, **ritonavir**, and **indinavir**, by modeling inhibitors that would fit into the active site of the enzyme. The enzyme structures were defined by x-ray crystallographic and molecular biologic studies. Proteases of other viruses are also targets for antiviral drugs.

The **neuraminidase of influenza** has also become a target for antiviral drugs. **Zanamivir** (**Relenza**) and **oseltamivir** (**Tamiflu**) act as enzyme inhibitors and, unlike amantadine and rimantadine, can inhibit influenza A and B.

Preventing the acquisition of the virus, preventing the spread of the virus, and promoting the antiviral immune response of the host also have therapeutic potential. For example, enveloped viruses are susceptible to certain lipid and detergent-like molecules that disperse or disrupt the envelope membrane, thereby preventing acquisition of the virus. Nonoxynol-9, a detergent-like component in birth control jellies, can inactivate HSV and HIV and prevent sexual acquisition of the virus. Antibodies, acquired naturally or by passive immunization (see Chapter 15), prevent both the acquisition and spread of the virus. Interferon, interferon inducers, and other immunomodulatory biologic response modifiers are agents that stimulate resolution of the infection by the host. Biologic response modifiers under investigation include adjuvants consisting of bacterial components, mismatched polynucleotides (e.g., Ampligen, poly rI:rC), and immunomodulatory chemicals. These agents stimulate the production and release of interferon and other lymphokines, which have antiviral activity and activate natural killer and killer cell immune responses.

Nucleoside Analogues

Most of the antiviral drugs approved by the U.S. Food and Drug Administration (FDA) (Table 47–2) are nucleoside analogues that inhibit viral polymerases. These drugs are generally activated by phosphorylation by cellular or viral kinases. Selective inhibition of viral replication occurs because (1) a drug can bind better to viral rather than cellular DNA polymerases or (2) a drug will be utilized more extensively than in uninfected cells because of the more rapid synthesis of DNA in the infected cells.

Acyclovir, Valacyclovir, Penciclovir, and Famciclovir

Acyclovir (**acycloguanosine**) differs from the nucleoside guanosine by having an acyclic (hydroxyethoxymethyl) side chain instead of a ribose or deoxyribose sugar. ACV has selective action against HSV and VZV, the herpesviruses that encode a thymidine kinase (Fig. 47–2). The viral thymidine kinase activates the drug by phosphorylation, and host cell enzymes complete the progression to the diphosphate form and, finally, to the triphosphate form. Because there is no initial phosphorylation in uninfected cells, there is no active drug to inhibit cellular DNA synthesis or to cause toxicity. The ACV triphosphate competes with the guanosine triphosphate to inhibit the polymerase and cause termination of the growing viral DNA chain, because there is no 3'-hydroxyl group on the ACV molecule to allow chain elongation. This inactivates the DNA polymerase. The minimal toxicity of ACV is also a result of a 100-fold or greater use by the viral DNA polymerase than by cellular DNA polymerases. **Resistance to acyclovir** develops upon mutation of either the thymidine kinase, so that activation of ACV cannot occur, or the DNA polymerase, to prevent ACV binding.

ACV is effective against HSV infections such as encephalitis, disseminated herpes, and other serious herpes diseases. The fact that it is not toxic to uninfected cells allows its use as a prophylactic treatment to prevent recurrent outbreaks, especially in immunosuppressed people. A recurrent episode may be prevented if it is treated within 48 hours of the stimulus of recurrence, before the onset of inflammatory responses. ACV inhibits the replication of HSV but cannot resolve the latent HSV infection.

ACV can also be used for the treatment of VZV infection, although higher doses are required. VZV is less sensitive to the agent because ACV is phosphorylated less efficiently by the VZV thymidine kinase. **Valacyclovir,** the valyl ester derivative of ACV, is more efficiently absorbed after oral administration and rapidly converted into ACV, increasing the bioavailability of ACV for the treatment of HSV and serious varicella or zoster disease.

Penciclovir inhibits HSV and VZV in the same way that ACV does but is concentrated and persists in the infected cells to a greater extent than ACV. Penciclovir also has some activity against the Epstein-Barr

TABLE 47–2. Antiviral Drug Therapies Approved by the U. S. Food and Drug Administration

Virus	Antiviral Drug	Trade Name
Herpes simplex virus	Acyclovir*	Zovirax
	Penciclovir	Denavir
	Adenosine arabinoside (ara-A, vidarabine)	Vira-A
	Iododeoxyuridine (idoxuridine)†	Stoxil
Varicella-zoster virus and herpes simplex virus	Valacyclovir	Valtrex
	Famciclovir	Famvir
Cytomegalovirus	Ganciclovir	Cytovene
	Phosphonoformate (foscarnet)	Foscavir
Human immunodeficiency virus		
Nucleoside analogue reverse transcriptase inhibitors	Azidothymidine (zidovudine)	Retrovir
	Dideoxyinosine (didanosine)	Videx
	Dideoxycytidine (zalcitabine)	Hivid
	Stavudine (d4T)	Zerit
	Lamivudine (3TC)	Epivir
Non-nucleoside reverse transcriptase inhibitors	Nevirapine	Viramune
	Delaviridine	Rescriptor
Protease inhibitors	Saquinavir	Invirase
	Ritanavir	Norvir
	Indinavir	Crixivan
	Nelfinavir	Viracept
Influenza A virus	Amantadine	Symmetrel
	Rimantadine	
Influenza A and B viruses	Zanamivir	Relenza
	Oseltamivir	Tamiflu
Hepatitis C virus	Interferon α	Roferon-A (interferon α-2a)
		Intron A (interferon α-2b)
Papillomavirus	Interferon α	
Respiratory syncytial virus, Lassa virus	Ribavirin	Virazole
Picornaviruses	Pleconaril	

*Also active against varicella-zoster virus.
†Topical use only.

virus and cytomegalovirus (CMV). **Famciclovir** is a prodrug derivative of penciclovir that is well absorbed orally and then is converted to the active drug in the liver or intestinal lining. Resistance to penciclovir and famciclovir develops in the same manner as that to acyclovir.

Ganciclovir

Ganciclovir (dihydroxypropoxymethyl guanine) differs from ACV in having a single hydroxymethyl group in the acyclic side chain (see Fig. 47–1). The remarkable result of this addition is that it confers considerable activity against CMV. CMV does not encode a thymidine kinase, but a viral-encoded protein kinase phosphorylates GCV. Once activated by phosphorylation,

GCV inhibits all herpesvirus DNA polymerases. The viral DNA polymerases have nearly 30 times greater affinity for the drug than the cellular DNA polymerase.

GCV is effective in the treatment of CMV retinitis and shows some efficacy in the treatment of CMV esophagitis, colitis, and pneumonia in patients with AIDS. It is currently available only for intravenous administration. Because the drug can cause bone marrow toxicity, its use is primarily limited to the treatment of CMV infections in patients with AIDS.

Interestingly, this potential toxicity has been used as the basis for the development of an antitumor therapy. In one application, an HSV thymidine kinase gene was incorporated into the cells of a brain tumor with the use of a retrovirus vector. The retrovirus replicated

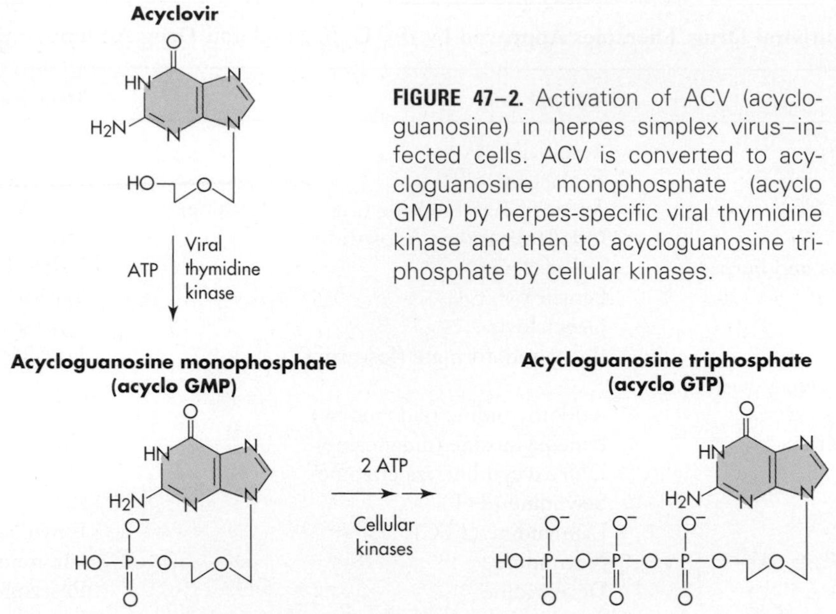

Acyclovir

FIGURE 47–2. Activation of ACV (acyclo-guanosine) in herpes simplex virus–infected cells. ACV is converted to acycloguanosine monophosphate (acyclo GMP) by herpes-specific viral thymidine kinase and then to acycloguanosine triphosphate by cellular kinases.

only in the growing cells of the tumor and the thymidine kinase was expressed only in the tumor cells, making the tumor cells susceptible to GCV.

Azidothymidine

Originally developed as an anticancer drug, **azidothymidine** was the first useful therapy for HIV infection. AZT (Retrovir), a nucleoside analogue of thymidine, inhibits the reverse transcriptase of HIV (see Fig. 47–1). Like other nucleosides, AZT must be phosphorylated, in this case by host cell enzymes. It lacks the 3′-hydroxyl necessary for DNA chain elongation and prevents cDNA synthesis. The selective therapeutic effect of AZT stems from the 100-fold lower sensitivity of the host cell DNA polymerase in comparison with the HIV reverse transcriptase.

Continuous oral AZT treatment is administered to HIV-infected people with depleted CD4 T-cell counts to prevent progression of disease. AZT treatment of pregnant HIV-infected women can reduce the likelihood of or prevent transmission of the virus to the baby. Side effects of AZT range from nausea to life-threatening bone marrow toxicity.

The same characteristic that makes HIV sensitive to AZT promotes the development of resistance. Specifically, the high error rate of the HIV polymerase creates extensive mutations and promotes the development of resistant strains. This problem is being addressed by the administration of multiple-drug therapy as initial therapy (highly active antiretroviral therapy [HAART]). It is more difficult for the HIV to develop resistance to multiple drugs, and any multiple-drug–resistant HIV strains are likely to be much weaker than the parent strains.

Dideoxyinosine, Dideoxycytidine, Stavudine, and Lamivudine

Several other nucleoside analogues have been approved as anti-HIV agents. **Dideoxyinosine** (didanosine) is a nucleoside analogue that is converted to dideoxyadenosine triphosphate (see Fig. 47–1). Like AZT, dideoxyinosine, **dideoxycytidine**, and **stavudine** (d4T) lack a 3′-hydroxyl group; they inhibit the HIV reverse transcriptase by preventing DNA chain elongation and inhibit HIV replication in a similar manner.

Lamivudine (2′-deoxy-3′-thiacytidine, 3TC) also has a modified sugar attached to the nucleoside base and prevents DNA chain elongation. These drugs are available for the treatment of AIDS unresponsive to AZT therapy or can be given in combination with AZT. Lamivudine is also active on the reverse transcriptase–like polymerase of hepatitis B virus.

Ribavirin

Ribavirin is an analogue of the nucleoside guanosine (see Fig. 47–1) but differs from guanosine in that its base ring is incomplete and open. Like other nucleoside analogues, ribavirin must be phosphorylated. The drug is active in vitro against a broad range of viruses.

Ribavirin monophosphate resembles guanosine monophosphate and inhibits nucleoside biosynthesis, mRNA capping, and other processes important to the replication of many viruses. Ribavirin depletes the cellular stores of guanine by inhibiting inosine monophosphate dehydrogenase, an enzyme important in the synthetic pathway of guanosine. It also prevents the synthesis of the mRNA 5′ cap by interfering with the guanylation and methylation of the nucleic acid base.

In addition, ribavirin triphosphate inhibits RNA polymerases and promotes hypermutation of the viral genome. Its multiple sites of action may explain the lack of ribavirin-resistant mutants of respiratory syncytial virus and influenza A virus.

Ribavirin is administered in an aerosol to children with severe respiratory syncytial virus bronchopneumonia and, potentially, to adults with severe influenza or measles. The drug may be effective for the treatment of influenza B, as well as Lassa, Rift Valley, Crimean-Congo, Korean, and Argentine hemorrhagic fevers, for which it is administered orally or intravenously. Ribavirin is also active against hepatitis C virus, especially in combination with interferon α.

Other Nucleoside Analogues

Idoxuridine, trifluorothymidine (see Fig. 47–1), and **fluorouracil** are analogues of thymidine. These drugs either (1) inhibit the biosynthesis of thymidine, a nucleotide essential for DNA synthesis, or (2) replace thymidine and become incorporated into the viral DNA. These actions inhibit further synthesis of the virus or cause extensive misreading of the genome, leading to mutation and inactivation of the virus. These drugs target cells in which extensive DNA replication is taking place, such as those infected with HSV.

Idoxuridine was the first anti-HSV drug approved for human use. It was at one time used for the topical treatment of herpes keratitis but has been replaced by trifluridine and other more effective, less toxic agents for this purpose. Fluorouracil is an antineoplastic drug that kills rapidly growing cells but has also been used for the topical treatment of warts caused by human papillomaviruses.

Adenine arabinoside was the principal antiviral drug used in the treatment of herpesvirus infections until ACV was introduced. Ara-A is a purine nucleoside analogue identical in structure to adenosine except that arabinose is substituted for ribose as the sugar moiety (see Fig. 47–1). This agent is phosphorylated by cellular enzymes (especially adenosine kinase), even in uninfected cells, and thus has a greater potential for causing toxicity than ACV. Although both cellular and viral DNA polymerases are inhibited by ara-A triphosphate, the viral enzyme is 6 to 12 times more sensitive. Resistance can develop as a result of the mutation of the viral DNA polymerase.

Many other nucleoside analogues that have antiviral activity are being investigated for clinical use against the herpesviruses, hepatitis B virus, and HIV. These compounds include modified pyrimidines such as bromovinyldeoxyuridine with a modified base, fluoroiodoaracytosine with a modified base and a 2-fluoro arabinose sugar instead of ribose, and 2-fluoromethylarauridine with the same modified sugar as fluoroio-doaracytosine. Researchers have also developed purine analogues that lack or have alternate sugar residues attached to the nucleoside base, similar in concept to ACV.

Non-Nucleoside Polymerase Inhibitors

Foscarnet and the related **phosphonoacetic acid (PAA)** are simple compounds that resemble pyrophosphate (Fig. 47–3). These drugs inhibit viral replication by binding to the pyrophosphate-binding site of the DNA polymerase to block nucleotide binding. PFA and PAA do not inhibit cellular polymerases at pharmacologic concentrations, but they can cause renal and other problems because of their ability to chelate divalent metal ions (e.g., calcium) and become incorporated into bone. PFA inhibits the DNA polymerase of all herpesviruses and the HIV reverse transcriptase without having to be phosphorylated by nucleoside kinases (e.g., thymidine kinase). PFA has been approved for the treatment of CMV retinitis in patients with AIDS.

Nevirapine, delavirdine, efavirenz, and other nonnucleoside reverse transcriptase inhibitors bind to sites on the enzyme different from the substrate. Because these drugs' mechanisms of action differ from those of the nucleoside analogues, the mechanism of HIV resistance to the agents is also different. As a result, these drugs may become very useful in combination with nucleoside analogues for the treatment of HIV infection.

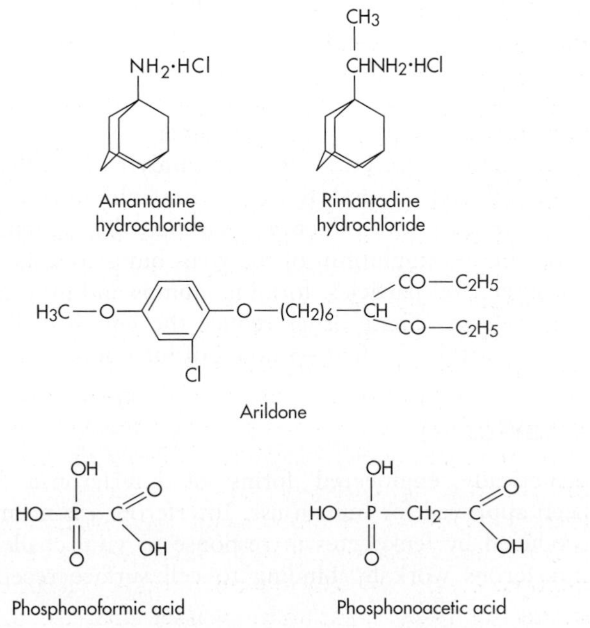

FIGURE 47–3. Structures of non-nucleoside antiviral drugs.

Protease Inhibitors

The unique structure of the HIV protease and its essential role in the production of a functional virion has made this enzyme a good target for antiviral drugs. **Saquinavir**, **indinavir**, **ritonavir**, **nelfinavir**, **amprenavir**, and other agents work by slipping into the hydrophobic active site of the enzyme to inhibit its action. As occurs with the other anti-HIV drugs, drug-resistant strains arise through mutation of the protease. The combination of a protease inhibitor with AZT and a second nucleoside analogue can reduce blood levels of HIV to undetectable levels. Development of resistance to a "cocktail" of anti-HIV drugs is also less likely than that to a single drug.

Anti-Influenza Drugs

Amantadine and **rimantadine** are amphipathic amine compounds with clinical efficacy against the influenza A virus but not the influenza B or other viruses (see Fig. 47–3). These drugs have several effects on influenza A replication. Both compounds are acidotrophic and concentrate in and buffer the contents of the endosomal vesicles involved in the uptake of the influenza virus. This effect can inhibit the acid-mediated change in conformation in the hemagglutinin protein that promotes the fusion of the viral envelope with cell membranes. However, the specificity for influenza A is due to its ability to bind to and block the proton channel formed by the M_2 matrix protein of the influenza A virus. Resistance is the result of an altered M_2 matrix or hemagglutinin protein.

Amantadine and rimantadine may be useful in ameliorating an influenza A infection if either agent is taken within 48 hours of exposure. They are also useful as a prophylactic treatment in lieu of vaccination. In addition, amantadine is an alternative therapy for Parkinson's disease. The principal toxic effect is on the central nervous system, with patients experiencing nervousness, irritability, and insomnia.

Zanamivir (**Relenza**) and **oseltamivir** (**Tamiflu**) inhibit influenza A and B as enzyme inhibitors of the neuraminidase of influenza. Without the neuraminidase, the hemagglutinin of the virus binds to sialic acid on other viral particles, forming clumps and preventing virus release. These drugs reduce the length of illness if taken within the first 48 hours of infection.

Interferon

Genetically engineered forms of interferon-α have been approved for human use. Interferon-α is normally produced by leukocytes in response to viral challenge. Interferons work by binding to cell surface receptors and initiating a cellular antiviral response. In addition, interferons stimulate the immune response and promote the immune clearance of viral infection.

The synthetic agent interferon α is active against many viral infections, including hepatitis A, B and C, HSV, papillomavirus, and rhinovirus. It has been approved for the treatment of condyloma acuminatum (genital warts, a presentation of papillomavirus) and hepatitis C. Natural interferon causes the influenza-like symptoms observed during many viremic and respiratory tract infections, and the synthetic agent has similar side effects during treatment. Interferon is discussed further in Chapter 14.

QUESTIONS

1. List the steps in viral replication that are poor targets for antiviral drugs. Why?

2. Which viruses can be treated with an antiviral drug? Distinguish the viruses treatable with an antiviral nucleoside analogue.

3. A mutation in the gene for which enzymes or proteins would confer resistance to the following antiviral drugs: ACV, ara-A, phosphonoformate, amantadine, AZT?

4. A patient has been exposed to influenza A virus and is in his third day of symptoms. He has heard that an anti-influenza drug is available and requests therapy. You tell him that therapy is not appropriate. To what therapeutic agents is the patient referring, and why did you decline to use the treatment?

BIBLIOGRAPHY

De Clercq E: In search of a selective antiviral chemotherapy, *Clin Microbiol Rev* 10:674–693, 1997.

Evans AS, Kaslow RA: *Viral infections of humans. Epidemiology and control*, ed, 4, New York, 1997, Plenum Medical Books.

Flint SE et al: *Principles of virology. Molecular biology, pathogenesis, and control*, Washington, DC, 2000, ASM Press.

Galasso GJ, Whitley RJ, Merigan TC: *Antiviral agents and human viral diseases*, ed 4, Philadelphia, 1997, Lippincott-Raven.

Hodinka RL: What clinicians need to know about antiviral drugs and viral resistance, *Infect Dis Clin North Am* 11: 945–967.

Richman DD, Whitley RJ, Hayden FG: *Clinical virology*, New York, 1997, Churchill Livingstone.

Specter S, Hodinka RL, Young SA: *Clinical virology manual*, ed 3, Washington, DC, 2000, ASM Press.

CHAPTER 48

Laboratory Diagnosis of Viral Diseases

The patient's history and symptoms provide the first clues to the diagnosis of a viral infection, often by excluding other types of infection (e.g., bacterial, fungal). Viral laboratory studies are performed to (1) confirm the diagnosis by identifying the viral agent of infection, (2) define the disease process, (3) monitor the disease epidemiologically, and (4) educate physicians and patients.

The following laboratory methods can be used to confirm clinical diagnosis:

1. Observation of virus-induced **cytopathologic effects** (**CPEs**) on cells.
2. Electron microscopic detection of viral particles.
3. Isolation and growth of the virus.
4. Detection of viral components (e.g., proteins, enzymes, nucleic acids).
5. Evaluation of the patient's immune response to the virus (**serology**).

The molecular and immunologic techniques used for many of these procedures are described in Chapters 17 and 18. Virus, viral antigens, and CPEs can be detected by means of cytologic examinations of clinical specimens or of tissue culture cells grown and infected in the laboratory (Box 48–1).

Cytology

The cytologic examination of specimens provides a rapid initial diagnosis for viral infections that produce a characteristic CPE. Characteristic CPEs include changes in cell morphology, cell lysis, vacuolation, syncytia (Fig. 48–1), and inclusion bodies. **Syncytia** are multinucleated giant cells formed by viral fusion of individual cells. Paramyxoviruses as well as herpes simplex, varicella-zoster, and human immunodeficiency viruses promote syncytia formation. **Inclusion bodies** constitute either histologic changes in the cells caused by viral components or virus-induced changes in cell structures. For example, Cowdry type A inclusions in single cells or in large syncytia (multiple cells fused together) are a characteristic finding in cells infected with herpes simplex virus (HSV) or varicella-zoster vi-

rus (VZV) (Fig. 48–2). Nuclear, owl's-eye inclusion bodies are found in the cells of tissues with cytomegalovirus (CMV) or in the sediment of urine from patients with the infection. Rabies may be detected through the finding of Negri bodies (rabies virus inclusions) in brain tissue (Fig. 48–3).

Electron Microscopy

Electron microscopy is not a standard clinical laboratory technique, but it can be used to detect and identify some viruses if sufficient viral particles are present. The addition of virus-specific antibody to a sample can cause viral particles to clump, thereby facilitating the detection and simultaneous identification of the virus (immunoelectron microscopy). This method is useful for the detection of enteric viruses, such as rotavirus, that are produced in abundance and have a characteristic morphology. Appropriately processed tissue from a biopsy or clinical specimen can also be examined for the presence of viral structures.

Viral Isolation and Growth

The "gold standard" for proving a viral etiology of a syndrome is the recovery and growth of the infecting agent. The patient's symptoms and travel history, the season of the year, and a presumptive diagnosis help determine the appropriate procedures to be used to isolate a viral agent (Table 48–1). For example, specimens of cerebrospinal fluid and urine are appropriate in a patient who has symptoms of central nervous system disease after parotitis, because the mumps virus that can cause such disease can be isolated in these specimens. A focal encephalitis with a temporal lobe localization preceded by headaches and disorientation suggests HSV infection, in which case biopsy of the brain should be performed to obtain tissue for cytologic studies and viral isolation. The development of meningitis symptoms during the summer indicates an enterovirus etiology, in which case cerebrospinal fluid, throat swab, and stool specimens should be collected.

The selection of the appropriate specimen for viral culture is often complicated because several viruses may cause the same clinical disease. For example, aseptic meningitis can be caused by many agents, so it may be necessary to obtain several types of specimens to identify the causal virus.

Specimens should be collected early in the acute phase of infection, before the virus ceases to be shed. For example, respiratory viruses may be shed for only 3 to 7 days, and shedding may lapse before the symptoms cease. HSV and VZV may not be recoverable from lesions more than 5 days after the onset of symptoms. It may be possible to isolate an enterovirus from the cerebrospinal fluid for only 2 to 3 days after the onset of the central nervous system manifestations. In addition, antibody produced in response to the infection may block the detection of virus.

The shorter the interval between the collection of a specimen and its delivery to the laboratory, the greater the potential for isolating a virus. The reasons are that many viruses are labile and that the samples are sus-

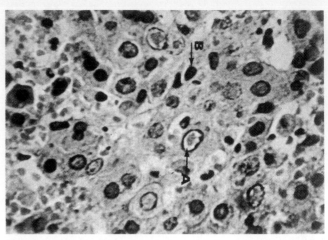

FIGURE 48–2. HSV-induced CPE. A biopsy specimen of an HSV-infected liver shows an eosinophilic Cowdry type A intranuclear inclusion body (*A*) surrounded by a halo and a ring of marginated chromatin at the nuclear membrane. An infected cell (*B*) exhibits a smaller condensed nucleus (pyknotic). (Courtesy of Dr. J.I. Pugh, St. Albans; from Emond RT, Rowland HAK: *A color atlas of infectious diseases*, ed 3, London, 1995, Mosby.)

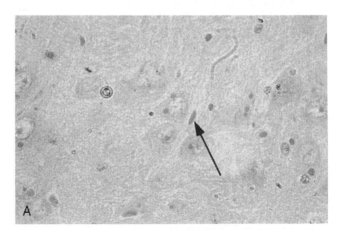

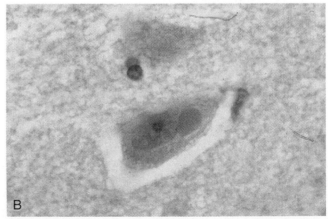

FIGURE 48–3. Negri bodies caused by rabies. *A*, A section of brain from a patient with rabies shows Negri bodies (*arrow*). *B*, Higher magnification from another biopsy specimen. (*A* from Hart C, Broadhead RL: *A color atlas of pediatric infectious diseases*, London, 1992, Wolfe.)

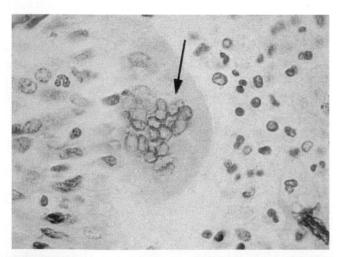

FIGURE 48–1. Syncytium formation by measles virus. Multinucleated giant cell (*arrow*) visible in a histologic section of lung biopsy tissue from a measles virus–induced giant cell pneumonia in an immunocompromised child. (From Hart C, Broadhead RL: *A color atlas of pediatric infectious diseases*, London, 1992, Wolfe.)

TABLE 48−1. Specimens for Viral Diagnosis

Common Pathogenic Viruses	Specimens for Culture	Comments
Respiratory Tract		
Adenovirus; influenza virus; enterovirus (picornavirus); rhinovirus; paramyxovirus; rubella virus; HSV	Nasal washing, throat swab, nasal swab, sputum	Enterovirus is also shed in stool
Gastrointestinal Tract		
Reovirus; rotavirus; adenovirus; Norwalk virus, calicivirus	Stool, rectal swab	Samples are analyzed by electron microscopy and antigen detection (ELISA); viruses are not cultured
Maculopapular Rash		
Adenovirus; enterovirus (picornavirus)	Throat swab, rectal swab	—
Rubella virus; measles virus	—	Rubella and measles viruses may be detected in urine
Vesicular Rash		
Coxsackievirus; echovirus; HSV; VZV	Vesicle fluid, scraping, or swab, enterovirus in stool	Initial diagnosis of HSV and VZV can be obtained from vesicle scraping (Tzanck smear)
Central Nervous System (Aseptic Meningitis, Encephalitis)		
Enterovirus (picornavirus)	Stool	—
Arboviruses (e.g., togaviruses, bunyavirus)	Rarely cultured	Diagnosis is by serologic tests
Rabies virus	Tissue, saliva, brain biopsy	Diagnosis is by immunofluorescence analysis for antigen
HSV; CMV; mumps virus; measles virus	Cerebrospinal fluid, brain immunofluorescence analysis	Virus isolation and antigen are assayed
Urinary Tract		
Adenovirus; CMV	Urine	CMV may be shed without apparent disease
Blood		
HIV; human T-cell leukemia virus; hepatitis B, C, and D viruses	Blood	Serologic antigen or antibody detection (ELISA), PCR and reverse transcriptase PCR are performed

CMV = cytomegalovirus; ELISA = enzyme-linked immunosorbent assay; HIV = human immunodeficiency virus; HSV = herpes simplex virus; PCR = polymerase chain reaction; VZV = varicella-zoster virus.

Data from Cherneskey MA, et al: *Cumitech 15: laboratory diagnosis of viral infections*, Washington, DC, 1982, American Society for Microbiology; and Hsiung GD: *Diagnostic virology*, New Haven, Conn, 1982, Yale University Press.

ceptible to bacterial and fungal overgrowth. Viruses are best transported and stored on ice and in special media that contain antibiotics and proteins such as serum albumin or gelatin. Significant losses in infectious titers occur when enveloped viruses (e.g., HSV, VZV, influenza virus) are kept at room temperature or frozen at 20°C. This is not a risk for nonenveloped viruses (e.g., adenoviruses, enteroviruses).

Viral Growth

Virus can be grown in tissue culture, embryonated eggs, or experimental animals (Box 48−2). Although embryonated eggs are still used for the growth of virus for some vaccines (e.g., influenza), they have been replaced by cell cultures for routine virus isolation in

BOX 48−2. Systems for the Propagation of Viruses

People
Animals: cows (e.g., Jenner's cowpox vaccine), chickens, mice, rats, suckling mice
Embryonated eggs
Organ culture
Tissue culture
    Primary
    Diploid cell line
    Tumor or immortalized cell line

BOX 48–3. Viral Cytopathologic Effects

Cell death
  Cell rounding
  Degeneration
  Aggregation
  Loss of attachments to substrate
Characteristic histologic changes: inclusion bodies in the
  nucleus or cytoplasm, margination of chromatin
Syncytia: multinucleated giant cells caused by virus-
  induced cell-cell fusion
Cell surface changes
  Viral antigen expression
  Hemadsorption (hemagglutinin expression)

clinical laboratories. Experimental animals are rarely used in clinical laboratories for the purpose of isolating viruses.

Cell Culture

Different types of tissue culture cells are used to grow viruses. **Primary cell cultures** are obtained by dissociating specific animal organs with trypsin or collagenase. The cells yielded by this method are then grown as monolayers (fibroblast or epithelial) or in suspension (lymphocyte) in artificial media supplemented with bovine serum or another source of growth factors. Primary cells can be dissociated with trypsin and passed or transferred to become secondary cell cultures. **Diploid cell lines** are cultures of a single cell type that are capable of being passed a large but finite number of times before they senesce, or undergo a significant change in their characteristics. **Tumor cell lines** and **immortalized cell lines,** which are initiated from patient tumors and by viruses or chemicals, respectively, consist of single cell types that can be passed continuously without senescing.

Primary monkey kidney cells are excellent for the recovery of myxoviruses, paramyxoviruses, many enteroviruses, and some adenoviruses. Human fetal diploid cells, which are generally fibroblastic cells, support the growth of a broad spectrum of viruses (e.g., HSV, VZV, CMV, adenoviruses, picornaviruses). HEp-2 cells, a continuous line of epithelial cells derived from a human cancer, are excellent for the recovery of respiratory syncytial virus, adenoviruses, and HSV. Many clinically significant viruses can be recovered in at least one of these cell cultures.

Viral Detection

A virus can be detected and initially identified through observation of the virus-induced CPE in the cell mon-

olayer (Box 48–3; Fig. 48–4). For example, a single virus may cause a cytopathologic focus (**plaque**). The type of cell culture, the characteristics of the CPE, and the rapidity of viral growth can be used to initially identify many clinically important viruses. This approach to identifying viruses is similar to that used in the identification of bacteria, which is based on the growth and morphology of colonies on selective differential media.

Some viruses grow slowly or not at all or do not readily cause a CPE in cell lines typically used in clinical virology laboratories. Some cause conditions that are hazardous to personnel. These viruses are most frequently diagnosed on the basis of serologic findings or through the detection of viral genomes or antigens.

Characteristic viral properties can also be used to identify viruses that do not have a classic CPE. For example, the rubella virus may not cause a CPE, but it does prevent (interfere with) the replication of picornaviruses in a process known as **heterologous interfer-**

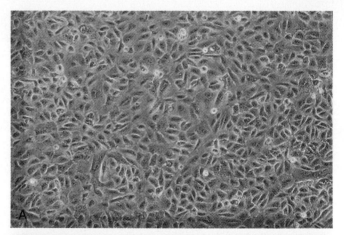
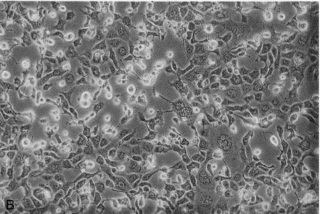

FIGURE 48–4. CPE of HSV infection. *A,* Uninfected Vero cells, an African green monkey kidney cell line. *B,* HSV-1–infected Vero cells showing rounded cells, multinucleated cells, and loss of the monolayer.

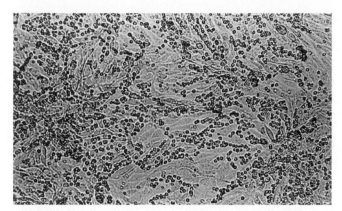

FIGURE 48–5. Hemadsorption of erythrocytes to cells infected with influenza viruses, mumps virus, parainfluenza viruses, or togaviruses, viruses that express a hemagglutinin on their surfaces that binds erythrocytes of selected animal species.

ence, which can be used to identify the rubella virus. Cells infected with the influenza virus, parainfluenza virus, mumps virus, and togavirus express a viral glycoprotein (hemagglutinin) that binds erythrocytes of defined animal species to the infected cell surface (**hemadsorption**) (Fig. 48–5). When released into the cell culture medium, such viruses can be detected from the agglutination of erythrocytes, a process termed **hemagglutination**. The strain of virus can then be identified from the specific antibody that blocks the hemagglutination, a process called **hemagglutination inhibition (HI)**.

One can quantitate a virus by determining one of the following titers:

1. **Tissue culture dose (TCD_{50})**: titer of virus that causes cytopathologic effects in tissue culture.
2. **Lethal dose (LD_{50})**: titer of virus that kills 50% of a set of test animals.
3. **Infectious dose (ID_{50})**: titer of virus that initiates a detectable symptom, antibody, or other response in 50% of a set of test animals.

The number of infectious viruses can also be evaluated with a count of the plaques produced by 10-fold dilutions of sample (**plaque-forming units**). The ratio of viral particles to plaque-forming units is always greater than 1, because numerous defective viral particles are produced during viral replication.

Interpretation of Culture Results

In general, the detection of any virus in host tissues, cerebrospinal fluid, blood, or vesicular fluid can be considered a highly significant finding. However, viral shedding may also be induced by an underlying condi-

tion (e.g., another infection, an immunosuppressed state, stress) and may therefore be unrelated to the disease symptoms. Certain viruses can be intermittently shed without causing symptoms in the affected person for periods ranging from weeks (enteroviruses in feces) to many months or years (HSV or CMV in the oropharynx and vagina; adenoviruses in the oropharynx and intestinal tract). Also, virus may not be isolated from a sample if the sample is improperly handled, contains neutralizing antibody, or is acquired before or after viral shedding.

Detection of Viral Proteins

Enzymes and other proteins are produced during viral replication and can be detected by biochemical, immunologic, and molecular biologic means (Box 48–4). The viral proteins can be separated by electrophoresis, and their patterns used to identify and distinguish different viruses. For example, the electrophoretically separated HSV-infected cell proteins and virion proteins exhibit different patterns for different types and strains of HSV-1 and HSV-2.

The detection and assay of characteristic enzymes or activities can identify and quantitate specific viruses. For example, the presence of reverse transcriptase in serum or cell culture indicates the presence of a retrovirus. Similarly, hemagglutination or hemadsorption can be used to easily assay the hemagglutinin produced by the influenza virus.

Antibodies can be used as sensitive and specific tools to detect, identify, and quantitate the virus and viral antigen in clinical specimens or cell cultures (immunohistochemistry). Specifically, monoclonal or monospe-

---

BOX 48–4. Assays for Viral Proteins and Nucleic Acids

Proteins

Protein patterns (electrophoresis)
Enzyme activities (e.g., reverse transcriptase)
Hemagglutination and hemadsorption
Antigen detection (e.g., indirect fluorescence, enzyme-linked immunosorbent assay, Western blot)

Nucleic Acids

Restriction endonuclease cleavage patterns
Electrophoretic mobilities of RNA for segmented RNA viruses (electrophoresis)
DNA genome hybridization in situ (cytochemistry)
Southern, Northern, and dot blots
Polymerase chain reaction (DNA)
Reverse transcriptase polymerase chain reaction (RNA)
Branched-chain DNA (DNA, RNA)

cific antibodies are useful for distinguishing among viral strains and mutants. Viral antigens on the cell surface or within the cell can be detected by **immunofluorescence** and **enzyme immunoassay (EIA)** (see Figs. 18–2 and 18–3). Virus or antigen released from infected cells can be detected by **enzyme-linked immunosorbent assay (ELISA)**, **radioimmunoassay (RIA)**, and **latex agglutination (LA)** (see Chapter 18 for definitions).

The detection of CMV can be enhanced through the use of a combination of cell culture and immunologic means. In this method, the clinical sample is centrifuged onto cells grown on a coverslip or the bottom of a shell vial. This step increases the efficiency of the method and accelerates virus entry into the cells on the coverslip or vial. The cells can then be analyzed with immunofluorescence or EIA for early viral antigens, which are detectable within 24 hours instead of the 7 to 14 days it takes for a CPE to become evident.

Detection of Viral Genetic Material

The genome structure and genetic sequence are major distinguishing characteristics of the family, type, and strain of virus (see Box 48–4). The electrophoretic patterns of RNA (influenza, reovirus) or restriction endonuclease fragment lengths from DNA viral genomes are like genetic fingerprints for these viruses. Different strains of HSV-1 and HSV-2 can be distinguished in this way by restriction fragment length polymorphism.

DNA probes with sequences complementary to specific regions of a viral genome can be used, like antibodies, as sensitive and specific tools for detecting a virus. These probes can detect the virus even in the absence of viral replication. DNA probe analysis is especially useful for detecting slowly replicating or nonproductive viruses, such as CMV and human papillomavirus. Specific viral genetic sequences in fixed, permeabilized tissue biopsy specimens can be detected by **in situ hybridization**.

Viral genomes can also be detected in clinical samples with the use of **dot blot** or **Southern blot analysis.** For the latter method, the viral genome or electrophoretically separated restriction endonuclease cleavage fragments of the genome are blotted onto nitrocellulose filters and then detected on the filter by their hybridization to DNA probes. Electrophoretically separated viral RNA (**Northern blot**–RNA:DNA probe hybridization) blotted onto a nitrocellulose filter can be detected in a similar manner. The DNA probes are detected with autoradiography or with fluorescent or EIA-like methods. Many viral probes and kits for detecting viruses are now commercially available.

DNA probes are especially useful for detecting and locating viral genomes in patient samples in which there is no CPE or in which the viral antigen cannot be detected using the specific immunologic tests available. DNA probes are also useful for studying the expression of specific viral genes in different cell types (see Fig. 17–3).

The **polymerase chain reaction (PCR)**, **reverse transcriptase PCR (RT-PCR)**, and **branched-chain DNA assays** are becoming very important for viral detection. Use of the appropriate primers for PCR can promote a million-fold amplification of a target sequence in a few hours. This technique is especially useful for detecting latent and integrated sequences of viruses such as retroviruses, herpesviruses, papillomaviruses, and other papovaviruses as well as the sequences of viruses present in low concentrations. RT-PCR uses the retroviral reverse transcriptase to convert viral RNA to DNA and allow PCR amplification of the viral nucleic acid sequences. This approach was very useful for identifying and distinguishing the Hantaviruses that caused the outbreak in New Mexico in 1993.

Branched-chain DNA assays quantitate viral DNA or RNA much like ELISA. The viral genome is captured by a complementary DNA sequence and then detected by another complementary DNA sequence that is attached to an extensively branched chain of DNA. Upon development, each of the branches elicits a reaction that amplifies the signal to detectable levels.

Viral Serology

The humoral immune response provides a history of a patient's infections. Serology can be used to identify the virus and its strain or serotype, evaluate the course of an infection, and determine whether it is a primary infection or a reinfection and whether it is acute or chronic. Serologic data about a viral infection are provided by the antibody type and titer and the nature of the antigenic targets. Serologic studies are used for the identification of viruses that are difficult to isolate and grow in cell culture as well as viruses that cause diseases of long duration (see Box 18–2).

The detection of **virus-specific immunoglobulin (Ig) M antibody**, which is present during the first 2 or 3 weeks of a primary infection, generally indicates a recent primary infection. **Seroconversion** is indicated by at least a **fourfold increase** in the antibody titer between the serum obtained during the acute phase of disease and that obtained at least 2 to 3 weeks later, during the convalescent phase. Reinfection or recurrence later in life causes an anamnestic (secondary or booster) response. Antibody titers may remain high in patients who suffer frequent recurrence of a disease (e.g., herpesviruses).

Because of the inherent imprecision of serologic assays based on twofold serial dilutions, a fourfold increase in the antibody titer between acute and convalescent sera is required to indicate seroconversion. For example, samples with 512 units and 1023 units of antibody would both give a signal on a 512-fold dilution but not on a 1024-fold dilution, and the titers of both would be reported as 512. On the other hand, samples with 1020 and 1030 units are not significantly different but would be reported as titers of 512 and 1024, respectively.

The course of a chronic infection can also be determined from a serologic profile. Specifically, the presence of antibodies to several key viral antigens and their titers can be used to identify the stage of disease due to certain viruses. This approach is especially useful for the diagnosis of viral diseases with slow courses (e.g., hepatitis B, infectious mononucleosis due to Epstein-Barr virus). In general, the first antibodies to be detected are directed against the antigens most available to the immune system (e.g., expressed on the virion or infected-cell surfaces). Later in the infection, when cells have been lysed by the infecting virus or the cellular immune response, antibodies directed against the intracellular viral proteins and enzymes are detected. For example, antibodies to the envelope and capsid antigens of Epstein-Barr virus are detected first. Then, during convalescence, antibodies to nuclear antigens, such as the Epstein-Barr virus nuclear antigen, are detected.

A serologic battery or panel consisting of assays for several viruses may be used for the diagnosis of certain diseases. Local epidemiologic factors, the time of year, and patient factors such as immunocompetence, travel history, and age influence the choice of virus assays to be included in a panel. For example, HSV and the viruses of mumps, western and eastern equine encephalitides, St. Louis encephalitis, and California encephalitis might be included in a panel of tests for central nervous system diseases.

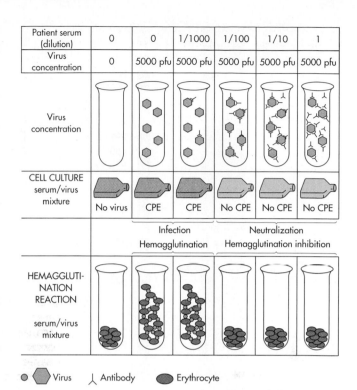

FIGURE 48–6. Neutralization, hemagglutination, and hemagglutination inhibition assays. In the assay shown, 10-fold dilutions of serum were incubated with virus. Aliquots of the mixture were then added to cell cultures or erythrocytes. In the absence of antibody, the virus infected the monolayer (indicated by CPE) and caused hemagglutination (i.e., formed a gel-like suspension of erythrocytes). In the presence of the antibody, infection was blocked (neutralization), and hemagglutination was inhibited, allowing the erythrocytes to pellet. The titer of antibody in the serum was 100. *pfu* = plaque-forming units.

Serologic Test Methods

The serologic tests used in virology are listed in Box 18–1 and described further in Chapter 18. **Neutralization** and **HI tests** assay antibody on the basis of its recognition of and binding to virus. The antibody coating of the virus blocks its binding to indicator cells (Fig. 48–6). Neutralization involves inhibition by the antibody of infection and cytopathologic effects of the virus in tissue culture cells. A neutralization antibody response is virus- and strain-specific. The response often develops with the onset of symptoms and persists for long periods. HI is used for the identification of viruses that can selectively agglutinate erythrocytes of various animal species (e.g., chicken, guinea pig, human). Antibody in serum prevents a standardized amount of virus from binding to and agglutinating erythrocytes.

The indirect fluorescent antibody test and solid-phase immunoassays such as **LA**, **ELISA**, and **RIA** are commonly used to detect and quantitate specific antibody-virus antigen immune complexes. These tests can detect both viral antigen and antiviral antibody. The ELISA test is used to screen the blood supply to exclude individuals who are seropositive for hepatitis B and C viruses and human immunodeficiency virus (HIV). Western blot analysis has become very important to confirm seroconversion and hence infection with the HIV. Patient antibody recognition of specific viral proteins separated by electrophoresis, transferred (blotted) onto a filter paper (e.g., nitrocellulose, nylon), and visualized with an enzyme-conjugated antihuman antibody confirms the ELISA-indicated diagnosis of HIV infection (Fig. 48–7).

Limitations to the Use of Serologic Methods

The presence of an antiviral antibody indicates previous infection but is not sufficient to indicate when the

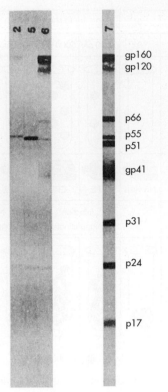

Strip	Interpretation	Bands present
2	Indeterminate	p24, p55, gp160
5	Indeterminate	p24, p55
6	Indeterminate	p24, gp41, p55, p66, gp120, gp160
7	Positive	p17, p24, p31, gp41, p51, p55, p66, gp120, gp160

FIGURE 48–7. Western blot analysis of HIV antigens and antibody. HIV protein antigens are separated by electrophoresis and blotted onto nitrocellulose paper strips. The strip is incubated with patient antibody, washed to remove the unbound antibody, and then reacted with enzyme-conjugated antihuman antibody and chromophoric substrate. Serum from an HIV-infected person binds and identifies the major antigenic proteins of HIV. Of the four sera shown, only serum 7 recognizes all the antigens and is definitively positive. (From Belshe RB, editor: *Textbook of human virology*, ed 2, St. Louis, 1991, Mosby.)

(e.g., parainfluenza and mumps express related antigens). Conversely, the antibody used in the assay may be too specific (many monoclonal antibodies) and may not recognize other viruses from the same family, giving a false-negative result (e.g., rhinovirus). A good understanding of the clinical symptoms and a knowledge of the limitations and potential problems with serologic assays aid in making the diagnosis.

QUESTIONS

1. Brain tissue is obtained at autopsy from a person who died of rabies. What procedures could be used to confirm the presence of rabies virus–infected cells in the brain tissue?

2. A cervical Papanicolaou smear is taken from a woman with a vaginal papilloma (wart). Certain types of papilloma have been associated with cervical carcinoma. What method or methods would be used to detect and identify the type of papilloma in the cervical smear?

3. A legal case would be settled by identification of the source of an HSV infection. Serum and viral isolates are obtained from the infected person and two contacts. What methods could be used to determine whether the person is infected with HSV-1 or HSV-2? What methods could be used to compare the type and strain of HSV obtained from each of the three people?

4. A 50-year-old man experiences flu-like symptoms. The figure below shows results of hemagglutination inhibition tests on serum specimens collected when the disease manifested (*Acute*) and 3 weeks later. The HI data for the current strain of influenza A (H3N2) are presented at *top right*. Hemagglutination is indicated by *filled circles*. Is the patient infected with the current strain of influenza A?

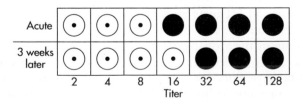

5. A policeman accidentally sticks his finger with a drug addict's syringe needle. He is concerned that he may be infected with HIV. Samples are taken from the policeman a month later for analysis. What assays would be appropriate to determine whether the man is infected with the virus? In this case, it may be too early to detect an antibody response to the virus. What procedures would be appropriate to assay for virus or viral components?

infection occurred. The finding of virus-specific IgM, a fourfold increase in the antibody titer between acute and convalescent sera, or specific antibody profiles is indicative of recent infection. False-positive or false-negative test results may also confuse the diagnosis. In addition, patient antibody may be bound with viral antigen (as occurs in patients with hepatitis B) in immune complexes, thereby preventing antibody detection. Serologic cross-reactions between different viruses may also confuse the identity of the infecting agent

BIBLIOGRAPHY

Forbes BA et al: *Bailey and Scott's diagnostic microbiology*, ed 10, St. Louis, 1998, Mosby.

Hsiung GD: *Diagnostic virology*, ed 3, New Haven, Conn, 1982, Yale.

Lennette EH, editor: *Laboratory diagnosis of viral infections*, ed 3, New York, 1999, Marcel Dekker.

Menegus MA: Diagnostic virology. In Belshe RB, editor: *Textbook of human virology*, ed 2, St. Louis, 1991, Mosby.

Specter S et al: *Clinical virology manual*, ed 3, Washington, DC, 2000, ASM Press.

Viruses in cell culture: Available at http://www.uct.ac.za/depts/mmi/stannard/linda.html

CHAPTER 49

Papovaviruses

The papovavirus family (Papovaviridae) consists of the **papillomaviruses** and **polyomaviruses** (Table 49–1). Papovaviruses are capable of causing lytic, chronic, latent, and transforming infections, depending on the host cell. Human papillomaviruses (HPVs) cause **warts**, and several genotypes are associated with human cancer (e.g., **cervical carcinoma**). BK and JC viruses, members of the Polyomavirus genus, usually cause asymptomatic infection but are associated with renal disease and **progressive multifocal leukoencephalopathy** (**PML**), respectively, in immunosuppressed people. Simian virus 40 (**SV40**) is the prototype polyomavirus. Although these two genera are in the same family, the viruses differ in size, antigenic determinants, and biologic properties.

The papovaviruses are small, nonenveloped icosahedral capsid viruses with double-stranded circular DNA genomes (Box 49–1). They encode proteins that promote cell growth. The promotion of cell growth facilitates lytic viral replication in a permissive cell type but *may oncogenically transform a cell that is nonpermissive.* The polyomaviruses, especially SV40, have been studied extensively as model oncogenic viruses.

Human Papillomaviruses

Structure and Replication

Classification of the HPVs is based on DNA sequence homology. At least 70 types have been identified and classified into 16 (A through P) groups. HPV can be distinguished further as **cutaneous HPV** or **mucosal HPV** on the basis of the susceptible tissue. Viruses in similar groups frequently cause similar types of warts.

The **icosahedral capsid** of HPV is 50 to 55 nm in diameter and consists of two structural proteins forming 72 capsomeres (Fig. 49–1). The HPV genome is **circular** and has approximately 8000 base pairs. The HPV DNA encodes seven or eight early genes (E1 to E8), depending on the virus, and two late or structural genes (L1 and L2). An upstream regulatory region (URR) contains the control sequences for transcription, the shared N-terminal sequence for the early proteins,

and the origin of replication. All the genes are located on one strand (the plus strand) (Fig. 49–2).

The steps in HPV replication parallel the differentiation of the skin or mucosal epithelium and depend heavily on the host cell's transcriptional machinery. The virus accesses the basal cell layer through breaks in the skin. The early genes of the virus stimulate cell growth and facilitate replication of the viral genome using the host cell DNA polymerase when the cells divide. The virus-induced cell growth causes the basal and the prickle cell layer (stratum spinosum) to thicken. As the basal cell differentiates, the specific nuclear factors expressed in the different layers and types of skin and mucosa promote transcription of the viral genes. The late genes encoding the structural proteins are expressed only in the terminally differentiated upper layer, disrupting the keratin, and the virus is shed with the dead cells of the upper layer. Expression of the viral genes correlates with the expression of specific keratins.

Pathogenesis

Papillomaviruses infect and replicate in the squamous epithelium of skin (**warts**) and mucous membranes (**genital**, **oral**, and **conjunctival papillomas**) to induce epithelial proliferation. The HPV types are very tissue-specific, causing different disease presentations. The

TABLE 49–1. Human Papovaviridae and Their Diseases

Virus	Disease
Papillomavirus	Warts
Polyomavirus	
BK virus	Renal disease*
JC virus	Progressive multifocal leukoencephalopathy*

*Disease occurs in immunosuppressed patients.

BOX 49–1. Unique Properties of Papovaviruses

Small icosahedral capsid virion.

Double-stranded circular DNA genome is replicated and assembled in the nucleus.

There are two major genera:

Papillomavirus: **HPV** types 1 to 58+ (as determined by genotype; types defined by DNA homology, tissue tropism, and association with oncogenesis).

Polyomavirus: SV40, **JC virus,** and **BK virus.**

Viruses have defined tissue tropisms determined by receptor interactions and the transcriptional machinery of the cell.

Viruses encode proteins that promote cell growth by binding to the cellular growth-suppressor proteins p53 and p105RB. Polyoma T antigen binds to p105RB and p53. **E6 binds to p53, and E7 binds to p105RB.**

Viruses can cause lytic infections in permissive cells but cause abortive, persistent, or latent infections or **immortalize (transform)** nonpermissive cells.

Integration often causes the E1 and E2 genes to be inactivated, thereby preventing viral replication without preventing expression of the E6 and E7 genes. The E6 and E7 proteins of HPV-16 and HPV-18 have been identified as **oncogenes,** because they bind and inactivate the cellular growth-suppressor (transformation-suppressor) proteins, p53 and p105 retinoblastoma gene product (p105RB). E6 binds the p53 protein and targets it for degradation, and E7 binds and inactivates p105RB. Without these brakes on cell growth, the cell is more susceptible to mutation, chromosomal aberrations, or the action of a co-factor and thereby develops into cancer.

The mechanism by which papillomas resolve is not known. However, it is known that cell-mediated immunity is an important factor, because immunosuppressed people have recurrences and more severe presentations of papillomavirus and other papovavirus infections.

Epidemiology

HPV resists inactivation and can be transmitted on fomites, such as the surfaces of counters or furniture, bathroom floors, and towels (Box 49–3). Asymptomatic shedding may promote transmission. HPV infection is acquired by (1) direct contact through small breaks in the skin or mucosa, (2) during sexual intercourse, (3) while an infant is passing through an infected birth canal, or (4) as the result of chewing warts (a childhood habit).

Common, plantar, and flat warts are most common in children and young adults. Laryngeal papillomas occur in young children and middle-aged adults.

Certain HPV types are sexually transmitted diseases common among sexually active people. Approximately 20 million people in the United States are infected with HPV, and the numbers are growing rapidly. HPV-16, HPV-18, and several other types are closely linked to cervical carcinoma, the second leading cause

wart develops as a result of virus stimulation of cell growth and thickening of the basal and prickle layers (stratum spinosum) as well as the stratum granulosum. **Koilocytes,** characteristic of papillomavirus infection, are enlarged keratinocytes with clear haloes around shrunken nuclei. It usually takes 3 to 4 months for the wart to develop. The viral infection remains local and generally regresses spontaneously but can recur (Fig. 49–3. The HPV pathogenic mechanisms are summarized in Box 49–2.

The oncogenic potential of HPV has been extensively studied. Viral DNA has been found in benign and malignant tumors, especially mucosal papillomas. HPV-16 and HPV-18 cause cervical papillomas and dysplasia, and *at least 85% of cervical carcinomas contain integrated HPV-DNA* rather than plasmid-like DNA.

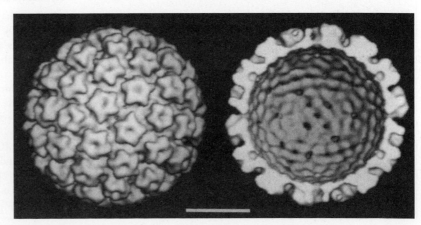

FIGURE 49–1. Computer reconstruction of cryoelectron micrographs of (human papillomavirus (HPV). *Left,* View of the surface of HPV shows 72 capsomeres arranged in an icosahedron. All the capsomeres (pentons and hexons) appear to form a head with a regular five-point–star shape. *Right,* Computer cross-section of the capsid shows the interaction of the capsomeres and channels in the capsid. (From Baker TS et al: Structures of bovine and human papillomaviruses: analysis by cryoelectron microscopy and three-dimensional image reconstruction. *Biophys J* 60:1445–1456, 1991.)

Genome is a double-stranded circular molecule.

E1 protein binds DNA at ori and promotes viral DNA replication and has helicase activity (like T antigen of SV-40). E2 protein binds DNA, helps E1, and activates viral mRNA synthesis.

E5-oncoprotein that activates the EGF receptor to promote growth. E4-disrupts cytokeratins to promote release. E6 and E7 of HPV-16 and HPV-18 can become immortalizing genes; HPV-16 is associated with human cervical cancer.

L1 and L2 gene products are late structural (capsid) proteins.

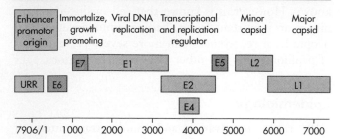

| Enhancer promotor origin | Immortalize, growth promoting | Viral DNA replication | Transcriptional and replication regulator | | Minor capsid | Major capsid |

FIGURE 49–2. Genome of human papillomavirus type HPV-16. DNA is normally a double-stranded circular molecule, but it is shown here in its linear form. E6 = oncogene protein that binds p53 and promotes its degradation; E7 = oncogene protein that binds p105RB (p105 retinoblastoma gene product); L1 = major capsid protein; L2 = minor capsid protein; rep ori = origin of replication; URR = upstream regulatory region. (Courtesy Tom Broker, MD, Baltimore.)

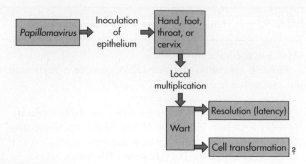

FIGURE 49–3. Progression of human papillomavirus infection.

of cancer death in women (approximately 500,000 deaths per year).

Clinical Syndromes

The clinical syndromes and the HPV types that cause them are summarized in Table 49–2.

Warts

A **wart** is a benign, self-limited proliferation of skin that regresses with time. Most people with HPV infection have the common types of the virus (HPV-1 through HPV-4), which infect keratinized surfaces, usually on the hands and feet (Fig. 49–4). Initial infection occurs in childhood or early adolescence. The incubation period before a wart develops may be as long as 3 to 4 months. The appearance of the wart (dome-shaped, flat, or plantar) depends on the HPV type and the infected site.

BOX 49–2. Disease Mechanisms of Papovaviruses

Papillomaviruses

Virus is acquired by **close contact** and infects the epithelial cells of the skin or mucous membranes.

Tissue tropism and disease presentation depend on the papillomavirus type.

Viral replication depends on the epithelial cell differentiation stage: It is persistent in the basal layer and active in differentiated keratinocytes.

Viruses cause benign outgrowth of cells into **warts.**

Warts resolve spontaneously, possibly as a result of immune response.

Certain types are associated with **dysplasia** that may become **cancerous** with the action of cofactors.

DNA of specific HPV types is present (integrated) in the tumor cell chromosomes.

Polyomaviruses (JC and BK Viruses)

Virus is probably acquired through the respiratory route and spread by viremia to the kidneys early in life.

Infections are **asymptomatic.**

Virus establishes **persistent** and **latent** infection in organs such as the kidneys and lungs.

In **immunocompromised** people, JC virus is activated, spreads to the brain, and causes progressive multifocal leukoencephalopathy **(PML),** a conventional slow virus disease.

In PML, JC virus partially transforms astrocytes and kills oligodendrocytes, causing characteristic lesions and sites of demyelination.

BK virus is ubiquitous but is not associated with serious disease.

BOX 49–3. **Epidemiology of Papovaviruses**

Disease/Viral Factors

Capsid virus is resistant to inactivation.
   Virus persists in host.
   Asymptomatic shedding is likely.

Transmission

Papillomavirus: **direct contact, sexual contact** (sexually transmitted disease) for certain virus types, or passage through infected birth canal for laryngeal papillomas (types 6 and 11).
   Polyomavirus: inhalation of infectious aerosols.

Who Is at Risk?

Papillomavirus: warts are common; sexually active people are at risk for infection with HPV types correlated with oral and genital cancers.
   Polyomavirus: ubiquitous; immunocompromised people at risk for progressive multifocal leukoencephalopathy.

Geography/Season

Viruses are found worldwide.
   There is no seasonal incidence.

Modes of Control

There are no modes of control.

Benign Head and Neck Tumors

Single oral papillomas are the most benign epithelial tumors of the oral cavity. They are pedunculated with a fibrovascular stalk, and their surface usually has a rough, papillary appearance. They can occur in people of any age group, are usually solitary, and rarely recur after surgical excision. **Laryngeal papillomas** are commonly associated with HPV-6 and HPV-11 and are the most common benign epithelial tumors of the larynx. Laryngeal papillomatosis can be life-threatening in children, however, because of the danger that the papillomas may obstruct the airway. Occasionally, papillomas may extend down the trachea and into the bronchi.

TABLE 49–2. **Clinical Syndromes Associated with Papillomaviruses**

Syndrome	HPV Types	
	Common	*Uncommon*
Cutaneous Syndromes		
Skin warts:		
Plantar wart	1	2, 4
Common wart	2, 4	1, 7, 26, 29
Flat wart	3, 10	27, 28, 41
Epidermodysplasia verruciformis	5, 8, 17, 20, 36	9, 12, 14, 15, 19, 21–25, 38, 46
Mucosal Syndromes		
Benign head and neck tumors:		
Laryngeal papilloma	6, 11	—
Oral papilloma	6, 11	2, 16
Conjunctival papilloma	11	—
Anogenital warts:		
Condyloma acuminatum	6, 11	1, 2, 10, 16, 30, 44, 45
Cervical intraepithelial neoplasia, cancer	16, 18	11, 31, 33, 35, 42–44

Modified from Balows A et al: *Laboratory diagnosis of infectious diseases: principles and practice*, vol 2, New York, 1988, Springer-Verlag.

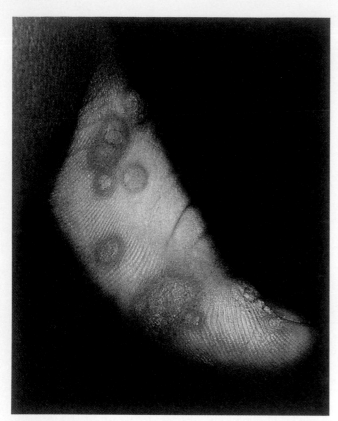

FIGURE 49–4. Common warts with thrombosed vessels *(black dots)*. (From Habif TP: *Clinical dermatology: a color guide to diagnosis and therapy,* St Louis, 1985, Mosby.)

Anogenital Warts

Genital warts (**condylomata acuminata**) occur almost exclusively on the squamous epithelium of the external genitalia and perianal areas. Approximately 90% are caused by HPV-6 and HPV-11. Anogenital lesions infected with these types of HPV rarely become malignant in otherwise healthy people.

Cervical Dysplasia and Neoplasia

HPV infection of the genital tract is now recognized as a common sexually transmitted disease. Cytologic changes characteristic of this viral infection (**koilocytotic cells**) are detected in approximately 5% of all **Papanicolaou-stained cervical smears** (Fig. 49–5). Infection of the female genital tract by HPV-16 and HPV-18 and, rarely, by other types of HPV is associated with intraepithelial cervical neoplasia and cancer. The first neoplastic changes noted on light microscopy are termed **dysplasia**. Approximately 40% to 70% of the mild dysplasias spontaneously regress.

Cervical cancer is thought to develop through a continuum of progressive cellular changes, from mild (cervical intraepithelial neoplasia [CIN I]) to moderate

neoplasia (CIN II) to severe dysplasia or carcinoma in situ. This sequence of events can occur over 1 to 4 years.

Laboratory Diagnosis

A wart can be confirmed microscopically on the basis of its characteristic histologic appearance, which consists of hyperplasia of the **prickle cells** and an excess production of keratin (**hyperkeratosis**) (Fig. 49–6). Papillomavirus infection can be detected in **Papanicolaou smears** by the presence of koilocytotic (vacuolated cytoplasm) squamous epithelial cells, which are rounded and occur in clumps (Table 49–3; see Fig. 49–5). **DNA molecular probes** and the **polymerase chain reaction (PCR)** are the methods of choice for establishing the diagnosis of HPV infection from cervical swabs and tissue specimens. Papillomaviruses do not grow in cell cultures, and tests for HPV antibodies are rarely used except in research surveys.

Treatment, Prevention, and Control

Warts spontaneously regress, but the regression may take many months to years. Warts are removed because of pain and discomfort, for cosmetic reasons, and to prevent spread to other parts of the body or to other people. They are removed through the use of surgical cryotherapy, electrocautery, or chemical means, although recurrences are common. Injection of interferon is also beneficial. Surgery may be necessary for the removal of laryngeal papillomas.

At present, the best way to prevent transmission of warts is to avoid coming in direct contact with infected

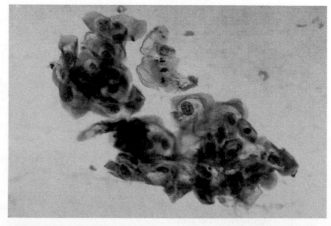

FIGURE 49–5. Papanicolaou stain of the exfoliated cervicovaginal squamous epithelial cells showing the perinuclear cytoplasmic vacuolization termed *koilocytosis* (vacuolated cytoplasm), characteristic of human papillomavirus infection. (×400.)

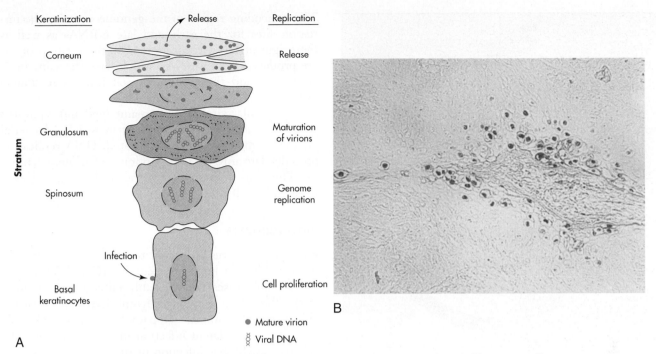

FIGURE 49-6. *A,* Comparison of normal skin and a papilloma (wart). Human papillomavirus (HPV) infection promotes the outgrowth of the basal layer, increasing the number of prickle cells (acanthosis). These changes cause the skin to thicken and promote the production of keratin (hyperkeratosis), thereby causing epithelial spikes to form (papillomatosis). Virus is produced in the granular cells close to the final keratin layer *B,* DNA probe analysis of an HPV-6–induced anogenital condyloma. A biotin-labeled DNA probe was localized by horseradish peroxidase–conjugated avidin conversion of a substrate to a chromogen precipitate. Dark staining is seen over the nuclei of koilocytotic cells. (*B* from Belshe RB, editor: *Textbook of human virology,* ed 2, St Louis, 1991, Mosby.)

tissue. Proper precautions (e.g., the use of condoms) can prevent the sexual transmission of HPV.

Polyomaviruses

The human polyomaviruses (**BK** and **JC viruses**) are ubiquitous but usually do not cause disease. They are difficult to grow in cell culture. SV40, a simian polyomavirus, and murine polyomaviruses in particular have been studied extensively as models of tumor-causing viruses.

Structure and Replication

The polyomaviruses are smaller (45 nm in diameter), contain less nucleic acid (5000 base pairs), and are less complex than the papillomaviruses (see Box 49–1). The genomes of BK virus, JC virus, and SV40 are closely related and are divided into early, late, and noncoding regions (Fig. 49–7). The early region on one strand codes for nonstructural **T** (**transformation**)

proteins (including **large T and small T antigens**), and the late region, which is on the other strand, codes for **three viral capsid proteins** (**VP1, VP2,** and **VP3**) (Box 49–4). The noncoding region contains the origin of DNA replication and transcriptional control sequences for both early and late genes.

TABLE 49–3. Laboratory Diagnosis of Papillomavirus Infections

Test	Detects
Cytology	Koilocytotic cells
In situ DNA probe analysis*	Viral nucleic acid
Polymerase chain reaction*	Viral nucleic acid
Southern blot hybridization	Viral nucleic acid
Immunofluorescent and immunoperoxidase staining	Viral structural antigens
Electron microscopy	Virus
Culture	Not useful

*Method of choice.

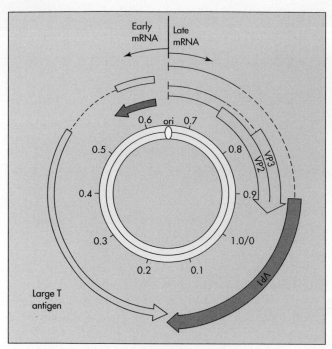

FIGURE 49-7. Genome of the SV40 virus. The genome is a prototype of that of other polyomaviruses and contains early, late, and noncoding regions. The noncoding region contains the star sequence for the early and late genes and for DNA replication *(ori).* The individual early and late messenger RNAs are processed from the larger nested transcripts. (Redrawn from Butel JS, Jarvis DL: The plasma-membrane form of SV40 large tumor antigen: biochemical and biological properties. *Biochem Biophys Acta* 865:171–195, 1986.)

After the virus enters a cell, the DNA is uncoated and delivered to the nucleus. The early genes encode the large T and small t antigens, proteins that promote cell growth. Viral replication requires the transcriptional and DNA replication machinery provided by a growing cell. The large T antigens of SV40, JC virus, and BK virus have several functions. For example, the T antigen of SV40 binds to DNA and controls early and late gene transcription as well as viral DNA replication. In addition, the T antigen binds to and inactivates the two major cellular growth-suppressor proteins, p53 and p105RB, promoting cell growth.

Like replication of the HPVs, replication of polyomavirus is highly dependent on host cell factors. Permissive cells allow the transcription of late viral messenger RNA (mRNA) and viral replication, which results in cell death. Some nonpermissive cells, however, allow only the early genes, including T antigen, to be expressed, promoting cell growth and potentially leading to oncogenic transformation of the cell.

The polyomavirus genome is used very efficiently.

The noncoding region of the genome contains the initiation sites for the early and late mRNAs as well as the origin of DNA replication. The three late proteins are produced from mRNAs, which have the same initiation site, and then are processed into three unique mRNAs.

The circular viral DNA is maintained and replicated bidirectionally, similar to the way in which a bacterial plasmid is maintained and replicated. DNA replication precedes late mRNA transcription and protein synthesis. The virus is assembled in the nucleus, and virus is released by cell lysis.

Pathogenesis

Each polyomavirus is limited to specific hosts and cell types within that host. For example, JC and BK viruses are human viruses that probably enter the respiratory tract, after which they infect lymphocytes and then the kidney with a minimal cytopathologic effect. The BK virus establishes latent infection in the kidney, and the JC virus establishes infection in the kidneys, in B cells, and in monocyte-lineage cells. Replication is blocked in immunocompetent people.

In immunocompromised patients, such as those with the acquired immunodeficiency syndrome (AIDS), reactivation of the virus in the kidney leads to viral shedding in the urine and potentially severe urinary tract infections (BK virus) or viremia and central nervous system infection (JC virus) (Fig. 49–8). JC virus crosses the blood-brain barrier by replicating in the endothelial cells of capillaries. An abortive infection of astrocytes results in partial transformation, yielding enlarged cells with abnormal nuclei resembling glioblastomas. Productive lytic infections of oligodendrocytes cause demyelination (see Box 49–3). Although SV40 and BK and JC viruses can cause tumors in hamsters, these viruses are not associated with any human tumors.

BOX 49-4. **Polyomavirus Proteins**

Early

Large T: Regulation of early and late messenger RNA transcription; DNA replication; cell growth promotion and transformation.
Small t: Viral DNA replication.

Late

VP1: Major capsid protein and viral attachment protein.
VP2: Minor capsid protein.
VP3: Minor capsid protein.

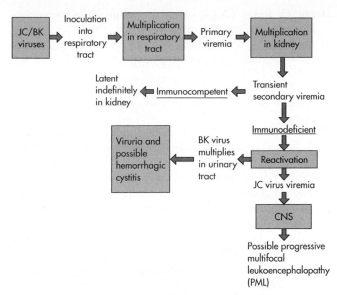

FIGURE 49–8. Mechanisms of spread of polyomaviruses within the body.

Epidemiology

Polyomavirus infections are ubiquitous, and most people are infected with both the JC and BK viruses by the age of 15 years (see Box 49–3). Respiratory transmission is the probable mode of spread. Latent infections can be reactivated in people whose immune systems are suppressed as a result of AIDS, organ transplantation, or pregnancy.

Early batches of polio vaccine were contaminated with SV40 that was undetected in the primary monkey cell cultures used to prepare the vaccine. Although many people were vaccinated with the contaminated vaccines, no SV40-related tumors have ever been reported.

Clinical Syndromes

Primary infection is virtually always asymptomatic. The BK and JC viruses are commonly found to be excreted in the urine of as many as 40% of immunocompromised patients. The viruses are also reactivated during pregnancy, but no effects on the fetus have been noted.

The ureteral stenosis observed in renal transplant recipients appears to be associated with BK virus, as is the hemorrhagic cystitis observed in bone marrow transplant recipients.

Progressive multifocal leukoencephalopathy (PML) is a rare syndrome. A subacute demyelinating disease that occurs in immunocompromised patients, including those with AIDS, PML is caused by the **JC virus**. As the name implies, patients may have multiple neurologic symptoms unattributable to a single anatomic lesion. Speech, vision, coordination, mentation, or a combination of these functions are impaired, followed by paralysis of the arms and legs and finally death. The cerebrospinal fluid is normal, however, and does not contain antibody to the JC virus.

Laboratory Diagnosis

PML is diagnosed through the histologic examination of brain tissue obtained by biopsy or at autopsy. Foci of demyelination surrounded by oligodendrocytes with inclusions adjacent to areas of demyelination are observed in such tissue. **Electron microscopy**, **polymerase chain reaction**, or **DNA probe analysis** can be used to detect virus in brain tissue. The term leukoencephalopathy refers to the presence of lesions in only the white matter. There is little if any inflammatory cell response. Magnetic resonance imaging or computed tomography may show evidence of lesions.

Urine cytologic tests can reveal the presence of JC or BK virus infection by revealing the existence of enlarged cells with dense basophilic intranuclear inclusions resembling those induced by cytomegalovirus. It is difficult to isolate BK and JC viruses in tissue cultures, and therefore this procedure is not routinely attempted.

Quicker methods of analysis now include in situ immunofluorescence, immunoperoxidase, DNA probe analysis, and PCR analysis of cerebrospinal fluid, urine, or biopsy material for the particular genetic sequences.

Treatment, Prevention, and Control

No specific treatment for polyomavirus infection is available, other than to decrease the immunosuppression responsible for allowing the polyomavirus to be reactivated and symptoms to occur. The ubiquitous nature of polyomaviruses and the lack of understanding of their modes of transmission make it unlikely that the primary infection can be prevented.

CASE STUDY AND QUESTIONS

■ A 25-year-old carpenter notices the appearance of several hyperkeratotic papules (warts) on the palm side of his index finger. They do not change in size and cause him only minimal discomfort. After a year, they spontaneously disappear.

1. Will this virus infection spread to other body sites?

2. After its disappearance, is the infection likely to be completely resolved or to persist in the host?

3. What viral, cellular, and host conditions regulate the replication of this virus and other HPVs?

4. How would the papillomavirus type causing this infection be identified?

5. Is it likely that this type of HPV is associated with human cancer? If not, which types are associated with cancers, and which cancers are they?

BIBLIOGRAPHY

Arthur RR et al: Association of BK viruria with hemorrhagic cystitis in recipients of bone marrow transplants, *N Engl J Med* 315:230–234, 1986.

Crum CP, Barber S, Roche JK: Pathobiology of papillomavirus-related cervical diseases, *Clin Microbiol Rev* 4:270–285, 1991.

Fields BN, Knipe DM, Howley PM, editors: *Virology*, ed 3, New York, 1996, Lippincott-Raven.

Gorbach SL, Bartlett JG, Blacklow NR, editors: *Infectious diseases*, ed 2, Philadelphia, 1997, WB Saunders.

Howley PM: Role of the human papillomaviruses in human cancer, *Cancer Res* 51(suppl 18):5019S–5022S, 1991.

Hseuh C, Reyes CV: Progressive multifocal leukoencephalopathy, *Am Fam Physician* 37:129–132, 1988.

Major EO et al: Pathogenesis and molecular biology of progressive multifocal leukoencephalopathy, *Clin Microbiol Rev* 5:49–73, 1992.

Mandell GL, Bennett JE, Dolin R: *Principles and practice of infectious diseases*, ed 5, New York, 2000, Churchill Livingstone.

Miller DM, Brodell RT: Human papillomavirus infection: treatment options for warts, *Am Fam Physician* 53:135–143, 1996.

Morrison EA: Natural history of cervical infection with human papillomavirus, *Clin Infect Dis* 18:172–180, 1994.

Papilloma virus NIAID fact sheet [on line]. Available at http://www.niaid.nih.gov/factsheets/stdhpv.htm

White DO, Fenner FJ: *Medical virology*, ed 4, New York, 1994, Academic Press.

zür-Hausen H: Viruses in human cancers, *Science* 254:1167–1173, 1991.

zür-Hausen H: Human pathogenic papillomaviruses, *Curr Top Microbiol Immunol* 186:1–274, 1994.

CHAPTER 50

Adenoviruses

Adenoviruses were first isolated in 1953 in a human adenoid cell culture. Since then, approximately 100 serotypes, at least 47 of which infect humans, have been recognized. All human serotypes are included in a single genus within the family Adenoviridae. On the basis of the findings from DNA homology studies and the hemagglutination patterns, all of the 47 serotypes have been classified into six subgroups (A through F) (Table 50–1). The viruses in each subgroup share many properties.

The first human adenoviruses to be identified, numbered 1 to 7, are the most common. Common disorders caused by the adenoviruses include **respiratory tract infection**, **conjunctivitis (pink eye)**, **hemorrhagic cystitis**, and **gastroenteritis**. Several adenoviruses have oncogenic potential in animals and for this reason have been extensively studied by molecular biologists. These studies have elucidated many viral and eukaryotic intracellular processes. For example, analysis of the gene for the adenovirus hexon protein led to the discovery of introns and the splicing of eukaryotic messenger RNAs (mRNAs). Adenovirus is also being used to deliver DNA for gene replacement therapy (e.g., cystic fibrosis).

Structure and Replication

Adenoviruses are double-stranded DNA viruses with a genome molecular mass of 20 to 25 $\times$ 10^6 Da. The adenovirus genome is a **linear, double-stranded DNA** with a **terminal protein** (molecular mass, 55 kDa) covalently attached at each 55′ end. The virions are **nonenveloped icosadeltahedrons** with a diameter of 70 to 90 nm (Fig. 50–1 and Box 50–1). The capsid comprises 240 capsomeres, which consist of hexons and pentons. The 12 pentons, which are located at each of the vertices, have a penton base and a fiber. The **fiber** contains the **viral attachment proteins** and can act as a hemagglutinin. The penton base and fiber are toxic to cells. The pentons and fibers also carry type-specific antigens.

The core complex within the capsid includes viral

TABLE 50–1. Illnesses Associated with Adenoviruses

Disease	Patient Population
Respiratory diseases:	
Febrile, undifferentiated upper respiratory tract infection	Infants, young children
Pharyngoconjunctival fever	Children, adults
Acute respiratory disease	Military recruits
Pertussis-like syndrome	Infants, young children
Pneumonia	Infants, young children
	Military recruits
	Immunocompromised patients
Other diseases:	
Acute hemorrhagic cystitis	Children, bone marrow transplant recipients
Epidemic keratoconjunctivitis	Any age; renal transplant recipients
Gastroenteritis	Infants, young children
Hepatitis	Liver transplant recipients or other immunocompromised individuals
Meningoencephalitis	Children, immunocompromised patients

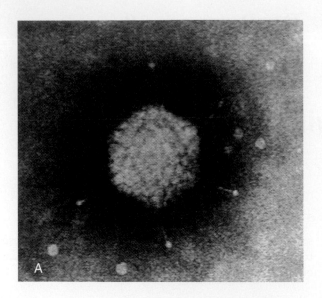

Adenovirus

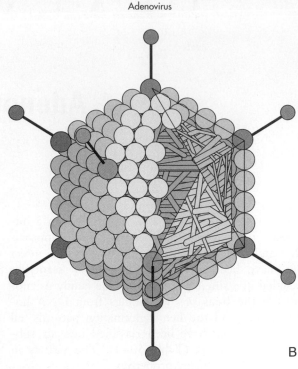

B

FIGURE 50–1. *A,* Electron micrograph of adenovirus virion with fibers. *B,* Model of adenovirus virion with fibers. (*A* from Valentine RC, Pereira HG: Antigens and structure of the adenovirus, *J Mol Biol* 13:13–20, 1965; *B* from Armstrong D, Cohen J: *Infectious diseases,* St Louis, 1999, Mosby.)

DNA and at least two major proteins. There are at least 11 polypeptides in the adenovirus virion, 9 of which have an identified structural function (Table 50–2).

A map of the adenovirus genome shows the locations of the viral genes (Fig. 50–2). The genes are transcribed from both DNA strands and in both directions at different times during the replication cycle. Genes for related functions are clustered together. Most of the RNA transcribed from the adenovirus genome is processed into several individual mRNAs in the nucleus. Early proteins promote cell growth and include a **DNA polymerase** that is involved in the replication of the genome. Adenovirus also encodes proteins that suppress host immune and inflammatory responses. Late proteins, which are synthesized after the onset of viral DNA replication, are primarily components of the capsid.

The replication of adenoviruses has been studied extensively in HeLa cell cultures. One virus cycle takes approximately 32 to 36 hours and produces 10,000 virions. Adenovirus binding to the cell surface occurs in two steps. The viral fiber proteins interact with a glycoprotein within the immunoglobulin superfamily of proteins (approximately 100,000 fiber receptors are present on each cell). This is the same receptor that is

for many coxsackie B viruses, which give its name, coxsackie adenovirus receptor (CAR). Then the penton base interacts with an αv integrin to promote internalization by receptor-mediated endocytosis in a clathrin-coated vesicle. The virus lyses the endosomal vesicle, and the capsid delivers the DNA genome to the nu-

---

BOX 50–1. Unique Features of Adenovirus

Naked icosadeltahedral capsid has **fibers** (viral attachment proteins) at vertices.

Linear double-stranded genome has 5′ terminal proteins.

Virus encodes proteins to promote messenger RNA and DNA synthesis, including its own **DNA polymerase.**

Human adenoviruses are grouped A through F by DNA homologies and by serotype (more than 42 types).

Serotype is mainly due to differences in the penton base and fiber protein, which determine the nature of tissue tropism and disease.

Virus causes **lytic, persistent,** and **latent** infections in humans, and some strains can **immortalize certain animal cells.**

TABLE 50-2. Major Adenovirus Proteins

Gene	Number	Molecular Mass (kDa$_2$)	Function
E1A*			Activates viral gene transcription
			Binds cellular growth suppressor: RB105 promotes transformation
			Deregulates cell growth
			Inhibits activation of interferon response elements
E1B			Binds cellular growth suppressor: p53 promotes transformation
			Blocks apoptosis
E2			Activates some promoters
			Terminal protein on DNA
			DNA polymerase
E3			Prevents tumor necrosis factor-α inflammation
E4			Limits viral cytopathologic effect
VA RNAs			Inhibit interferon response
Capsid			
	II	120	Hexon protein
			Contains family antigen and some serotyping antigens
	III	85	Penton base protein
			Toxic to tissue culture cells
	IV	62	Fiber
			Responsible for attachment and hemagglutination; contains some serotyping antigens
	VI	24	
	VIII	13	Hexon-associated proteins
	IX	12	Penton-associated proteins
	IIIa	66	
Core			
	V	48	Core protein 1: DNA-binding protein
	VII	18	Core protein 2: DNA-binding protein

*Early genes encode several messenger RNA and proteins by alternative splicing patterns.

E = early; RB = retinoblastoma gene product; VA = virus-associated.

cleus. The penton and fiber proteins of the capsid are toxic to the cell and can inhibit cellular macromolecular synthesis.

Early transcriptional events lead to the formation of gene products that can stimulate cell growth and promote viral DNA replication. As is the case for the papovaviruses, several adenovirus mRNAs share the same promoter and initial sequences but are produced through the splicing out of different introns. Transcription of the early gene E1, processing of the primary transcript (splicing out of introns to yield three mRNAs), and translation produce the transactivator proteins required for transcription of the other early proteins. Other early proteins include more DNA-binding proteins, the DNA polymerase, and proteins to help the virus escape the immune response. The **E1A** and **E1B** proteins stimulate cell growth by binding to the cellular growth-suppressor proteins **p53** (E1A) and **RB** (retinoblastoma gene product) (E1B). In permissive cells, stimulation of cell division facilitates transcription

and replication of the genome, but this activity ultimately causes cell death. In nonpermissive cells, the virus establishes latency and the genome remains in the nucleus. For rodent cells, the E1A and E1B may promote cell growth without cell death and, therefore, oncogenesis.

Viral DNA replication occurs in the nucleus and is mediated by a viral DNA polymerase from both strands of the DNA. The polymerase uses a primer consisting of a 55 kDa viral protein (terminal protein) and a cytosine monophosphate.

Late gene transcription starts after DNA replication. Most of the individual late mRNAs are generated from a large (83% of the genome) primary RNA transcript encoded by the right strand of the genome, which is processed into individual mRNAs.

Capsid proteins are produced in the cytoplasm and then transported to the nucleus for viral assembly. Empty procapsids first assemble, and then the viral DNA and core proteins enter the capsid through an

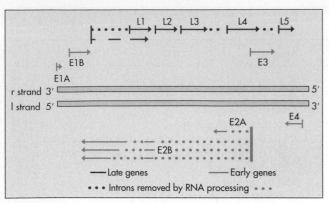

FIGURE 50–2. Simplified genome map of adenovirus type 2. Genes are transcribed from both strands (l and r) in opposite directions. The early genomes are transcribed from four promoter sequences and generate several messenger RNAs. All of the late genes are transcribed from one promoter sequence. Alternative splicing patterns of primary RNA transcripts produce the full repertoire of viral proteins. The splicing pattern for only the E2 transcript is shown as an example. E = Early protein; L = late protein. (Modified from Jawetz E et al, editors: *Review of medical microbiology*, ed 17, Norwalk, Conn, 1987, Appleton & Lange.)

opening at one of the vertices. Cleavage of several of the capsid proteins and of the terminal protein attached to the DNA causes the particle to mature into a stable and infectious virion. Replication and the assembly process are inefficient and error-prone; only one infectious unit is produced per 11 to 2300 particles. DNA, protein, and numerous defective particles accumulate in nuclear inclusion bodies. The virus remains in the cell until the cell degenerates and lyses.

Pathogenesis and Immunity

Adenoviruses are capable of causing lytic (e.g., mucoepithelial cells), latent (e.g., lymphoid and adenoid cells), and transforming (hamster, not human) infections. These viruses infect epithelial cells lining the oropharynx as well as the respiratory and enteric organs (Box 50-2). Viremia may occur after local replication of the virus, with subsequent spread to visceral organs (Fig. 50-3). This dissemination is more likely to occur in immunocompromised patients than in immunocompetent people. The viral fiber proteins determine the target cell specificity among adenovirus serotypes. The toxic activity of the penton base protein can result in inhibition of cellular mRNA transport and protein synthesis, cell rounding, and tissue damage.

The virus has a propensity to become **latent** in lymphoid and other tissue, such as adenoids, tonsils, and Peyer's patches, and can be reactivated in patients who are in an immunosuppressed state or have been

BOX 50–2. Disease Mechanisms of Adenoviruses

Virus is spread by **aerosol, close contact,** or **fecal-oral** means to establish pharyngeal infection. Fingers spread virus to eyes.

Virus infects **mucoepithelial cells** in the respiratory tract, gastrointestinal tract, and conjunctiva or cornea, causing cell damage directly.

Disease is determined by the tissue tropism of the specific group or serotype of the virus strain.

Virus **persists** in lymphoid tissue (e.g., tonsils, adenoids, Peyer's patches).

Antibody is important for prophylaxis and resolution.

infected with other agents. Although certain adenoviruses (groups A and B) can transform and are **oncogenic in rodent cells**, adenovirus transformation of human cells has not been observed. The time course of adenovirus infection is shown in Figure 50–4).

The histologic hallmark of adenovirus infection is a dense, central intranuclear inclusion within an infected epithelial cell that consists of viral DNA and protein (Fig. 50–5). These inclusions may resemble those seen in cells infected with cytomegalovirus, but adenovirus does not cause cellular enlargement (cytomegaly). Mononuclear cell infiltrates and epithelial cell necrosis are seen at the site of infection.

Antibody is important for resolving lytic adenovirus infections and protects the person from reinfection with the same serotype but not other serotypes. Cell-mediated immunity is important in limiting virus out-

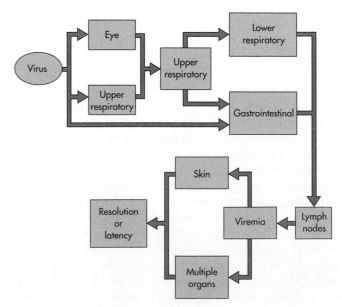

FIGURE 50–3. Mechanism of adenovirus spread within the body.

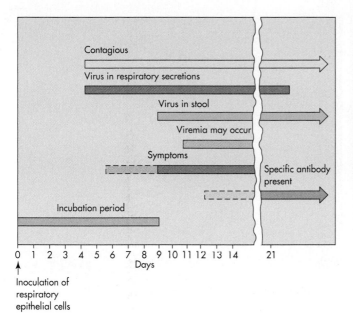

FIGURE 50–4. Time course of adenovirus respiratory infection.

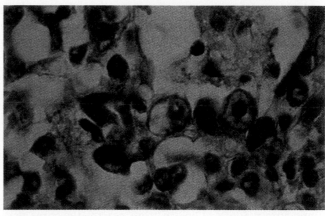

FIGURE 50–5. Histologic appearance of adenovirus-infected cells. Inefficient assembly of virions yields dark basophilic nuclear inclusion bodies containing DNA, proteins, and capsids.

growth, as borne out by the fact that immunosuppressed people suffer recurrent disease.

Adenovirus encodes several early proteins that help the virus **avoid immune defenses**. For example, during viral replication, short RNA segments are produced (virus-associated [VA] RNAs); one of these segments forms a double-stranded duplex and blocks activation of the enzymes of the interferon-induced antiviral state. In addition, a 19 kDa early protein binds to the heavy chain of class I major histocompatibility (MHC) antigen and prevents it from reaching the cell membrane, thus preventing the cell from presenting antigenic targets to cytotoxic T cells. Several proteins inhibit the induction of inflammation by tumor necrosis

factor, limiting the immunopathologic effect and the severity of the disease symptoms.

Epidemiology

Adenovirus virions resist drying, detergents, gastrointestinal tract secretions (acid, protease, and bile), and even mild chlorine treatment (Box 50–3). They can therefore be spread by the fecal-oral route, by fingers, by fomites (including towels and medical instruments), and in poorly chlorinated swimming pools.

Adenoviruses are spread exclusively by human-to-human transmission, mainly by respiratory or fecal-oral contact, with no apparent animal reservoirs for the virus. Close interaction among people, as occurs in classrooms and military barracks, promotes spread of the virus. Adenoviruses may be shed intermittently and over long periods from the pharynx and especially in

---

BOX 50–3. Epidemiology of Adenoviruses

Disease/Viral Factors

Capsid virus is resistant to inactivation by gastrointestinal tract and drying.

    Disease symptoms may resemble those of other respiratory virus infections.

    Virus may cause asymptomatic shedding.

Transmission

Direct contact via respiratory droplets and fecal matter, on hands, on fomites (e.g., towels, contaminated medical instruments), close contact, and inadequately chlorinated swimming pools.

Who Is at Risk?

Children younger than 14 years.

    People in daycare centers, military training camps, and swimming clubs.

Geography/Season

Virus is found worldwide.

    There is no seasonal incidence.

Modes of Control

Live vaccine for serotypes 4 and 7 is available for military use.

feces. Most infections are asymptomatic, a feature that greatly facilitates their spread in the community.

Adenoviruses 1 through 7 are the most prevalent serotypes. From 5% to 10% of cases of pediatric respiratory tract disease are caused by adenovirus types 1, 2, 5, and 6, and the infected children shed virus for months after infection. Serotypes 4 and 7 seem especially able to spread among military recruits because of their close proximity and rigorous lifestyle.

Clinical Syndromes

Adenoviruses primarily infect children and less commonly infect adults. Disease from reactivated virus occurs in immunocompromised children and adults. Several distinct clinical syndromes are associated with adenovirus infection (see Table 50–1).

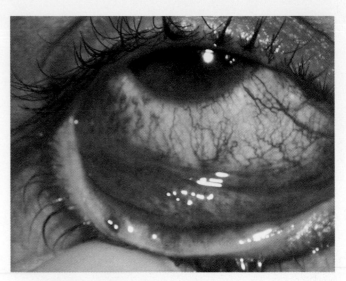

FIGURE 50–6. Conjunctivitis caused by adenovirus.

Acute Febrile Pharyngitis and Pharyngoconjunctival Fever

Adenovirus causes **pharyngitis**, which is often accompanied by **conjunctivitis (pink eye) (pharyngoconjunctival fever)**. Pharyngitis alone occurs in young children, particularly those younger than 3 years, and may mimic streptococcal infection. Affected patients have mild flu-like symptoms, including nasal congestion, cough, coryza, malaise, fever, chills, myalgia, and headache, that may last 3 to 5 days. Pharyngoconjunctival fever occurs more often in outbreaks involving older children.

Acute Respiratory Tract Disease

Acute respiratory tract disease is a syndrome consisting of fever, cough, pharyngitis, and cervical adenitis. It occurs primarily among military recruits infected with adenovirus serotypes 4 and 7.

Other Respiratory Tract Diseases

Adenoviruses cause coldlike symptoms, laryngitis, croup, and bronchiolitis. They can also cause a pertussis-like illness in children and adults that consists of a prolonged clinical course and true viral pneumonia.

Conjunctivitis and Epidemic Keratoconjunctivitis

Adenoviruses cause a follicular conjunctivitis in which the mucosa of the palpebral conjunctiva becomes pebbled or nodular and both conjunctivae (palpebral and bulbar) become inflamed (Fig. 50–6). Such conjunctivitis may occur sporadically or in outbreaks that can be traced to a common source. Swimming pool conjunctivitis is a familiar example of a common-source adeno-

virus infection. Epidemic keratoconjunctivitis may be an occupational hazard for industrial workers. The most striking such epidemic occurred in people working in the naval shipyards of Pearl Harbor, where it caused more than 10,000 cases during 1941 and 1942. Irritation of the eye by a foreign body, dust, debris, and the like is a risk factor for the acquisition of this infection.

Gastroenteritis and Diarrhea

Adenovirus is a major cause of acute viral gastroenteritis; 15% of the cases of gastroenteritis in hospitalized patients are caused by this virus. Adenovirus serotypes 40, 41, and 42 have been grouped as enteric adenoviruses (group F) and appear to be responsible for episodes of diarrhea in infants. These enteric adenoviruses do not replicate in the same tissue culture cells as other adenoviruses and rarely cause fever or respiratory tract symptoms.

Other Manifestations

Adenovirus has also been associated with a pertussis-like illness, intussusception in young children, acute hemorrhagic cystitis with dysuria and hematuria in young boys, musculoskeletal disorders, and genital and skin infections.

Systemic Infection in Immunocompromised Patients

Immunocompromised patients are at risk for serious adenovirus infections, although not as much as they are for infections caused by herpesviruses. Adenoviral disease in immunocompromised patients include pneumonia and hepatitis. Infection can originate from exogenous or endogenous (reactivation) sources.

Laboratory Diagnosis

The isolation of most adenovirus types is best accomplished in cell cultures derived from epithelial cells (e.g., primary human embryonic kidney cells, continuous [transformed] lines such as HeLa and human epidermal carcinoma cells). Within 2 to 20 days, the virus causes a lytic infection with characteristic inclusion bodies. Recovery of virus from cell culture requires an average of 6 days.

For the results of virus isolation to be significant, the isolate should be obtained from a site or secretion relevant to the disease symptoms. Isolation of adenovirus from the throat of a patient with pharyngitis is usually diagnostic if laboratory findings eliminate other common causes of pharyngitis, such as *Streptococcus pyogenes*.

Immunoassays, including fluorescent antibody and enzyme-linked immunosorbent assays, the polymerase chain reaction (PCR), and DNA probe analysis, can be used to detect, type, and group the virus in clinical samples and tissue cultures. Enzyme immunoassay, PCR, DNA probe analysis, and immunoelectron microscopy are used to identify enteric adenovirus serotypes 40, 41, and 42, which do not grow readily in available cell cultures. The characteristic intranuclear inclusions can be seen in infected tissue during histologic examination. However, such inclusions are rare and must be distinguished from those produced by cytomegalovirus. Serologic testing is rarely used except for epidemiologic purposes or to confirm the significance of a fecal or upper respiratory tract isolate by identifying its serotype.

Treatment, Prevention, and Control

There is no known treatment for adenovirus infection. Live oral vaccines have been used to prevent infections with adenovirus types 4 and 7 in military recruits but are not used in civilian populations. The widespread use of live adenovirus vaccines is unlikely, because members of some species of the adenovirus family are oncogenic. However, genetically engineered subunit vaccines could be prepared and used in the future.

Gene Replacement Therapy

Adenoviruses have been used and are being considered for more applications of gene delivery for correction of several human diseases, including immune deficiencies (e.g., adenosine deaminase deficiency), cystic fibrosis, lysosomal storage diseases, and even cancer. The virus is inactivated by deletion or mutation of the E1 and other viral genes (e.g., E2, E4). The appropriate gene is inserted into the genome, replacing this DNA, and is controlled by an appropriate promoter. The resultant virus vector must be grown in a cell that expresses the missing viral functions (E1, E4) and can complement the deficiency to allow production of virus. Adenovirus types 4 and 7 have been used most extensively since attenuated (vaccine) strains have been developed.

CASE STUDY AND QUESTIONS

■ A 7-year-old boy attending summer camp complains of sore throat, headache, cough, red eyes, and tiredness and is sent to the infirmary. His temperature is 40°C. Within hours, other campers and counselors visit the infirmary with similar symptoms. Symptoms last for 5 to 7 days. All the patients have gone swimming in the camp pond. More than 50% of the people in the camp complain of symptoms similar to those in the initial case. The Public Health Department identifies the agent as adenovirus serotype 3.

1. Toward which adenovirus syndrome do the symptoms point?

2. An outbreak as large as this indicates a common source of infection. What was the most likely source or sources? What were the most likely routes by which the virus was spread?

3. What physical properties of the virus facilitate its transmission?

4. What precautions should the camp owners take to prevent other outbreaks?

5. What sample or samples would have been used by the Public Health Department to identify the infectious agent, and what tests would be required to diagnose the infection?

BIBLIOGRAPHY

Balows A, Hausler WJ Jr, Lennette EH, editors: *Laboratory diagnosis of infectious diseases: principles and practice*, vol 2, New York, 1988, Springer-Verlag.

Belshe RB, editor: *Textbook on human virology*, ed 2, St Louis, 1991, Mosby.

Benihoud K, Yeh P, Perricaudet M: Adenovirus vectors for gene delivery, *Curr Opin Biotechnol* 10:440–447, 1999.

Doerfleur W, Böhm P, editors: The molecular repertoire of adenoviruses parts I, II, III, *Curr Top Microbiol Immunol* 199, 1995.

Fields BN, Knipe DM, Howley PM, editors: *Virology*, ed 3, New York, 1996, Lippincott-Raven.

Ginsberg HS: *The adenoviruses*, New York, 1984, Plenum.

Gorbach SL, Bartlett JG, Blacklow NR, editors: *Infectious diseases*, ed 2, Philadelphia, 1997, WB Saunders.

Mandell GL, Bennett JE, Dolin R: *Principles and practice of infectious diseases*, ed 5, New York, 2000, Churchill Livingstone.

Robbins PD, Ghivizzani SC: Viral vectors for gene therapy, *Pharmacol Ther* 80:35–47, 1998.

White DO, Fenner FJ: *Medical virology*, ed 4, New York, 1994, Academic.

C H A P T E R   5 1

Human Herpesviruses

The human herpesviruses are grouped into three subfamilies on the basis of differences in viral characteristics (genome structure, tissue tropism, cytopathologic effect, and site of latent infection) as well as the pathogenesis of the disease and disease manifestation (Table 51–1). The human herpesviruses are herpes simplex viruses (HSV) types 1 and 2, varicella-zoster virus (VZV), Epstein-Barr virus (EBV), cytomegalovirus (CMV), human herpesvirus 6 (HHV6), human herpesvirus 7 (HHV7), and the recently discovered human herpesvirus 8 (HHV8) associated with Kaposi's sarcoma.

The herpesviruses are an important group of large DNA viruses with the following features in common: virion morphology, basic mode of replication, and capacity to establish latent and recurrent infections. Cell-mediated immunity is also important for controlling infection with these viruses and causing symptoms. Herpesviruses encode proteins and enzymes that facilitate the replication and interaction of the virus with the host. The herpesviruses can cause lytic, persistent, latent/recurrent, and, in the case of EBV, immortalizing infections (Box 51–1).

Herpesvirus infections are common, and the viruses are **ubiquitous**. Although these viruses usually cause benign disease, especially in children, they can also cause significant morbidity and mortality, especially in immunosuppressed people. Fortunately, the herpesviruses encode targets for antiviral agents. The U.S. Food and Drug Administration (FDA) has approved a live-virus vaccine for VZV.

Structure of Herpesviruses

The herpesviruses are **large, enveloped** viruses that contain **double-stranded DNA**. The virion is approximately 150 nm in diameter and has the characteristic morphology shown in Figure 51–1. The DNA core is surrounded by an **icosadeltahedral capsid** containing 162 capsomeres. This is enclosed by a glycoprotein-containing envelope. Herpesviruses encode several glycoproteins for viral attachment, fusion, and for escaping immune control. The space between the envelope and the capsid, called the tegument, contains viral proteins and enzymes that help initiate replication. As enveloped viruses, the herpesviruses are sensitive to acid, solvents, detergents, and drying.

Herpesviral genomes are linear, double-stranded DNA but they differ in size and gene orientation (Fig. 51–2). Direct or inverted repeat sequences bracket unique regions of the genome (unique long [U_L], unique short [U_S]), allowing circularization and recombination within the genome. Recombination among inverted repeats of HSV, CMV, and VZV allows large portions of the genome to switch the orientation of their U_L and U_S gene segments with respect to each other.

Replication of the Herpesviruses

Herpesvirus replication is initiated by the interaction of viral glycoproteins with cell surface receptors (see Fig. 6–14). The tropism of some herpesviruses (e.g., EBV) is restricted as a result of the tissue-specific expression of their receptors. The nucleocapsid is then released into the cytoplasm through fusion of the envelope with the plasma membrane. Enzymes and transcription factors are carried into the cell in the tegument of the virion. The nucleocapsid docks with the nuclear membrane and delivers the genome into the nucleus, where the genome is transcribed and replicated.

Transcription of the viral genome and viral protein synthesis proceeds in a coordinated and regulated manner in three phases:

1. **Immediate early proteins** (α), consisting of DNA-binding proteins important for the regulation of gene transcription.
2. **Early proteins** (β), consisting of more transcription factors and enzymes, including the DNA polymerase.
3. Late **proteins** (γ), consisting mainly of structural proteins, which are generated after viral genome replication has begun.

The viral genome is transcribed by the cellular

TABLE 51–1. Properties Distinguishing the Herpesviruses

Subfamily	Virus	Primary Target Cell	Site of Latency	Means of Spread
Alphaherpesvirinae				
Human herpesvirus 1	Herpes simplex type 1	Mucoepithelial cells	Neuron	Close contact
Human herpesvirus 2	Herpes simplex type 2	Mucoepithelial cells	Neuron	Close contact (sexually transmitted disease)
Human herpesvirus 3	Varicella-zoster virus	Mucoepithelial cells	Neuron	Respiratory and close contact
Gammaherpesvirinae				
Human herpesvirus 4	Epstein-Barr virus	B cells and epithelial cells	B cell	Saliva (kissing disease)
Human herpesvirus 8	Kaposi's sarcoma–related virus	Lymphocyte and other cells	?	Close contact (sexual), saliva?
Betaherpesvirinae				
Human herpesvirus 5	Cytomegalovirus	Monocyte, lymphocyte, and epithelial cells	Monocyte, lymphocyte, and ?	Close contact, transfusions, tissue transplant, and congenital
Human herpesvirus 6	Herpes lymphotropic virus	T cells and ?	T cells and ?	Respiratory and close contact?
Human herpesvirus 7	Human herpesvirus 7	T cells and ?	T cells and ?	?

? indicates that other cells may also be the primary target or site of latency.

DNA-dependent RNA polymerase *and is regulated by viral-encoded and cellular nuclear factors. The interplay of these factors determines whether the infection is lytic, persistent, or latent.* Cells that promote latent infection transcribe only specific genes without genome replication. Progression to early and late gene expression results in cell death and lytic infection.

Replication of the viral genome is performed by the viral-encoded DNA polymerase. Viral-encoded scavenging enzymes provide deoxyribonucleotide substrates for the polymerase and are targets of antiviral drugs.

These and other viral enzymes facilitate replication of the virus in nongrowing cells that lack sufficient deoxyribonucleotides and enzymes for viral DNA synthesis (e.g., neurons).

Empty procapsids assemble in the nucleus, are filled with DNA, acquire an envelope at the nuclear or Golgi membrane, and exit the cell by exocytosis or by lysis of the cell. Transcription, protein synthesis, glycoprotein processing, and exocytotic release from the cell are performed by cellular machinery. The replication of HSV is discussed in more detail as the prototype of the herpesviruses.

BOX 51–1. Unique Features of Herpesviruses

Herpesviruses have large, enveloped icosadeltahedral capsids containing **double-stranded DNA genomes.**

Herpesviruses encode many proteins that regulate messenger RNA and DNA synthesis and the shutoff of the host cell DNA, RNA, and protein synthesis.

Herpesviruses encode enzymes **(DNA polymerase)** that promote viral DNA replication and that are good targets for **antiviral drugs.**

DNA replication and assembly occur in the nucleus; virus buds from nuclear membrane and is released by exocytosis and cell lysis.

Herpesviruses can cause **lytic, persistent, latent,** and, for Epstein-Barr virus, **immortalizing infections.**

Herpesviruses are ubiquitous.

Cell-mediated immunity is required for control.

Herpes Simplex Virus

HSV was the first human herpesvirus to be recognized. The name herpes is derived from a Greek word meaning "to creep." "Cold sores" were described in antiquity, and their viral etiology was established in 1919.

The two types of herpes simplex virus, HSV-1 and HSV-2, share many characteristics, including DNA homology, antigenic determinants, tissue tropism, and disease symptoms. However, they can still be distinguished from differences in these properties.

Structure

The HSV genome is large enough to encode approximately 80 proteins. Only half of the proteins are required for viral replication; the others facilitate the

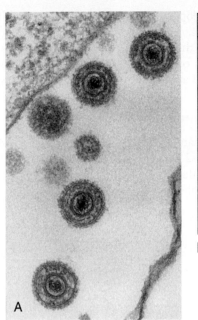

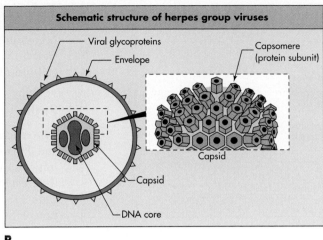

FIGURE 51–1. Electron micrograph *(A)* and general structure *(B)* of the herpesviruses. The DNA genome of the herpesvirus in the core is surrounded by an icosadeltahedral capsid and an envelope. Glycoproteins are inserted into the envelope. *(A from Armstrong D, Cohen J: Infectious diseases,* St Louis, 1999, Mosby.)

virus's interaction with different host cells and the immune response. The HSV genome encodes enzymes, including a DNA-dependent DNA polymerase and scavenging enzymes such as deoxyribonuclease, thymidine kinase, ribonucleotide reductase, and protease. Ribonucleotide reductase converts ribonucleotides to deoxyribonucleotides, and thymidine kinase phosphorylates the deoxyribonucleotides to provide substrates for replication of the viral genome. The substrate specificities of these enzymes and the DNA polymerase differ significantly from those of their cellular analogues and thus represent potentially good targets for antiviral chemotherapy.

HSV encodes at least 11 glycoproteins that serve as viral attachment proteins (gB, gC, gD, gH), fusion proteins (gB), structural proteins, immune escape proteins (gC, gE, gI), and other functions. For example, the C3 component of the complement system binds to gC and is depleted from serum. The Fc portion of immunoglobulin G (IgG) binds to a gE/gI complex, thereby camouflaging the virus and virus-infected cells. These actions reduce the antiviral effectiveness of antibody.

Replication

HSV can infect most types of human cells and even cells of other species. The virus generally causes lytic infections of fibroblasts and epithelial cells and latent infections of neurons (see Fig. 6–14 for diagram).

HSV-1 binds initially to heparan sulfate, a proteoglycan found on the outside of many cell types, and then interacts with a receptor protein at the cell surface. HveC (herpes virus entry mediator C) is a member of the immunoglobulin protein family similar to the polio virus receptor, and is found on most cells and neurons. The major route by which HSV penetrates the host cell is through fusion at the cell surface membrane. Upon fusion, the virion releases a protein that promotes the initiation of viral gene transcription, a viral-encoded protein kinase, and cytotoxic proteins into the cytoplasm.

The **immediate early gene products** include DNA-binding proteins, which stimulate DNA synthesis and promote the transcription of the early viral genes. During a latent infection of neurons, the only region of the genome to be transcribed generates the **latency-associated transcripts (LATs)**, but these RNAs are not translated into protein. Viral replication does not proceed further until the cell is activated.

The **early proteins** include the DNA-dependent polymerase and a thymidine kinase. As catalytic proteins, relatively few copies of these enzymes are required to promote replication. Other early proteins inhibit the production and initiate the degradation of cellular messenger RNA (mRNA) and DNA. Expres-

Herpesvirus
genomes

Number of
isomeric
forms

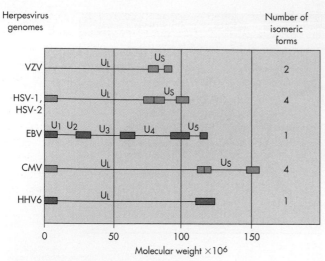

FIGURE 51–2. Herpesvirus genomes. The genomes of the herpesvirus are doubled-stranded DNA. The length and complexity of the genome differ for each virus. Inverted repeats in herpes simplex virus (HSV), varicella-zoster virus (VZV), and cytomegalovirus (CMV) allow the genome to recombine with itself to form isomers. Large genetic repeat sequences are *boxed*. The genomes of HSV and CMV have two sections, the unique long (U_L) and the unique short (U_S), each of which is bracketed by two sets of inverted repeats of DNA. The inverted repeats facilitate the replication of the genome but also allow the U_L and U_S regions to invert independently of each other to yield four different genomic configurations, or isomers. VZV has only one set of inverted repeats and can form two isomers. Epstein-Barr virus (EBV) exists in only one configuration, with several unique regions surrounded by direct repeats. *Purple* indicates direct repeat DNA sequences; *green* indicates inverted repeated DNA sequences. HHV6 = human herpesvirus 6.

sion of the early and late genes generally leads to cell death.

The genome is replicated as soon as the polymerase is synthesized. Circular, end-to-end concatameric forms of the genome are made initially. Later in the infection, the DNA is replicated by a rolling circle mechanism to produce a linear string of genomes that, in concept, resembles a roll of toilet paper. The concatamers cleave into individual genomes as the DNA is sucked into a procapsid.

Genome replication triggers transcription of the late genes by which the structural proteins are encoded. Many copies of these proteins are required. The capsid proteins are then transported to the nucleus, where they are assembled into empty procapsids and filled with DNA. The glycoproteins are synthesized and then receive the high-mannose, *N*-linked glycan precursor in the endoplasmic reticulum. Thereafter, the glycoproteins diffuse to the contiguous nuclear membrane. DNA-containing capsids associate with and bud from

viral glycoprotein-modified portions of the nuclear membrane. Final processing of the viral glycoproteins occurs in the Golgi apparatus. The virus is released by exocytosis or cell lysis. The virus is also spread by cell-cell fusion and through intracellular bridges.

Pathogenesis and Immunity

The mechanisms involved in the pathogenesis of HSV-1 and HSV-2 are very similar (Box 51–2). Both viruses initially infect and replicate in mucoepithelial cells and then establish latent infection of the innervating neurons. HSV generally causes disease at the site of infection. HSV-1 is usually associated with infections above the waist, and HSV-2 with infections below the waist (Fig. 51–3), consistent with the means of spread for these viruses. Other differences between HSV-1 and HSV-2 are those in growth characteristics and antigenicity; also, HSV-2 has a greater potential to cause viremia with the associated systemic "flu"-like symptoms.

HSV can cause **lytic** infections of most cells, persistent infections of lymphocytes and macrophages, and **latent** infection of neurons. Cytolysis generally results from the virus-induced inhibition of cellular macromolecular synthesis, the degradation of host cell DNA, membrane permeation, cytoskeletal disruption, and senescence of the cell. In addition, changes in the nuclear structure and margination of the chromatin occur, and **Cowdry type A acidophilic intranuclear inclusion bodies** are produced. Many strains of HSV also initiate **syncytia** formation. In tissue culture, HSV rapidly kills cells.

HSV initiates infection through mucosal membranes or breaks in the skin. The virus replicates in the cells at the base of the lesion and infects the innervating neuron, traveling by retrograde transport to the ganglion (the trigeminal ganglia for oral HSV and the

---

BOX 51–2. **Disease Mechanisms for Herpes Simplex Viruses**

Disease is initiated by direct contact and depends on infected tissue (e.g., oral, genital, brain).

Virus causes direct cytopathologic effects.

Virus avoids antibody by cell-to-cell spread (syncytia).

Virus establishes latency in neurons (hides from immune response).

Virus is reactivated from latency by stress or immune suppression.

Cell-mediated immunity is *required* for resolution with limited role for antibody.

Cell-mediated immunopathologic effects contribute to symptoms.

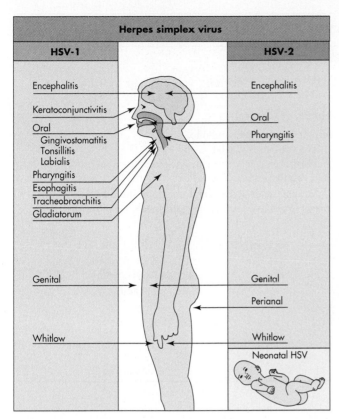

FIGURE 51–3. Disease syndromes of herpes simplex virus (HSV). HSV-1 and HSV-2 can infect the same tissues and cause similar diseases but have a predilection for the sites and diseases indicated.

sacral ganglia for genital HSV). The virus then returns to the initial site of infection and may be inapparent or may produce **vesicular lesions**. The vesicle fluid contains infectious virions. Tissue damage is caused by a combination of viral pathology and immunopathology. The lesion generally heals without producing a scar.

Interferon and natural killer cells may be sufficient to limit the progression of the infection. *T-helper 1 (TH1)-associated delayed-type hypersensitivity and cytotoxic killer T-cell responses are required to kill infected cells and resolve the current disease.* The immunopathologic effects of the cell-mediated and inflammatory responses are also a major cause of the symptoms. Antibody directed against the glycoproteins of the virus neutralizes extracellular virus, limiting its spread. However, the virus can escape such antibody neutralization and clearance by direct cell-to-cell spread and latent infection of the neuron. In addition, the virion and virus-infected cells express antibody (Fc) and complement receptors that weaken these humoral defenses. In the absence of functional cell-mediated immunity, HSV infection is more severe and may disseminate to the vital organs and the brain.

Latent infection occurs in neurons and results in no detectable damage. A **recurrence** can be activated by various stimuli (e.g., stress, trauma, fever, sunlight [ultraviolet B]). In this event, the virus travels back down the nerve, causing lesions to develop at the dermatome and at the same spot each time. The stress triggers reactivation by promoting replication of the virus in the nerve, by transiently depressing cell-mediated immunity, or by inducing both processes. The virus can be reactivated despite the presence of antibody. However, recurrent infections are generally less severe, more localized, and of shorter duration than the primary episodes because of the existence of memory immune responses.

Epidemiology

Because HSV can establish latency with the potential for asymptomatic recurrence, the infected person is a lifelong source of contagion (Box 51–3). As an enveloped virus, HSV is very labile and is readily inactivated by drying, detergents, and the conditions of the gastrointestinal tract. Although HSV can infect animal cells, HSV infection is exclusively a human disease.

HSV is transmitted in vesicle fluid, saliva, and vaginal secretions (the "**mixing and matching of mucous membranes**" [**MMMM**]). Both types of HSV can cause oral and genital lesions. HSV-1 is usually spread by oral contact (kissing) or through the sharing of glasses, toothbrushes, or other saliva-contaminated items. HSV-1 infection of the fingers or body can result from mouth-to-skin contact, with the virus in this case entering through a break in the skin. Autoinoculation may also cause infection of the eyes.

HSV-1 infection is common. More than 90% of people living in underdeveloped areas have the antibody to HSV-1 by 2 years of age. This finding may result from crowded living conditions or poor hygiene.

HSV-2 is spread mainly by sexual contact or autoinoculation or from an infected mother to her infant at birth. Depending on a person's sexual practices and hygiene, HSV-2 may infect the genitalia, anorectal tissues, or oropharynx. The virus may then cause symptomatic or asymptomatic primary infection or recurrences. Neonatal infection usually results from the excretion of HSV-2 from the cervix during vaginal delivery but can occur from an ascending *in utero* infection during a primary infection of the mother. Neonatal infection results in disseminated and neurologic disease with severe consequences.

Initial infection with HSV-2 occurs later in life than infection with HSV-1 and correlates with increased sexual activity. The current statistics indicate that 5 of every 12 adults in the United States are infected with HSV-2, amounting to approximately 45 million individuals with up to 1 million newly infected people per year.

BOX 51–3. Epidemiology of Herpes Simplex Virus (HSV)

Disease/Viral Factors

Virus causes lifelong infection.

  Recurrent disease is source of contagion.

  Virus may cause asymptomatic shedding.

Transmission

Virus is transmitted in saliva, in vaginal secretions, and by contact with lesion fluid (mixing and matching of mucous membranes).

  Virus is transmitted orally and sexually and by placement into eyes and breaks in skin.

  HSV-1 is generally transmitted orally; HSV-2 is generally transmitted sexually.

Who Is at Risk?

Children and sexually active people: at risk for classic presentations of HSV-1 and HSV-2, respectively.

  Physicians, nurses, dentists, and others in contact with oral and genital secretions: at risk for infections of fingers (herpetic whitlow).

  Immunocompromised people and neonates: at risk for disseminated, life-threatening disease.

Geography/Season

Virus is found worldwide.

  There is no seasonal incidence.

Modes of Control

Antiviral drugs are available.

  No vaccine is available.

  Health care workers should wear gloves to prevent herpetic whitlow.

  Patients with active genital lesions should refrain from intercourse until lesions are completely reepithelialized.

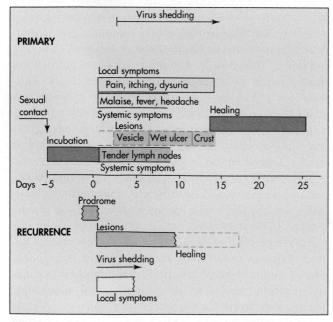

FIGURE 51–4. Clinical course of genital herpes infection. The time course and symptoms of primary and recurrent genital infection with herpes simplex virus type 2 (HSV-2) are compared. *Top,* Primary infection. *Bottom,* Recurrent disease. (Data from Corey L et al: Genital herpes simplex virus infections: clinical manifestations, course, and complications. *Ann Intern Med* 98:958–973, 1983.)

HSV-2 is seroepidemiologically associated with human cervical cancer, possibly as a co-factor with human papillomavirus or another infectious agent. Partial inactivation of the HSV-2 genome with ultraviolet light allows the virus to immortalize cells in tissue culture.

Clinical Syndromes

HSV-1 and HSV-2 are common human pathogens that can cause painful but benign manifestations and recurrent disease. In the classic manifestation, the lesion is a clear vesicle on an erythematous base ("dewdrop on a rose petal") and then progresses to pustular lesions, ulcers, and crusted lesions (Fig. 51–4). However, **both viruses can cause significant morbidity and mortality on infection of the eye or brain and on disseminated infection in an immunosuppressed person or a neonate.**

Oral herpes can be caused by HSV-1 or HSV-2. Primary herpetic gingivostomatitis in toddlers and children is almost always caused by HSV-1, whereas young adults may be infected with HSV-1 or HSV-2. The lesions begin as clear vesicles that rapidly ulcerate. These whitish areas may be widely distributed throughout the mouth, involving the palate, pharynx, gingivae, buccal mucosa, and tongue (Fig. 51–5).

People may experience recurrent mucocutaneous HSV infection (**cold sores, fever blisters**) (Fig. 51–6) even though they never had clinically apparent primary infection. The lesions usually occur at the corners of

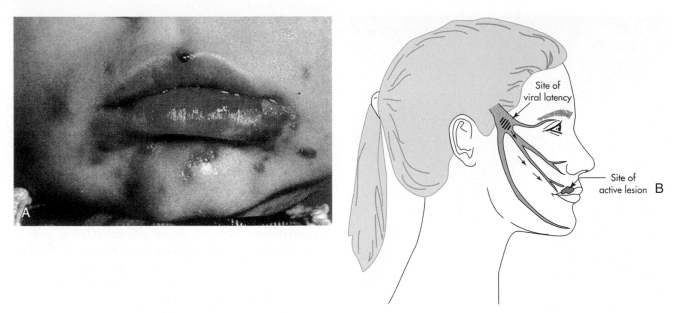

FIGURE 51–5. *A,* Primary herpes gingivostomatitis. *B,* Herpes simplex virus estab-
lishes latent infection and can recur from the trigeminal ganglia. (*A* from Hart CA,
Broadhead RL: *A color atlas of pediatric infectious diseases,* London, 1992, Wolfe;
B modified from Straus SE: Herpes simplex virus and its relatives. In Schaechter
M, Eisenstein BI, Medoff G, editors: *Mechanisms of microbial disease,* ed 2,
Baltimore, 1993, Williams & Wilkins.)

the mouth or next to the lips. The virus is generally
activated from the trigeminal ganglia. As noted earlier,
the symptoms of a recurrent episode are less severe,
more localized, and of shorter duration than those of a
primary episode. **Herpes pharyngitis** is becoming a
prevalent diagnosis in young adults with sore throats.
Severe HSV stomatitis, resembling a primary gingivo-

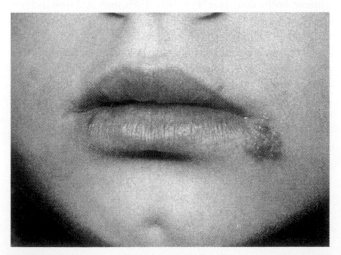

FIGURE 51–6. Cold sore of recurrent herpes labialis. It is
less severe than that of primary disease. (From Hart CA,
Broadhead RL: *A color atlas of pediatric infectious diseases,* London, 1992, Wolfe.)

stomatitis, may occur in patients who are immunosuppressed.

Herpetic keratitis is almost always limited to one
eye. It can cause recurrent disease, leading to permanent scarring, corneal damage, and blindness.

Herpetic whitlow is an infection of the finger, and
herpes gladiatorum is an infection of the body. The
virus establishes infection through cuts or abrasions in
the skin. Herpetic whitlow often occurs in nurses or
physicians who attend patients with HSV infections, in
thumb-sucking children (Fig. 51–7), and in people
who have genital HSV infections. Herpes gladiatorum
is often acquired during wrestling or rugby.

Eczema herpeticum is acquired by children with
active eczema. The underlying disease promotes the
spread of the infection along the skin and potentially
to the adrenal glands, liver, and other organs.

Genital herpes is usually caused by HSV-2 but can
also be caused by HSV-1 (responsible for 10% of genital infections). Most primary genital infections are
asymptomatic. When present, the lesions vary in number and are usually painful. In male patients, the lesions typically develop on the glans or shaft of the
penis and occasionally in the urethra. In female patients, the lesions may be seen on the vulva, vagina,
cervix, perianal area, or inner thigh and are frequently
accompanied by itching and a mucoid vaginal discharge. In patients of both sexes, a primary infection
may be accompanied by fever, malaise, myalgia, and

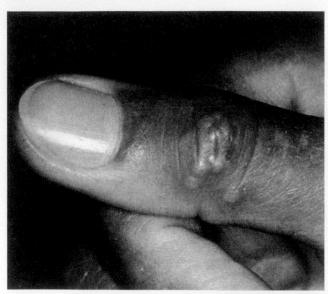

FIGURE 51-7. Herpetic whitlow. (From Emond RTD, Rowland HAK: *A color atlas of infectious diseases,* ed 3, London, 1995, Mosby.)

inguinal adenitis, which are symptoms related to a transient viremia. HSV proctitis is a painful disease in which the lesions are found in the lower rectum and anus. The symptoms and time course of primary and recurrent genital herpes are compared in Figure 51-4.

Recurrent genital HSV disease is shorter in duration and less severe than the primary episode. In approximately 50% of patients, recurrences are preceded by a characteristic prodrome of burning or tingling in the area in which the lesions eventually erupt. Episodes of recurrence may be as frequent as every 2 to 3 weeks or may be infrequent. Unfortunately, any infected person may shed virus asymptomatically. Such individuals may be important vectors for spread of this virus.

Herpes encephalitis is an acute febrile disease that is usually caused by HSV-1. The lesions are generally limited to one of the temporal lobes. The viral pathology and immunopathology cause the destruction of the temporal lobe and give rise to erythrocytes in the cerebrospinal fluid, seizures, focal neurologic abnormalities, and other characteristics of viral encephalitis. HSV is the most common viral cause of sporadic encephalitis and engenders significant morbidity and mortality even in patients who receive appropriate treatment. The disease occurs at all ages and at any time of the year. **HSV meningitis** is most often a complication of genital HSV-2 infection, and symptoms resolve on their own.

HSV infection in the neonate is a devastating and usually fatal disease caused most often by HSV-2. It may be acquired in utero but more commonly is contracted either during passage of the infant through the genital canal because the mother is shedding herpesvi-

rus at the time of delivery or postnatally from family members or hospital personnel. Because cell-mediated immune response is not yet developed in the neonate, HSV disseminates to the liver, lung, and other organs as well as to the central nervous system. The baby initially appears septic, and vesicular lesions may be present. Progression of the infection to the CNS results in death, mental retardation, or neurologic disability, even with treatment.

Laboratory Diagnosis

Cytology and Histology

Characteristic cytopathologic effects (CPEs) can be identified in a **Tzanck smear** (a scraping of the base of a lesion), Papanicolaou smear, or biopsy specimen (Table 51-2). Brain biopsy provides a definitive diagnosis for herpes encephalitis. CPEs include syncytia, "ballooning" cytoplasm, and Cowdry type A intranuclear inclusions (see Fig. 48-2). A definitive diagnosis can be made by demonstrating viral antigen (using immunofluorescence or the immunoperoxidase method) or DNA (using in situ hybridization or polymerase chain reaction [PCR]) in the tissue or vesicle fluid.

Virus Isolation

Virus isolation is the most definitive assay for the diagnosis of HSV infection. Virus can be obtained from vesicles but not crusted lesions. Specimens are collected by aspiration of the lesion fluid or by application of a cotton swab to the vesicles and direct inoculation of the sample into cell cultures.

HSV produces CPEs within 1 to 3 days in HeLa cells, HEp-2 cells, human embryonic fibroblasts, and rabbit kidney cells. Infected cells become enlarged and appear ballooned (see Fig. 48-4). Some isolates induce fusion of neighboring cells, giving rise to multinucleated giant cells (syncytia). A new, sensitive approach to isolation and identification uses a cell line that expresses β-galactosidase upon HSV infection (enzyme-linked viral inducible system [ELVIS]). Addition of a chromophoric substrate allows detection of enzyme in the infected cells.

HSV isolates can be typed by biochemical, biologic, nucleic acid, or immunologic methods. The restriction endonuclease cleavage patterns of the DNA of HSV-1 and HSV-2 are unique and allow unequivocal typing of the isolates. HSV type-specific DNA probes, specific DNA primers for PCR and antibodies are also available for detecting and differentiating HSV-1 and HSV-2.

Serology

Serologic procedures are useful only for diagnosing a primary HSV infection and for epidemiologic studies.

TABLE 51–2. Laboratory Diagnosis of Herpes Simplex Virus (HSV) Infections

Approach	Test/Comment
Direct microscopic examination of cells from base of lesion	**Tzanck smear** shows **multinucleated giant cells** and **Cowdry type A inclusion bodies.**
Cell culture	HSV replicates and causes identifiable cytopathologic effect in most cell cultures.
Assay of tissue biopsy, smear, or vesicular fluid for HSV antigen	Enzyme immunoassay, immunofluorescent stain, in situ DNA probe analysis, and polymerase chain reaction (PCR).
HSV type distinction (HSV-1 vs. HSV-2)	Type-specific antibody, DNA maps of restriction enzyme fragments, sodium dodecyl sulfate–gel protein patterns, DNA probe analysis, and PCR.
Serology	Serology is not useful except for epidemiology.

They are not useful for diagnosing recurrent disease because a significant rise in antibody titers does not usually accompany recurrent disease.

Treatment, Prevention, and Control

HSV encodes several target enzymes for antiviral drugs (Box 51–4) (see Chapter 47). Most antiherpes drugs are nucleotide analogues and other inhibitors of the viral DNA polymerase, an enzyme essential for viral replication and the best antiviral drug target. Treatment prevents or shortens the course of primary or recurrent disease. None of the drug treatments can eliminate latent infection.

The prototype FDA-approved anti-HSV drug is **acyclovir (ACV)**. **Valacyclovir** (the valyl ester of ACV), **penciclovir,** and **famciclovir** (a derivative of penciclovir) are related to ACV in their mechanisms of action but have different pharmacologic properties. Vidarabine (adenosine arabinoside [Ara A]), idoxuridine (iododeoxyuridine), and trifluridine, also FDA-approved for treatment of HSV, are less effective.

ACV is the most-prescribed anti-HSV drug. Phosphorylation of ACV and penciclovir by the viral **thymidine kinase** activates the drug as a substrate for the viral **DNA polymerase**. These drugs are then incorporated into and **prevent the elongation of the viral DNA** (see Fig. 47–2). These drugs (1) are relatively nontoxic, (2) are effective in treating serious presentations of HSV disease and first episodes of genital herpes, and (3) are also used for prophylactic treatment.

The most prevalent form of resistance to these

BOX 51–4. Antiviral Treatments Approved by the U.S. Food and Drug Administration for Herpesvirus Infections

Herpes Simplex 1 and 2
Acyclovir
Penciclovir
Valacyclovir
Famciclovir
Adenosine arabinoside
Iododeoxyuridine
Trifluridine

Varicella-Zoster Virus
Acyclovir
Famciclovir
Valacyclovir
Varicella-zoster immune globulin (VZIG)
Zoster immune plasma (ZIP)
Live vaccine

Epstein-Barr Virus
None

Cytomegalovirus
Ganciclovir*
Foscarnet*

* Also inhibits herpes simplex and varicella-zoster viruses.

drugs results from mutations that inactivate the thymidine kinase, thereby preventing conversion of the drug to its active form. Mutation of the viral DNA polymerase also produces resistance. Fortunately, resistant strains appear to be less virulent.

Ara A is less soluble, less potent, and more toxic than ACV. Trifluridine, penciclovir, and ACV have replaced iododeoxyuridine as topical agents for the treatment of herpetic keratitis. Tromantadine, an amantadine derivative, is approved for topical use in countries other than the United States. It works by inhibiting penetration and syncytia formation. Various nonprescription treatments may be effective for specific individuals.

HSV-1 is transmitted most often from an active mucocutaneous lesion, so avoidance of direct contact with lesions reduces the risk of infection. Unfortunately, the symptoms may be inapparent, and thus, the virus can be transmitted unknowingly. Physicians, nurses, dentists, and technicians must be especially careful when handling potentially infected tissue or fluids. The wearing of gloves can prevent the acquisition of infections of the fingers (herpetic whitlow). People with recurrent herpetic whitlow disease are very contagious and can spread the infection to patients. The virus is readily disinfected by washing with soap.

Patients who have a history of genital HSV infection must be instructed to refrain from sexual intercourse while they have prodromal symptoms or lesions and to resume sexual intercourse only after lesions are completely reepithelialized because virus may be transmitted from lesions that have crusted over. Condoms may be useful and are undoubtedly better than nothing but may not be fully protective.

A pregnant woman who has active genital HSV infection or who is asymptomatically shedding the virus in the vagina at term may transmit HSV to the neonate if the infant is delivered vaginally. Such transmission can be prevented by cesarean section.

No vaccine is currently available for HSV. However, killed, subunit, vaccinia hybrid, and DNA vaccines are being developed to prevent acquisition of the virus or to treat infected people. The glycoprotein D is being utilized in several subunit vaccines. Disabled infectious single-cycle (DISC) vaccines are being developed that utilize live, defective mutant viruses lacking essential genes. Upon administration, the vaccine virus produces noninfectious virions.

Varicella-Zoster Virus

VZV causes **chickenpox (varicella)** and, with recurrence, causes herpes **zoster, or shingles**. VZV shares many characteristics with HSV, including (1) the ability to establish latent infection of neurons and recurrent disease, (2) the importance of cell-mediated immunity in controlling and preventing serious disease, and (3) the characteristic blister-like lesions. Like HSV, VZV encodes a **thymidine kinase** and is susceptible to **antiviral drugs**. Unlike HSV, VZV is spread predominantly by the **respiratory route**. Viremia occurs after local replication of the virus in the respiratory tract, leading to the formation of skin lesions over the entire body.

Structure and Replication

VZV has the smallest genome of the human herpesviruses. VZV replicates slower and in fewer types of cells than HSV. Human diploid fibroblasts in vitro and epithelial and epidermal cells in vivo support productive VZV replication. VZV establishes a latent infection of neurons, like HSV.

Pathogenesis and Immunity

Primary VZV infection begins in the mucosa of the respiratory tract and then progresses via the blood stream and lymphatic system to the cells of the reticuloendothelial system (Box 51–5 and Figs. 51–8 and 51–9). A secondary viremia occurs after 11 to 13 days and spreads the virus throughout the body and to the skin. The virus causes a dermal vesiculopustular rash that develops in successive crops. Fever and systemic symptoms occur with the rash.

The virus becomes latent in the dorsal root or cranial nerve ganglia after the primary infection. The virus can be reactivated in older adults or in patients with impaired cellular immunity. On reactivation, the

---

BOX 51–5. Disease Mechanisms of Varicella-Zoster Virus (VZV)

Initial replication is in the respiratory tract.

VZV infects epithelial cells and fibroblasts.

VZV can form syncytia and spread directly from cell to cell.

Virus is spread by viremia to skin and causes lesions in successive crops.

VZV can escape antibody clearance, and cell-mediated immune response is essential to control infection. Disseminated, life-threatening disease can occur in immunocompromised people.

Virus establishes latent infection of neurons, usually dorsal root and cranial nerve ganglia.

Herpes zoster is a recurrent disease; it results from virus replication along the entire dermatome.

Herpes zoster may result from depression of cell-mediated immunity and other mechanisms of viral activation.

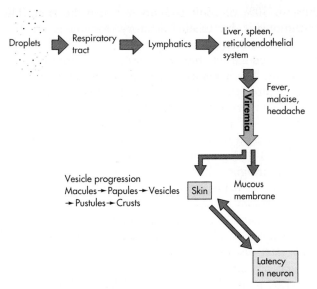

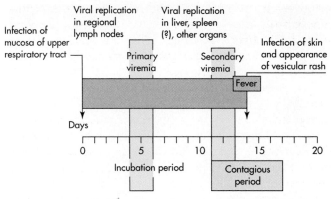

FIGURE 51–8. Mechanism of spread of varicella-zoster virus (VZV) within the body. VZV initially infects the respiratory tract and is spread by the reticuloendothelial system and by viremia to other parts of the body.

FIGURE 51–9. Time course of varicella (chickenpox). The course in young children, as presented in this figure, is generally shorter and less severe than that in adults.

virus replicates and is released along the neural pathways to the skin, causing a vesicular rash along the entire dermatome known as herpes zoster, or shingles.

Antibody is important in limiting the viremic spread of VZV, but cell-mediated immunity is essential for limiting the progression of and resolving the disease. The virus causes more disseminated and more serious disease in the absence of cell-mediated immunity (e.g., in children with leukemia) and may recur on immunosuppression. Waning of the immune response later in life may allow VZV to recur and cause herpes zoster.

Although important for protection, cell-mediated immune responses contribute to the symptomatology. An overzealous response in adults is responsible for causing more extensive cell damage and a more severe manifestation (especially in the lung) in primary infection than that seen in children.

Epidemiology

VZV is extremely communicable, with rates of infection exceeding 90% among susceptible household contacts (Box 51–6). The disease is spread principally by the respiratory route but may also be spread through contact with skin vesicles. Patients are contagious before and during symptoms. More than 90% of adults in developed countries have the VZV antibody. Herpes zoster results from the reactivation of a patient's latent

---

BOX 51–6. Epidemiology of Varicella-Zoster Virus

Disease/Viral Factors

Virus causes lifelong infection.
  Recurrent disease is source of contagion.

Transmission

Virus is transmitted mainly by respiratory droplets but also by direct contact.

Who Is at Risk?

Children (age 5–9): mild classic disease.
  Teens and adults: at risk for more severe disease with potential pneumonia.
  Immunocompromised people and newborns: at risk for life-threatening pneumonia, encephalitis, and progressive-disseminated varicella.
  Elderly and immunocompromised people: at risk for recurrent disease (herpes zoster [shingles]).

Geography/Season

Virus is found worldwide.
  There is no seasonal incidence.

Modes of Control

Antiviral drugs are available.
  Immunity is lifelong.
  Varicella-zoster immunoglobulin is available for immunocompromised people and staff exposed to virus as well as newborns of mothers showing symptoms within 5 days of birth.
  Live vaccine (Oka strain) is available.

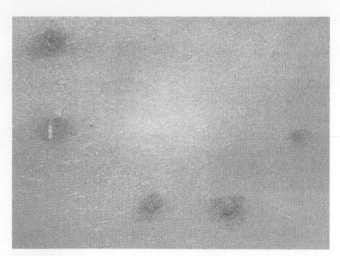

FIGURE 51–10. Characteristic rash of varicella in all stages of its evolution. (From Hart CA, Broadhead RL: *A color atlas of pediatric infectious diseases,* London, 1992, Wolfe.)

virus. The disease develops in approximately 10% to 20% of the population infected with VZV, and the incidence rises with age. Herpes zoster lesions contain viable virus and therefore may be a source of varicella infection in a nonimmune person (child).

Clinical Syndromes

Varicella (**chickenpox**) is one of the five **classic childhood exanthems** (along with rubella, roseola, fifth disease, and measles). The disease results from a primary infection with VZV; it is usually a mild disease of childhood and is normally symptomatic, although asymptomatic infection may occur (see Fig. 51–9). Varicella is characterized by fever and a maculopapular rash that appear after an incubation period of about 14 days (Fig. 51–10). Within hours, each maculopapular lesion forms a thin-walled vesicle on an erythematous base ("dewdrop on a rose petal") that measures approximately 2 to 4 mm in diameter. This vesicle is the hallmark of varicella. Within 12 hours, the vesicle becomes pustular and begins to crust, after which scabbed lesions appear. Successive crops of lesions appear for 3 to 5 days, and at any given time, all stages of skin lesions can be observed.

The rash is generalized, is more severe on the trunk than on the extremities, and is notably present on the scalp, to distinguish it from many other diseases. The lesions itch and cause scratching, which may lead to bacterial superinfection and scarring. Lesions on the mucous membrane typically occur in the mouth, conjunctivae, and vagina.

Primary infection is usually more severe in adults than in children. **Interstitial pneumonia** may occur in 20% to 30% of adult patients and may be fatal. The pneumonia is due to inflammatory reactions at the primary site of infection.

As noted earlier, **herpes zoster** (*zoster* means "belt" or "girdle") is a recurrence of a latent varicella infection acquired earlier in the patient's life. Severe pain in the area innervated by the nerve usually precedes the appearance of the chickenpox-like lesions. The rash is usually limited to a dermatome and resembles varicella (Fig. 51–11). A chronic pain syndrome called **postherpetic neuralgia**, which can persist for months to years, occurs in as many as 30% of patients older than 65 years in whom herpes zoster develops.

VZV infection in immunocompromised patients or neonates can result in serious, progressive, and potentially fatal disease. Defects of cell-mediated immunity in such patients increase the risk for dissemination of the virus to the lungs, brain, and liver, which may be fatal. The disease may occur in response to a primary exposure to varicella or because of recurrent disease.

Laboratory Diagnosis

Cytology

The CPEs in VZV-infected cells are similar to those seen in HSV-infected cells and include Cowdry type A intranuclear inclusions and syncytia. These cells may be seen in skin lesions, respiratory specimens, or organ biopsy specimens. Syncytia may also be seen in Tzanck smears of scrapings of a vesicle's base. A direct fluorescent antibody to membrane antigen (FAMA) test can also be used to examine skin lesion scrapings or biopsy specimens for membrane antigens. Antigen detection and PCR are more sensitive than virus isolation as a means of diagnosing VZV infection.

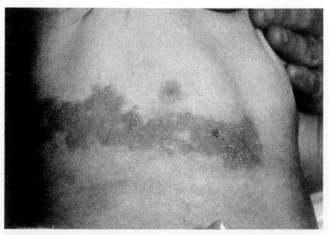

FIGURE 51–11. Herpes zoster ("shingles") in a thoracic dermatome.

Virus Isolation

It is difficult to isolate VZV in cell cultures, because the virus is labile during transport to the laboratory and replicates poorly in vitro. Cultures of material from skin lesions that are crusted over (5 or more days after onset) are usually negative for the virus. Human diploid fibroblasts can support VZV replication and exhibit a CPE similar to that seen in HSV-infected cells, but after a longer incubation period.

Serology

Serologic tests that detect antibodies to VZV are used to screen people for immunity to VZV. However, antibody levels are normally low, so sensitive tests such as immunofluorescence and enzyme-linked immunosorbent assay (ELISA) must be performed to detect the antibody. A significant increase in antibody level can be detected in people experiencing herpes zoster.

Treatment, Prevention, and Control

Treatment may be appropriate for adults and immunocompromised patients with VZV infections and for people with shingles, but no treatment is usually necessary for children with varicella. **ACV, famciclovir,** and **valacyclovir** have been approved for the treatment of VZV infections. The VZV DNA polymerase is much less sensitive to ACV treatment than the HSV enzyme, requiring large doses of ACV or the improved pharmacodynamics of famciclovir and valacyclovir (see Box 51–4).

As with other respiratory viruses, it is difficult to limit the transmission of VZV. Because VZV infection in children is generally mild and induces lifelong immunity, exposure of children to VZV early in life is often encouraged. However, high-risk people (e.g., immunosuppressed children) should be protected from exposure to VZV.

Immunosuppressed patients susceptible to severe disease may be protected from serious disease through the administration of **varicella-zoster immunoglobulin (VZIG)**. VZIG is prepared through the pooling of plasma from seropositive people. It is ineffective, however, as a therapy for patients suffering from active varicella or herpes zoster disease.

A **live attenuated vaccine** for VZV (Oka strain) has been licensed for use in the United States and is administered after 2 years of age, on the same schedule as the measles, mumps, and rubella (MMR) vaccine. The vaccine induces the production of protective antibody and cell-mediated immunity. It is effective as a prophylactic treatment in people even after exposure to VZV. Most significantly, the vaccine promotes protection in immunodeficient children.

Epstein-Barr Virus

EBV has developed into the ultimate B-lymphocyte parasite, and the diseases it causes reflect this association. EBV was discovered through electron-microscopic observation of characteristic herpes virions in biopsy specimens of a B-cell neoplasm, African Burkitt's lymphoma (AfBL). Its association with infectious mononucleosis was discovered accidentally when serum collected from a laboratory technician convalescing from infectious mononucleosis was found to contain the antibody that recognized AfBL cells. This finding was later confirmed in a large serologic study performed on college students.

EBV causes **heterophile antibody-positive infectious mononucleosis** and has been causally associated with **AfBL (endemic Burkitt's lymphoma)**, **Hodgkin's disease**, and **nasopharyngeal carcinoma**. EBV has also been associated with B-cell lymphomas in patients with acquired or congenital immunodeficiencies. **EBV is a mitogen for B cells and immortalizes B cells** in tissue culture.

Structure and Replication

EBV is a member of the Gammaherpesvirinae with a very limited host range and a **tissue tropism** defined by the limited cellular expression of its receptor. This receptor is also **the receptor for the C3d component of the complement system (also called CR2 or CD21)**. It is expressed on B cells of humans and New World monkeys and on some epithelial cells of the oropharynx and nasopharynx. EBV also uses class II major histocompatibility complex (MHC) molecules as a co-receptor.

EBV infection has the following three potential outcomes:

1. EBV can replicate in B cells or epithelial cells permissive for EBV replication.
2. EBV can cause latent infection of B cells in the presence of competent T cells.
3. EBV can stimulate and immortalize B cells. B cells are semipermissive for EBV replication.

EBV encodes more than 70 proteins, different groups of which are expressed for the different types of infections.

Permissive cells allow the transcription and translation of the ZEBRA transcriptional activator protein, which activates the early genes of the virus and the lytic cycle. After synthesis of the DNA polymerase and replication of DNA, the viral capsid and glycoproteins are synthesized. They include gp350/220 (related glycoproteins of 350,000 and 220,000 Da), which is the viral attachment protein, and gp85 (85,000 Da). The viral proteins produced during a productive infection are serologically defined and grouped as **early antigen (EA)**, **viral capsid antigen (VCA)**, and the glycoproteins of the **membrane antigen (MA)** (Table 51–3).

During nonpermissive infection of B cells, the cells contain a small number of circular, plasmid-like EBV genomes that replicate only during cell division. Select immediate early genes are expressed; they include **Epstein-Barr nuclear antigens (EBNAs)** 1, 2, 3A, 3B, and 3C; latent proteins (**LPs**); **latent membrane proteins (LMPs) 1 and 2**; and two small Epstein-Barr–encoded RNA (EBER) molecules, EBER-1 and EBER-2. The EBNAs and LPs are DNA-binding proteins that are essential for establishing and maintaining the infection (EBNA-1), immortalization (EBNA-2), and other purposes. The LMPs are membrane proteins with oncogene-like activity. These proteins stimulate the growth of and immortalize the B cell. EBV establishes latency in memory B cells in which only the EBNA-1 and LMP-2 are expressed, maintaining the genome in the cells but with minimal potential for immune recognition of the infected cell.

Pathogenesis and Immunity

EBV has adapted to the human B cell and manipulates and uses the different phases of B-cell development to establish lifelong infection of the individual and still promote its transmission. The diseases of EBV result from either an overactive immune response (infectious mononucleosis) or the lack of an effective immune response (lymphoma).

The productive infection of B cells and epithelial cells of the oropharynx, such as tonsils (Box 51–7 and Fig. 51–12), promotes virus shedding into saliva to transmit the virus to other hosts and establishes a viremia to spread the virus to other B cells in lymphatic tissue and blood.

EBV acts as a B-cell mitogen. The virus's proteins activate B-cell growth and also prevent apoptosis (programmed cell death). As a result, more B cells contain the EBV genome. In vitro, these actions result in immortalization of the cells and the development of B-lymphoblastoid cell lines as a result of the absence of T cells to control the virus-induced proliferation. In vivo, B-cell proliferation occurs and is indicated by the

TABLE 51–3. Markers of Epstein-Barr Virus (EBV) Infection

Name	Abbreviation	Characteristics	Biologic Association	Clinical Association
EBV nuclear antigens	EBNAs	Nuclear	EBNAs are nonstructural antigens and are the first antigens to appear; EBNAs are seen in all infected and transformed cells, and bind to cell DNA.	Anti-EBNA develops late in infection.
Early antigen	EA-R	Only cytoplasmic	EA-R appears before EA-D; its appearance is first sign that infected cell has entered lytic cycle.	Anti–EA-R is seen in Burkitt's lymphoma.
	EA-D	Diffuse in cytoplasm and nucleus	—	Anti–EA-D is seen in infectious mononucleosis.
Viral capsid antigen	VCA	Cytoplasmic	VCA is a late antigen; it is found in virus producer cells.	Anti-VCA immunoglobulin M is transient; anti-VCA immunoglobulin G is persistent.
Lymphocyte-defined membrane antigen	LYDMA	—	LYDMA is not found on Burkitt's lymphoma cells; it is found on cells infected in vitro and on nonproducer cells.	LYDMA is not detectable by antibody.
Membrane antigen	MA	Cell surface	MAs are the envelope glycoproteins.	Same as VCA.
Heterophile antibody		Recognition of Paul-Bunnell antigen on sheep, horse, or bovine erythrocytes	EBV-induced B-cell proliferation promotes production of heterophile antibody.	Early symptom occurs in more than 50% of patients.

BOX 51−7. Disease Mechanisms of Epstein-Barr Virus

Virus in saliva initiates infection of oral epithelia and spreads to B cells in lymphatic tissue.

There is productive infection of epithelial and B cells.

Virus promotes growth of B cells (immortalizes).

T cells kill and limit B-cell outgrowth and promote latency in B cells. T cells are *required for controlling infection*. Antibody role is limited.

T-cell response (lymphocytosis) contributes to symptoms of **infectious mononucleosis.**

There is causative association with lymphoma in immunosuppressed people and African children living in malarial regions (African Burkitt's lymphoma) and with nasopharyngeal carcinoma in China.

spurious production of an IgM antibody to the Paul-Bunnell antigen, termed the heterophile antibody (see later discussion of serology). The B-cell proliferation is usually controlled by T cells, but continued B-cell proliferation in conjunction with the effects of other co-factors may result in the development of lymphoma.

During productive infection, antibody is first developed against the components of the virion, VCA and MA, and later against the EA. After resolution of the infection (lysis of the productively infected cells), anti-body against the nuclear antigens (EBNAs) is produced. T cells are essential for limiting the proliferation of EBV-infected B cells and controlling the disease (Fig. 51−13). The T cells respond to viral antigenic peptides and B-cell markers of proliferation. EBV counteracts some of the protective action of TH1 CD4 T-cell responses by producing an interleukin-10 analogue (BCRF-1) during productive infection that inhibits the protective TH1 CD4 T-cell responses and also stimulates B-cell growth.

Infectious mononucleosis results from a "civil war" between the EBV-infected B cells and the protective T cells. The classic **lymphocytosis** (increase in mononuclear cells) associated with infectious mononucleosis results mainly from the activation and proliferation of T cells. These appear as **atypical lymphocytes** (also called **Downey cells**) (Fig. 51−14). They increase in number in the peripheral blood during the second week of infection, accounting for 10% to 80% of the total white blood cell count at this time. The large T-cell response causes the swelling of lymph glands, spleen, and liver that appears later in the disease. Children have a less active immune response to EBV infection and therefore have very mild disease.

On resolution of active disease, the virus persists in approximately 1 memory B cell per milliliter of blood for the person's life. EBV may be reactivated when the memory B cell is activated (especially in the tonsils or oropharynx) and may be shed in saliva.

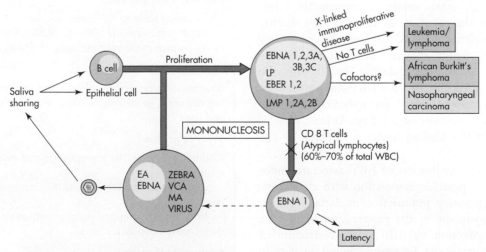

FIGURE 51−12. Progression of Epstein-Barr virus (EBV) infection. Infection may result in lytic, latent, or immortalizing infection, which can be distinguished on the basis of production of virus and expression of different viral proteins and antigens. T cells limit the outgrowth of the EBV-infected cells and maintain the latent infection. EA = early antigen; EBER = Epstein-Barr–encoded RNA; EBNA = Epstein-Barr nuclear antigen; LMP = latent membrane protein; LP = latent protein; MA = membrane antigen; VCA = viral capsid antigen; ZEBRA = peptide encoded by the Z gene region.

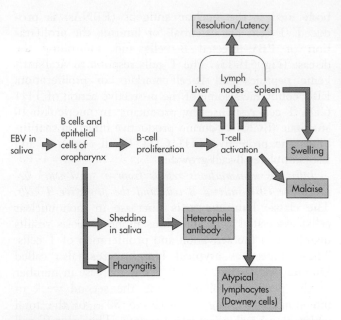

FIGURE 51–13. Pathogenesis of Epstein-Barr virus (EBV). EBV is acquired by close contact between persons through saliva and infects the B cells. The resolution of the EBV infection and many of the symptoms of infectious mononucleosis result from the activation of T cells in response to the infection.

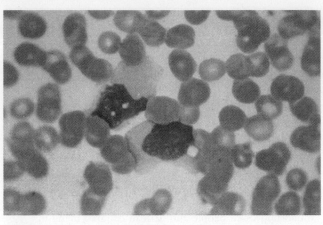

FIGURE 51–14. Atypical T-cell (Downey cell) characteristic of infectious mononucleosis. The cells have a more basophilic and vacuolated cytoplasm than normal lymphocytes, and the nucleus may be oval, kidney-shaped, or lobulated. The cell margin may seem to be indented by neighboring red blood cells.

may appear as polyclonal and monoclonal B-cell lymphomas. Such people are also at high risk for a productive infection in the form of **hairy oral leukoplakia**.

Epidemiology

EBV is transmitted in saliva (Box 51–8). More than 90% of EBV-infected people intermittently shed the virus for life, even when totally asymptomatic. Children can acquire the virus at an early age by sharing contaminated drinking glasses. *Children generally have subclinical disease.* Saliva sharing between adolescents and young adults often occurs during kissing; thus, the nickname "the kissing disease" for EBV mononucleosis. Disease in these people may go unnoticed or may manifest in varying degrees of severity. At least 70% of the population of the United States is infected by age 30.

The geographic distribution of EBV-associated neoplasms indicates a possible association with co-factors. The immunosuppressive potential of malaria has been suggested as a co-factor in the progression of chronic or latent EBV infection to AfBL. The restriction of nasopharyngeal carcinoma to people living in certain regions of China indicates a possible genetic predisposition to the cancer or the presence of co-factors in the food or environment.

Transplant recipients, patients with the acquired immunodeficiency syndrome (AIDS), and genetically immunodeficient people are at high risk for lymphoproliferative disorders initiated by EBV. These disorders

---

BOX 51–8. **Epidemiology of Epstein-Barr Virus**

Disease/Viral Factors

Virus causes lifelong infection.
  Recurrent disease is cause of contagion.
  Virus may cause asymptomatic shedding.

Transmission

Transmission occurs via saliva, close oral contact ("kissing disease"), or sharing of items such as toothbrushes and cups.

Who Is at Risk?

Children, who may be asymptomatic or may have mild symptoms.
  Teenagers and adults: at risk for infectious mononucleosis.
  Immunocompromised people: at highest risk for life-threatening neoplastic disease.

Geography/Season

Infectious mononucleosis has worldwide distribution.
  There is causative association with African Burkitt's lymphoma in malarial belt of Africa.
  There is no seasonal incidence.

Modes of Control

There are no modes of control.

Clinical Syndromes

Heterophile Antibody-Positive Infectious Mononucleosis

Like infections caused by other herpesviruses, EBV infection in a child is much milder than infection in an adolescent or adult. In fact, infection in children is usually subclinical. Infectious mononucleosis is characterized by high fever, malaise, pharyngitis, lymphadenopathy (swollen glands), and, often, hepatosplenomegaly. A rash may occur, especially after ampicillin treatment. The major complaint of people with infectious mononucleosis is fatigue (Fig. 51–15). The disease is rarely fatal in healthy people but can cause serious complications resulting from neurologic disorders, laryngeal obstruction, or rupture of the spleen. Neurologic complications include meningoencephalitis and the Guillain-Barré syndrome. Heterophile-negative "mononucleosis" may be caused by CMV if the patient is 25 years or older.

Chronic Disease

EBV can cause cyclic recurrent disease in some people. These patients experience chronic tiredness and may also have low-grade fever, headaches, and sore throat. This disorder is different from chronic fatigue syndrome, which has another etiology.

Epstein-Barr Virus–Induced Lymphoproliferative Diseases

On infection with EBV, people lacking T-cell immunity are likely to suffer life-threatening polyclonal leukemia-like B-cell proliferative disease and lymphoma instead of infectious mononucleosis. People with congenital deficiencies of T-cell function are likely to suffer life-threatening X-linked lymphoproliferative disease. One such X-linked genetic defect in a T-cell gene (SLAM [signaling lymphocyte activation molecule]–associated protein) prevents the T cell from controlling B-cell growth, induced by antigen or EBV. Transplant recipients undergoing immunosuppressive treatment are at high risk for **post-transplant lymphoproliferative** disease instead of infectious mononucleosis after exposure to the virus or on reactivation of latent virus. Similar diseases are seen in patients with AIDS.

African Burkitt's lymphoma (endemic lymphoma) is a poorly differentiated monoclonal B-cell lymphoma of the jaw and face that is endemic in children living in the malarial regions of Africa. The tumors contain EBV DNA sequences but express only the EBNA-1 viral antigen. Virions can occasionally be seen on electron micrographs of infected material. In addition to EBV DNA, the tumor cells contain chromosomal translocations that juxtapose the *C-myc* oncogene to a very active promoter such as an immunoglobulin gene promoter [t(8;14), t(8;22), t(8;2)]. The tumor cells are also relatively invisible to immune control. It is not known how malaria acts to promote EBV involvement with AfBL. EBV is also associated with Burkitt's lymphomas in people living in other parts of the world but to a much smaller extent. Many **Hodgkin's lymphomas** can also be attributed to EBV.

As noted earlier, **nasopharyngeal carcinoma** is endemic in Asia, occurs in adults, and contains EBV DNA within the tumor cells. Unlike Burkitt's lymphoma, in which the tumor cells are derived from lymphocytes, the tumor cells of nasopharyngeal carcinoma are of epithelial origin.

Hairy Oral Leukoplakia

Hairy oral leukoplakia is an unusual manifestation of a productive EBV infection of epithelial cells characterized by lesions of the mouth. It is an opportunistic manifestation that occurs in patients with AIDS.

Laboratory Diagnosis

EBV-induced infectious mononucleosis is diagnosed on the basis of the symptoms, the finding of atypical lym-

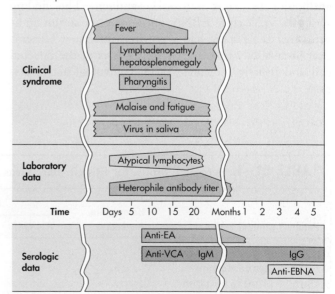

FIGURE 51–15. Clinical course of infectious mononucleosis and laboratory findings of those with the infection. Epstein-Barr virus (EBV) infection may be asymptomatic or may produce the symptoms of mononucleosis. The incubation period can last as long as 2 months. EA = Early antigen; VCA = viral capsid antigen.

phocytes, and the presence of **lymphocytosis** (mononuclear cells constituting 60% to 70% of the white blood cell count with 30% atypical lymphocytes), heterophile antibody, and antibody to viral antigens. Virus isolation is not practical. DNA probe analysis and immunofluorescent identification of viral antigens are used to detect evidence of infection.

Atypical lymphocytes are probably the earliest detectable indication of an EBV infection. These cells appear with the onset of symptoms and disappear with resolution of the disease.

Heterophile antibody results from the nonspecific, mitogen-like activation of B cells by EBV and the production of a wide repertoire of antibodies. These antibodies include an IgM heterophile antibody that recognizes the Paul-Bunnell antigen on sheep, horse, and bovine erythrocytes but not that on guinea pig kidney cells. The heterophile antibody response can usually be detected by the end of the first week of illness and lasts for as long as several months. It is an excellent indication of EBV infection in adults but is not as reliable in children or infants. The horse cell (Monospot) test and ELISA are rapid and widely used for the detection of the heterophile antibody.

Serologic tests for antibody to viral antigens are useful to confirm the diagnosis and when the results of heterophile antibody tests are questionable (see Fig. 51–15; Table 51–4). EBV infection is indicated by the finding of any of the following: (1) IgM antibody to the VCA, (2) the presence of VCA antibody and the absence of EBNA antibody, or (3) elevation of antibodies to VCA and early antigen. The finding of both VCA and EBNA antibodies in serum indicates that the person had a previous infection. Generation of antibody to EBNA requires lysis of the infected cell and usually indicates T-cell control of active disease.

Treatment, Prevention, and Control

No effective treatment or vaccine is available for EBV disease (see Box 51–4). The ubiquitous nature of the virus and the potential for asymptomatic shedding make control of infection difficult. However, infection elicits lifelong immunity. Therefore, the best means of preventing infectious mononucleosis is exposure to the virus early in life, because the disease is more benign in children.

Cytomegalovirus

CMV is a common human pathogen, infecting 0.5% to 2.5% of all newborns and approximately 50% of the adult population in developed countries. It is the most common viral cause of **congenital defects**. CMV becomes particularly important as an **opportunistic pathogen in immunocompromised patients**.

Structure and Replication

CMV is a member of the Betaherpesvirinae and is considered lymphotropic. It has the largest genome of the human herpesviruses. In contrast to the traditional definition of *virus*, which states that a virion particle contains DNA or RNA, studies now indicate that CMV carries mRNA into the cell in the virion particle to facilitate infection. Human CMV replicates only in human cells. Fibroblasts, epithelial cells, macrophages, and other cells are permissive for CMV replication. CMV establishes latent infection in mononuclear lymphocytes, the stromal cells of the bone marrow, and other cells.

Pathogenesis and Immunity

The pathogenesis of CMV is similar to that of other herpesviruses in many respects (Box 51–9). CMV

TABLE 51–4. Serologic Profile for Epstein-Barr Virus (EBV) Infections

Patient's Clinical Status	Heterophile Antibodies	EBV-Specific Antibodies				Comment
		VCA-IgM	VCA-IgG	EA	EBNA	
Susceptible	−	−	−	−	−	—
Acute primary infection	+	+	+	±	−	—
Chronic primary infection	−	−	+	+	−	—
Past infection	−	−	+	−	+	—
Reactivation infection	−	−	+	+	+	EA restricted or diffuse
Burkitt's lymphoma	−	−	+	+	+	EA restricted only
Nasopharyngeal carcinoma	−	−	+	+	+	EA diffuse only

EA = early antigen; EBNA = Epstein-Barr nuclear antigen; Ig = immunoglobulin; VCA = viral capsid antigen.
Modified from Balows A et al, editors: *Laboratory diagnosis of infectious diseases: principles and practices*, New York, 1988, Springer-Verlag.

BOX 51−9. **Disease Mechanisms of Cytomegalovirus (CMV)**

CMV is acquired from blood, tissue, and most body secretions.

CMV causes productive infection of epithelial and other cells.

CMV establishes latency in T cells, macrophages, and other cells.

Cell-mediated immunity is required for resolution and contributes to symptoms. Role of antibody is limited.

Suppression of cell-mediated immunity allows recurrence and severe presentation.

CMV generally causes subclinical infection.

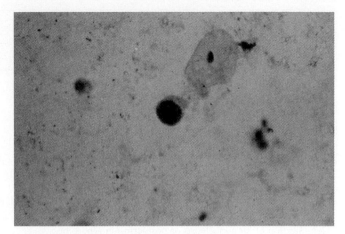

FIGURE 51−16. Cytomegalovirus-infected cell with basophilic nuclear inclusion body.

readily establishes persistent and latent infections, usually without causing definable symptoms, in mononuclear leukocytes and in organs such as the kidneys and heart. The virus is reactivated by immunosuppression (e.g., corticosteroids, infection with human immunodeficiency virus) and possibly by allogeneic stimulation (i.e., the host response to transfused or transplanted cells). Cell-mediated immunity is essential for resolving and controlling the outgrowth of CMV infection.

In most cases, the virus replicates and is shed without causing symptoms (Table 51−5). Replication of CMV in ductal epithelial cells promotes excretion of the virus in most body fluids. CMV is highly cell-associated and is transmitted by infected cells, including lymphocytes and leukocytes (Fig. 51−16). Virus can be transmitted in cells to different organs of the body or to other individuals by means of blood transfusions and organ transplants. Activation and replication of the virus in the kidney and secretory glands promote its secretion in urine and bodily secretions, including semen and milk.

Epidemiology and Clinical Syndromes

CMV can be isolated from urine, blood, throat washings, saliva, tears, breast milk, semen, stool, amniotic

fluid, vaginal and cervical secretions, and tissues obtained for transplantation (Table 51−6 and Box 51−10). The congenital, oral, and sexual routes, blood transfusion, and tissue transplantation are the major means by which CMV is transmitted. CMV disease is an opportunistic disorder, rarely causing symptoms in the immunocompetent host but engendering serious disease in the immunodeficient person, such as a patient with AIDS or a neonate (Fig. 51−17).

Congenital Infection

CMV is the most prevalent viral cause of congenital disease. A significant percentage (0.5% to 2.5%) of all newborns in the United States are infected with CMV at birth, and a large percentage of babies are infected within the first months of life. Approximately 10% of affected newborns (4000 per year) show clinical evidence of disease, such as microcephaly, intracerebral calcification, hepatosplenomegaly, and rash (**cytomegalic inclusion disease**). Unilateral or bilateral hearing loss and mental retardation are common consequences of congenital CMV infection. The risk for serious birth defects is extremely high for infants born to mothers who underwent primary CMV infections during their pregnancies.

Fetuses are infected by virus in the mother's blood (primary infection) or by virus ascending from the cervix (after a recurrence). The symptoms of congenital infection are less severe or can be prevented by the immune response of a seropositive mother. Congenital CMV infection is best documented by isolation of the virus from the infant's urine during the first week of life.

Perinatal Infection

In the United States, as many as 20% of pregnant women harbor CMV in the cervix at term and are

TABLE 51−5. **Sources of Cytomegalovirus Infection**

Age Group	Source
Neonate	Transplacental transmission, intrauterine infections, cervical secretions
Baby or child	Body secretions: breast milk, saliva, tears, urine
Adult	Sexual transmission (semen), blood transfusion, organ graft

TABLE 51–6. Cytomegalovirus Syndromes

Tissue	Children/Adults	Immunosuppressed Patients
Predominant presentation	Asymptomatic	**Disseminated disease, severe disease**
Eyes	—	Chorioretinitis
Lungs	—	Pneumonia, pneumonitis
Gastrointestinal tract	—	Esophagitis, colitis
Nervous system	Polyneuritis, myelitis	Meningitis and encephalitis, myelitis
Lymphoid system	Mononucleosis syndrome, post-transfusion syndrome	Leukopenia, lymphocytosis
Major organs	Carditis,* hepatitis*	Hepatitis
Neonates	**Deafness, mental retardation**	—

* Complication of mononucleosis or postperfusion syndrome.

likely to experience reactivation of the virus during pregnancy. Approximately half the neonates born through an infected cervix acquire CMV infection and become excreters of the virus at 3 to 4 weeks of age. Neonates may also acquire CMV from maternal milk or colostrum. Perinatal infection causes no clinically evident disease in healthy full-term infants.

Another means by which neonates can acquire CMV is through blood transfusions. Of the seronegative babies who are exposed to blood from seropositive donors, 13.5% acquire CMV infection in the immediate postnatal period. Significant clinical infection may occur in premature infants who acquire CMV from transfused blood, pneumonia and hepatitis being the major manifestations.

Infection in Children and Adults

Only 10% to 15% of adolescents are infected with CMV, but this number increases to 50% by 35 years of age. CMV is a **sexually transmitted disease**. It has been isolated from the cervix of 13% to 23% of women at venereal disease clinics, and the titer of the CMV in semen is the highest of that in any body secretion. CMV is more prevalent among people in low socioeconomic brackets living in crowded conditions and in people living in underdeveloped countries.

BOX 51–10. Epidemiology of Cytomegalovirus Infection

Disease/Viral Factors

Virus causes lifelong infection.
   Recurrent disease is source of contagion.
   Virus may cause asymptomatic shedding.

Transmission

Transmission occurs via blood, organ transplants, and all secretions (urine, saliva, semen, cervical secretions, breast milk, and tears).
   Virus is transmitted orally and sexually, in blood transfusions, in tissue transplants, in utero, at birth, and by nursing.

Who Is at Risk?

Babies.
   Babies of mothers who experience seroconversion during term: at high risk for congenital defects.
   Sexually active people.
   Blood and organ recipients.
   Burn patients.
   Immunocompromised people: symptomatic and recurrent disease.

Geography/Season

Virus is found worldwide.
   There is no seasonal incidence.

Modes of Control

Antiviral drugs are available for patients with acquired immunodeficiency syndrome.
   Screening potential blood and organ donors for cytomegalovirus reduces transmission of virus.

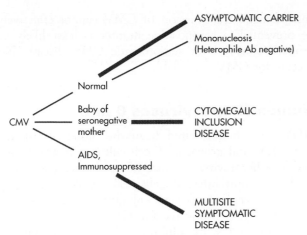

FIGURE 51-17. Outcomes of cytomegalovirus (CMV) infections. The outcome of CMV infection depends very heavily on the immune status of the patient.

Although most CMV infections acquired in young adulthood are asymptomatic, patients may show a **heterophile-negative mononucleosis syndrome**. The symptoms of CMV disease are similar to those of EBV infection but with less severe pharyngitis and lymphadenopathy (see Fig. 51-17). Although CMV infection promotes a T-cell outgrowth (atypical lymphocytosis) similar to that seen in EBV infection, heterophile antibody is not present. Absence of this antibody reflects the differences in the target cell and the action of the viruses on the target cell. CMV disease should be suspected in a patient who has heterophile-negative mononucleosis or in whom there are signs of hepatitis but results of tests for hepatitis A, B, and C are negative.

Transmission via Transfusion and Transplantation

Transmission of CMV by blood most often results in an asymptomatic infection; if symptoms are present, they typically resemble those of mononucleosis. Fever, splenomegaly, and atypical lymphocytosis usually begin 3 to 5 weeks after transfusion. Pneumonia and mild hepatitis may also occur. CMV may also be transmitted by organ transplantation (e.g., kidneys, bone marrow), and CMV infection is often reactivated in transplant recipients during periods of intense immunosuppression.

Infection in the Immunocompromised Host

CMV is a prominent opportunistic infectious agent. In immunocompromised people, it causes symptomatic primary or recurrent disease (see Table 51-6).

CMV disease of the lung (**pneumonia and pneumonitis**) is a common outcome in immunosuppressed patients and can be fatal if not treated. In addition,

CMV often causes **retinitis** in patients who are severely immunodeficient (e.g., in as many as 10% to 15% of patients with AIDS). Interstitial pneumonia and encephalitis may also be caused by CMV but may be difficult to distinguish from infections caused by other opportunistic agents. CMV **colitis or esophagitis** may develop in as many as 10% of patients with AIDS. CMV esophagitis may mimic candidal esophagitis. A smaller percentage of immunocompromised patients may experience CMV infection of the gastrointestinal tract. Patients with CMV colitis usually have diarrhea, weight loss, anorexia, and fever. CMV is also responsible for the **failure of many kidney transplants**.

Laboratory Diagnosis

Histology

The histologic hallmark of CMV infection is the **cytomegalic cell**, which is an **enlarged cell** (25 to 35 mm) that contains a dense, **central, "owl's-eye," basophilic intranuclear inclusion body** (Table 51-7; see Fig. 51-16). Such infected cells may be found in any tissue of the body and in urine and are thought to be epithelial in origin. The inclusions are readily seen with Papanicolaou or hematoxylin-eosin staining.

Immune and DNA Probe Techniques

A rapid, sensitive diagnosis can be obtained by histologic means through the use of antibodies (especially monoclonal), DNA probes, and PCR to directly detect the CMV antigens and the genome in tissues or fluids (see Figure 17-3). Enzyme immunoassay and fluorescence methods detect the probes.

TABLE 51-7. Laboratory Tests for Diagnosing Cytomegalovirus Infection

Test	Finding
Cytology and histology*	"Owl's-eye" inclusion body
	Antigen detection
	In situ DNA probe hybridization
	Polymerase chain reaction (PCR)
Cell culture	Cytologic effect in human diploid fibroblasts
	Immunofluorescence detection of early antigens
	PCR
Serology	Primary infection

*Samples taken for analysis include urine, saliva, blood, bronchoalveolar lavage specimens, and tissue biopsy specimens.

Culture

Culture has generally been regarded as the definitive method for detecting CMV infection. It is especially reliable in immunocompromised patients, who often have high titers of virus in their secretions. For example, in the semen of patients with AIDS, titers of viable virus may be greater than 10^6.

CMV grows only in diploid fibroblast cell cultures and must be maintained for at least 4 to 6 weeks because the characteristic CPE develops very slowly in specimens with very low titers of the virus. More rapid results may be achieved by culture amplification of a specimen. In this procedure, specimens are inoculated by centrifuging in a shell vial seeded with diploid fibroblast cells. Specimens are examined after 1 to 2 days of incubation by indirect immunofluorescence for the presence of either immediate early antigen or a combination of immediate early antigen and early antigen.

Serology

Seroconversion is usually an excellent marker for primary CMV infection. Titers of CMV-specific IgM antibody may be very high in patients with AIDS. However, CMV-specific IgM antibody may also develop during the reactivation of CMV and is therefore not a dependable indicator of primary infection.

Treatment, Prevention, and Control

Ganciclovir (dihydroxypropoxymethyl guanine) and **foscarnet** (phosphonoformic acid) have been approved by the FDA for the treatment of CMV infections and are especially useful for immunosuppressed patients (see Box 51–4). Ganciclovir is structurally similar to ACV; it is phosphorylated and activated by a CMV enzyme, inhibits the viral DNA polymerase, and causes DNA chain termination (see Chapter 47). Ganciclovir is more toxic than ACV. Ganciclovir can be used to treat severe CMV infections in immunocompromised patients. Foscarnet is a simple molecule that inhibits the viral DNA polymerase by mimicking the pyrophosphate portion of nucleotide triphosphates. It has been approved as an alternative to ganciclovir.

CMV is spread mainly by the sexual, tissue transplantation, and transfusion routes, and spread by these means is preventable. Semen is a major vector for the sexual spread of CMV to both heterosexual and homosexual contacts. The use of condoms or abstinence would limit viral spread. Transmission of the virus can also be reduced through the screening of potential blood and organ donors for CMV seronegativity. Screening is especially important for donors of blood transfusions to be given to infants. Although congenital and perinatal transmission of CMV cannot effectively be prevented, a seropositive mother is least likely to produce a baby with symptomatic CMV disease. No vaccine for CMV is available.

Human Herpesviruses 6 and 7

HHV6 was first isolated from the blood of patients with AIDS and grown in T-cell cultures. It was identified as a herpesvirus because of its characteristic morphology within infected cells. Like EBV and CMV, HHV6 is lymphotropic and ubiquitous. At least 45% of people are seropositive for HHV6 by age 2 years, and almost 100% by adulthood. In 1988, HHV6 was serologically associated with a common disease of children, **exanthema subitum**, commonly known as **roseola**.

HHV7 was isolated in a similar manner from the T cells of a patient with AIDS who was also infected with HHV6. However, HHV7 remains an orphan virus with no disease association.

Pathogenesis and Immunity

HHV6 infection occurs very early in life, indicating that it must be shed and spread readily. It is present in the saliva of most adults and is spread by oral secretions.

HHV6 replicates in the salivary glands, the source of virus secreted in saliva. HHV6 establishes a latent infection in T cells and monocytes but may be activated and may replicate upon mitogen stimulation of the cells. Cells in which the virus is replicating appear large and refractile and have occasional intranuclear and intracytoplasmic inclusion bodies. T-cell leukemia cell lines also support replication of the virus. Resting lymphocytes and lymphocytes of normal immune people are resistant to infection.

Like the replication of EBV and CMV, the replication of HHV6 is controlled by cell-mediated immunity. The virus is likely to become activated in patients with AIDS or other lymphoproliferative and immunosuppressive disorders.

Clinical Syndromes

Exanthema subitum, or roseola, is one of the five classic childhood exanthems previously mentioned (Fig. 51–18). It is characterized by the rapid onset of high fever of a few days' duration, which is followed by a generalized rash that lasts only 24 to 48 hours. The presence of infected T cells or the activation of delayed-type hypersensitivity T cells in the skin may be the cause of the rash. The disease is effectively controlled and resolved by cell-mediated immunity, but

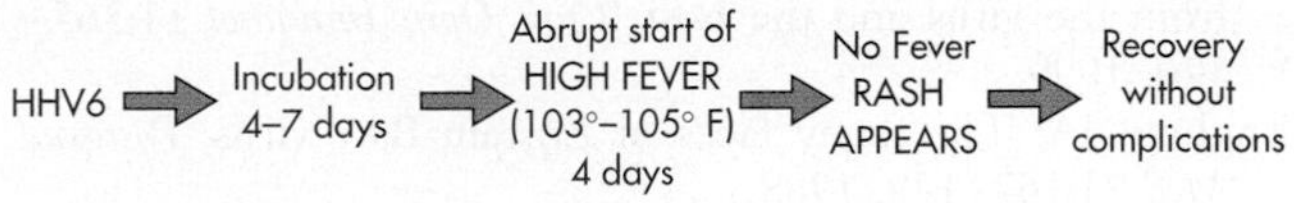

FIGURE 51–18. Time course of symptoms of exanthema subitum (roseola) caused by human herpesvirus 6 (HHV6). Compare these symptoms and this time course with those of fifth disease, which is caused by parvovirus B19 (see Chapter 53).

the virus establishes a lifelong latent infection of T cells.

HHV6 may also cause a mononucleosis syndrome and lymphadenopathy and may be a co-factor in the pathogenesis of AIDS.

Other Human Herpesviruses

Human Herpesvirus 8

HHV8 DNA sequences were discovered in biopsy specimens of **Kaposi's sarcoma**, **primary effusion lymphoma** (a rare type of B-cell lymphoma), **and multicentric Castleman's disease** through the use of PCR analysis. Kaposi's sarcoma is one of the characteristic opportunistic diseases associated with AIDS. Genome sequence analysis showed that the virus was unique and a member of the Gammaherpesvirinae (like EBV). HHV8 infects B cells but also null cells as well as vascular endothelial, perivascular spindle, and other cells.

HHV8 encodes several proteins with homology to human proteins that promote the growth and prevent apoptosis of the infected and surrounding cells. These proteins include an interleukin-6 homologue (growth and antiapoptosis), a Bcl-2 analogue (antiapoptosis), chemokines, and a chemokine receptor. These proteins can promote the growth and development of polyclonal Kaposi's sarcoma cells in patients with AIDS and others. HHV8 DNA is present and is associated with peripheral blood lymphocytes, most likely B cells, in approximately 10% of immunocompetent people. HHV8 is limited to certain geographic areas (Italy, Greece, Africa) and to patients with AIDS. The virus is most likely a sexually transmitted disease but may be spread by other means.

Herpesvirus simiae (B virus) (the simian counterpart of HSV), is indigenous to Asian monkeys. The virus is transmitted to humans by monkey bites or saliva or even by tissues and cells widely used in virology laboratories. Once infected, a human may have pain, localized redness, and vesicles at the site of the virus's entrance. An encephalopathy develops and is frequently fatal; most people who survive have serious brain damage. Virus isolation or serologic tests can be used to establish the diagnosis of B-virus infections.

| CASE STUDY AND QUESTIONS |

■ A 2-year-old child with fever for 2 days has not been eating and has been crying often. On examination, the physician notes that the mucous membranes of the mouth are covered with numerous shallow, pale ulcerations. A few red papules and blisters are also observed around the border of the lips. The symptoms worsen over the next 5 days and then slowly resolve, with complete healing after 2 weeks.

1. The physician suspects that this is an HSV infection. How would the diagnosis be confirmed?
2. How could you determine whether this infection was caused by HSV-1 or HSV-2?
3. What immune responses were most helpful in resolving this infection, and when were they activated?
4. HSV escapes complete immune resolution by causing latent and recurrent infections. What was the site of latency in this child, and what might promote future recurrences?
5. What were the most probable means by which the child was infected with HSV?
6. Which antiviral drugs are available for the treatment of HSV infections? What are their targets? Were they indicated for this child? If not, why not?

■ A 17-year-old high school student has had low-grade fever and malaise for several days, followed by sore throat, swollen cervical lymph nodes, and increasing fatigue. The patient also notes some discomfort in the left upper quadrant of the abdomen. The sore throat, lymphadenopathy, and fever gradually resolve over the next 2 weeks, but the patient's full energy level does not return for another 6 weeks.

1. What laboratory tests would confirm the diagnosis of EBV-induced infectious mononucleosis and distinguish it from CMV infection?
2. To what characteristic diagnostic feature of the disease does *mononucleosis* refer?
3. What causes the swollen glands and fatigue?
4. Who is at greatest risk for a serious outcome of an EBV infection? What is the outcome? Why?

BIBLIOGRAPHY

Belshe RB: *Textbook of human virology*, ed 2, St Louis, 1991, Mosby.

Fields BN, Knipe DM, Howley PM, editors: *Virology*, ed 3, New York, 1996, Lippincott-Raven.

Garcia-Blanco MA, Cullen BR: Molecular basis of latency in pathogenic human viruses, *Science* 254:815–820, 1991.

Gorbach SL, Bartlett JG, Blacklow NR, editors: *Infectious diseases*, ed 2, Philadelphia, 1997, WB Saunders.

Mandell GL, Bennett JE, Dolin R: *Principles and practice of infectious diseases*, ed 5, New York, 2000, Churchill Livingstone.

McGeoch DJ: The genomes of the human herpesviruses: contents, relationships and evolution, *Annu Rev Microbiol* 43:235–265, 1989.

White DO, Fenner FJ: *Medical virology*, ed 4, New York, 1994, Academic.

Herpes Simplex Virus

Arbesfeld DM, Thomas I: Cutaneous herpes simplex infections, *Am Fam Physician* 43:1655–1664, 1991.

Dawkins BJ: Genital herpes simplex infections, *Prim Care* 17:95–113, 1990.

Herpes simplex virus: NIAID fact sheet [on line]. Available at http://www.niaid.nih.gov/factsheets/stdherp.htm

Landy HJ, Grossman JH III: Herpes simplex virus, *Obstet Gynecol Clin North Am* 16:495–515, 1989.

Rouse BT: Herpes simplex virus: pathogenesis, immunobiology and control, *Curr Top Microbiol Immunol* 179:1–179, 1992.

Wald A: New therapies and prevention strategies for genital herpes, *Clin Infect Dis* 28(suppl 1):S4–S13, 1999.

Whitley RJ, Kimberlin DW, Roizman B: Herpes simplex virus: state of the art clinical article, *Clin Infect Dis* 26:541–555, 1998.

Varicella-Zoster Virus

Arvin AM, Moffat JF, Redman R: Varicella-zoster virus: aspects of pathogenesis and the host response to natural infection and varicella vaccine, *Adv Virus Res* 46:263–309, 1996.

Croen KD, Strauss SE: Varicella zoster latency, *Annu Rev Microbiol* 45:265–282, 1991.

Ostrove JM: Molecular biology of varicella zoster virus, *Adv Virus Res* 38:45–98, 1990.

White CJ: Varicella-zoster virus vaccine, *Clin Infect Dis* 24:753–761; quiz 762–763, 1997.

Epstein-Barr Virus

Basgoz N, Preiksaitis JK: Post-transplant lymphoproliferative disorder, *Infect Dis Clin North Am* 9:901–923, 1995.

Cohen JI: The biology of Epstein-Barr virus: lessons learned from the virus and the host, *Curr Opin Immunol* 11:365–370, 1999.

Englund JA: The many faces of Epstein-Barr virus, *Postgrad Med* 83:167–179, 1988.

Faulkner GC, Krajewski AS, Crawford DH: The ins and outs of EBV infection, *Trends Microbiol* 8:185–189, 2000.

Khanna R, Burrows SR, Moss DJ: Immune regulation in EBV-associated diseases, *Microbiol Rev* 59:387–405, 1995.

Sugden B: EBV's open sesame, *Trends Biochem Sci* 17:239–240, 1992.

Thorley-Lawson DA: Epstein-Barr virus and the B cell: that's all it takes, *Trends Microbiol* 4:204–208, 1996.

Thorley-Lawson DA, Babcock GJ: A model for persistent infection with Epstein-Barr virus: the stealth virus of human B cells, *Life Sci* 65:1433–1453, 1999.

Cytomegalovirus and Human Herpesviruses 6, 7, and 8

Ablashi DV et al: Human herpesvirus-6 (HHV6) (short review), *In Vivo* 5:193–200, 1991.

Bigoni B et al: Human herpesvirus 8 is present in the lymphoid system of healthy persons and can reactivate in the course of AIDS, *J Infect Dis* 173:542–549, 1996.

Gnann JW Jr, Pellett PE, Jaffe HW: Human herpesvirus 8 and Kaposi's sarcoma in persons infected with human immunodeficiency virus, *Clin Infect Dis* 30:S72–S76, 2000.

McDougall JK: Cytomegalovirus, *Curr Top Microbiol Immunol* 154:1–279, 1990.

Pellet PE, Black JB, Yamamoto Y: Human herpesvirus 6: the virus and the search for its role as a human pathogen, *Adv Virol* 41:1–52, 1992.

Plachter B, Sinzger C, Jahn G: Cell types involved in replication and distribution of human cytomegalovirus, *Adv Virus Res* 46:197–264, 1996.

Proceedings of a conference on pathogenesis of cytomegalovirus diseases, *Transplant Proc* 23(suppl 3):1–182, 1991.

Stoeckle MY: The spectrum of human herpesvirus 6 infection: from roseola infantum to adult disease, *Annu Rev Med* 51:423–430, 2000.

Wyatt LS, Frenkel N: Human herpesvirus 7 is a constitutive inhabitant of adult human saliva, *J Virol* 66:3206–3209, 1992.

Yamanishi K et al: Identification of human herpesvirus-6 as a causal agent for exanthema subitum, *Lancet* 1:1065–1067, 1988.

CHAPTER 52

Poxviruses

The poxviruses include the human viruses **variola (smallpox)** (Orthopoxvirus) and **molluscum contagiosum** (Molluscipoxvirus) as well as some viruses that naturally infect animals but can cause incidental infection in humans (**zoonosis**). Many of these viruses share antigenic determinants with smallpox, allowing the use of an animal poxvirus for a human vaccine.

In 18th century England, smallpox accounted for 7% to 12% of all deaths and the deaths of one third of children. However, the development of the first live vaccine in 1796 and the later worldwide distribution of this vaccine led to the eradication of smallpox by 1980. As a result, reference stocks of smallpox virus in two World Health Organization (WHO) laboratories were destroyed in 1996 after an international agreement to do so had been reached. Stocks of the virus still exist in the United States and in Russia.

It is still important, however, to study the poxvirus family for the following reasons:

1. The mechanisms of spread of variola virus within the body represent a model for the spread of other viral infections.
2. Poxviruses other than variola virus cause human disease.
3. Vaccinia and other poxviruses have excellent potential as vectors for hybrid vaccines, which contain and express the genes of other infectious agents.

Structure and Replication

The structure of the vaccinia virus and the way in which the virus replicates are representative of the structure and replication of other poxviruses. Poxviruses are the largest viruses, almost visible on light microscopy (Box 52–1). They measure 230 × 300 nm and are ovoid to brick-shaped with a complex morphology (Fig. 52–1). The poxvirus virion particle must carry many enzymes, including a DNA-dependent RNA polymerase, to allow viral replication to occur in the cytoplasm. The viral genome consists of a large double-stranded, linear DNA that is fused at both ends. The genome of vaccinia virus consists of 86,000 base pairs (molecular weight, approximately 120×10^6 Da).

The replication of poxviruses is unique among the DNA-containing viruses, in that the entire multiplication cycle takes place within the host cell cytoplasm (Fig. 52–2). As a result, *poxviruses must encode the enzymes required for messenger RNA (mRNA) and DNA synthesis as well as activities that other DNA viruses normally obtain from the host cell.*

After binding to a cell surface receptor, the poxvirus outer envelope fuses with cellular membranes, either at the cell surface or within the cell. Early gene transcription is initiated upon removal of the outer membrane. The virion core contains a specific transcriptional activator and all the enzymes necessary for transcription, including a multisubunit RNA polymerase, as well as enzymes for polyadenylate addition and capping. Among the early proteins produced is an uncoating protein (uncoatase) that removes the core membrane, thereby liberating viral DNA into the cell cytoplasm. Viral DNA then replicates in electron-dense cytoplas-

---

BOX 52–1. Unique Properties of Poxviruses

Poxviruses are the largest, most complex viruses.

Poxviruses have complex, oval to brick-shaped morphology with internal structure.

Poxviruses have a linear, double-stranded DNA genome with fused ends.

Poxviruses are **DNA viruses that replicate in the cytoplasm.**

Virus encodes and carries all proteins necessary for mRNA synthesis.

Virus also encodes proteins for functions such as DNA synthesis, nucleotide scavenging, and immune escape mechanisms.

Virus is assembled in inclusion bodies (Guarnieri's bodies), where it acquires its outer membranes.

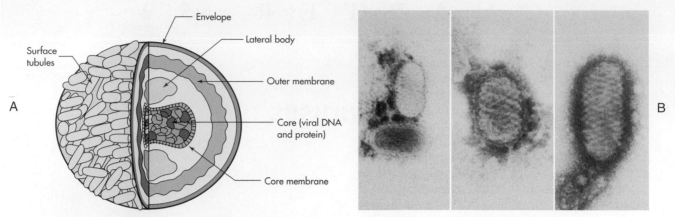

FIGURE 52–1. *A,* Structure of the vaccina virus. Within the virion, the core assumes the shape of a dumbbell because of the large lateral bodies. Virions have a double membrane; the "outer membrane" assembles around the core in the cytoplasm, and the envelope is acquired on exit from the cell. *B,* Electron micrographs of orf virus. Notice its complex structure.

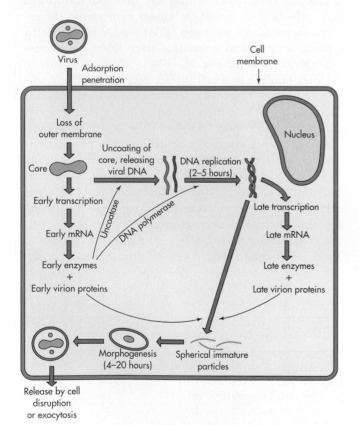

FIGURE 52–2. Replication of vaccina virus. The core is released into the cytoplasm, where virion enzymes initiate transcription. A viral-encoded "uncoatase" enzyme then causes the release of DNA. Viral polymerase replicates the genome, and late transcription occurs. DNA and protein are assembled into cores with the core membrane. An outer membrane shrouds the core containing the lateral bodies and the enzymes required for infectivity. The virion buds through the plasma membrane or is released by cell lysis. mRNA = messenger RNA.

mic inclusions (Guarnieri's inclusion bodies) referred to as factories. Late viral mRNA is translated into structural and virion proteins. In poxviruses, unlike other viruses, the membranes assemble around the core factories. About 10,000 viral particles are produced per infected cell and are released upon cell lysis.

The vaccinia and canarypox viruses are being used as expression vectors to produce live recombinant/hybrid vaccines for more virulent infectious agents (Fig. 52–3). In this process, the foreign gene, which encodes the immunizing molecule, and specific poxvirus gene sequences are added to a plasmid. This recombinant plasmid is inserted into a host cell, which is then infected with the poxvirus. The foreign gene is incorporated into the "rescuing" poxvirus genome because of the homologous viral sequences included on the plasmid. Immunization with the recombinant poxvirus results from expression of the foreign gene and its presentation to the immune response almost as if by infection with the other agent. Experimental vaccines for human immunodeficiency virus, hepatitis B, influenza, and other viruses have been prepared using these techniques. The potential for producing other vaccines in this manner is unlimited.

Pathogenesis and Immunity

Smallpox virus was inhaled and then replicated in the upper respiratory tract (Fig. 52–4). Dissemination occurred via lymphatic and cell-associated viremic spread. Internal and dermal tissues were inoculated after a second, more intense viremia, causing the characteristic "pocks." Molluscum contagiosum and the other poxviruses, however, are acquired through direct contact with lesions and do not spread extensively.

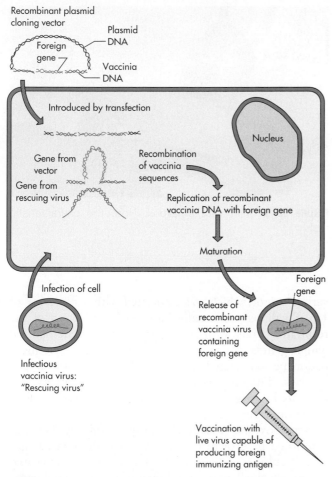

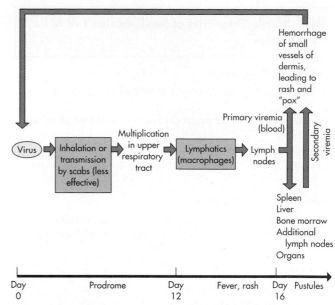

FIGURE 52–4. Spread of smallpox within the body. The virus enters and replicates in the respiratory tract without causing symptoms or contagion. The virus infects macrophages, which enter the lymphatic system and carry the virus to regional lymph nodes. The virus then replicates and initiates a viremia, causing the infection to spread to the spleen, bone marrow, lymph nodes, liver, and all organs, followed by the skin (rash). A secondary viremia causes the development of additional lesions throughout the host, followed by death or recovery with or without sequelae. Recovery from smallpox was associated with prolonged immunity and lifelong protection.

FIGURE 52–3. Vaccinia virus as an expression vector for the production of live recombinant vaccines. (Modified from Piccini A, Paoletti E: Vaccinia: virus, vector, vaccine, *Adv Virus Res* 34:43–64, 1988.)

The poxviruses encode many proteins that facilitate their replication and pathogenesis in the host. They include proteins that initially stimulate host cell growth and then lead to cell lysis and viral spread. Molluscum contagiosum causes a wartlike lesion rather than a lytic infection.

Cell-mediated immunity is essential for resolving a poxvirus infection. However, poxviruses encode activities that help the virus evade immune control. These include the cell-to-cell spread of the virus to avoid antibody and proteins that impede the interferon, complement, and inflammatory responses. The disease mechanisms of poxviruses are summarized in Box 52–2.

Epidemiology

The natural hosts for most of the poxviruses important to humans are vertebrates other than humans (e.g., cow, sheep, goats). The viruses infect humans only through accidental or occupational exposure (zoonosis). The exceptions are molluscum contagiosum and smallpox viruses.

Smallpox (variola) was very contagious and, as just noted, was spread primarily by the respiratory route. It was also spread less efficiently through close contact with dried virus on clothes or other materials. Despite the severity of the disease and its tendency to spread,

---

BOX 52–2. **Disease Mechanisms of Poxvirus**

Smallpox was initiated by respiratory tract infection and was spread mainly by the lymphatic system and cell-associated viremia.

Molluscum contagiosum and **zoonoses** are transmitted by contact.

Virus may cause initial stimulation of cell growth and then cell lysis.

Virus encodes immune escape mechanisms.

Cell-mediated immunity and humoral immunity are important for resolution.

BOX 52–3. Properties of Smallpox that Led to Its Eradication

Viral Characteristics

Exclusive human host range (no animal reservoirs or vectors).

Single serotype (immunization protected against all infections).

Animal and human poxviruses share antigenic determinants ("safe" live vaccines prepared from animal poxviruses).

Disease Characteristics

Consistent disease presentation with visible pustules (identification of sources of contagion allowed quarantine and vaccination of contacts).

Vaccine

Stable, inexpensive, easy-to-administer vaccine.
Presence of scar indicating successful vaccination.

Public Health Service

Successful worldwide WHO program combining vaccination and quarantine.

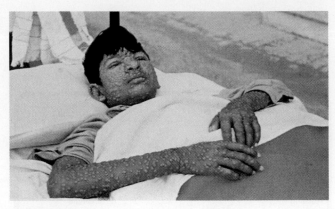

FIGURE 52–5. Child with smallpox. Note the characteristic rash.

---

several factors contributed to its elimination, as listed in Box 52–3.

Clinical Syndromes

The diseases associated with poxviruses are listed in Table 52–1.

Smallpox

The two variants of smallpox were variola major, which was associated with a mortality of 15% to 40%, and variola minor, which was associated with a mortality of 1%. Smallpox was usually initiated by infection of the respiratory tract with subsequent involvement of local lymph glands, which in turn led to viremia. The incubation period ranged from 5 to 17 days and averaged 12 days. The symptoms and course of the disease are presented in Figure 52–4, and the characteristic rash is shown in Figure 52–5.

Smallpox was usually diagnosed clinically but was confirmed by growth of the virus in embryonated eggs or cell cultures. Characteristic lesions (pocks) appeared on the chorioallantoic membrane of embryonated eggs.

Smallpox was the first disease to be controlled by immunization, and its eradication is one of the greatest triumphs of medical epidemiology. Eradication resulted from a massive WHO campaign to vaccinate all susceptible people, especially those exposed to anyone with the disease, and thereby interrupt the chain of human-to-human transmission. The campaign began in 1967 and succeeded. The last case of naturally acquired

---

TABLE 52–1. Diseases Associated with Poxviruses

Virus	Disease	Source	Location
Variola	Smallpox (now extinct)	Humans	Extinct
Vaccinia	Used for smallpox vaccination	Laboratory product	—
Orf	Localized lesion	Zoonosis—sheep, goats	Worldwide
Cowpox	Localized lesion	Zoonosis—rodents, cats, cows	Europe
Pseudocowpox	Milker's nodule	Zoonosis—dairy cows	Worldwide
Monkeypox	Generalized disease	Zoonosis—monkeys, squirrels	Africa
Bovine papular stomatitis virus	Localized lesion	Zoonosis—calves, beef cattle	Worldwide
Tanapox	Localized lesion	Rare zoonosis—monkeys	Africa
Yabapox	Localized lesion	Rare zoonosis—monkeys, baboons	Africa
Molluscum contagiosum	Many skin lesions	Humans	Worldwide

Modified from Balows A et al, editors: *Laboratory diagnosis of infectious diseases: principles and practice,* vol 2, New York, 1988, Springer-Verlag.

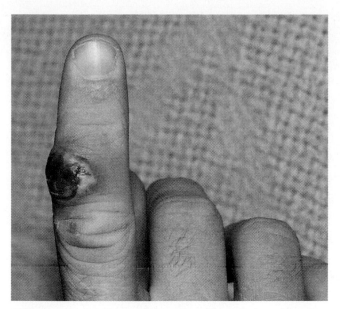

FIGURE 52–6. Orf lesion on the finger of a taxidermist. (Courtesy Joe Meyers, MD, Akron, Ohio.)

Orf, Cowpox, and Monkeypox

Human infection with the orf (poxvirus of sheep and goat) or cowpox (vaccinia) virus is usually an occupational hazard resulting from direct contact with the lesions on the animal. A single nodular lesion usually forms on the point of contact, such as the fingers, hand, or forearm, and are hemorrhagic (cowpox) or granulomatous (orf or pseudocowpox) (Fig. 52–6). Vesicular lesions frequently develop and then regress in 25 to 35 days, generally without scar formation. The lesions may be mistaken for anthrax. The virus can be grown in culture or seen directly with electron microscopy but is usually diagnosed from the symptoms and patient history.

More than 100 cases of illnesses resembling smallpox have been attributed to the monkeypox virus. All have occurred in western and central Africa, especially Zaire.

infection was reported in 1977, and eradication of the disease was acknowledged in 1980.

Variolation, an early approach to immunization, involved the inoculation of susceptible people with the virulent smallpox pus. It was first performed in the Far East and later in England. Cotton Mather introduced the practice to America. Variolation was associated with a fatality rate of approximately 1%, a better risk than that associated with smallpox itself. In 1796, Jenner developed and then popularized a vaccine using the less virulent cowpox virus, which shares antigenic determinants with smallpox.

As the eradication program neared its goal, it became apparent that the rate of serious reactions to vaccination (see the discussion of vaccinia) exceeded the risk of infection in the developed world. Therefore, smallpox vaccination began to be discontinued in the 1970s and was totally discontinued after 1980.

Vaccinia

Vaccinia, a form of cowpox, was used for the smallpox vaccine. The vaccination procedure consisted of scratching live virus into the patient's skin and then observing for the development of vesicles and pustules to confirm a "take." As the incidence of smallpox waned, however, it became apparent that there were more complications related to vaccination than cases of smallpox. Several of these complications were severe and even fatal. They included encephalitis and progressive infection (vaccinia necrosum), the latter occurring occasionally in immunocompromised patients who were inadvertently vaccinated.

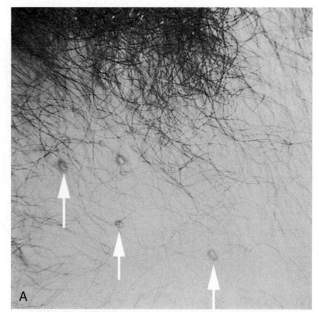

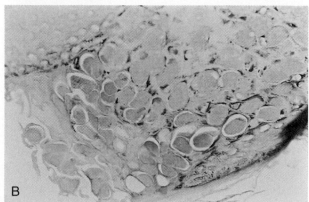

FIGURE 52–7. Molluscum contagiosum. *A,* Skin lesion. *B,* Microscopic view; epidermis is filled with molluscum bodies (×100).

Molluscum Contagiosum

The lesions of molluscum contagiosum differ significantly from pox lesions in being nodular to wartlike (Fig. 52–7*A*). They begin as papules and then become pearl-like, umbilicated nodules that are 2 to 10 mm in diameter and have a central caseous plug that can be readily expressed (squeezed out). They are most common on the trunk, genitalia, and proximal extremities and usually occur in a cluster of 5 to 20 nodules. The incubation period for molluscum contagiosum is 2 to 8 weeks, and the disease is spread by direct contact (e.g., sexual contact, wrestling) or fomites (e.g., towels). The disease is more common in children than adults but its incidence is increasing in sexually active individuals.

The diagnosis of molluscum contagiosum is confirmed histologically by the finding of very characteristic large, eosinophilic cytoplasmic inclusions (molluscum bodies) in epithelial cells (Fig. 52–7*B*). These bodies can be seen in biopsy specimens or in the expressed caseous core of a nodule. The molluscum contagiosum virus cannot be grown in tissue culture or animal models.

Lesions of molluscum contagiosum disappear in 2 to 12 months, presumably as a result of immune responses. The nodules can be removed by curettage (scraping) or the application of liquid nitrogen or iodine solutions.

QUESTIONS

1. The structure of poxviruses is more complex than that of most other viruses. What problems does this complexity create for viral replication?

2. Poxviruses replicate in the cytoplasm. What problems does this feature create for viral replication?

3. How does the immune response to smallpox infection in an immunologically naive person differ from that in a vaccinated person? When is antibody present in each case? What stage or stages of viral dissemination are blocked in each case?

4. What characteristics of smallpox facilitated its elimination?

5. Vaccinia virus is being used as a vector for the development of hybrid vaccines. Why is vaccinia virus well suited to this task? Which infectious agents would be appropriate for a vaccinia hybrid vaccine, and why?

BIBLIOGRAPHY

Belshe RB, editor: *Textbook of human virology*, ed 2, St Louis, 1991, Mosby.

Fenner F: A successful eradication campaign: global eradication of smallpox, *Rev Infect Dis* 4:916–930, 1982.

Fields BN, Knipe DM, Howley PM, editors: *Virology*, ed 3, New York, 1996, Lippincott-Raven.

Gorbach SL, Bartlett JG, Blacklow NR, editors: *Infectious diseases*, ed 2, Philadelphia, 1997, WB Saunders.

Mandell GL, Bennett JE, Dolin R. *Principles and practice of infectious diseases*, ed 5, New York, 2000, Churchill Livingstone.

Moyer RW, Turner PC, editors: Poxviruses, *Curr Top Microbiol Immunol* 163:1–211, 1990.

Piccini A, Paoletti E: Vaccinia: virus, vector, vaccine, *Adv Virus Res* 34:43–64, 1988.

White DO, Fenner FJ: *Medical virology*, ed 4, New York, 1994, Academic.

CHAPTER 53

Parvoviruses

The Parvoviridae are the smallest of the DNA viruses. Their small size and limited genetic repertoire make them more dependent than any other DNA virus on the host cell or the presence of a helper virus to replicate. Only one member of the Parvoviridae, **B19**, a member of the Parvovirus genus, is known to cause human disease.

B19 normally causes **erythema infectiosum**, or **fifth disease**, a mild febrile exanthematous disease that occurs in children. It goes by the latter name because it was the fifth of the childhood exanthems (the first four being varicella, rubella, roseola, and measles). B19 is also responsible for episodes of **aplastic crisis in patients with chronic hemolytic anemia** and is associated with **acute polyarthritis** in adults. Intrauterine infection of a fetus may cause abortion.

Other parvoviruses, such as RA-1 (isolated from a person with rheumatoid arthritis) and fecal parvoviruses, have not been shown to cause human disease. Feline and canine parvoviruses do not cause human disease and are preventable with vaccination of the pet.

Adeno-associated viruses (AAVs) are members of the Dependovirus genus in the family Parvoviridae. They commonly infect humans but replicate only in association with a second "helper" virus, usually an adenovirus. Dependoviruses neither cause illness nor modify infection by their helper viruses. These properties and the propensity of AAVs to integrate into the host chromosome has made genetically modified AAVs candidates for use in **gene replacement therapy**. A third genus of the family, Densovirus, infects only insects.

Structure and Replication

The parvoviruses are extremely small (18 to 26 nm in diameter) and have a nonenveloped, icosahedral capsid (Box 53–1 and Fig. 53–1). The B19 virus genome contains one linear, single-stranded DNA molecule with a molecular mass of 1.5 to 1.8×10^6 Da (5,500 bases in length) (Box 53–2). Plus or minus DNA strands are packaged separately into virions. Three structural, one major nonstructural, and several smaller proteins are encoded by the plus-stranded genome. Only one serotype of B19 is known to exist.

B19 virus replicates in mitotically active cells and prefers cells of the erythroid lineage, such as fresh human bone marrow cells, erythroid cells from fetal liver, and erythroid leukemia cells (Fig. 53–2). After binding to the erythrocyte blood group P antigen (globoside) and its internalization, the virion is uncoated, and the single-stranded DNA genome is delivered to the nucleus. Factors available only during the S phase of the cell's growth cycle and cellular DNA polymerases are required to generate a complementary DNA strand.

The double-stranded DNA version of the virion genome is required for transcription and replication. Inverted repeat sequences of DNA at both ends of the genome facilitate viral DNA synthesis. These ends fold back and hybridize with the genome to create a primer for the cell's DNA polymerase. Messenger RNA (mRNA) for the nonstructural regulatory and structural capsid proteins is generated from the same promoter by differential splicing of the primary transcript. Viral proteins synthesized in the cytoplasm then return to the nucleus, where the virion is assembled. The nuclear and cytoplasmic membrane degenerates, and the virus is released upon cell lysis.

Pathogenesis and Immunity

B19 targets and is cytolytic for erythroid precursor cells (Box 53–3). B19 disease is determined by the direct killing of these cells and the subsequent immune response to the infection (rash and arthralgia).

Studies performed in volunteers suggest that B19 virus first replicates in the nasopharynx or upper respiratory tract, then spreads by viremia to the bone marrow and elsewhere, where it replicates and kills erythroid precursor cells (Fig. 53–3). The disease has a **biphasic course**.

The *initial febrile stage is the infectious stage*. During this time, erythrocyte production is stopped for ap-

---

BOX 53–1. **Unique Properties of Parvoviruses**

Smallest DNA virus
Naked icosahedral capsid
Single-stranded DNA genome
Requirement of growing cells (B19) or helper virus (dependovirus) for replication

---

BOX 53–2. **Parvovirus Genome**

Single-stranded linear DNA genome.
    Approximately 5.5 kilobases in length.
    Plus and minus strands packaged into separate B19 virions with approximately equal frequency.
    Ends of the genome have inverted repeats that hybridize to form hairpin loops and a primer for DNA synthesis.

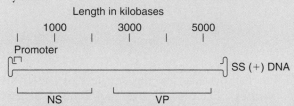

    Coding region for B19 on plus strand.
    Separate coding regions for nonstructural (NS) and structural proteins (VP) transcribed from one promoter.

---

proximately 1 week as a result of the viral killing of erythroid precursor cells. A large viremia occurs within 8 days of infection and is accompanied by nonspecific flu-like symptoms. Large numbers of virus are also released into oral and respiratory secretions. Antibody stops the viremia and is important for resolution of the disease but contributes to the symptoms.

The *second, symptomatic stage appears to be immune-mediated.* The rash and arthralgia seen in this stage coincide with the appearance of virus-specific antibody, the disappearance of detectable B19 virus, and the formation of immune complexes.

Hosts with chronic hemolytic anemia (e.g., sickle cell anemia) who are infected with B19 are at risk for a life-threatening reticulocytopenia, which is referred to as an **aplastic crisis**. The reticulocytopenia results from the combination of (1) B19 depletion of the red blood cell precursors and (2) shortened life span of the erythrocytes caused by the underlying anemia.

Epidemiology

As much as 65% of the adult population is infected with B19 by 40 years of age (Box 53–4). Erythema infectiosum is most common in children and adolescents aged 4 to 15 years, and it tends to occur in late

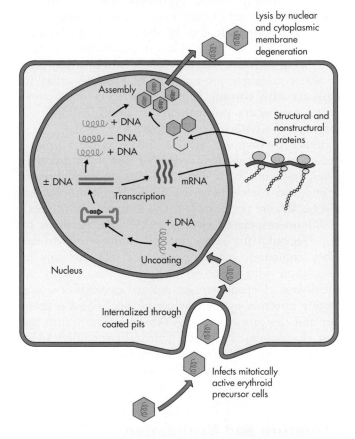

FIGURE 53–2. Postulated replication of parvovirus (B19) based on information from related viruses (minute virus of mice). The internalized parvovirus delivers its genome to the nucleus, where the single-stranded (plus or minus) DNA is converted to double-stranded DNA by host factors and DNA polymerases present only in growing cells. Transcription, replication, and assembly occur in the nucleus. Virus is released by cell lysis.

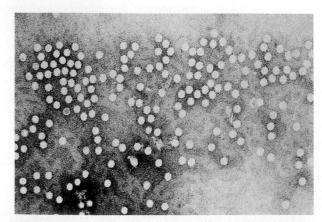

FIGURE 53–1. Electron micrograph of parvovirus. Parvoviruses are small (18 to 26 nm), nonenveloped viruses with single-stranded DNA. (Courtesy Centers for Disease Control and Prevention, Atlanta.)

BOX 53-3. Disease Mechanisms of B19 Parvovirus

Virus is spread by **respiratory** and **oral** secretions.
   Virus **infects mitotically active erythroid precursor** cells in bone marrow and establishes lytic infection.
   Virus establishes large **viremia** and can **cross the placenta.**
   Antibody is important for resolution and prophylaxis.
Virus causes **biphasic disease:**
   Initial phase is related to viremia:
      Flu-like symptoms and viral shedding.
   Later phase is related to immune response:
      Circulating immune complexes of antibody and virions that do not fix complement.
      Result: erythematous maculopapular rash, arthralgia, and arthritis.
   Depletion of erythroid precursor cells and destabilization of erythrocytes initiate **aplastic crisis in people with chronic anemia.**

BOX 53-4. Epidemiology of B19 Parvovirus Infection

Disease/Viral Factors

Capsid virus is resistant to inactivation.
   Contagious period precedes symptoms.
   Virus crosses placenta and infects fetus.

Transmission

Respiratory droplets.

Who Is at Risk?

Children, especially elementary school age: erythema infectiosum (fifth disease).
   Parents of children with B19 infection.
   Pregnant women: fetal infection and disease.
   People with chronic anemia: aplastic crisis.

Geography/Season

Virus is found worldwide.
   Fifth disease is more common in late winter and spring.

Modes of Control

There are no modes of control.

---

winter and spring. Arthralgia and arthritis are likely to occur in adults. The virus is most probably transmitted by respiratory droplets and oral secretions. Parenteral transmission of the virus by blood-clotting factor concentrate has also been described.

Clinical Syndromes

B19 virus is the cause of erythema infectiosum (fifth disease) (Box 53–5). Infection starts with an unremarkable prodromal period, during which the person is contagious. Infection of a normal host may cause either no noticeable symptoms or fever and nonspecific symptoms, such as sore throat, malaise, and myalgia as well

as a slight decrease in hemoglobin levels (Fig. 53–4). This period is followed by a distinctive rash on the cheeks, which appear to have been slapped. The rash then usually spreads, especially to exposed skin such as the arms and legs (Fig. 53–5), and then subsides over 1 to 2 weeks. Relapse of the rash is common.

B19 infection in adults causes polyarthritis. Arthritis of the hands, wrists, knees, and ankles predominates. The rash may precede the arthritis but often does not occur. B19 infection of immunocompromised people may result in chronic disease.

The most serious complication of parvovirus infection is the aplastic crisis that occurs in patients with chronic hemolytic anemia (e.g., sickle cell anemia). Infection in these people causes a transient reduction in

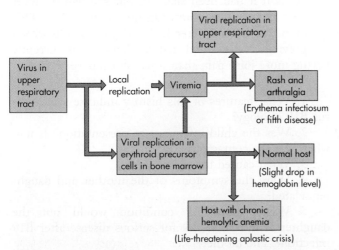

FIGURE 53–3. Mechanism of spread of parvovirus within the body.

BOX 53-5. Clinical Consequences of Parvovirus (B19) Infection

Mild flu-like illness (fever, headache, chills, myalgia, malaise).
   Erythema infectiosum (fifth disease).
   Aplastic crisis in people with chronic anemia.
   Arthropathy (polyarthritis: symptoms in many joints).
   Risk of fetal loss as a result of B19 virus crossing the placenta, causing anemia-related disease but not congenital anomalies.

erythropoiesis in the bone marrow. The reduction results in a transient reticulocytopenia that lasts 7 to 10 days and a decrease in hemoglobin level. An aplastic crisis is accompanied by fever and nonspecific symptoms, such as malaise, myalgia, chills, and itching. A maculopapular rash with arthralgia and some joint swelling may also be present.

B19 infection of a seronegative mother increases the risk for fetal death. The virus can infect the fetus and kill erythrocyte precursors, causing anemia and congestive heart failure (**hydrops fetalis**). Infection of seropositive pregnant women often has no adverse effect on the fetus. There is no evidence that B19 causes congenital abnormalities (see Box 53–5).

Laboratory Diagnosis

The diagnosis of erythema infectiosum is usually based on the clinical presentation. For B19 disease to be definitively diagnosed, however, specific immunoglobulin M (IgM) or viral DNA must be detected (e.g., to distinguish the rash of B19 from that of rubella in a pregnant woman). Enzyme-linked immunosorbent assays (ELISAs) for B19 IgM and IgG are available. The polymerase chain reaction (PCR) is a very sensitive method for detecting the B19 genome in clinical samples but requires adequate controls. Virus isolation is not performed.

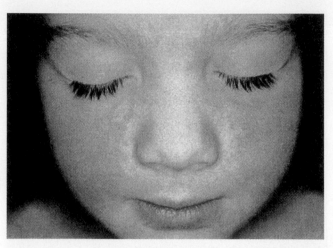

FIGURE 53–5. A "slapped cheek" appearance is typical of the rash for erythema infectiosum. (From Hart CA, Broadhead RL: *A color atlas of pediatric infectious diseases,* London, 1992, Wolfe.)

Treatment, Prevention, and Control

No specific antiviral treatment or means of control is available. Vaccines are available for dog and cat parvoviruses.

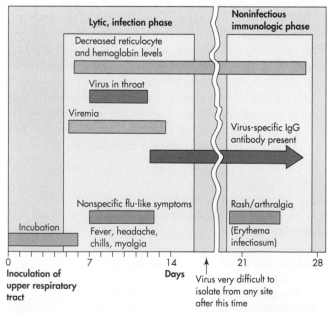

FIGURE 53–4. Time course of parvovirus (B19) infection. B19 causes biphasic disease: first, an initial, lytic infection phase characterized by febrile, flu-like symptoms and then a noninfectious immunologic phase characterized by a rash and arthralgia.

CASE STUDY AND QUESTIONS

■ Mrs. Doe brought her daughter to the pediatrician with the complaint of a rash. The daughter's face appeared as if it had been slapped, but she had no fever or other notable symptoms. On questioning, Mrs. Doe reported that her daughter had had a mild cold within the previous 2 weeks and that she herself was currently having more joint pain than usual and was very tired.

1. What features of this history indicate a parvovirus B19 etiology?
2. Was the child infectious at presentation? If not, when was she contagious?
3. What caused the symptoms?
4. Were the symptoms of the mother and daughter related?
5. What underlying condition would put the daughter at increased risk for serious disease after B19 infection? The mother?
6. Why is quarantine a poor means of limiting the spread of B19 parvovirus?

BIBLIOGRAPHY

Anderson LJ: Human parvoviruses, *J Infect Dis* 161:603–608, 1990.

Anderson MJ: Parvoviruses. In Belshe RB, editor: *Textbook of human virology*, ed 2, St Louis, 1991, Mosby.

Balows A, Hausler WJ Jr, Lennette EH, editors: *Laboratory diagnosis of infectious diseases: principles and practice*, vol 2, New York, 1988, Springer-Verlag.

Berns KI: *The parvoviruses*, New York, 1984, Plenum.

Berns KI: Parvovirus replication, *Microbiol Rev* 54:316–329, 1990.

Brown KE, Young NS: Parvovirus B19 in human disease, *Annu Rev Med* 48:59–67, 1997.

Chorba T et al: The role of parvovirus B19 in aplastic crisis and erythema infectiosum (fifth disease), *J Infect Dis* 154:383–393, 1986.

Fields BN, Knipe DM, Howley PM, editors: *Virology*, ed 3, New York, 1996, Lippincott-Raven.

Gorbach SL, Bartlett JG, Blacklow NR, editors: *Infectious diseases*, ed 2, Philadelphia, 1997, WB Saunders.

Mandell GL, Bennett JE, Dolin R: *Principles and practice of infectious diseases*, ed 5, New York, 2000, Churchill Livingstone.

Naides SJ et al: Rheumatologic manifestations of human parvovirus B19 infection in adults, *Arthritis Rheum* 33:1297–1309, 1990.

Török TJ: Parvovirus B19 and human disease, *Adv Intern Med* 37:431–455, 1992.

Ware RE: Parvovirus infections. In Krugman SK et al: *Infectious diseases of children*, ed 10, St Louis, 1998, Mosby.

White DO, Fenner FJ: *Medical virology*, ed 4, New York, 1994, Academic.

Picornaviruses

Picornaviridae is one of the largest families of viruses and includes some of the most important human and animal viruses (Box 54–1). As the name indicates, these viruses are **small** (*pico*) **RNA** viruses that have a **naked capsid** structure. The family has more than 230 members that are divided into five genera: Enterovirus, Rhinovirus, Heparnavirus, Cardiovirus, and Aphthovirus. The enteroviruses are distinguished from the rhinoviruses by the stability of the capsid at pH 3, the optimum temperature for growth, the mode of transmission, and the diseases caused (Box 54–2).

At least 72 serotypes of human enteroviruses exist, including the polioviruses, coxsackieviruses, and echoviruses. Hepatitis A virus was included in this group, but has been reclassified as a hepatovirus in the Heparnavirus genus, and is discussed separately in Chapter 62. The capsids of these viruses are *very resistant to harsh environmental conditions* (sewage systems) and the conditions in the gastrointestinal tract, a fact that facilitates their transmission by the fecal-oral route. However, even though they may initiate infection in the gastrointestinal tract, the enteroviruses rarely cause enteric disease. Infections are usually asymptomatic. Several different disease syndromes may be caused by a specific serotype of enterovirus. Likewise, several different serotypes may cause the same disease, depending on the target tissue affected. The best-known and most-studied picornavirus is poliovirus, of which there are three serotypes.

Coxsackieviruses are named after the town of Coxsackie, New York, where they were first isolated. They are divided into two groups, A and B, on the basis of certain biologic and antigenic differences and are further subdivided into numeric serotypes on the basis of additional antigenic differences.

The name **echovirus** is derived from **e**nteric **c**ytopathic **h**uman **o**rphan, because these agents were not initially thought to be associated with clinical disease. Now 32 serotypes are recognized. Since 1967, newly isolated enteroviruses have been distinguished numerically.

The human rhinoviruses consist of at least 100 serotypes and are the major cause of the common cold. They are *sensitive to acidic pH and replicate poorly at temperatures above 33°C*. This sensitivity usually limits rhinoviruses to causing upper respiratory tract infections.

Structure

The plus-strand RNA of the picornaviruses is surrounded by an **icosahedral capsid** approximately 30 nm in diameter. The icosahedral capsid has 12 pentameric vertices, each of which is composed of five protomeric units of proteins. The protomers are made of four virion polypeptides (VP1 to VP4). VP2 and VP4 are generated by the cleavage of a precursor, VP0. VP4 in the virion solidifies the structure, but it is not generated until the genome is incorporated into the capsid. This protein is released on binding of the virus to the cellular receptor. The capsids are stable in the presence of heat and detergent and, except for the rhinoviruses, are also stable in acid. The capsid structure is so regular that paracrystals of virions often form in infected cells (Figs. 54–1 and 54–2).

The **genome of the picornaviruses resembles a messenger RNA** (mRNA) (Fig. 54–3). It is a single strand of plus-sense RNA of approximately 7400 bases that has a poly A at the 3′ end and a small protein, VPg (22 to 24 amino acids), attached to the 5′ end. The poly A sequence enhances the infectivity of the RNA, and the VPg may be important in packaging the genome into the capsid and initiating viral RNA synthesis. *The naked picornavirus genome is sufficient to infect a cell.*

The genome encodes a polyprotein that is proteolytically cleaved to produce the enzymatic and structural proteins of the virus. In addition to the capsid proteins and VPg, the picornaviruses encode at least two proteases and an RNA-dependent RNA polymerase. Poliovirus also produces a protease that degrades the 200,000-Da cap-binding protein of eukaryotic ribosomes, thereby blocking the translation of most cellular mRNA.

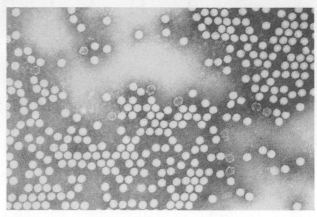

FIGURE 54–1. Electron micrograph of poliovirus. (Courtesy Centers for Disease Control and Prevention, Atlanta.)

Replication

The specificity of the picornavirus interaction for cellular receptors is the major determinant of the target tissue tropism and disease (see Fig. 6–12). The VP1 proteins at the vertices of the virion contain a canyon structure to which the receptor binds. The site of binding is protected from antibody neutralization. Pleconaril and related antiviral compounds contain a 3-methylisoxazole group that binds to the floor of this canyon and alters its conformation to prevent the uncoating of the virus.

The picornaviruses can be categorized according to their cell surface receptor specificity. The receptors for polioviruses and rhinoviruses are members of the immunoglobulin superfamily of proteins. Their primary function is to promote normal and immunologic cell-to-cell interactions. At least 80% of the rhinoviruses and several serotypes of coxsackievirus recognize intercellular adhesion molecule 1 (ICAM-1), which is expressed on epithelial cells, fibroblasts, and endothelial cells. Poliovirus binds to a different molecule that has a similar structure. Expression of the poliovirus receptor is a primary determinant of the limited cell tropism of poliovirus infection.

On binding to the receptor, the VP4 is released and the virion weakened.

The genome is then injected directly across the membrane through a channel created at one of the vertices of the virion. The genome binds directly to ribosomes despite the lack of a 5′ cap structure. The ribosomes recognize a unique internal RNA loop in the genome. A polyprotein containing all the viral protein sequences is synthesized within 10 to 15 minutes of infection. This polyprotein is cleaved by viral proteases encoded in it. The viral RNA-dependent RNA polymerase generates a negative-strand RNA template from which the new mRNA/genome and templates can be synthesized. The amount of viral mRNA increases rapidly in the cell, with the number of viral RNA molecules reaching 400,000 per cell.

Several picornaviruses inhibit cellular RNA and protein synthesis during infection. For example, cleavage of the 200,000-Da cap-binding protein of the ribosome by a poliovirus protease prevents most cellular mRNA from binding to the ribosome. Permeability changes induced by picornaviruses also reduce the ability of cellular mRNA to bind to the ribosome. In addition, viral mRNA can outcompete cellular mRNA for the factors required in protein synthesis. These activities contribute to the cytopathologic effect of the virus on the target cell.

As the viral genome is being replicated and translated, the structural proteins VP0, VP1, and VP3 are cleaved from the polyprotein by a viral-encoded protease and assembled into subunits. A total of 5 **subunits** associate into **pentamers**, and 12 **pentamers** associate to form the **procapsid**. After insertion of the genome,

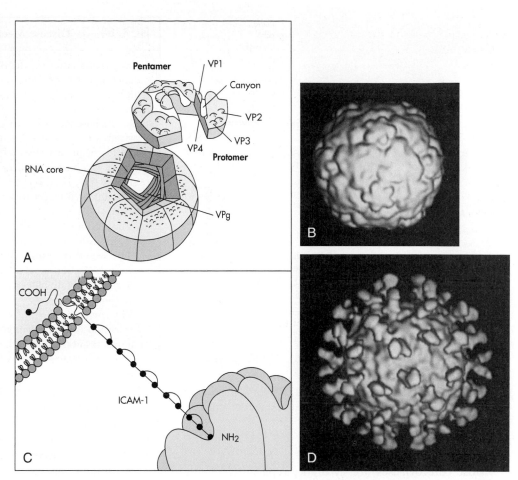

FIGURE 54–2. *A,* Structure of the human rhinovirus and its interaction with the ICAM-1 receptor-binding canyon surrounding the starlike structure at the vertices. *B,* Cryoelectron microscopy computer-generated reconstruction of the human rhinovirus 16. *C,* Interaction of ICAM-1 molecule with the virion. *D,* Cryoelectron microscopy reconstruction of the interaction of a soluble form of ICAM-1 with human rhinovirus 16. *Note:* There is one ICAM-1 per capsomere. ICAM-1 = intercellular adhesion molecule 1. (*B* and *D* courtesy Tim Baker, Purdue University.)

VP0 is cleaved into VP2 and VP4 to complete the **capsid.** The virion is usually released upon cell lysis.

Enteroviruses

Pathogenesis and Immunity

Contrary to their name, enteroviruses do not usually cause enteric disease but are transmitted by the fecal-oral route. The diseases produced by the enteroviruses are determined mainly by differences in tissue tropism

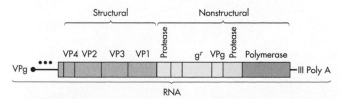

FIGURE 54–3. Structure of the picornavirus genome. The genome is translated as a polyprotein, which is cleaved by viral-encoded proteases into individual proteins. g^r = guanidine resistance marker (a genetic locus involved in the initiation of RNA synthesis); Poly A = polyadenylate.

and the cytolytic capacity of the virus (Fig. 54–4; Box 54–3). Poliovirus has one of the narrowest tissue tropisms, recognizing a receptor expressed on anterior horn cells of the spinal cord, dorsal root ganglia, motor neurons, skeletal muscle cells, lymphoid cells, and few other cells. Coxsackieviruses and echoviruses recognize receptors expressed on more cell types and tissues and cause a broader spectrum of diseases (Table 54–1). Receptors for these enteroviruses are present on cells of the central nervous system, heart, lung, pancreas, mucosa, and other tissues.

The upper respiratory tract, the oropharynx, and the intestinal tract are the portals of entry for enteroviruses. The virions are impervious to stomach acid, proteases, and bile. Viral replication is initiated in the mucosa and lymphoid tissue of the tonsils and pharynx, and the virus later infects lymphoid cells of Peyer's patches underlying the intestinal mucosa. Primary viremia spreads the virus to receptor-bearing target tissues, where a second phase of viral replication may occur, resulting in symptoms and a secondary viremia. In the case of poliovirus, the virus crosses the blood-brain barrier or gains access to the brain by infecting skeletal muscle and traveling up the innervating nerves to the brain, like the rabies virus (see Chapter 58).

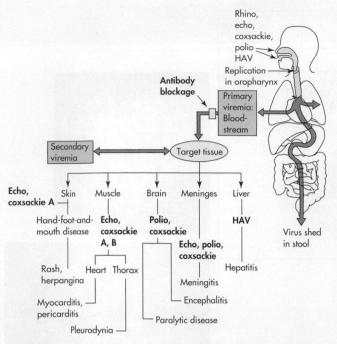

BOX 54−3. **Disease Mechanisms of Picornaviruses**

Enteroviruses enter via the oropharynx, intestinal mucosa, or upper respiratory tract and infect the underlying lymphatic tissue; rhinoviruses are restricted to the upper respiratory tract.

In the absence of serum antibody, enterovirus spreads by viremia to cells of a receptor-bearing target tissue.

Different picornaviruses bind to different receptors, many of which are members of the immunoglobulin superfamily (i.e., ICAM-1).

The infected target tissue determines the subsequent disease.

Viral, rather than immune, pathologic effects are usually responsible for causing disease symptoms.

The secretory antibody response is transitory but can prevent the initiation of infection.

Serum antibody blocks viremic spread to target tissue, preventing symptoms.

Enterovirus is shed in feces for long periods.

Infection is often asymptomatic or causes mild flu-like or upper respiratory tract disease.

FIGURE 54−4. Pathogenesis of enterovirus infection. The target tissue infected by the enterovirus determines the predominant disease caused by the virus. Rhino = rhinovirus; echo = echovirus; coxsackie = coxsackievirus; polio = poliovirus; HAV = hepatitis A virus.

Most enteroviruses are cytolytic, replicating rapidly and causing direct damage to the target cell. The hepatitis A virus is the exception, because it is not very cytolytic. The kinetics of the immune response to hepatitis A correlate with the appearance of symptoms, indicating immunopathogenesis.

Viral shedding from the oropharynx can be detected for a short time before symptoms begin, whereas viral production and shedding from the intestine may last for 30 days or longer, even in the presence of a humoral immune response.

Antibody is the major protective immune response to the enteroviruses. Secretory antibody can prevent the initial establishment of infection in the oropharynx and gastrointestinal tract, and serum antibody prevents viremic spread to the target tissue and, therefore, disease. The

TABLE 54−1. **Summary of Clinical Syndromes Associated with Major Enterovirus Groups**

Syndrome	Occurrence	Polioviruses	Coxsackie A Viruses	Coxsackie B Viruses	Echoviruses
Paralytic disease	Sporadic	+	+	+	+
Encephalitis, meningitis	Outbreaks	+	+	+	+
Carditis	Sporadic		+	+	+
Neonatal disease	Outbreaks			+	+
Pleurodynia	Outbreaks			+	
Herpangina	Common		+		
Hand-foot-and-mouth disease	Common		+		
Rash disease	Common		+	+	+
Acute hemorrhagic conjunctivitis	Epidemics		+		
Respiratory tract infections	Common	+	+	+	+
Undifferentiated fever	Common	+	+	+	+
Diarrhea, gastrointestinal disease	Uncommon				+
Diabetes, pancreatitis	Uncommon			+	
Orchitis	Uncommon			+	
Disease in immunodeficient patients	—	+	+		+
Congenital anomalies	Uncommon		+	+	

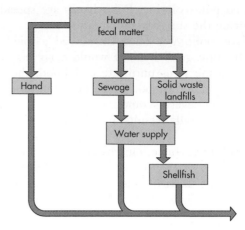

FIGURE 54–5. Transmission of enteroviruses. The capsid structure is resistant to mild sewage treatment, salt water, detergents, and temperature changes, allowing these viruses to be transmitted by fecal-oral routes and on hands.

BOX 54–4. Epidemiology of Enterovirus Infections

Disease/Viral Factors

(Nature of disease correlates with specific enterovirus types and age of person.)

Infection is often asymptomatic, with viral shedding.

Virion is resistant to environmental conditions (detergents, acid, drying, mild sewage treatment, and heat).

Transmission

Fecal-oral route: poor hygiene, dirty diapers (especially in daycare settings).

Ingestion via contaminated food and water.

Contact with infected hands and fomites.

Inhalation of infectious aerosols.

Who Is at Risk?

Young children: at risk for polio (asymptomatic or mild disease).

Older children and adults: at risk for polio (asymptomatic to paralytic disease).

Newborns and neonates: at highest risk for serious coxsackievirus and enterovirus disease.

Geography/Season

Viruses have worldwide distribution; wild-type polio is virtually eradicated in developed countries because of vaccination program.

Disease is more common in summer.

Modes of Control

For polio, live oral polio vaccine (trivalent OPV) or inactivated trivalent polio vaccine (IPV) is administered.

For other enteroviruses, there is no vaccine; good hygiene limits spread.

---

time course for antibody development after an infection with a live vaccine is presented in Figure 54–10.

Cell-mediated immunity is not usually involved in protection but may play a role in pathogenesis. Hepatitis A virus is the exception, in that T cells are also important for the resolution of the disease. T cells also appear to contribute to the pathogenesis of coxsackie B virus–induced myocarditis in mice.

Epidemiology

The enteroviruses are exclusively human pathogens (Box 54–4). As the name implies, these viruses are primarily spread by the **fecal-oral** route. **Asymptomatic shedding** can occur for up to a month, putting virus into the environment. Poor sanitation and crowded living conditions foster transmission of the viruses (Fig. 54–5). Sewage contamination of water supplies can result in enterovirus epidemics. Outbreaks of enterovirus disease are seen in schools and daycare

settings. Summer is the major season for such disease. The coxsackieviruses and echoviruses may also be spread in aerosol droplets and cause respiratory tract infections.

With the success of the polio vaccines, the wild-type poliovirus has been eliminated from the Western Hemisphere (Fig. 54–6) but not from the world. Paralytic polio is still prevalent in areas where the vaccine is not available and in communities where vaccination is contrary to religious beliefs or other teachings. A small but significant number of vaccine-related cases of polio result from the reversion of the live vaccine virus and its reestablishing neurovirulence. This development has prompted a change to promote the use of the

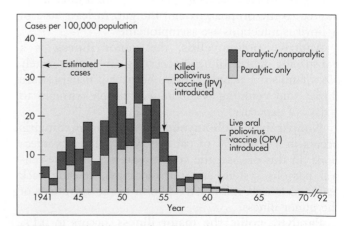

FIGURE 54–6. Incidence of polio in the United States. Killed (inactivated) poliovirus vaccine (IPV) was introduced in 1955 and live (oral) poliovirus vaccine (OPV) in 1961 and 1962. (Courtesy Centers for Disease Control: *Immunization against disease: 1972,* Washington, DC, 1973, U.S. Government Printing Office.)

inactivated polio vaccine. Polioviruses are spread most often during the summer and autumn.

Paralytic polio was once considered a middle-class disease because good hygiene would delay exposure of a person to the virus until late childhood, the adolescent years, or adulthood, when infection would produce the most severe symptoms. Infection during early childhood generally results in asymptomatic or very mild disease.

Like poliovirus infection, coxsackie A virus disease is generally more severe in adults than in children. However, coxsackie B virus and some of the echoviruses (especially echovirus 11) can be particularly harmful to infants.

Clinical Syndromes

The clinical syndromes produced by the enteroviruses are determined by several factors, including (1) viral serotype, (2) infecting dose, (3) tissue tropism, (4) portal of entry, (5) patient's age, gender, and state of health, and (6) pregnancy. The incubation period for enterovirus disease varies from 1 to 35 days, depending on the virus, the target tissue, and the person's age. Viruses that affect oral and respiratory sites have the shortest incubation periods.

Poliovirus Infections

Wild-type polio infections are becoming rarer because of the success of the polio vaccines (see Fig. 54–6). As noted earlier, however, vaccine-associated cases of polio do occur, and some populations remain unvaccinated, putting them at risk for infection. Poliovirus may cause one of the following four outcomes in unvaccinated people, depending on the progression of the infection (Fig. 54–7):

Asymptomatic illness results if the viral infection is limited to the oropharynx and the gut. At least 90% of poliovirus infections are asymptomatic.

Abortive poliomyelitis, the **minor illness**, is a nonspecific febrile illness occurring in approximately 5% of infected people. Fever, headache, malaise, sore throat, and vomiting occur in such people within 3 to 4 days of exposure.

Nonparalytic poliomyelitis or **aseptic meningitis** occurs in 1% to 2% of patients with poliovirus infections. In this disease, the virus progresses into the central nervous system and the meninges, causing back pain and muscle spasms in addition to the symptoms of the minor illness.

Paralytic polio, the major illness, occurs in 0.1% to 2.0% of persons with poliovirus infections and is the most severe outcome. It appears 3 to 4 days after the minor illness has subsided, thereby producing a biphasic illness. In this disease, the virus spreads from

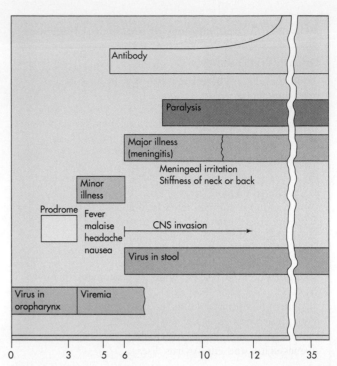

FIGURE 54–7. Progression of poliovirus infection. Infection may be asymptomatic or may progress to minor or major disease. CNS = central nervous system.

the blood to the **anterior horn cells** of the spinal cord and the motor cortex of the brain. The severity of the paralysis is determined by the extent of the neuronal infection and which neurons are affected. Spinal paralysis may involve one or more limbs, whereas bulbar (cranial) paralysis may involve a combination of cranial nerves and even the medullary respiratory center.

Paralytic poliomyelitis is characterized by an asymmetrical flaccid paralysis with no sensory loss. Poliovirus type 1 is responsible for 85% of the cases of paralytic polio. Reversion of the attenuated vaccine virus types 2 and 3 to virulence can cause vaccine-associated disease.

The degree of paralysis varies, in that it may involve only a few muscle groups (e.g., one leg) or there may be complete flaccid paralysis of all four extremities. The paralysis may then progress over the first few days and may result in complete recovery, residual paralysis, or death. Most recoveries occur within 6 months, but as long as 2 years may be required for complete remission.

Bulbar poliomyelitis can be more severe, may involve the muscles of the pharynx, vocal cords, and respiration, and may result in death in 75% of patients. Iron lungs, chambers that provided external respiratory compression, were used during the 1950s to assist the breathing of patients with such polio disease. Before vaccination programs, iron lungs filled the wards of children's hospitals.

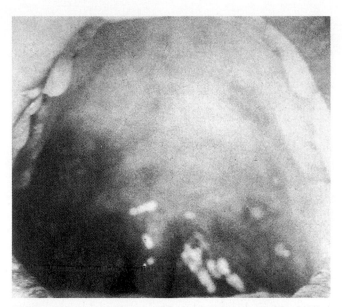

FIGURE 54–8. Herpangina. Characteristic discrete vesicles are seen on the anterior tonsillar pillars. (Courtesy Dr. GDW McKendrick. From Lambert HP et al: *Infectious diseases illustrated*, London, 1982, Gower.)

Postpolio syndrome is a sequela of poliomyelitis that may occur much later in life (30 to 40 years later) in 20% to 80% of the original victims. Affected people suffer a deterioration of the originally affected muscles. Poliovirus is not present, but the syndrome is believed to result from a loss of neurons in the initially affected nerves.

Coxsackievirus and Echovirus Infections

Several clinical syndromes may be caused by either a coxsackievirus or an echovirus (e.g., aseptic meningitis), but certain illnesses are specifically associated with coxsackieviruses. Coxsackie A viruses are associated with diseases involving vesicular lesions (e.g. herpangina), whereas coxsackie B viruses (**B for** *body*) are most frequently associated with myocarditis and pleurodynia. These viruses can also cause a polio-like paralytic disease. The most common result of infection is lack of symptoms or a mild upper respiratory tract or flu-like disease.

Herpangina is caused by several types of coxsackie A virus and is not related to a herpesvirus infection. Fever, sore throat, pain on swallowing, anorexia, and vomiting characterize this disorder. The classic finding is vesicular ulcerated lesions around the soft palate and uvula (Fig. 54–8). Less typically, the lesions affect the hard palate. The virus can be recovered from the lesions or from feces. The disease is self-limited and requires only symptomatic management.

Hand-foot-and-mouth disease is a vesicular exanthem usually caused by coxsackievirus A16. The name is descriptive because the main features of this infec-tion consist of vesicular lesions on the hands, feet, mouth, and tongue (Fig. 54–9). The patient is mildly febrile, and the illness subsides in a few days.

Pleurodynia (Bornholm's disease), also known as the devil's grip, is an acute illness in which patients have a sudden onset of fever and unilateral low thoracic, pleuritic chest pain that may be excruciating. Abdominal pain and even vomiting may also occur, and muscles on the involved side may be extremely tender. Pleurodynia lasts an average of 4 days but may relapse after the condition has been asymptomatic for several days. Coxsackie B virus is the causative agent.

Myocardial and **pericardial infections** caused by coxsackie B virus occur sporadically in older children and adults but are most threatening in newborns. Neonates with these infections have febrile illnesses and sudden and unexplained onset of heart failure. Cyanosis, tachycardia, cardiomegaly, and hepatomegaly occur. Electrocardiographic changes are found in patients with myocarditis. The mortality associated with the infection is high, and autopsy typically reveals the involvement of other organ systems, including the brain, liver, and pancreas. Acute benign pericarditis affects young adults but may be seen in older people. The symptoms resemble those of myocardial infarction with fever.

Viral (aseptic) meningitis is an acute febrile illness accompanied by headache and signs of meningeal irritation, including nuchal rigidity. Petechiae or a rash may occur in patients with enteroviral meningitis. Recovery is usually uneventful, unless the illness is associated with encephalitis (meningoencephalitis) or occurs in children younger than 1 year. Outbreaks of picorna-

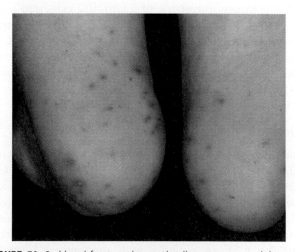

FIGURE 54–9. Hand-foot-and-mouth disease caused by coxsackie A virus. Lesions initially appear in the oral cavity and then develop within 1 day on the palms and, as seen here, soles. (From Habif TP: *Clinical dermatology: a color guide to diagnosis and therapy*, ed 3, St. Louis, 1996, Mosby.)

virus meningitis (echovirus 11) occur each year during the summer and autumn.

Fever, rash, and **common cold–like symptoms** may occur in patients infected with echoviruses or coxsackieviruses. The eruptions are usually maculopapular but may occasionally be petechial or even vesicular. The petechial type of eruption must be differentiated from that of meningococcemia. The symptoms of enteroviral infection are less intense for the child than meningococcemia. Coxsackieviruses A21 and A24 and echoviruses 11 and 20 can cause rhinovirus-like, cold-like symptoms.

Other Enterovirus Diseases

Enterovirus 70 and a variant of coxsackievirus A24 have been associated with an extremely contagious ocular disease, **acute hemorrhagic conjunctivitis**. The infection causes subconjunctival hemorrhages and conjunctivitis. The disease has a 24-hour incubation period and resolves within 1 or 2 weeks. Some strains of coxsackie B virus and echovirus can be transmitted transplacentally to the fetus. Infection of the fetus or an infant by this or another route may produce severe disseminated disease. Coxsackie B virus infections of the pancreas have been suspected of causing insulin-dependent diabetes as a result of the destruction of the islets of Langerhans.

Laboratory Diagnosis

Clinical Chemistry

Cerebrospinal fluid (CSF) from poliovirus or enterovirus aseptic meningitis reveals a predominantly lymphocytic pleocytosis (presence of 25 to 500 cells/mm³). In contrast with bacterial meningitis, the CSF in viral meningitis lacks neutrophils, and the glucose level is usually normal or slightly low. The CSF protein level is normal to slightly elevated. The CSF is rarely positive for the virus.

Culture

Polioviruses may be isolated from the patient's pharynx during the first few days of illness, from the feces for as long as 30 days, but from the CSF only rarely. The virus grows well in monkey kidney tissue culture. Coxsackieviruses and echoviruses can usually be isolated from the throat and stool during infection and often from the CSF in patients with meningitis. Virus is rarely isolated in patients with myocarditis, however, because the symptoms occur several weeks after the initial infection. The coxsackie B viruses can be grown on primary monkey or human embryo kidney cells. Many strains of coxsackie A virus do not grow in tissue

culture, however, and must still be grown in suckling mice. The specific type of enterovirus can be determined through the use of specific antibody and antigen assays (e.g., neutralization, immunofluorescence, enzyme-linked immunosorbent assay [ELISA]) or reverse transcriptase–polymerase chain reaction (RT-PCR) detection of specific viral RNA.

Serology is used to confirm an enterovirus infection through detection of specific immunoglobulin (Ig) M or the finding of a fourfold increase in the antibody titer between the time of the acute illness and the period of convalescence. This approach may not be practical for detection of echovirus and coxsackievirus because of their many serotypes, unless a specific virus is suspected.

Treatment, Prevention, and Control

A new antiviral drug, pleconaril, is available on a limited basis. The drug inhibits the penetration of picornaviruses into the cell. It must be administered early in the course of the infection.

The prevention of paralytic poliomyelitis is one of the triumphs of modern medicine. By 1979, infections with the wild-type poliovirus disappeared from the United States, with the number of cases of polio decreasing from 21,000 per year in the prevaccine era to 18 in unvaccinated patients in 1977. Like smallpox, polio has been targeted for elimination. Health care delivery to underdeveloped countries is more difficult, and for this reason, wild-type viral disease still exists in Africa, the Middle East, and Asia. New worldwide vaccination programs have been developed to reach the goal.

The two types of poliovirus vaccine are (1) **inactivated polio vaccine (IPV)**, developed by Jonas Salk, and (2) **live attenuated oral polio vaccine (OPV)**, developed by Albert Sabin. Both vaccines incorporate the three strains of polio, are stable, are relatively inexpensive, and induce a protective antibody response (Fig. 54–10). The IPV was proven effective in 1955, but the oral vaccine has been used instead because of its ease of delivery and its capacity to elicit lifelong immunity (Table 54–2). New recommendations now involve the use of the IPV for initial immunizations of babies because of its safety.

The OPV was *attenuated* (i.e., rendered less virulent) by passage in human or monkey cell cultures. Attenuation yielded a virus that can replicate in the oropharynx and intestinal tract but cannot infect neuronal cells. A mixed blessing of the live vaccine strain is that it is shed in feces for weeks and may be spread to close contacts. The spread will immunize or reimmunize close contacts, thus promoting mass immunization. The major drawbacks of the live vaccine are that (1) the vaccine virus may infect an immunologically com-

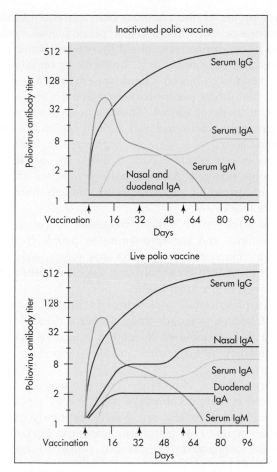

FIGURE 54–10. Serum and secretory antibody response to intramuscular inoculation of inactivated polio vaccine and to live attenuated oral polio vaccine. Note the presence of secretory IgA induced by the live polio vaccine. (Redrawn from Ogra P et al: Viral vaccination via the mucosal routes, *Rev Infect Dis* 2:352–369, 1980 ©1980, University of Chicago Press.)

promised individual and (2) there is a remote potential for the virus to revert to its virulent form and cause paralytic disease. The incidence of paralytic disease is estimated to be 1 per 4 million doses administered (versus 1 in 100 people infected with the wild-type poliovirus).

Children should receive the IPV at 2, 4, and 15 months and then at 4 to 6 years of age. Alternatively, the first two doses of IPV can be followed by OPV. The IPV has been administered instead of the OPV in several European countries for many years, with good results.

There are no vaccines for coxsackieviruses or echoviruses. Transmission of these viruses can presumably be reduced by improvements in hygiene and living conditions.

Rhinoviruses

Rhinoviruses are the most important cause of the **common cold** and upper respiratory tract infections. Such infections are self-limited, however, and do not cause serious disease. More than 100 serotypes of rhinovirus have been identified. At least 80% of the rhinoviruses have a common receptor that is also used by some of the coxsackieviruses. This receptor has been identified as ICAM-1, a member of the immunoglobulin superfamily, which is expressed on epithelial, fibroblast, and B-lymphoblastoid cells.

Pathogenesis and Immunity

Unlike the enteroviruses, rhinoviruses are **unable to replicate in the gastrointestinal tract** (see Box 54–3). The rhinoviruses are **labile to acidic pH**. Also,

TABLE 54–2. Advantages and Disadvantages of Polio Vaccines

Vaccine	Advantages	Disadvantages
Live (oral polio vaccine)	Effective Lifelong immunity Induction of secretory antibody response similar to that of natural infection Spread of attenuated virus circulating to contacts promotes indirect immunization (herd immunity) Ease of administration No need for repeated booster vaccine	Risk of vaccine-associated poliomyelitis in vaccine recipients or contacts Spread of vaccine to contacts without their consent Not safe for administration to immunodeficient patients
Inactivated polio vaccine	Effective Good stability during transport and in storage Safe administration in immunodeficient patients No risk of vaccine-related disease	Lack of induction of secretory antibody Booster vaccine needed for lifelong immunity Injection more painful than oral administration Higher community immunization levels needed than with live vaccine

they **grow best at 33°C**, a feature that may partly account for their predilection for the cooler environment of the nasal mucosa. Infection can be initiated by as little as one infectious viral particle. During the peak of illness, nasal secretions contain concentrations of 500 to 1000 infectious virions per milliliter. The virus enters through the nose, mouth, or eyes and initiates infection of the upper respiratory tract, including the throat. Most viral replication occurs in the nose, and the onset and the severity of the symptoms correlate with the time of viral shedding and the quantity (titer) of virus shed. Infected cells release bradykinin and histamine, which cause a "runny nose."

Interferon, which is generated in response to the infection, may limit the progression of the infection and contribute to the symptoms. Interestingly, the release of cytokines during inflammation can promote the spread of the virus by enhancing the expression of ICAM-1 viral receptors.

Immunity to rhinoviruses is transient and is unlikely to prevent subsequent infection because of the numerous serotypes of the virus. Both nasal secretory IgA and serum IgG antibody are induced by a primary rhinovirus infection and can be detected within a week of infection. The secretory IgA response dissipates quickly, and immunity begins to wane approximately 18 months after infection. Cell-mediated immunity is not likely to play an important role in controlling rhinovirus infections.

Epidemiology

Rhinoviruses cause at least half of all upper respiratory tract infections (Box 54–5). Other agents that cause the symptoms of the common cold are enteroviruses, coronaviruses, adenoviruses, and parainfluenza viruses. Rhinoviruses can be transmitted by two mechanisms, as aerosols and on fomites (e.g., by hands or on contaminated inanimate objects). Hands appear to be the major vector, and direct person-to-person contact is the predominant mode of spread. These nonenveloped viruses are extremely stable and can survive on such objects for many hours.

Rhinoviruses produce clinical illness in only half of the people infected. Asymptomatic people are also capable of spreading the virus, even though they may produce less virus.

Rhinovirus "colds" most frequently occur in the early autumn and the late spring in people living in temperate climates. These peaks may reflect social patterns (e.g., return to school and daycare) rather than any change in the virus itself.

Rates of infection are highest in infants and children. Children younger than 2 years "share" their colds with their families. Secondary infections occur in approximately 50% of family members, especially other children.

Many different rhinovirus serotypes may be found in a given community during a specific cold season, but the predominant strains are usually the newly categorized serotypes. This pattern indicates the existence of a gradual antigenic drift (mutation), similar to that seen for the influenza virus.

Clinical Syndromes

Common cold symptoms caused by rhinoviruses cannot readily be distinguished from those caused by other viral respiratory pathogens (e.g., enteroviruses, paramyxoviruses, coronaviruses). An upper respiratory tract infection usually begins with sneezing, which is soon followed by rhinorrhea (runny nose). The rhinorrhea increases and is then accompanied by symptoms of nasal obstruction. Mild sore throat also occurs, along with headache and malaise. The illness peaks in 3 to 4 days, but the cough and nasal symptoms may persist for 7 to 10 days or longer. Fever and rigors sometimes accompany rhinovirus infections.

Laboratory Diagnosis

The clinical syndrome of the common cold is usually so characteristic that laboratory diagnosis is unnecessary. Virus can be obtained from nasal washings. Rhinoviruses are grown in human diploid fibroblast cells (e.g., WI-38) at 33°C. Virus is identified by the typical cytopathologic effect and the demonstration of acid lability. Serotyping is rarely necessary but can be performed with the use of pools of specific neutralizing sera. The performance of serologic testing to document rhinovirus infection is not practical.

BOX 54–5. **Epidemiology of Rhinovirus Infections**

Disease/Viral Factors

Virion is resistant to drying and detergents.
  Replication occurs at optimum temperature of 33°C and cooler temperatures.

Transmission

Direct contact via infected hands and fomites.
  Inhalation of infectious droplets.

Who Is at Risk?

People of all ages.

Geography/Season

Virus is found worldwide.
  Disease is more common in early autumn and late spring.

Modes of Control

Washing hands and disinfecting contaminating object help prevent spread.

Treatment, Prevention, and Control

There are many over-the-counter remedies for the common cold. Nasal vasoconstrictors may provide relief, but their use may be followed by rebound congestion and a worsening of symptoms. Rigorous studies of vitamin C therapy have not shown it to be efficacious.

Pleconaril inhibits rhinovirus replication but has not proved therapeutically useful in controlling rhinovirus infections. The intranasal administration of interferon can block infection for a short time after a known exposure, but its long-term use (e.g., throughout the "cold season") could cause symptoms at least as bad as those of the rhinovirus infection. Experimental antiviral drugs similar to pleconaril, such as arildone, rhodanine, disoxaril, and their analogues, contain a 3-methylisoxazole group that inserts into the base of the receptor-binding canyon and blocks uncoating of the virus. Enviroxime inhibits the viral RNA–dependent RNA polymerase. A polypeptide receptor analogue based on the ICAM-1 protein structure may have potential as an antiviral drug.

Rhinovirus is not a good candidate for a vaccine program. The multiple serotypes, the apparent antigenic drift in rhinoviral antigens, the requirement for secretory IgA production, and the transience of the antibody response pose major problems for the development of vaccines. In addition, the benefit-to-risk ratio would be very low because rhinoviruses do not cause significant disease.

Hand washing and the disinfection of contaminated objects are the best means of preventing the spread of the virus. The impregnation of facial tissues with antiviral chemicals has been attempted, but the product was not a commercial success.

CASE STUDY AND QUESTIONS

■ A 6-year-old girl was brought to the doctor's office at 4:30 PM because she had a sore throat, had been unusually tired, and was napping excessively. Her temperature was 39°C. She had an erythematous throat with enlarged tonsils and a faint rash on her back. At 10:30 PM, the patient's mother reported that the child had vomited three times, continued to nap excessively, and complained of a headache when awake.

The doctor examined the child at 11:30 PM and noted that she was lethargic and aroused only when her head was turned, complaining that her back hurt. Her CSF contained no red blood cells, but there were 28 white blood cells/mm³, half polymorphonuclear neutrophils and half lymphocytes. The glucose and protein levels in the CSF were normal, and Gram stain of a specimen of CSF showed no bacteria.

1. What were the key signs and symptoms in this case?
2. What was the differential diagnosis?
3. What signs and symptoms suggested an enterovirus infection?
4. How would the diagnosis be confirmed?
5. What were the most likely sources and means of infection?
6. What were the target tissue and mechanism of pathogenesis?

BIBLIOGRAPHY

Ansardi D et al: Poliovirus assembly and encapsidation of genomic RNA, *Adv Virus Res* 46:2–70, 1996.

Fields BN et al, editors: *Virology*, ed 3, New York, 1996, Lippincott-Raven.

Levandowski RA: Rhinoviruses. In Belshe RB, editor: *Textbook of human virology*, ed 2, St Louis, 1991, Mosby.

McKinlay MA et al: Treatment of the picornavirus common cold by inhibitors of viral uncoating and attachment, *Ann Rev Microbiol* 46:635–654, 1992.

Melnick JL: Live attenuated poliovaccines. In Plotkin SA, Martin EA, editors: *Vaccines*, Philadelphia, 1988, WB Saunders.

Moore M, Morens DM: Enteroviruses including polioviruses. In Belshe RB, editor: *Textbook of human virology*, ed 2, St. Louis, 1991, Mosby.

Racaniello VR: Picornaviruses, *Curr Top Microbiol Immunol* 161:1–192, 1990.

Ren R, Racaniello VR: Human poliovirus receptor gene expression and poliovirus tissue tropism in transgenic mice, *J Virol* 66:296–304, 1992.

Robbins FC: Polio: historical. In Plotkin SA, Martin EA, editors: *Vaccines*, Philadelphia, 1988, WB Saunders.

Salk J, Drucker J: Noninfectious poliovirus vaccine. In Plotkin SA, Martin EA, editors: *Vaccines*, Philadelphia, 1988, WB Saunders.

Tracy S, Chapman NM, Mahy BWJ: Coxsackie B viruses. *Current Topics in Microbiology and Immunology*, Vol 223, Berlin, 1997, Springer-Verlag.

Wilfert CM et al: Enteroviruses and meningitis, *Pediatr Infect Dis* 2:333–341, 1983.

C H A P T E R 5 5

Paramyxoviruses

The Paramyxoviridae include the following genera: *Morbillivirus*, *Paramyxovirus*, and *Pneumovirus* (Table 55–1). Human pathogens within the morbilliviruses include the **measles** virus; within the paramyxoviruses, the **parainfluenza** and **mumps** viruses; and within the pneumoviruses, the **respiratory syncytial virus** (RSV). Their virions have similar morphologies and protein components, and they share the capacity to induce **cell-cell fusion** (syncytia formation and multinucleated giant cells). A new group of highly pathogenic paramyxoviruses including two zoonosis-causing viruses, **Nipah virus** and **Hendra virus**, was identified in 1998 following an outbreak of severe encephalitis in Malaysia and Singapore.

The major diseases these agents cause are well known. Measles virus causes a potentially serious generalized infection characterized by a maculopapular rash (**rubeola**). Parainfluenza viruses cause upper and lower respiratory tract infections, primarily in children, including pharyngitis, croup, bronchitis, bronchiolitis, and pneumonia. Mumps virus causes a systemic infection whose most prominent clinical manifestation is parotitis. RSV causes mild upper respiratory tract infections in children and adults but can cause life-threatening pneumonia in infants.

Measles and mumps viruses have *only one serotype*, and protection is provided by an effective **live vaccine**. In the United States and other developed countries, successful vaccination programs using the live attenuated measles and mumps vaccines have made measles and mumps rare. In particular, these programs have led to the virtual elimination of the serious sequelae of measles.

Structure and Replication

Paramyxoviruses consist of **negative-sense, single-stranded RNA** (5 to 8 × 10⁶ Da) in a helical nucleocapsid surrounded by a pleomorphic **envelope** of approximately 156 to 300 nm (Fig. 55–1). They are similar in many respects to orthomyxoviruses but are larger and do not have the unique segmented genome of the influenza viruses (Box 55–1). Although significant homology exists among paramyxovirus genomes, the order of the protein-coding regions differs for each genus. The gene products of the measles virus are listed in Table 55–2.

The nucleocapsid consists of the negative-sense, single-stranded RNA associated with the nucleoprotein (**NP**), polymerase phosphoprotein (**P**), and large (**L**) protein. The L protein is the RNA polymerase, the P protein facilitates RNA synthesis, and the NP protein helps maintain genomic structure. The nucleocapsid associates with the matrix (**M**) protein at the base of the lipid envelope. The virion envelope contains two glycoproteins, a fusion (**F**) protein, which promotes fusion of the viral and host cell membranes, and a viral attachment protein (hemagglutinin-neuraminidase [**HN**], hemagglutinin [**H**], or **G** protein) (see Box 55–1). The F protein must be activated by proteolytic cleavage, which produces F_1 and F_2 glycopeptides held together by a disulfide bond, to express membrane-fusing activity.

Replication of the paramyxoviruses is initiated by the binding of the HN, H, or G protein on the virion envelope to sialic acid on the cell surface glycolipids. A major receptor for measles virus is CD46 (membrane cofactor protein, MCP); this receptor is present on most cell types and protects the cell from complement by regulating complement activation. The F protein promotes fusion of the envelope with the plasma membrane. Paramyxoviruses are also able to induce cell-cell fusion, thereby creating multinucleated giant cells (syncytia).

The replication of the genome occurs in a manner similar to that of other negative-strand RNA viruses (i.e., rhabdoviruses). The RNA polymerase is carried into the cell as part of the nucleocapsid. Transcription, protein synthesis, and replication of the genome all occur in the host cell's cytoplasm. The genome is transcribed into individual messenger RNAs (mRNAs) and a full-length positive-sense RNA template. New genomes associate with the L, N, and NP proteins to form nucleocapsids, which associate with the M pro-

TABLE 55–1. Paramyxoviridae

Genus	Human Pathogen
Morbillivirus	Measles virus
Paramyxovirus	Parainfluenza viruses 1 to 4
	Mumps virus
Pneumovirus	Respiratory syncytial virus

BOX 55–1. Unique Features of the Paramyxoviridae

Large virion consists of a negative RNA genome in a helical nucleocapsid surrounded by an envelope containing a viral attachment protein (HN, parainfluenza and mumps virus; H, measles virus; and G, respiratory syncytial virus [RSV]) and a fusion glycoprotein (F).

The three genera can be distinguished by the activities of the viral attachment protein: HN of paramyxovirus and mumps virus has hemagglutinin and neuraminidase, and H of measles virus has hemagglutinin activity, but G of RSV lacks these activities.

Virus replicates in the cytoplasm.

Virions penetrate the cell by fusion with and exit by budding from the plasma membrane.

Viruses induce cell-cell fusion, causing multinucleated giant cells.

Paramyxoviridae are transmitted in respiratory droplets and initiate infection in the respiratory tract.

Cell-mediated immunity causes many of the symptoms but is essential for control of the infection.

teins on viral glycoprotein–modified plasma membranes. The glycoproteins are synthesized and processed like cellular glycoproteins. Mature virions then bud from the host cell plasma membrane and exit the cell. Replication of the paramyxoviruses is represented by the RSV infectious cycle shown in Figure 55–2.

Measles Virus

Measles is one of the five classic childhood exanthems, along with rubella, roseola, fifth disease, and chickenpox. Historically, measles was one of the most common and unpleasant viral infections with potential sequelae. Before 1960, the rash, high fever, cough, conjunctivitis, and coryza affected more than 90% of the population younger than 20 years. Since the use of the live vaccine began in 1993, fewer than 1000 cases

have been reported in the United States. Measles is still one of the most prominent causes of disease (30 to 40 million cases per year) and death (1 to 2 million per year) worldwide in unvaccinated populations.

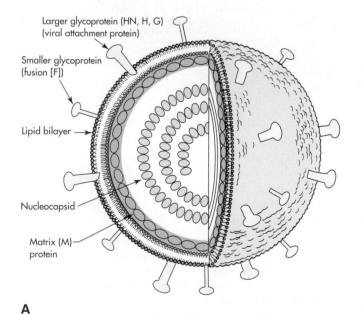

A

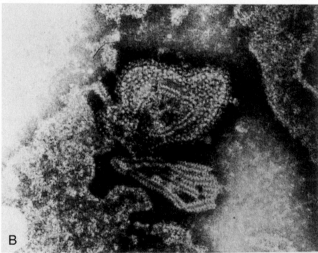

B

FIGURE 55–1. *A,* Model of paramyxovirus. The helical nucleocapsid—consisting of negative-sense, single-stranded RNA and the P protein, nucleoprotein (NP), and large (L) protein—associates with the matrix (M) protein at the envelope membrane surface. The nucleocapsid contains RNA transcriptase activity. The envelope contains the viral attachment glycoprotein (hemagglutinin-neuraminidase [HN], hemagglutinin [H], or G protein [G]) and the fusion (F) protein. *B,* Electron micrograph of a disrupted paramyxovirus showing the helical nucleocapsid. (*A* redrawn from Jawetz E, Melnick JL, Adelberg EA: *Review of medical microbiology,* ed 17, Norwalk, Conn, 1987, Appleton & Lange; *B* courtesy Centers for Disease Control and Prevention, Atlanta.)

TABLE 55–2. Viral-Encoded Proteins of Measles Virus

Gene Products*	Virion Location	Function
Nucleoprotein (NP)	Major internal protein	Protection of viral RNA
Polymerase phosphoprotein (P)	Association with nucleoprotein	Possible part of transcription complex
Matrix (M)	Inside virion envelope	Assembly of virions
Fusion factor (F)	Transmembranous envelope glycoprotein	Factor active in fusion of cells, hemolysis, and viral entry
Hemagglutinin-neuraminidase (HN): hemagglutinin (H); glycoprotein (G)	Transmembranous envelope glycoprotein	Viral attachment proteins
Large protein (L)	Association with nucleoprotein	Polymerase

*In order of transcription.
Modified from Fields BN, editor: *Virology*, New York, 1985, Raven.

Pathogenesis and Immunity

Measles is known for its propensity to cause cell fusion, leading to the formation of giant cells (Box 55–2). As a result, the virus can pass directly from cell to cell and escape antibody control. Inclusions occur most commonly in the cytoplasm and are composed of incomplete viral particles. Infection usually leads to cell lysis, but persistent infections without lysis can occur in certain cell types (e.g., human brain cells).

Measles is **highly contagious** and is transmitted from person to person by **respiratory droplets** (Fig. 55–3). Local replication of virus in the respiratory tract precedes its spread to the lymphatic system and viremia. The wide dissemination of the virus causes infection of the conjunctiva, respiratory tract, urinary tract, small blood vessels, lymphatic system, and the central nervous system. During the incubation period, measles causes a decrease in eosinophils and lymphocytes, including B and T cells, and a depression of their response to activation (mitogens). *The characteristic measles rash is caused by immune T cells targeted to measles-infected endothelial cells lining small blood vessels.* Recovery follows the rash in most patients, who then have **lifelong immunity** to the virus. The time course of measles infection is shown in Figure 55–4.

Measles can cause encephalitis in three ways: direct infection of neurons, a postinfectious encephalitis, which is believed to be immune mediated, and subacute sclerosing panencephalitis (SSPE) caused by a defective variant of measles generated during the acute disease. The SSPE virus acts as a slow virus and causes cytopathologic effect in neurons and symptoms many years after acute disease.

Cell-mediated immunity is responsible for most of the symptoms and is essential for the control of measles infection. T-cell–deficient children who are infected with measles have an atypical presentation consisting of a **giant cell pneumonia without a rash.**

Immunocompromised patients with measles may not be able to resolve the infection, resulting in death.

Epidemiology

The development of effective vaccine programs has made measles a rare disease in the United States. In areas without a vaccine program, epidemics tend to occur in 1- to 3-year cycles, when a sufficient number of susceptible people has accumulated. Many of these cases occur in preschool-aged children who have not been vaccinated and who live in large urban areas. The incidence of infection peaks in the winter and spring. Measles is still common in people living in developing countries and is the most significant cause of death in children 1 to 5 years of age in several countries.

Measles, which can be spread in respiratory secretions before and after the onset of characteristic symptoms, is one of the most contagious infections known

---

BOX 55–2. Disease Mechanisms of Measles Virus

Virus infects epithelial cells of respiratory tract.

Virus spreads systemically in lymphocytes and by **viremia.**

Virus replicates in cells of conjunctivae, respiratory tract, urinary tract, lymphatic system, blood vessels, and central nervous system.

Rash is caused by T-cell response to virus-infected epithelial cells lining capillaries.

Cell-mediated immunity is essential to control infection; antibody is not sufficient because of measles' ability to spread cell to cell.

Sequelae in central nervous system may result from immunopathogenesis (postinfectious measles encephalitis) or development of defective mutants (subacute sclerosing panencephalitis).

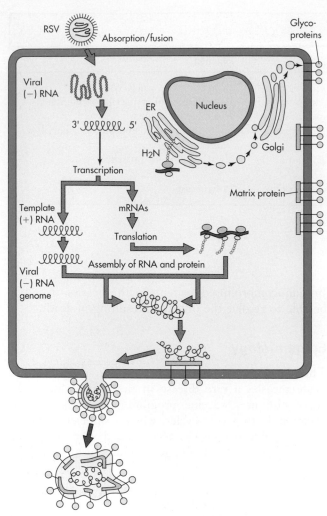

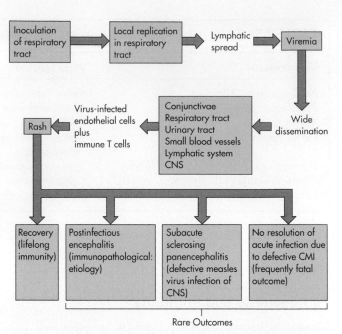

FIGURE 55–3. Mechanisms of spread of the measles virus within the body and the pathogenesis of measles. CNS = central nervous system; CMI = cell-mediated immunity.

to 1962. A 15-fold increase in the incidence of measles was noted between 1989 and 1991 in the United States, however, resulting mainly from poor compliance with vaccination programs.

FIGURE 55–2. Replication of paramyxoviruses. The virus binds to glycolipids or proteins and fuses with the cell surface. Individual mRNAs for each protein and a full-length template are transcribed from the genome. Replication occurs in the cytoplasm. The nucleocapsid associates with matrix and glycoprotein-modified plasma membranes and leaves the cell by budding. (−) = Negative sense; (+) = positive sense; ER = endoplasmic reticulum. (Redrawn from Balows A, Hausler WJ Jr, Lennette-EH: *Laboratory diagnosis of infectious diseases: principles and practice*, New York, 1988, Springer-Verlag.)

(Box 55–3). In a household, approximately 85% of exposed susceptible people become infected, and 95% of these people develop clinical disease.

The measles virus has only one serotype and infects only humans, and infection usually manifests as symptoms. These properties facilitated the development of an effective vaccine program. Once vaccination was introduced, the yearly incidence of measles dropped dramatically in the United States, from 300 to 1.3 per 100,000 (U.S. statistics for 1981 to 1988). This change represented a 99.5% reduction in the incidence of the infection from that in the prevaccination period 1955

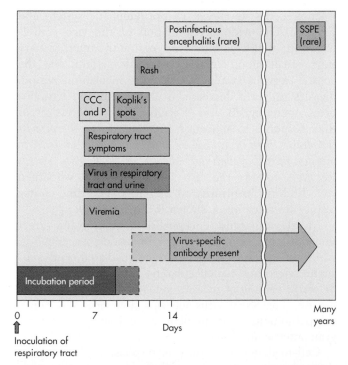

FIGURE 55–4. Time course of measles virus infection. Characteristic prodrome symptoms are cough, conjunctivitis, coryza, and photophobia (CCC and P), followed by the appearance of Koplik's spots and rash. SSPE = Subacute sclerosing panencephalitis.

BOX 55−3. Epidemiology of Measles

Disease/Viral Factors

Virus has large virion that is easily inactivated by dryness and acid.
Contagion period precedes symptoms.
Host range is limited to humans.
Only one serotype exists.
Immunity is lifelong.

Transmission

Inhalation of large-droplet aerosols.

Who Is at Risk?

Unvaccinated people.
Immunocompromised people, who have more serious outcomes.

Geography/Season

Virus is found worldwide.
Virus is endemic from autumn to spring, possibly because of crowding indoors.

Modes of Control

Live attenuated vaccine (Schwartz or Moraten variants of Edmonston B strain) can be administered.
Immune serum globulin can be administered after exposure.

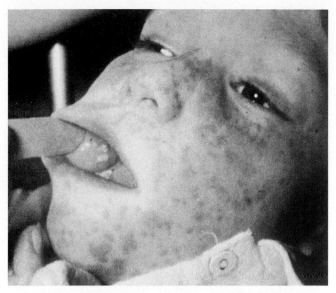

FIGURE 55−5. Koplik's spots in the mouth and exanthem. Koplik's spots usually precede the measles rash and may be seen for the first day or two after the rash appears. (Courtesy Dr. J.I. Pugh, St. Albans; from Emond RTD, Rowland HAK: *A color atlas of infectious diseases,* ed 3, London, 1995, Mosby.)

Clinical Syndromes

Measles is a serious febrile illness (Table 55−3). The incubation period lasts 7 to 13 days, and the prodrome starts with **high fever** and CCC and P—**cough, coryza, and conjunctivitis**, in addition to **photophobia**. The disease is most infectious at this time.

After 2 days of illness, the typical mucous membrane lesions, known as **Koplik's spots** (Fig. 55−5), appear. They are seen most commonly on the buccal mucosa across from the molars, but they may appear on other mucous membranes as well, including the conjunctivae and the vagina. The lesions, which last 24 to 48 hours, are usually small (1 to 2 mm) and are best described as grains of salt surrounded by a red halo. Their appearance in the mouth establishes with certainty the diagnosis of measles.

Within 12 to 24 hours of the appearance of Koplik's spots, the **exanthem** of measles starts below the ears and spreads over the body. The **rash is maculopapular** and usually very extensive, and often the lesions become confluent. The rash, which takes 1 or 2 days to cover the body, fades in the same order in which it appeared over the body. The fever is highest and the patient the sickest on the day the rash appears (Fig. 55−6).

TABLE 55−3. Clinical Consequences of Measles Virus Infection

Disorder	Symptoms
Measles	Characteristic maculopapular rash, cough, conjunctivitis, coryza, photophobia, Koplik's spots *Complications:* otitis media, croup, bronchopneumonia, and encephalitis
Atypical measles	Rash (most prominent in distal areas); possible vesicles, petechiae, purpura, or urticaria
Subacute sclerosing panencephalitis	Central nervous system manifestations (e.g., personality, behavior, and memory changes; myoclonic jerks; spasticity; and blindness)

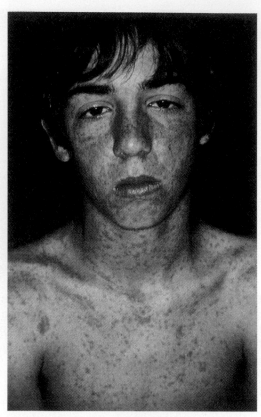

FIGURE 55–6. Measles rash. (From Habif TP: *Clinical dermatology: Color guide to diagnosis and therapy*, St Louis, 1985, Mosby.)

Pneumonia, which can also be a serious complication, accounts for 60% of the deaths caused by measles. The mortality associated with pneumonia, like the incidence of the other complications associated with measles, is higher in the setting of malnutrition and is inversely proportional to age. **Bacterial superinfection** is common in patients with pneumonia due to the measles virus.

One of the most feared complications of measles is **encephalitis**, which may occur in as many as 0.5% of those infected and may be fatal in 15% of cases. Encephalitis can rarely result during acute disease, but usually begins 7 to 10 days after the onset of illness. **This post-infectious encephalitis** is due to immunopathologic reactions, is associated with demyelination of neurons, and occurs more often in older children and adults.

Atypical measles occurred in people who received the older inactivated measles vaccine and were subsequently exposed to the wild measles virus. It may also rarely occur in those vaccinated with the attenuated virus vaccine. Prior sensitization with insufficient protection enhances the immunopathologic response to the challenge by wild measles virus. The illness begins abruptly and is a more intense presentation of measles.

Subacute sclerosing panencephalitis (SSPE) is an extremely serious, very late neurologic sequela of measles that afflicts about 7 in every 1 million patients. The incidence of SSPE has decreased markedly as the result of the measles vaccination programs.

This disease occurs when a defective measles virus persists in the brain and acts as a slow virus. The virus can replicate and spread directly from cell to cell but is not released. SSPE is most prevalent in children who were initially infected when younger than 2 years and occurs approximately 7 years after clinical measles. The patient demonstrates changes in personality, behavior, and memory, followed by myoclonic jerks, blindness, and spasticity. Unusually high levels of measles antibodies are found in the blood and cerebrospinal fluid of patients with SSPE.

The immunocompromised and malnourished child is at highest risk for severe outcome of measles. **Giant cell pneumonia without rash** occurs in children lacking T-cell immunity. Severe bacterial superinfection and pneumonia occur in malnourished children, with up to 25% mortality.

Laboratory Diagnosis

The clinical manifestations of measles are usually so characteristic that it is rarely necessary to perform laboratory tests to establish the diagnosis. The measles virus is difficult to isolate and grow, although it can be grown in primary human or monkey cell cultures. Respiratory tract secretions, urine, blood, and brain tissue are the recommended specimens. It is best to collect respiratory and blood specimens during the prodromal stage and up until 1 to 2 days after the appearance of the rash.

Measles antigen can be detected with immunofluorescence in pharyngeal cells or urinary sediment, but this test is not generally available. Characteristic cytopathologic effects, including multinucleated giant cells with cytoplasmic and nuclear inclusion bodies, can be seen in Giemsa-stained cells taken from the upper respiratory tract and urinary sediment.

Antibody, especially immunoglobulin (Ig) M, can be detected when the rash is present. Measles infection can be confirmed by the finding of seroconversion or a fourfold increase in the titer of measles-specific antibodies between sera obtained during the acute stage and the convalescent stage.

Treatment, Prevention, and Control

A live attenuated measles vaccine, in use since 1963, has been responsible for a significant reduction in the incidence of measles in the United States. The current Schwartz or Moraten attenuated strains of the original Edmonston B vaccine are being used in the United States. Live attenuated vaccine is given to all children at 2 years of age, in combination with mumps and rubella vaccines (**MMR vaccine**) (Box 55–4). Although immunization is successful in more than 95% of vaccinees, revaccination is required in most states for children before grade school or junior high school. As noted earlier, a killed measles vaccine, which was introduced in 1963, was not protective, and its use was subsequently discontinued because recipients were at risk for the more serious atypical measles presentation upon infection.

Hospitals in areas experiencing endemic measles may wish to vaccinate or check the immune status of their employees to decrease the risk of nosocomial transmission.

Exposed susceptible people who are immunocompromised should be given immune globulin to lessen the risk and severity of clinical illness. This product is most effective if given within 6 days of exposure. No specific antiviral treatment is available for measles.

Parainfluenza Viruses

Parainfluenza viruses, which were discovered in the late 1950s, are respiratory viruses that usually cause **mild coldlike symptoms** but can also cause **serious respiratory tract disease**. Four serologic types within the parainfluenza genus are human pathogens. Types 1, 2, and 3 are second only to RSV as important causes of severe lower respiratory tract infection in infants and young children. They are especially associated with **laryngotracheobronchitis (croup)**. Type 4 causes only mild upper respiratory tract infection in children and adults.

Pathogenesis and Immunity

Parainfluenza viruses infect epithelial cells of the upper respiratory tract (Box 55–5). The virus replicates more rapidly than measles and mumps viruses and can cause giant cell formation and cell lysis. Unlike measles and

---

BOX 55–4. Measles-Mumps-Rubella (MMR) Vaccine

Composition: live attenuated viruses
   Measles: Schwartz or Moraten substrains of Edmonston B strain
   Mumps: Jeryl Lynn strain
   Rubella: RA/27-3 strain
   Vaccination schedule: at 15–24 months and at 4–6 years or before junior high school
   Efficiency: 95% lifelong immunization with a single dose

Data from update on adult immunization, *MMWR Morb Mortal Wkly Rep* 40(RR-12), 1991.

BOX 55–5. Disease Mechanisms of Parainfluenza Viruses

There are four serotypes of viruses.
Infection is **limited to respiratory tract**; upper respiratory tract disease is most common, but significant disease can occur with lower respiratory tract infection.
Parainfluenza viruses are not systemic and do *not* cause viremia.
Diseases include **coldlike** symptoms, **bronchitis** (inflammation of bronchial tubes), and **croup** (laryngotracheobronchitis).
Infection induces protective immunity of short duration.

---

mumps viruses, the parainfluenza viruses rarely cause viremia. The viruses generally stay in the upper respiratory tract, causing only coldlike symptoms. In approximately 25% of cases, the virus spreads to the lower respiratory tract, and in 2% to 3%, disease may take the severe form of laryngotracheobronchitis.

The cell-mediated immune response both causes cell damage and confers protection. Ig A responses are protective but short-lived. Multiple serotypes and the short duration of immunity after natural infection make reinfection common, but the reinfection disease is milder, suggesting at least partial immunity.

Epidemiology

Parainfluenza viruses are ubiquitous, and infection is common (Box 55–6). The virus is transmitted by person-to-person contact and respiratory droplets. Primary infections usually occur in infants and children younger than 5 years. Reinfections occur throughout life, indicating that immunity is short-lived. Infections with parainfluenza viruses 1 and 2, the major causes of croup, tend to occur in the autumn, whereas parainfluenza virus 3 infections occur throughout the year. All of these viruses spread readily within hospitals and can cause outbreaks in nurseries and pediatric wards.

Clinical Syndromes

Parainfluenza viruses 1, 2, and 3 may cause respiratory tract syndromes ranging from a **mild coldlike upper respiratory tract infection** (coryza, pharyngitis, mild bronchitis, wheezing, and fever) to **bronchiolitis** and **pneumonia**. Older children and adults generally experience milder infections than those seen in young children, although pneumonia may occur in the elderly.

A parainfluenza virus infection in infants may be more severe than infections in adults, causing bronchiolitis, pneumonia, and, most notably, croup (laryngotracheobronchitis). **Croup** results in subglottal swell-

---

BOX 55–6. Epidemiology of Parainfluenza Virus Infections

Disease/Viral Factors

Virus has large virion that is easily inactivated by dryness and acid.

Contagion period precedes symptoms and may occur in absence of symptoms.

Host range is limited to humans.

Reinfection can occur later in life.

Transmission

Inhalation of large-droplet aerosols.

Who Is at Risk?

Children: at risk for mild disease and croup.

Adults: at risk for reinfection with milder symptoms.

Geography/Season

Virus is ubiquitous and worldwide.

Incidence is seasonal.

Modes of Control

There are no modes of control.

---

ing, which may close the airway. Hoarseness, a "seal bark" cough, tachypnea, tachycardia, and suprasternal retraction develop in infected patients after a 2- to 6-day incubation period. Most children recover within 48 hours. The principal differential diagnosis is epiglottitis due to *Haemophilus influenzae*.

Laboratory Diagnosis

Parainfluenza virus is isolated from nasal washings and respiratory secretions and grows well in primary monkey kidney cells. Like other paramyxoviruses, the virions are labile during transit to the laboratory. The presence of virus-infected cells in aspirates or in cell culture is indicated by the finding of syncytia and is identified with immunofluorescence. Like the hemagglutinin of the influenzaviruses, the hemagglutinin of the parainfluenza viruses promotes hemadsorption and hemagglutination. The serotype of the virus can be determined through the use of specific antibody to block hemadsorption or hemagglutination (hemagglutination inhibition).

Treatment, Prevention, and Control

Treatment of croup consists of the administration of nebulized cold or hot steam and careful monitoring of the upper airway. On rare occasions, intubation may become necessary. No specific antiviral agents are available.

Vaccination with killed vaccines is ineffective, possibly because they fail to induce local secretory antibody and appropriate cellular immunity. No live attenuated vaccine is available.

Mumps Virus

Mumps virus is the cause of acute, benign viral **parotitis** (painful swelling of the salivary glands). Mumps is rarely seen in countries that promote use of the live vaccine, which is administered with the measles and rubella live vaccines.

Mumps virus was isolated in embryonated eggs in 1945 and in cell culture in 1955. The virus is most closely related to parainfluenza virus 2, but there is no cross-immunity with the parainfluenza viruses.

Pathogenesis and Immunity

The mumps virus, of which only one serotype is known, causes a lytic infection of cells (Box 55–7). The virus initiates infection in the epithelial cells of the upper respiratory tract and infects the parotid gland either by way of Stensen's duct or by means of a viremia. The virus is spread by the viremia throughout the body to the testes, ovary, pancreas, thyroid, and other organs. Infection of the central nervous system, especially the meninges, with symptoms (meningoencephalitis) occurs in as many as 50% of those infected (Fig. 55–7). Inflammatory responses are mainly responsible for the symptoms. The time course of human infection is shown in Figure 55–8. Immunity is lifelong.

Epidemiology

Mumps, like measles, is a very communicable disease with only one serotype, and it infects only humans (Box 55–8). In the absence of vaccination programs, infection occurs in 90% of people by age 15 years. The virus is spread by direct person-to-person contact

---

BOX 55–7. Disease Mechanisms of Mumps Virus

Virus infects epithelial cells of respiratory tract.

Virus spreads systemically by viremia.

Infection of parotid gland, testes, and central nervous system occurs.

Principal symptom is swelling of parotid glands due to inflammation.

Cell-mediated immunity is essential for control of infection and is responsible for causing portion of symptoms. Antibody is not sufficient because of virus's ability to spread cell to cell.

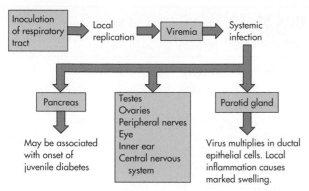

FIGURE 55–7. Mechanism of spread of mumps virus within the body.

and respiratory droplets. The virus is present in respiratory secretions for as long as 7 days before clinical illness occurs and often does not produce symptoms, so it is virtually impossible to control the spread of the virus. Living or working in close quarters promotes the spread of the virus, and the incidence of the infection is greatest in the winter and spring.

Clinical Syndromes

Mumps infections are often asymptomatic. Clinical illness manifests as a parotitis that is almost always bilateral and accompanied by fever. Onset is sudden. Oral examination reveals redness and swelling of the ostium of Stensen's duct. The swelling of other glands (epididymo-orchitis, oophoritis, mastitis, pancreatitis, and thyroiditis) and meningoencephalitis may occur a few days after the onset of the viral infection but can occur in the absence of parotitis. The swelling resulting from mumps orchitis may cause sterility. Mumps virus involves the central nervous system in approximately 50% of patients; and 10% of those affected may exhibit clinical evidence of such an infection.

Laboratory Diagnosis

Virus can be recovered from saliva, urine, the pharynx, secretions from Stensen's duct, and cerebrospinal fluid. Virus is present in saliva for approximately 5 days after the onset of symptoms and in urine for as long as 2 weeks. Mumps virus grows well in monkey kidney cells, causing the formation of multinucleated giant cells. The hemadsorption of guinea pig erythrocytes also occurs on virus-infected cells, due to the viral hemagglutinin.

A clinical diagnosis can be confirmed by serologic testing. A fourfold increase in the virus-specific antibody level or the detection of mumps-specific IgM antibody indicates active infection. Enzyme-linked immunosorbent assay, immunofluorescence tests, and hemagglutination inhibition can be used to detect the mumps virus, antigen, or antibody.

Treatment, Prevention, and Control

Vaccines provide the only effective means for preventing the spread of mumps infection. Since the introduc-

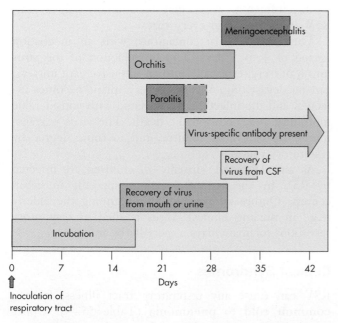

FIGURE 55–8. Time course of mumps virus infection.

tion of the live attenuated vaccine (Jeryl Lynn vaccine) in the United States in 1967 and its administration as part of the MMR vaccine, the yearly incidence of the infection has declined from 76 to 2 per 100,000. Antiviral agents are not available.

Respiratory Syncytial Virus

RSV, first isolated from a chimpanzee in 1956, is a member of the Pneumovirus genus. It is the most common cause of **fatal acute respiratory tract infection** in infants and young children. It infects virtually everyone by 4 years of age, and reinfections occur throughout life, even among the elderly.

The major structural difference between RSV and the other paramyxoviruses is that the RSV has a smaller nucleocapsid. It also lacks hemagglutinin and neuraminidase activities.

Pathogenesis and Immunity

RSV produces an infection that is localized to the respiratory tract (Box 55–9). As the name suggests, RSV induces syncytia. The pathologic effect of RSV is mainly due to direct viral invasion of the respiratory epithelium, which is followed by immunologically mediated cell injury. Necrosis of the bronchi and bronchioles leads to the formation of "plugs" of mucus, fibrin, and necrotic material within smaller airways. The narrow airways of young infants are readily obstructed by such "plugs." Natural immunity does not prevent reinfection, and vaccination with killed vaccine appears to enhance the severity of subsequent disease.

Epidemiology

RSV is very prevalent in young children, and 65% to 98% of children in daycare centers are infected by age

---

> **BOX 55–9.** Disease Mechanisms of Respiratory Syncytial Virus
>
> Virus causes localized infection of respiratory tract.
> Virus does not cause viremia or systemic spread.
> Pneumonia results from cytopathologic spread of virus (including syncytia).
> Bronchiolitis is most likely mediated by host's immune response.
> Narrow airways of young infants are readily obstructed by virus-induced pathologic effects.
> Maternal antibody does not protect infant from infection.
> Natural infection does not prevent reinfection.
> Improper vaccination increases severity of disease.

> **BOX 55–10.** Epidemiology of Respiratory Syncytial Virus
>
> **Disease/Viral Factors**
>
> Virus has large virion that is easily inactivated by dryness and acid.
> Contagion period precedes symptoms and may occur in absence of symptoms.
> Host range is limited to humans.
>
> **Transmission**
>
> Inhalation of large-droplet aerosols.
>
> **Who Is at Risk?**
>
> Infants: lower respiratory tract infection (bronchiolitis and pneumonia).
> Children: spectrum of disease—mild to pneumonia.
> Adults: reinfection with milder symptoms.
>
> **Geography/Season**
>
> Virus is ubiquitous and is found worldwide.
> Incidence is seasonal.
>
> **Modes of Control**
>
> Immune globulin is available for infants at high risk.
> Aerosol ribavirin is available for infants with serious disease.

---

3 years (Box 55–10). As many as 25% to 33% of these cases involve the lower respiratory tract, and 1% are severe enough to necessitate hospitalization (occurring in as many as 95,000 children in the United States each year).

RSV infections almost always occur in the winter. Unlike influenza, which may occasionally skip a year, RSV epidemics occur every year.

The virus is very contagious, with an incubation period of 4 to 5 days. The introduction of the virus into a nursery, especially into an intensive care nursery, can be devastating. Virtually every infant becomes infected, and the infection is associated with considerable morbidity and, occasionally, death. The virus is transmitted on hands, by fomites, and to some degree by respiratory routes.

As already noted, virtually all children are infected by RSV by the age of 4 years, especially in urban centers. Outbreaks may also occur among the elderly (e.g., in nursing homes). Virus is shed in respiratory secretions for many days, especially by infants.

Clinical Syndromes

RSV can cause any respiratory tract illness, from a **common cold** to **pneumonia** (Table 55–4). Upper respiratory tract infection with prominent rhinorrhea

TABLE 55–4. Clinical Consequences of Respiratory Syncytial Virus Infection

Disorder	Age Group Affected
Bronchiolitis, pneumonia, or both	Fever, cough, dyspnea, and cyanosis in children younger than 1 year
Febrile rhinitis and pharyngitis	Children
Common cold	Older children and adults

("runny nose") is most common in older children and adults. A more severe lower respiratory tract illness, **bronchiolitis**, may occur in infants. Because of inflammation at the level of the bronchiole, there is air trapping and decreased ventilation. Clinically, the patient usually has low-grade fever, tachypnea, tachycardia, and expiratory wheezes over the lungs. Bronchiolitis is usually self-limited, but it can be a frightening disease to observe in an infant. It may be fatal in premature infants, individuals with underlying lung disease, and the immunocompromised.

Laboratory Diagnosis

RSV is difficult to isolate in cell culture. Commercially available immunofluorescence and enzyme immunoassay tests are available for direct detection of the viral antigen in infected cells and nasal washings. The finding of seroconversion or a fourfold or greater increase in the antibody titer can substantiate the diagnosis.

Treatment, Prevention, and Control

In otherwise healthy infants, treatment is supportive, consisting of the administration of oxygen, intravenous fluids, and nebulized cold steam. **Ribavirin**, a guanosine analogue, is approved for the treatment of patients predisposed to a more severe course (e.g., premature or immunocompromised infants). It is administered by inhalation (nebulization).

Passive immunization with anti-RSV immunoglobulin is available for premature infants. Infected children must be isolated. Control measures are required for hospital staff caring for infected children to avoid transmitting the virus to uninfected patients. These measures include hand-washing and the wearing of gowns, goggles, and masks.

No vaccine is currently available for RSV prophylaxis. A previously available vaccine containing inactivated RSV caused recipients to have more severe RSV infection when subsequently exposed to the live virus.

This development is thought to have resulted from the mounting of a heightened immunologic response at the time of exposure to the wild virus.

Nipah and Hendra Viruses

A new paramyxovirus, Nipah virus, was isolated from patients following an outbreak of severe encephalitis in Malaysia and Singapore in 1998. Nipah virus is more closely related to the Hendra virus, discovered in 1994 in Australia, than to other paramyxoviruses. Both viruses have broad host ranges, including pigs, man, dogs, horses, cats, and other mammals. For Nipah virus, the reservoir is a fruit bat (flying fox). The virus is amplified in pigs and spread to humans. The human is an accidental host for these viruses, but the outcome of human infection is severe. Of the 269 cases occurring in 1999, 108 were fatal.

CASE STUDY AND QUESTIONS

■ An 18-year-old college freshman complained of a cough, runny nose, and conjunctivitis. The physician in the campus health center noticed small white lesions inside the patient's mouth. The next day, a confluent red rash covered his face and neck.

1. What clinical characteristics of this case were diagnostic for measles?
2. Are any laboratory tests readily available to confirm the diagnosis? If so, what are they?
3. Is there a possible treatment for this patient?
4. When was this patient contagious?
5. Why is this disease not common in the United States?
6. Provide several possible reasons for this person's susceptibility to measles at 18 years of age.

A 13-month-old child had a runny nose, mild cough, and low-grade fever for several days. The cough got worse and sounded like "barking." The child made a wheezing sound when agitated. The child appeared well except for the cough. A lateral radiograph of the neck showed a subglottic narrowing.

1. What is the specific and common name for these symptoms?
2. What other agents would cause a similar clinical presentation (differential diagnosis)?
3. Are there readily available laboratory tests to confirm this diagnosis? If so, what are they?
4. Was there a possible treatment for this child?
5. When was this child contagious, and how was the virus transmitted?

BIBLIOGRAPHY

Balows A et al: *Laboratory diagnosis of infectious diseases: principles and practice*, New York, 1988, Springer-Verlag.

Belshe RB, editor: *Textbook of human viruses*, ed 2, St Louis, 1991, Mosby.

Centers for Disease Control: Public-sector vaccination efforts in response to the resurgence of measles among preschool-aged children: United States, 1989–1991, MMWR Morb Mortal Wkly Rep 41:522–525, 1992.

Fields BN et al, editors: *Virology*, ed 3, New York, 1996, Lippincott-Raven.

Galinski MS: Paramyxoviridae: transcription and replication, *Adv Virus Res* 40:129–163, 1991.

Hart CA, Broadhead RL: *Color atlas of pediatric infectious diseases*, St Louis, 1992, Mosby.

Hinman AR: Potential candidates for eradication, *Rev Infect Dis* 4:933–939, 1982.

Katz SL et al: *Krugman's infectious diseases of children*, ed 10, St Louis, 1998, Mosby.

ter Meulen V, Billeter MA: Measles virus, *Curr Top Microbiol Immunol* 191:1–196, 1995.

White DO, Fenner F: *Medical virology*, ed 4, San Diego, 1994, Academic.

CHAPTER 56

Orthomyxoviruses

Influenza A, B, and C viruses are the only members of the Orthomyxoviridae family, and only influenza A and B viruses cause significant human disease. The orthomyxoviruses are **enveloped and have a segmented negative-sense RNA genome**. The segmented genome of these viruses facilitates the development of new strains through the mutation and reassortment of the gene segments among different human and animal strains of virus. This genetic instability is responsible for the annual **epidemics (mutation: drift)** and **periodic pandemics (reassortment: shift)** of influenza infection worldwide.

Influenza is one of the most prevalent and significant viral infections. There are even descriptions of influenza **epidemics (local dissemination)** that occurred in ancient times. Probably the most famous influenza **pandemic (worldwide)** is the one that swept the world in 1918 to 1919, killing 20 million people. In fact, more people died of influenza during this time than in the battles of World War I. Pandemics due to novel influenza viruses occurred in 1918, 1947, 1957, 1968, and 1977, but, fortunately, none has occurred since. New virus strains have been detected since the last pandemic, including a limited outbreak in Hong Kong in 1997 ("chicken flu"). Fortunately, prophylaxis, in the form of vaccines and antiviral drugs, is now available for people at risk for serious outcomes.

Influenza viruses are respiratory viruses that cause respiratory symptoms and the classic flu-like symptoms, fever, malaise, headache, and myalgia (body aches). The term *flu*, however, has been mistakenly used to refer to many other respiratory and viral infections (e.g., "intestinal flu").

Structure and Replication

Influenza virions are pleomorphic, appearing spherical or tubular (Box 56–1 and Fig. 56–1) and ranging in diameter from 80 to 120 nm. The envelope contains two glycoproteins, **hemagglutinin (HA)** and **neuraminidase (NA)**, and is internally lined by the **matrix (M_1)** and **membrane (M_2)** proteins. The genome of

---

---

the influenza A and B viruses consists of **eight different helical nucleocapsid segments**, each of which contains a negative-sense RNA associated with the **nucleoprotein (NP)** and the **transcriptase (RNA polymerase components: PB1, PB2, PA)** (Table 56–1). Influenza C has only seven genomic segments.

The genomic segments in the influenza A virus range from 890 to 2340 bases. All the proteins are encoded on separate segments, with the exception of the nonstructural proteins (NS_1 and NS_2) and the M_1 and M_2 proteins, which are transcribed from one segment each.

The **HA** forms a spike-shaped trimer; each unit is activated by a protease and is cleaved into two subunits held together by a disulfide bond (see Fig. 6–8). The HA has several functions: It is the viral attachment protein, binding to sialic acid on epithelial cell surface receptors; it promotes fusion of the envelope to the

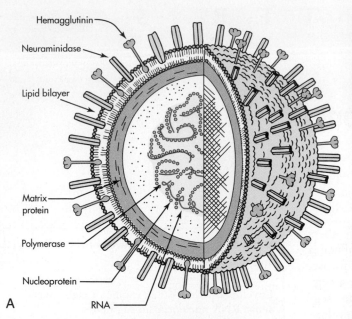

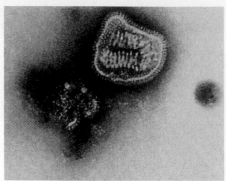

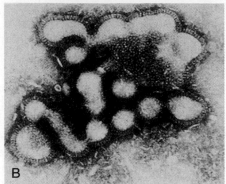

FIGURE 56–1. *A,* Model of influenza A virus. *B,* Electron micrographs of influenza A virus. (*A* from Kaplan MM, Webster RG: The epidemiology of influenza, *Sci Am* 237:88–106, 1977; *B* from Balows A et al, editors: *Laboratory diagnosis of infectious diseases: principles and practice,* vol 2, Heidelberg, 1988, Springer-Verlag.)

TABLE 56–1. **Products of Influenza Gene Segments**

Segment*	Protein	Function
1	PB2	Polymerase component
2	PB1	Polymerase component
3	PA	Polymerase component
4	HA	Hemagglutinin, viral attachment protein, fusion protein, target of neutralizing antibody
5	NP	Nucleocapsid
6	NA	Neuraminidase (cleaves sialic acid and promotes virus release)
7†	M_1	Matrix protein: viral structural protein (interacts with nucleocapsid and envelope, promotes assembly)
	M_2	Membrane protein (forms membrane channel and target for amantadine, facilitates uncoating and HA production)
8†	NS_1	Nonstructural protein (inhibits cellular messenger RNA translation)
	NS_2	Nonstructural protein (important but unknown function)

* Listed in decreasing order of size.
† Encodes two messenger RNAs.

cell membrane; it hemagglutinates (binds and aggregates) human, chicken, and guinea pig red blood cells; and it elicits the protective neutralizing antibody response. Mutation-derived changes in HA are responsible for the minor ("drift") and major ("shift") changes in antigenicity. *Shifts occur only with influenza A virus, and the different HAs are designated H1, H2, and so on.*

The **NA** glycoprotein forms a tetramer and has enzyme activity. The NA cleaves the sialic acid on glycoproteins, including the cell receptor. Cleavage of the sialic acid on virion proteins prevents clumping and facilitates the release of virus from infected cells sufficiently such that NA is a target for two antiviral drugs, **zanamivir** (**Relenza**) and **oseltamivir** (**Tamiflu**). The NA of influenza A virus also undergoes antigenic changes, and major differences acquire the designations N1, N2, and so on.

The M_1, M_2, and **NP** proteins are type-specific and are therefore used to differentiate among influenza A, B, and C viruses. The M_1 proteins line the inside of the virion and promote assembly. The M_2 protein forms a proton channel in membranes and promotes uncoating and viral release. The M_2 of influenza A is a target for the antiviral drugs amantadine and rimantadine.

Viral replication begins with the binding of HA to specific sialic acid structures on cell surface glycoproteins (Fig. 56–2). The virus is then internalized into a coated vesicle and transferred to an endosome. Acidification of the endosome causes the HA to bend over and expose hydrophobic fusion-promoting regions of the protein. The viral envelope then fuses with the endosome membrane. The M_2 protein promotes acidification of the envelope contents to break the interaction between the M_1 protein and the NP to allow uncoating and delivery of the nucleocapsid into the cytoplasm. The nucleocapsid travels to the nucleus, where it is transcribed into messenger RNA (mRNA).

The influenza transcriptase (PA, PB1, PB2) uses host cell mRNA as a primer for viral mRNA synthesis. In so doing, it steals the methylated cap region of the RNA, the sequence required for efficient binding to ribosomes. All the genomic segments are transcribed into 5' capped, 3' polyadenylated (poly A) mRNA for individual proteins, except the segments for the M and NS proteins, which are each differentially spliced (using cellular enzymes) to produce two different mRNAs. The mRNAs are translated into protein in the cytoplasm. The HA and NA glycoproteins are processed by the endoplasmic reticulum and Golgi apparatus. The M_2 protein inserts into cellular membranes. Its proton channel prevents acidification of Golgi and other vesicles, thus preventing acid-induced folding and inactivation of the HA within the cell. The HA and NA are then transported to the cell surface.

Positive-sense RNA templates for each segment are

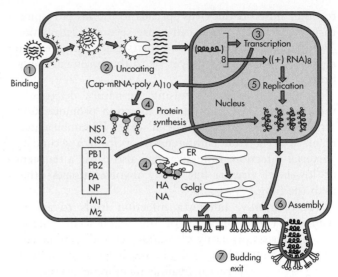

FIGURE 56–2. Replication of influenza A virus. After binding (1) to sialic acid–containing receptors, influenza is endocytosed and fuses (2) with the vesicle membrane. Unlike for most other RNA viruses, transcription (3) and replication (5) of the genome occur in the nucleus. Viral proteins are synthesized (4), helical nucleocapsids form and associate (6) with $M_1 M_2$, and the protein-lined membranes containing HA and NA glycoproteins. (7) The virus buds from the plasma membrane. (+) = Positive sense; ER = endoplasmic reticulum.

produced, and the negative-sense RNA genome is replicated in the nucleus. The genomic segments are then transported to the cytoplasm and associate with polymerase and NP proteins to form nucleocapsids, which interact with the M_1 protein lining plasma membrane sections containing M_2, HA, and NA. The genomic segments are enveloped in a random manner, with 11 segments per virion. This process produces a small number of virions with a complete genome and numerous defective particles. The particles are antigenic and can cause interference, which may limit the progression of the infection. The virus buds selectively from the apical surface of the cell as a result of the preferential insertion of the HA in this membrane. Virus is released about 8 hours after infection.

Pathogenesis and Immunity

Influenza initially establishes a local upper respiratory tract infection (Box 56–2). To do so, the virus first targets and kills mucus-secreting, ciliated, and other epithelial cells, causing the loss of this primary defense system. NA facilitates the development of the infection by cleaving sialic acid residues of the mucus, thereby providing access to tissue. Preferential release of the virus at the apical surface of epithelial cells and into the lung promotes cell-to-cell spread and transmission to other hosts. If the virus spreads to the lower respiratory tract, the infection can cause severe desquamation (shedding) of bronchial or alveolar epithelium down to a single-cell-thick basal layer or to the basement membrane.

In addition to compromising the natural defenses of the respiratory tract, influenza infection promotes bacterial adhesion to the epithelial cells. Pneumonia may result from a viral pathogenesis or from a secondary bacterial infection. Influenza may also cause a transient or low-level viremia but rarely involves tissues other than the lung.

Histologically, influenza infection leads to an inflammatory cell response of the mucosal membrane, which consists primarily of monocytes and lymphocytes and few neutrophils. Submucosal edema is present. Lung tissue may reveal hyaline membrane disease, alveolar emphysema, and necrosis of the alveolar walls (Fig. 56–3).

Recovery is associated with the production of interferon and the mounting of cell-mediated immune responses. T-cell responses are important for effecting recovery and immunopathogenesis. However, influenza infection depresses macrophage and T-cell function, hindering immune resolution. Interestingly, recovery often precedes detection of antibody in serum or secretions.

Protection against reinfection is primarily associated with the development of antibodies to HA, but antibodies to NA are also protective. The antibody re-

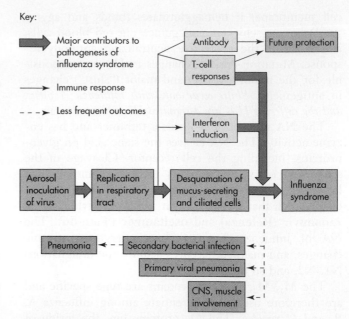

FIGURE 56–3. Pathogenesis of influenza A virus. The symptoms of influenza are caused by viral pathologic and immunopathologic effects, but the infection may promote secondary bacterial infection. *CNS* = central nervous system.

sponse is specific for each strain of influenza, but the cell-mediated immune response is more general and is capable of reacting to influenza strains of the same type (influenza A or B virus). Antigenic targets for T-cell responses include peptides from HA but also from the nucleocapsid proteins (NP, PB2) and M_1 protein, which are not as variable.

The symptoms and time course of the disease are determined by the interferon and T-cell responses and the extent of the epithelial tissue loss. Influenza is normally a self-limited disease that rarely involves organs other than the lung. *Many of the classic "flu" symptoms (e.g., fever, malaise, headache, and myalgia) are associated with interferon induction.* Repair of the compromised tissue is initiated within 3 to 5 days of the start of symptoms but may take as long as a month. The time course of influenza virus infection is illustrated in Figure 56–4.

Epidemiology

Strains of influenza A virus are classified by the following four characteristics:

1. Type (A, B, and C).
2. Place of original isolation.
3. Date of original isolation.
4. Antigen (HA and NA).

For example, a current strain of influenza virus might be designated A/Bangkok/1/79 (H3N2), meaning that it is an influenza A virus that was first isolated in

---

BOX 56–2. **Disease Mechanisms of Influenza A and B Viruses**

Virus can establish infection of upper and lower respiratory tract.

Systemic symptoms are due to the interferon and lymphokine response to the virus. Local symptoms are due to epithelial cell damage, including ciliated and mucus-secreting cells.

Interferon and cell-mediated immune responses (NK [natural killer] and T-cell) are important for immune resolution and immunopathogenesis.

Infected people are predisposed to bacterial superinfection because of the loss of natural barriers and exposure of the binding sites on epithelial cells.

Antibody is important for future protection against infection and is specific for defined epitopes on HA and NA proteins.

The HA and NA of influenza A virus can undergo **major (reassortment: shift)** and **minor (mutation: drift)** antigenic changes to ensure the presence of immunologically naive, susceptible people.

Influenza B virus undergoes only minor antigenic changes.

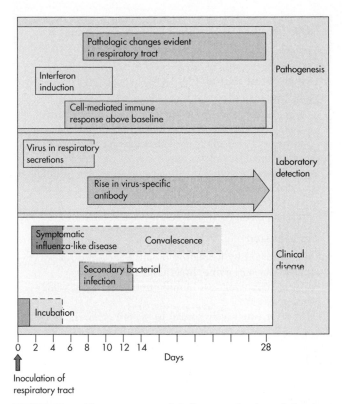

FIGURE 56–4. Time course of influenza A virus infection. The classic "flu syndrome" occurs early. Later, pneumonia may result from bacterial pathogenesis, viral pathogenesis, or immunopathogenesis.

Bangkok in January 1979 and contains HA (H3) and NA (N2) antigens.

Strains of influenza B are designated by (1) type, (2) geography, and (3) date of isolation (e.g., B/Singapore/3/64), but without specific mention of HA or NA antigens because influenza B does not undergo antigenic shift and pandemics like influenza A.

New influenza A strains are generated through mutation and reassortment. The genetic diversity of influenza A is fostered by its segmented genomic structure and ability to infect and replicate in humans and many animal species **(zoonose),** including birds and pigs. Hybrid viruses are created by co-infection of a cell with different strains of influenza A virus, allowing the genomic segments to randomly associate into new virions. An exchange of the HA glycoproteins may generate a new virus that can infect an immunologically naive human population. For example, an H1N1 duck virus and an H3N2 human virus infected pigs, reassortants were isolated from the pig, and the resulting virus was able to infect humans (Fig. 56–5).

This type of reassortment is postulated to be the source of pathogenic human strains. Because of the high population density and proximity of humans, pigs, chickens, and ducks in China, this country is thought to be a breeding ground for new reassortant viruses and the source of many of the pandemic strains of influenza. In 1997, an A/Hong Kong/156/97 (H5N1) strain was isolated from at least 18 humans and caused 6 deaths. The virus resembled a chicken virus, A/Chicken/Hong Kong/258/97 (H5N1), leading to the destruction of all 1.6 million chickens in Hong Kong to destroy the potential source of the virus.

Minor antigenic changes resulting from mutation of the HA and NA genes are called **antigenic drift**. This

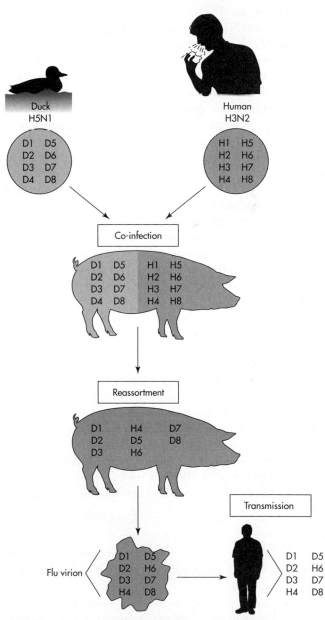

FIGURE 56–5. Example of reassortment of genomic fragments of influenza A virus. Diagram of the origin of a new human virus with a shift from H3N2 to H1N1. Pigs were infected with a duck influenza virus and another set of pigs, with the human influenza virus. At some time, a pig underwent mixed infection with both viruses. The resulting virus created by reassortment of the viral gene segments could be transmitted to and infect humans.

process occurs every 2 to 3 years, causing local outbreaks of influenza A and B infection. Major antigenic changes (**antigenic shift**) result from the reassortment of genomes among different strains, including animal strains. This process occurs only with the influenza A virus. Such changes are often associated with the occurrence of pandemics.

Antigenic shifts occur infrequently, taking place on average every 10 years (Table 56–2). For example, the prevalent influenza A virus in 1947 was the H1N1 subtype. In 1957, there was a shift in both antigens, resulting in an H2N2 subtype. H3N2 appeared in 1968, and H1N1 reappeared in 1977. The reappearance of H1N1 is probably due to the infection of seronegative members of the population younger than 30 years, who were susceptible to the virus. Prior exposure and an anamnestic antibody response protected the members of the population older than 30 years. *In contrast to influenza A, influenza B is predominantly a human virus and does not undergo antigenic shift.*

The changing antigenic nature of influenza ensures a large proportion of immunologically naive, susceptible people (especially children) in the population (Box 56–3). An influenza outbreak can be readily detected from the increased absenteeism in schools and work and the number of emergency department visits. During the winter, influenza outbreaks occur annually in temperate climates. Fortunately, influenza virus is present in a community for only a short time (4 to 6 weeks).

Influenza infection is spread readily via small airborne droplets expelled during talking, breathing, and coughing. The virus can also survive on countertops for as long as a day.

The most susceptible population is children, and school-aged children are most likely to spread the infection. Contagion precedes symptoms and lasts for a long time, especially in children. Children, immunosuppressed people (including pregnant women), the elderly, and people with heart and lung ailments (including smokers) are at highest risk for more serious disease, pneumonia, or other complications of infection.

TABLE 56–2. **Influenza Pandemics Resulting from Antigenic Shift**

Year of Pandemic	Influenza A Subtype
1918	$H_{sw}N1$; probable swine flu strain
1947	H1N1
1957	H2N2; Asian flu strain
1968	H3N2; Hong Kong flu strain
1977	H1N1

BOX 56–3. **Epidemiology of Influenza A and B Viruses**

Disease/Viral Factors

Influenza is enveloped and inactivated by detergents.

Segmented genome facilitates major genetic changes, especially on HA and NA proteins.

Influenza A infects many vertebrate species, including other mammals and birds.

Co-infection with animal and human strains of influenza can generate very different virus strains by genetic reassortment.

Transmission of virus often precedes symptoms.

Transmission

Virus is spread by inhalation of small aerosol droplets expelled during talking, breathing, and coughing.

Virus likes cool, less humid atmosphere (e.g., winter heating season).

Virus is extensively spread by school children.

Who Is at Risk?

Seronegative people.

Adults: classic "flu syndrome."

Children: asymptomatic to severe respiratory tract infections.

High-risk groups: elderly, immunocompromised people, and people with underlying cardiac or respiratory problems (including people with asthma and smokers).

Geography/Season

There is worldwide occurrence: epidemics are local; pandemics are worldwide.

Disease is more common in winter.

Modes of Control

Amantadine, rimantadine, zanamivir, and oseltamivir have been approved for prophylaxis or early treatment.

Killed vaccine contains predicted yearly strains of influenza A and B viruses.

Extensive surveillance of influenza A and B outbreaks is conducted to identify the new strains that should be incorporated into new vaccines. The prevalence of a particular strain of influenza A or B virus changes each year and reflects the particular immunologic naiveté of the population at that time. Surveillance also extends into the animal populations because of the possible presence of recombinant animal influenza A strains that can cause human pandemics.

Clinical Syndromes

Depending on the degree of immunity to the infecting strain of virus and other factors, infection may range from asymptomatic to severe. Patients with underlying

TABLE 56–3. Diseases Associated with Influenza Virus Infection

Disorder	Symptoms
Acute influenza infection in adults	Rapid onset of fever, malaise, myalgia, sore throat, and nonproductive cough
Acute influenza infection in children	Acute disease similar to that in adults but with higher fever, gastrointestinal tract symptoms (abdominal pain, vomiting), otitis media, myositis, and more frequent croup

Complications of influenza virus infection	Primary viral pneumonia
	Secondary bacterial pneumonia
	Myositis and cardiac involvement
	Neurologic syndromes:
	    Guillain-Barré syndrome
	    Encephalopathy
	    Encephalitis
	    Reye's syndrome

cardiorespiratory disease, people with immune deficiency (even that associated with pregnancy), and smokers are more prone to have a severe case.

After an incubation period of 1 to 4 days, the "flu syndrome" begins with a brief prodrome of malaise and headache lasting a few hours. The prodrome is followed by the additional abrupt onset of fever, severe myalgia, and usually a nonproductive cough. The illness persists for approximately 3 days, and unless a complication occurs, recovery is complete within 7 to 10 days. Influenza in young children resembles other severe respiratory tract infections, causing bronchiolitis, croup, otitis media, and, rarely, febrile convulsions (Table 56–3). Complications of influenza include bacterial pneumonia, myositis, and Reye's syndrome. The central nervous system can also be involved. Influenza B disease is similar to influenza A disease.

Influenza may directly cause pneumonia, but it more commonly promotes a secondary bacterial superinfection that leads to bronchitis or pneumonia. The tissue damage caused by progressive influenza virus infection of alveoli can be extensive, leading to hypoxia and bilateral pneumonia. Secondary bacterial infection usually involves *Streptococcus pneumoniae*, *Haemophilus influenzae*, or *Staphylococcus aureus*. In these infections, sputum usually is produced and becomes purulent.

Although generally the infection is limited to the lung, some strains of influenza can spread to other sites in certain people. For example, myositis (inflammation of muscle) may occur in children. Encephalopathy, although rare, may accompany an acute influenza illness and may be fatal. Postinfluenza encephalitis occurs 2 to

3 weeks after recovery from influenza. It is associated with evidence of inflammation and is rarely fatal.

Reye's syndrome is an acute encephalitis that affects children and occurs after a variety of acute febrile viral infections, including varicella as well as influenza B and A diseases. Children given salicylates (aspirin) are at increased risk for this syndrome. In addition to encephalopathy, hepatic dysfunction is present. The mortality rate may be as high as 40%.

Laboratory Diagnosis

The occurrence of the characteristic symptoms of influenza in a person during a community outbreak of the infection is often sufficient to "clinch" the diagnosis. Laboratory methods can distinguish influenza from other respiratory viruses and identify its type and strain (Table 56–4).

Influenza viruses are obtained from respiratory secretions. The virus is generally isolated in primary monkey kidney cell cultures or the Madin-Darby canine kidney cell line. Nonspecific cytopathologic effects may be noted within as few as 2 days (average, 4 days). Before the cytopathologic effects develop, the addition of guinea pig erythrocytes may reveal **hemadsorption** (the adherence of these erythrocytes to HA-expressing infected cells) (see Fig. 48–5). The addition of influ-

TABLE 56–4. Laboratory Diagnosis of Influenza Virus Infection

Test	Detects
Cell culture in primary monkey kidney or Madin-Darby canine kidney cells	Presence of virus, limited cytopathologic effects
Hemadsorption to infected cells	Presence of HA protein on cell surface
Hemagglutination	Presence of virus in secretions
Hemagglutination inhibition	Type and strain of influenza virus or specificity of antibody
Antibody inhibition of hemadsorption	Identification of influenza type and strain
Immunofluorescence, ELISA	Influenza virus antigens in respiratory secretions or tissue culture
Serology: hemagglutination inhibition, hemadsorption inhibition, ELISA, immunofluorescence, complement fixation	Seroepidemiology

ELISA = Enzyme-linked immunosorbent assay.

enza virus–containing media to erythrocytes promotes the formation of a gel-like aggregate due to **hemagglutination**. Hemagglutination and hemadsorption are not specific to influenza viruses, however; parainfluenza and other viruses also exhibit these properties.

Specific identification of the influenza virus requires immunologic tests, such as immunofluorescence or inhibition of hemadsorption, or hemagglutination (hemagglutination inhibition [HI]) with specific antibody (see Chapter 48). Enzyme immunoassay or immunofluorescence can be used to detect viral antigen in exfoliated cells, respiratory secretions, or cell culture and are more sensitive assays. Serologic studies do not aid in the diagnosis of an influenza infection and are generally used for epidemiologic purposes.

Treatment, Prevention, and Control

Hundreds of millions of dollars are spent on acetaminophen, antihistamines, and similar drugs to relieve the symptoms of influenza. The antiviral drug **amantadine** and its analogue **rimantadine** inhibit an uncoating step of the influenza A virus but do not affect the influenza B or C virus. The target for their action is the M_2 protein. **Zanamivir** and **oseltamivir** inhibit both influenza A and B as enzyme inhibitors of the neuraminidase. Without the neuraminidase, the hemagglutinin of the virus binds to sialic acid on other viral particles to form clumps, thereby preventing virus release. Zanamivir is inhaled, whereas oseltamivir is taken orally as a pill. These drugs are effective for prophylaxis and for treatment during the first 24 to 48 hours after the onset of influenza A illness. Treatment cannot prevent the later host-induced immunopathogenic stages of the disease.

The airborne spread of influenza is almost impossible to limit. However, the best way to control the virus is through immunization. Natural immunization, which results from prior exposure, is protective for long periods. A killed-virus vaccine representing the "strains of the year" and antiviral drug prophylaxis can also prevent infection.

Killed (formalin-inactivated) influenza vaccine is available every year. Killed whole-virus vaccines are prepared from virus grown in embryonated eggs and then chemically inactivated. Detergent-treated virion preparations and HA- and NA-containing detergent extracts of virus are also available. Ideally, the vaccine incorporates antigens of the A and B influenza strains that will be prevalent in the community during the upcoming winter. For instance, the trivalent influenza vaccine used in 1992 and 1993 consisted of inactivated A/Texas/91–like (H1N1), A/Beijing/89–like (H3N2),

and B/Panama/90–like virus strains. Vaccination is routinely recommended for the elderly and people with chronic pulmonary or heart disease.

CASE STUDY AND QUESTIONS

■ In late December, a 22-year-old man suddenly experienced headache, myalgia, malaise, dry cough, and a fever. He basically felt "lousy." After a couple of days, he had a sore throat, his cough had worsened, and he started to feel nauseated and vomited. Several of his family members had experienced similar symptoms during the previous 2 weeks.

1. In addition to influenza, what other agents could cause similar symptoms (differential diagnosis)?

2. How would the diagnosis of influenza be confirmed?

3. Amantadine is effective against influenza. What is its mechanism of action? Will it be effective for this patient? For uninfected family members or contacts?

4. When was the patient contagious, and how was the virus transmitted?

5. What family members were at greatest risk for serious disease and why?

6. Why is influenza so difficult to control even when there is a national vaccination program?

BIBLIOGRAPHY

Cox NJ, Subbarao K: Global epidemiology of influenza: past and present, *Annu Rev Med* 51:407–421, 2000.

Fields BN, Knipe DM, Howley PM, editors: *Virology*, ed 3, New York, 1996, Lippincott-Raven.

Hay AJ et al: Influenza viruses. In Belshe RB, editor: *Textbook of human virology*, ed 2, St Louis, 1991, Mosby.

Helenius A: Unpacking the incoming influenza virus, *Cell* 69: 577–578, 1992.

Influenza: NIAID fact sheet [on line]. Available at http://www.niaid.nih.gov/spotlight/flu00/default.htm

Laver WG, Bischofberger N, Webster RG: Disarming flu viruses, *Sci Am* 280:78–87, 1999.

Laver WG, Bischofberger N, Webster RG : The origin and control of pandemic influenza, *Perspect Biol Med* 43:173–192, 2000.

Stuart-Harris C: The epidemiology and prevention of influenza, *Am Sci* 69:166–172, 1981.

Webster RG: Predictions for future human influenza pandemics, *J Infect Dis* 176(suppl 1):S14–S19, 1997.

Webster RG et al: Evolution and ecology of influenza viruses, *Microbiol Rev* 56:152–179, 1992.

CHAPTER 57

Reoviruses

The **Reoviridae** consist of the orthoreoviruses, rotaviruses, orbiviruses, and coltiviruses (Table 57–1). The name reovirus was proposed in 1959 by Albert Sabin for a group of respiratory and enteric viruses that were not associated with any known disease process (*r*espiratory, *e*nteric, *o*rphan). The Reoviridae are nonenveloped viruses with **double-layered protein capsids** containing **10 to 12 segments of the double-stranded RNA genomes**. These viruses are stable over wide pH and temperature ranges and in airborne aerosols. The orbiviruses and coltiviruses are spread by arthropods and are arboviruses.

The **orthoreoviruses**, also referred to as mammalian reoviruses or simply reoviruses, were first isolated in the 1950s from the stools of children. They are the prototype of this virus family, and the molecular basis of their pathogenesis has been studied extensively. In general, these viruses cause asymptomatic infections in humans.

Rotaviruses cause **human infantile gastroenteritis**, a very common disease. In fact, rotaviruses account for approximately 50% of all cases of diarrhea in children requiring hospitalization because of dehydration (70,000 cases per year in the United States). In underdeveloped countries, rotaviruses may be responsible for as many as 1 million deaths each year from uncontrolled viral diarrhea.

Structure

Rotaviruses and reoviruses share many structural, replicative, and pathogenic features. Reoviruses and rotaviruses have an icosahedral morphology with a double-layered capsid (60 to 80 nm in diameter) (Box 57–1; Fig. 57–1) and a double-stranded segmented genome (**"double:double"**). The name rotavirus is derived from the Latin word *rota*, meaning "wheel," which refers to the virion's appearance in negative-stained electron micrographs (Fig. 57–2). Proteolytic cleavage of the outer capsid (as occurs in the gastrointestinal tract) activates the virus for infection and produces an **intermediate/infectious subviral particle (ISVP)**.

The outer capsid is composed of structural proteins (Fig. 57–3), which surround a nucleocapsid core that includes enzymes for RNA synthesis and 10 (reo) or 11 (rota) different double-stranded RNA genomic segments. Like the influenza virus capsid, the reovirus and rotavirus capsids are randomly filled with more than 10 or 11 genome segments to generate virions with a complete set of different segments. In addition, **reassortment of gene segments** can occur and thus create hybrid viruses.

Interestingly, rotaviruses resemble enveloped viruses in that they (1) have glycoproteins that act as the viral attachment proteins, (2) acquire but then lose an envelope during assembly, and (3) appear to have a fusion protein activity that promotes direct penetration of the target cell membrane.

The genomic segments of rotaviruses and reoviruses encode structural and nonstructural proteins. The genomic segments of reovirus, the proteins they encode, and their functions are summarized in Table 57–2; those of rotavirus are summarized in Table 57–3. Core proteins include enzymatic activities required for the transcription of messenger RNA (mRNA). They include a 5′-methyl guanosine mRNA capping enzyme and an RNA polymerase. The $\sigma 1$ protein (reo) and VP4 (rota) are located at the vertices of the capsid and extend from the surface like spike proteins. They have several functions, including hemagglutination and viral attachment, and they elicit neutralizing antibodies. VP4 is activated by protease cleavage, exposing a structure similar to that of the fusion proteins of paramyxoviruses. Its cleavage is necessary for productive entry of the virus into cells. The viral attachment proteins, $\sigma 3$ of reoviruses and VP7 of rotaviruses, elicit neutralizing antibody.

Replication

The replication of reoviruses and rotaviruses starts with ingestion of the virus (Fig. 57–4). The virion outer capsid protects the inner nucleocapsid and core from the environment, especially the acidic environment of

TABLE 57–1. Reoviridae Responsible for Human Disease

Virus	Disease
Orthoreovirus*	Mild upper respiratory tract illness, gastrointestinal tract illness, biliary atresia
Orbivirus/coltivirus	Febrile illness with headache and myalgia (zoonosis)
Rotavirus	Gastrointestinal tract illness, respiratory tract illness (?)

* Reovirus is the common name for the family Reoviridae and for the specific genus *Orthoreovirus*.

the gastrointestinal tract. The complete virion is then partially digested in the gastrointestinal tract and presumably activated by protease cleavage and loss of the external capsid proteins (σ3/VP7) and cleavage of the σ1/VP4 protein to produce the ISVP. The σ1/VP4 protein at the vertices of the ISVP binds to sialic acid–containing glycoproteins on epithelial and other cells, which include the β-adrenergic receptor for reovirus. The ISVP of rotavirus appears to penetrate through the target cell membrane directly. Whole virions of reovirus and rotavirus can be taken up by receptor-mediated endocytosis; however, this is a dead-end pathway for rotavirus.

The ISVP releases the core into the cytoplasm, and the enzymes in the core initiate mRNA production. The **double-stranded RNA always remains in the core.** Transcription of the genome occurs in two

BOX 57–1. Unique Features of Reoviridae

Double-layered capsid virion (60 to 80 nm) has icosahedral symmetry containing 10 to 12 **double-stranded genomic segments** (depending on the virus) (double:double).

Virion is **resistant** to environmental and gastrointestinal conditions (e.g., detergents, acidic pH, drying).

Rotavirus and orthoreovirus virions are activated by mild proteolysis to intermediate/infectious subviral particles (ISVPs), increasing their infectivity.

Inner capsid contains a complete transcription system, including enzymes for 5′ capping and polyadenylate addition.

Viral replication occurs in the cytoplasm. Double-stranded RNA remains in the inner core.

Rotavirus inner capsid aggregates in the cytoplasm and then buds into the endoplasmic reticulum, acquiring its outer capsid and a membrane, which is then lost.

Virus is released by cell lysis.

phases, early and late, before replication of the genome. Each of the negative-sense (−) RNA strands is used as a template by virion core enzymes, which synthesize individual mRNAs complete with a 5′-methyl guanosine cap and a 3′-polyadenylate tail. The mRNA then leaves the core and is translated. (This is similar in concept to negative-strand RNA viruses.) Later, virion proteins and positive-sense (+) RNA segments associate together into corelike structures that aggregate into large cytoplasmic inclusions. The (+) RNA segments are copied to produce (−) RNAs in the new cores, replicating the double-stranded genome. The new cores either generate more (+) RNA or are assembled into virions.

The assembly processes for reovirus and rotavirus differ. In the assembly of reovirus, the outer capsid proteins associate with the core, and the virion leaves the cell upon cell lysis. Assembly of rotavirus resembles that of an enveloped virus, in that the rotavirus cores associate with the NS28 viral protein on the outside of the endoplasmic reticulum (ER) and, upon budding into the ER, acquire its VP7 outer capsid protein. The membrane is lost in the ER, and the virus leaves the cell during cell lysis. Reovirus inhibits cellular macromolecular synthesis within 8 hours of infection.

Orthoreoviruses (Mammalian Reoviruses)

The orthoreoviruses are ubiquitous. The virions are very stable and have been detected in sewage and river water. The mammalian reoviruses occur in three serotypes, referred to as reovirus types 1, 2, and 3; these serotypes are based on neutralization and hemagglutination-inhibition tests. All three serotypes share a common complement-fixing antigen.

Pathogenesis and Immunity

Orthoreoviruses do not cause significant disease in humans. However, studies of reovirus disease in mice have advanced our understanding of the pathogenesis of viral infections in humans. Depending on the reovirus strain, the virus can be neurotropic or viscerotropic in mice. The functions and virulence properties of the reovirus proteins were identified through comparison of the activities of interstrain hybrid viruses that differ in only one genomic segment (encoding one protein). With this approach, the new activity is attributable to the genomic segment from the other virus strain.

After ingestion and proteolytic production of the ISVP, the orthoreoviruses bind to M cells in the small intestine, which then transfer the virus to the lymphoid tissue of Peyer's patches lining the intestines. The viruses then replicate and initiate a viremia. Although the virus is cytolytic in vitro, it causes few if any symptoms before entering the circulation and producing in-

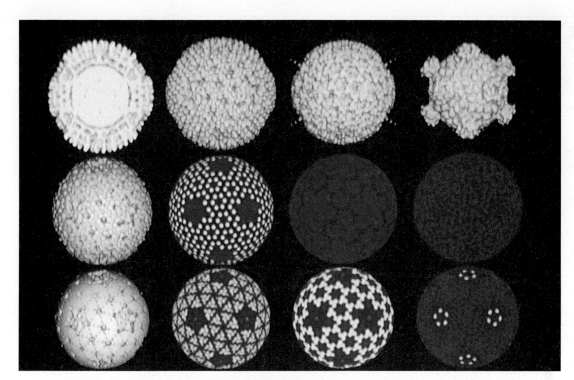

FIGURE 57–1. Computer reconstruction of cryoelectron micrograph of human reovirus type 1 (Lang). *Top left to right,* Cross section of virion, intermediate/infectious subviral particle (ISVP), and core particle. The ISVP and core particles are generated by proteolysis of the virion and play important roles in the replication cycle. *Center and bottom,* Computer-generated images of the virions at different radii after the outer layers of features have been shaved off. The colors help one visualize the symmetry and molecular interactions within the capsid. (Courtesy Tim Baker, Purdue University.)

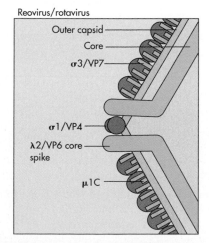

FIGURE 57–2. Structure of reovirus/rotavirus core and outer proteins. σ1/VP4, viral attachment protein; σ3/VP7, major capsid component; λ2/VP6, major inner capsid protein; μ1C, minor outer capsid protein. (Redrawn from Sharpe AH, Fields BN: Pathogenesis of viral infections: basic concepts derived from the reovirus model, *N Engl J Med* 312: 486–497, 1985.)

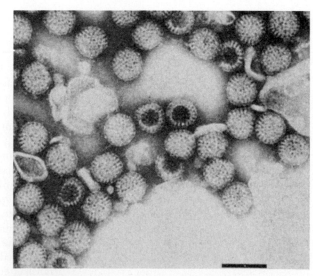

FIGURE 57–3. Electon micrograph of rotavirus. *Bar* = 100 nm. (From Fields BN et al, eds: *Virology,* New York, Raven, 1985.)

TABLE 57–2. Functions of Reovirus Gene Products

Genomic Segments (Molecular Weight, Da)	Protein	Function (If Known)
Large segments (2.8 × 10⁶)		
1	λ3 (inner capsid)	Polymerase
2	λ2 (outer capsid)	Capping enzyme
3	λ1 (inner capsid)	Transcriptase component
Medium segments (1.4 × 10⁶)		
1	μ2 (inner capsid)	—
2	μ1C (outer capsid)	Cleaved from μ1, complexes with σ3, promotes entry
3	μNS	Promotes viral assembly*
Small segments (0.7 × 10⁶)		
1	σ1 (outer capsid)	Viral attachment protein, hemagglutinin, determines tissue tropism†
2	σ2 (inner capsid)	Facilitates viral RNA synthesis
3	σNS	Facilitates viral RNA synthesis
4	σ3 (outer capsid)	Major component of outer capsid with μ1C

* Proteins are not found in the virion.
   † Neutralizing antibodies.
   Modified from Field BN et al, editors: *Virology*, ed 3, New York, 1996, Lippincott-Raven.

fection at a distant site. In the mouse model, the outer capsid protein responsible for causing hemagglutinin activity (σ1) also facilitates viral spread to the mesenteric lymph nodes and determines whether the virus is neurotropic.

Mice, and presumably humans, mount protective humoral and cellular immune responses to outer capsid proteins. Although orthoreoviruses are normally lytic, they can also establish persistent infection in cell culture.

Epidemiology

As already mentioned, the orthoreoviruses have been found worldwide. Seroprevalence studies suggest that most people are probably infected during childhood,

TABLE 57–3. Functions of Rotavirus Gene Products

Gene Segment	Protein (Location)	Function
1	VP1 (inner capsid)	Polymerase
2	VP2 (inner capsid)	Transcriptase component
3	VP3 (inner capsid)	mRNA capping
4	VP4 (outer capsid spike protein at vertices of virion)	Activation by protease to VP5 and VP8 in ISVP, hemagglutinin, viral attachment protein
5	NSP1 (NS53)	RNA binding
6	VP6 (inner capsid)	Major structural protein of inner capsid, binding to NS28 at ER to promote assembly of outer capsid
7	NSP3 (NS34)	RNA binding
8	NSP2 (NS35)	RNA binding
9	VP7 (outer capsid)	Type-specific antigen, major outer capsid component that is glycosylated in ER and facilitates attachment and entry
10	NSP4 (NS28)	Glycosylated protein in ER that promotes inner capsid binding to ER, transient envelopment, and addition of outer capsid
11	NSP5 (NS26)	RNA binding

ER = endoplasmic reticulum; ISVP = intermediate/infectious subviral particle.
   Modified from Field BN et al, editors: *Virology*, ed 3, New York, 1996, Lippincott-Raven.

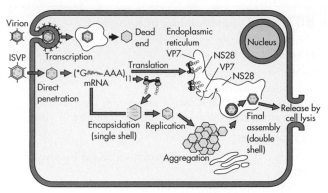

FIGURE 57–4. Replication of rotavirus. Rotavirus virions are activated by protease (e.g., in the gastrointestinal tract) to an intermediate/infectious subviral particle (ISVP). The ISVP binds, penetrates the cell, and loses its outer capsid. The inner capsid contains the enzymes for mRNA transcription using the (±) strand as a template. Some mRNA segments are transcribed early; others are transcribed later. Enzymes in the virion cores attach 5' cap (*G) and poly A (AA) to mRNA. VP7 and NS28 are synthesized as glycoproteins and expressed in the endoplasmic reticulum. (+) RNA is mRNA and is also enclosed into inner capsids as a template to replicate the ± segmented genome. The capsids aggregate and "dock" onto the NS28 protein in the endoplasmic reticulum, acquiring VP7 and its outer capsid and an envelope. The virus loses the envelope and leaves the cell on cell lysis.

because approximately 75% of adults have the antibody. Antibody is also detected in most animals, including chimpanzees and monkeys. It is not known whether animals are a reservoir for human infections.

Clinical Syndromes

Orthoreoviruses infect people of all ages, but linking specific diseases to these agents has been difficult. Most infections are thought to be asymptomatic or are so mild that they go undetected. Thus far, these viruses have been linked to common cold–like mild upper respiratory tract illness (low-grade fever, rhinorrhea, pharyngitis), gastrointestinal tract disease, and biliary atresia.

Laboratory Diagnosis

Human orthoreovirus infection can be detected through assay of the viral antigen or RNA in clinical material, virus isolation, or serologic assays for virus-specific antibody. Throat, nasopharyngeal, and stool specimens from patients with suspected upper respiratory tract or diarrheal disease are used as samples. Human orthoreoviruses can be isolated using mouse L-cell fibroblasts, primary monkey kidney cells, and HeLa cells. Serologic assays can be performed for epidemiologic purposes.

Treatment, Prevention, and Control

Orthoreovirus disease is mild and self-limited. For this reason, treatment has not been necessary, and prevention and control measures have not been investigated.

Rotaviruses

Rotaviruses are common agents of infantile diarrhea worldwide. The rotaviruses are a large group of gastroenteritis-causing viruses found in many different mammals and birds.

Rotavirus virions are relatively stable at room temperature and to treatment with detergents, at pH extremes of 3.5 to 10, and even with repeated freezing and thawing. Infectivity is enhanced by proteolytic enzymes such as trypsin.

Human and animal rotaviruses are divided into serotypes, groups, and subgroups. Serotypes are distinguished primarily from the VP7 outer capsid protein and, to a lesser extent, from the VP4 minor outer capsid protein. Groups are determined primarily on the basis of the antigenicity of VP6 and the electrophoretic mobility of the genomic segments. Seven groups (A to G) of human and animal rotaviruses have been identified on the basis of the VP6 inner capsid protein. Human disease is caused by group A and, occasionally, group B and C rotaviruses.

Pathogenesis and Immunity

The rotavirus can survive the acidic environment in a buffered stomach or in a stomach after a meal (Box 57–2). Viral replication occurs after adsorption to columnar epithelial cells covering the villi of the small intestine. Approximately 8 hours after infection, cytoplasmic inclusions are seen that contain newly synthesized proteins and RNA. As many as 10^{10} viral particles per gram of stool may be released during disease. Studies of the small intestine, either of experimentally infected animals or in biopsy specimens from infants, show shortening and blunting of the microvilli and mononuclear cell infiltration into the lamina propria.

BOX 57–2. **Disease Mechanisms of Rotavirus**

Virus is spread by the **fecal-oral route** and possibly the respiratory route.

Cytolytic and toxin-like action on the intestinal epithelium causes loss of electrolytes and prevents readsorption of water.

Disease can be significant in infants younger than 24 months but asymptomatic in adults.

Large amounts of virus are released during the diarrheal phase.

Like cholera, rotavirus infection prevents the absorption of water, causing a net secretion of water and loss of ions, which together result in a watery diarrhea. The NSP4 protein of rotavirus may act in a toxin-like manner to promote calcium ion influx into enterocytes, release of neuronal activators, and a neuronal alteration in water absorption. The loss of fluids and electrolytes can lead to severe dehydration and even death if therapy does not include electrolyte replacement.

Immunity to infection requires the presence of antibody, primarily immunoglobulin (Ig) A, in the lumen of the gut. Actively or passively acquired antibody (including antibody in colostrum and mother's milk) can lessen the severity of disease but does not consistently prevent reinfection. In the absence of antibody, the inoculation of even small amounts of virus causes infection and diarrhea. Infection in infants and small children is generally symptomatic, whereas that in adults is usually asymptomatic.

Epidemiology

Rotaviruses are ubiquitous worldwide, with 95% of children infected by 3 to 5 years of age (Box 57–3). Rotaviruses are assumed to be passed from person to person by the **fecal-oral route**. Maximal shedding of the virus occurs 2 to 5 days after the start of diarrhea but can occur without symptoms. The virus survives well on fomites such as furniture and toys as well as on hands, because it can withstand drying. Although domestic animals are known to harbor serologically related rotaviruses, they are not believed to be a common source of human infection. Outbreaks occur in preschools and daycare centers and among hospitalized infants.

Rotaviruses are **one of the most common causes of serious diarrhea in young children** worldwide, accounting for 600,000 deaths due to dehydration per year. Most children have been infected by the virus by 4 years of age. In North America, outbreaks occur annually during the autumn, winter, and spring. More severe disease occurs in severely malnourished children. Rotavirus diarrhea is a very contagious, severe life-threatening disease for infants in developing countries, and it occurs year-round.

Clinical Syndromes

Rotavirus is a major cause of gastroenteritis. The incubation period for rotavirus diarrheal illness is estimated to be 48 hours. The major clinical findings in hospitalized patients are **vomiting**, **diarrhea**, **fever**, and **dehydration**. Fecal leukocytes and blood in stool do not occur in this form of diarrhea. Rotavirus gastroenteritis is a self-limited disease, and recovery is generally complete and without sequelae. However, the infection may prove fatal in infants who live in developing coun-

---

> **BOX 57–3.** **Epidemiology of Rotavirus**
>
> **Disease/Viral Factors**
>
> Capsid virus is resistant to environmental and gastrointestinal conditions.
>> Large amounts of virus are released in fecal matter.
>> Asymptomatic infection can result in release of virus.
>
> **Transmission**
>
> Virus is transmitted in fecal matter, especially in daycare settings.
>> Respiratory transmission may be possible.
>
> **Who Is at Risk?**
>
> *Rotavirus Type A*
>
> Infants younger than 24 months of age: at risk for infantile gastroenteritis with potential dehydration.
>> Older children and adults: at risk for mild diarrhea.
>> Undernourished people in underdeveloped countries: at risk for diarrhea, dehydration, and death.
>
> *Rotavirus Type B*
>
> Infants, older children, and adults in China: at risk for severe gastroenteritis.
>
> **Geography/Season**
>
> Virus is found worldwide.
>> Disease is more common in autumn, winter, and spring.
>
> **Modes of Control**
>
> Hand washing and isolation of known cases are modes of control.
>> Experimental live vaccines use bovine or monkey rotavirus.

---

tries and who are malnourished and dehydrated before the infection.

Laboratory Diagnosis

The clinical findings in patients with rotavirus infection resemble those of other viral diarrheas (e.g., Norwalk virus). Most patients have large quantities of virus in stool, making the direct detection of viral antigen the method of choice for diagnosis. Enzyme immunoassay and latex agglutination are quick, easy, and relatively inexpensive ways to detect rotavirus in stool. Viral particles in specimens can also be readily detected on electron microscopy.

The cell culture of rotavirus is difficult and not reliable for diagnostic purposes. Serologic studies are primarily used for research and epidemiologic purposes. Because so many people have rotavirus-specific antibody, a fourfold rise in antibody titer is necessary for the diagnosis of recent infection or active disease.

Treatment, Prevention, and Control

No specific antiviral therapy is available for a rotavirus infection. The morbidity and mortality associated with rotavirus diarrhea result from dehydration and electrolyte imbalance. The purpose of supportive therapy is to replace fluids so that the blood volume and electrolyte and acid-base imbalances are corrected.

Rotavirus vaccines have been developed to protect children, especially those in underdeveloped countries, from potentially fatal disease. Vaccines have been prepared from animal rotaviruses, such as the rhesus monkey rotavirus and the Nebraska calf diarrhea virus. These vaccines share antigenic determinants with human rotaviruses, do not cause disease in humans, and afford protection against infection. Rhesus-human reassortant vaccines have also been prepared. One such vaccine was approved by the U.S. Food and Drug Administration (FDA) but was recalled because of the incidence of intussusception. The vaccines may not protect against all serotypes of rotavirus.

Rotaviruses are acquired very early in life. Their ubiquitous nature make it difficult to limit the spread of the virus and infection. Hospitalized patients with disease must be isolated, however, to limit spread of the infection to other susceptible patients.

Coltiviruses and Orbiviruses

The coltiviruses and orbiviruses infect vertebrates and invertebrates. The coltiviruses cause Colorado tick fever and related human disease. The orbiviruses mainly cause disease in animals, including blue tongue disease of sheep, African horse sickness, and epizootic hemorrhagic disease of deer.

Colorado tick fever, an acute disease characterized by fever, headache, and severe myalgia, was originally described in the 19th century and is now believed to be one of the most common tick-borne viral diseases in the United States. Although hundreds of infections occur annually, the exact number is not known because Colorado tick fever is not a reportable disease.

The structure and physiology of the coltiviruses and orbiviruses are similar to those of the other Reoviridae, with the following major exceptions:

1. The outer capsid of the orbiviruses has no discernible capsomeric structure, even though the inner capsid is icosahedral.
2. The virus causes viremia, infects erythrocyte precursors, and remains in the mature red blood cells protected from the immune response.
3. The orbivirus life cycle includes both vertebrates and invertebrates (insects).

Colorado tick fever viruses have 12 double-stranded RNA genomic segments, and orbiviruses have 10.

Pathogenesis

Colorado tick fever virus infects erythroid precursor cells without severely damaging them. The virus remains within the cells, even after they mature into red blood cells; this factor protects the virus from clearance. The resulting viremia can persist for weeks or months, even after symptomatic recovery. Both of these factors promote transmission of the virus to the tick vector.

Serious hemorrhagic disease can result from the infection of vascular endothelial and vascular smooth muscle cells and pericytes, thereby weakening capillary structure. The weakness leads to leakage and hemorrhage and, potentially, hypotension and shock. Neuronal infection can lead to meningitis and encephalitis.

Epidemiology

Colorado tick fever occurs in western and northwestern areas of the United States and western Canada, where the wood tick *Dermacentor andersoni* is distributed (elevations of 4000 to 10,000 feet) (Fig. 57–5). Ticks acquire the virus by feeding on a viremic host and subsequently transmit the virus in saliva when feeding on a new host. Natural hosts of this virus constitute many mammals, including squirrels, chipmunks, rabbits, and deer. Human disease is observed during the spring, summer, and autumn, seasons when humans are more likely to invade the habitat of the tick.

Clinical Syndromes

Colorado tick fever virus generally causes mild or subclinical infection. The symptoms of the acute disease resemble those of dengue fever. After a 3- to 6-day incubation period, symptomatic infections start with

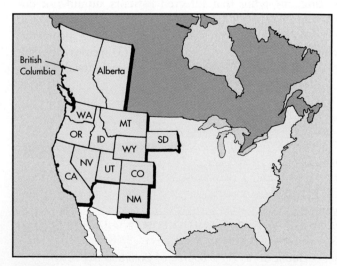

FIGURE 57–5. Geographic distribution of Colorado tick fever.

the sudden onset of fever, chills, headache, photophobia, myalgia, arthralgia, and lethargy (Fig. 57–6). Characteristics of the infection include a biphasic fever and conjunctivitis, and possibly lymphadenopathy, hepatosplenomegaly, and a maculopapular or petechial rash. A leukopenia involving both neutrophils and lymphocytes is an important hallmark of the disease. Children occasionally have a more severe hemorrhagic disease. Colorado tick fever must be differentiated from Rocky Mountain spotted fever, a tick-borne rickettsial infection characterized by a rash, because the latter disease may require antibiotic treatment.

Laboratory Diagnosis

A diagnosis of Colorado tick fever can be established through the direct detection of viral antigens, virus isolation, or serologic tests. The best, most rapid method is detection of viral antigen on the surfaces of erythrocytes in a blood smear through the use of immunofluorescence. Laboratory tests may be available through state Public Health departments or the Centers for Disease Control and Prevention.

The titers of antibody in acute and convalescent specimens must be compared for a serologically based diagnosis to be rendered, because subclinical infections can occur and antibody may persist for a lifetime. Specific IgM is present for about 45 days after the onset of illness, and its detection is also presumptive evidence of an acute or a very recent infection. Immunofluorescence is the best technique, but complement fixation, neutralization, and enzyme immunoassay are also used to detect Colorado tick fever antibody.

Treatment, Prevention, and Control

No specific treatment is available for Colorado tick fever. The disease is generally self-limited, indicating that supportive care is sufficient. The viremia is long-lasting, implying that infected patients should not donate blood soon after recovery. Prevention consists of (1) avoiding tick-infested areas, (2) using protective clothing and tick repellents, and (3) removing ticks before they bite. Unlike tick-borne rickettsial disease,

in which prolonged feeding is required for the bacteria to be transmitted, the coltivirus from the tick's saliva can enter the blood stream rapidly. A formalinized Colorado tick fever vaccine has been developed and evaluated, but because of the mildness of the disease, its distribution to the general public is not warranted.

CASE STUDY AND QUESTIONS

■ A 6-month-old boy was seen in the emergency department in January after 2 days of persistent watery diarrhea and vomiting accompanied by a low-grade fever and mild cough. The infant appeared dehydrated and required hospitalization. The patient attended a daycare center.

1. In addition to rotavirus, what other viral agents must be considered in the differential diagnosis of this infant's disease? What agents would need consideration if the patient were a teenager or an adult?
2. How would the diagnosis of rotavirus have been confirmed?
3. How was the virus transmitted? How long was the patient contagious?
4. Who was at risk for serious disease?

BIBLIOGRAPHY

Balows A et al, editors: *Laboratory diagnosis of infectious diseases: principles and practice*, New York, 1988, Springer-Verlag.

Bellamy AR, Both GW: Molecular biology of rotaviruses, *Adv Virol* 38:1–44, 1990.

Belshe RB, editor: *Textbook of human virology*, ed 2, St Louis, 1991, Mosby.

Blacklow NR, Greenberg HB: Viral gastroenteritis, *N Engl J Med* 325:252–264, 1991.

Christensen ML: Human viral gastroenteritis, *Clin Microbiol Rev* 2:51–89, 1989.

Feigin RD, Cherry JD, editors: *Textbook of pediatric infectious disease*, ed 4, Philadelphia, 1998, WB Saunders.

Fields BN et al, editors: *Virology*, ed 3, New York, 1996, Lippincott-Raven.

Joklik WK, editor: *The Reoviridae*, New York, 1983, Plenum.

Nibert ML et al: Mechanisms of viral pathogenesis: distinct forms of reovirus and their roles during replication in cells and host, *J Clin Invest* 88:727–734, 1991.

Ramig RF: Rotaviruses, *Curr Top Microbiol Immunol* 185:1–380, 1994.

Sharpe AH, Fields BN: Pathogenesis of viral infections: basic concepts derived from the reovirus model, N Engl J Med 312:486–497, 1985.

Tyler KL, Oldstone MBA, editors: Reoviruses. *Current Topics in Microbiology and Immunology*, vol 233, Berlin, New York, 1998, Springer.

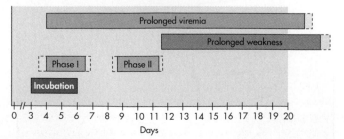

FIGURE 57–6. Time course of Colorado tick fever.

C H A P T E R   5 8

Rhabdoviruses

The members of the family Rhabdoviridae (from the Greek word *rhabdos*, meaning "rod") include pathogens for a variety of mammals, fish, birds, and plants. The family contains *Vesiculovirus* (vesicular stomatitis viruses [VSVs]); *Lyssavirus* (rabies and rabies-like viruses), an unnamed genus constituting the plant rhabdovirus group; and other ungrouped rhabdoviruses of mammals, birds, fish, and arthropods.

Rabies virus is the most significant pathogen of the rhabdoviruses. Until Louis Pasteur developed the killed-rabies vaccine, a bite from a "mad dog" always led to the characteristic symptoms of **hydrophobia** and certain death.

Physiology, Structure, and Replication

Rhabdoviruses are simple viruses encoding only five proteins and appearing as **bullet-shaped, enveloped virions** with a diameter of 50 to 95 nm and length of 130 to 380 nm (Box 58–1, Fig. 58–1). Spikes composed of a trimer of the glycoprotein (G) cover the surface of the virus. The viral attachment protein, G protein generates neutralizing antibodies. The G protein of the vesicular stomatitis virus is a simple glycoprotein with *N*-linked glycan. This G protein has been used as the prototype for studying eukaryotic glycoprotein processing.

Within the envelope, the **helical nucleocapsid** is coiled symmetrically into a cylindrical structure, giving it the appearance of striations (see Fig. 58–1). The nucleocapsid is composed of one molecule of **single-stranded, negative-sense RNA** and the nucleoprotein (N), plus large (L) and nonstructural (NS) proteins. The matrix (M) protein lies between the envelope and the nucleocapsid. The N protein is the major structural protein of the virus. It protects the RNA from ribonuclease digestion and maintains the RNA in a configuration acceptable for transcription. The L and NS proteins constitute the RNA-dependent RNA polymerase.

The replicative cycle of VSV is the prototype for the rhabdoviruses and other negative-strand RNA viruses (see Fig. 6–13). The viral G protein attaches to the host cell and is internalized by endocytosis. The viral envelope then fuses with the membrane of the endosome upon acidification of the vesicle. This uncoating releases the nucleocapsid to be released into the cytoplasm, where replication takes place.

The RNA-dependent RNA polymerase associated with the nucleocapsid transcribes the viral genomic RNA, producing five individual messenger RNAs (mRNAs). These mRNAs are then translated into the five viral proteins. The viral genomic RNA is also transcribed into a full-length positive-sense RNA template that is used to generate new genomes. The G protein is synthesized by membrane-bound ribosomes, processed by the Golgi apparatus, and delivered to the cell surface in membrane vesicles. The M protein associates with the G protein–modified membranes.

Assembly of the virion occurs in two phases, (1) assembly of the nucleocapsid in the cytoplasm and (2) envelopment and release at the cell plasma membrane. The genome associates with the N protein and then with the polymerase proteins L and NS to form the nucleocapsid. Association of the nucleocapsid with the M protein at the plasma membrane induces coiling into its condensed form. The virus then buds through the plasma membrane and is released when the entire nucleocapsid is enveloped. Cell death and lysis occur after infection with most rhabdoviruses, with the important exception of rabies virus, which produces little discernible cell damage.

Pathogenesis and Immunity

Only the pathogenesis of rabies virus infection is discussed here (Box 58–2). Rabies infection usually results from the bite of a rabid animal. Rabies infection of the animal causes secretion of the virus in the animal's saliva and promotes aggressive behavior ("mad dog"), which in turn promotes transmission of the virus. The virus can also be transmitted through the inhalation of aerosolized virus (as may be found in bat caves), in transplanted infected tissue (e.g., cornea), and by inoculation through intact mucosal membranes.

Virus may directly infect nerve endings by binding to nicotinic acetylcholine or ganglioside receptors of neurons or muscle at the site of inoculation. The virus remains at the site for days to months (Fig. 58–2) before progressing to the central nervous system (CNS). Rabies virus travels by retrograde axoplasmic transport to the dorsal root ganglia and to the spinal cord. Once the virus gains access to the spinal cord, the brain becomes rapidly infected. The affected areas are the hippocampus, brain stem, ganglionic cells of the pontine nuclei, and Purkinje cells of the cerebellum. The virus then disseminates from the CNS via afferent neurons to highly innervated sites, such as the skin of the head and neck, **salivary glands,** retina, cornea, nasal mucosa, adrenal medulla, renal parenchyma, and pancreatic acinar cells. After the virus invades the brain and spinal cord, an encephalitis develops, and neurons degenerate. Despite the extensive CNS involvement and impairment of CNS function, little histopathologic change can be observed in the affected tissue other than the presence of Negri bodies (see later).

With rare exception (three known cases), rabies is fatal once clinical disease is apparent. The length of the incubation period is determined by (1) the concentration of the virus in the inoculum, (2) the proximity of the wound to the brain, (3) the severity of the

wound, (4) the host's age, and (5) the host's immune status.

In contrast to other viral encephalitis syndromes, rabies rarely causes inflammatory lesions. Neutralizing antibodies are not apparent until after the clinical disease is well-established. Little antigen is released, and the infection probably remains hidden from the immune response. Cell-mediated immunity appears to play little or no role in protection against rabies virus infection.

Antibody can block the spread of virus to the CNS and to the brain if administered or generated during the incubation period. *The incubation period is usually long enough to allow generation of a therapeutic protective antibody response after active immunization with the killed rabies vaccine.*

Epidemiology

Rabies is the **classic zoonotic infection,** spread from animals to humans (Box 58–3). It is endemic in a variety of animals worldwide, except in Australia. Rabies is maintained and spread in two ways: In urban rabies, dogs are the primary transmitter, and in sylvatic (forest) rabies, many species of wildlife can serve as the transmitter. In the United States, rabies is more prevalent in cats because they are not vaccinated. Virus-containing aerosols, bites, and scratches from infected bats also spread the disease. The principal reservoir for

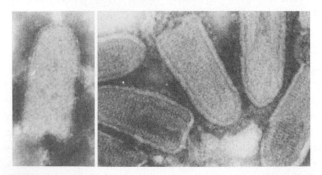

FIGURE 58–1. Rhabdoviridae seen by electron microscopy: rabies virus (*left*) and vesicular stomatitis virus (*right*). (From Fields BN: *Virology,* New York, 1985, Raven.)

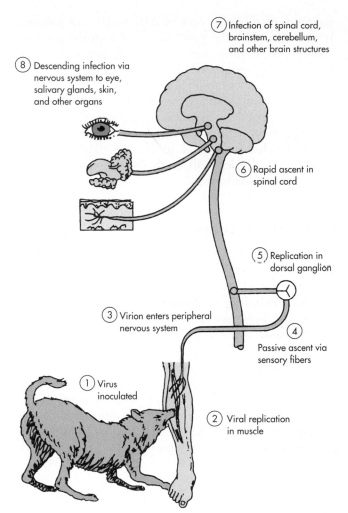

⑦ Infection of spinal cord, brainstem, cerebellum, and other brain structures

⑧ Descending infection via nervous system to eye, salivary glands, skin, and other organs

⑥ Rapid ascent in spinal cord

⑤ Replication in dorsal ganglion

③ Virion enters peripheral nervous system

④ Passive ascent via sensory fibers

① Virus inoculated

② Viral replication in muscle

FIGURE 58–2. Pathogenesis of rabies virus infection. Numbered steps describe the sequence of events. (Redrawn from Belshe RB, editor: *Textbook of human virology*, ed 2, St Louis, 1991, Mosby.)

BOX 58–3. **Epidemiology of Rabies Virus**

Disease/Viral Factors

Virus induced aggressive behavior in animals promotes virus spread.
    Disease has long, asymptomatic incubation period.

Transmission

 Zoonosis:
        Reservoir: wild animals.
        Vector: wild animals and unvaccinated dogs and cats.
    Source of virus:
    Major: saliva in bite of rabid animal.
    Minor: aerosols in bat caves containing rabid bats.

Who Is at Risk?

Veterinarians and animal handlers.
    Person bitten by a rabid animal.
    Inhabitants of countries with no pet vaccination program.

Geography/Season

Virus is found worldwide, except in some island nations.
    There is no seasonal incidence.

Modes of Control

Vaccination program is available for pets.
    Vaccination is available for at-risk personnel.
    Vaccination programs have been implemented to control rabies in forest mammals.

---

rabies in most of the world, however, is the dog. In Latin America and Asia, this feature is a problem because of the existence of many stray, unvaccinated dogs and the absence of rabies-control programs. These two factors are responsible for thousands of rabies cases in dogs each year in these countries.

Because of the excellent vaccination program in the United States, sylvatic rabies accounts for most of the cases of animal rabies in this country. Statistics for animal rabies are collected by the Centers for Disease Control and Prevention, which in 1999 recorded more than 8000 documented cases of rabies in skunks, raccoons, bats, and farm animals, in addition to dogs and cats (Fig. 58–3). Badgers and foxes are also major carriers of rabies in Western Europe. In South America, vampire bats transmit rabies to cattle, resulting in losses of millions of dollars each year.

The distribution of human rabies approximates the distribution of animal cases in each country. It is estimated that rabies accounts for at least 25,000 deaths annually in India, where the virus is transmitted by dogs in 96% of cases. In Latin America, cases of human rabies primarily result from contact with rabid dogs in urban areas. In Indonesia, an outbreak of more than 200 human cases of rabies in 1999 promoted the killing of more than 40,000 dogs on the islands. The incidence of human rabies in the United States is approximately 1 case per year because of effective dog vaccination programs and limited human contact with skunks, raccoons, and bats; even so, annual costs for rabies prevention exceed $300 million.

Clinical Syndromes

Rabies is virtually always fatal unless treated by vaccination. After a long but highly variable incubation period, the prodrome phase of rabies ensues (Table 58–1). The patient has symptoms such as fever, malaise, headache, pain or paresthesia (itching) at the site of the bite, gastrointestinal symptoms, fatigue, and anorexia. The prodrome usually lasts 2 to 10 days, after which the neurologic symptoms specific to rabies appear. **Hydrophobia** (fear of water), the most characteristic

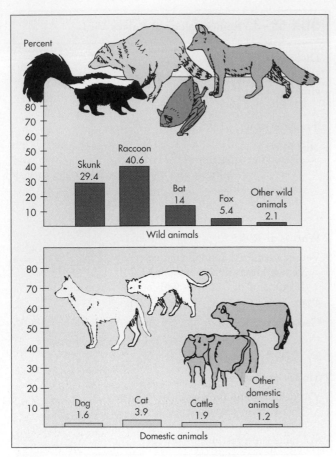

FIGURE 58–3. Distribution of animal rabies in the United States, 1999. The percentages relate to the total number of cases of animal rabies. (Data from Krebs JW et al: *JAVMA* 217:1799–1811, 2000.)

symptom of rabies, occurs in 20% to 50% of patients. It is triggered by the pain associated with the patient's attempts to swallow water. Focal and generalized seizures, disorientation, and hallucinations are also common during the neurologic phase. From 15% to 60% of patients exhibit paralysis as the only manifestation of rabies. The paralysis may lead to respiratory failure.

The patient becomes comatose after the neurologic phase, which lasts from 2 to 10 days. This phase almost universally leads to death due to neurologic and pulmonary complications.

Laboratory Diagnosis

The occurrence of neurologic symptoms in a person who has been bitten by an animal generally establishes the diagnosis of rabies. Unfortunately, **evidence of infection, including symptoms and the detection of antibody, does not occur until it is too late for intervention.** Laboratory tests are usually performed to confirm the diagnosis and to determine whether a suspected individual or animal is rabid (post mortem).

The diagnosis of rabies is made through detection of viral antigen in the CNS or skin, isolation of the virus, and serologic findings. The hallmark diagnostic finding has been the detection of intracytoplasmic inclusions consisting of aggregates of viral nucleocapsids (**Negri bodies**) in affected neurons (see Fig. 48–3). Although their finding is diagnostic of rabies, Negri bodies are seen in only 70% to 90% of brain tissue from infected humans.

Antigen detection using immunofluorescence has become the most widely used method for diagnosing ra-

TABLE 58–1. Progression of Rabies Disease

Disease Phase	Symptoms	Time (days)	Viral Status	Immunologic Status
Incubation phase	Asymptomatic	60–365 after bite	Low titer, virus in muscle	—
Prodrome phase	Fever, nausea, vomiting, loss of appetite, headache, lethargy, pain at site of bite	2–10	Low titer, virus in CNS and brain	—
Neurologic phase	Hydrophobia, pharyngeal spasms, hyperactivity, anxiety, depression CNS symptoms: loss of coordination, paralysis, confusion, delirium	2–7	High titer, virus in brain and other sites	Detectable antibody in serum and CNS
Coma	Coma: cardiac arrest, hypotension, hypoventilation, secondary infections	0–14	High titer, virus in brain and other sites	—
Death	—	—	—	—

CNS = central nervous system.

bies. Brain biopsy or autopsy material, impression smears of corneal epithelial cells, and skin biopsy material from the nape of the neck are the specimens most commonly used for this procedure.

Rabies can also be grown in cell culture or intracerebrally inoculated infant mice. Inoculated cell cultures or brain tissues are subsequently examined with direct immunofluorescence.

Rabies antibody titers in serum and cerebrospinal fluid are usually measured with a rapid fluorescent focus inhibition test. Antibody usually is not detectable until late in the disease, however.

Treatment and Prophylaxis

Clinical rabies is almost always fatal unless treated. Once the symptoms have appeared, little other than supportive care can be given.

Postexposure prophylaxis is the only hope for preventing overt clinical illness in the affected person. Although human cases of rabies are rare, appoximately 20,000 people receive rabies prophylaxis each year in the United States alone. Prophylaxis should be initiated for anyone exposed by bite or by contamination of an open wound or mucous membrane to the saliva or brain tissue of an animal suspected to be infected with the virus, unless the animal is tested and shown not to be rabid.

The first protective measure is local treatment of the wound. The wound should be washed immediately with soap and water, detergent, or another substance that inactivates the virus. The World Health Organization Expert Committee on Rabies also recommends the instillation of antirabies serum around the wound.

Subsequently, immunization with vaccine in combination with administration of one dose of human rabies immunoglobulin (HRIG) or equine antirabies serum is recommended. Passive immunization with HRIG provides antibody until the patient produces antibody in response to the vaccine. A series of five immunizations is then administered over the course of a month. The slow course of rabies disease allows active immunity to be generated in time to afford protection.

The rabies vaccine is a killed-virus vaccine prepared through the chemical inactivation of rabies-infected tissue culture human diploid cells (HDCV) or fetal rhesus lung cells. These vaccines cause fewer negative reactions than the older vaccines (Semple and Fermi), which were prepared in the brains of adult or suckling animals. The HDCV is administered intramuscularly on the day of exposure and then on days 3, 7, 14, and 28.

Preexposure vaccination of animal workers, laboratory workers who handle potentially infected tissue, and people traveling to areas where rabies is endemic should be performed. HDCV administered intramuscu-

larly or intradermally in three doses is recommended and provides 2 years of protection.

Ultimately, the prevention of human rabies hinges on the effective control of rabies in domestic and wild animals. Its control in domestic animals depends on the removal of stray and unwanted animals and the vaccination of all dogs and cats. A variety of attenuated oral vaccines have also been used successfully to immunize foxes. A live recombinant vaccinia virus vaccine expressing the rabies virus G protein is in use in the United States. This vaccine, which is injected into a bait and parachuted into the forest, successfully immunizes raccoons, foxes, and other animals.

CASE STUDY AND QUESTIONS

■ An 11-year-old boy was brought to a hospital in California after falling; his bruises were treated, and he was released. The following day he refused to drink water with his medicine, and he became more anxious. That night, he began to act up and hallucinate. He also was salivating and had difficulty breathing. Two days later, he had a fever of 40.8°C (105.4°F) and experienced two episodes of cardiac arrest. Although rabies was suspected, no remarkable data were obtained from a computed tomographic image of the brain or cerebrospinal fluid analysis. A skin biopsy from the nape of the neck was negative for viral antigen on day 3 but was positive for rabies on day 7. The patient's condition continued to deteriorate, and he died 11 days later. When the parents were questioned, it was learned that the boy had been bitten on the finger by a dog 6 months earlier while on a trip to India.

1. What clinical features of this case suggested rabies?

2. Why does rabies have such a long incubation period?

3. What treatment should have been given immediately after the dog bite? As soon as the diagnosis was suspected?

4. How do the clinical aspects of rabies differ from those of other neurologic viral diseases?

BIBLIOGRAPHY

Anderson LJ et al: Human rabies in the United States, 1960–1979: epidemiology, diagnosis, and prevention, *Ann Intern Med* 100:728–735; 1984.

Baer GM et al: Rhabdoviruses. In Fields BN, Knipe DM, editors: *Virology*, New York, 1990, Raven.

Fields BN et al, editors: *Virology*, ed 3, New York, 1996, Lippincott-Raven.

Fishbein DB: Rabies, *Infect Dis Clin North Am* 5:53–71, 1991.

Krebs JW et al: Rabies surveillance in the United States during 1999. *JAVMA* 217:1799–1811, 2000. (Available online at www.cdc.gov/ncidod/dvrd/rabies/Professional/Surveillance99/index.htm)

Immunization Practices Advisory Committee: Rabies prevention: supplementary statement on the preexposure use of human diploid cell rabies vaccine by the intradermal route, *MMWR Morb Mortal Wkly Rep* 35:767–768, 1986.

Plotkin SA: Rabies: State of the Art Clinical Article. *Clin Infect Dis* 30:4–12,2000.

Rabies vaccine, absorbed: a new rabies vaccine for use in humans, *MMWR Morb Mortal Wkly Rep* 37:217–218, 223, 1988.

Rabies virus: NIAID fact sheet. Available online at http://www.cdc.gov/ncidod/dvrd/rabies/Professional/professi.htm

Robinson PA: Rabies virus. In Belshe RB, editor: *Textbook of human virology*, ed 2, St. Louis, 1991, Mosby.

Steele JH: Rabies in the Americas and remarks on the global aspects, *Rev Infect Dis* 10(suppl 4):S585–S597, 1988.

Warrell DA, Warrell MJ: Human rabies and its prevention: an overview, *Rev Infect Dis* 10(suppl 4):S726–S731, 1988.

Winkler WG, Bogel K: Control of rabies in wildlife, *Sci Am* 266:86–92, 1992.

Wunner WH et al: The molecular biology of rabies viruses, *Rev Infect Dis* 10(suppl 4):S771–S784, 1988.

Togaviruses and Flaviviruses

The members of the Togaviridae and Flaviviridae families are enveloped, positive, single-stranded RNA viruses (Box 59–1). Alphavirus and Flavivirus are discussed together because of similarities in the diseases that they cause as well as in epidemiology. Most are transmitted by arthropods and are therefore **arboviruses** (*arthropod-borne viruses*). They differ in size, morphology, gene sequence, and replication.

The togaviruses can be classified into the following major genera (Table 59–1): Alphavirus, Rubivirus, and Arterivirus. No known arteriviruses cause disease in humans, so this genus is not discussed further. **Rubella** virus is the only member of the Rubivirus group; it is discussed separately, however, because its disease manifestation (*German measles*) and its means of spread differ from those of the alphaviruses. The Flaviviridae include the flaviviruses, pestivirus, and hepatitis C and G viruses; hepatitis C and G are discussed in Chapter 62.

Alphaviruses and Flaviviruses

The alphaviruses and flaviviruses were classified as arboviruses because they are usually spread by arthropod vectors. These viruses have a very **broad host range**, including vertebrates (e.g., mammals, birds, amphibians, reptiles) and invertebrates (e.g., mosquitoes, ticks). Diseases spread by animals or with an animal reservoir are called **zoonoses**. Examples of pathogenic alphaviruses and flaviviruses are listed in Table 59–2. The hepatitis C and G viruses are classified as flaviviruses on the basis of their genomic structure. They are not likely to prove to be arboviruses.

Structure and Replication of Alphaviruses

The alphaviruses are similar to the picornaviruses in having an **icosahedral capsid** and a positive-sense, single-strand RNA genome that resembles messenger RNA (mRNA). They differ from picornaviruses by being slightly larger (45 to 75 nm in diameter) and are surrounded by an **envelope** (Latin *toga*, "cloak"). In addition, the togavirus genome encodes **early** and **late proteins**. The envelope consists of lipids obtained from the host cell membranes and glycoprotein spikes that protrude from the surface of the virion.

Alphaviruses have two or three glycoproteins that associate to form a single spike. The COOH-terminus of the glycoproteins is anchored in the capsid, forcing the envelope to wrap tightly ("shrink-wrap") and take on the shape of the capsid (Fig. 59–1). The capsid proteins of all the alphaviruses are similar in structure and are antigenically cross-reactive. The envelope glycoproteins express unique antigenic determinants that distinguish the different viruses and also express antigenic determinants that are shared by a group, or "complex," of viruses.

The alphaviruses attach to specific receptors expressed on many different cell types from many different species (Fig. 59–2). The host range for these viruses includes vertebrates, such as humans, monkeys, horses, birds, reptiles, and amphibians, and invertebrates, such as mosquitoes and ticks. However, the individual viruses have different tissue tropisms, accounting somewhat for the different disease presentations.

The virus enters the cell by means of receptor-mediated endocytosis (see Fig. 59–2). The viral envelope then fuses with the membrane of the endosome

---

BOX 59–1. Unique Features of Togaviruses and Flaviviruses

Viruses have enveloped single-stranded positive-sense RNA.

Togavirus replication includes early (nonstructural) and late (structural) protein synthesis.

Togaviruses replicate in the cytoplasm and bud at the plasma membranes.

Flaviviruses replicate in the cytoplasm and bud at internal membranes.

TABLE 59–1. Togaviruses and Flaviviruses

Virus Group	Human Pathogens
Togaviruses	
Alphavirus	Arboviruses
Rubivirus	Rubella virus
Pestivirus	None
Arterivirus	None
Flaviviruses	Arboviruses
Hepaciviridae	Hepatitis C virus

a polyprotein, which is subsequently cleaved by proteases into four nonstructural early proteins (NSPs 1 through 4). Each of these proteins contains a protease activity and an RNA-dependent RNA polymerase. A full-length, 42S, negative-sense RNA is synthesized as a template for replication of the genome, and more 42S positive-sense mRNA is produced. In addition, a 26S mRNA, corresponding to one third of the genome, is transcribed from the template. The 26S RNA encodes the capsid (C) and envelope (E1 through E3) proteins. Late in the replication cycle, viral mRNA can account for as much as 90% of the mRNA in the infected cell. The abundance of late mRNAs allows the production of a large amount of the structural proteins required for packaging the virus.

The structural proteins are produced by protease cleavage of the late polyprotein that was produced from the 26S mRNA. The C protein is translated first and is cleaved from the polyprotein (see Fig. 59–2). A signal sequence is then made that associates the nascent polypeptide with the endoplasmic reticulum. Thereafter, envelope glycoproteins are translated, gly-

upon acidification of the vesicle to deliver the capsid and genome into the cytoplasm.

Once released into the cytoplasm, the alphavirus genomes bind to ribosomes as mRNA. The alphavirus genome is translated in early and late phases. The initial two thirds of the alphavirus RNA is translated into

TABLE 59–2. Arboviruses

Disease	Vector	Host	Distribution	Disease
Alphaviruses				
Sindbis*	*Aedes* and other mosquitoes	Birds	Africa, Australia, India	Subclinical
Semliki Forest*	*Aedes* and other mosquitoes	Birds	East and West Africa	Subclinical
Venezuelan equine encephalitis	*Aedes, Culex*	Rodents, horses	North, South, and Central America	Mild systemic; severe encephalitis
Eastern equine encephalitis	*Aedes, Culiseta*	Birds	North and South America, Caribbean	Mild systemic; encephalitis
Western equine encephalitis	*Culex, Culiseta*	Birds	North and South America	Mild systemic; encephalitis
Chikungunya	*Aedes*	Humans, monkeys	Africa, Asia	Fever, arthralgia, arthritis
Flaviviruses				
Dengue*	*Aedes*	Humans, monkeys	Worldwide, especially tropics	Mild systemic; break-bone fever, dengue hemorrhagic fever, and dengue shock syndrome
Yellow fever*	*Aedes*	Humans, monkeys	Africa, South America	Hepatitis, hemorrhagic fever
Japanese encephalitis	*Culex*	Pigs, birds	Asia	Encephalitis
West Nile encephalitis	*Culex*	Birds	Africa, Europe, Central Asia, North America	Fever, encephalitis, hepatitis
St. Louis encephalitis	*Culex*	Birds	North America	Encephalitis
Russian spring-summer encephalitis	*Ixodes* and *Dermacentor* ticks	Birds	Russia	Encephalitis
Powassan encephalitis	*Ixodes* ticks	Small mammals	North America	Encephalitis

* Prototypical viruses.

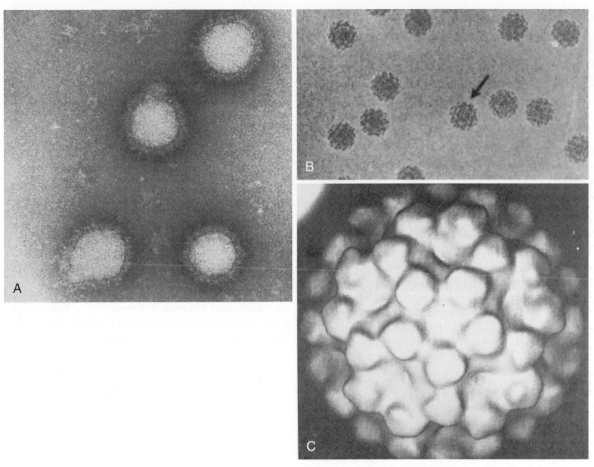

FIGURE 59–1. Alphavirus morphology. *A,* The outline of the envelope and the glycoprotein spikes of the Sindbis virus are visualized by negative staining. *B,* More detail on the morphology of the virion is obtained from electron microscopy. *C,* Surface representation of the Sindbis virus obtained by image processing of the cryoelectron micrographs indicates that the envelope is held tightly and conforms to the shape and symmetry of the capsid. (From Fuller SD: The T_4 envelope of Sindbis virus is organized by interaction with a complementary T_3 capsid, *Cell* 48: 923–934, 1987.)

cosylated, and cleaved from the remaining portion of the polyprotein to produce the E1, E2, and E3 glycoprotein spikes. The E3 is released from most alphavirus glycoprotein spikes. The glycoproteins are processed by the normal cellular machinery in the endoplasmic reticulum and Golgi apparatus and are also acetylated and acylated with long-chain fatty acids (see Fig. 59–2). Alphavirus glycoproteins are then transferred efficiently to the plasma membrane.

The C proteins associate with the genomic RNA soon after their synthesis and form an icosahedral capsid. Once this step is completed, the capsid associates with portions of the membrane expressing the viral glycoproteins. The alphavirus capsid has binding sites for the C-terminus of the glycoprotein spike, which pulls the envelope tightly around itself in a manner like shrink-wrapping (see Figs. 59–1 and 59–2). Alphavi-

ruses are released upon budding from the plasma membrane.

Structure and Replication of Flaviviruses

The flaviviruses also have a positive-strand RNA genome and an envelope. However, the virions of the flavivirus are slightly smaller than those of an alphavirus (37 to 50 nm in diameter), the RNA does not have a polyadenylate sequence, and the virus lacks a visible capsid structure in the virion. Most of the flaviviruses are serologically related, and antibodies to one virus may neutralize another virus.

The attachment and penetration by the flaviviruses occur in the same way as described for the alphaviruses, but the flaviviruses can also attach to the Fc receptors on macrophages, monocytes, and other cells

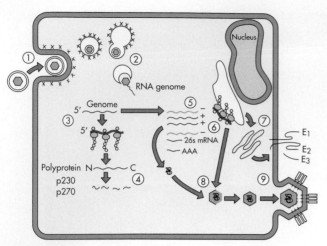

FIGURE 59–2. Replication of a togavirus. Semliki Forest virus. 1, Semliki Forest virus binds to cell receptors, is shuttled into a coated pit, and is internalized in a coated vesicle. 2, The virus is transferred to an endosome, and the viral envelope fuses with the endosomal membrane on acidification to release the nucleocapsid into the cytoplasm. 3, Ribosomes bind to the positive-sense RNA genome, and the p230 or p270 (full-length) early polyproteins are made. 4, The polyproteins are cleaved to produce nonstructural proteins 1 to 4 (NSP1 to NSP4), which include a polymerase to transcribe the genome into a negative-sense RNA template. 5, The template is used to produce a full-length 42S positive-sense mRNA genome and a late 26S mRNA for the structural proteins. 6, The C (capsid) protein is translated first, exposing a protease cleavage site and then a signal peptide for association with the endoplasmic reticulum. 7, The E glycoproteins are then synthesized, glycosylated, processed in the Golgi apparatus, and transferred to the plasma membrane. 8, The capsid proteins assemble on the 42S genomic RNA and then associate with regions of cytoplasmic and plasma membranes containing the E1, E2, and E3 spike proteins. 9, Budding from the plasma membrane releases the virus.

when the virus is coated with antibody. The antibody actually enhances the infectivity of these viruses by providing new receptors for the virus and by promoting viral uptake into these target cells.

The major differences between alphaviruses and flaviviruses are in the organization of their genomes and their mechanisms of protein synthesis. The entire flavivirus genome is translated into a single polyprotein, in a manner more similar to the process for picornaviruses than for alphaviruses (Fig. 59–3). As a result, there is no temporal distinction in the translation of the different viral proteins. The polyprotein produced from the yellow fever genome contains four nonstructural proteins, including a protease and an RNA-dependent RNA polymerase, plus the capsid and envelope structural proteins.

Unlike in the alphavirus genome, the structural genes are at the 5' end of the flavivirus genome. As a

result, the portions of the polyprotein containing the structural (not the catalytic) proteins are synthesized first and with the greatest efficiency. This arrangement may allow the production of more structural proteins, but it decreases the efficiency of nonstructural protein synthesis and the initiation of viral replication. This feature of flaviviruses may contribute to the lag prior to detection of their replication.

Another distinction of the flaviviruses is that they acquire their envelope by budding into intracellular vesicles rather than at the cell surface. The virus is then released by exocytosis or cell lysis mechanisms. This route is less efficient, and the virus may remain cell-associated.

Pathogenesis and Immunity

Because the arboviruses are acquired from the bite of an arthropod such as a mosquito, a knowledge of the course of infection in both the vertebrate host and the invertebrate vector is important for an understanding of the diseases. These viruses can cause lytic or persistent infections of both vertebrate and invertebrate hosts (Box 59–2). Infections of invertebrates are usually persistent, with continued virus production.

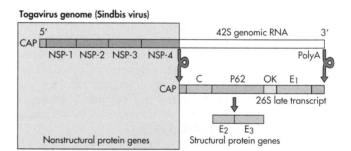

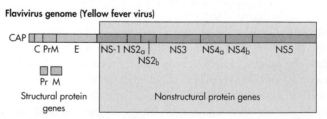

FIGURE 59–3. Comparison of the togavirus (alphavirus) and flavivirus genomes. Alphavirus: The enzymatic activities are translated from the 5' end of the input genome, promoting their early rapid translation. The structural proteins are translated later from a smaller mRNA transcribed from the genomic template. Flavivirus: The genes for the structural proteins of the flaviviruses are at the 5' end of the genome/mRNA, and only one species of polyprotein is made, which represents the entire genome. Poly A = polyadenylate. (Redrawn, with permission, from Hahn CS et al: Flavivirus genome organization, expression, and replication, *Annu Rev Microbiol* 44:649–688, © 1990 by Annual Reviews www.AnnualReviews.org.)

BOX 59–2. Disease Mechanisms of Togaviruses and Flaviviruses

Viruses are cytolytic, except for rubella.
 Viruses establish systemic infection and viremia.
 Viruses are good inducers of interferon, which can account for the flu-like symptoms of infection.

Viruses, except rubella and hepatitis C, are arboviruses.
 Flaviviruses can infect cells of the monocyte-macrophage lineage. Non-neutralizing antibody can enhance flavivirus infection via Fc receptors on the macrophage.

	Flu-like Syndrome	Encephalitis	Hepatitis	Hemorrhage	Shock
Dengue	+		+	+	+
Yellow fever	+		+	+	+
St. Louis encephalitis	+	+			
West Nile encephalitis	+	+			
Venezuelan encephalitis	+	+			
Western equine encephalitis	+	+			
Eastern equine encephalitis	+	+			
Japanese encephalitis	+	+			

The death of an infected cell results from a combination of virus-induced insults. The large amount of viral RNA produced upon the replication and transcription of the genome blocks cellular mRNA from binding to ribosomes. Increased permeability of the target cell membrane and changes in ion concentrations can alter enzyme activities and favor the translation of viral mRNA over cellular mRNA. The displacement of cellular mRNA from the protein synthesis machinery prevents rebuilding and maintenance of the cell and is a major cause of the death of the virus-infected cell. Some alphaviruses, such as western equine encephalitis (WEE) virus, make a nucleotide triphosphatase that degrades deoxyribonucleotides, depleting even the substrate pool for DNA production.

Female mosquitoes acquire the alphaviruses and flaviviruses by taking a blood meal from a **viremic vertebrate host**. *A sufficient viremia must be maintained in the vertebrate host to allow acquisition of the virus by the mosquito.* The virus then infects the epithelial cells of the midgut of the mosquito, spreads through the basal lamina of the midgut to the circulation, and infects the salivary glands. The virus sets up a persistent infection and replicates to high titers in these cells. The salivary glands can then release virus into the saliva. Not all arthropod species support this type of infection, however. For example, the normal vector for the WEE virus is the *Culex tarsalis* mosquito, but certain strains of virus are limited to the midgut of this mosquito, cannot infect its salivary glands, and therefore cannot be transmitted to humans.

On biting a host, the female mosquito regurgitates virus-containing saliva into the victim's blood stream. The virus then circulates freely in the host's plasma and comes into contact with susceptible target cells, such as the endothelial cells of the capillaries, monocytes, and macrophages.

The nature of alphavirus and flavivirus disease is determined primarily by (1) the specific tissue tropisms of the individual virus type, (2) the concentration of infecting virus, and (3) individual responses to the infection. These viruses are associated with **mild systemic disease**, **encephalitis**, **arthrogenic disease**, or **hemorrhagic disease**.

The initial viremia produces systemic symptoms such as fever, chills, headaches, backaches, and other flu-like symptoms within 3 to 7 days of infection. Some of these symptoms can be attributed to the effects of the interferon produced in response to the viremia and infection of host cells. The viremia is considered a mild systemic disease, and most viral infections do not progress beyond this point.

After replication in cells of the monocyte-macrophage system, a secondary viremia may result. This viremia can produce sufficient virus to infect target organs such as the brain, liver, skin, and vasculature, depending on the tissue tropism of the virus (Fig. 59–4). The virus gains access to the brain by infecting the endothelial cells lining the small vessels of the brain or the choroid plexus.

The primary target cells of the flaviviruses are of the monocyte-macrophage lineage. Although these cells are found throughout the body and may have different characteristics, they express Fc receptors for antibody and release cytokines upon challenge. Flavivirus infection is enhanced 200- to 1000-fold by non-neutralizing antiviral antibody that promotes binding of the virus to the Fc receptors and its uptake into the cell.

Immune Response

Both humoral immunity and cellular immunity are elicited and are important to the control of primary infection and the prevention of future infections with the alphaviruses and flaviviruses.

Replication of the alphaviruses and flaviviruses pro-

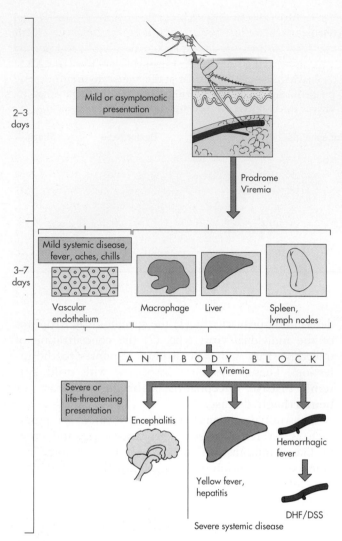

2–3
days

Mild or asymptomatic
presentation

Prodrome
Viremia

3–7
days

Mild systemic disease,
fever, aches, chills

Vascular
endothelium

Macrophage   Liver

Spleen,
lymph nodes

A N T I B O D Y   B L O C K

Viremia

Severe or
life-threatening
presentation

Encephalitis

Hemorrhagic
fever

Yellow fever,
hepatitis

DHF/DSS

Severe systemic disease

FIGURE 59–4. Disease syndromes of the alphaviruses and flaviviruses. Primary viremia may be associated with mild systemic disease. Most infections are limited to this. If sufficient virus is produced during the secondary viremia to escape immune protection and to reach critical target tissues, severe systemic disease or encephalitis may result. For dengue virus, rechallenge with another strain can result in severe dengue hemorrhagic fever (DHF), which can cause dengue shock syndrome (DSS) because of the loss of fluids from the vasculature.

duces a double-stranded RNA replicative intermediate that is a good inducer of interferon-α and interferon-β. The interferon is released into the blood stream and limits replication of the virus; it also stimulates the immune response but, in doing so, causes the rapid onset of the flu-like symptoms characteristic of mild systemic disease.

Circulating immunoglobulin (Ig) M is produced within 6 days of infection, followed by the production of IgG. The antibody blocks the viremic spread of the virus and the subsequent infection of other tissues. Im-

munity to one flavivirus can provide some protection against infection with other flaviviruses through recognition of the type common antigens expressed on all viruses in the family. Cell-mediated immunity is also important in controlling the primary infection.

Immunity to these viruses is a double-edged sword. A non-neutralizing antibody can enhance the uptake of flaviviruses into macrophages and other cells that express Fc receptors. Such an antibody can be generated to a related strain of virus in which the neutralizing epitope is not expressed or is different. Inflammation resulting from the cell-mediated immune response can destroy tissues and significantly contribute to the pathogenesis of encephalitis. Hypersensitivity reactions, such as delayed-type hypersensitivity, the formation of immune complexes with virions and viral antigens, and the activation of complement, can also occur. They can weaken the vasculature and cause it to rupture, leading to hemorrhagic symptoms. Immune responses to a related strain of dengue virus that do not prevent infection can promote immunopathogenesis, leading to dengue hemorrhagic fever or dengue shock syndrome.

Epidemiology

Alphaviruses and most flaviviruses are prototypical arboviruses (Box 59–3). To be an arbovirus, the virus must be able to (1) infect both vertebrates and invertebrates, (2) initiate a sufficient viremia in a vertebrate host for a sufficient time to allow acquisition of the virus by the invertebrate vector, and (3) initiate a persistent productive infection of the salivary gland of the invertebrate to provide virus for the infection of other host animals. **Humans are usually "dead-end" hosts**, in that they cannot spread the virus back to the vector because they do not maintain a persistent viremia. If the virus is not in the blood, the mosquito cannot acquire it. A full cycle of infection occurs when the virus is transmitted by the arthropod vector and amplified in a susceptible, immunologically naive host (**reservoir**) that allows the reinfection of other arthropods (Fig. 59–5). The vectors, natural hosts, and geographic distribution of representative alphaviruses and flaviviruses are listed in Table 59–2.

These viruses are usually restricted to a specific arthropod vector, its vertebrate host, and their ecologic niche. The most common vector is the mosquito, but some arboviruses are also spread by ticks and sandflies. Even in a tropical region overrun with mosquitoes, the spread of these viruses is still restricted to a specific genus of mosquitoes. Not all arthropods can act as good vectors for each virus. For example, *Culex quinquefasciatus* is resistant to infection by the WEE virus (alphavirus) but is an excellent vector for St. Louis encephalitis virus (flavivirus).

Birds and small mammals are the usual reservoir

mosquito vector, they risk being infected by the virus. Pools of standing water, drainage ditches, and trash dumps in cities can also provide breeding grounds for mosquitoes such as *Aedes aegypti*, the vector for yellow fever, dengue, and chikungunya. An increase in the population of these mosquitoes therefore puts the human population at risk for infection. Health departments in many areas monitor birds and mosquitoes caught in traps for arboviruses and initiate control measures, such as insecticide spraying, when necessary.

Urban outbreaks of arbovirus infections occur when the reservoirs for the virus are humans or urban animals. Humans can be reservoir hosts for yellow fever, dengue, and chikungunya viruses (see Fig. 59–5).

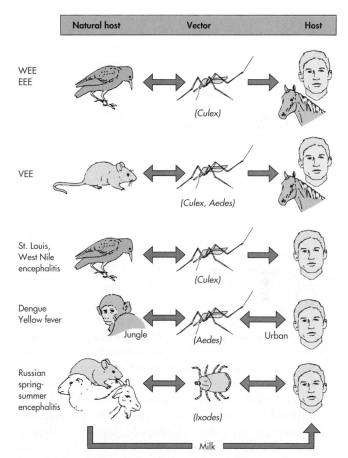

FIGURE 59–5. Patterns of alphavirus and flavivirus transmission. The cycle of arbovirus transmission maintains and amplifies the virus in the environment. Host-vector relationships that can provide this cycle are indicated by the *double arrow.* "Dead-end" infections with no transmission of the virus back to the vector are indicated by the single arrow. For St. Louis encephalitis, yellow fever, and dengue viruses, humans are not dead-end hosts and support an urban cycle. The Russian spring-summer encephalitis virus can be transmitted to humans by a tick bite and in milk form from infected goats. EEE = eastern equine encephalitis; VEE = Venezuelan equine encephalitis.

hosts for the alphaviruses and flaviviruses, but reptiles and amphibians can also act as hosts. A large population of viremic animals can develop in these species to continue the infection cycle of the virus. A 1999 epidemic of West Nile encephalitis virus in New York City was marked by the unusual deaths of captive birds at the Bronx Zoo as well as of crows, blue jays, and other wild birds. Representative birds and *Culex pipiens* mosquitoes in the region were demonstrated to be positive for the viral genome through the use of reverse transcriptase–polymerase chain reaction (RT-PCR) testing.

Arbovirus diseases occur during the summer months and rainy seasons, when the arthropods breed and the arboviruses are cycled among a host reservoir (birds), an arthropod (e.g., mosquitoes), and human hosts. This cycle maintains and increases the amount of virus in the environment. In the winter, the vector is not present to maintain the virus. The virus may either (1) persist in arthropod larvae or eggs or in reptiles or amphibians that remain in the locale or (2) migrate with the birds and then return during the summer.

When humans travel into the ecologic niche of the

These viruses are maintained by *Aedes* mosquitoes in a **sylvatic** or **jungle cycle**, in which monkeys are the natural host, and also in an **urban cycle**, in which humans are the host. *A. aegypti*, a vector for each of these viruses, is a household mosquito. It breeds in pools of water, open sewers, and other accumulations of water in cities. The occurrence of numerous inapparent infections in high-density populations provides enough viremic human hosts for the continued spread of these viruses. St. Louis encephalitis and West Nile encephalitis viruses are maintained in an urban environment because their vectors, *Culex* mosquitoes, breed in stagnant water, including puddles and sewage, and the reservoir group includes common city birds like crows.

Clinical Syndromes

More humans are infected with alphaviruses and flaviviruses than show significant, characteristic symptoms. The incidence of arbovirus disease is sporadic. Alphavirus disease is usually characterized as low-grade disease, and **flu-like symptoms** (chills, fever, rash, aches) correlate with systemic infection during the initial viremia. Eastern equine encephalitis (EEE), WEE, and Venezuelan equine encephalitis (VEE) virus infections can progress to **encephalitis** in humans. The equine encephalitis viruses are usually more of a problem to livestock than to humans. An affected human may experience fever, headache, and decreased consciousness 3 to 10 days after infection. Unlike herpes simplex virus encephalitis, the disease generally resolves without sequelae, but there is the possibility of paralysis, mental disability, seizures, and death. The name **chikungunya** (Swahili for "that which bends up") refers to the crippling arthritis associated with serious disease due to infection with these viruses. Although predominant in South America and western Africa, this disease may spread to the United States because of the return of the *A. aegypti* mosquito, its vector.

Most infections with flaviviruses are relatively benign, but serious **aseptic meningitis** and **encephalitic** or **hemorrhagic disease** can occur. The encephalitis viruses include St. Louis, West Nile, Japanese, Murray Valley, and Russian spring-summer viruses. Symptoms and outcomes are similar to those of the togavirus encephalitides. Hundreds to thousands of cases of St. Louis encephalitis virus disease are noted in the United States annually.

The hemorrhagic viruses are dengue and yellow fever viruses. **Dengue virus** is a major worldwide problem, with up to 100 million cases of dengue fever and 250,000 cases of **dengue hemorrhagic fever (DHF)** occurring per year. The incidence of the more serious DHF has quadrupled since 1985. Dengue fever is also known as **break-bone fever**; the symptoms and signs consist of high fever, headache, rash, and back and bone pain that last 6 to 7 days. On rechallenge with another of the four related strains, dengue can also cause DHF and **dengue shock syndrome (DSS)**. Non-neutralizing antibody promotes uptake of the virus into macrophages, which causes memory T cells to become activated, release inflammatory cytokines, and initiate hypersensitivity reactions. These reactions result in weakening and rupture of the vasculature, internal bleeding, and loss of plasma, leading to shock symptoms and internal bleeding. In 1981 in Cuba, dengue-2 virus infected a population previously exposed to dengue-1 virus between 1977 and 1980, leading to an epidemic in which there were more than 100,000 cases of DHF/DSS and 168 deaths.

Yellow fever infections are characterized by severe systemic disease, with degeneration of the liver, kidney, and heart as well as hemorrhage. Liver involvement causes the jaundice from which the disease gets its name, but massive gastrointestinal hemorrhages ("black vomit") may also occur. The mortality rate associated with yellow fever during epidemics is as high as 50%.

Laboratory Diagnosis

The alphaviruses and flaviviruses can be grown in both vertebrate and mosquito cell lines, but most are difficult to isolate. Infection can be detected through the use of cytopathologic studies, immunofluorescence, and the hemadsorption of avian erythrocytes. Detection and characterization can be performed by **reverse transcriptase-polymerase chain reaction** testing of genomic RNA or viral mRNA in blood or other samples. After isolation, the viral RNA can also be distinguished by the finding of RNA "fingerprints" of the genomic RNA. Monoclonal antibodies to the individual viruses have become a useful tool for distinguishing the individual species and strains of viruses.

A variety of serologic methods can be used to diagnose infections, including hemagglutination inhibition, enzyme-linked immunosorbent assays, and latex agglutination. The presence of specific IgM or a fourfold increase in titer between acute and convalescent sera is used to indicate a recent infection. The serologic cross-reactivity among viruses limits distinction of the actual viral species in many cases.

Treatment, Prevention, and Control

No treatments exist for arbovirus diseases other than supportive care.

The easiest means of preventing the spread of any arbovirus is elimination of its vector and breeding grounds. After 1900, when Walter Reed and his colleagues discovered that yellow fever was spread by *A. aegypti*, the number of cases was reduced from 1400 to none within 2 years purely through control of the mosquito population. Many Public Health departments monitor the bird and mosquito populations in a region for arboviruses and periodically spray to reduce the mosquito population. Avoidance of the breeding grounds of a mosquito vector is also a good preventive measure.

A live vaccine against yellow fever virus and killed vaccines against EEE, WEE, Japanese, and Russian spring-summer encephalitis viruses are available. These vaccines are meant for people working with the virus or at risk for contact. A live vaccine against VEE virus is available but only for use in domestic animals. A vaccine against dengue virus has not been developed because of the potential risk for immune enhancement of the disease upon subsequent challenge.

The yellow fever vaccine is prepared from the 17D strain isolated from a patient in 1927 and grown for long periods in monkeys, mosquitoes, embryonic tissue culture, and embryonated eggs. The vaccine is administered intradermally and elicits lifelong immunity to yellow fever and, possibly, other cross-reacting flaviviruses.

Rubella Virus

Rubella virus has the same structural properties and mode of replication as the other togaviruses. Unlike the other togaviruses, rubella is a **respiratory virus** and **does not cause readily detectable cytopathologic effects**.

Rubella is one of the five **classic childhood exanthems**, with measles, roseola, fifth disease, and chickenpox the other four. Rubella, meaning "little red" in Latin, was first distinguished from measles and other exanthems by German physicians; thus the common name for the disease, **German measles**. An astute Australian ophthalmologist, Norman McAlister Gregg, recognized in 1941 that maternal rubella infection was the cause of congenital cataracts. Maternal rubella infection has since been correlated with several other **severe congenital defects**. This finding prompted the development of a unique program to vaccinate children to prevent infection of pregnant women and neonates.

Pathogenesis and Immunity

Rubella virus is not cytolytic but does have limited cytopathologic effects in certain cell lines, such as Vero and RK13. The replication of rubella prevents (in a process known as **heterologous interference**) the replication of superinfecting picornaviruses. This property allowed the first isolations of rubella virus in 1962.

Rubella infects the upper respiratory tract and then spreads to local lymph nodes, which coincides with a period of lymphadenopathy (Fig. 59–6). This stage is followed by establishment of viremia, which spreads

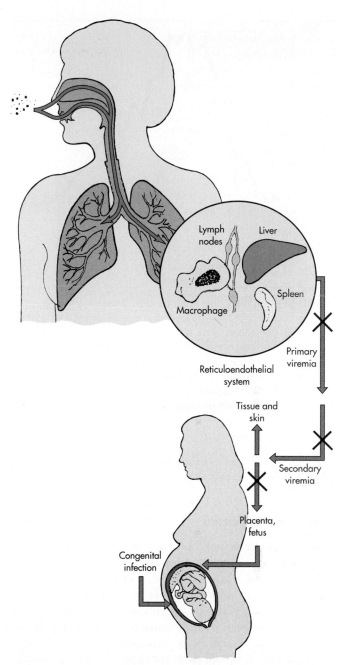

FIGURE 59–6. Spread of rubella virus within the host. Rubella enters and infects the nasopharynx and lung and then spreads to the lymph nodes and monocyte-macrophage system. The resulting viremia spreads the virus to other tissues and the skin. Circulating antibody can block the transfer of virus at the indicated points (X). In an immunologically deficient pregnant woman, the virus can infect the placenta and spread to the fetus.

the virus throughout the body. Infection of other tissues and the characteristic mild rash result. The prodromal period lasts approximately 2 weeks (Fig. 59–7). The person can shed virus in respiratory droplets dur-

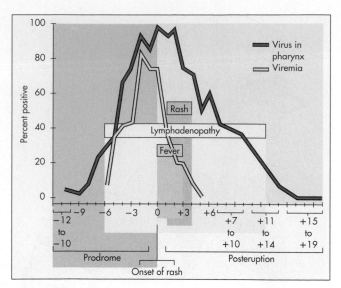

FIGURE 59–7. Time course of rubella disease. Rubella production in the pharynx precedes the appearance of symptoms and continues throughout the course of the disease. The onset of lymphadenopathy coincides with the viremia. Fever and rash occur later. The person is infectious as long as the virus is produced in the pharynx. (Redrawn from Plotkin SA: Rubella vaccine. In Plotkin SA, Mortimer EA, editors: *Vaccines,* Philadelphia, 1988, WB Saunders.)

ing the prodromal period and for as long as 2 weeks after the onset of the rash.

Immune Response

Antibody is generated after the viremia, and its appearance correlates with the appearance of the rash. The antibody limits viremic spread, but cell-mediated immunity plays an important role in resolving the infection. Only one serotype of rubella exists, and natural infection produces lifelong protective immunity. Most important, serum antibody in a pregnant woman prevents spread of the virus to the fetus. *Immune complexes most likely cause the rash and arthralgia associated with rubella infection.*

Congenital Infection

Rubella infection in a pregnant woman can result in serious congenital abnormalities in the child. If the mother does not have antibody, the virus can replicate in the placenta and spread to the fetal blood supply and throughout the fetus. Rubella can replicate in most tissues of the fetus. The virus may not be cytolytic, but the normal growth, mitosis, and chromosomal structure of the fetus's cells can be altered by the infection. The alterations can lead to improper development of the fetus, small size of the infected baby, and the **tera-**

togenic effects associated with congenital rubella infection. The nature of the disorder is determined by (1) the tissue affected and (2) the stage of development disrupted.

The virus may persist in tissues, such as the lens of the eye, for 3 to 4 years and may be shed up to a year after birth. The presence of the virus during the development of the baby's immune response may even have a tolerative effect on the system, preventing effective clearance of the virus after birth. Immune complexes that produce further clinical abnormalities may also form in the neonate or infant.

Epidemiology

Humans are the only host for rubella (Box 59–4). The virus is spread in respiratory secretions and is generally acquired during childhood. Spread of virus prior to or in the absence of symptoms and crowded conditions, such as those in daycare centers, promote contagion.

Approximately 20% of women of childbearing age escape infection during childhood and are susceptible to infection unless vaccinated. Programs in many states in the United States test expectant mothers for antibodies to rubella.

Before the development and use of the rubella vaccine, cases of rubella in school children would be reported every spring, and major epidemics of rubella occurred at regular 6- to 9-year intervals. The severity of the 1964 to 1965 epidemic in the United States is indicated in Table 59–3. Congenital rubella occurred in as many as 1% of all the children born in cities such as Philadelphia during this epidemic. Since the development of the vaccine, however, the incidence of ru-

---

BOX 59–4. **Epidemiology of Rubella Virus**

Disease/Viral Factors

Rubella infects only humans.
  Virus causes asymptomatic disease.
  There is one serotype.

Transmission

Respiratory route.

Who Is at Risk?

Children: mild exanthematous disease.
  Adults: more severe disease with arthritis or arthralgia.
  Neonates younger than 20 weeks: congenital defects.

Modes of Control

Live attenuated vaccine is administered as part of measles, mumps, and rubella (MMR) vaccine.

TABLE 59–3. Estimated Morbidity Associated with the 1964–1965 U.S. Rubella Epidemic

Clinical Events	Number Affected
Rubella cases	12,500,000
Arthritis-arthralgia	159,375
Encephalitis	2,084
Deaths	
Excess neonatal deaths	2,100
Other deaths	60
Total deaths	2,160
Excess fetal wastage	6,250
Congenital rubella syndrome	
Deaf children	8,055
Deaf-blind children	3,580
Mentally retarded children	1,790
Other congenital rubella syndrome symptoms	6,575
Total congenital rubella syndrome	20,000
Therapeutic abortions	5,000

From National Communicable Disease Center: *Rubella surveillance*, U.S. Department of Health, Education and Welfare, No 1, June 1969.

bella and congenital rubella is now less than 1 and 0.1 per 100,000 pregnancies, respectively.

Clinical Syndromes

Rubella disease is normally benign in children. After a 14- to 21-day incubation period, the symptoms in children consist of a 3-day **maculopapular** or **macular rash** and swollen glands (Fig. 59–8). Infection in adults, however, can be more severe and include problems such as bone and joint pain (arthralgia and arthritis) and (rarely) thrombocytopenia or postinfectious encephalopathy. Immunopathologic effects resulting from cell-mediated immunity and hypersensitivity reactions are a major cause of the more severe forms of rubella in adults.

Congenital disease is the most serious outcome of rubella infection. The fetus is at major risk until the 20th week of pregnancy. Maternal immunity to the virus resulting from prior exposure or vaccination prevents spread of the virus to the fetus. The most common manifestations of congenital rubella infection are cataracts, mental retardation, and deafness (Box 59–5; see Table 59–3). The mortality in utero and within the first year after birth is high for affected babies.

Laboratory Diagnosis

Isolation of the rubella virus is difficult and rarely attempted. The diagnosis is usually confirmed by the

FIGURE 59–8. Close-up of the rubella rash. Small erythematous macules are visible. (From Hart CA, Broadwell RL: *A color atlas of pediatric infectious disease,* London, 1992, Wolfe.)

presence of anti–rubella-specific IgM. A fourfold increase in specific IgG antibody titer between acute and convalescent sera is also used to indicate a recent infection. Antibodies to rubella are assayed early in pregnancy to determine the immune status of the woman; this test is required in many states.

When isolation of the virus is necessary, the virus is usually obtained from urine and is detected as interference with replication of echovirus 11 in primary African green monkey kidney cell cultures.

Treatment, Prevention, and Control

No treatment has been found for rubella. The best means of preventing rubella is vaccination with the live cold-adapted RA27/3 vaccine strain of virus (Fig. 59–9). The live rubella vaccine is usually administered with the measles and mumps vaccines (**MMR vaccine**) at 24 months of age. The triple vaccine is included routinely in well-baby care. Vaccination promotes both humoral and cellular immunity.

The primary reason for the rubella vaccination program is to prevent congenital infection by decreasing the number of susceptible people in the population, especially children. As a result, there are fewer sero-

BOX 59–5. Prominent Clinical Findings in Congenital Rubella Syndrome

Cataracts and other ocular defects
Heart defects
Deafness
Intrauterine growth retardation
  Failure to thrive
    Mortality within the first year
Microcephaly
  Mental retardation

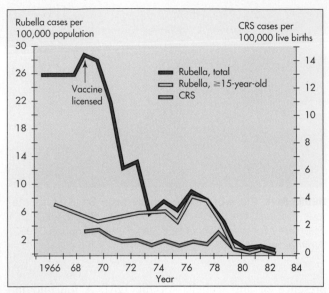

FIGURE 59–9. Effect of rubella virus vaccination on the incidence of rubella and congenital rubella syndrome (CRS). (Redrawn from Williams MN, Preblud SR: Current trends: rubella and congenital rubella—United States, 1983, MMWR Morbid Mortal Wkly Rep 33:237–247, 1984.)

negative mothers and smaller chance that they will be exposed to the virus from contact with the children. Because only one serotype for rubella exists and humans are the only reservoir, vaccination of a large proportion of the population can significantly reduce the likelihood of exposure to the virus.

CASE STUDY AND QUESTIONS

■ A 27-year-old businessman experienced a high fever, serious retro-orbital headache, and severe joint and back pain 5 days after he and his family returned from a trip to Malaysia. The symptoms lasted for 4 days, and then a rash appeared on his palms and soles that lasted for 2 days.

At the same time, the man's 5-year-old son experienced mild flu-like symptoms and then collapsed after 2 to 5 days. The boy's hands were cold and clammy, his face was flushed, and his body was warm. There were petechiae on his forehead and ecchymoses elsewhere. He bruised very easily. He was breathing rapidly and had a weak rapid pulse. He then rapidly recovered after 24 hours.

1. What features of these cases pointed to the diagnosis of dengue virus infection?
2. Of what significance was the trip to Malaysia?
3. What was the source of infection in the father and son?
4. What were the significance of and the pathogenic basis for the petechiae and ecchymoses in the child?

■ Two weeks after returning from a trip to Mexico, a 25-year-old man had arthralgia (joint aches) and a mild rash that started on his face and spread to his body. He recalled that he had felt as if he had the flu a few days before the onset of the rash. The rash disappeared in 4 days.

1. What features of this case pointed to the diagnosis of rubella infection?
2. Why is it significant that the symptoms started after a trip outside the United States?
3. What precaution could the man have taken to prevent this infection?
4. How was this infection transmitted?
5. Who was at risk for a serious outcome of this infection?
6. If this disease is normally mild in children, why is their immunization so important?

BIBLIOGRAPHY

Belshe RB, editor: *Textbook of human virology*, ed 2, St. Louis, 1991, Mosby.

Fields BN et al, editors: *Virology*, ed 3, New York, 1996, Lippincott-Raven.

Monath TP: Yellow fever vaccine. In Plotkin SA, Orenstein WA, editors: *Vaccines*, ed 3, Philadelphia, 1999, WB Saunders.

Hahn CS et al: Flavivirus genome organization, expression, and replication, *Annu Rev Microbiol* 44:649–688, 1990.

Johnson RT: *Viral infections of the nervous system*, New York, 1982, Raven.

Koblet H: The "merry-go-round": alphaviruses between vertebrate and invertebrate cells, *Adv Virus Res* 38:343–403, 1990.

Plotkin SA: Rubella vaccine. In Plotkin SA, Monath TP, editors: *Vaccines*, ed 3, Philadelphia, 1999, WB Saunders.

Stollar V: Approaches to the study of vector specificity for arboviruses: model systems using cultured mosquito cells. In Maramorosch K et al, editors: *Advances in virus research*, vol 33, New York, 1987, Academic.

Tsai TF: Arboviral infections in the United States, *Infect Dis Clin North Am* 5:73–102, 1991.

West Nile virus: NIAID fact sheet: Available at http://www.niaid.nih.gov/factsheets/westnile.htm/

CHAPTER 60

Bunyaviridae

The Bunyaviridae constitute a "supergroup" of at least **200 enveloped, segmented, negative-strand RNA viruses**. The supergroup is further broken down into the following four genera on the basis of structural and biochemical features: Bunyavirus, Phlebovirus, Nairovirus, and Hantavirus (Table 60–1). Most of the Bunyaviridae are **arboviruses** (*ar*thropod-*bo*rne) that are spread by mosquitoes, ticks, or flies and are endemic to the environment of the vector. The **hantaviruses** are the exception; they are carried by **rodents**.

Structure

The bunyaviruses are roughly spherical particles 90 to 120 nm in diameter (Box 60–1). The envelope of the virus contains two glycoproteins (G1 and G2) and encloses three unique negative-strand RNAs, the large (**L**), medium (**M**), and small (**S**) RNAs that are associated with the protein to form nucleocapsids (Table 60–2). The genome segments for the La Crosse and related California encephalitis viruses are circular. The nucleocapsids include the RNA-dependent RNA polymerase (L protein) and two nonstructural proteins (NS_s, NS_m) (Fig. 60–1). Unlike other negative-strand RNA viruses, the Bunyaviridae **do not have a matrix protein**. The five genera of Bunyaviridae are distinguished by differences in (1) the number and sizes of the virion proteins, (2) the lengths of the L, M, and S strands of the genome, and (3) their transcription.

Replication

The Bunyaviridae replicate in the same way as the enveloped, negative-strand viruses. Specifically, after interaction of the G1 glycoprotein with cell surface receptors, the virus is internalized by endocytosis and fuses with endosomal membranes on acidification of the vesicle. The release of the nucleocapsid into the cytoplasm allows mRNA and protein synthesis to begin.

The M strand encodes the NS_m nonstructural protein and the G1 (viral attachment) and G2 proteins, and the L strand encodes the L protein (polymerase) (see Table 60–2). The S strand of RNA encodes two nonstructural proteins, N and NS_s.

Replication of the genome by the L protein also provides new templates for transcription, thereby increasing the rate of mRNA synthesis. The glycoproteins are then synthesized and glycosylated in the endoplasmic reticulum, after which they are transferred to the Golgi apparatus but not translocated to the plasma membrane. Virions are assembled by budding into the Golgi apparatus and are released by cell lysis or exocytosis.

Pathogenesis

As **arboviruses,** Bunyaviridae possess many of the same pathogenic mechanisms as the togaviruses and flaviviruses (Box 60–2). For example, the virus is spread by an arthropod vector and is injected into the blood, initiating a viremia. Progression past this stage to secondary viremia and further dissemination of the virus can deliver the virus to target sites typically involved in that particular viral disease, such as the central nervous system, liver, kidney, and vascular endothelium.

Many Bunyaviridae cause neuronal and glial damage and cerebral edema, leading to encephalitis. In certain viremic infections (e.g., Rift Valley fever), hepatic necrosis may occur. In others (e.g., Crimean-Congo hem-

---

BOX 60–1. Unique Features of Bunyaviruses

There are at least 200 related viruses in 5 genera that share a common morphology and basic components.
   Virion is enveloped with three (L, M, S) negative RNA nucleocapsids but no matrix proteins.
   Virus replicates in the cytoplasm.
   Virus can infect humans and arthropods.
   Virus in arthropod can be transmitted to its eggs.

TABLE 60–1. Notable Bunyaviridae Genera*

Genus	Members	Insect Vector	Pathologic Conditions	Vertebrate Hosts
Bunyavirus	Bunyamwera virus, California encephalitis virus, La Crosse virus, Oropouche virus; 150 members	Mosquito	Febrile illness, encephalitis, febrile rash	Rodents, small mammals, primates, marsupials, birds
Phlebovirus	Rift Valley fever virus, sandfly fever virus; 36 members	Fly	Sandfly fever, hemorrhagic fever, encephalitis, conjunctivitis, myositis	Sheep, cattle, domestic animals
Nairovirus	Crimean-Congo hemorrhagic fever virus; 6 members	Tick	Hemorrhagic fever	Hares, cattle, goats, seabirds
Uukuvirus	Uukuniemi virus; 7 members	Tick	—	Birds
Hantavirus	Hantaan virus	None	Hemorrhagic fever with renal syndrome, adult respiratory distress syndrome	Rodents
	Sin Nombre	None	Hantavirus pulmonary syndrome, shock, pulmonary edema	Deer mouse

* An additional 35 viruses possess several common properties with Bunyaviridae but are as yet unclassified.

orrhagic fever and Hantaan hemorrhagic disease), the primary lesion involves the leakage of plasma and erythrocytes through the vascular endothelium. In the latter infection, these changes are most prominent in the kidney and are accompanied by hemorrhagic necrosis of the kidney. Unlike most other bunyaviruses, the hantavirus initiates infection and remains in the lung, where it causes hemorrhagic tissue destruction and lethal pulmonary disease.

Epidemiology

Most bunyaviruses are transmitted by infected mosquitoes, ticks, or *Phlebotomus* flies to rodents, birds, and larger animals (Box 60–3). The animals then become the **reservoirs** for the virus, thereby continuing the cycle of infection. Humans are infected when they en-

ter the environment of the insect vector (Fig. 60–2). Transmission occurs during the summer, but unlike many other arboviruses, many of the Bunyaviridae can survive a winter in the ova of the mosquito and remain in a locale.

Many of the members of this virus family are found in South America, southeastern Europe, Southeast Asia, and Africa and bear the exotic names of their ecological niches. Viruses of the **California encephalitis virus group** (e.g., La Crosse virus) are spread by mosquitoes that are found in the forests of North America (Fig. 60–3). Up to 150 cases of encephalitis occur during the summer each year in the United States, but most infections are asymptomatic. These viruses are spread mainly by *Aedes triseriatus* and by *Culiseta*, which breeds in the water in tree holes and discarded tires.

The hantaviruses do not have an arthropod vector but are maintained in a rodent species specific for each

TABLE 60–2. Genome and Proteins of California Encephalitis Virus

Genome*	Proteins
L	RNA polymerase, 170 kDa
M	Spike glycoprotein, 75 kDa
	Spike glycoprotein, 65 kDa
	Nonstructural protein, 15 to 17 kDa
S	Nucleocapsid protein, 25 kDa
	Nucleocapsid protein, 10 kDa

* Negative-strand RNA.

BOX 60–2. Disease Mechanisms for Bunyaviruses

Virus is acquired from an arthropod bite (e.g., mosquito)
  Initial viremia may cause flu-like symptoms.
  Establishment of secondary viremia may allow virus access to specific target tissues, including the central nervous system, organs, and vascular endothelium.
  Antibody is important in controlling viremia; interferon and cell-mediated immunity may prevent the outgrowth of infection.

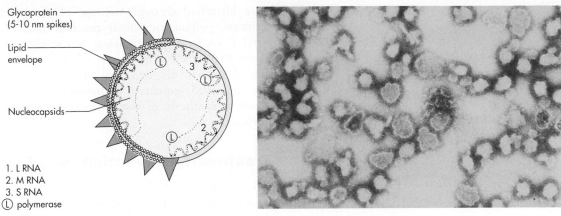

FIGURE 60–1. *A*, Model of bunyavirus particle. *B*, Electron micrograph of La Crosse variant of bunyavirus. Note the spike proteins at the surface of the virion envelope. (*A* redrawn from Fraenkel-Conrat H, Wagner RR, editors: *Comprehensive virology*, vol 14, New York, 1979, Plenum; *B* courtesy Centers for Disease Control and Prevention, Atlanta.)

virus. Humans are infected by close contact with rodents or through the inhalation of aerosolized rodent urine. In May 1993, an outbreak of **hantavirus pulmonary syndrome** occurred in the Four Corners area of New Mexico. The outbreak is attributed to increased contact with the deer mouse vector during a season of unusually high rainfall, greater availability of food, and rise in the rodent population. The Sin Nombre and Convict Creek virus strains were isolated from the victims and rodents. Since this incident, hantavirus has been associated with other outbreaks of respiratory tract disease.

Clinical Syndromes

Bunyaviridae, which are mosquito-borne viruses, usually cause a nonspecific febrile flu-like illness related to the viremia (see Table 60–1) that is indistinguishable from illnesses caused by other viruses. The incubation period for these illnesses is about 48 hours, and the fevers last approximately 3 days. Most patients with infections, even those infected by agents known to cause severe disease (e.g., Rift Valley fever virus, La Crosse virus), have mild illness.

Encephalitis illnesses (e.g., La Crosse virus) are

BOX 60–3. **Epidemiology of Bunyavirus Infections**

Disease/Viral Factors

Virus is able to replicate in mammalian and arthropod cells.

Virus is able to pass into ovary and infect arthropod eggs, allowing virus to survive during winter.

Transmission

Via arthropods through break in skin. California encephalitis group: *Aedes* mosquito.

Aedes mosquitoes are daytime feeders and live in forest.

Aedes mosquitoes lay eggs in small pools of water trapped in places such as trees and tires.

Who Is at risk?

People in habitat of arthropod vector.

California encephalitis group: campers, forest rangers, woodsmen.

Geography/Season

Disease incidence correlates with distribution of vector.

Disease is more common in summer.

Modes of Control

Elimination of vector or vector's habitat.

Avoidance of vector's habitat.

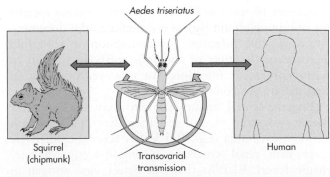

FIGURE 60–2. Transmission of La Crosse (California) encephalitis virus.

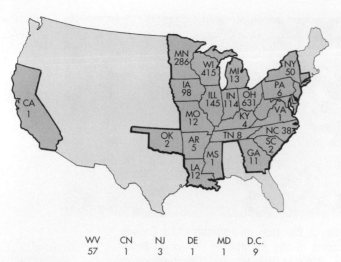

FIGURE 60–3. Distribution of California encephalitis, 1964 to 1989. (Redrawn from Tsai TF: Arboviral infections in the United States. *Infect Dis Clin North Am* 5:73–102, 1991.)

sudden in onset after an incubation period of approximately 1 week, and symptoms at this time consist of fever, headache, lethargy, and vomiting. Seizures occur in 50% of patients with encephalitis, usually early in the illness. Signs of meningitis may also be present. The illness lasts an average of 7 days. Death occurs in less than 1% of patients, but seizure disorders may occur as sequelae in as much as 20%.

Hemorrhagic fevers such as Rift Valley fever are characterized by petechial hemorrhages, ecchymosis, epistaxis, hematemesis, melena, and bleeding of the gums. Death occurs in as many as half of patients with hemorrhagic phenomena. The **hantavirus pulmonary syndrome** is a terrible disease consisting of a prodrome of fever and muscle aches, followed rapidly by interstitial pulmonary edema, respiratory failure, and death within days.

Laboratory Diagnosis

Serologic tests are generally performed to confirm a diagnosis of bunyavirus infection. Virus neutralization assays can be used to identify the virus. Assays specific for immunoglobulin (Ig) M are useful in the documentation of acute infection. Seroconversion or a fourfold increase in the titer of the IgG antibody is used to document recent infection, but cross-reactions within viral genera are common.

Enzyme-linked immunosorbent assay (ELISA) may detect antigen in clinical specimens from patients with an intense viremia (e.g., Rift Valley fever, hemorrhagic fever with renal syndrome, Crimean-Congo hemorrhagic fever). ELISAs that can detect viral antigen in mosquitoes have been developed.

The Sin Nombre and Convict Creek hantaviruses were identified through the use of the reverse transcriptase–polymerase chain reaction (RT-PCR) test. Viral RNA from patient tissue was converted to complementary DNA with the use of the reverse transcriptase of a retrovirus, and then DNA primers representing conserved sequences of hantaviruses were used to promote synthesis of the characteristic hantavirus sequences.

Treatment, Prevention, and Control

No specific therapy for infections of the Bunyaviridae is available. Human disease is prevented by interruption of the contact between humans and the vector, whether arthropod or mammal. Arthropod vectors are controlled by (1) eliminating the growth conditions for the vector, (2) spraying with insecticide, (3) installing netting or screening at windows and doors, (4) wearing protective clothing, and (5) controlling the tick infestation of animals. Rodent control minimizes the transmission of many viruses, especially hantaviruses. Rift Valley fever vaccines have been developed for use in humans and animals (sheep and cattle).

CASE STUDY AND QUESTIONS

■ A 15-year-old summer camp counselor in Ohio suddenly complained of a headache, nausea, and vomiting; she had a fever and experienced a stiff neck. She was admitted to the hospital, where a spinal tap and examination of cerebrospinal fluid revealed inflammatory cells. She became lethargic over the next day but became alert again after 4 to 5 days.

1. The physician suspected La Crosse encephalitis virus as the agent. What clues pointed to La Crosse virus?

2. What other agents would also be considered in the differential diagnosis?

3. How was the patient infected?

4. How would the transmission of this agent be prevented?

5. How could the local public health department determine the prevalence of La Crosse virus in the environment of the summer camp? What samples would they obtain and how would they test them?

BIBLIOGRAPHY

Bishop DHL, Shope RE: Bunyaviridae. In Fraenkel-Conrat H, Wagner RR, editors: *Comprehensive virology*, vol 14, New York, 1979, Plenum.

Fields BN, Knipe DM, Howley PM, editors: *Virology*, ed 3, New York, 1996, Lippincott-Raven.

Kolakofsky D: Bunyaviridae, *Curr Top Microbiol Immunol* 169: 1–256, 1991.

McKee KT, LeDuc JW, Peters CJ: Hantaviruses. In Belshe RB, editor: *Textbook of human virology*, ed 2, St. Louis, 1991, Mosby.

Peters CJ, LeDuc JW: Bunyaviruses, phleboviruses and related viruses. In Belshe RB, editor: *Textbook of human virology*, ed 2, St. Louis, 1991, Mosby.

Peters CJ, Simpson GL, Levy H: Spectrum of hantavirus infection: hemorrhagic fever with renal syndrome and hantavirus pulmonary syndrome, *Annu Rev Med* 50:531–545, 1999.

Tsai TF: Arboviral infections in the United States, *Infect Dis Clin North Am* 5:73–102, 1991.

Wrobel S: Serendipity, science and a new hantavirus, *FASEB J* 9:1247–1254, 1995.

CHAPTER 61

Retroviruses

he retroviruses are probably the most studied group of viruses in molecular biology. These viruses are **enveloped, positive-strand RNA** viruses with a unique morphology and means of replication. In 1970, Baltimore and Temin showed that the retroviruses encode an **RNA-dependent DNA polymerase (reverse transcriptase)** and replicate through a DNA intermediate. The DNA copy of the viral genome is then integrated into the host chromosome to become a cellular gene. This discovery, which earned the Nobel Prize, contradicted the central dogma of molecular biology—that genetic information passed from DNA to RNA and then to protein.

The first retrovirus to be isolated was the Rous sarcoma virus, shown by Peyton Rous to produce solid tumors (sarcomas) in chickens. Like most retroviruses, the Rous sarcoma virus proved to have a very limited host and species range. Cancer-causing retroviruses have since been isolated from other animal species and are classified as RNA tumor viruses or **oncornaviruses.** Many of these viruses alter cellular growth by expressing analogues of cellular growth–controlling genes **(oncogenes).** Not until 1981, however, when Robert Gallo and his associates isolated human T-lymphotropic virus (HTLV-1) from a person with adult human T-cell leukemia, was a human retrovirus isolated and associated with human disease.

In the late 1970s and early 1980s, an unusual number of young homosexual men, Haitians, heroin addicts, and hemophiliacs in the United States (the initial "4H club" of risk groups) were noted to be dying of normally benign opportunistic infections. Their symptoms defined a new disease, the **acquired immunodeficiency syndrome (AIDS).** However, as is now known, AIDS proved not to be limited to these groups but can occur in anyone exposed to the virus. Now approximately 35 million men, women, and children around the world are living with the virus that causes AIDS. Montagnier and associates in Paris and Gallo and colleagues in the United States reported the isola-

TABLE 61–1. Classification of Retroviruses

Subfamily	Characteristics	Examples
Oncovirinae	Are associated with cancer and neurologic disorders	—
B	Have eccentric nucleocapsid core in mature virion	Mouse mammary tumor virus
C	Have centrally located nucleocapsid core in mature virion	Human T-lymphotropic virus* (HTLV-1, HTLV-2, HTLV-5), Rous sarcoma virus (chickens)
D	Have nucleocapsid core with cylindrical form	Mason-Pfizer monkey virus
Lentivirinae	Have slow onset of disease: cause neurologic disorders and immunosuppression; are viruses with D-type, cylindrical nucleocapsid core	Human immunodeficiency virus* (HIV-1, HIV-2), visna virus (sheep), caprine arthritis/encephalitis virus (goats)
Spumavirinae	Cause no clinical disease but characteristic vacuolated "foamy" cytopathology	Human foamy virus*
Endogenous viruses	Have retrovirus sequences that are integrated into human genome	Human placental virus

*Also classified as complex retroviruses because of the requirement for accessory proteins for replication.

tion of the human immunodeficiency virus (HIV-1) from patients with lymphadenopathy and AIDS. A variant of HIV-1, designated **HIV-2,** was isolated later and is prevalent in West Africa. HIV appears to have evolved since the 1930s from a simian virus and then rapidly spread through Africa and the world by an increasingly mobile population.

Our understanding of the retroviruses has paralleled progress in molecular biology. In turn, the retroviruses have provided a major tool for molecular biology, the reverse transcriptase enzyme, and through the study of viral oncogenes have also provided a means of advancing our understanding of cell growth, differentiation, and oncogenesis.

The three subfamilies of human retroviruses are the **Oncovirinae,** or oncovirus (HTLV-1, HTLV-2, HTLV-5); the **Lentivirinae** (HIV-1, HIV-2); and the **Spumavirinae** (Table 61–1). Although a spumavirus was the first human retrovirus to be isolated, no such virus has been associated with human disease. **Endogenous retroviruses,** the ultimate parasite, have integrated, are transmitted vertically, and may take up as much as 1% of the human chromosome. Although they may not produce virions, their gene sequences have been detected in many animal species and in humans.

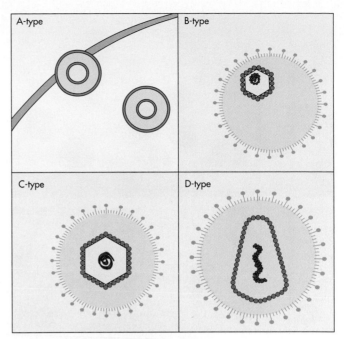

FIGURE 61–1. Morphologic distinction of retrovirions. The morphology and position of the nucleocapsid core are used to classify the viruses. A-type particles are immature intracytoplasmic forms that bud through the plasma membrane into mature B-type, C-type, and D-type particles.

Classification

The retroviruses are classified by the diseases they cause, tissue tropism and host range, virion morphology, and genetic complexity (see Table 61–1). The **oncoviruses** include the only retroviruses that can *immortalize or transform target cells.* These viruses are also categorized by the morphology of their core and capsid as type A, B, C, or D, as seen in electron micrographs (Fig. 61–1; see Table 61–1). The **lentiviruses** *are slow viruses associated with neurologic and immunosuppressive diseases.* The spumaviruses, represented by a foamy virus, cause a distinct cytopathologic effect but, as already noted, do not seem to cause clinical disease.

Structure

The retroviruses are roughly spherical, enveloped RNA viruses with a diameter of 80 to 120 nm (Fig. 61–2 and Box 61–1). The envelope contains viral glycoproteins and is acquired by budding from the plasma membrane. The **envelope surrounds a capsid that contains two identical copies of the positive-strand RNA genome** inside an electron-dense core. The virion also contains 10 to 50 copies of the **reverse transcriptase and integrase enzymes** and **two cellular transfer RNA** (tRNAs). These tRNAs are base-paired to each copy of the genome to be used as a primer for the reverse transcriptase. The morphology of the core differs for different viruses and is used as a means of classifying the retroviruses (see Fig. 61–1). The HIV virion core resembles a truncated cone (Fig. 61–3).

The retrovirus genome has a 5′ cap and is polyadenylated at the 3′ end (Fig. 61–4 and Table 61–2). Although the genome resembles a messenger RNA (mRNA), it is not infectious because it does not encode a polymerase that can directly generate more mRNA. The genome of the **simple retroviruses** *consists of three major genes that encode polyproteins* for the following enzymatic and structural proteins of the virus: **gag** (group-specific antigen, *capsid proteins*), **pol** (*polymerase, protease,* and *integrase*), and **env** (envelope, *glycoproteins*). At each end of the genome are **long-terminal repeat (LTR)** sequences. The LTR sequences contain promoters, enhancers, and other gene sequences used for binding different cellular transcription factors. Oncogenic viruses may also contain a growth-regulating oncogene that may replace other sequences. The **complex retroviruses,** HTLV, and the lentiviruses (including HIV) also *encode several regulatory proteins* that require more complex transcriptional processing (splicing) than the simple retroviruses.

The viral glycoproteins are produced by proteolytic cleavage of the polyprotein encoded by the env gene. The size of the glycoproteins differs for each group of viruses. For example, the (glycoprotein) gp62 of

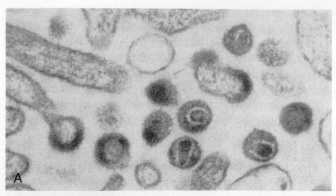

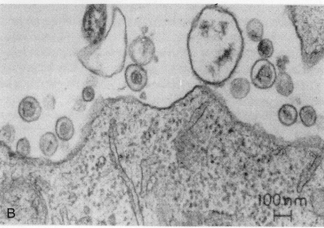

B   100 nm

FIGURE 61-2. Electron micrographs of two retroviruses. *A,* Human immunodeficiency virus. Note the cone-shaped nucleocapsid in several of the virions. *B,* Human T-lymphotropic virus. Note the C-type morphology characterized by a central symmetrical nucleocapsid. (From Belshe RB, editor: *Textbook of human virology,* ed 2, St Louis, 1991, Mosby.)

BOX 61-1. Unique Characteristics of Retroviruses

Virus has an **enveloped** spherical virion that is 80 to 120 nm in diameter and that encloses a capsid containing **two** copies of the **positive-strand RNA** genome (approximately 9 kilobases for HIV and HTLV).

RNA-dependent DNA polymerase **(reverse transcriptase)** and integrase enzymes are carried in the virion.

Virus receptor is the initial determinant of tissue tropism.

Replication proceeds through a DNA intermediate, termed the provirus.

The provirus **integrates** randomly into the host chromosome and becomes a cellular gene.

Transcription of the genome is regulated by the interaction of host transcription factors with promoter and enhancer elements in the long-terminal repeat (LTR) portion of the genome.

Simple retroviruses encode gag, pol, and env genes. **Complex viruses** also encode accessory genes (e.g., tat, rev, nef, vif, vpu for HIV).

Virus assembles and buds from the plasma membrane.

Final morphogenesis of HIV *requires* protease cleavage of gag and gag-pol polypeptides after envelopment.

HIV = human immunodeficiency virus; HTLV = human T-lymphotropic virus.

HTLV-1 is cleaved into a gp46 and p21, and the *gp160 of HIV is cleaved into gp41 and gp120.* These glycoproteins form lollipop-like trimer spikes that are visible on the surface of the virion. The larger of the glycoproteins binds to cell surface receptors, initially determines the tissue tropism of the virus, and is recognized by neutralizing antibody. The smaller subunit (gp41 in HIV) forms the lollipop stick and promotes cell-cell fusion. The gp120 of HIV is extensively glycosylated, and *its antigenicity and receptor specificity can drift during the course of a chronic HIV infection.* These factors impede immune clearance of the virus.

Replication

Replication of the human retroviruses (HIV and HTLV) starts with binding of the viral glycoprotein spikes to **the CD4 surface receptor protein** (Fig. 61–5). Initially, the gp120 of HIV binds mainly to the CD4 molecule expressed on cells of the macrophage lineage (e.g., macrophage, dendritic cells, microglial cells) (M-tropic) as well as a second receptor, a 7-transmembrane G-protein–coupled chemokine receptor **(CCR5 on macrophages).** Later in the course of disease, the virus changes and binds to CD4 on helper T cells (T-tropic) and a different chemokine receptor, **fusin [CXCR4]** (Fig. 61–6). Chemokines are

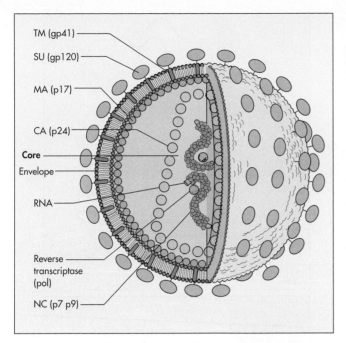

FIGURE 61–3. Cross section of human immunodeficiency virus. The enveloped virion contains two identical RNA strands, RNA polymerase, integrase, and two transfer RNAs (tRNAs) base-paired to the genome within the protein core. This is surrounded by proteins and a lipid bilayer. The envelope spikes are the glycoprotein (gp) 120 attachment protein and gp41 fusion protein. (Redrawn from Gallo RC, Montagnier L: Aids in 1988, *Sci Am* 259:41–51, 1988.)

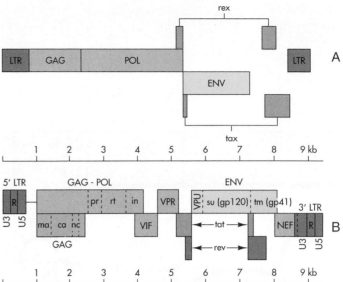

FIGURE 61–4. Genomic structure of human retroviruses. *A*, Human T-lymphotropic virus (HTLV-1). *B*, Human immunodeficiency virus (HIV-1). The genes are defined in Table 61–2 and Figure 61–7. Unlike the other genes of these viruses, production of the messenger RNA for tax and rex (HTLV-1) and tat and rev (HIV) requires excision of two intron units. HIV-2 has a similar genome map. The vpu for HIV-2 is termed *vpx*. LTR = long-terminal repeat. Protein nomenclature for HIV: ma = matrix protein; ca = capsid protein; nc = nucleocapsid protein; pr = protease; rt = reverse transcriptase; in = integrase; su = surface glycoprotein component; tm = transmembrane glycoprotein component. (Redrawn from Belshe RB, editor: *Textbook of human virology*, ed 2, St Louis, 1991, Mosby.)

TABLE 61–2. Retrovirus Genes and Their Function

Gene	Virus	Function
gag	All	Group-specific antigen: core and capsid proteins
pol	All	Polymerase: reverse transcriptase, protease, integrase
env	All	Envelope: glycoproteins
tax	HTLV	Transactivation of viral and cellular genes
tat	HIV-1	Transactivation of viral and cellular genes
rex	HTLV	Regulation of RNA splicing and promotion of export to cytoplasm
rev	HIV-1	Regulation of RNA splicing and promotion of export to cytoplasm
nef	HIV-1	Alteration of cell activation signals; progression to AIDS (essential)
vif	HIV-1	Virus infectivity, promotion of assembly
vpu	HIV-1	Facilitation of release of virus, decrease of cell surface CD4
vpr (vpx*)	HIV-1	Transport of complementary DNA to nucleus, arresting of cell growth
LTR	All	Promoter, enhancer elements

*In HIV-2.

HIV = human immunodeficiency virus; HTLV = human T-lymphotropic virus; LTR = long-terminal repeat (sequence).

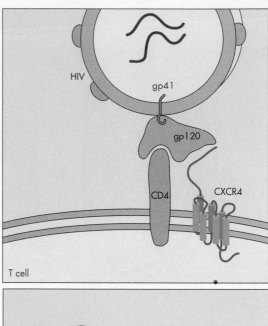

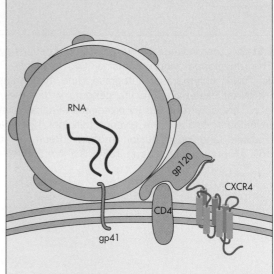

FIGURE 61–6. Target cell binding of human immunodeficiency virus. (Redrawn from Balter M: AIDS research: new hope in HIV disease, *Science* 274:1988, 1996.)

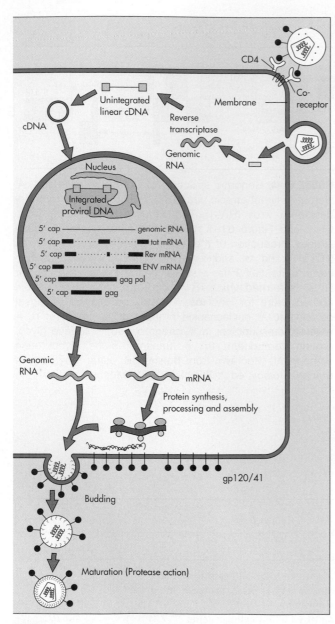

FIGURE 61–5. The life cycle of human immunodeficiency virus (HIV). HIV binds to CD4 and chemokine co-receptors and enters by fusion. The genome is reverse transcribed into DNA in the cytoplasm and integrated into the nuclear DNA. Transcription and translation of the genome occur in a fashion similar to that of human T-lymphotropic virus (HTLV-1) (see Fig. 61–7). The virus assembles at the plasma membrane and matures after budding from the cell. cDNA = complementary DNA. (Redrawn from Fauci AS: The human immunodeficiency virus: infectivity and mechanisms of pathogenesis, *Science* 239:617–622, 1988.)

small peptides involved in promoting inflammatory responses and chemotaxis. A small percentage of people are resistant to infection because they are genetically deficient in these co-receptors. HIV enters the cell by fusion of the envelope with the cellular plasma membrane; other retroviruses may enter the cell by receptor-mediated endocytosis.

Once released into the cytoplasm, the reverse transcriptase uses the virion tRNA as a primer and synthesizes a complementary, negative-strand DNA. The reverse transcriptase also acts as a ribonuclease H, degrades the RNA genome, and then synthesizes the positive strand of DNA **(complementary DNA)** (Fig. 61–7). During the synthesis of the virion DNA **(provirus),** sequences from each end of the genome (U3 and

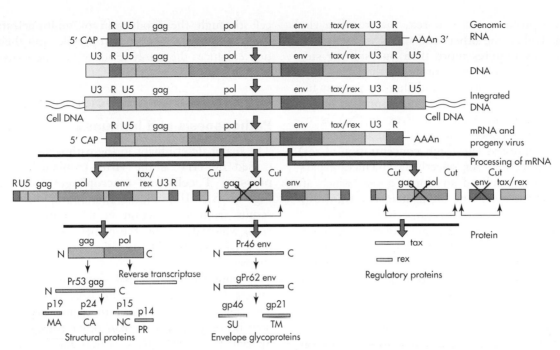

FIGURE 61–7. Transcription and translation of human T-lymphotropic virus (HTLV-1). (A similar but more complex approach is used for human immunodeficiency virus [HIV].). All HTLV-1 and HIV messenger RNA (mRNA) initiate and include the 5′ end of the genome. The mRNA for tax and rex requires excision of two sequences, the gag-pol and env sequences. The other mRNAs, including the env mRNA, require excision of one sequence. Translation of these mRNAs produces polyproteins, which are subsequently cleaved. Gene nomenclature: gag = group antigen gene; pol = polymerase; env = envelope glycoprotein gene; tax = transactivator; rex = regulator of splicing. Protein nomenclature: MA = matrix; CA = capsid; NC = nucleocapsid; PR = protease; SU = surface component; TM = transmembrane component of envelope glycoprotein; N = amino terminus; C = carboxyl terminus of peptide. Prefixes: p = protein; PR = precursor polyprotein; gp = glycoprotein; gPr = glycosylated precursor polyprotein.

U5) are duplicated, thus attaching the LTRs to both ends. This process creates sequences necessary for integration and *creates enhancer and promoter sequences within the LTR for the regulation of transcription.* The DNA copy of the genome is larger than the original RNA.

Reverse transcriptase is very error-prone. For example, the error rate for the reverse transcriptase from HIV is 1 error per 2000 base pairs, or approximately 5 errors per genome (HIV, 9000 base pairs). This genetic instability of HIV is responsible for promoting the generation of new strains of virus during a person's disease, a property that may alter the pathogenicity of the virus and promote immune escape.

The double-stranded complementary DNA is then delivered to the nucleus and spliced into the host chromosome with the aid of a virus-encoded, virion-carried enzyme, **integrase.** HIV and other lentiviruses produce an abundance of nonintegrated circular DNA, which is not transcribed efficiently but may have a role in the cytopathogenesis of the virus.

Once integrated, the viral DNA is transcribed as a cellular gene by the host RNA polymerase II. Transcription of the genome produces a full-length RNA, which for simple retroviruses is processed to produce several mRNAs containing either the gag, gag-pol, or env gene sequences. The full-length transcripts of the genome can also be assembled into new virions.

Because the virus acts as a cellular gene, its replication depends on the extent of methylation of the viral DNA, on the cell's growth rate, but mostly on the ability of the cell to activate the enhancers and promoter sequences encoded in the LTR region. Stimulation of the cell by mitogens, certain lymphokines, or infection with exogenous viruses (e.g., herpesviruses) produces transcription factors that also bind to the LTR and can activate transcription of the virus. Viral oncogenes (if present) promote cell growth and as a result stimulate transcription and viral replication. *The efficiency of viral transcription is the second major determinant of retroviral tissue tropism and the host range of the virus.*

HTLV and HIV are complex retroviruses. HTLV-1

encodes two proteins, **tax** and **rex,** that regulate viral replication. Unlike the other viral mRNAs, the mRNA for tax and rex requires more than one splicing step. The rex gene encodes two proteins that bind to a structure on the viral mRNA and thereby prevent further splicing and promote mRNA transport to the cytoplasm. The doubly spliced tax/rex mRNA is expressed early (low concentration of rex), and structural proteins are expressed late (high concentration of rex). Late in the infection, rex selectively enhances expression of the singly spliced structural genes, which are required in abundance. The tax protein is a **transcriptional activator** and enhances transcription of the viral genome from the promoter gene sequence in the 5′ LTR. Tax also activates other genes, including interleukin-2 (IL-2), IL-3, granulocyte-macrophage colony-stimulating factor, and the receptor for IL-2. Activation of these genes promotes the growth of the infected T cell.

HIV replication is regulated by as many as six **"accessory" gene products** (see Table 61–2). The **tat,** like tax, is a transactivator of the transcription of viral and cellular genes. The **rev** acts like the rex protein. The **nef** protein reduces cell surface CD4 expression, alters T-cell signaling pathways, regulates the cytotoxicity of the virus, and is required to maintain high viral loads. The nef protein appears to be essential for causing the infection to progress to AIDS. The **vif** protein promotes assembly and maturation. The **vpu** reduces cell surface CD4 expression and enhances virion release. The **vpr** (vpx in HIV-2) is required to give the virus a growth advantage. HIV is also under cellular control, and activation of the T cell by a mitogen or antigen also activates the virus.

The proteins translated from the gag, gag-pol, and env mRNAs are synthesized as polyproteins and are subsequently cleaved to functional proteins (see Fig. 61–7). The viral glycoproteins are synthesized, glycosylated, and processed by the endoplasmic reticulum and Golgi apparatus. These glycoproteins are then cleaved into a membrane-spanning and an extracellular region and associate to form trimers that migrate to the plasma membrane.

The gag and the gag-pol polyproteins are acylated and then bind to the plasma membrane containing the envelope glycoprotein. The association of two copies of the genome and cellular transfer RNA molecules promotes budding of the virion. After its envelopment and release from the cell, the viral protease cleaves the gag and gag-pol polyproteins. This action releases the reverse transcriptase and forms the virion core and is required for the production of infectious virions. This requirement makes the protease a target for antiviral drugs.

The envelopment and release of retroviruses occur at the cell surface. HIV can also spread from cell to cell through the production of multinucleated giant cells, or syncytia. Syncytia are fragile, and their formation enhances the cytolytic activity of the virus.

Human Immunodeficiency Virus
Pathogenesis and Immunity

The major determinant in the pathogenesis and disease caused by HIV is the **virus tropism for CD4-expressing T cells and macrophages** (Box 61–2 and Fig. 61–8). HIV-induced immunosuppression (AIDS) results from a reduction in the number of CD4 T cells, which decimates the helper and delayed-type hypersensitivity (DTH) functions of the immune response.

During vaginal or anal sexual intercourse, HIV-1 infects Langerhans dendritic cells in the epithelium, and these can then travel to lymph nodes. Anal sex may be of greater risk than other routes of infection. Special T cells bearing a greater number of co-receptors for the virus are separated by only a single layer of cells from the colon. On injection of virus into blood, the virus is likely to infect dendritic and other monocyte-macrophage lineage cells. Macrophage-lineage cells express both the CCR5 and CXCR4 chemokine receptors and can be infected by M-tropic and T-tropic HIV. The virus reaches the lymph node within 2 days of infection, and there the CD4 T cells are infected. Macrophages are persistently infected with HIV and are probably the major reservoirs and means of distribution of HIV.

Continuous replication of the virus occurs in the lymph nodes, with subsequent release of the virus and infected T cells into the blood. Reductions in the numbers of CD4 T cells may result from HIV-induced cytolysis, cytotoxic T-cell immune cytolysis, or the natural terminal differentiation of T cells, which would occur in response to the large HIV antigen challenge.

BOX 61–2. **Disease Mechanisms of HIV**

Human immunodeficiency virus primarily infects CD4 T cells and cells of the macrophage lineage (e.g., monocytes, macrophages, alveolar macrophages of the lung, dendritic cells of the skin, and microglial cells of the brain).

Virus causes lytic infection of CD4 T cells and persistent low-level productive infection of macrophage lineage cells.

Virus causes syncytia formation, with cells expressing large amounts of CD4 antigen (T cells) with subsequent lysis of the cells.

Virus alters T-cell and macrophage cell function.

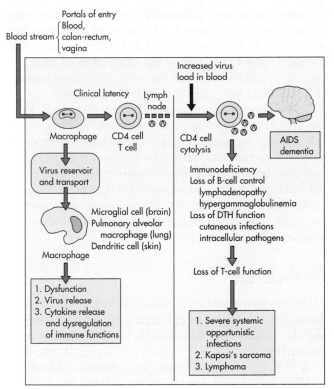

FIGURE 61-8. Pathogenesis of human immunodeficiency virus (HIV). HIV causes lytic and latent infection of CD4 T cells and persistent infection of cells of the monocyte macrophage family and disrupts neurons. The outcomes of these actions are immunodeficiency and acquired immunodeficiency syndrome (AIDS) dementia. DTH = delayed-type hypersensitivity. (Redrawn from Fauci AS: The human immunodeficiency virus: infectivity and mechanisms of pathogenesis, *Science* 239:617–622, 1988.)

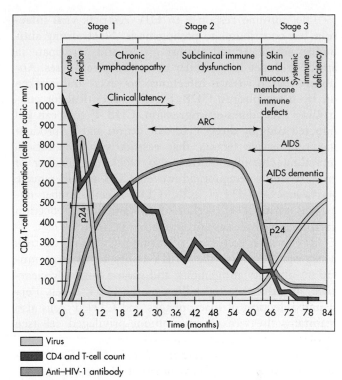

FIGURE 61-9. Time course and stages of human immunodeficiency virus (HIV) disease. A long clinical latency period follows the initial mononucleosis-like symptoms. The progressive decrease in the number of CD4 T cells, even during the latency period, allows opportunistic infections to occur. The stages (World Health Organization and Centers for Disease Control and Prevention) in HIV disease are defined by the CD4 T-cell levels and occurrence of opportunistic diseases. ARC = acquired immunodeficiency syndrome (AIDS)-related complex. (Redrawn from Redfield RR, Buske DS: HIV infection: the clinical picture, *Sci Am* 259:90–98, 1988, updated 1996.)

The increased release of virus into the blood as the numbers of CD4 cells decrease correlates directly with the development of the symptoms of AIDS (Fig. 61–9).

HIV induces several cytopathologic effects that may kill the infected T cell (Table 61–3). These include an accumulation of nonintegrated circular DNA copies of the genome, increased permeability of the plasma membrane, syncytia formation, and induction of apoptosis (programmed cell death). The relative ability of HIV to kill the target cell correlates with the amount of CD4 expressed by the cell. Macrophages may be spared the cytolytic action of HIV because they express less CD4 than T cells. The accessory proteins of HIV are important for replication and virulence. As noted earlier, the nef protein appears to be essential for promoting the progression of HIV infection to AIDS. Individuals infected with natural mutants of nef and primates infected with the simian immunodeficiency virus, which lacks nef, have lived beyond their expected lifetimes.

TABLE 61–3. Means of HIV Escape from the Immune System

Characteristic	Function
Infection of lymphocytes and macrophages	Inactivation of key element of immune defense
Inactivation of CD4 helper cells	Loss of activator of the immune system and delayed-type hypersensitivity
Antigenic drift of gp120	Evasion of antibody detection
Heavy glycosylation of gp120	Evasion of antibody detection

The immune response to HIV restricts viral infection but contributes to pathogenesis. Neutralizing antibodies are generated against gp120 and participate in antibody-dependent cellular cytotoxicity responses. Antibody-coated virus is infectious, however, and is taken up by macrophages. CD8 T cells are critical for controlling HIV disease progression. CD8 T cells can kill infected cells by direct cytotoxic action and by producing suppressive factors that restrict viral replication, including chemokines that also block the binding of virus to its co-receptor. However, CD8 T cells require activation by CD4 T cells, CD8 T-cell number decreases with CD4 T-cell number, and their reduction correlates with disease progression to AIDS.

HIV has several ways of escaping immune control. Most significant are the virus's ability to undergo mutation, alter its antigenicity and escape antibody clearance, and the targeted killing of the CD4 T cell. Persistent infection of macrophages and CD4 T cells also maintains the virus in an immune-privileged cell (see Table 61–3).

The course of HIV disease parallels the CD4 T-cell numbers and the amount of virus in the blood (see Fig. 61–9). Initially, there is a large burst of virus production and viremia, which corresponds to the occurrence of a mononucleosis-like syndrome. Virus levels in the blood decrease during a clinically latent period, but viral replication continues in the lymph nodes. Late in the disease, virus levels in the blood increase, CD4 levels are significantly decreased, the structure of the lymph nodes is destroyed, and the patient becomes immunosuppressed.

The central role of the CD4 helper T cells in the initiation of an immune response and DTH is indicated by the extent of immunosuppression induced by HIV infection (Fig. 61–10). Activated CD4 T cells initiate immune responses by the release of cytokines required for the activation of macrophages, other T cells, B cells, and natural killer cells. When CD4 T cells are unavailable or not functional, antigen-specific immune responses (especially cellular immune responses) are incapacitated, and humoral responses are uncontrolled. The loss of the CD4 T cells responsible for producing DTH allows the outgrowth of many of the opportunistic intracellular infections characteristic of AIDS (e.g., fungi and intracellular bacteria).

In addition to immunosuppressive disorders, HIV can also cause neurologic abnormalities. The microglial cell and macrophage are the predominant cell types of a brain infected with HIV, but neurons and glial cells may also be infected. Infected monocytes and microglial cells may release neurotoxic substances or chemotactic factors that promote inflammatory responses in the brain. Direct cytopathologic effects of the virus on neurons are also possible.

Epidemiology

AIDS was first noted in homosexual men in the United States but has spread in epidemic proportions throughout the population (Box 61–3). In 1999, it was estimated that 15,000 HIV infections occurred per day, with 95% occurring in developing countries (according to UNAIDS-WHO data) (Figs. 61–11 and 61–12).

HIV is thought to be derived from simian immunodeficiency virus, and, in fact, HIV-2 is similar to simian immunodeficiency virus. The initial human infection occurred in Africa in the 1930s but went unnoticed in rural areas. The migration of infected people to the cities after the 1960s brought the virus into population centers, and cultural acceptance of prostitution promoted its transmission throughout the population.

Transmission

The presence of **HIV in the blood, semen, and vaginal secretions** of infected people and **the long asymptomatic period of infection** are factors that have promoted the spread of the disease through sexual

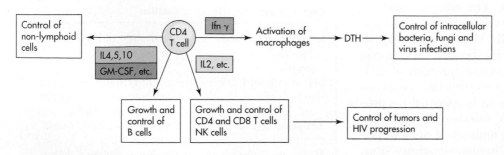

FIGURE 61–10. CD4 T cells have a critical role in the regulation of the human immune response by mediating the release of soluble factors and the delayed-type hypersensitivity (DTH) response toward intracellular pathogens. Human immunodeficiency virus–induced loss of the CD4 T cells results in loss of the functions shown, especially the DTH responses and the lymphokine control of immune responses

BOX 61–3. Epidemiology of HIV Infections

Disease Viral Factors

Enveloped virus is easily inactivated and must be transmitted in body fluids.

Disease has a long prodromal period.

Virus can be shed before development of identifiable symptoms.

Transmission

Virus is present in blood, semen, and vaginal secretions.
See Table 61–4 for modes of transmission.

Who Is at Risk?

Intravenous drug abusers; sexually active people with many partners (homosexual and heterosexual); prostitutes; newborns of human immunodeficiency virus–positive mothers.

Blood and organ transplant recipients and hemophiliacs: before 1985 (pre-screening programs).

Geography Season

There is an expanding epidemic worldwide.
There is no seasonal incidence.

Modes of Control

Antiviral drugs limit progression of disease.

Vaccines for prevention and treatment are in trials.

Safe, monogamous sex helps limit spread.

Sterile injection needles should be used.

Large-scale screening programs have been developed for blood for transfusions, organs for transplants, and clotting factors used by hemophiliacs.

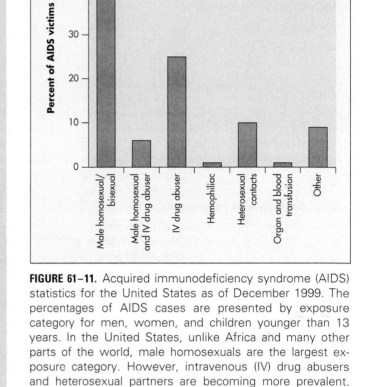

FIGURE 61–11. Acquired immunodeficiency syndrome (AIDS) statistics for the United States as of December 1999. The percentages of AIDS cases are presented by exposure category for men, women, and children younger than 13 years. In the United States, unlike Africa and many other parts of the world, male homosexuals are the largest exposure category. However, intravenous (IV) drug abusers and heterosexual partners are becoming more prevalent. (From the Centers for Disease Control and Prevention: *HIV/AIDS surveillance report,* available at www.cdc.gov/hiv/stats/hasrlink.htm)

contact and exposure to contaminated blood and blood products (Table 61–4). The virus can also be transmitted perinatally to newborns. HIV is *not,* however, transmitted by casual contact, touching, hugging, kissing, coughing, sneezing, insect bites, water, food, utensils, toilets, swimming pools, or public baths.

Populations at Highest Risk

Sexually active people (homosexual and heterosexual), intravenous drug abusers and their sexual partners, and the newborns of HIV-positive mothers are at highest risk for HIV infections, with black and Hispanic persons disproportionally represented in the HIV-positive population.

As already noted, AIDS was initially described in young, promiscuous homosexual men and is still prevalent in the gay community. Anal intercourse is an efficient means of viral transmission. However, heterosexual transmission by vaginal intercourse and intravenous drug abuse have become the major routes by which HIV is being spread in the population. The prevalence

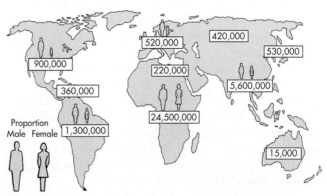

FIGURE 61–12. Estimated cumulative global distribution of human immunodeficiency virus (HIV) infections as of the end of 1999. The estimated cumulative global total of HIV-infected adults in 1996 was about 34.3 million. Infection rates vary widely in different regions of the world. The highest rates are in sub-Saharan Africa. (Modified from the World Health Organization report, June 2000 www.unaids.org/hivaidsinfo)

TABLE 61–4. Transmission of HIV Infection

Routes	Specific Transmission
Known Routes of Transmission	
Inoculation in blood	Transfusion of blood and blood products
	Needle sharing among intravenous drug abusers
	Needlestick, open wound, and mucous membrane exposure in health care workers
	Tattoo needles
Sexual transmission	Anal and vaginal intercourse
Perinatal transmission	Intrauterine transmission
	Peripartum transmission
	Breast milk
Routes Not Involved in Transmission	
Close personal contact	Household members
	Health care workers not exposed to blood

of HIV in drug abusers stems from sharing contaminated syringe needles, a common practice in "shooting galleries." In New York City alone, more than 80% of intravenous drug abusers are positive for the HIV antibody, and these people are now the major source of heterosexual and congenital transmission of the virus.

Before 1985, people receiving blood transfusions or organ transplants and hemophiliacs receiving clotting factors from pooled blood were at high risk for HIV infection. Now, however, screening of the blood supply in the United States has practically eliminated the danger of HIV's being transmitted in blood transfusions. Hemophiliacs who receive pooled clotting factors are protected further by the proper handling of the factor (prolonged heating) to kill the virus.

Health care workers are at risk for HIV infection from accidental needlesticks or cuts or through the exposure of broken skin and mucosal membranes to contaminated blood. Fortunately, studies of needlestick victims have shown that seroconversion occurs in fewer than 1% of those exposed to HIV-positive blood. Tattoo needles and contaminated inks are other potential means by which HIV can be transmitted.

Geographic Distribution

HIV-1 infections are spreading worldwide, with the largest number of AIDS cases in sub-Saharan Africa but with a growing number of cases in Asia, the United States, and the rest of the world (see Fig. 61–12). HIV-2 is more prevalent in Africa (especially West

Africa) than in the United States. Heterosexual transmission is the major means of spread of HIV-1 and HIV-2 in Africa, and both men and women are equally affected by these viruses. HIV-2 produces a disease similar to but less severe than AIDS.

Clinical Syndromes

AIDS is one of the most devastating epidemics ever recorded. Most HIV-infected people will become symptomatic, and the overwhelming majority of these will ultimately succumb to the disease. HIV disease progresses from an asymptomatic infection to profound immunosuppression, referred to as full-blown AIDS (see Fig. 61–9). The diseases related to AIDS mainly

TABLE 61–5. Indicator Diseases of AIDS*

Infection	Disease
Opportunistic infections	
Protozoal	Toxoplasmosis of the brain
	Cryptosporidiosis with diarrhea
	Isosporiasis with diarrhea
Fungal	Candidiasis of the esophagus, trachea, and lungs
	Pneumocystis carinii pneumonia
	Cryptococcosis (extrapulmonary)
	Histoplasmosis (disseminated)
	Coccidioidomycosis (disseminated)
Viral	Cytomegalovirus disease
	Herpes simplex virus infection (persistent or disseminated)
	Progressive multifocal leukoencephalopathy
	Hairy leukoplakia caused by Epstein-Barr virus
Bacterial	_Mycobacterium avium-intracellulare_ complex (disseminated)
	Any "atypical" mycobacterial disease
	Extrapulmonary tuberculosis
	Salmonella septicemia (recurrent)
	Pyogenic bacterial infections (multiple or recurrent)
Opportunistic neoplasias	Kaposi's sarcoma
	Primary lymphoma of the brain
	Other non-Hodgkin's lymphomas
Others	HIV wasting syndrome
	HIV encephalopathy
	Lymphoid interstitial pneumonia

*Manifestations of HIV infection–defining acquired immunodeficiency syndrome according to criteria of Centers for Disease Control and Prevention.

HIV = human immunodeficiency virus.

Modified from Belshe RB, editor: _Textbook of human virology,_ ed 2, St Louis, 1991, Mosby.

consist of opportunistic infections, cancers, and the direct effects of HIV on the central nervous system (Table 61–5). Although rare, there are cases of long-term survivors. Some of these result from infection with HIV strains that lack a functional nef protein. Resistance to the virus correlates with a lack of expression of the chemokine co-receptor for the virus.

The initial symptoms following HIV infection (2 to 4 weeks after infection) may resemble those of influenza or infectious mononucleosis, with an "aseptic" meningitis or a rash occurring up to 3 months after infection. As in mononucleosis, the symptoms stem from immune responses triggered by a widespread infection of lymphoid cells. These symptoms subside spontaneously after 2 to 3 weeks and are followed by a period of asymptomatic infection or a persistent generalized lymphadenopathy that may last for several years. During this period, the virus is replicating in the lymph nodes.

Deterioration of the immune response is indicated by increased susceptibility to opportunistic pathogens, especially those controlled by CD4 T-cell DTH responses (e.g., yeasts, herpesviruses, or intracellular bacteria). The onset of symptoms correlates with a reduction in the number of CD4 T cells to less than 450/μL and increased levels of virus and protein p24 in the blood. Full-blown AIDS occurs when the CD4 T-cell counts are less than 200/μL and involves the onset of more significant diseases, including HIV wasting syndrome (weight loss and diarrhea for more than 1 month) and the occurrence of indicator diseases such as **Kaposi's sarcoma** or specific opportunistic diseases, especially *Pneumocystis carinii* **pneumonia**, *Mycobacterium avium-intracellulare* **complex** infection, and **severe cytomegalovirus disease** (see Table 61–5).

AIDS may be manifested in several different ways, including lymphadenopathy and fever, opportunistic infections, malignancies, and AIDS-related dementia.

Lymphadenopathy and Fever

Lymphadenopathy and fever can occur, and this combination of clinical findings has been called the **AIDS-related complex (ARC)**. It is a process that develops insidiously and may be accompanied by weight loss and malaise. These findings may persist indefinitely or may progress. Symptoms may also include opportunistic infections, diarrhea, night sweats, and fatigue. The wasting disease is termed "slim disease" in Africa.

Opportunistic Infections

Normally benign infections caused by agents such as *Candida albicans* and other fungi, DNA viruses capable of recurrent disease, parasites, and intracellularly growing bacteria cause significant disease after the HIV de-

pletion of CD4 T cells. *P. carinii* pneumonia is a major sign of AIDS. Oral candidiasis (thrush), cerebral toxoplasmosis, and cryptococcal meningitis also often occur, as do prolonged and severe infections caused by the herpesviruses (e.g., herpes simplex virus; varicellazoster virus; Epstein-Barr virus [hairy leukoplakia of the mouth, Epstein-Barr virus–associated lymphomas]; cytomegalovirus [especially retinitis, pneumonia, and bowel disease]; and papovaviruses [JC virus causing progressive multifocal leukoencephalopathy]). Tuberculosis and other mycobacterial diseases and diarrhea caused by common pathogens (*Salmonella*, *Shigella*, and *Campylobacter* species) and uncommon agents (cryptosporidia, mycobacteria, *Amoeba* species) are also frequent problems.

Malignancies

The most notable malignancy to develop in patients with AIDS is the human herpesvirus-8 virus–associated Kaposi's sarcoma, an otherwise benign skin cancer that disseminates to involve visceral organs in immunodeficient patients. Non-Hodgkin's lymphoma and Epstein-Barr virus–related lymphomas are also prevalent.

Dementia Related to Acquired Immunodeficiency Syndrome

AIDS-related dementia may result from HIV infection of the microglial cells and neurons of the brain. Patients with this condition may undergo a slow deterioration of their intellectual abilities and other signs of a neurologic disorder, similar to the signs of the early stages of Alzheimer's disease. Neurologic deterioration could also result from infection with one of the many opportunistic infections.

Laboratory Diagnosis

Tests for HIV infection are performed for one of three reasons: to identify those with the infection so that antiviral drug therapy can be initiated, to identify carriers who may transmit infection to others (specifically blood or organ donors, pregnant women, and sex partners), and to confirm the diagnosis of AIDS (Table 61–6). The chronic nature of the disease allows the use of serologic tests to document HIV infection. Unfortunately, serologic tests cannot identify recently infected people. HIV is very difficult to culture, and culture is not routinely performed. The finding of the p24 viral antigen, the reverse transcriptase enzyme, or viral RNA in blood samples indicates the presence of recent infection or late-stage disease (see Fig. 61–9). Viral RNA in blood can be detected by the reverse transcriptase–polymerase chain reaction and branched-chain DNA methods. Blood levels of viral RNA are

TABLE 61–6. Laboratory Analysis for HIV

Test	Purpose
Serology	
Enzyme-linked im-munosorbent assay	Initial screening
Latex agglutination	Initial screening
Western blot analysis	Confirmation test
Immunofluorescence	Confirmation test
Virion RNA RT-PCR	Detection of virus in blood
Branched-chain DNA	Detection of virus in blood
p24 antigen	Early marker of infection
Isolation of virus	Test not readily available
CD4:CD8 T-cell ratio	Correlate of human immu-nodeficiency virus disease

RT-PCR = reverse transcriptase–polymerase chain reaction.

also useful as a monitor for the success of antiviral drug therapy.

Serology

Enzyme-linked immunosorbent assays (ELISAs) or agglutination procedures are used for routine screening. The ELISA test, however, can yield false-positive results and will not detect a recent infection. More specific procedures, such as the Western blot analysis, are subsequently used to confirm seropositive results. The Western blot assay (see Fig. 48–7), on the other hand, determines the presence of antibody to the viral antigens (p24 or p31) and glycoproteins (gp41 and gp120/160). HIV antibody may develop slowly, taking 4 to 8 weeks in most patients; however, it may take 6 months or more in as much as 5% of those infected (see Fig. 61–9).

Immunologic Studies

The status of an HIV infection can be implied from an analysis of the T-cell subsets. The absolute number of CD4 lymphocytes and the ratio of helper to inducer lymphocytes (CD4:CD8 ratio) are abnormally low in HIV-infected people. The particular concentration of CD4 lymphocytes identifies the stage of AIDS.

Treatment, Prevention, and Control

Treatment

An extensive effort to develop antiviral drugs and vaccines effective against HIV has been initiated worldwide. The principal (as of summer 2000) anti-HIV therapies are listed in Box 61–4. The anti-HIV drugs approved by the U.S. Food and Drug Administration can be classified as **nucleoside analogue reverse transcriptase inhibitors, non-nucleoside reverse transcriptase inhibitors, or protease inhibitors.** Azidothymidine (AZT), dideoxyinosine (ddI), and dideoxycytidine (ddC) and the other nucleotide analogues are phosphorylated by cellular enzymes, inhibit the reverse transcriptase, and after incorporation into DNA cause chain termination. Non-nucleoside reverse transcriptase inhibitors (nevirapine) inhibit the enzyme by other mechanisms. Protease inhibitors block the morphogenesis of the virion by inhibiting the cleavage of the gag and gag-pol polyproteins. This prevents activation of the virion.

Other anti-HIV drugs being developed include different nucleotide analogues and other inhibitors of reverse transcriptase, receptor antagonists (CD4 and gp120 analogues), inhibitors of tat function (Ro 24-7429), glycoprotein glycosylation inhibitors, interferon and interferon inducers, and antisense DNA to essential genome sequences.

In the current guidelines, AZT is recommended for the treatment of asymptomatic or mildly symptomatic people with CD4 counts of less than $500/\mu L$ and for the treatment of infected pregnant women to reduce

BOX 61–4. Potential Antiviral Therapies for HIV Infection

Nucleoside Analogue Reverse Transcriptase Inhibitors

Azidothymidine (AZT) (Zidovudine)
Dideoxycytidine (ddC) (Zalcitabine)
Dideoxyinosine (ddI) (Didanosine)
d4T (Stavudine)
3TC (Lamivudine)
ABC (Abacavir)

Non-nucleoside Reverse Transcriptase Inhibitors

Nevirapine (Viramune)
Delavirdine (Rescriptor)
Efavirenz (Sustiva)

Protease Inhibitors

Saquinavir (Invirase/Fortovase)
Ritonavir (Norvir)
Indinavir (Crixivan)
Nelfinavir (Viracept)
Amprenavir (Agenerase)

Highly Active Antiretroviral Therapy (HAART) (Combination)

Indinavir/AZT/3TC
Ritonavir/AZT/3TC
Nelfinavir/AZT/3TC
Nevirapine/AZT/ddI
Nevirapine/indinavir/3TC

the likelihood of transmission of the virus to the fetus. The significant toxic side effects associated with high-dose AZT therapy can be minimized by administering AZT early in the disease and in smaller, repeated doses. Unfortunately, the high mutation rate of HIV promotes the development of resistance to these drugs. A cocktail of several antiviral drugs (e.g., AZT, 3TC, protease inhibitor) termed **highly active antiretroviral treatment** (HAART), each with different mechanisms of action, has less potential to breed resistance and has become a recommended therapy. Multidrug therapy can reduce blood levels of virus to nearly zero and reduce morbidity and mortality in many patients with advanced AIDS. Although HAART is a difficult drug regimen, many patients return to nearly normal on this therapy.

Education

The principal way in which HIV infection can be controlled is by educating the population about the methods of transmission and the measures that may curtail viral spread. For instance, monogamous relationships, the practice of safe sex, and the use of condoms reduce the possibility of exposure. Because contaminated needles are a major source of HIV in intravenous drug abusers, people must be taught that needles must not be shared. The reuse of contaminated needles in clinics was the source of outbreaks of AIDS in the former Soviet bloc and other countries. In some places, efforts have been launched to provide sterile equipment to intravenous drug abusers.

Blood and Blood Product Screening

Potential blood donors are screened before they donate blood, and blood products are screened before use. People testing positive for HIV must not donate blood. People who anticipate a future need for blood, such as those awaiting elective surgery, should consider donating blood beforehand. To limit the worldwide epidemic, blood screening must be initiated in underdeveloped nations as well.

Infection Control

The infection-control procedures for HIV infection are the same as those for hepatitis B virus. They include the use of universal blood and body fluid precautions, which were founded on the assumption that all patients are infectious for HIV and other blood-borne pathogens. The precautions include wearing protective clothing (e.g., gloves, mask, gown) and using other barriers to prevent exposure to blood products. Contaminated surfaces should be disinfected with 10% household bleach, 70% ethanol or isopropanol, 2% glutaraldehyde, 4% formaldehyde, or 6% hydrogen peroxide. Washing laundry in hot water with detergent should be sufficient to inactivate HIV.

Vaccine Development

No vaccine against HIV is available despite several trials. A successful vaccine would prevent acquisition of the virus by adults and transmission of the virus to infants of HIV-positive mothers; it would also block the progression of the disease.

Most HIV vaccines being investigated use gp120 or its precursor, gp160, as the immunogen. The gene for this protein has been cloned, expressed in different eukaryotic cell systems (e.g., yeast, baculovirus), and developed as a subunit vaccine. The env gene has also been incorporated into the vaccinia virus to create a hybrid vaccine. Specific epitopes and T-cell antigens are also being investigated as possible peptide vaccines. DNA vaccines consisting of eukaryotic expression vectors (plasmids) containing the gene for gp160 or other HIV genes is the newest approach to immunization.

The development of a vaccine against HIV is, however, fraught with several problems unique to the virus. For instance, initial protection would require the production of secretory antibody to prevent sexual transmission and acquisition of the virus. Both antibody and cell-mediated immunity are necessary to protect against HIV infection. In addition, the antigenicity of the virus changes readily through mutation. A further problem is that the virus can be spread through syncytia and remains latent, thereby hiding from antibody. HIV also infects and inactivates the cells required to initiate an immune response. Testing of the vaccine would be a problem because HIV is a human disease and long-term follow-up is required to monitor the efficacy of the vaccine.

Human T-Lymphotropic Virus and Other Oncogenic Retroviruses

The Oncovirinae were originally called the *RNA tumor viruses* and have been associated with the development of leukemias, sarcomas, and lymphomas in many animals. These viruses are not cytolytic. The members of this family are distinguished by the mechanism of cell transformation and thus the length of the latency period between infection and the development of disease (Table 61–7).

The **sarcoma and acute leukemia viruses** have incorporated cellular genes (**protooncogenes**) encoding growth-controlling factors into their genome. These include genes that encode growth hormones, growth hormone receptors, protein kinases, guanosine triphosphate–binding proteins, and nuclear DNA-binding proteins. These viruses can cause transformation and

TABLE 61–7. Mechanisms of Retrovirus Oncogenesis

Disease	Speed	Effect
Acute leukemia or sarcoma	Fast: oncogene	Direct effect Provision of growth-enhancing proteins
Leukemia	Slow: transactivation	Indirect effect Transactivation protein (tax) or long-terminal repeat promoter sequences that enhance expression of cellular growth genes

are highly oncogenic. *No human virus of this type has been identified.*

At least 35 different viral oncogenes have been identified (Table 61–8). Transformation results from the overproduction or altered activity of the growth-stimulating oncogene product. Increased cell growth then promotes transcription, which also promotes viral replication. Incorporation of the oncogene into many of these viruses causes the coding sequences for the gag, pol, or env genes to be replaced, such that most of these viruses are defective and require helper viruses for replication. Many of these viruses remain endogenous and are transmitted vertically through the germ line of the animal.

The **leukemia viruses,** including HTLV-1, are competent in terms of replication but cannot transform cells in vitro. They cause cancer after a **long latency period** of at least 30 years. The leukemia viruses pro-

mote cell growth in more indirect ways than the oncogene-encoding viruses. Specifically, a transcriptional regulator, tax, is produced and is capable of activating promoters in the LTR region and specific cellular genes (including growth-controlling and cytokine genes such as IL-2 and granulocyte-macrophage colony-stimulating factor [GM-CSF]) to promote the outgrowth of that cell. Alternatively, by integrating near cellular growth-controlling genes, the enhancer and promoter gene sequences encoded in the viral LTR region can promote the expression of growth-stimulating proteins. Uncontrolled cell growth may be sufficient to transform the cell neoplastically or may promote other genetic aberrations over a long period. These viruses are also associated with non-neoplastic neurologic disorders and other diseases. For example, HTLV-1 causes **adult acute T-cell lymphocytic leukemia (ATLL)** and **HTLV-1–associated myelopathy (tropical spastic paraparesis),** a nononcogenic neurologic disease.

The human oncoviruses include HTLV-1, HTLV-2, and HTLV-5, but only HTLV-1 has been definitively associated with disease (i.e., ATLL). HTLV-2 was isolated from atypical forms of hairy cell leukemia, and HTLV-5 was isolated from a malignant cutaneous lymphoma. HTLV-1 and HTLV-2 share as much as 50% homology.

Pathogenesis and Immunity

HTLV-1 is cell-associated and is spread in cells after blood transfusion, sexual intercourse, or breast-feeding. The virus enters the blood stream and infects the CD4 helper and DTH T cells. These T cells have a tendency to reside in the skin, thus contributing to the symptoms of ATLL. Neurons also express a receptor for HTLV-1.

HTLV is competent for replication, with the gag, pol, and env genes transcribed, translated, and proc-

TABLE 61–8. Representative Examples of Oncogenes

Function	Oncogene	Virus
Tyrosine kinase	*src*	Rous sarcoma virus
	abl	Abelson murine leukemia virus
	fes	ST feline sarcoma virus
Growth factor receptors	*erb*-B (EGF receptor)	Avian erythroblastosis virus
	erb-A (thyroid hormone receptor)	Avian erythroblastosis virus
Guanosine triphosphate–binding proteins	Ha-*ras*	Harvey murine sarcoma virus
	Ki-*ras*	Kirsten murine sarcoma virus
Nuclear proteins	*myc*	Avian myelocytomatosis virus
	myb	Avian myeloblastosis virus
	fos	Murine osteosarcoma virus FBJ
	jun	Avian sarcoma virus 17

Based on data from Jawetz E et al: *Medical microbiology,* ed 18, Los Altos, Calif, 1989, Appleton & Lange.

essed as described earlier. In addition to its action on viral genes, the tax protein transactivates the cellular genes for the T-cell growth factor, IL-2 and its receptor (IL-2R), which activates growth in the infected cell. The virus may remain latent or may replicate slowly for many years but may also induce the clonal outgrowth of particular T-cell clones. There is a long latency period (approximately 30 years) before the onset of leukemia.

Although the virus can induce a polyclonal outgrowth of T cells, the HTLV-1–induced adult T-cell leukemia is usually monoclonal. Chromosomal aberrations and rearrangements in the T-cell antigen receptor β gene may accumulate in the HTLV growth-stimulated cells, and it may be this that causes the leukemia.

Antibodies are elicited to the gp46 and other proteins of HTLV-1. HTLV-1 infection also causes immunosuppression.

Epidemiology

HTLV-1 is transmitted and acquired by the same routes as HIV. It is endemic in southern Japan and is also found in the inhabitants of the Caribbean and among blacks in the southeastern United States. In the endemic regions of Japan, the children acquire HTLV-1 in breast milk from their mothers, whereas the adults are infected sexually. The number of seropositive people in some regions of Japan may be as high as 35% (Okinawa), with the mortality resulting from leukemia double that in other regions. Intravenous drug abuse and blood transfusion are becoming the most prominent means of transmitting the virus in the United States. In the United States, the high-risk groups for HTLV-1 infection are the same as those for HIV infection, and the seroprevalence of HTLV-1 is approaching that of HIV.

Clinical Syndromes

HTLV infection is usually asymptomatic but can progress to ATLL in approximately 1 in 20 persons over a 30- to 50-year period. ATLL caused by HTLV-1 is a neoplasia of the CD4 helper T cells that can be acute or chronic. The malignant cells have been termed "flower cells" because they are pleomorphic and contain lobulated nuclei. In addition to an elevated white blood cell count, this form of ATLL is characterized by skin lesions similar to those seen in another leukemia, Sézary's syndrome. ATLL is usually fatal within a year of diagnosis, regardless of treatment.

Laboratory Diagnosis

HTLV-1 infection is detected using ELISA to find virus-specific antigens in blood, using reverse transcrip-

tase–polymerase chain reaction for viral RNA, or using ELISA serologically to detect specific antibodies.

Treatment, Prevention, and Control

A combination of AZT and interferon-α has been effective in some patients with ATLL. However, no particular treatment has been approved for the management of HTLV-1 infection.

The measures used to limit the spread of HTLV-1 are the same as those used to limit the transmission of HIV. Sexual precautions, screening of the blood supply, and increased awareness of the potential risks and diseases all are ways to prevent transmission of the virus. Maternal infection of children is very difficult to control, however. The use of routine screening procedures for HTLV would limit spread of the virus, but such measures have not been instituted.

Endogenous Retroviruses

Different retroviruses have integrated into and become a part of the chromosomes of humans and animals. In fact, retrovirus sequences may make up at least 1% of the human genome. Complete and partial provirus sequences with gene sequences similar to those of HTLV, mouse mammary tumor virus, and other retroviruses can be detected in humans. These endogenous viruses generally lack the ability to replicate because of deletions or the insertion of termination codons or because they are poorly transcribed. One such retrovirus can be detected in placental tissue and is activated by pregnancy. This virus may facilitate placental function.

CASE STUDY AND QUESTIONS

■ A 28-year-old man had several complaints. He had a bad case of thrush (oral candidiasis) and low-grade fever, had serious bouts of diarrhea, had lost 20 pounds in the past year without dieting, and, most seriously, complained of difficulty breathing. His lungs showed a bilateral infiltrate on radiographic examination, characteristic of *P. carinii* pneumonia. A stool sample was positive for *Giardia* organisms. He was a heroin addict and admitted to sharing needles at a "shooting gallery."

1. What laboratory tests should have been done to support and confirm a diagnosis of HIV infection and AIDS?
2. How did this man acquire the HIV infection? What are other high-risk behaviors for HIV infection?
3. What was the immunologic basis for the in-

creased susceptibility of this patient to opportunistic infections?

    4. What precautions should have been taken in handling samples from this patient?

    5. Several forms of HIV vaccines are being developed. What are possible components of an HIV vaccine? Who would be appropriate recipients of an HIV vaccine?

BIBLIOGRAPHY

AIDS: Ten years later, *FASEB J* 5:2338–2455, 1991.

Anderson RM: Understanding the AIDS pandemic, *Sci Am* 266: 58–66, 1992.

Antiretroviral therapy for HIV infection in 1996: consensus statement, *JAMA* 276:146–154, 1996.

Arts EJ, Wainberg MA: Human immunodeficiency virus type 1 reverse transcriptase and early events in reverse transcription, *Adv Virus Res* 46:99–166, 1996.

Caldwell JC, Caldwell P: The African AIDS epidemic, *Sci Am* 274, March 1996.

Carpenter CC et al: Antiretroviral therapy in adults: updated recommendations of the International AIDS Society—USA Panel, *JAMA* 283:381–390, 2000.

Centers for Disease Control and Prevention: Guidelines for prevention of transmission of human immunodeficiency virus and hepatitis B virus to health-care and public-safety workers, *MMWR* 38:S–6, 1989.

Dewhurst S, da Cruz RLW, Whetter L: 2000. Bioscience. Pathogenesis and treatment of HIV-1 infection: recent developments (Y2K update). Available at http://bioscience.org/2000/v5/d/dewhurst/fulltext.htm

Fauci AS: The human immunodeficiency virus: infectivity and mechanisms of pathogenesis, *Science* 239:617–622, 1988.

Fields BN, Knipe DM, Howley PM, editors: *Virology*, ed 3, New York, 1996, Lippincott-Raven.

Hehlmann R: Human retroviruses. In Belshe RB, editor: *Textbook of human virology*, ed 2, St Louis, 1991, Mosby.

Hehlmann R, Erfle V: Introduction to retroviruses: human retroviruses. In Belshe RB, editor: *Textbook of human virology*, ed 2, St Louis, 1991, Mosby.

Kräusslich HG: Morphogenesis and maturation of retroviruses, *Curr Top Microbiol Immunol* 214:1–344, 1996.

Löwer R: The pathogenic potential of endogenous retroviruses: facts and fantasies, *Trends Microbiol* 7:350–356, 1999.

Ng VL, McGrath MS: Human T-cell leukemia virus involvement in adult T-cell leukemia, *Cancer Bull* 40:276–280, 1988.

Oldstone MBA, Vitkovic L: HIV and dementia, *Curr Top Microbiol Immunol* 202:1–279, 1995.

Pantaleo G, Fauci AS: Immunopathology of HIV infection, *Annu Rev Microbiol* 50:825–854, 1996.

The new face of AIDS, *Science* 272:1879–1890, 1996.

The science of AIDS 1989: readings from Scientific American, New York, 1989, Scientific American Books.

Williams AO: *AIDS: an African perspective*, Boca Raton, Fla, 1992, CRC.

World Health Organization UNAIDS: HIV/AIDS Information and Data: Available at http://www.unaids.org/hivaidsinfo/

HIV/AIDS Web Sites

General information available at www.aegis.com
    http://hivinsite.ucsf.edu
    http://www.niaid.nih.gov/spotlight/hiv00/default.htm
NIAID fact sheet
    http://www.niaid.nih.gov/publications/aidsfact.htm#G
Treatment options: Available at www.hivatis.org

CHAPTER 62

Hepatitis Viruses

At least six viruses, A through E and a newly discovered G, are considered hepatitis viruses (Table 62–1). Although the target organ for each of these viruses is the liver, they differ greatly in their structure, mode of replication, and mode of transmission and in the course of the disease they cause. **Hepatitis A virus (HAV)** and **Hepatitis B virus (HBV)** are the best known, but three **non-A, non-B hepatitis (NANBH)** viruses **(C, G, and E)** have been described, as has **hepatitis D virus (HDV)**, the delta agent. Additional non-A, non-B agents also exist.

Each of the hepatitis viruses infects and damages the liver, causing the classic **icteric symptoms of jaundice and the release of liver enzymes.** The specific virus causing the disease can be distinguished by the course, nature, and serology of the disease. These viruses are readily spread because infected people are contagious before, or even without, showing symptoms.

Hepatitis A, which is sometimes known as infectious hepatitis, (1) is caused by a picornavirus, an RNA virus; (2) is spread by the fecal-oral route; (3) has an incubation period of approximately 1 month, after which icteric symptoms start abruptly; (4) does not cause chronic liver disease; and (5) rarely causes fatal disease.

Hepatitis B, previously known as serum hepatitis, (1) is caused by a hepadnavirus with a DNA genome; (2) is spread parenterally by blood or needles, by sexual contact, and perinatally; (3) has a median incubation period of approximately 3 months, after which icteric symptoms start insidiously; (4) is followed by chronic hepatitis in 5% to 10% of patients; and (5) is causally associated with primary hepatocellular carcinoma (PHC). More than one third of the world's population has been infected with HBV, resulting in 1 to 2 million deaths per year. The incidence of HBV is decreasing, however, especially in infants, because of the development and use of the HBV subunit vaccine.

NANBH viruses include hepatitis C, G, E, and other undefined hepatitis viruses. **Hepatitis C virus (HCV)** is also widely prevalent, with more than 170 million carriers of the disease. HCV is spread by the same routes as HBV but usually causes chronic disease. HCV is a flavivirus with an RNA genome. **Hepatitis G virus** is also a flavivirus and causes chronic infections. **Hepatitis E virus** (HEV) is an enteric virus, and its disease resembles HAV.

Hepatitis D, or delta hepatitis, is unique in that it requires actively replicating HBV as a "helper virus" and occurs only in patients who have active HBV infection. HBV provides an envelope for HDV RNA and its antigen or antigens. Delta agent exacerbates the symptoms caused by HBV.

Hepatitis A Virus

HAV causes infectious hepatitis and is spread by the fecal-oral route. HAV infections often result from consumption of contaminated water, shellfish, or other food. HAV is a picornavirus that was called enterovirus 72, but it has been placed into a new genus, Heparnavirus, on the basis of its unique genome.

Structure

HAV has a 27-nm, **naked icosahedral capsid** surrounding a **positive-sense, single-stranded RNA** genome consisting of approximately 7470 nucleotides (Fig. 62–1). The HAV genome has a VPg protein attached to the 5' end and polyadenosine attached to the 3' end. The capsid is even more stable than other picornaviruses to acid and other treatments (Box 62–1). There is only one serotype of HAV.

Replication

HAV replicates like other picornaviruses (see Chapter 54). It interacts specifically with a receptor expressed on liver cells and a few other cell types. Unlike other picornaviruses, however, HAV is not cytolytic and is released by exocytosis. Laboratory isolates of HAV have been adapted to growth in primary and continuous monkey kidney cell lines, but clinical isolates are difficult to grow in cell culture.

TABLE 62–1. Comparative Features of Hepatitis Viruses

Feature	Hepatitis A	Hepatitis B	Hepatitis C	Hepatitis D	Hepatitis E
Common name	"Infectious"	"Serum"	"Non-A, non-B–post-transfusion"	"Delta agent"	"Enteric non-A, non-B"
Virus structure	Picornavirus; capsid, RNA	Hepadnavirus; envelope, DNA	Flavivirus; envelope, RNA	Viroid-like; envelope, circular RNA	*Calicivirus*-like; capsid, RNA
Transmission	Fecal-oral	Parenteral, sexual	Parenteral, sexual	Parenteral, sexual	Fecal-oral
Onset	Abrupt	Insidious	Insidious	Abrupt	Abrupt
Incubation period (days)	15–50	45–160	14–180	15–64	15–50
Severity	Mild	Occasionally severe	Usually subclinical; 80% chronicity	*Co-infection* with HBV occasionally severe; *superinfection* with HBV often severe	Normal patients, mild; pregnant women, severe
Mortality	<0.5%	1%–2%	~4%	High to very high	Normal patients, 1%–2%; pregnant women, 20%
Chronicity/carrier state	No	Yes	Yes	Yes	No
Other disease associations	None	Primary hepatocellular carcinoma, cirrhosis	Primary hepatocellular carcinoma, cirrhosis	Cirrhosis, fulminant hepatitis	None
Laboratory diagnosis	Symptoms and anti-HAV IgM	Symptoms and serum levels of HBsAg, HBeAg, and anti-HBc IgM	Symptoms and anti-HCV ELISA	Anti-HDV ELISA	—

ELISA = enzyme-linked immunosorbent assay; HAV = hepatitis A virus; HCV = hepatitis C virus; HDV = hepatitis D virus; IgM = immunoglobulin M.

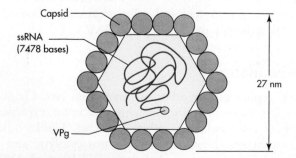

FIGURE 62–1. The picornavirus structure of hepatitis A virus. The icosahedral capsid is made up of four viral polypeptides (VP1 to VP4). Inside the capsid is a single-stranded, positive-sense RNA (ssRNA) that has a genomic viral protein (VPg) on the 5' end.

BOX 62–1. Characteristics of Hepatitis A Virus

Stable to:
    Acid at pH 1
    Solvents (ether, chloroform)
    Detergents
    Salt water, ground water (months)
    Drying (stable)
    Temperature
      4°C: weeks
      56°C for 30 minutes: stable
      61°C for 20 minutes: partial inactivation
Inactivated by:
    Chlorine treatment of drinking water
    Formalin (0.35%, 37°C, 72 hours)
    Peracetic acid (2%, 4 hours)
    β-Propiolactone (0.25%, 1 hour)
    Ultraviolet radiation (2 μW/cm^2/min)

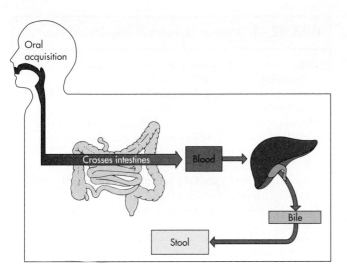

FIGURE 62–2. Spread of hepatitis A virus within the body.

Pathogenesis

HAV is ingested and probably enters the blood stream through the oropharynx or the epithelial lining of the intestines to reach its target, the parenchymal cells of the liver (Fig. 62–2). The virus can be localized by immunofluorescence in hepatocytes and Kupffer's cells. Virus is produced in these cells and is released into the bile and from there into the stool. Virus is shed in large quantity into the stool approximately 10 days before symptoms of jaundice appear or antibody can be detected.

HAV replicates slowly in the liver without producing apparent cytopathic effects. Although interferon limits viral replication, natural killer cells and cytotoxic T cells are required to lyse infected cells. Antibody, complement, and antibody-dependent cellular cytotoxicity also facilitate clearance of the virus and induction of immunopathology. Icterus, resulting from damage to the liver, occurs when antibody is detected and cell-mediated immune responses to the virus occur. Antibody protection against reinfection is lifelong.

The liver pathology caused by HAV infection is indistinguishable histologically from that caused by HBV. It is most likely caused by immunopathology and not virus-induced cytopathology. However, unlike HBV, HAV cannot initiate a chronic infection and is not associated with hepatic cancer.

Epidemiology

Approximately 40% of acute cases of hepatitis are caused by HAV (Box 62–2). The virus spreads readily in a community because most infected people are contagious before symptoms occur and 90% of infected children and 25% to 50% of infected adults have **inapparent but productive** infections.

The virus is released into stool in high concentra-

tions and is spread via the **fecal-oral route:** in contaminated water, in food, and by dirty hands. HAV is resistant to detergents, acid (pH of 1), and temperatures as high as 60°C, and it can survive for many months in fresh water and salt water. Raw or improperly treated sewage can taint the water supply and contaminate shellfish. Shellfish, especially clams, oysters, and mussels, are important sources of the virus because they are efficient filter feeders and can therefore concentrate the viral particles, even from dilute solutions. This is exemplified by an epidemic of HAV that occurred in Shanghai, China, in 1988, when 300,000 people were infected with the virus as the result of eating clams obtained from a polluted river.

HAV outbreaks usually originate from a common source (e.g., water supply, restaurant, daycare center). Daycare settings are a major source for spread of the virus among classmates and their parents. A further problem is posed by the fact that because the children and personnel in daycare centers may be transient, the number of contacts at risk for HAV infection from a single daycare center can be great.

A relatively high incidence of HAV infection is di-

BOX 62–2. Epidemiology of Hepatitis A Virus and Hepatitis E Virus

Disease/Viral Factors

Capsid viruses are strongly resistant to inactivation.
Contagious period extends from before to after symptoms.
Virus may cause asymptomatic shedding.

Transmission

Virus can be transmitted via fecal-oral route.
Ingestion of contaminated food and water can cause infection.
HAV in shellfish is from sewage-contaminated water.
Virus can be transmitted by food handlers, daycare workers, and children.

Who Is at Risk?

People in overcrowded, unsanitary areas.
Children: mild disease, possibly asymptomatic; daycare centers; major source of spread of HAV.
Adults: abrupt-onset hepatitis.
Pregnant women: high mortality associated with HEV.

Geography/Season

Virus is found worldwide.
There is no seasonal incidence.

Means of Control

Good hygiene.
HAV: passive antibody protection for contacts.
Killed vaccine.

HAV = hepatitis A virus; HEV = hepatitis E virus.

rectly related to poor hygienic conditions and over-crowding. Most people infected with HAV in developing countries are children who have mild illness and then lifelong immune protection against reinfection. In the populations of more highly developed countries, infection occurs later in life. The seropositivity rate of adults ranges from a low of 13% of the adult population in Sweden to a high of 88% in Taiwan and 97% in Yugoslavia, with a 41% to 44% rate in the United States.

Clinical Syndromes

The symptoms caused by HAV are very similar to those caused by HBV and stem from immune-mediated damage to the liver. As already noted, disease in children is generally milder than that in adults and is usually asymptomatic. The **symptoms occur abruptly** 15 to 50 days after exposure and intensify for 4 to 6 days before the icteric (jaundice) phase (Fig. 62–3). Initial symptoms include fever, fatigue, nausea, loss of appetite, and abdominal pain. Jaundice is observed in 2 of 3 adults but in only 1 or 2 of 10 children. Symptoms generally wane during the jaundice period. Viral shedding in the stool precedes the onset of symptoms by approximately 14 days but stops before the cessation of symptoms. Complete recovery occurs 99% of the time.

Fulminant hepatitis in HAV infection occurs in 1 to 3 persons per 1000 and is associated with an 80% mortality rate. Liver failure is associated with encephalopathy. Unlike HBV, immune complex–related symptoms (e.g., arthritis, rash) rarely occur in people with HAV disease.

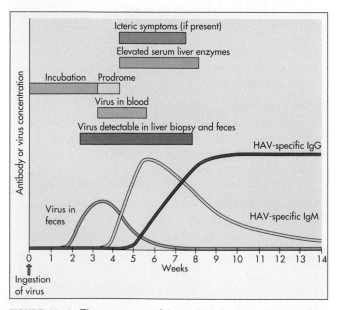

FIGURE 62–3. Time course of hepatitis A virus (HAV) infection.

Laboratory Diagnosis

The diagnosis of HAV infection is generally made on the basis of the time course of the clinical symptoms, the identification of a known infected source, and, most reliably, the results yielded by specific serologic tests. The best way to demonstrate an acute HAV infection is by finding anti-HAV immunoglobulin M, as measured by an enzyme-linked immunosorbent assay (ELISA) or radioimmunoassay. Virus isolation is not routinely performed because efficient tissue culture systems for growing the virus are not available.

Treatment, Prevention, and Control

The spread of HAV is reduced by interrupting the fecal-oral spread of the virus. This is accomplished by avoiding potentially contaminated water or food, especially uncooked shellfish. Proper hand washing, especially in daycare centers, mental hospitals, and other care facilities, is vitally important. Chlorine treatment of drinking water is generally sufficient to kill the virus.

Prophylaxis with immune serum globulin given before or early in the incubation period (i.e., less than 2 weeks after exposure) is 80% to 90% effective in preventing clinical illness.

A **killed HAV vaccine** has been approved by the U.S. Food and Drug Administration and is available for use in children and adults at high risk for infection, especially travelers to endemic regions. A live HAV vaccine has been developed in China. There is only one serotype of HAV, and HAV infects only humans, factors that help ensure the success of an immunization program.

Hepatitis B Virus

HBV is the major member of the **hepadnaviruses.** Other members of this family (Box 62–3) include woodchuck, ground squirrel, and duck hepatitis viruses. These viruses have limited tissue tropisms and host ranges. HBV infects the liver and, to a lesser extent, the kidneys and pancreas of only humans and chimpanzees. Advances in molecular biology have made it possible to study HBV despite the limited host range of the virus and the lack of a cell culture system in which to grow it.

Structure

HBV is a small, enveloped DNA virus with several unusual properties (Fig. 62–4). Specifically, the **genome is a small, circular, partly double-stranded DNA** of only 3200 bases. Although a DNA virus, it encodes a **reverse transcriptase** and replicates through an **RNA intermediate.**

The virion, also called the **Dane particle,** is 42 nm in diameter. The virions are unusually stable for an enveloped virus. They resist treatment with ether, a low pH, freezing, and moderate heating. These characteristics assist transmission from one person to another and hamper disinfection.

The HBV **virion includes a polymerase** with reverse transcriptas and ribonuclease H activity, and a P protein attached to the genome, which is surrounded by the **hepatitis B core antigen (HBcAg)** and an envelope containing the glycoprotein **hepatitis B surface antigen (HBsAg). A hepatitis B e antigen (HBeAg)** protein is a minor component of the virion. The HBeAg and HBcAg proteins share most of their protein sequence. However, the HBeAg is processed differently by the cell, is primarily secreted into serum, does not self-assemble like a capsid antigen, and expresses different antigenic determinants.

HbsAg-containing particles are released into the serum of infected people and outnumber the actual virions. These particles can be spherical (but smaller than the Dane particle) or filamentous (see Fig. 62–4). They are immunogenic and were processed into the first commercial vaccine against HBV.

HBsAg, originally termed the Australia antigen, includes three glycoproteins (L, M, and S) encoded by the same gene and read in the same frame but translated into protein from different AUG start codons. The S (gp27; 24 to 27 kDa) glycoprotein is completely contained in the M (gp36; 33 to 36 kDa) glycoprotein, which is contained in the L (gp42; 39 to 42 kDa) glycoprotein; all share the same C-terminal amino acid sequences. All three forms of HBsAg are found in the virion. The S glycoprotein is the major component of HBsAg particles. It self-associates into 22-nm spherical particles that are released from the cells. The filamentous particles of HBsAg found in serum contain mostly S but also small amounts of the M and L glycoproteins and other proteins and lipids. The L glycoprotein is an essential component for virion assembly and promotes filament formation and the retention of these structures in the cell. The glycoproteins of HBsAg contain the group-specific (termed a) and type-specific determinants of HBV (termed d or y and w or r). Combinations of these antigens (e.g., ady, adw) result in eight subtypes of HBV that are useful epidemiologic markers.

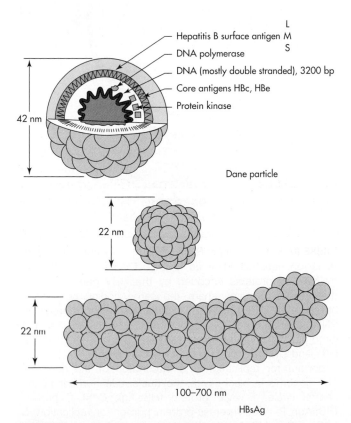

Hepatitis B surface antigen
DNA polymerase
DNA (mostly double stranded), 3200 bp
Core antigens HBc, HBe
Protein kinase

L
M
S

42 nm

Dane particle

22 nm

22 nm

100–700 nm

HBsAg

FIGURE 62–4. Hepatitis B virus (Dane particle) and hepatitis B surface antigen (HBsAg) particles. The spherical HBsAg consists mainly of the S form of HBsAg with some M. The fiber HBsAg has S, M, and L forms. bp = Base pair; L = gp42; M = gp36; S = gp27.

Replication

The replication of HBV is unique for several reasons (see Box 62–1). First, HBV has a distinctly defined tropism for the liver. Its small genome also necessitates economy, as illustrated by the pattern of its transcription and translation. In addition, *HBV replicates through an RNA intermediate and produces and releases antigenic decoy particles (HBsAg)* (Fig. 62–5).

The attachment of HBV to hepatocytes is mediated by the HBsAg glycoproteins. Although the actual receptor and mechanism of entry are not known, it is known that HBsAg binds to polymerized human serum albumin and other serum proteins, and this interaction may target the virus to the liver.

On penetration into the cell, the partial DNA strand

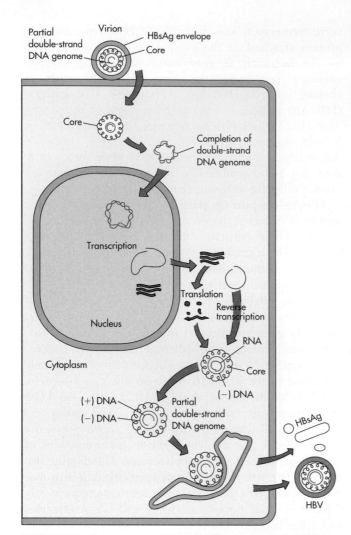

larger than the genome. It encodes the HBc and HBe antigens, the polymerase, and a protein primer for DNA replication and acts as the template for replication of the genome. The HBe and HBc are related proteins that are translated from different in-phase start codons of closely related mRNA. This causes differences in their processing, structure, and distribution in the cell and virion. Similarly, the 2100-base mRNA encodes the small and medium glycoproteins from dif-

FIGURE 62–5. Proposed pathway for the replication of hepatitis B virus. After entry into the hepatocyte and uncoating of the nucleocapsid core, the partially double-stranded DNA genome is completed by enzymes in the core and then delivered to the nucleus. Transcription of the genome produces four messenger RNAs (mRNAs), including an mRNA larger than the genome (3500 bases). The mRNA then moves to the cytoplasm and is translated into protein. Core proteins assemble around the 3500-base mRNA, and negative-sense DNA is synthesized by a reverse transcriptase activity in the core. The RNA is then degraded as a positive-sense (+) DNA is synthesized. The core is enveloped before completion of the positive-sense DNA and then released by exocytosis.

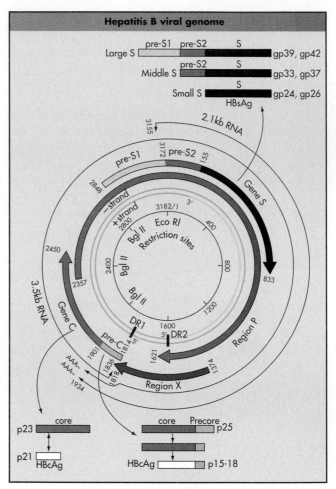

FIGURE 62–6. Messenger RNA (mRNA) transcripts and proteins of hepatitis B virus (HBV). Diagram depicts the mRNA and proteins encoded by the HBV genome. Note that several proteins share the same coding sequences but start at different AUG codons and that different mRNAs overlap. The 3500-base transcript is larger than the genome and is the template for replication of the genome. DR1 and DR2 are direct repeat sequences of DNA and are important for replication and integration of the genome. The genome is black, with the nucleotide number in the central circle. E = E protein (HBeAg); C = C protein (HBcAg); P = polymerase-protein primer for replication; S = S protein (HBsAg); l = large glycoprotein; m = medium glycoprotein; s = small glycoprotein; X = X protein; AAA = 3' polyA at end of mRNA. (From Armstrong D, Cohen J: *Infectious diseases,* St Louis, 1999, Mosby).

of the genome is completed by being formed into a complete double-stranded DNA circle, and the genome is delivered to the nucleus. Transcription of the genome is controlled by cellular transcription elements found in hepatocytes. The DNA is transcribed into three major classes (2100, 2400, and 3500 bases) and two minor classes (900 bases) of overlapping messenger RNAs (mRNAs) (Fig. 62–6). The 3500-base mRNA is

ferent in-phase start codons. The 2400-base mRNA, which encodes the large glycoprotein, overlaps the 2100-base mRNA. The 900-base mRNA encodes the X protein, which promotes viral replication as a transactivator of transcription and as a protein kinase.

Replication of the genome begins with production of the larger-than-genome, 3500-base mRNA. This is packaged into the core nucleocapsid that contains the RNA-dependent DNA polymerase. This polymerase has **reverse transcriptase** and ribonuclease H activity but lacks the integrase activity of the retrovirus enzyme. The 3500-base RNA acts as a template, and negative-strand DNA is synthesized on a protein primer, which remains covalently attached to the 5' end. After this, the RNA is degraded by the ribonuclease H activity as the positive-strand DNA is synthesized from the negative-sense DNA template. However, this process is interrupted by envelopment of the nucleocapsid at HBsAg-containing membranes of the endoplasmic reticulum or the Golgi apparatus, thereby capturing genomes containing RNA-DNA circles with different lengths of RNA. Continued degradation of the remainder of the RNA in the virion yields a partly double-stranded DNA genome. The virion is then released from the hepatocyte by exocytosis and not by cell lysis.

The entire genome can also be integrated into the host cell chromatin. HBsAg, but not other proteins, can often be detected in the cytoplasm of cells containing integrated HBV DNA. The significance of the integrated DNA in the replication of the virus is not known, but integrated viral DNA has been found in hepatocellular carcinomas.

Pathogenesis and Immunity

HBV can cause acute or chronic, symptomatic or asymptomatic disease. Which of these occurs seems to be determined by the person's immune response to the infection (Fig. 62–7). *Detection of both the HBsAg and the HBeAg components of the virion in the blood indicates the existence of an ongoing active infection.* HBsAg particles continue to be released into the blood even after virion release has ended and until the infection is resolved.

The major source of infectious virus is blood, but HBV can be found in semen, saliva, milk, vaginal and menstrual secretions, and amniotic fluid. The most efficient way to acquire HBV is through injection of the virus into the blood stream (Fig. 62–8). Common but less efficient routes of infection are sexual contact and birth.

The virus starts to replicate within 3 days of its acquisition, but as already noted, symptoms may not be observed for 45 days or longer, depending on the infectious dose, the route of infection, and the person. The virus replicates in hepatocytes with minimal cyto-

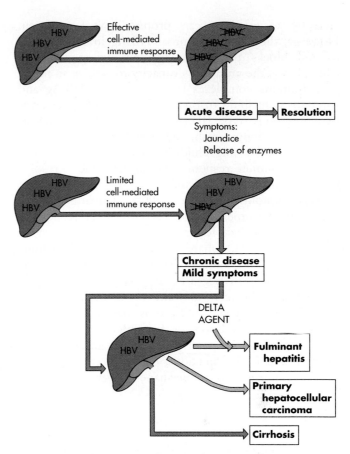

FIGURE 62–7. Major determinants of acute and chronic hepatitis B virus (HBV) infection. HBV infects the liver but does not cause direct cytopathology. Cell-mediated immune lysis of infected cells produces the symptoms and resolves the infection. Insufficient immunity can lead to chronic disease. Chronic HBV disease predisposes a person to more serious outcomes. *Purple arrows* indicate symptoms; *green arrows* indicate a possible outcome.

pathic effect, after which infection proceeds for a relatively long time without causing liver damage (i.e., elevation of liver enzyme levels) or symptoms. During this time, copies of the HBV genome integrate into the hepatocyte chromatin and remain latent. Intracellular buildup of filamentous forms of HBsAg can produce the ground-glass hepatocyte cytopathology characteristic of HBV infection.

Cell-mediated immunity and inflammation are responsible for causing the symptoms and effecting resolution of the HBV infection by eliminating the infected hepatocyte. Interferon most likely initiates the response by enhancing major histocompatibility complex antigen expression and the display of peptides from the HBs, HBc, and HBe antigens to cytotoxic killer T cells. Epitopes from the HBc antigen are prominent T-cell antigens. An insufficient T-cell response to the infection generally results in the occurrence of mild symptoms, an inability to resolve the infection, and the development of chronic hepatitis (see Fig. 62–7). Antibody (as generated by vaccination) can protect against infection. However, the large amount of HBsAg in serum binds to and blocks the action of neutralizing antibody, which limits the antibody's capacity to resolve an infection. Immune complexes formed between HBsAg and anti-HBs contribute to the development of hypersensitivity reactions (type III), leading to problems such as vasculitis, arthralgia, rash, and renal damage.

Infants and young children have an immature cell-mediated immune response and are less able to resolve the infection, but they suffer less tissue damage and milder symptoms. As many as 90% of infants infected perinatally become chronic carriers. Viral replication persists in these people for long periods.

During the acute phase of infection, the liver parenchyma shows degenerative changes consisting of cellular swelling and necrosis, especially in hepatocytes surrounding the central vein of a hepatic lobule. The inflammatory cell infiltrate is mainly composed of lymphocytes. Resolution of the infection allows the parenchyma to regenerate. Fulminant infections, activation of chronic infections, or co-infection with the delta agent can lead to permanent liver damage and cirrhosis.

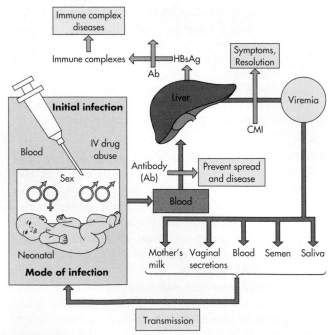

FIGURE 62–8. Spread of hepatitis B virus (HBV) in the body. Initial infection with HBV occurs through injection, heterosexual and homosexual sex, and birth. The virus then spreads to the liver, replicates, induces a viremia, and is transmitted in various body secretions in addition to blood to start the cycle again. Symptoms are caused by cell-mediated immunity (CMI) and immune complexes between antibody and hepatitis B surface antigen (HBsAg). IV = intravenous.

Epidemiology

In the United States, more than 300,000 persons are infected with HBV each year, resulting in 4000 deaths. However, even more people are infected in underdeveloped nations, with as much as 15% of the **population infected during birth or childhood.** High rates of seropositivity are observed in Italy, Greece, Africa, and Southeast Asia (Fig. 62–9). In some areas of the world (southern Africa and southeastern Asia), the seroconversion rate is as high as 50%. PHC, a long-term sequela of the infection, is also endemic in these regions.

The many asymptomatic chronic carriers with virus in blood and other body secretions foster the spread of the virus. In the United States, 0.1% to 0.5% of the general population are chronic carriers, but this is very low in comparison with many areas of the world. Carrier status may be lifelong.

The virus is spread by sexual, parenteral, and perinatal routes. Transmission occurs through contaminated blood and blood components by transfusion, needle sharing, acupuncture, ear piercing, or tattooing and through very close personal contact involving the exchange of semen, saliva, and vaginal secretions (e.g., sex, childbirth) (see Fig. 62–8). Medical personnel are at risk in accidents involving needlesticks or sharp instruments. People at particular risk are listed in Box 62–4. Sexual promiscuity and drug abuse are major risk factors for HBV infection. HBV can be transmitted to babies through contact with the mother's blood at birth and in mother's milk. Babies born to chronic HBV-positive mothers are at highest risk for infection. Serologic screening of donor units in blood banks has greatly reduced the risk of acquisition of the virus from contaminated blood or blood products. Safer sex habits adopted to prevent HIV transmission and the administration of the HBV vaccine have also been responsible for decreasing the transmission of HBV.

One of the major concerns about HBV is its association with PHC. This type of carcinoma probably accounts for 250,000 to 1 million deaths per year worldwide; in the United States, approximately 5000 deaths per year are attributed to PHC.

Clinical Syndromes

Acute Infection

As already noted, the clinical presentation of HBV in children is less severe than that in adults, and infection may even be asymptomatic. Clinically apparent illness occurs in as many as 25% of those infected with HBV (Figs. 62–10 to 62–12).

HBV infection is characterized by a **long incubation period and an insidious onset.** Symptoms during the prodromal period may include fever, malaise, and

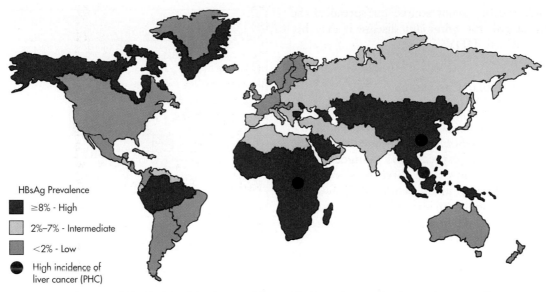

HBsAg Prevalence

■ ≥8% - High

▨ 2%–7% - Intermediate

▨ <2% - Low

● High incidence of liver cancer (PHC)

FIGURE 62–9. Worldwide prevalence of hepatitis B carriers and primary hepatocellular carcinoma. (Courtesy Centers for Disease Control and Prevention, Atlanta.)

anorexia, followed by nausea, vomiting, abdominal discomfort, and chills. The classic icteric symptoms of liver damage (e.g., jaundice, dark urine, pale stools) follow soon thereafter. Recovery is indicated by a decline in the fever and renewed appetite.

Fulminant hepatitis occurs in approximately 1% of icteric patients and may be fatal. It is marked by more severe symptoms and indications of severe liver damage, such as ascites and bleeding.

HBV infection can promote hypersensitivity reactions that are due to immune complexes of HBsAg and antibody. These may produce rash, polyarthritis, fever, acute necrotizing vasculitis, and glomerulonephritis.

Chronic Infection

Chronic hepatitis occurs in 5% to 10% of people with HBV infections, usually after mild or inapparent initial disease. It may be detected only by finding elevated liver enzyme levels on a routine blood chemistry profile, but as many as 10% of patients with chronic hepatitis may develop cirrhosis and liver failure. Chronically

---

BOX 62–4. **High-Risk Groups for Hepatitis B Virus Infection**

People from endemic regions (i.e., China, parts of Africa, Alaska, Pacific Islands)

Babies of mothers with chronic hepatitis B virus

Intravenous drug abusers

People with multiple sex partners: homosexual and heterosexual

Hemophiliacs and other patients requiring blood and blood product treatments

Health care personnel who have contact with blood

Residents and staff members of institutions for the mentally retarded

Hemodialysis patients and blood and organ recipients

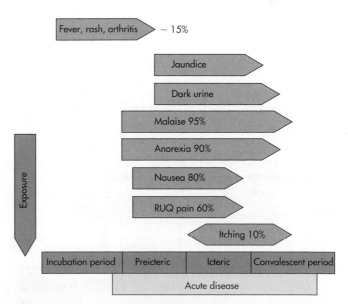

Fever, rash, arthritis   ~ 15%

Jaundice

Dark urine

Malaise 95%

Anorexia 90%

Nausea 80%

RUQ pain 60%

Itching 10%

Exposure

| Incubation period | Preicteric | Icteric | Convalescent period |

Acute disease

FIGURE 62–10. Symptoms of typical acute viral hepatitis B infection are correlated with the four clinical periods of this disease. RUQ = right upper quadrant. (Redrawn from Hoofnagle JH: *Lab Med* 14:705–716, 1983.)

infected people are the major source for spread of the virus and are at risk for fulminant disease if they become co-infected with HDV.

Primary Hepatocellular Carcinoma

The World Health Organization estimates that 80% of all cases of PHC can be attributed to chronic HBV infections. The HBV genome is integrated into these PHC cells, and the cells express HBV antigens. PHC is usually fatal and is one of the three most common causes of cancer mortality in the world. In Taiwan, at least 15% of the population are HBV carriers, and nearly half die of PHC or cirrhosis. PHC may become the first vaccine-preventable human cancer.

HBV may induce PHC by promoting continued liver repair and cell growth in response to tissue damage or by integrating into the host chromosome and stimulating cell growth directly. Such integration could stimulate genetic rearrangements or juxtapose viral promoters next to cellular growth–controlling genes. Alternatively, a protein encoded by the HBV X gene may transactivate (turn on) the transcription of cellular proteins and stimulate cell growth. The presence of the HBV genome may allow a subsequent mutation to promote carcinogenesis. The latency period between HBV infection and PHC may be as short as 9 years or as long as 35 years.

Laboratory Diagnosis

The initial diagnosis of hepatitis can be made on the basis of the clinical symptoms and the presence of liver enzymes in the blood (see Fig. 62–12). However, the

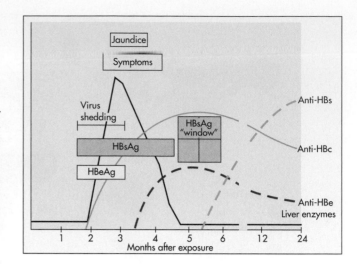

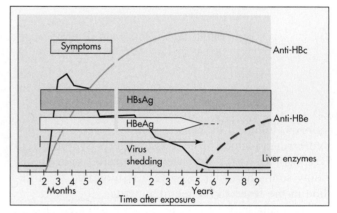

FIGURE 62–12. *A,* The serologic events associated with the typical course of acute hepatitis B disease. *B,* Development of the chronic hepatitis B virus carrier state. Routine serodiagnosis is difficult during the hepatitis B surface antigen (HBsAg) window when HBs and anti-HBs are undetectable. Anti-HBs-antibody to HBsAg; anti-HBc-antibody to HBcAg; anti-HBe-antibody to HBeAg. (Redrawn from Hoofnagle JH: *Annu Rev Med* 32:1–11, 1981.)

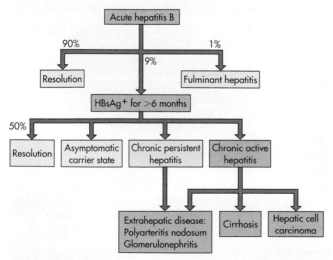

FIGURE 62–11. Clinical outcomes of acute hepatitis B infection. (Redrawn from White DO, Fenner F: *Medical virology,* ed 3, New York, 1986, Academic Press.)

serology of HBV infection describes the course and the nature of the disease (Table 62–2). Acute and chronic HBV infections can be distinguished by the presence of HBsAg and HBeAg in the serum and the pattern of antibodies to the individual HBV antigens.

HBsAg, HBcAg, and HBeAg are secreted into the blood during viral replication. The detection of HBeAg is the best correlate to the presence of infectious virus. A chronic infection can be distinguished by the continued finding of HBeAg, HBsAg, or both and a lack of detectable antibody to these antigens.

During the symptomatic phase of infection, detection of antibodies to HBeAg and HBsAg is obscured because the antibody is complexed with antigen in the serum. The best way to diagnose a recent acute infection, especially during the period when neither HBsAg

TABLE 62–2. Interpretation of Serologic Markers of Hepatitis B Virus Infection

Serologic Reactivity	Disease State					Healthy State	
	Early (Presymptomatic)	*Early Acute*	*Acute*	*Chronic*	*Late Acute*	*Resolved*	*Vaccinated*
Anti-HBc	−	−	−*	+	+/−	+	−
Anti-HBe	−	−	−	−	+/−	+/−†	−
Anti-HBs	−	−	−	−	−	+	+
HBeAg	−	+	+	+	−	−	−
HBsAg	+	+	+	+	+	−	−
Infectious virus	+	+	+	+	+	−	−

*Anti-HBc IgM should be present.
 †Anti-HBe may be negative after chronic disease.
 HBeAg = hepatitis Be antigen; HBsAg = hepatitis B surface antigen.

nor anti-HBs can be detected (the window), is to measure immunoglobulin M (IgM) anti-HBc.

Treatment, Prevention, and Control

No specific treatment exists for HBV infection. Interferon-α may be effective for treating a chronic HBV infection. **Hepatitis B immune globulin** may be administered within a week of exposure and to newborn infants of HBsAg-positive mothers. Drugs targeted at the polymerase, such as the human immunodeficiency virus reverse transcriptase inhibitor lamivudine, and the anti–herpes simplex virus drug famciclovir, show some efficacy and are being tested in human trials for HBV treatment.

Transmission of HBV in blood or blood products has been greatly reduced by screening donated blood for the presence of HBsAg and anti-HBc. Additional efforts to prevent transmission of HBV consist of avoiding intimate personal contact with a carrier of HBV and avoiding the lifestyles that facilitate spread of the virus. Household contacts and sexual partners of HBV carriers are at increased risk, as are patients undergoing hemodialysis, recipients of pooled plasma products, health care workers exposed to blood, and babies born of HBV-carrier mothers.

Vaccination is recommended for infants, children, and especially people in high-risk groups (see Box 62–4). Vaccination is useful even after exposure for newborns of HBsAg-positive mothers and people accidentally exposed either percutaneously or permucosally to blood or secretions from an HBsAg-positive person. Immunization of mothers should decrease the incidence of transmission to babies and older children, thus also reducing the number of chronic HBV carriers. Prevention of chronic HBV will reduce the incidence of PHC.

The HBV vaccines are subunit vaccines. The initial HBV vaccine was derived from the 22-nm HBsAg particles in human plasma obtained from chronically infected people. The current vaccine was genetically engineered and is produced by the insertion of a plasmid containing the S gene for HBsAg into a yeast, *Saccharomyces cerevisiae*.

The vaccine must be given in a series of three injections, with the second and third given 1 and 6 months after the first. More than 95% of individuals receiving the full three-dose course will develop protective antibody. The single serotype and limited host range (humans) help ensure the success of an immunization program.

The procedures of limiting exposure to HBV are described by the objectives of **universal blood and body fluid precautions.** Gloves are required for handling blood and body fluids; wearing protective clothing and eyeglasses may also be necessary. Special care should be taken with needles and sharp instruments. HBV-contaminated materials can be disinfected with 10% bleach solutions, but unlike most enveloped viruses, HBV is not inactivated by detergents.

Hepatitis C and G Viruses

Hepatitis C virus was identified by molecular biologic means in 1989 by screening infected chimpanzee blood for a viral RNA. The viral RNA was converted to DNA, its proteins were expressed, and antibodies from people with NANBH were then used to detect the viral proteins. These studies led to the development of ELISA and other tests for detection of the virus, which still cannot be grown in tissue culture.

HCV is the predominant cause of NANBH virus infections and was the major cause of post-transfusion hepatitis before routine screening of the blood supply for HCV. There are more than 170 million carriers of HCV in the world and more than 4 million in the

United States. HCV is transmitted by means similar to HBV but has an even greater potential for establishing persistent, chronic hepatitis. The chronic hepatitis often leads to cirrhosis and potentially to hepatocellular carcinoma. The significance of the HCV epidemic has become more apparent with the development of laboratory screening procedures.

Structure and Replication

Although HCV has never been isolated, its properties classify it as the only member of the Hepaciviridae, in the **Flaviviridae** family. It is 30 to 60 nm in diameter, with a **positive-sense RNA genome,** and is **enveloped.** The genome of HCV (9100 nucleotides) encodes 10 proteins, including 2 glycoproteins (E1, E2) that undergo variation during infection due to hypervariable regions within their genes. There are six major groups of variants (clades), which differ in their worldwide distribution.

HCV infects only humans and chimpanzees. It binds to cells using the CD81 surface receptor or coats itself with low-density lipoprotein or very-low-density lipoprotein and then uses their receptor for uptake into hepatocytes. The virus replicates like other flaviviruses but remains in the endoplasmic reticulum and is cell-associated. HCV proteins inhibit apoptosis and interferon-α action by binding to the tumor necrosis factor receptor (TNFR) and to protein kinase R (PKR). These actions prevent the death of the host cell and promote persistent infection.

Pathogenesis

The ability of HCV to remain cell-associated and prevent host cell death promotes persistent infection but results in liver disease later in life. Cell-mediated immunopathology is responsible mainly for producing the tissue damage. It has been suggested that the continual liver repair and induction of cell growth occurring during chronic HCV infection, especially in cirrhotic livers, are predisposing factors in the development of PHC. Antibody to HCV is not protective, and findings yielded by experimental infection of chimpanzees indicate that immunity to HCV may not be lifelong.

Epidemiology

HCV is **transmitted primarily in infected blood** and sexually. Intravenous drug abusers, transfusion and organ recipients, and hemophiliacs receiving factors VIII or IX are at highest risk for infection (Box 62–5). Almost all (>90%) human immunodeficiency virus–infected individuals who are or were intravenous drug users are infected with HCV. HCV is especially prevalent in southern Italy, Spain, central Europe, Japan,

---

BOX 62–5. Epidemiology of Hepatitis B, C, and D Viruses

Disease/Viral Factors

Enveloped virus is labile to drying. HBV is less sensitive to detergents than other enveloped viruses.
Virus is shed during asymptomatic periods.
Virus causes chronic disease with potential shedding.

Transmission

In blood, semen, and vaginal secretions (HBV: saliva and mother's milk).
Via transfusion, needlestick injury, shared drug paraphernalia, sex, and breast-feeding.

Who Is at Risk?

Children: mild asymptomatic disease with establishment of chronic infection.
Adults: insidious onset of hepatitis.
HBV-infected people co-infected or superinfected with HDV: abrupt, more severe symptoms with possible fulminant disease.
Adults with chronic HBV or HCV: at high risk for primary hepatocellular carcinoma.

Geography/Season

Viruses are found worldwide.
There is no seasonal incidence.

Modes of Control

Avoidance of high-risk behavior.
HBV: **vaccine** and screening of blood supply.

HBV = hepatitis B virus; HCV = hepatitis C virus; HDV = hepatitis D virus.

---

and parts of the Middle East (e.g., almost 20% of Egyptian blood donors are HCV-positive). The **high incidence of chronic asymptomatic infections** promotes the spread of the virus in the population. Screening procedures have led to a reduction in the levels of transmission by blood transfusion and organ donation, but transmission by other routes is prevalent.

Clinical Syndromes

HCV causes three types of disease (Fig. 62–13): acute hepatitis with resolution of the infection and recovery in 15% of cases, chronic persistent infection with possible progression to disease much later in life for 70%, and severe rapid progression to cirrhosis in 15% of patients. A viremia can be detected within 1 to 3 weeks of a transfusion of HCV-contaminated blood. The viremia lasts 4 to 6 months in people with an acute infection and longer than 10 years in those with a persistent infection. In its acute form, HCV infection is similar to acute HAV and HBV infection, but the

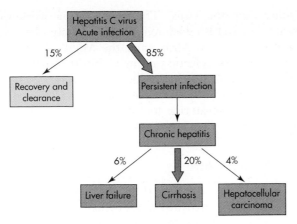

FIGURE 62–13. Outcomes of hepatitis C virus infection.

inflammatory response is less intense, and the symptoms are usually milder. More commonly (>80%), the initial disease is asymptomatic but establishes chronic persistent disease. The chronic persistent disease often progresses to chronic active hepatitis within 10 to 15 years and to cirrhosis (20% of chronic cases) and liver failure (20% of cirrhotic cases) after 20 years. Alcohol is a co-factor for HCV-induced cirrhosis. HCV promotes the development of hepatocellular carcinoma after 30 years in up to 5% of chronically infected patients.

Laboratory Diagnosis

The diagnosis and detection of HCV infection are based on ELISA recognition of antibody. Seroconversion occurs within 7 to 31 weeks of infection. However, antibody is not always present in viremic people. ELISA is used for screening the blood supply from normal donors but may not be sufficient for immunocompromised patients and those receiving hemodialysis. Reverse transcriptase–polymerase chain reaction, branched-chain DNA, and other genetic techniques can detect HCV RNA in seronegative people and have become key tools in the diagnosis of HCV infection.

Treatment, Prevention, and Control

Recombinant interferon-α alone or with ribavarin is the only known treatment for HCV.

Hepatitis G Virus

Hepatitis G virus resembles HCV in many ways. HGV is a flavivirus, is transmitted in blood, and has a predilection for chronic hepatitis disease. HGV is identified by detection of the genome by reverse transcriptase–polymerase chain reaction or other RNA detection methods.

Hepatitis D Virus

Approximately 15 million people in the world are infected with HDV (delta agent), and the virus is responsible for causing 40% of the **fulminant hepatitis** infections. HDV is unique in that it uses HBV and target cell proteins to replicate and produce its one protein. It is a viral parasite, proving that "even fleas have fleas." **HBsAg is essential for packaging the virus.** The delta agent resembles plant virus satellite agents and viroids in its size, genomic structure, and requirement for a helper virus for replication (Fig. 62–14).

Structure and Replication

The **HDV RNA genome is very small** (approximately 1700 nucleotides), and unlike other viruses, the single-stranded RNA is circular and forms a rod shape as a result of its extensive base pairing. The virion is approximately the same size as the HBV virion (35 to 37 nm in diameter). The genome is surrounded by the delta antigen core, which in turn is surrounded by an HBsAg-containing envelope. The **delta antigen** exists as a small (24 kDa) or large (27 kDa) form; the small form is predominant.

The delta agent binds to and is internalized by hepatocytes in the same manner as HBV because it has HBsAg in its envelope. The transcription and replication processes of the HDV genome are unusual. The host cell's RNA polymerase II makes an RNA copy, replicates the genome, and makes mRNA. The genome then forms an RNA structure called a **ribozyme,** which cleaves the RNA circle to produce an mRNA. The gene for the delta antigen is mutated by a cellular

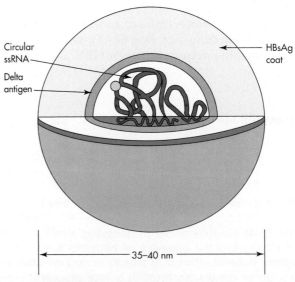

FIGURE 62–14. The delta hepatitis virion.

enzyme (double-stranded RNA–activated adenosine deaminase) during infection, thereby allowing production of the large delta antigen. Production of this antigen limits replication of the virus and cell destruction, thus promoting persistent infection. The genome becomes wrapped in an envelope containing the delta antigen, and HBsAg and the virus is then released from the cell.

Pathogenesis

Similar to HBV, the delta agent is spread in blood, semen, and vaginal secretions. However, it can replicate and cause disease only in people with active HBV infections. Because the two agents are transmitted by the same routes, a person can be **co-infected** with HBV and the delta agent. A person with chronic HBV can also be **superinfected** with the delta agent. More rapid, severe progression occurs in HBV carriers superinfected with HDV than in people co-infected with HBV and the delta agent, because during co-infection HBV must first establish its infection before HDV can replicate (Fig. 62–15), whereas superinfection of an HBV-infected person allows the delta agent to replicate immediately.

Replication of the delta agent results in cytotoxicity and liver damage. Persistent delta agent infection is often established in HBV carriers. Although antibodies are elicited against the delta agent, protection probably stems from the immune response to HBsAg because it is the external antigen and viral attachment protein for HDV. Unlike HBV disease, damage to the liver occurs as a result of the direct cytopathic effect of the delta agent combined with the underlying immunopathology of the HBV disease.

Epidemiology

The delta agent infects children and adults with underlying HBV infection (see Box 62–5), and people who are persistently infected with both HBV and HDV are a source for the virus. The agent has a worldwide distribution and is endemic in southern Italy, the Amazon Basin, parts of Africa, and the Middle East. Epidemics of HDV infection occur in North America and Western Europe, usually in illicit drug users.

HDV is spread by the same routes as HBV, and the same groups are at risk for infection, with parenteral drug abusers and hemophiliacs at highest risk.

Clinical Syndromes

The delta agent increases the severity of HBV infections. Fulminant hepatitis is more likely to develop in people infected with the delta agent than in those infected with the other hepatitis viruses. This type of hepatitis can result in hepatic encephalopathy (with altered mental capacity) and massive hepatic necrosis, which is fatal in 80% of cases. Chronic infection with the delta agent can occur in people with chronic HBV.

Laboratory Diagnosis

The only way to determine the presence of the agent is by detecting the delta antigen or antibodies. ELISA and radioimmunoassay procedures are available for doing this. The delta antigen can be detected in the blood during the acute phase of disease in a detergent-treated serum sample.

Treatment, Prevention, and Control

There is no known specific treatment for HDV hepatitis. Because the delta agent depends on HBV for replication and is spread by the same routes, prevention of infection with HBV prevents HDV infection. Immunization with HBV vaccine protects against subsequent deltavirus infection. If a person has already acquired HBV, delta agent infection may be prevented by halting illicit intravenous drug use and avoiding HDV-contaminated blood products.

Hepatitis E Virus

HEV (E-NANBH) (the E stands for "enteric" or "epidemic") is predominantly spread by the fecal-oral route, especially in contaminated water (see Box 62–2). It resembles calicivirus or the Norwalk agent in size (27 to 34 nm) and structure. Although HEV is found throughout the world, it is most problematic in developing countries. Epidemics have been reported in India, Pakistan, Nepal, Burma, North Africa, and Mexico.

The symptoms and course of HEV disease are similar to those of HAV disease; it causes only acute disease. However, the symptoms for HEV may occur later than those of HAV disease, and response to serum immunoglobulin G may be poor. The mortality

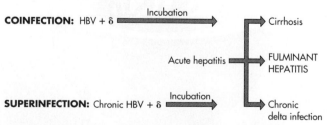

FIGURE 62–15. Consequences of deltavirus infection. Deltavirus (δ) requires the presence of hepatitis B virus (HBV) infection. Superinfection of a person already infected with HBV (carrier) causes more rapid, severe progression than co-infection (*shorter arrow*).

rate associated with HEV disease is 1% to 2%, approximately 10 times that associated with HAV disease. HEV infection is especially serious in pregnant women (mortality rate of approximately 20%).

CASE STUDIES AND QUESTIONS

■ A 55-year-old man (**patient A**) was admitted to the hospital with fatigue, nausea, and abdominal discomfort. He had a slight fever, his urine was dark yellow, and his abdomen was distended and tender. He had returned from a trip to Thailand within the previous month.

A 28-year-old woman (**patient B**) was admitted to the hospital complaining of vomiting, abdominal discomfort, nausea, anorexia, dark urine, and jaundice. She admitted that she was a former heroin addict and that she had shared needles. She was also 3 months pregnant.

A 65-year-old man (**patient C**) was admitted with jaundice, nausea, and vomiting 6 months after undergoing coronary artery bypass grafting.

1. What clinical or epidemiologic clues would have assisted in the diagnosis of hepatitis A, B, and C?

2. What laboratory tests would have been helpful in distinguishing the different hepatitis infections?

3. What was the most likely means of viral acquisition in each case?

4. What personal and public health precautions should have been taken to prevent the transmission of virus in each case?

5. Which of the patients was susceptible to chronic disease?

6. What laboratory tests distinguish acute from chronic HBV disease?

7. How can HBV disease be prevented? Treated?

BIBLIOGRAPHY

Blum HE, Gerok W, Vyas GN: The molecular biology of hepatitis B virus, *Trends Genet* 5:154–158, 1989.

Bradley DW, Krawczynski K, Kane MA: Hepatitis E. In Belshe RB, editor: *Textbook of human virology*, ed 2, St Louis, 1991, Mosby.

Catalina G, Navarro V: Hepatitis C: a challenge for the generalist. *Hosp Prac* 35:97–108, 2000.

Fallows DA, Goff AP: Hepadnaviruses: current models of RNA encapsidation and reverse transcription, *Adv Virus Res* 46:167–196, 1996.

Fields BN, Knipe DM, Howley PM, editors: *Virology*, ed 3, New York, 1996, Lippincott-Raven.

Frosner G: Hepatitis A virus. In Belshe RB, editor: *Textbook of human virology*, ed 2, St Louis, 1991, Mosby.

Hadler SC, Fields HA: Hepatitis delta virus. In Belshe RB, editor: *Textbook of human virology*, ed 2, St Louis, 1991, Mosby.

Hagedorn CH, Rice CM: The hepatitis C viruses, *Curr Top Microbiol Immunol* 242:1–380, 2000.

Hepatitis NIAID fact sheet: Available at http://www.niaid.nih.gov/publications/hepatitis.htm

Hoofnagle JH: Type A and type B hepatitis, *Lab Med* 14: 705–716, 1983.

Lennette EH, Halonen P, Murphy FA, editors: *Laboratory diagnosis of infectious diseases: principles and practice*, New York, 1988, Springer-Verlag.

Lutwick LI: Hepatitis B virus. In Belshe RB, editor: *Textbook of human virology*, ed 2, St Louis, 1991, Mosby.

Mason WS, Seeger C, editors: Hepadnaviruses: molecular biology and pathogenesis, *Curr Top Microbiol Immunol* 162: 1–206, 1991.

Plageman PGW: Hepatitis C virus, *Arch Virol* 120:165–180, 1991.

Reyes GR, Baroudy BM: Molecular biology of NANBH agents: hepatitis C and hepatitis E viruses, *Adv Virus Res* 40:57–102, 1991.

Robinson W, Koike K, Will H, editors: *Hepadnavirus*, New York, 1987, Liss.

Tam AW et al: Hepatitis E virus: molecular cloning and sequencing of the full-length viral genome, *Virology* 185: 120–131, 1991.

CHAPTER 63

Unconventional Slow Viruses: Prions

The unconventional slow viruses cause spongiform encephalopathies, which are slow neurodegenerative diseases. These disorders include the human diseases **kuru, Creutzfeldt-Jakob disease (CJD), Gerstmann-Sträussler-Scheinker (GSS) disease,** and **fatal familial insomnia (FFI)** and the animal diseases **scrapie, bovine spongiform encephalopathy (BSE) (mad cow disease), chronic wasting disease (in mule, deer, and elk),** and **transmissible mink encephalopathy** (Box 63–1). Since the late 1990s, there have been outbreaks of BSE and a rapid progressing form of CJD affecting younger people (40 years) in the United Kingdom. **CJD, FFI, and GSS disease are also genetic human disorders**.

Slow virus agents are filterable and can transmit disease but otherwise do not conform to the standard definition of a virus (Table 63–1). Unlike conventional viruses, these agents apparently have no virion structure or genome, elicit no immune response, and are extremely resistant to inactivation by heat, disinfectants, and radiation. The slow virus agent appears to be a modified host protein known as a **prion (a small proteinaceous infectious particle)**, which can transmit the disease.

After long incubation periods, these agents cause damage to the central nervous system that leads to a subacute spongiform encephalopathy. The long incubation period, which can last 30 years in humans, has made study of these agents difficult. Carlton Gajdusek won the Nobel Prize for showing that kuru has an infectious etiology and also for developing a method for analyzing the agent. The major breakthroughs came when the kuru agent was transmitted to monkeys and with the recognition that the scrapie agent from sheep induced a characteristic cytopathologic effect in hamsters long before the disease was evident. These studies provided a useful means for assaying slow virus agents and identifying their biologic properties.

Structure and Physiology

The slow virus agents were suspected to be viruses because they can pass through filters that block the passage of particles more than 100 nm in diameter and still transmit disease. Unlike viruses, the agents are resistant to a wide range of chemical and physical treatments, such as formaldehyde, ultraviolet radiation, and heat to 80°C.

The prototype of these agents is scrapie, which has been adapted so that it can infect hamsters. Scrapie-infected hamsters have scrapie-associated fibrils in their brains. These fibrils are infectious and contain the prion.

The prion, which lacks detectable nucleic acids, consists of aggregates of a protease-resistant, hydrophobic glycoprotein, which for scrapie is termed PrP^{Sc} (scrapie prion protein) (27,000 to 30,000 Da). Humans and other animals encode a protein PrP^{C} (cellular prion protein) that is closely related to PrP^{Sc} in its protein sequence but differs in many of its other properties (Table 63–2). Differences in post-translational modifications cause the two proteins to behave very differently. PrP^{Sc} is protease-resistant, aggregates into amyloid rods (fibrils), is found in cytoplasmic vesicles in the cell, and is secreted. The normal PrP^{C}, on the other hand, is protease-sensitive and appears on the cell surface.

Many theories have been proposed to explain how an aberrant protein could cause disease. Stanley Prusiner was awarded the Nobel Prize in 1997 for showing that the PrP^{Sc} is sufficient to cause disease. PrP^{Sc} binds to the normal PrP^{C} on the cell surface, causing it to be processed into PrP^{Sc}, to be released from the cell, and to be aggregated as amyloid-like plaques in the brain. The cell then replenishes the PrP^{C}, and the cycle continues. The human version of the PrP^{Sc} is encoded on chromosome 20. The fact that these plaques consist of host protein may explain the lack of an immune response to these agents in patients with the spongiform encephalopathies.

Pathogenesis

Spongiform encephalopathy describes the appearance of the vacuolated neurons as well as their loss of function

BOX 63–1. Slow Virus Diseases

Human

Kuru
Creutzfeldt-Jakob disease (CJD)
Gerstmann-Sträussler-Scheinker (GSS disease)
Fatal familial insomnia (FFI)

Animal

Scrapie (sheep and goats)
Transmissible mink encephalopathy
Bovine spongiform encephalopathy (mad cow disease)
Chronic wasting disease (mule, deer, and elk)

TABLE 63–2. Comparison of Scrapie Prion Protein (PrP^{Sc}) and (Normal) Cellular Prion Protein (PrP^{C})

	PrP^{Sc}	PrP^{C}
Structure	Globular	Extended
Protease resistance	Yes	No
Presence in scrapie fibrils	Yes	No
Location in or on cells	Cytoplasmic vesicles	Plasma membrane
Turnover	Days	Hours

and the lack of an immune response or inflammation (Box 63–2). Vacuolation of the neurons, the formation of amyloid-containing plaques and fibrils, a proliferation and hypertrophy of astrocytes, and the fusion of neurons and adjacent glial cells are observed (Fig. 63–1). The PrP^{Sc} is taken up by neurons and phagocytic cells but is difficult to degrade, a feature that may contribute to the vacuolation of the brain tissue. In addition, prions reach high concentrations in the brain, further contributing to the tissue damage. Prions can also be isolated from tissue other than the brain, but only the brain shows any disease. No inflammation or immune response to the agent is generated, distinguishing this disease from a classic viral encephalitis. A

protein marker (14-3-3 brain protein) can be detected in the cerebrospinal fluid of symptomatic individuals.

The incubation period for CJD and kuru may be as long as 30 years, but once the symptoms become evident, the patient dies within a year.

Epidemiology

CJD is transmitted predominantly by (1) injection, (2) transplantation of contaminated tissue (e.g., corneas), (3) contact with contaminated medical devices (e.g., brain electrodes), and (4) possibly in food (Box 63–3). CJD, FFI, and GSS disease are also inheritable, and families with genetic histories of these diseases have been identified. The diseases are rare but occur worldwide.

Kuru, however, was limited to a very small area of the New Guinea highlands. The name of the disease means "shivering" or "trembling," and the disease was related to the cannibalistic practices of the Fore tribe of New Guinea. Before Gajdusek intervened, it was the custom of these people to eat the bodies of their de-

TABLE 63–1. Comparison of Classic Viruses and Prions

	Virus	Prion
Filterable, infectious agents	Yes	Yes
Presence of nucleic acid	Yes	No?
Defined morphology (electron microscopy)	Yes	No
Presence of protein	Yes	Yes
Disinfection by:		
Formaldehyde	Yes	No
Proteases	Some	No
Heat (80°C)	Most	No
Ionizing and ultraviolet radiation	Yes	No
Disease		
Cytopathologic effect	Yes	No
Incubation period	Depends on virus	Long
Immune response	Yes	No
Interferon production	Yes	No
Inflammatory response	Yes	No

BOX 63–2. Pathogenic Characteristics of Slow Viruses

No cytopathologic effect in vitro.
　Long doubling time of at least 5.2 days.
　Long incubation period.
　Cause vacuolation of neurons (spongiform), amyloid-like plaques, gliosis.
　Symptoms that include loss of muscle control, shivering, tremors, dementia.
　Lack of antigenicity.
　Lack of inflammation.
　Lack of immune response.
　Lack of interferon production.

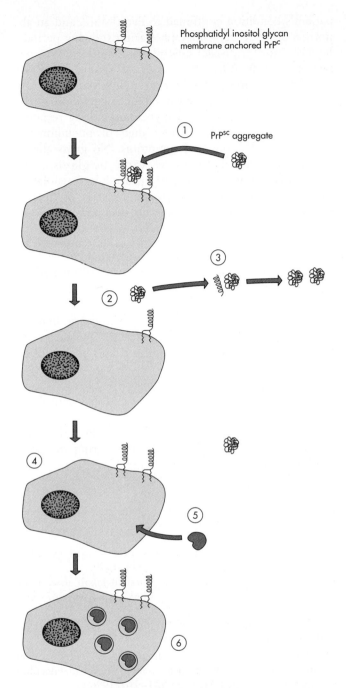

FIGURE 63–1. Model for proliferation of prions. PrPᶜ is a normal cellular protein that is anchored in the cell membrane by phosphatidyl inositol glycan. PrPˢᶜ is a hydrophobic globular protein that aggregates with itself and with PrPᶜ on the cell surface (1). This causes the release of PrPᶜ (2) and its conversion to PrPˢᶜ (3). The cell synthesizes new PrPᶜ (4), and the cycle is repeated. A form of PrPˢᶜ is internalized by neurons (5) and accumulates (6), giving the cell a spongiform appearance. Other models have been proposed.

BOX 63–3. **Epidemiology of Disease Caused by Slow Viruses**

Disease/Viral Factors

Agents are impervious to standard viral disinfection procedures.

Diseases have very long incubation periods, as long as 30 years.

Transmission

Transmission is via **infected tissue**, or syndrome **may be inherited.**

Infection occurs through cuts in skin, transplantation of contaminated tissues (e.g., cornea), use of contaminated medical devices (e.g., brain electrodes), and potentially through ingestion of infected tissue.

Who Is at Risk?

Women and children of the Fore tribe in New Guinea were at risk for kuru.

Surgeons, transplant and brain surgery patients, others are at risk for CJD and GSS disease.

Geography/Season

GSS disease and CJD have sporadic occurrence worldwide.

There is no seasonal incidence.

Modes of Control

No treatments are available.

Cessation of ritual cannibalism has led to the disappearance of kuru.

For GSS disease and CJD, neurosurgical tools and electrodes should be disinfected in 5% hypochlorite solution or 1.0 M sodium hydroxide or autoclaved at 15 psi for 1 hour.

CJD = Creutzfeldt-Jakob disease, GSS = Gerstman-Straüssler-Scheinker.

---

ceased kinsmen. When Gajdusek began his study, he noted that women and children in particular were the most susceptible to the disease, and he deduced that the reasons were that the women and children pre-

pared the food and they were given the less desirable viscera and brains to eat. Their risk for infection was higher because they handled the contaminated tissue, making it possible for the agent to be introduced through the conjunctiva or cuts in the skin, and they ingested the neural tissue, which contains the highest concentrations of the kuru agent. Cessation of this cannibalistic custom has stopped the spread of kuru.

An epidemic of mad cow disease in the United Kingdom and the unusual incidence of CJD in younger people (younger than 45 years) prompted concern that contaminated beef was the source of this new variant of CJD. The association between the bovine and human diseases has not been proved, however.

Clinical Syndromes

As already noted, the slow virus agents cause a progressive, degenerative neurologic disease with a long

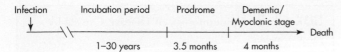

FIGURE 63–2. Progression of transmissible Creutzfeldt-Jakob disease.

incubation period but with rapid progression to death after the onset of symptoms (Fig. 63–2). The spongiform encephalopathies are characterized by a loss of muscle control, shivering, myoclonic jerks and tremors, loss of coordination, rapidly progressive dementia, and death.

Laboratory Diagnosis

There are no methods for directly detecting virus in tissue through the use of electron microscopy, antigen detection, or nucleic acid probes. Also, no serologic tests can detect viral antibody. The diagnosis must be made on clinical grounds, with confirmation by the characteristic histologic changes in brain tissue described in the section on pathogenesis. Demonstration of a proteinase K–resistant form of PrP in a Western blot using antibody to PrP can confirm a case of CJD.

Treatment, Prevention, and Control

No treatment exists for kuru or CJD. The causative agents are also impervious to the disinfection procedures used for other viruses, including formaldehyde, detergents, and ionizing radiation. Autoclaving at 15 psi for 1 hour instead of 20 minutes or treatment with 5% hypochlorite solution or 1.0 M sodium hydroxide can be used for decontamination. Because these agents can be transmitted on instruments and brain electrodes, such items should be carefully disinfected before being reused.

CASE STUDY AND QUESTIONS

■ A 70-year-old woman complained of severe headaches and appeared dull and apathetic with a constant tremor in the right hand. One month later, she experienced memory loss and moments of confusion. The patient's condition continued to deteriorate, and an abnormal electroencephalograph tracing showing periodic biphasic and triphasic slow-wave complexes was obtained at 2 months after onset of symptoms. By 3 months, the patient was in a coma-like state. She also had occasional spontaneous clonic twitching of the arms and legs and a startle myoclonic jerking response to a loud noise. The patient died of pneumonia 4 months after the onset of symptoms. No gross abnormalities were noted at autopsy. Astrocytic gliosis of the cerebral cortex with fibrils and intracellular vacuolation throughout the cerebral cortex were seen on microscopic examination. There was no swelling and no inflammation.

1. What viral neurologic diseases would have been considered in the differential diagnosis formulated on the basis of the symptoms described? What other diseases?

2. What key features of the postmortem findings were characteristic of the diseases caused by unconventional slow virus agents (spongiform encephalopathies, prions)?

3. What key features distinguish the unconventional slow virus diseases from more conventional neurologic viral diseases?

4. What precautions should the pathologist have taken for protection against infection during the postmortem examination?

BIBLIOGRAPHY

Belay ED: Transmissible spongiform encephalopathies in humans, *Annu Rev Microbiol* 53:283–314, 1999.

Brown P, et al: Diagnosis of Creutzfeld-Jakob disease by Western blot identification. N Engl J Med 314:547–551, 1986.

Fields BN et al, editors: *Virology*, ed 3, New York, 1996, Lippincott-Raven.

Hsich G, et al: The 14-3-3 brain protein in cerebrospinal fluid as a marker for transmissible spongiform encephalopathies. N Engl J Med 335:924–930, 1996.

Manson JC: Understanding transmission of the prion diseases, *Trends Microbiol* 7:465–467, 1999.

Prusiner SB: Molecular biology and genetics of neurodegenerative diseases caused by prions, *Adv Virus Res* 41:241–280, 1992.

Prusiner SB: Prions, prions, prions, *Curr Top Microbiol Immunol* 207:1–162, 1996.

CHAPTER 64

Miscellaneous Viruses

Coronaviruses

Coronaviruses are named for the solar corona–like appearance (the surface projections) of their virions when viewed with an electron microscope (Fig. 64–1). Coronaviruses are the second most prevalent cause of the **common cold** (rhinovirus is the first). Electron microscopy findings have also linked coronaviruses to gastroenteritis in children and adults. Only two strains of virus have been isolated from humans; however, other strains are believed to exist.

Structure and Replication

Coronaviruses are **enveloped virions** with a long **positive (+) RNA** genome. Virions measure 80 to 160 nm (Box 64–1). The glycoproteins on the surface of the envelope appear as club-shaped projections that are 20 nm long and 5 to 11 nm wide. The virion is normally sensitive to acid, ether, and drying, but some strains are capable of traversing the gastrointestinal tract.

The large plus-stranded RNA genome (27,000 to 30,000 bases) associates with the N protein to form a helical nucleocapsid. Protein synthesis occurs in two phases similar to that of the togaviruses. The genome is translated to produce an RNA-dependent RNA polymerase (L [225,000 Da]). The polymerase generates a negative-sense template RNA. The L protein then uses the template RNA to replicate new genomes and produce **individual messenger RNAs (mRNAs)** encoding the other viral proteins.

Virions contain the glycoproteins E1 (20,000 to 30,000 Da) and E2 (160,000 to 200,000 Da) and a core nucleoprotein (N [47,000 to 55,000 Da]); some strains also contain a hemagglutinin-neuraminidase (E3 [120,000 to 140,000 Da]) (Table 64–1). The E2 glycoprotein is responsible for mediating viral attachment and membrane fusion and is the target of neutralizing antibodies. The E1 glycoprotein is a transmembrane matrix protein. The replication scheme for coronaviruses is shown in Figure 64–2.

Pathogenesis and Clinical Syndromes

Coronaviruses inoculated into the respiratory tracts of human volunteers have been found to infect epithelial cells. Infection remains localized to the upper respiratory tract because the *optimum temperature for viral growth is 33°C to 35°C* (Box 64–2).

The virus is most likely spread by aerosols and in large droplets (e.g., sneezes). Coronaviruses cause an upper respiratory tract infection similar to the colds caused by rhinoviruses but with a longer incubation period (average, 3 days). The infection may exacerbate a preexisting chronic pulmonary disease, such as asthma and bronchitis, and on rare occasions may cause pneumonia.

Infections occur mainly in infants and children. Coronavirus disease appears either sporadically or in outbreaks in the winter and spring. Usually, one strain predominates in an outbreak. Findings from serologic studies show that coronaviruses cause approximately 10% to 15% of upper respiratory tract infections and pneumonias in humans. Antibodies to coronaviruses are uniformly present by adulthood, but reinfections are common despite the preexisting serum antibodies.

Coronavirus-like particles have also been seen in electron micrographs of stool specimens obtained from adults and children with diarrhea and gastroenteritis and infants with neonatal necrotizing enterocolitis.

Laboratory Diagnosis

Laboratory tests are not routinely performed to diagnose coronavirus infections. However, enzyme-linked immunosorbent assay (ELISA) can be used to evaluate acute and convalescent sera. Elcctron microscopy has also been used to detect coronavirus-like particles in stool specimens.

Treatment, Prevention, and Control

Control of the respiratory transmission of coronaviruses would be difficult and is probably unnecessary

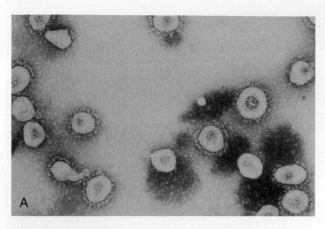

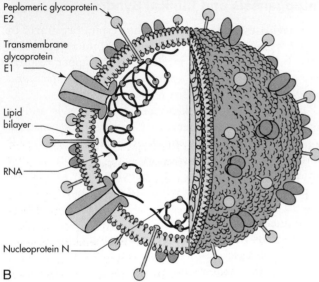

Peplomeric glycoprotein E2

Transmembrane glycoprotein E1

Lipid bilayer

RNA

Nucleoprotein N

B

FIGURE 64–1. *A,* Electron micrograph of the human respiratory coronavirus. (×90,000.) *B,* Model of a coronavirus. The viral nucleocapsid is a long, flexible helix composed of the positive-strand genomic RNA and many molecules of the phosphorylated nucleocapsid protein N. The viral envelope consists of a lipid bilayer derived from the intracellular membranes of the host cell and two viral glycoproteins (E1 and E2). (*A,* Courtesy Centers for Disease Control and Prevention, Atlanta; *B,* redrawn from Fields BF, Knipe DM, editors: *Virology,* New York, 1985, Raven.)

because of the mildness of the infection. No vaccine or specific antiviral therapy is available.

Calicivirus and Other Small, Round Gastroenteritis Viruses

Norwalk agent was discovered on electron microscopic examination of stool samples from adults during an epidemic of acute gastroenteritis in Norwalk, Ohio. Norwalk agent is a **calcivirus,** which is a member of a group of small, round gastroenteritis viruses that include the **astroviruses** and unclassified viruses bearing the names of the geographic locations where they were identified (Box 64–3).

Structure and Replication

Caliciviruses, including Norwalk virus, are approximately the same size as picornaviruses. Their **positive-sense RNA genome** (approximately 7500 bases) is contained in a 27-nm **naked capsid** consisting of one 60,000-Da capsid protein. Norwalk virions are round with a ragged outline, whereas other calicivirions have cup-shaped indentations and a six-pointed star shape. The virions of the astroviruses have a five- or six-

TABLE 64–1. Major Human Coronavirus Proteins

Proteins	Molecular Weight (kDa)	Location	Functions
E2 (peplomeric glycoprotein)	160–200	Envelope spikes (peplomer)	Binding to host cells; fusion activity
H1 (hemagglutinin protein)	60–66	Peplomer	Hemagglutination
N (nucleoprotein)	47–55	Core	Ribonucleoprotein
E1 (matrix glycoprotein)	20–30	Envelope	Transmembrane protein
L (polymerase)	225	Infected cell	Polymerase activity

Modified from Balows A et al, editors: *Laboratory diagnosis of infectious diseases: principles and practice,* New York, 1988, Springer-Verlag.

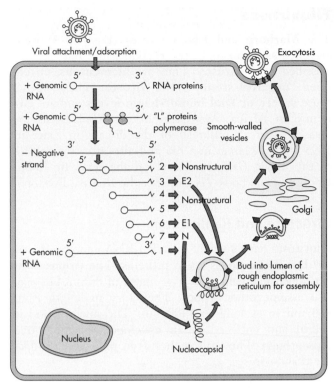

FIGURE 64-2. Replication of human coronaviruses. The E2 glycoprotein interacts with receptors on epithelial cells, the virus fuses or is endocytosed into the cell, and the genome is released into the cytoplasm. Protein synthesis is divided into early and late phases similar to that in the togaviruses. The genome binds to ribosomes, and an RNA-dependent RNA polymerase is translated. This enzyme generates a full-length, negative-sense RNA template for the production of new virion genomes and six individual mRNAs for the other coronavirus proteins. The genome associates with rough endoplasmic reticulum membranes modified by virion proteins and buds into the lumen of the rough endoplasmic reticulum. Vesicles that contain virus migrate to the cell membrane and are released by exocytosis. (Redrawn from Balows A et al, editors: *Laboratory diagnosis of infectious diseases: principles and practice,* New York, 1988, Springer-Verlag.)

pointed star shape on the surface but no indentations. Antibodies from seropositive people can also be used to distinguish these viruses.

Caliciviruses and astroviruses can be grown in cell culture, but the Norwalk viruses cannot. These viruses replicate in the cytoplasm, with release of viral particles on cell destruction.

Pathogenesis

The virus compromises the function of the intestinal brush border, preventing proper absorption of water and nutrients. Although no histologic changes occur in the gastric mucosa, gastric emptying may be delayed.

BOX 64-2. Disease Mechanisms of Human Coronaviruses

Virus infects epithelial cells of upper respiratory tract.
Virus replicates best at 33°C to 35°C; therefore, it is restricted to upper respiratory tract.
Reinfection occurs in presence of serum antibodies.
Enveloped virus may be able to survive the gastrointestinal tract.

Examination of jejunal biopsy specimens from human volunteers infected with caliciviruses has revealed the existence of blunted villi, cytoplasmic vacuolation, and infiltration with mononuclear cells, but viral particles are not detected on electron micrographs of epithelial cells.

Epidemiology

Norwalk and related viruses typically cause outbreaks of gastroenteritis as a result of a common source of contamination (e.g., water, shellfish, food service). These viruses are transmitted mainly by the fecal-oral but possibly by airborne routes. Outbreaks in developed countries may occur year-round and have been described in schools, resorts, hospitals, nursing homes, restaurants, and cruise ships. Common-source outbreaks can often be traced to a careless, infected food handler. The importance of these agents is indicated by the fact that almost 10% of all outbreaks of gastroenteritis and almost 60% of those that are nonbacterial in origin are attributed to Norwalk-like viruses. Immunity is generally short-lived at best and may not be protective.

Approximately 3% of the cases of gastroenteritis in children in daycare centers in the United States are

---

BOX 64-3. Characteristics of Small, Round Gastroenteritis Viruses*

Viruses are small capsid viruses distinguishable by **capsid** morphology.
Viruses are resistant to environmental pressure: detergents, drying, and acid.
Viruses are transmitted by **fecal-oral** route in contaminated water and food.
Viruses cause **outbreaks of gastroenteritis.**
Disease resolves after 48 hours without serious consequences.

*Includes Norwalk agent and other caliciviruses.

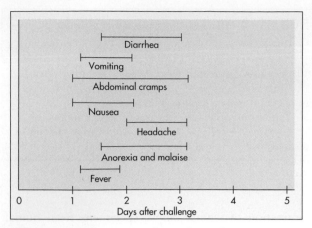

FIGURE 64–3. Response to ingestion of Norwalk virus. Symptoms vary in severity.

attributed to caliciviruses. As many as 70% of children have antibodies to the astroviruses by age 7 years.

Clinical Syndromes

Norwalk and related viruses cause symptoms similar to those caused by the rotaviruses. Infection causes **diarrhea with nausea and vomiting**, especially in children (Fig. 64–3). Bloody stools do not occur. Fever may occur in as many as one third of the patients. The incubation period is 24 to 48 hours, and the illness resolves within 12 to 60 hours without problems. Astroviruses cause diarrhea without vomiting and are less likely to cause disease in adults.

Laboratory Diagnosis

Immunoelectron microscopy can be used to concentrate and identify the virus from stool. The addition of an antibody directed against the suspected agent causes the virus to aggregate, thereby facilitating recognition. Radioimmunoassay (RIA) and ELISA have been developed to detect the virus and viral antigen.

Serology is the method used to identify most infections. Antibody to the Norwalk agent may be detected by RIA or ELISA. Antibodies to the other calicivirus-like agents are more difficult to detect.

Treatment, Prevention, and Control

No specific treatment for infection with the calicivirus or other small, round gastroenteritis viruses is available. Bismuth subsalicylate may reduce the severity of the gastrointestinal symptoms. Outbreaks may be minimized by handling food carefully and by maintaining the purity of the water supply.

Filoviruses

The **Marburg** and **Ebola** viruses (Fig. 64–4) were classified as members of the rhabdoviridae but are now classified as **filoviruses**. They are **filamentous, enveloped, negative-strand RNA viruses**. These agents cause **severe or fatal hemorrhagic fevers** and are **endemic in Africa**. Awareness of the Ebola virus increased after an outbreak of the disease in Zaire in 1995 and in Gabon in 1996 and also after the release of the movie *Outbreak*, based on the book by Robin Cook, and the book *The Hot Zone* by Richard Preston.

Structure and Replication

Filoviruses have a single-stranded RNA genome (4.5×10^6 Da) that encodes seven proteins. The virions form enveloped filaments with a diameter of 80 nm but may also assume other shapes. They vary in length from 800 nm to as long as 1400 nm. The nucleocapsid is helical and enclosed in an envelope containing one glycoprotein. The virus replicates in the cytoplasm like the rhabdoviruses.

Pathogenesis

The filoviruses replicate efficiently, producing large amounts of virus and causing extensive tissue necrosis in parenchymal cells of the liver, spleen, lymph nodes, and lungs. The breakdown of endothelial cells leading to vascular injury can be attributed to the ebola glycoprotein. Strains with mutations in this protein eliminate the hemorrhagic component of disease. The widespread hemorrhage that occurs in affected patients causes edema and hypovolemic shock.

Epidemiology

Marburg virus infection was first detected among laboratory workers in Marburg, Germany, who had been

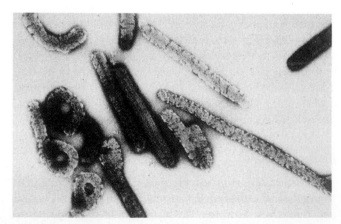

FIGURE 64–4. Electron micrograph of the Ebola virus. (Courtesy Centers for Disease Control and Prevention, Atlanta.)

exposed to tissues from apparently healthy African green monkeys. Rare cases of Marburg virus infection have been seen in Zimbabwe and Kenya.

Ebola virus was named for the river in the Democratic Republic of Congo (formerly Zaire) where it was discovered. Outbreaks of Ebola virus disease have occurred in the Democratic Republic of Congo and the Sudan. During an outbreak, the Ebola virus is so lethal that it eliminates the susceptible population before it can be spread extensively. However, in rural areas of central Africa as much as 18% of the population have antibody to this virus, indicating that subclinical infections do occur.

These viruses may be endemic in wild monkeys but can be spread from monkeys to humans and between humans. Contact with the animal reservoir or direct contact with infected blood or secretions can spread the disease. These viruses have been transmitted by accidental injection and through the use of contaminated syringes. Health care workers tending the sick and monkey handlers may be at risk.

Clinical Syndromes

Marburg and Ebola viruses are the most severe causes of viral hemorrhagic fevers. The illness usually begins with flu-like symptoms such as headache and myalgia. Nausea, vomiting, and diarrhea occur within a few days; a rash also may develop. Subsequently, hemorrhage from multiple sites, especially the gastrointestinal tract, and death occur in as many as 90% of patients with clinically evident disease. The 1995 outbreak in Kikwit, Congo, killed 245 people.

Laboratory Diagnosis

All specimens from patients with a suspected filovirus infection must be handled with extreme care to prevent accidental infection. Handling of these viruses requires **level 4 isolation** procedures that are not routinely available. Marburg virus may grow rapidly in tissue culture (Vero cells), but animal (e.g., guinea pig) inoculation may be necessary to recover Ebola virus.

Infected cells have large eosinophilic cytoplasmic inclusion bodies. Viral antigens can be detected in tissue by direct immunofluorescence analysis, and fluids by ELISA. Reverse transcriptase–polymerase chain reaction (RT-PCR) amplification of the viral genome in secretions can be used to confirm the diagnosis.

Immunoglobulin (Ig) G and IgM antibody to filovirus antigens can be detected by immunofluorescence, ELISA, or RIA.

Treatment, Prevention, and Control

Antibody-containing serum and interferon therapies have been tried in patients with filovirus infections.

Infected patients should be quarantined, and contaminated animals should be sacrificed. Handling of the viruses or contaminated materials requires very stringent (level 4) isolation procedures.

Arenaviruses

The arenaviruses include **lymphocytic choriomeningitis (LCM)** and **hemorrhagic fever viruses** such as the **Lassa, Junin,** and **Machupo** viruses. These viruses cause persistent infections in specific rodents and can be transmitted to humans as **zoonoses**.

Structure and Replication

Arenaviruses are seen in electron micrographs as **pleomorphic, enveloped viruses** (diameter, 120 nm) that have a **sandy appearance** (the name comes from the Greek word *arenosa*, meaning "sandy") because of the **ribosomes in the virion** (Box 64–4). Although functional, the ribosomes do not seem to serve a purpose. Virions contain a beaded nucleocapsid with **two single-stranded RNA circles** (S, 2400 nucleotides; L, 3400 to 4800 nucleotides) and a transcriptase. The L strand is a negative-sense RNA and encodes the polymerase. The S strand encodes the nucleoprotein (N protein) and the glycoproteins but is **ambisense**. Whereas the mRNA for the N protein is transcribed directly from the ambisense S strand, the mRNA for the glycoprotein is transcribed from a full-length template of the genome. As a result, the glycoproteins are produced as late proteins after genome replication. Arenaviruses replicate in the cytoplasm and acquire their envelope by budding from the host cell plasma membrane.

Arenaviruses readily cause persistent infections. This may result from inefficient transcription of the glycoprotein genes and thus poor virion assembly.

Pathogenesis

Arenaviruses are able to infect macrophages and possibly cause the release of mediators of cell and vascular

---

BOX 64–4. **Characteristics of Arenaviruses**

Virus has **enveloped** virion with two **circular, negative RNA** genome segments (L, S). Virion appears **sandy because of ribosomes.**

S genome segment is ambisense.

Arenavirus infections are zoonoses, establishing persistent infections in rodents.

Pathogenesis of arenavirus infections is largely attributed to T-cell immunopathogenesis.

damage. Tissue destruction is significantly exacerbated by T-cell–induced immunopathologic effects. Persistent infection of rodents results from neonatal infection and the induction of immune tolerance. The incubation period for arenavirus infections averages 10 to 14 days.

Epidemiology

Most arenaviruses, except for the virus that causes LCM, are found in the tropics of Africa and South America. The arenaviruses infect specific rodents and are endemic to the rodents' habitats. Chronic asymptomatic infection is common in these animals and leads to a chronic viremia and long-term viral shedding in saliva, urine, and feces. Humans may become infected through the inhalation of aerosols, the consumption of contaminated food, or contact with fomites. Bites are not a usual mechanism of spread.

The virus that causes LCM infects hamsters and house mice (*Mus musculus*). In Washington, D.C., it was found in 20% of mice. LCM disease in the United States is associated with contact with pet hamsters and with the animals in rodent-breeding facilities. Lassa fever virus infects *Mastomys natalensis*, an African rodent. The Lassa fever virus is spread from human to human through contact with infected secretions or body fluids, but the viruses that cause LCM or other hemorrhagic fevers are rarely if ever spread in this way.

In California during 1999 and 2000, three cases of fatal hemorrhagic disease were found to be caused by the Whitewater Arroyo arenavirus. This virus is normally found in the white-throated wood rat, so its occurrence in humans constitutes a newly emergent disease. The disease association was made by a special RT-PCR assay.

Clinical Syndromes

Lymphocytic Choriomeningitis

The name of the virus that causes LCM suggests that meningitis is a typical clinical event, but actually, LCM causes a febrile illness with flu-like myalgia more often than meningeal illness. It is estimated that approximately 25% of infected persons exhibit clinical evidence of a central nervous system infection. The meningeal illness, if it occurs, may be subacute and persist for several months. Perivascular mononuclear infiltrates may be seen in neurons of all sections of the brain and in the meninges of an affected patient.

Lassa and Other Hemorrhagic Fevers

Lassa fever, which is endemic to West Africa, is the best known of the hemorrhagic fevers caused by an arenavirus. Other agents, however, such as the Junin and Machupo viruses, cause similar syndromes in the inhabitants of different geographic areas (Argentina and Bolivia, respectively).

Clinical illness is characterized by fever, coagulopathy, petechiae, and occasional visceral hemorrhage as well as liver and spleen necrosis, but not vasculitis. Hemorrhage and shock also occur, as does occasional cardiac and liver damage. In contrast to LCM, hemorrhagic fevers cause no lesions in the central nervous system. Pharyngitis, diarrhea, and vomiting may be prevalent, especially in patients with Lassa fever. Death occurs in as many as 50% of those with Lassa fever and in a smaller percentage of those infected with the other arenaviruses that cause hemorrhagic fevers. The diagnosis is suggested by recent travel to endemic areas.

Laboratory Diagnosis

An arenavirus infection is usually diagnosed on the basis of serologic findings. These viruses are too dangerous for routine isolation. Throat specimens can yield arenaviruses; urine is a source for the Lassa fever virus but not for the LCM virus. The risk of infection is substantial for laboratory workers handling body fluids. Therefore, if the diagnosis is suspected, laboratory personnel should be so warned, and specimens processed only in facilities that specialize in the isolation of contagious pathogens (**level 3 for LCM and level 4 for Lassa fever and other arenaviruses**).

Treatment, Prevention, and Control

The antiviral drug **ribavirin** has limited activity against arenaviruses and can be used to treat Lassa fever. However, supportive therapy is usually all that is available for patients with arenavirus infections.

These rodent-borne infections can be prevented by limiting contact with the vector. For example, improved hygiene to limit contact with mice reduced the incidence of LCM in Washington, D.C. In the geographic areas where hemorrhagic fever occurs, trapping rodents and carefully storing food may decrease exposure to the virus.

The incidence of laboratory-acquired cases can be reduced if samples submitted for arenavirus isolation are processed in at least level 3 or 4 biosafety facilities and not in the usual clinical virology laboratory.

CASE STUDIES AND QUESTIONS

■ A 58-year-old woman complained of flu-like symptoms, severe headache, stiff neck, and photophobia.

She was lethargic and had a mild fever. The cerebrospinal fluid specimen contained 900 white blood cells per mL, mostly lymphocytes, and LCM virus. She recovered after a week. Her home was infested with gray mice (*Mus musculus*).

1. What were the significant symptoms of this disease?

2. How was the virus transmitted?

3. What type of immune response is most important in controlling this infection?

■ Several adults complained of serious diarrhea, nausea, vomiting, and a mild fever 2 days after visiting Le Café Grease. The symptoms were too severe to result from food poisoning or a routine gastroenteritis but lasted only 24 hours.

1. What characteristics distinguished this disease from a rotavirus infection?

2. What was the most likely means of viral transmission?

3. What physical characteristics of the virus allowed it to be transmitted by these means?

4. What public health measures could be followed to prevent such outbreaks?

BIBLIOGRAPHY

Balows A, Hausler WJ Jr, Lennette EH: *Laboratory diagnosis of infectious diseases: principles and practice*, New York, 1988, Springer-Verlag.

Belshe RB, editor: *Textbook of human virology*, ed 2, St Louis, 1991, Mosby.

Bishop RF: Other small virus-like particles in humans. In Tyrrell DAJ, Kapikian AZ, editors: *Virus infections of the gastrointestinal tract*, New York, 1982, Marcel Dekker.

Blacklow NR, Greenberg HB: Viral gastroenteritis, *N Engl J Med* 325:252–264, 1991.

Christensen ML: Human viral gastroenteritis, *Clin Microbiol Rev* 2:51–89, 1989.

Fields BN, Knipe DM, Howley PM, editors: *Virology*, ed 3, New York, 1996, Lippincott-Raven.

Klenk HD: Marburg and ebola viruses, *Current topics in microbiology and immunology*, vol 235, Berlin, New York, 1999, Springer-Verlag.

Oldstone MBA: Arenaviruses, *Curr Top Microbiol Immunol* 133:1–116, 134:1–242, 1987.

Preston R: *The hot zone*, New York, 1994, Random House.

Sodhi A: Ebola virus disease, *Postgrad Med* 99:75–76, 1996.

ter Meulen V, Siddell S, Wege H, editors: *Biochemistry and biology of coronaviruses*, New York, 1981, Plenum.

Xi JN et al: Norwalk virus genome cloning and characterization, *Science* 250:1580–1583, 1990.

C H A P T E R   6 5

Role of Viruses in Disease

Most viral infections cause mild or no symptoms and do not require extensive treatment. The common cold, influenza, flu-like syndromes, and gastroenteritis are common viral diseases. Other viral infections, which target essential tissues and organs, are very cytolytic, or induce immunopathologic effects, can cause serious and even life-threatening disease. In general, the symptoms and severity of a viral infection are determined by the following factors:

1. The patient's ability to prevent or rapidly resolve the infection before the virus can reach important organs or cause significant damage.
2. The target tissue and virulence of the virus.
3. The ability of the body to repair the damage.

Previous chapters stressed the viral characteristics that promote disease. In this chapter, viral diseases are discussed with respect to their symptoms, the organ system they target, and the host factors that influence their presentation.

Viral Diseases

The major sites of viral disease are the respiratory tract; the gastrointestinal tract; the epithelial, mucosal, and endothelial linings of the skin, mouth, and genitalia; the lymphoid tissue; the liver and other organs; and the central nervous system (CNS) (Fig. 65–1). The examples given in this chapter represent more common causes of disease.

Oral and Respiratory Tract Infections

The oropharynx and respiratory tract are the **most common sites** of viral infection and disease (Table 65–1). The viruses are spread in respiratory droplets and aerosols, food and water, and saliva; by close contact; and on hands. Similar respiratory symptoms may be caused by several different viruses. For example, bronchiolitis may be caused by respiratory syncytial or parainfluenza virus. Alternatively, one virus may cause different symptoms in different people. For example, influenza virus may cause a mild upper respiratory tract infection in one person and life-threatening pneumonia in another.

Many viral infections start in the oropharynx or respiratory tract, infect the lung, and spread without causing significant symptoms. *Varicella-zoster* virus (VZV) and the *measles* virus initiate infection in the lung and can cause pneumonia but generally cause systemic infections resulting in an exanthem (rash). Other viruses that establish primary infection of the oropharynx or respiratory tract and then progress to other sites are *rubella, mumps, enteroviruses,* and several human herpesviruses—*herpes simplex virus* (HSV), *VZV, Epstein-Barr* virus (EBV), *cytomegalovirus* (CMV), and *human herpesvirus 6* (HHV6).

The symptoms and severity of a respiratory viral disease depend on the nature of the virus, the site of infection (upper or lower respiratory tract), and the immune status and the age of the person. Conditions such as cystic fibrosis and smoking, which compromise the ciliated and mucoepithelial barriers to infection, increase the risk of serious disease.

Pharyngitis and oral disease are common viral presentations. Most enteroviruses infect the oropharynx and then progress by way of a viremia to other target tissues. For example, symptoms such as acute-onset pharyngitis, fever, and oral vesicular lesions are characteristic of *coxsackie A virus* infections (herpangina, hand-foot-and-mouth disease) and some *coxsackie B virus* and *echovirus* infections. *Adenovirus* and the early stages of *EBV* disease are characterized by sore throat and tonsillitis with an exudative membrane and then *EBV* infects B lymphocytes to cause infectious mononucleosis. *HSV* causes local primary infections of the oral mucosa and face (gingivostomatitis) and then establishes a latent neuronal infection that can recur in the form of herpes labialis (cold sores, fever blisters). HSV is also a common cause of pharyngitis. Vesicular lesions on the buccal mucosa (Koplik's spots) are an early diagnostic feature of *measles* infection.

Although upper respiratory tract viral infections, including the common cold and pharyngitis, are generally benign, they still account for at least 50% of ab-

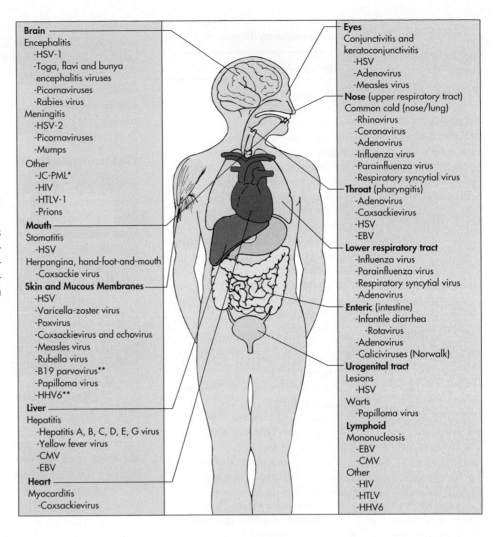

FIGURE 65–1. Major target tissues of viral disease. (*) indicates progressive multifocal leukoencephalopathy. Infection by viruses indicated by (**) results in an immune-mediated rash.

Brain
Encephalitis
  -HSV-1
  -Toga, flavi and bunya encephalitis viruses
  -Picornaviruses
  -Rabies virus
Meningitis
  -HSV-2
  -Picornaviruses
  -Mumps
Other
  -JC-PML*
  -HIV
  -HTLV-1
  -Prions

Mouth
Stomatitis
  -HSV
Herpangina, hand-foot-and-mouth
  -Coxsackie virus

Skin and Mucous Membranes
  -HSV
  -Varicella-zoster virus
  -Poxvirus
  -Coxsackievirus and echovirus
  -Measles virus
  -Rubella virus
  -B19 parvovirus**
  -Papilloma virus
  -HHV6**

Liver
Hepatitis
  -Hepatitis A, B, C, D, E, G virus
  -Yellow fever virus
  -CMV
  -EBV

Heart
Myocarditis
  -Coxsackievirus

Eyes
Conjunctivitis and keratoconjunctivitis
  -HSV
  -Adenovirus
  -Measles virus
Nose (upper respiratory tract)
Common cold (nose/lung)
  -Rhinovirus
  -Coronavirus
  -Adenovirus
  -Influenza virus
  -Parainfluenza virus
  -Respiratory syncytial virus
Throat (pharyngitis)
  -Adenovirus
  -Coxsackievirus
  -HSV
  -EBV
Lower respiratory tract
  -Influenza virus
  -Parainfluenza virus
  -Respiratory syncytial virus
  -Adenovirus
Enteric (intestine)
  -Infantile diarrhea
    -Rotavirus
  -Adenovirus
  -Caliciviruses (Norwalk)
Urogenital tract
Lesions
  -HSV
Warts
  -Papilloma virus
Lymphoid
Mononucleosis
  -EBV
  -CMV
Other
  -HIV
  -HTLV
  -HHV6

senteeism from schools and the workplace. *Rhinoviruses* and *coronaviruses* are the predominant causes of upper respiratory tract infections. A runny nose (rhinitis) followed by congestion, cough, sneezing, conjunctivitis, headache, and sore throat are typical symptoms of the common cold. Other causes of the common cold and pharyngitis are specific serotypes of *echoviruses* and *coxsackieviruses, adenoviruses, influenza viruses, parainfluenza viruses,* and *respiratory syncytial virus.*

Tonsillitis, laryngitis, and croup (laryngotracheobronchitis) may accompany certain respiratory tract viral infections. HSV and coxsackie A viruses may also involve the tonsils, but with vesicular lesions. Laryngitis (adults) and croup (children) are caused by inflammatory responses to the viral infection that cause the trachea to narrow below the vocal cords (subglottic area). This narrowing causes loss of voice; a hoarse, barking cough; and the risk, especially in young children, for a blocked airway and choking. Children infected with *parainfluenza* viruses are especially at risk for croup.

Lower respiratory tract viral infections can also result in more serious disease. Symptoms of such infections include bronchiolitis (inflammation of the bronchioles), pneumonia, and related diseases. The *parainfluenza* and *respiratory syncytial viruses* are major problems for infants and children but cause only asymptomatic infections or common cold symptoms in adults. Parainfluenza 3 virus and especially respiratory syncytial virus infections are major causes of life-threatening pneumonia or bronchiolitis in infants younger than 6 months. Infection with these viruses does not provide lifelong immunity.

Influenza virus is probably the best known and most feared of the common respiratory viruses, with the annual introduction of new strains of virus ensuring the presence of immunologically naive victims. Children are universally susceptible to new strains of virus, whereas older people may have been immunized during a prior outbreak of the annual strain. Despite such immunization, the elderly are especially susceptible to new strains of virus, because they may not be able either to mount a sufficient primary immune response to the new strain of influenza virus or to repair the

TABLE 65–1. Oral and Respiratory Diseases

Disease	Etiologic Agent
Common cold (including pharyngitis)	Rhinovirus*
	Coronavirus*
	Influenza viruses
	Parainfluenza viruses
	Respiratory syncytial virus
	Adenovirus
	Enteroviruses
Pharyngitis	Herpes simplex virus
	Epstein-Barr virus
	Adenovirus*
	Coxsackie A virus* (herpangina, hand-foot-and-mouth disease) and other enteroviruses
Croup, tonsillitis, laryngitis, and bronchitis (children younger than 2 years)	Parainfluenza virus 1*
	Parainfluenza virus 2
	Influenza virus
	Adenovirus
	Epstein-Barr virus
Bronchiolitis	Respiratory syncytial virus* (infants)
	Parainfluenza virus 3* (infants and children)
	Parainfluenza viruses 1 and 2
Pneumonia	Respiratory syncytial virus* (infants)
	Parainfluenza virus* (infants)
	Influenza virus*
	Adenovirus
	Varicella-zoster virus (primary infection of adults or immunocompromised hosts)
	Cytomegalovirus (infection of immunocompromised host)
	Measles

*Most common causal agents.

tissue damage caused by the disease. Other possible viral agents of pneumonia are *adenovirus*, *paramyxoviruses*, and *primary VZV* infections of adults.

Flu-Like and Systemic Symptoms

Many viral infections cause classic **flu-like symptoms (fever, malaise, anorexia, headache, and body aches)**, side effects due to host responses to the infection. During the viremic phase, many viruses induce the release of interferon and cytokines. In addition to the respiratory viruses, flu-like symptoms may accompany infections by arboencephalitis viruses, HSV type 2 (HSV-2), and other viruses.

Arthritis and other inflammatory diseases may result from immune hypersensitivity responses induced by the infection or immune complexes containing viral antigen. For example, *B19 parvovirus* infection of adults, *rubella*, and infection with *several other togaviruses* elicit arthritis. Immune complex disease that is associated with *chronic hepatitis B virus* (HBV) can result in various presentations, including arthritis and nephritis.

Gastrointestinal Tract Infections

Infections of the gastrointestinal tract can result in gastroenteritis, vomiting, diarrhea, or no symptoms (Box 65–1). *Norwalk virus, caliciviruses, astroviruses, adenoviruses, reoviruses,* and *rotaviruses* infect the small intestine but not the colon, damaging the epithelial lining and the absorptive villi. This damage leads to the malabsorption of water and an electrolyte imbalance. The resultant diarrhea in older children and adults is generally self-limited and can be treated with rehydration and restoration of the electrolyte balance. These viruses, especially rotavirus, are major problems for adults and children in regions where there is drought and starvation.

Viral gastroenteritis has a more significant effect on infants and may necessitate hospitalization. The extent of tissue damage and consequent loss of fluids and electrolytes is a more significant problem for infants. *Rotavirus* and *adenovirus serotypes 40* and *41* are the major causes of infantile gastroenteritis.

Fecal-oral spread of the enteric viruses is promoted by poor hygiene and is especially prevalent in daycare centers. *Norwalk virus* and *calicivirus* outbreaks affecting older children and adults are generally linked to a common contaminated food or water source. Vomiting usually accompanies diarrhea in patients infected with the Norwalk virus and rotavirus. Although enteroviruses (picornaviruses) are spread by the fecal-oral route, they usually cause only mild or no gastrointestinal symptoms. Instead, these viruses establish a vire-

BOX 65–1. Gastrointestinal Viruses

Infants

Rotavirus A*
Adenovirus 40, 41
Coxsackie A24 virus

Infants, Children, and Adults

Norwalk virus
Calicivirus
Astrovirus
Rotavirus B (outbreaks in China)
Reovirus

*Most common cause.

TABLE 65–2. Viral Exanthems	
Condition	Etiologic Agent
Rash	
Rubeola	Measles virus
German measles	Rubella virus
Roseola infantum	Human herpesvirus 6
Erythema infectiosum	Human parvovirus B19
Boston exanthem	Echovirus 16
Infectious mononu-cleosis	Epstein-Barr virus, cy-tomegalovirus
Vesicles	
Oral or genital herpes	Herpes simplex virus*
Chickenpox/shingles	Varicella-zoster virus*
Hand-foot-and-mouth disease, herpangina	Coxsackie A virus*
Papillomas	
Warts	Papillomavirus*
Molluscum	Molluscum conta-giosum

*Most common cause.

endothelial cell lining of the vasculature, possibly compromising the structure of the blood vessel. Viral or immune cytolysis may then lead to greater permeability or rupture of the vessel, producing a hemorrhagic rash with petechiae (pinpoint hemorrhages under the skin) and ecchymoses (massive bruises) and hence internal bleeding, the loss of electrolytes, and shock.

Infections of the Eye

Infections of the eye result from direct contact with a virus or from viremic spread (Box 65–2). Conjunctivitis (pinkeye) is a normal feature of many childhood infections and is a characteristic of infections caused by specific *adenovirus serotypes (3, 4a, and 7)*, the *measles virus*, and the *rubella virus*. Keratoconjunctivitis caused by *adenovirus (8, 19a, and 37)*, *HSV*, or *VZV* involves the cornea and can cause severe damage. *Enterovirus 70* and *coxsackie A24 viruses* can cause an acute hemorrhagic conjunctivitis. Cataracts are classic features of babies born with *congenital rubella syndrome*. Chorioretinitis is associated with *CMV infection* in newborns

mia, spread to other target organs, and then cause clinical disease.

Exanthems and Hemorrhagic Fevers

Virus-induced skin disease (Table 65–2) can result from infection through the mucosa or small cuts or abrasions in the skin (*HSV*), as a secondary infection after establishment of a *viremia (VZV and smallpox)*, or as a result of the inflammatory response mounted against viral antigens (*parvovirus B19*). The major classifications of viral rashes are maculopapular, vesicular, nodular, and hemorrhagic. **Macules** are flat, colored spots. **Papules** are slightly raised areas of the skin and may result from immune or inflammatory responses rather than the direct effects of the virus. **Nodules** are larger, raised areas of the skin. **Vesicular lesions** are blisters and are likely to contain virus. *Papillomaviruses* cause warts, and *molluscum contagiosum* causes wartlike growths (nodules) by stimulating the growth of skin cells.

The classic childhood exanthems are roseola infantum (*exanthem subitum [HHV6]*), fifth disease (erythema infectiosum *[parvovirus B19]*), and, in unvaccinated children, *varicella*, *measles*, and *rubella*. The rash follows a viremia and is accompanied by fever. Rashes are also caused by *enterovirus infections*, *dengue*, and other infections caused by flaviviruses or alphaviruses. They also are occasionally seen in patients with infectious mononucleosis.

The *yellow fever virus*, *dengue virus*, and other *hemorrhagic fever viruses* establish a viremia and infect the

BOX 65–2. Infections of the Organs and Tissues
Liver
Hepatitis A,* B,* C,* G, D, and E viruses
Yellow fever virus
Epstein-Barr virus
Hepatitis in the neonate or immunocompromised person:
Cytomegalovirus
Herpes simplex virus
Varicella-zoster virus
Rubella virus (congenital rubella syndrome)
Heart
Coxsackie B virus
Kidney
Cytomegalovirus
Muscle
Coxsackie B virus (pleurodynia)
Glands
Cytomegalovirus
Mumps virus
Eye
Herpes simplex virus
Adenovirus*
Measles virus
Rubella virus
Enterovirus 70
Coxsackie A24 virus

*Most common cause.

(congenital) as well as in immunosuppressed people (e.g., those with acquired immunodeficiency syndrome [AIDS]).

Infections of the Organs and Tissues

Infection of the major organs may cause significant disease or may result in further spread or secretion of the virus (see Box 65–2). The symptoms may arise from tissue damage or inflammatory responses.

The liver is a prominent target for many viruses that reach the liver by means of a viremia or the mononuclear phagocyte (reticuloendothelial) system. The liver acts as a source for a secondary viremia but can also be damaged by the infection. The classic symptoms of hepatitis result from infections with *hepatitis A, B, C, G, D, and E viruses* and *yellow fever virus* and are often associated with *EBV infectious mononucleosis* and *CMV infections*. The liver is also a major target in *disseminated HSV infection* of neonates and infants.

The heart and other muscles are also susceptible to viral infection and damage. *Coxsackievirus* can cause myocarditis or pericarditis in newborns, children, and adults. *Coxsackie B* virus can infect muscle and cause pleurodynia (Bornholm's disease). Other viruses (e.g., *influenza virus, CMV*) may also infect the heart.

Infection of the secretory glands, accessory sexual organs, and mammary glands results in contagious spread of the virus (*CMV*). An inflammatory response to the infection, as occurs in *mumps* (parotitis, orchitis), may be the cause of the symptoms. CMV infection of the kidney and reactivation are problems for immunosuppressed people and a predominant reason for kidney transplant failure.

Infections of the Central Nervous System

Viral infections of the brain and CNS may cause the most serious viral diseases because of the importance of the CNS and its very limited capacity to repair damage (Box 65–3). Tissue damage is usually caused by a combination of viral pathogenesis and immunopathogenesis. Most neurotropic viral infections do not result in disease, however, because the virus does not reach the brain or does not cause sufficient tissue damage to produce symptoms.

Virus may spread to the CNS in blood (*arboviruses*) or in macrophages (*human immunodeficiency virus [HIV]*); it may spread from a peripheral infection of the neurons (olfactory), or it may first infect skin (*HSV*) or muscle (*rabies*) and then progress to the innervating neurons. The virus may have a predilection for certain sites in the brain. For example, the temporal lobe is targeted in *HSV encephalitis*, Ammon's horn in *rabies*, and the anterior horn of the spinal cord and motor neurons in *paralytic poliomyelitis*.

BOX 65–3. **Central Nervous System Infections**

Meningitis

Enteroviruses
   Echoviruses
   Coxsackievirus*
   Poliovirus
Herpes simplex virus 2
Adenovirus
Mumps virus
Lymphocytic choriomeningitis virus
Epstein-Barr virus
Arboencephalitis viruses

Paralysis

Poliovirus
Enteroviruses 70 and 71
Coxsackie A7 virus

Encephalitis

Herpes simplex virus 1*
Varicella-zoster virus
Arboencephalitis viruses*
Rabies virus
Coxsackie A and B viruses
Polioviruses

Postinfectious Encephalitis (Immune-Mediated)

Measles virus
Mumps virus
Rubella virus
Varicella-zoster virus
Influenza viruses

Other

JC virus (progressive multifocal leukoencephalopathy [in immunosuppressed people])
Measles variant (subacute sclerosing panencephalitis)
Prion (encephalopathy)
Human immunodeficiency virus (AIDS [acquired immunodeficiency syndrome] dementia)
Human T-cell lymphotrophic virus 1 (tropical spastic paraparesis)

*Most common cause.

Viral infections of the CNS are usually distinguished from bacterial infections by the finding of mononuclear cells, low numbers of polymorphonuclear leukocytes, and normal or slightly reduced levels of glucose in the cerebrospinal fluid. Immunoassay detection of specific antigen, polymerase chain reaction (PCR) detection of viral genomes or messenger RNA (mRNA), or isolation of the virus from a cerebrospinal fluid or biopsy specimen confirms the diagnosis and identifies the viral agent. The season of the year also facilitates the diagnosis, in that *enteroviral* and *arboviral* diseases generally occur during the summer, whereas *HSV* encephalitis and other viral syndromes may be observed year-round.

Aseptic meningitis is caused by an inflammation and swelling of the meninges enveloping the brain and spinal cord in response to infection with *enteroviruses* (especially *echoviruses* and *coxsackieviruses*), *HSV-2*, the *mumps virus*, or the *lymphocytic choriomeningitis virus*. The disease is usually self-limited and, unlike bacterial meningitis, resolves without sequelae unless the virus gains access to and infects neurons or the brain (**me-**

ningoencephalitis). The viruses gain access to the meninges by means of a viremia.

Encephalitis and **myelitis** result from a combination of viral pathogenesis and immunopathogenesis in brain tissue and neurons and either are fatal or cause significant damage and permanent neurologic sequelae. *HSV, VZV, rabies virus, California encephalitis viruses, West Nile* and *St. Louis encephalitis viruses*, and *measles virus* are potential causes of encephalitis. *Poliovirus* and several *other enteroviruses* cause paralytic disease (myelitis).

HSV and VZV are ubiquitous and usually cause asymptomatic latent infections of the CNS but can also cause encephalitis. Most arboencephalitis virus infections result in flu-like symptoms rather than encephalitis. Postmeasles encephalitis and subacute sclerosing panencephalitis were rare sequelae of measles in the prevaccine era.

Other virus-induced neurologic syndromes are *HIV* dementia, *human T-lymphotropic virus type 1 (HTLV-1)* tropical spastic paraparesis, *JC papovavirus*–induced, progressive multifocal leukoencephalopathy (PML) in immunosuppressed people, and the *prion*-associated spongiform encephalopathies (kuru, Creutzfeldt-Jakob disease, Gerstmann-Sträussler-Scheinker disease). PML and the spongiform encephalopathies have long incubation periods (slow viruses).

Hematologic Diseases

Lymphocytes and macrophages are not very permissive for viral replication but are targets for several viruses that establish persistent infections. Transient viral replication of *EBV, HIV,* or *CMV* elicits a large T-cell response, resulting in **mononucleosis-like syndromes**. In addition, *CMV, measles virus,* and *HIV* infections of T cells are immunosuppressive. HIV reduces the numbers of CD4 helper and delayed-type hypersensitivity T cells, further compromising the immune system. *HTLV-1* infection causes little disease on infection but may lead to **adult T-cell leukemia** or tropical spastic paraparesis much later in life.

Macrophages and cells of the macrophage lineage can be infected by many viruses. Macrophages act as vehicles for spreading the virus throughout the body, because viruses replicate inefficiently in them and the cells are generally not lysed by the infection. This process promotes persistent and chronic infections. The macrophage is the primary target cell for the *dengue virus*. Non-neutralizing antibody can promote uptake of dengue virus and *HIV* into the cell through Fc receptors. Macrophages and cells of the macrophage lineage infected with *HIV* provide a reservoir for the virus and access to the brain. AIDS dementia is thought to result from the actions of HIV-infected microglial cells in the brain.

Sexually Transmitted Viral Diseases

Sexual transmission is a major route for the spread of *papillomavirus, HSV, CMV, HIV, HTLV-1, HBV, hepatitis C virus (HCV),* and *hepatitis D virus (HDV)* (Box 65–4). Such viruses establish chronic and latent-recurrent infections, with asymptomatic shedding into the semen and vaginal secretions. These viral properties foster dissemination via a route of transmission that is used relatively infrequently and might be avoided during symptomatic disease. The viruses can also be transmitted neonatally or perinatally to infants. *Papillomaviruses* and *HSV* establish local primary infections with recurrent disease at the same site. Lesions and asymptomatic shedding are sources for sexual transmission and for perinatal transmission to the newborn. *CMV* and *HIV* enter the blood stream and infect lymphoid cells, whereas *the hepatitis viruses* are delivered to the liver. CMV, HIV, and the hepatitis viruses are present in blood, semen, and vaginal secretions, in which the virus can be transmitted to sexual partners and neonates.

Viruses Spread by Transfusion and Transplantation

HBV, HCV, HDV, HIV, HTLV-1, and *CMV* are transmitted by blood and organ transplants. These viruses are also present in semen and therefore are sexually transmitted. The chronic nature of the infection, the persistent asymptomatic release of the virus, or the infection of macrophages and lymphocytes promotes transmission by these routes. Screening of the blood supply for *HBV, HCV* and *HIV* has controlled transmission of these viruses in blood transfusions. Large-scale procedures for screening the other viruses have not been developed, so the risk remains for the spread of HTLV and CMV by these routes.

Syndromes of Possible Viral Etiology

Several diseases either produce symptoms or have epidemiologic or other characteristics that resemble those

---

BOX 65–4. **Sexually Transmitted Viruses**

Human papillomavirus 6, 11, 42
Human papillomavirus 16 and 18 (associated with human cervical carcinoma)
Herpes simplex virus (predominantly HSV-2)
Cytomegalovirus
Hepatitis B, C, and D viruses
Human immunodeficiency virus
Human T-cell lymphotrophic virus 1

of viral infections or may be the sequelae of viral infections (e.g., inflammatory responses to a persistent viral infection). They include **multiple sclerosis, Kawasaki disease, arthritis, diabetes,** and **chronic fatigue syndrome**.

Chronic and Potentially Oncogenic Infections

Chronic infections occur when the immune system has difficulty resolving the infection. *The DNA viruses* (except parvovirus and poxvirus) and the *retroviruses* cause latent infections with the potential for recurrence. *CMV* and other herpesviruses; *hepatitis B, C,* and *D viruses*; and *retroviruses* cause chronic productive infections.

HBV, HCV, EBV, HHV8, papillomavirus, and *HTLV-1* are associated with **human cancers**. *EBV, papillomavirus,* and *HTLV-1* can immortalize cells; after immortalization, cofactors, chromosomal aberrations, or both enable a clone of virus-containing cells to grow out into a cancer. EBV normally causes infectious mononucleosis but is also associated with African Burkitt's lymphoma, Hodgkin's lymphoma, and nasopharyngeal carcinoma; *HTLV-1* is associated with human adult T-cell leukemia. Many *papillomaviruses* induce a simple hyperplasia characterized by the development of a wart; however, several other strains of papillomaviruses have been associated with human cancers (e.g., *type 16 and 18 associated with cervical carcinoma*). Direct viral action or the chronic cell damage and repair in livers infected by *HBV* or *HCV* may result in a tumorigenic event leading to hepatocellular carcinoma. *HSV-2* has been associated with human cervical carcinoma, most likely as a cofactor. Immunosuppression in patients who have AIDS, patients undergoing cancer chemotherapy, or transplant recipients also promotes lymphomagenesis by *EBV. HHV8* infection produces many cytokines to stimulate cell growth, and in AIDS patients, this growth can progress to *Kaposi's sarcoma*.

Development of a worldwide vaccine program for HBV not only would reduce the spread of viral hepatitis but also would prevent the occurrence of primary hepatocellular carcinoma. The development of a vaccine for EBV and papillomavirus should also reduce the incidence of their associated cancers.

Infections in Immunocompromised Patients

Patients with **deficient cell-mediated immunity** are generally more susceptible to infection with enveloped viruses (especially the *herpesviruses, measles virus,* and even the *vaccinia virus* used for smallpox vaccinations) and to recurrences of infections with latent viruses (*herpesviruses* and *papovaviruses*). Severe T-cell deficiencies also affect the antiviral antibody response. Cell-mediated immunodeficiencies can be congenital or acquired. They may result from genetic defects (e.g., Duncan's disease, DiGeorge's syndrome, Wiskott-Aldrich syndrome), leukemia or lymphoma, infections (e.g., AIDS), or immunosuppressive therapy.

Viruses cause atypical and more severe presentations in immunosuppressed people. For example, infections with herpesviruses (*HSV, CMV, VZV*), which are normally benign and localized, can progress locally or can disseminate and cause visceral and neurologic infections that may be life-threatening. A *measles* infection can cause a giant cell (syncytial) pneumonia rather than the characteristic rash.

People with immunoglobulin A deficiency or hypogammaglobulinemia (antibody deficiency) have more problems with *respiratory and gastrointestinal viruses*. Hypogammaglobulinemic people are more likely to suffer significant disease after infection by viruses that progress by viremia, including the *live polio vaccine, echovirus,* and *VZV*.

Congenital, Neonatal, and Perinatal Infections

The development and growth of the fetus are so ordered and rapid that a viral infection may damage or prevent the appropriate formation of important tissues, leading to miscarriage or congenital abnormalities. Infection may occur in utero (prenatal) (*rubella, parvovirus B19, CMV, HIV*), during transit through the birth canal (neonatal) (*HSV-2, HBV, CMV*), or soon after birth (postnatal) (*HIV, CMV, HBV, HSV, coxsackie B virus, echovirus*).

Neonates depend on the mother's immunity to protect them from viral infections. They receive maternal antibodies through the placenta and then in the mother's milk. This type of passive immunity can remain effective for 6 months to a year after birth. Maternal antibodies can (1) protect against spread of virus to the fetus during a viremia (e.g., *rubella, B19*), (2) protect against many enteric and respiratory tract viral infections, and (3) reduce the severity of other viral diseases after birth. Nevertheless, because the cell-mediated immune system is not mature at birth, newborns are susceptible to viruses that spread by cell-to-cell contact (e.g., *HSV, VZV, CMV, HIV*).

Rubella virus and *CMV* are examples of **teratogenic viruses** that can cause congenital infection and severe congenital abnormalities. *HIV* infection that is acquired in utero or from mother's milk initiates a chronic infection leading to lymphadenopathy, failure to thrive, or encephalopathy within 2 years of birth. *HSV* can be acquired during passage through an infected birth canal and result in life-threatening disseminated disease.

Nosocomial infection of newborns can result in a similar outcome. If *parvovirus B19* is acquired in utero, it can cause spontaneous abortion.

Infection Control

Infection control is essential in hospital and health care settings. The spread of respiratory viruses is the most difficult to prevent. Viral spread can be controlled in the following ways:

1. Limiting personnel contact with sources of infection (i.e., wearing gloves, mask, goggles; using quarantine).
2. Improving hygiene, sanitation, and disinfection.
3. Ensuring that all personnel are immunized against common diseases.
4. Educating all personnel regarding points 1, 2, and 3 and in the ways to decrease high-risk behaviors.

Methods for disinfection differ for each virus and depend on its structure. Most viruses are inactivated by 70% ethanol, 10% chlorine bleach, 2% glutaraldehyde, 4% formaldehyde, or autoclaving (as described in "Guidelines for prevention of transmission of human immunodeficiency virus and hepatitis B virus to health-care and public-safety workers," issued in 1989 by the Centers for Disease Control and Prevention [CDC]). Most enveloped viruses do not require such rigorous treatment and are inactivated by soap and detergents. Other means of disinfection are also available.

Special "universal" precautions are required for the handling of human blood; that is, all blood should be assumed to be contaminated with HIV or HBV and should be handled with caution. In addition to these procedures, special care must be taken with syringe needles and surgical tools contaminated with blood to prevent needlesticks and cuts. Specific guidelines are available from the CDC.

Control of an outbreak usually requires identification of the source or reservoir of the virus, followed by cleanup, quarantine, immunization, or a combination of these measures. The first step in controlling an outbreak of gastroenteritis or hepatitis A is identification of the food, water, or possibly daycare center that is the source of the outbreak.

Education programs can promote compliance with immunization programs and help people change lifestyles associated with viral transmission. Such programs have had a significant impact in reducing the prevalence of vaccine-preventable diseases such as smallpox, polio, measles, mumps, and rubella. It is hoped that educational programs will also promote changes in lifestyles and habits that restrict the spread of the bloodborne and sexually transmitted HBV and HIV.

QUESTIONS

1. What disinfection procedures are sufficient for inactivating the following viruses: HAV, HBV, HSV, and rhinovirus?
2. What precautions should health care workers take to protect themselves from infection with the following viruses: HBV, influenza A virus, HSV (whitlow), and HIV?
3. What predisposing conditions would exacerbate an infection with influenza A virus, VZV, or rotavirus?
4. Describe and compare the nature and mechanism of exanthem development for measles, VZV, HSV (primary and recurrence), and yellow fever.
5. A kidney transplant recipient undergoing immunosuppressive therapy has a lymphoma that regresses in response to a reduction in immunosuppressive therapy. The lymphoma cells are found to contain EBV. How might EBV be involved in this lymphoma? Why does the lymphoma regress in response to the reduction in the immunosuppressive therapy? For what other viral infections would this person be at increased risk during the immunosuppressive therapy?

BIBLIOGRAPHY

Belshe RB, editor: *Textbook of human virology*, ed 2, St Louis, 1991, Mosby.

Ellner PD, Neu HC: *Understanding infectious disease*, St Louis, 1992, Mosby.

Emond RTD, Rowland HAK: *Color atlas of infectious diseases*, ed 2, St Louis, 1987, Mosby.

Gorbach SL, Bartlett JG, Blacklow NR: *Infectious diseases*, Philadelphia, 1992, WB Saunders.

Guidelines for prevention of transmission of human immunodeficiency virus and hepatitis B virus to health-care and public-safety workers, *MMWR Morb Mortal Wkly Rep* 38(suppl 6):1-37, 1989.

Hart CA, Broadhead RL: *Color atlas of pediatric infectious diseases*, St Louis, 1992, Mosby.

Haukenes G, Haaheim LR, Pattison JR: *A practical guide to clinical virology*, New York, 1989, John Wiley & Sons.

Katz SL, Gershon AA, Hotez PJ: *Krugman's infectious diseases of children*, ed 10, St Louis, 1998, Mosby.

Mandell GL, Bennett JE, Dolin R: *Principles and practice of infectious disease*, ed 3, New York, 1990, Churchill Livingstone.

Mims CA, White DO: *Viral pathogenesis and immunology*, Cambridge, Mass, 1984, Blackwell.

Shulman ST, Phair JP, Sommers HM: *The biologic and clinical basis of infectious diseases*, ed 4, Philadelphia, 1992, WB Saunders.

White DO, Fenner FJ: *Medical virology*, ed 4, Orlando, Fla, 1994, Academic.

All the virology on the Worldwide Web and specific viruses. Available at http://www.virology.net/

Mycology

CHAPTER 66

Mechanisms of Fungal Pathogenesis

Fungi are extremely common in nature, where they exist as free-living saprobes. They are major pathogens of plants and frequently damage foods and other commodities. They often reside on body surfaces as transient environmental colonizers but obtain no obvious benefit from this relationship. Because they are ubiquitous, they are occasionally cultured from clinical specimens. Determining their role in an infection, however, may be difficult. The effects of fungi on humans are numerous. Three major categories are of medical importance (Box 66–1).

Mycotoxicoses

Fungi are metabolically versatile organisms and sources of innumerable secondary metabolites such as alkaloids and other toxic compounds. The mycotoxicoses are most often the result of the accidental or recreational ingestion of fungi that produce these compounds. The source of the toxin is determined through the patient's clinical history. Unfortunately, because the patient is often comatose or delirious, a history cannot be obtained. When the fungi are ingested, emesis (vomiting) should be induced, and supportive measures consistent with the physiologic signs exhibited by the patient should be instituted. The clinical situation and laboratory diagnosis are complicated when fungal material has been injected intravenously.

Ergot Alkaloids

The pharmacologic properties of ergot alkaloids, which are produced when grain is infected with *Claviceps purpurea*, have been known throughout history. During the Middle Ages, epidemics known as St. Anthony's fire were associated with the consumption of bread and other bakery products made with contaminated rye and other grains. Symptoms consisted of **inflammation** of the infected tissues (cellular response to injury) followed by **necrosis** (cell death), and **gangrene** (death of large masses of tissue). Pharmacologically, the ergot alkaloids produce an α-adrenergic blockade, which in-

hibits certain responses to epinephrine and 5-hydroxytryptamine. These inhibited responses create marked peripheral vasoconstriction that, if not corrected, restricts the blood flow, resulting in necrosis and gangrene.

Another property of the ergot alkaloids is their ability to directly stimulate smooth muscle contraction. They have been used as **oxytocic agents,** promoting labor during childbirth by increasing the force and frequency of uterine contractions. The ergot alkaloids also affect the central nervous system by stimulating the hypothalamus and other sympathetic portions of the midbrain.

Psychotropic Agents

Toxic metabolites produced by fungi have been used by primitive tribes for religious, magical, and social purposes. In the 20th century, problems involving toxins of fungi were seen with the recreational use of psychotropic agents such as psilocybin and psilocin, as well as the semisynthetic derivative lysergic acid diethylamide (LSD).

Aflatoxins

Among the mycotoxicoses, contamination with *Aspergillus flavus* has had a profound economic impact on society. Toxic metabolites produced by these fungi resulted in the outbreak of Turkey X disease in the early 1960s in England, which nearly destroyed the turkey industry. Turkey poults consumed contaminated feed and developed lethargy, anorexia, and muscle weakness followed by spasms and death. Postmortem studies of the animals demonstrated gross hemorrhage and necrosis of the liver. Further histopathologic examination showed parenchymal cell degeneration and extensive proliferation of the bile duct epithelial cells. Through biochemical and pharmacologic studies, the etiologic agents of the disease were shown to be *A. flavus* toxins that belonged to a group of compounds known as the **bisfuranocoumarin metabolites**. These compounds, called aflatoxins, have become known as potent carcinogens, but they have not been shown to play a specific role in human carcinogenesis.

Other Mycotoxicoses

Several other mycotoxicoses that have caused human illness have also been described. Two of these are yellow rice toxicosis in Japan and alimentary toxic aleukia in the former Soviet Union.

Hypersensitivity Diseases

One index used to measure the level of air pollution is the fungal spore count, because fungal spores are ubiquitous in nature, supply a good indication of environmental contamination, and carry medical relevance. Airborne spores and other fungal elements constantly bombard people. They can be an antigenic stimulus and may induce, depending on an individual's immunologic status, hypersensitivity from the production of immunoglobulins or sensitized lymphocytes.

Clinical manifestations of **hypersensitivity pneumonitis** include rhinitis, bronchial asthma, alveolitis, and various forms of atrophy. Growth of the fungus in the tissues is not required for the development of hypersensitivity, however, and clinical manifestations of the disease are seen only in sensitized persons after subsequent exposure to the fungus, its metabolites, or other cross-reactive materials. Symptomatic patients can have their skin tested with various crude and purified fungal extracts **(allergens)** to identify the allergen or allergens responsible for the hypersensitivity.

Colonization and Diseases

Virtually all of the fungal organisms implicated in human disease processes are free-living. In general, people have a high level of innate immunity to fungi. Most fungal infections are mild and self-limited. Intact skin serves as a primary barrier to any infection caused by fungi that primarily colonize the superficial, cutaneous, and subcutaneous layers of skin. Mucosal surfaces discourage colonization by organisms that cause pulmonary infections. Fatty acid content, pH, epithelial turnover, and the normal bacterial flora of the skin appear to contribute to host resistance. Humoral factors such as transferrin restrict the growth of several fungi by limiting the amount of available iron, but the role they play in resistance has not been established.

A few fungi can cause disease in otherwise healthy people. Once established, the infection can be classified according to the tissue layers infected (Box 66–2).

Fungal diseases of another category have gained significance because of their association with the acquired immunodeficiency syndrome (AIDS) and the more common use of immunosuppressive therapy. These diseases can be the result of infection with low pathogenic potential and produce disease only under unusual circumstances, mostly involving host debilitation. Fungi once thought to be innocuous saprobes have gained prominence as etiologic agents of disease because of many medical advances. Some circumstances that lead to infection by these fungi are (1) changes in the normal intestinal flora resulting from the use of broad-spectrum antibacterial drugs, (2) debilitation of the host by the use of therapeutic measures (e.g., cytotoxins, x-ray irradiation, steroids, and other immunosuppressive drugs), and (3) alteration of the host's immune system by underlying endocrine disorders (e.g., uncontrolled diabetes mellitus, suppression such as that caused by AIDS).

Fungal infections that occur only because of compromising situations are categorized as **opportunistic mycoses.** If they are not rapidly diagnosed and aggressively managed and if the underlying disorders are not controlled, the infections become life-threatening. Organisms that can be etiologic agents of opportunistic mycoses include *Candida albicans,* a yeast that is part of the normal flora of the mouth, buccal mucosa, gastrointestinal tract, and vaginal vault; *Malassezia furfur,* a lipophilic yeast often isolated from areas rich in sebaceous glands; and other environmental fungi (e.g., *Aspergillus* species and *Mucor* species).

Characteristics of Fungal Pathogenesis

A great deal is known about the molecular and genetic basis of bacterial virulence and factors that contribute to plant pathogenesis. However, there is a paucity of information concerning the genes and the genetic factors that control and influence the virulence of human fungal pathogens. Generally, healthy, immunocompetent people have a high innate resistance to fungi, even though they are constantly exposed to the infectious propagules produced by these organisms. Infection and disease occur when there are disruptions in the protective barriers of the skin and mucous membranes or when defects in the immune system allow fungi to penetrate, colonize, and reproduce in the host.

Although most exposures are accidental, many fungi that cause disease have developed mechanisms that ease their survival and reproduction within this hostile environment. For example, **dermatophytes** (colonizers of the skin, hair, and nails) elaborate the enzyme keratinase, which hydrolyzes the structural protein keratin. Yeasts of the genus *Candida* become filamentous when they invade tissues, but the role of morphogenesis in virulence is unknown. Several agents that cause systemic mycoses are dimorphic; they are molds in nature but adapt to a unicellular morphology when they parasitize tissues. Those that cannot undergo the transition from mold to yeast, such as has been shown for *Histoplasma capsulatum*, are not virulent. *Cryptococcus neoformans* elaborates an acidic mucopolysaccharide capsule, a virulence factor.

The characteristics of human fungal pathogens allow them to be categorized into groups according to the primary tissues that they colonize. The agents causing superficial infections (**superficial mycoses**), for example, tend to grow only on the outermost layers of the skin or cuticle of the hair shaft, rarely inducing an immune reaction. The **cutaneous mycoses** (dermatophytes) are also limited to keratinized tissues of the epidermis, hair, and nails, but the fungi that cause cutaneous mycoses have greater invasive properties, and they may, depending on the species involved, evoke a highly inflammatory reaction from the host. The fungi that cause **subcutaneous mycoses** generally have a low degree of infectivity, and infections by these organisms are usually associated with some form of traumatic injury. All the **systemic mycoses** involve the respiratory tract, and the agents possess unique morphologic features that contribute to their ability to survive within the host.

BIBLIOGRAPHY

Cutler JE: Putative virulence factors of *Candida albicans*, *Annu Rev Microbiol* 454:187–218, 1991.

Lincoff G, Mitchel DH: *Toxic and hallucinogenic mushroom poisoning*, New York, 1977, Van Nostrand Reinhold.

Maresca B, Kobayashi GS: HSPs in fungal infections. In van Eden W, Young D, editors: *Stress proteins in medicine*, New York, 1996, Marcel Dekker.

Perfect, JR: Fungal virulence genes as target for antifungal chemotherapy, *Antimicrob Agents Chemother* 40:1577–1583, 1996.

CHAPTER 67

Antifungal Agents

The etiologic agent and the tissues involved in fungal disease as well as the immune status of the patient must be considered when selecting a therapeutic strategy for infection management. The fungal pathogens that colonize humans and cause disease have features that allow them to be categorized into groups according to the primary tissues that they colonize (see Box 66–2). These facts and the immunologic status of the patient dictate the best clinical approach for disease management.

The agents causing superficial infections tend to grow only on the outermost layers of the skin or on the cuticles of the hair shafts, rarely inducing an immune reaction. These infections cause minimal destructive disease, are cosmetic in nature, and are readily diagnosed. In general, excellent clinical responses result from the use of topical antifungals combined with attentive personal hygiene.

The agents causing cutaneous infections (tineas or dermatophytes) are limited to keratinized tissues of the epidermis, hair, and nails. However, they have greater invasive properties than the agents that cause superficial infections, and they may, depending on the species involved, cause chronic disease or evoke a highly inflammatory reaction from the host. Although these infections respond well to topical agents, systemic therapy may occasionally be required, particularly with widespread involvement of the skin, scalp, or nails (see the later description of griseofulvin).

The agents that cause subcutaneous disease generally have a low degree of infectivity, and infections caused by these organisms are usually associated with some form of traumatic injury. The strategies used to treat the infection depend on the organism and the degree of tissue involvement. The drug of choice in treating lymphocutaneous sporotrichosis, for example, is a saturated solution of potassium iodide. Some forms of chromoblastomycosis, depending on the etiologic agent, respond to high doses of orally administered 5-fluorocytosine (see the later discussion of 5-fluorocytosine). Other infections in this group are refractory to antifungal therapy and may require amputation or surgical excision of the involved area.

All systemic fungal agents of disease involve the respiratory tract, and they have unique morphologic features that appear to contribute to the organism's ability to survive within the host. Depending on the immune status of the patient and other underlying host factors, these diseases can be life-threatening. They require rapid diagnosis and aggressive therapy with systemic antifungal compounds.

Whereas a large number of antibiotics are available to treat bacterial infections, only a few exist for therapy of systemic fungal infections. Several reasons can be given for this difference. There is not a great impetus for the development of antifungal agents because systemic fungal infections are less common than bacterial infections. Furthermore, fungal cells, like mammalian cells, are eukaryotic, and compounds that are highly specific for fungal cells but nontoxic to the parasitized host cells are difficult to develop.

The antifungals now used in treating systemic fungal infections fall into three major classes of compounds: polyenes, azoles, and nucleoside analogues (Table 67–1). The polyenes affect cytosolic membranes, the azole derivatives inhibit ergosterol biosynthesis, and the fluorinated pyrimidine analogue 5-fluorocytosine interferes with DNA and RNA synthesis. The increasing incidence of life-threatening fungal infections has created a need to develop newer antifungals that are safer and more effective. This is particularly important in patients with acquired immunodeficiency syndrome (AIDS), other immunosuppressed patients who are receiving radiation or chemotherapy for various cancers, or patients who are candidates for organ transplantation. In most cases, the patient's defective immunity must be corrected for antifungal treatment to be successful.

Antifungals Used to Treat Systemic Infections

Polyenes

The polyenes are secondary metabolites produced by various species of *Streptomyces*. More than 150 have

TABLE 67–1. Antifungal Agents and Primary Sites of Activity

Agent	Target
Polyenes (e.g., amphotericin B, nystatin)	Membrane sterols (bind to ergosterol)
Azole derivatives (e.g., miconazole, ketoconazole, fluconazole, itraconazole)	Ergosterol biosynthesis (inhibit cytochrome P-450–dependent enzymes)
Nucleoside analogues (e.g., 5-fluorocytosine)	DNA and RNA synthesis (inhibit synthesis)
Grisans (e.g., griseofulvin)	Microtubules (inhibits microtubular function)
Allylamines (e.g., naftifine, terbinafine)	Squalene epoxidase
Thiocarbamates (e.g., tolnaftate, tolciclate)	Squalene epoxidase
Morpholines (e.g., amorolfine)	Ergosterol biosynthesis (inhibit Δ^{14}-reductase and Δ^7-Δ^8-isomerase)
Potassium iodide (e.g., saturated solution)	Unknown (possibly activates lysosomal enzymes and breaks down granulomas)

been isolated and chemically characterized. They are cyclic macrolide lactones containing a variable number of hydroxyls and from two to seven conjugated double bonds (Fig. 67–1). These compounds are classified by their amount of ring structure unsaturation (e.g., diene, triene, tetraene, pentaene, hexaene, heptaene). Although the mechanism of their action is complex, it is based primarily on the ability of these compounds to bind to sterols in the cytosolic membranes of susceptible cells. Because fungal membranes contain ergosterol, mammals contain cholesterol, plants contain sitosterol, and certain protozoa contain ergosterol, all are susceptible to the action of polyenes. This fact is the basis for the toxicity of these compounds when they are used to treat patients with systemic fungal infections.

Amphotericin B, a heptaene macrolide, is the only clinically useful polyene because its potency for damage is greater for fungal cells than for mammalian cells (Fig. 67–1*A*). It is selective because it preferentially binds to ergosterol-containing membranes rather than cholesterol-containing membranes. Although the structural aspects of the polyene-sterol binding are unclear, experimental evidence indicates that the amphotericin B molecule inserts into the cytoplasmic membrane of susceptible cells. Several molecules of the drug orient themselves parallel to the acyl side chains of the membrane phospholipids to form a cylindrical channel (Fig. 67–2). The pores that are formed by amphotericin B increase the permeability of the membrane in a dose-dependent manner, leading to leakage of essential ions from the cytosol at low concentrations and destruction of the cell at high doses. Amphotericin B also has

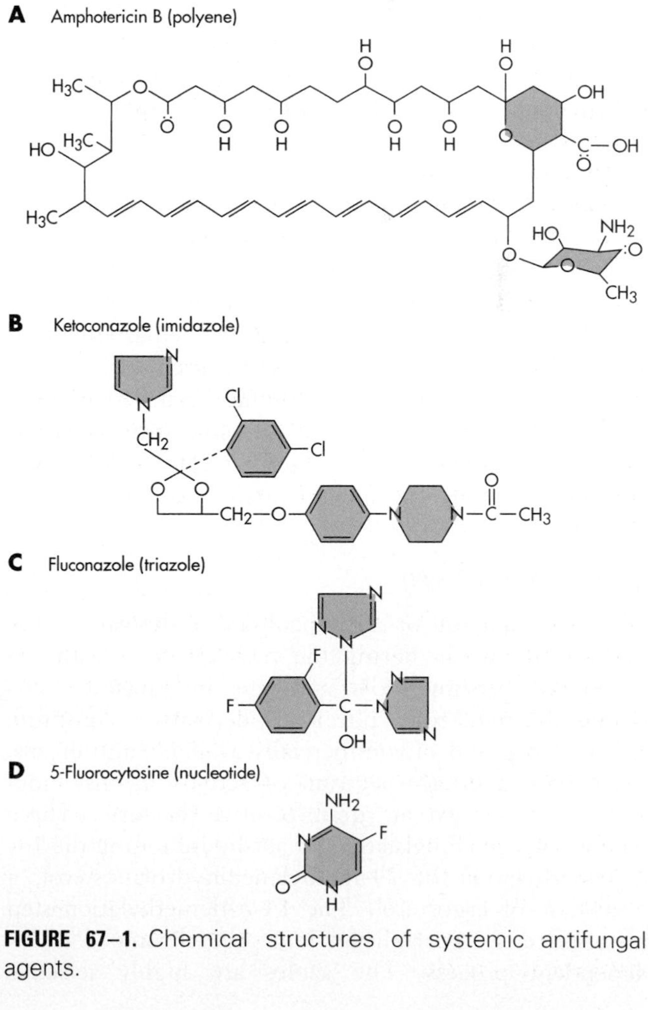

FIGURE 67–1. Chemical structures of systemic antifungal agents.

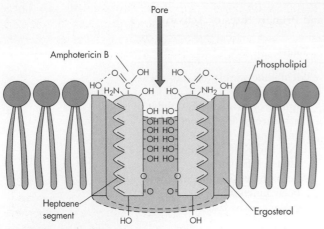

FIGURE 67–2. Mechanism of action of amphotericin B.

immunomodulatory properties that may have a role in its biologic activity in vivo. Amphotericin B is insoluble in water at pH 6 to 7. A mixture of amphotericin B, deoxycholate, and phosphate buffer is used clinically. In aqueous solutions, amphotericin B dissociates from deoxycholate and forms, depending on its concentration, self-associated or monomeric species. When injected intravenously, it interacts with plasma proteins and binds to cholesterol in lipoproteins, whereupon it is delivered mainly to tissues of the liver, spleen, lungs, and kidneys.

Nystatin (formerly called fungicidin) is a structural analogue of amphotericin B. The only difference between the two polyenes is the stretch of conjugated double bonds. The nystatin ring is interrupted to yield a diene-tetraene chromophore. Nystatin resembles amphotericin B in its permeabilizing and lethal effects on eukaryotic cells; however, little research has investigated its potential use as a systemic agent. At present, it is available only in topical, cream, suspension, or suppository form, primarily for the treatment of mucocutaneous, oropharyngeal, and vaginal candidiasis.

Azole Derivatives

The development of antifungal azole derivatives has progressed rapidly during the past 20 years with the advent of benzimidazole and the antiparasitic compound thiabendazole. The azole derivatives constitute the largest group of commercially available antifungals. They have a broad spectrum of activity against fungi and, to some extent, gram-positive bacteria. These compounds are fungistatic and act by inhibiting the 14-α-demethylation of 24-methylenedihydrolanosterol, a precursor of ergosterol. The 14-α-demethylation step in ergosterol biosynthesis is a cytochrome P-450–dependent process. The azoles are highly selective

and act by binding to the heme moiety of cytochrome P-450, thereby interfering with certain mixed oxidase reactions. As a result, synthesis of ergosterol is blocked and 14-α-methyl sterols accumulate.

These compounds are divided into two major groups characterized by five-membered azole rings with an *N*-linked methyl group derived by the addition of various halogenated phenyl or other complex chemical groups. The imidazoles (e.g., clotrimazole, miconazole, econazole, ketoconazole) (Fig. 67–1*B*) are derivatives that have two nitrogens in the ring, and the triazoles (e.g., fluconazole, itraconazole, terconazole) (Fig. 67–1*C*) are those with three nitrogens in the ring.

Nucleoside Analogues

5-Fluorocytosine (Fig. 67–1*D*) is a polar fluorinated pyrimidine that has a narrow spectrum of activity. It is used orally for the treatment of systemic infections caused by specific fungi mainly in the *Candida*, *Cryptococcus*, and *Aspergillus* genera and by certain fungi that cause chromoblastomycosis. It is well absorbed from the gastrointestinal tract, has low protein binding, is metabolically stable, and exhibits high bioavailability in humans. Unfortunately, it has a narrow spectrum of antifungal activity and rapidly induces resistance in susceptible organisms. In susceptible fungi, 5-fluorocytosine is taken up by a cytosine permease and is rapidly deaminated to 5-fluorouracil. This compound is then converted to either 5-fluorouridylic acid monophosphate, which inhibits RNA function, or 5-fluorodeoxyuridine monophosphate, a potent inhibitor of DNA synthesis.

Antifungals Used to Treat Dermatophyte Infections

Griseofulvin, an orally administered antifungal agent used to manage dermatophyte infections, is a grisan derivative produced by *Penicillium griseofulvum* (Fig. 67–3*A*). Griseofulvin interacts specifically with the tubulin of susceptible fungi, acting as a mitotic poison. The exact mechanism of action is unknown, but it appears to alter the function of tubulin rather than to disaggregate or assemble tubulin subunits. Griseofulvin is active against dermatophytes but inactive against *Candida albicans* and the agents causing systemic mycoses. The mechanism of resistance appears to be lack of uptake, because griseofulvin reacts in vitro with tubulins isolated from various sources (e.g., mammalian, dermatophyte, and amphibian cells).

The allylamines include the topical agent naftifine and the orally active antifungal agent terbinafine. The allylamines inhibit squalene epoxidase, a complex,

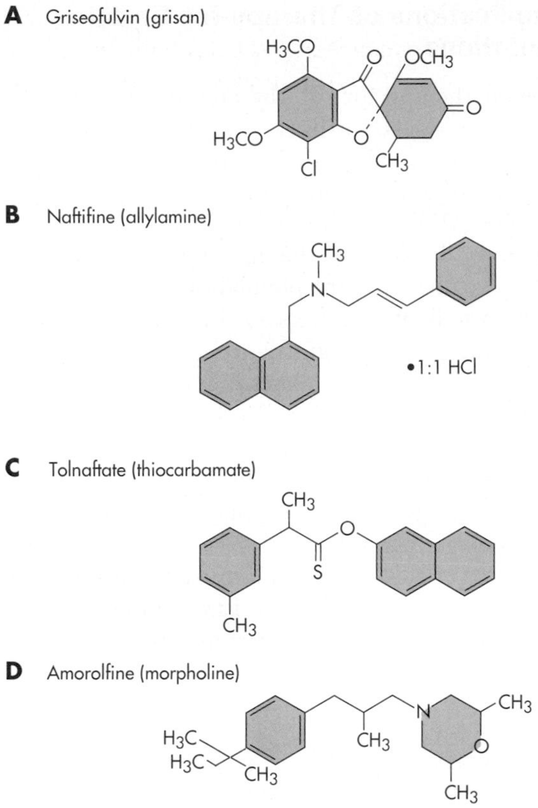

A Griseofulvin (grisan)

B Naftifine (allylamine)

•1:1 HCl

C Tolnaftate (thiocarbamate)

D Amorolfine (morpholine)

FIGURE 67–3. Chemical structures of agents used primarily for dermatophyte infections.

membrane-bound system that requires phospholipids and oxygen as a source of reducing equivalents (Fig. 67–3*B*). These compounds are highly active in vitro against dermatophytes and are effective against filamentous and dimorphic fungi but not against yeasts.

Tolnaftate and tolciclate are thiocarbamates whose mechanisms of action are similar to those of the allylamines (Fig. 67–3*C*). They inhibit ergosterol biosynthesis in dermatophytes at the level of squalene epoxidase but are less active against yeasts. They are used topically in the management of dermatophyte infections.

Amorolfine, a morpholine derivative, is highly active against dermatophytes and moderately active against yeasts, but its response in filamentous fungi is variable (Fig. 67–3*D*). Amorolfine has no effect on DNA, RNA, protein, or carbohydrate synthesis, but it appears to inhibit Δ^{14}-reductase and Δ^7-Δ^8-isomerase in the pathway of ergosterol biosynthesis.

Other preparations, such as those containing 10-undecenoic (undecylenic acid), caprylic, or propionic acid as active ingredients, have also been used in the management of ringworm infections. These compounds do not have fungicidal properties, and their

role in eradicating fungi from the skin has not been established. Appropriate hygienic practices in addition to the use of preparations containing these compounds are undoubtedly important to favorable clinical responses.

Future Considerations

Identification of Novel Targets for the Development of Agents

The development of antifungals has primarily focused on the cytostolic membrane. Unfortunately, the antifungals in use are toxic to host cells or are fungistatic and have a limited spectrum of activity. Clearly, there is a need to look for other targets. The cell wall is a major constituent of the fungal envelope. It determines the shape of the cell, serves as a protective permeability barrier to large molecules, and is essential for survival of the fungus. The fungal wall structure is multilayered and composed mainly of glucan, mannoproteins, and chitin. Chitin and β-glucans are absent in host cells and unique to fungi. Thus, the cell wall is an attractive target for antifungal drug development, and several efforts have been made to design compounds that interfere with its synthesis. Polyoxins are analogues of uridine diphosphate-N-acetyglucosamine, a class of compounds that are specific competitive inhibitors of chitin synthase. Antifungal activity has been demonstrated in vitro against *C. albicans*, but only a limited number of studies have been conducted in vivo. There is some question about uptake of these analogues by medically important fungi. As a result, development of the polyoxins has not progressed. The nikkomycins, a related group of compounds that are structurally similar to the polyoxins, are more promising. Like the polyoxins, nikkomycin Z is a competitive inhibitor of chitin synthase. It is highly effective against murine coccidioidomycosis, blastomycosis, and histoplasmosis and prolongs the life of mice infected with *C. albicans*.

Efforts have been made to find compounds that inhibit the synthesis of β-glucan. Echinocandin B, a compound that was discovered about 20 years ago, is very effective against yeast. It is a cyclic lipopeptide metabolite produced by *Aspergillus nidulans*. Cilofungin (LY121019), a recently synthesized compound, is a derivative of echinocandin B that is produced by enzymatic deacylation using *Actinoplanes utahensis* with *p*-octyl-oxobenzoic acid. It is less toxic and more potent than its parent compound. Promising results with cilofungin in vitro and in vivo have led to clinical trials for invasive candidiasis and esophageal disease. Unfortunately, its development has been abandoned because of toxicity from the vehicle used for its delivery. To meet the pressing need for novel agents that are spe-

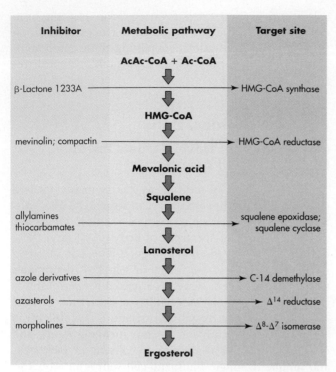

Inhibitor	Metabolic pathway	Target site
	AcAc-CoA + Ac-CoA	
β-Lactone 1233A		HMG-CoA synthase
	HMG-CoA	
mevinolin; compactin		HMG-CoA reductase
	Mevalonic acid	
	Squalene	
allylamines thiocarbamates		squalene epoxidase; squalene cyclase
	Lanosterol	
azole derivatives		C-14 demethylase
azasterols		Δ^{14} reductase
morpholines		Δ^{8}-Δ^{7} isomerase
	Ergosterol	

FIGURE 67–4. Metabolic pathway of ergosterol biosynthesis in fungi and potential target sites for development of novel antifungals. AcAc-CoA = acetoacetyl coenzyme A; Ac-CoA = acetyl coenzyme A; HMG-CoA = β-hydroxy-β-methylglutaryl coenzyme A.

cific, fungicidal, and nontoxic to patients, newer antifungal agents are continually being sought and are in various stages of development. At present, one major focus of investigations deals with developing inhibitors of various enzymes in ergosterol biosynthesis (Fig. 67–4).

In Vitro Susceptibility Testing

Paralleling the development and discovery of newer antifungal compounds has been the increasing use of these agents to treat the growing number of common and exotic fungal infections. This situation has brought about demands for in vitro antifungal testing methods that will accurately predict in vivo activity. Unfortunately, in vitro susceptibility testing with fungi has not yet been standardized, and the results of the current tests thus are not always predictive of clinical responses, particularly with the azole derivatives and, to some extent, 5-fluorocytosine. Efforts are being expended to develop standardized methods for in vitro susceptibility testing and to develop animal models of infection to evaluate these agents.

Complications of Therapy for Certain Populations

Although therapy for life-threatening fungal infections is far from ideal, progress has been made. Despite these advances, significant problems still exist in the treatment of fungal infections, particularly in patients who have AIDS or who are otherwise severely immunosuppressed. None of the agents in use appears to be curative in these patient populations. Lifelong suppressive therapy is often necessary to prevent recurrence of disease but poses a significant problem for these patients because they are taking numerous medications to suppress the AIDS virus and other opportunistic organisms. Some of the available antifungals may interact with these drugs. In patients being treated with combinations of drugs, monitoring plasma levels and relevant pharmacologic parameters may be necessary so that adverse drug effects can be minimized. Another complication of therapy is drug-resistant fungi, which may explain the emergence of recurrent disease.

QUESTIONS

1. What is the current thought on the mechanism of action of amphotericin B?

2. How do the azoles work?

3. How does 5-fluorocytosine work? What major problem is encountered with its use?

4. If you were to design an antifungal agent that specifically targeted fungi, what strategy would you use?

BIBLIOGRAPHY

Anker van den JN, Popele van NML, Sauer PJJ: Antifungal agents in neonatal candidiasis, *Antimicrob Agents Chemother* 39:1391–1397, 1995.

Georgopapadakou NH, Walsh TJ: Antifungal agents: chemotherapeutic targets and immunological strategies, *Antimicrob Agents Chemother* 40:279–291, 1996.

Ghanmoum MA, Rice LB: Mode of action, mechanisms of resistance, and correlation of these mechanisms with bacterial resistance, *Clin Microbiol Rev* 12:501–517, 1999.

Graybill JR, Patterson TF: Antifungal agents and antifungal susceptibility testing. In Ajello L, Hay RJ, editors: *Topley and Wilson's microbiology and microbial diseases*, vol 4, *Medical mycology*, London, 1998, Arnold.

Perfect JR: Fungal virulence genes as targets for antifungal chemotherapy, *Antimicrob Agents Chemother* 40:1577–1583, 1996.

C H A P T E R 6 8

Laboratory Diagnosis of Fungal Diseases

Diagnostic Procedures

The diagnosis of fungal infections caused by primary pathogens (e.g., *Histoplasma capsulatum*, *Blastomyces dermatitidis*, *Coccidioides immitis*, *Paracoccidioides brasiliensis*, *Cryptococcus neoformans*) can be made microscopically from visualization of the parasitic phase of the organism in clinical specimens or from growth of the organism from tissues taken from the lesion. Diagnosis is more complicated when the fungal infections are caused by ubiquitous opportunistic agents (e.g., *Aspergillus*, *Candida*, and *Mucor* species), because these fungi, which are common in the environment, are frequently found as contaminants in the cultures. In this case, isolates of the same organism must be cultured repeatedly from lesion specimens that have been sampled at different times. The validity of the isolates is further supported when fungal elements are seen in material taken from the site of infection.

The methods used in collecting and handling clinical specimens are considerably important in the isolation and identification of fungi. The sampling procedures vary according to the area and type of tissue involved. Although selective media are available for the isolation and culture of most pathogenic fungi, it is important to use sterile techniques whenever possible, especially with skin surfaces, nails, and hair that may be contaminated with saprobic fungi, bacteria, dirt, and epithelial debris. These sterile techniques are as follows:

1. The skin surface is swabbed with 70% ethanol and allowed to air-dry before sampling.
2. The surface is scraped to remove skin scales or hair that contain the fungus.
3. The specimen is treated with 10% potassium hydroxide to destroy tissue elements.

A portion of the treated specimen should be examined microscopically to determine whether hyphal elements are present. Because fungi contain chitin and various complex polysaccharides in their cell wall, they are refractory to the alkali treatment, making them easy to visualize with light microscopy (Fig. 68–1). Several histologic procedures that specifically stain fungi in tissue sections, such as the use of Gomori's methenamine silver and periodic acid–Schiff stains, are based on the presence of chitin and polysaccharides in their cell wall.

When an infectious etiology is suspected, a portion of diseased tissue should be submitted to the pathologist for microscopic examination. Fungi can be stained preferentially because of the polysaccharide-rich properties of their cell walls. Preferential staining tells the clinician only whether fungi are present in the tissue. For definitive identification of the organism, the fungi must be cultured on suitable media and incubated at 25°C to 30°C. Specimens taken from the blood, from the cerebrospinal fluid, and by surgical biopsy must be examined microscopically and cultured rapidly, because desiccation, autolytic processes, and bacterial contamination can make the specimen unsuitable for diagnostic procedures.

A variety of media support the growth of fungi. **Sabouraud's dextrose agar,** which is composed of 4% dextrose, 1% peptone, and 2% agar adjusted to a pH of 5.5, is the medium most conventionally used in diagnostic laboratories for the growth of fungi. It is selective for the growth of fungi because of its acidic pH and high sugar concentration. Unfortunately, saprobic fungi grow rapidly on this medium and often overgrow the surface, obscuring any pathogens that might be present. Therefore, a medium containing 2% glucose, 1% neopeptone, and 2% agar that is supplemented with cycloheximide and chloramphenicol and adjusted to a pH of 7.0 is often used for the primary isolation of dermatophytes and other pathogens. Chloramphenicol inhibits most bacteria, and cycloheximide inhibits the growth of most saprobic fungi. Some pathogens, such as *C. neoformans*, do not grow on this latter medium. Furthermore, the parasitic phase of

FIGURE 68–1. Skin scraping treated with 10% potassium hydroxide. Fungi are refractory to alkali treatment and appear as septate hyphal fragments.

some primary pathogens, such as *H. capsulatum*, does not grow on this medium at 37°C, so all cultures should be incubated at 25°C to 30°C. Because the number of opportunistic fungal infections caused by saprobic fungi has increased tremendously, clinical specimens taken from deep tissues should be cultured on media with and without antibiotics.

In general, the techniques used for the laboratory identification of yeast are similar to those used to identify bacteria. These techniques are based on the biochemical and physiologic properties of the organism. Gram stain, however, plays no role in identifying fungi, because all fungi are gram-positive. Yeasts are unicellular, grow rapidly, and can be uniformly suspended in broth. On the other hand, molds are filamentous, produce specialized conidia, and grow slowly. They are identified microscopically according to the size and shape of the conidia and the way they develop. The morphologic features of specialized structures (e.g., chlamydospores, hyphae) also aid in the identification of molds. Identification of fungi requires a basic understanding and knowledge of different morphologic features of fungi. (See Chapters 69 through 71 and the Bibliography in this chapter for detailed descriptions of their identifying features.)

Progression of Medical Mycology

The study of fungi is in the process of transition, and advances in medicine have placed a great deal of importance on the organisms' role in human infections. Traditionally, medical mycology was almost entirely descriptive and taxonomically oriented, a result of its close and historical associations with botany and dermatology. At present, medical mycology is enjoying a period of rapid growth and interest. Fungi are being used as models for the elucidation of many molecular, genetic, and biologic processes common to all living things. They are also being used as models to study cellular differentiation and adaptation, particularly host-parasite interactions. The need for rapid identification of fungi in clinical material has been partially met with the development of specific molecular probes, and there is now an emphasis on discovering newer antifungal agents and novel therapeutic strategies to treat the growing number of fungal infections.

QUESTIONS

1. Fungi can be visualized in tissue sections by specific staining methods. What is the basis behind this technique?
2. Why are cultures for fungi held for at least 4 weeks before they are discarded as negative, whereas cultures for bacteria are usually discarded after 2 to 5 days?
3. The laboratory procedure used to identify yeasts differs from that for molds. Why?
4. When clinical material is processed, why are media with and without antibiotics used?
5. In contrast to bacteria, why is it unnecessary to use 1000× magnification to visualize fungi in clinical material?
6. Why is a strong alkaline solution used to treat tissue specimens when the presence of fungi is suspected?
7. In certain situations, fungal cultures are incubated at 25°C and 37°C. Why?

BIBLIOGRAPHY

Goodman NL, Roberts GD: Laboratory diagnosis. In Ajello L, Hay RJ, editors: *Topley and Wilson's microbiology and microbial diseases*, vol 4. *Medical mycology*, London, 1998, Arnold.

Kawasaki M, Aoki M: Application of molecular biological techniques to medical mycology. In Ajello L, Hay RJ, editors: *Topley and Wilson's microbiology and microbial diseases*, vol 4, *Medical mycology*, London, 1998, Arnold.

Larone DH: *Medically important fungi: a guide to identification*, ed 3, Washington, DC, 1995, American Society for Microbiology.

Merz WG, Roberts GD: Algorithms for detection and identification of fungi. In Ajello L, Hay RJ, editors: *Topley and Wilson's microbiology and microbial diseases*, vol 4, *Medical mycology*, London, 1998, Arnold.

Wilson ML: General principles of specimen collection and transport, Clin Infect Dis 22:766–777, 1996.

CHAPTER 69

Superficial, Cutaneous, and Subcutaneous Mycoses

Fungal infections can be classified according to the tissues that are initially colonized (see Box 66–2). Infections are classified as follows:

1. **Superficial mycoses**, limited to the outermost layers of the skin and hair.
2. The **cutaneous mycoses**, including infections that are deeper in the epidermis and its integuments, the hair and nails.
3. The **subcutaneous mycoses**, involving the dermis, subcutaneous tissues, muscle, and fascia.

In general, intact skin and mucosal surfaces serve as barriers to infection caused by superficial, cutaneous, and subcutaneous mycoses. Fatty acid content, pH, epithelial turnover of the skin, and normal bacterial flora contribute to host resistance. The mucosa and the ciliary action of cells lining the respiratory tract help eliminate organisms that are accidentally inhaled. Humoral factors such as transferrin restrict the growth of several fungi in vitro by limiting the amount of available iron. Such factors may restrict the growth of dermatophytes to the outer layers of skin.

Superficial Mycoses

Superficial fungal infections are usually cosmetic problems that are easily diagnosed and treated. Four infections belonging to this classification are pityriasis versicolor and tinea nigra, both involving the skin, and black piedra and white piedra, both involving the hair (Fig. 69–1). Skin infections are limited to the outermost layers of the stratum corneum. Hair infections involve only the cuticle.

In general, these superficial fungal organisms do not elicit a cellular response from the host because they colonize tissues that are not living. Furthermore, these infections cause no physical discomfort. They are generally brought to the attention of the physician as an incidental finding or for cosmetic reasons. They are easy to diagnose, and specific therapeutic measures usually result in good clinical responses (Table 69–1).

Etiology, Clinical Syndromes, and Diagnosis

Pityriasis Versicolor

Pityriasis versicolor (see Fig. 69–1A) is caused by *Malassezia furfur* (*Pityrosporum orbiculare*), a lipophilic, yeastlike organism. The organism is found in areas of the body that are rich in sebaceous glands, and it is part of the normal flora of the skin. The organism requires a medium supplemented with saturated or unsaturated fatty acids to support its growth. It grows as a budding yeast, although the hyphal form is occasionally seen.

The lesions of pityriasis versicolor occur most commonly on the upper torso, arms, and abdomen as discrete, hyperpigmented or hypopigmented macular lesions (Fig. 69–2). They scale very easily, giving the affected area a dry, chalky appearance. On rare occasions, the lesions take on a papular (elevated) appearance, and in some cases in which the hair follicle is involved, the lesions can cause folliculitis.

Clinical diagnosis of pityriasis versicolor is made microscopically from visualization of the characteristic "spaghetti and meatballs" appearance of the organism in potassium hydroxide–treated specimens (Fig. 69–3). Cultures are not routinely performed to confirm the diagnosis, because *M. furfur* requires a special medium containing fatty acids.

Tinea Nigra

The etiologic agent of tinea nigra (see Fig. 69–1B), *Exophiala werneckii*, is a dimorphic fungus that produces melanin, which gives it a brown to black color. On primary isolation from clinical material, it grows as a yeast with many cells in various stages of cell division, producing characteristic two-celled oval structures (Fig. 69–4). As the colony ages, elongated hyphae develop, and in older cultures, mycelia and conidia predominate.

The clinical manifestations of tinea nigra are usually asymptomatic and consist of well-demarcated macular

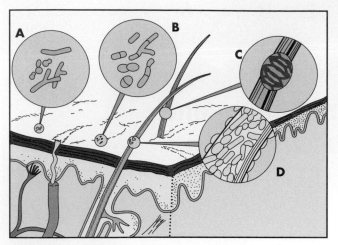

FIGURE 69–1. Schematic illustration of superficial fungal infection and tissue involvement. *A,* Pityriasis versicolor. *B,* Tinea nigra. *C,* Black piedra. *D,* White piedra.

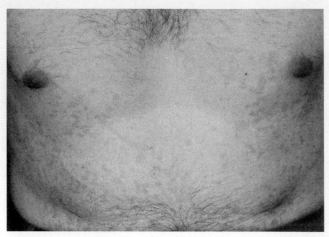

FIGURE 69–2. Clinical presentation of pityriasis versicolor.

TABLE 69–1. Features of the Organisms Causing Superficial Mycoses

Organism	Disease	Tissue	Clinical Features	Diagnostic Procedures
Malassezia furfur	Pityriasis versicolor	Skin	Hyperpigmented or hypopigmented macular lesions that scale readily, giving it chalky-branny appearance, and that occur most frequently on the upper torso of the body	Direct microscopic examination of skin scrapings treated with alkali stain* reveals fungal elements having the classic "spaghetti and meatballs" appearance Cultures not routinely performed to confirm the diagnosis Organism requires fatty acid–supplemented medium for growth
Exophiala werneckii	Tinea nigra	Skin	Gray to black, well-demarcated macular lesions most frequently occurring on the palms	Direct microscopic examination of skin scrapings treated with alkali stain* Culture on Sabouraud's dextrose agar yields pigmented (brown to black) yeasts and hyphae (dimorphic)
Piedraia hortae	Black piedra	Hair	Hard, gritty, brown to black concretions that develop along the hair shaft and that house the sexual phase (asci and ascospores) of the fungus	Direct microscopic examination of hairs Culture yields asexual phase of the fungus
Trichosporon beigelii	White piedra	Hair	Soft, white to creamy yellow granules that form a sleevelike collarette along the hair shaft	Direct microscopic examination of hairs Culture on Sabouraud's dextrose agar Growth is dimorphic: hyphae, arthroconidia, and blastoconidia

*A useful alkaline dye containing clearing agent can be made from Parker Super Quink permanent blue-black ink by adding 10 g of potassium hydroxide/100 mL of ink. The solution is centrifuged to sediment the amorphous precipitate that forms. The clear blue supernatant should be decanted and stored in a plastic container to prevent insoluble carbonate precipitates from forming.

From Swartz JH, Medrek TF: Rapid contrast stain as a diagnostic aid for fungous infections. *Arch Dermatol* 99:494–497, 1969.

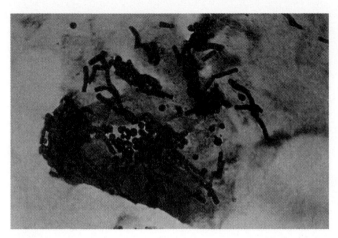

FIGURE 69–3. Skin scrapings stained with periodic acid–Schiff stain showing typical yeastlike and hyphal fragments of *Malassezia furfur,* the etiologic agent at pityriasis versicolor.

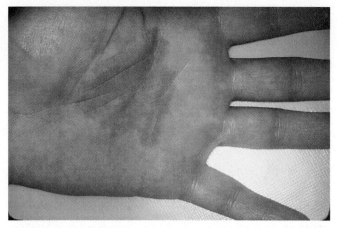

FIGURE 69–5. Clinical presentation of tinea nigra. Note the dark pigmentation in the center of the palm.

lesions (discolored spots on the skin that are not raised above the surface) that enlarge by peripheral extension (Fig. 69–5). The brown to black lesions are most often seen on the palms and soles but may occur on other areas of the body.

The diagnosis is made through visualization of the characteristic darkly pigmented, yeastlike cells and hyphal fragments during microscopic examination of potassium hydroxide–treated scrapings taken from the affected areas; it is confirmed by culture of the organism.

Black Piedra

The cause of black piedra (see Fig. 69–1*C*), a superficial hair infection, is *Piedraia hortae,* an organism that exists in the perfect (**teleomorphic**) state when it colonizes the hair shaft. Cultures from clinical material

usually yield only the asexual (**anamorphic**) state of the fungus, which consists of slow-growing, brown to reddish black mycelia. The teleomorphic state is a state in which asci, which contain spindle-shaped ascospores, develop within specialized structures. This state is occasionally found in older cultures.

The major clinical feature of black piedra is the presence of hard nodules, found along the infected hair shaft (Fig. 69–6). The nodules have a hard, carbonaceous consistency and contain asci. The differential diagnosis includes the nits of pediculosis and abnormal hair growth.

The infection is easily diagnosed with microscopic examination of affected hairs.

White Piedra

White piedra (see Fig. 69–1*D*), an infection of the hair, is caused by the yeastlike organism *Trichosporon*

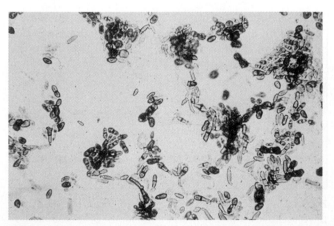

FIGURE 69–4. Yeastlike cells of *Exophiala werneckii,* the causative agent of tinea nigra.

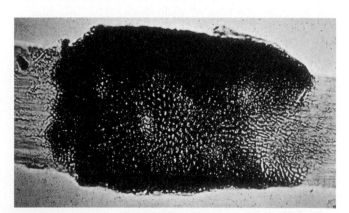

FIGURE 69–6. Hair infected with *Piedraia hortae.* The hard black nodule contains asci and ascospores, the sexual phase of the fungus.

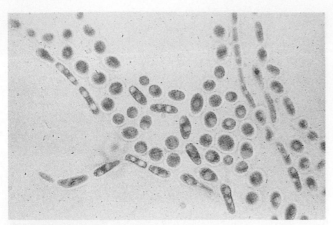

FIGURE 69–7. Hyphae, arthroconidia, and blastospores of *Trichosporon beigelii*. The dimorphic characteristics of the agent of white piedra are shown.

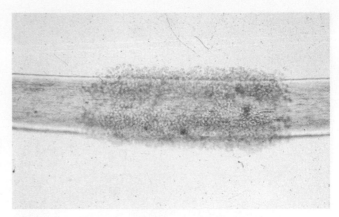

FIGURE 69–8. Clinical presentation of white piedra.

beigelii (Fig. 69–7). The organism grows well on all laboratory media except those containing cycloheximide, an antibiotic used in some media (e.g., Mycosel agar) for the selective isolation of most pathogenic fungi. Young cultures are white and have a pasty consistency. As the culture ages, colonies develop deep, radiating furrows and become yellow and creamy. Microscopic examination reveals septate hyphae that fragment rapidly to form arthroconidia (see Fig. 69–7). The arthroconidia rapidly become round, and many cells form blastoconidia.

White piedra affects the hair of the scalp, mustache, and beard. It is characterized by the development of a soft, pasty, cream-colored growth along infected hair shafts (Fig. 69–8). The growth occurs as a sleeve or collarette around the hair shaft and consists of mycelia that rapidly fragment into arthroconidia.

The organism is identified from results of various biochemical tests and its ability to assimilate certain carbohydrates. The differential diagnosis includes trichomycosis axillaris (caused by *Corynebacterium tenuis*) and includes the nits of pediculosis. The infection is diagnosed through microscopic examination of infected hairs and confirmed by culture of the organism.

Treatment

These four infections—pityriasis versicolor, tinea nigra, black piedra, and white piedra—generally are cosmetic and easily diagnosed. When proper therapy is instituted, the infections respond well, with no consequences. The general approach to treating pityriasis versicolor and tinea nigra is removal of the organism from the skin. This is accomplished by the topical use of keratolytic agents (chemicals that lyse keratin). Preparations containing selenium disulfide, hyposulfite, thiosulfate, or salicylic acid remove the organism, but the

disease may recur. Topical preparations containing miconazole nitrate, an antifungal agent that inhibits ergosterol synthesis (see Chapter 67), are used effectively in eradicating the disease.

Effective therapy of hair infections caused by *P. hortae* and *T. beigelii* is achieved by shaving or cropping the infected hairs close to the scalp surface. These infections will not recur if the patient practices proper personal hygiene.

Cutaneous Mycoses

The cutaneous mycoses are diseases of the skin, hair, and nails. They are generally restricted to the keratinized layers of the integument and its appendages (Fig. 69–9). Unlike the superficial infections, cutaneous in-

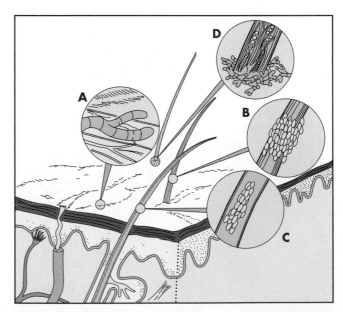

FIGURE 69–9. Schematic of tissues colonized by dermatophytes. *A,* Stratum corneum infection. *B,* Ectothrix hair infection. *C,* Endothrix hair infection. *D,* Favic hair infection.

fections may evoke various cellular immune responses, causing pathologic changes in the host that may be expressed in the deeper tissues of the skin. The severity of the response appears to be directly related to the immune status of the host and the strain or species of fungus involved in the infection.

The term *dermatophyte* has been used traditionally to describe these agents. However, the suffix *-phyte*, which implies that these organisms are plants, is misleading, because fungi are not phylogenetically related to plants. Nevertheless, for historical reasons, *dermatophyte* is used in this section to refer to the organisms causing these diseases.

The clinical manifestations of these diseases are also referred to as ringworm or tinea. *Tinea* comes from Latin and means "worm" or "moth." It describes the serpentine (snakelike) and annular (ringlike) lesions on the skin that resemble a worm burrowing at the margin (Fig. 69–10). A modifying term indicates the anatomic site involved: tinea pedis, feet; tinea capitis, scalp; tinea manus, hands; tinea unguium, nails; and tinea corporis, body. In some cases, the cutaneous mycoses are given special names that indicate the clinical appearance of the infection or the origin of the organism causing the disease. For example, favus (the Latin word for "honeycomb"), which is caused by *Trichophyton schoenleinii*, has a honeycomb appearance, and tokelau (from the name of a South Pacific atoll) is caused by *Trichophyton concentricum*, which is geographically restricted to the Pacific islands of Oceania, Southeast Asia, and Central and South America.

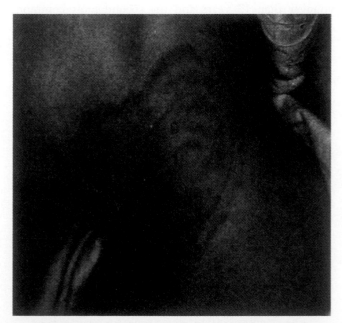

FIGURE 69–10. Clinical presentation of tinea corporis.

BOX 69–1. Asexual (Anamorphic) State of Selected Dermatophytes*

Microsporum	*Trichophyton*
M. audouinii	T. concentricum
M. canis	T. equinum
M. cookei	T. mentagrophytes var. interdigitale
M. equinum	T. rubrum
M. fulvum	T. schoenleinii
M. gallinae	T. tonsurans
M. gypseum	T. verrucosum
M. nanum	T. violaceum

Epidermophyton

E. floccosum

*At present, 41 species of dermatophytes are recognized as etiologic agents of disease.

Etiology

The cutaneous mycoses are caused by a homogeneous group of closely related organisms known as the **dermatophytes**. Although more than 100 species have been described, only about 40 are considered valid, and less than half of these are associated with human disease (Box 69–1). In the anamorphic state, they are classified in three genera (*Microsporum*, *Trichophyton*, and *Epidermophyton*) according to their sporulation patterns (Fig. 69–11), certain morphologic features of development, and nutritional requirements. The teleomorphic states of some organisms belonging to the genera *Microsporum* and *Trichophyton* are known. They are all Ascomycetes and have been reclassified in the genus *Arthroderma*. As yet, the sexual phase of *Epidermophyton* organisms has not been observed.

Ecology and Epidemiology

The isolation of different species of dermatophytes varies markedly from one ecological niche to another. Some species are commonly isolated from the soil and have been grouped as **geophilic dermatophytes**. Other species have been found most often in association with domestic and wild animals and birds. These are referred to as **zoophilic dermatophytes**. A third group, the **anthropophilic dermatophytes**, has been found almost exclusively in association with humans and their habitats. Box 69–2 summarizes the groupings of the various species that are common throughout the world.

The clinical purpose of identifying species of dermatophytes is to determine the possible source of infection. There are also some considerations of prognostic value. The anthropophilic group tends to cause chronic infections that may be difficult to cure. The

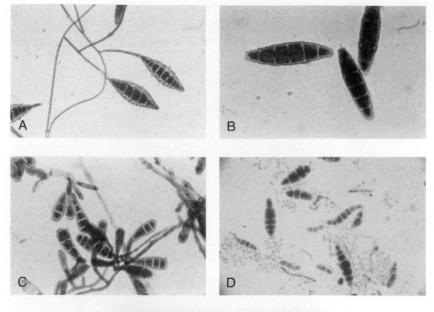

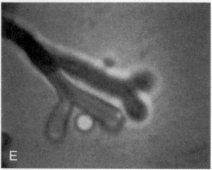

FIGURE 69–11. Sporulation pattern and identifying features of some dermatophytes. *A,* Macroconidia of *Microsporum canis. B,* Macroconidia of *Microsporum gypseum. C,* Macroconidia of *Epidermophyton floccosum. D,* Microconidia and macroconidia of *Trichophyton mentagrophytes. E,* Favic chandelier of *Trichophyton schoenleinii.*

zoophilic and geophilic dermatophytes tend to cause inflammatory lesions that respond well to therapy and may occasionally heal spontaneously.

Some species of dermatophytes are endemic in certain parts of the world and have a limited geographic distribution. *Trichophyton yaoundei, Trichophyton gourvilii,* and *Trichophyton soudenense* are geographically restricted to Central and West Africa; *Microsporum ferrugineum* predominates in Japan and its surrounding areas; and *T. concentricum* is confined to islands in the South Pacific and a small area of Central and South America. However, the increasing mobility of the world's population is disrupting several of these patterns. In recent times, *Trichophyton tonsurans* has replaced *Microsporum audouinii* as the principal agent of tinea capitis in the United States because of the mass migration of individuals from Mexico and other Latin American countries where *T. tonsurans* predominates. Less understood are the epidemics of ringworm that occasionally occur.

The prevalence of dermatophytes and the incidence of disease are difficult to determine because the disorders are not reportable. Fragmentary surveys from epidemiologic studies and case reports indicate that the cutaneous mycoses are among the most common among human diseases. Reports estimate that they are the third most common skin disorder in children younger than 12 years and the second most common in older populations. The occurrence of these diseases varies with age, gender, ethnic group, and cultural and social habits of the population.

The incidence of the cutaneous mycoses and the clinical manifestations of disease among various age groups depend on the anatomic site of involvement and the dermatophyte species involved in disease. Tinea capitis is a problem of the pediatric population until puberty, when it spontaneously ceases to be a major infectious disorder. Tinea pedis, however, which is rarely a disease in childhood, gradually becomes the predominant infection with age and remains so into adulthood.

The incidence of tinea capitis in black children in the United States is disproportionately high. In India, tinea capitis occurs more often in the native children than in Europeans, whereas the Europeans have a higher incidence of tinca pedis. Clinical surveys conducted during the war in Southeast Asia revealed that people from the United States had a higher incidence of tinea pedis caused by *Trichophyton mentagrophytes* than the native population. The indigenous population appeared to be highly susceptible to a distinctive strain of *Trichophyton rubrum*. Tinea capitis, tinea pedis, and tinea cruris are more common in men than women. Tinea unguium (infections of the nail plate) of the hand is more common in women, but the same disorder on the feet is seen more often in men.

The reasons for these differences are poorly understood. The incidence of cutaneous mycoses is related to customs associated with the type of clothing and footwear worn. Studies on institutionalized populations and family outbreaks of dermatophyte infections indicate that close and crowded living conditions are a factor in the spread of infections. There is evidence that natural resistance to these infections exists in certain individuals. Certain humoral factors are fungistatic, and cell-mediated immunity appears to be important in resistance to dermatophyte infections.

Pathogenesis

A delicate balance appears to operate between the host and parasite in dermatophyte infections. Some fungi show an evolutionary development toward a parasitic existence. Those that have achieved a high level of coexistence with humans also exhibit a degree of specificity for the tissues that are colonized. These fungi are often referred to as **keratinophilic fungi** because they can use keratin as a substrate. Keratinases have been isolated from some of these fungi, but keratin is not an essential metabolite for them. The tissues containing

this protein are highly selective for the growth of dermatophytes, but the reason is unknown. As versatile as these fungi may appear, they seem unable to invade organs other than the keratinized layers of skin, hair, and nails.

Laboratory Diagnosis

The diagnosis of dermatophyte disease requires that fungal elements be seen in clinical specimens of the lesion or that they be confirmed by culture of the organism. Skin and nail scrapings or hair taken from areas suspected to be infected are examined microscopically. The procedure for processing these specimens is similar to those described previously for examining clinical material from superficial fungal infections. The specimen is treated with an alkali solution to clear the epithelial cells and other debris. Dermatophytes resist the caustic solution and appear as branching, septate hyphal elements in specimens taken from cutaneous lesions or nails. Examination of fungal elements in infected hair reveals spores inside the hair shaft (**endothrix infection**) (Fig. 69–12*A*) or surrounding it (**ectothrix infection**) (Fig. 69–12*B*).

An exception to this type of sporulation is the hair infection caused by *T. schoenleinii*. Disease due to this organism is called favus, and the infected hair has a waxy mass of hyphal elements (scutulum) surrounding the base of the hair follicle at the scalp line. Microscopic examination of the hair reveals degenerated hyphal elements coursing throughout the hair shaft (see Fig. 69–9*D*). Such hairs are called favic and are diagnostic of the infection.

Direct microscopic examination of clinical material confirms only the diagnosis of a fungal infection. Cultures must be performed to identify the specific etiologic agent.

The skin surface harbors many bacterial species and saprobic fungi as part of the normal flora or transient colonizers. Thus, media such as Sabouraud's dextrose agar are not routinely used for primary culture, because these organisms overgrow the culture and inhibit the growth of the more slow-growing dermatophytes. For this reason, selective media containing antibiotics are recommended for culturing of specimens from the skin. A medium commonly used for the isolation of dermatophytes from clinical material contains cycloheximide to suppress saprobic fungal growth and chloramphenicol to inhibit the growth of bacteria. Clinical material is seeded directly onto the medium and is incubated at 25°C. Dermatophytes and most pathogenic fungi grow well on this medium when incubated at 25°C, whereas saprobic fungi and bacteria are inhibited.

Cultures are examined periodically, and all fungi that grow are identified by microscopic examination and physiologic tests. In general, the mycelia of these

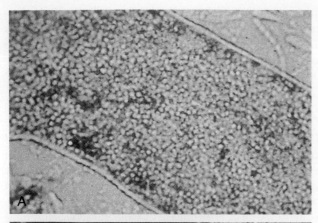

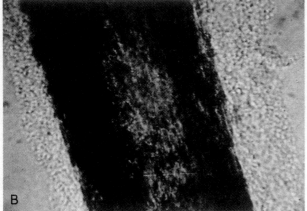

FIGURE 69–12. Fungal infections of the hair. *A*, Endothrix infection. *B*, Ectothrix infection.

fungi are undifferentiated, and species identification is based primarily on the conidia produced (Table 69–2). The conidia may be large (5 to 100 × 6 to 8 μm) and multicellular (macroconidia), or they may be small (3 × 10 μm) and unicellular (microconidia).

In addition to conidia, some dermatophytes produce spiral hyphae, chlamydospores, nodular bodies, racquet hyphae, and chandeliers. These structures are produced commonly by some species of dermatophytes and in-

TABLE 69–2. General Characteristics of Macroconidia and Microconidia of Dermatophytes

Genus	Macroconidia	Microconidia
Microsporum	Numerous, thick-walled, rough*	Rare
Epidermophyton	Numerous, smooth-walled	Absent
Trichophyton	Rare, thin-walled, smooth	Abundant†

* *M. audouinii* is an exception.
† *T. schoenleinii* is an exception.

frequently by others; however, they should not be considered distinguishing features of the species. Figure 69–11 illustrates the identifying features of some dermatophytes. All cultures are routinely held for 4 weeks before being discarded as "negative."

Treatment

The clinical nature of the dermatophyte infections frequently poses a challenge to the clinician. Skin infections generally are approached conservatively with topical treatment. The discovery of azole derivatives as effective antifungal agents has provided several new drugs that can be used topically (e.g., miconazole, clotrimazole, econazole). All of the azole derivatives appear to work by interfering with the cytochrome P-450 dependent enzyme systems at the demethylation step from lanosterol to ergosterol.

For hair infections, griseofulvin, a secondary metabolite of the fungus *Penicillium griseofulvum*, is a safe, effective drug prescribed orally for the management of tinea capitis. This compound is fungistatic and appears to work by affecting the microtubular system of fungi. It interferes with the mitotic spindle and cytoplasmic microtubules. The molecular action of griseofulvin is different from that of other inhibitors, such as colchicine and the vinca alkaloids, which bind to receptors on tubulin and inactivate the free subunits of microtubules.

Subcutaneous Mycoses

The subcutaneous mycoses comprise a wide spectrum of fungal infections characterized by the development of lesions, usually at sites of trauma where the organism is implanted in the tissue (Fig. 69–13). The infections initially involve the deeper layers of the dermis, subcutaneous tissue, or bone. Most infections have a chronic and insidious growth pattern that eventually extends into the epidermis and are expressed clinically as lesions on the skin surface.

This group of infections has several features in common. The patient can usually remember trauma (e.g., a splinter, a thorn, a bite, the implantation of other foreign bodies) at the infection sites, after which lesions developed. The infections occur on parts of the body that are most prone to trauma (e.g., feet, legs, hands, arms, buttocks). The etiologic agents are commonly found in the soil or on decaying vegetation.

Several bacterial infections (e.g., actinomycotic mycetoma, botryomycosis, atypical acid-fast disease) mimic the subcutaneous fungal infections. It is extremely important to establish the etiologic agent, because most of the bacterial infections can be managed with antibiotics. Finally, with one or two exceptions, the subcutaneous mycoses are difficult to treat, and

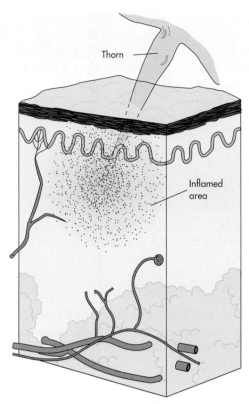

FIGURE 69–13. Schematic of tissue level colonized primarily by agents causing subcutaneous mycoses. The fungus gains access to the deeper layers of skin by traumatic implantation. The organisms implicated in these disease processes are usually common fungi found in the soil.

surgical intervention (e.g., excision or amputation) may be indicated.

Etiology and Clinical Syndromes

Most subcutaneous fungal infections, with the exception of lymphocutaneous sporotrichosis, are rare and are considered exotic in the United States and other highly developed countries. The diseases less frequently or rarely seen are chromoblastomycosis, phaeohyphomycosis, chronic subcutaneous zygomycosis, and eumycotic mycetoma. Two diseases, lobomycosis and rhinosporidiosis, are considered to be caused by fungi, but culture fails to isolate the etiologic agent.

The causative agents are a heterogeneous group of organisms with low pathogenic potential that are commonly isolated from soil or decaying vegetation. The clinical manifestations of these diseases appear to results from an interplay between the etiologic agent and host responses. In general, patients who experience disease have no underlying immunologic defect.

Lymphocutaneous Sporotrichosis

Lymphocutaneous sporotrichosis, a chronic infection characterized by nodular and ulcerative lesions, devel-

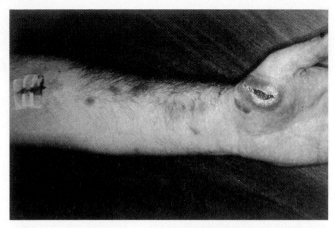

FIGURE 69–14. Clinical case of lymphocutaneous sporotrichosis. The characteristic pattern of lesions along the lymphatic system that drain the site of the original lesion is shown.

ops along the lymphatic glands that drain the primary site of inoculation (Fig. 69–14). Other infrequently seen forms of sporotrichosis are fixed cutaneous lesions, primary and secondary pulmonary sporotrichosis, and disseminated disease. The etiologic agent is the dimorphic fungus *Sporothrix schenckii*.

Chromoblastomycosis

Chromoblastomycosis is characterized by the development of verrucous (warty) nodules that appear at sites of inoculation (Fig. 69–15). As lesions progress, they appear to vegetate and take on a cauliflower-like appearance. The organisms responsible for chromoblastomycosis are common soil inhabitants collectively called the **dematiaceous fungi**. The term *dematiaceous* is used to describe fungi that have brown to black melanin pigments in their cell walls (see also the section on tinea nigra).

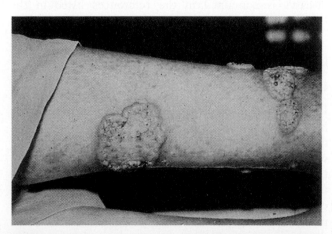

FIGURE 69–15. Clinical case of chromoblastomycosis. The characteristic verrucous vegetative lesions are illustrated.

Phaeohyphomycosis

Phaeohyphomycosis is actually a heterogeneous group of cutaneous diseases caused by various dematiaceous fungi. The most common form described is phaeohyphomycotic cyst. The disease does not exhibit the intense hyperplasia seen in chromoblastomycosis, and when organisms are seen during histopathologic examination of tissue, they usually appear as pigmented, septate hyphal fragments.

The taxonomy of the dematiaceous agents is undergoing careful scrutiny, and as yet, complete agreement has not been reached. The dematiaceous fungi most often associated with chromoblastomycosis are *Fonsecaea pedrosoi*, *Fonsecaea compacta*, *Cladosporium carrionii*, and *Phialophora verrucosa*. These organisms are identified according to the pattern and type of sporulation exhibited by the isolate. In many cases, the isolate may exhibit more than one pattern of sporulation; for this reason, confusion and conflicts often arise concerning the correct taxonomic placement of the organism.

Similar taxonomic problems exist in the identification of agents implicated in phaeohyphomycosis, for which about 40 different organisms have been identified. Included in this large number of etiologic agents are some rare fungi that undoubtedly reflect the exotic nature of some of these clinical entities.

Eumycotic Mycetoma

The term *mycetoma* is clinically descriptive and includes a wide spectrum of manifestations of the skin and deeper tissues of the dermis and subcutaneous tissues. The disease is characterized by indolent, deforming, swollen lesions that contain numerous draining sinus tracts.

Other Subcutaneous Mycoses

Zygomycosis, lobomycosis, and rhinosporidiosis are rare clinical entities. A detailed description of these diseases is contained in the references listed in the Bibliography at the end of this chapter.

Laboratory Diagnosis

Lymphocutaneous Sporotrichosis

In tissue and in cultures incubated at 37°C, *S. schenckii* is a budding yeast cell. Cultures incubated at 25°C develop as delicate, radiating colonies that appear within 3 to 5 days on most media. The colonies are initially moist and white; they slowly take on a brown to black pigmentation with prolonged incubation. Microscopic examination reveals delicate branching hyphae about 2 μm in diameter, with numerous conidia developing in a rosette pattern at the ends of conidio-

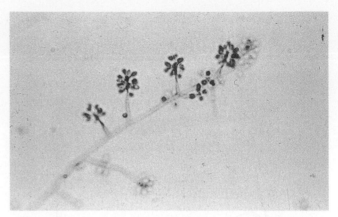

FIGURE 69-16. Microscopic examination illustrating the rosette pattern of conidia in *Sporothrix schenckii*.

phores (Fig. 69–16). Laboratory confirmation is established by conversion of the mycelial growth to yeast morphology through subculture at 37°C.

Chromoblastomycosis

The diagnosis of chromoblastomycosis is usually made through histopathologic examination of clinical material taken from the lesions. A characteristic tissue response of the disease is pseudoepitheliomatous hyperplasia, an epithelial overgrowth caused by an abnormal multiplication in the number of normal cells in normal arrangement in the tissue. In addition to the histopathologic features, copper-colored, spherical cells in various stages of cell division are seen (Fig. 69–17). These structures, called "sclerotic" or **Medlar bodies**, are the tissue forms of the fungus.

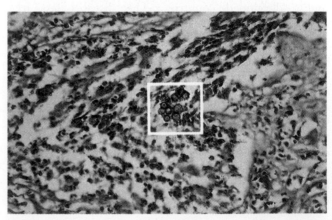

FIGURE 69-17. Tissue section taken from a case of chromoblastomycosis. The characteristic "sclerotic" cells are shown.

Eumycotic Mycetoma

Examination of the purulent fluid from the sinus tracts in eumycotic mycetoma often reveals small grains of fungal tissue. These elements may be white, brown, yellow, or black and can be well-demonstrated on histopathologic examination of lesion biopsy specimens (Fig. 69–18). The etiologic agents causing these diseases consist of various bacteria belonging to the genera *Actinomyces*, *Nocardia*, *Streptomyces*, and *Actinomadura* as well as a whole host of fungi, including *Pseudallescheria boydii* and *Madurella grisea*. It is important to establish the cause of the disease by culturing specimens, because the clinical management of the infection varies according to the causative organism.

Treatment

Subcutaneous lymphangitic sporotrichosis responds dramatically to a saturated solution of potassium iodide given orally. Adverse side effects include gastrointestinal upset and dermatologic problems, which are rapidly reversed by discontinuation of therapy. Extracutaneous sporotrichosis invariably requires systemic therapy with amphotericin B.

Cautery and surgical removal of early lesions are used in the treatment of chromoblastomycosis; however, most patients who seek help have advanced disease. The extensive tissue involvement is often not amenable to surgical intervention and requires chemotherapy. The drug of choice for treating chromoblastomycosis is 5-fluorocytosine. This drug, which is given orally, acts by inhibiting RNA and DNA synthesis.

As stated previously, the clinical treatment of eumycotic mycetoma varies with the causative agent. In the case of actinomycotic mycetomas, several antibacterial antibiotics can be used. For example, infections by

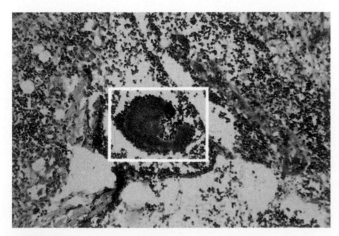

FIGURE 69–18. Histopathologic section of tissue taken from mycetoma. A microcolony (often referred to as a *granule*) is illustrated.

Actinomyces israelii respond to high doses of penicillin, and those by *Nocardia asteroides* respond to sulfa drugs and streptomycin. However, if a fungal organism is the causative agent and the disease is extensive, the physician frequently resorts to total excision of the lesion or amputation of an affected limb, because antifungal therapy in general is unsuccessful.

CASE STUDIES AND QUESTIONS

■ The school nurse was informed that three first-grade boys had scaly, patchy alopecia. She examined them for nits but found none, so she sent them home with instructions for them to be seen by their pediatrician. The pediatrician confirmed that nits were not the problem.

1. What should the pediatrician have done to confirm the diagnosis of tinea capitis?
2. Should their siblings and the rest of the classroom have been examined?
3. What are some interesting epidemiologic, clinical, and pathophysiologic features of tinea capitis, tinea pedis, and tineas due to anthropophilic, zoophilic, and geophilic fungi?

■ Two healthy construction laborers were seen by a dermatologist after developing painless bilateral ulcerative lesions along the lymphatics of their forearms. On examination, both patients were afebrile. The dermatologist noted regional lymphadenopathy, and the lesions extended up the lymphatics as tender erythematous subcutaneous nodules, some of which were fluctuant. Histories taken from the patients revealed that these lesions began to appear 2 to 3 weeks after the two laborers had demolished an attic as part of an urban renewal project. Both stated that they got splinters from carrying salvaged wood from the rafters. They also commented that bats and pigeons had roosted in the attic and that a lot of dust was raised during the salvage.

1. What was the most likely diagnosis, and how should the diagnosis have been confirmed?
2. What generalizations can you make about subcutaneous mycotic infections?
3. What are the therapeutic strategies used in the various subcutaneous mycoses?

BIBLIOGRAPHY

Larone DH: *Medically important fungi: a guide to identification*, ed 2, New York, 1987, Elsevier Science.

Martin AG, Kobayashi GS: Superficial fungus infection: dermatophytosis, tinea nigra, piedra. In Friedman IM et al: *Fitzpatrick's dermatology in general medicine*, ed 5, New York, 1999, McGraw-Hill.

Padhye A, Weitzman I: The dermatophytes. In Ajello L,

Hay RJ, editors: *Topley and Wilson's microbiology and microbial diseases*, vol 4. *Medical mycology*, London, 1998, Arnold.

Rebell G, Taplin D: *Dermatophytes: their recognition and identification*, Coral Gables, Fla, 1979, University of Miami.

CHAPTER 70

Systemic Mycoses

The organisms classified as systemic mycotic agents are inherently virulent and cause disease in healthy humans. Five fungi are included in this group: *Histoplasma capsulatum, Blastomyces dermatitidis, Paracoccidioides brasiliensis, Coccidioides immitis*, and *Cryptococcus neoformans*. Each of these fungi exhibits biochemical and morphologic features that enable it to evade host defenses.

Four of these pathogens (*H. capsulatum, B. dermatitidis, P. brasiliensis*, and *C. immitis*) are dimorphic. They grow as filamentous molds as saprobes and in culture at 25°C; however, when they infect humans or are cultured at 37°C, they transform to a unicellular morphology (Fig. 70–1*A* to *D*). Tissue infections caused by *H. capsulatum, B. dermatitidis*, and *P. brasiliensis* are characterized by the presence of budding yeast cells (Fig. 70–1*A* to *C*), whereas *C. immitis* infections are characterized by the presence of spherules (sporangium-like structures filled with endospores) (Fig. 70–1*D*).

Unlike the dimorphic pathogens, *C. neoformans* is monomorphic, growing as a yeast within infected tissue and culture at 25°C or 37°C (Fig. 70–1*E*). A characteristic feature of *C. neoformans* is that it possesses an acidic mucopolysaccharide capsule.

The primary focus of infection for the systemic fungi is the lung. In most cases, the respiratory infections are asymptomatic or of very short duration, resolve rapidly without therapy, and are accompanied by a high degree of specific resistance to reinfection in the host. In some cases, the infection spreads to a secondary organ. Each organism exhibits its own characteristic pattern of secondary organ involvement. The secondary spread of systemic disease frequently causes the patient to seek medical attention. The etiologic agent and the host's immune status determine the severity of infection. The infection can be life-threatening if therapy is not rapidly instituted and the underlying disorder not corrected for patients whose immune status is compromised because of underlying disease or immunosuppressive therapy. In addition, immunosuppression may cause reactivation of latent infection.

Four of the systemic mycoses (histoplasmosis, blastomycosis, paracoccidioidomycosis, and coccidioidomycosis) tend to be restricted to particular geographic regions. However, the ease of travel and increases in reactivation of disease are starting to blur these distinctions.

Histoplasmosis

Histoplasmosis results from **inhalation** of conidia or hyphal fragments of *H. capsulatum* (Fig. 70–2). It occurs worldwide and is particularly common in midwestern United States (Fig. 70–3). In most cases, it is asymptomatic, but in about 5% of the cases, clinical symptoms of an acute pneumonia occur, followed less often by a progressive disseminated disease. Histoplasmosis is also known as Darling's disease, reticuloendothelial cytomycosis, cave disease, and spelunker's disease (Box 70–1).

Morphology

The mold phase of *H. capsulatum* is characterized by thin, branching, septate hyphae that produce microconidia and tuberculate macroconidia (Fig. 70–4). The parasitic or tissue phase of *H. capsulatum* is a small, budding yeast cell that is 2 to 5 μm in diameter and found almost exclusively within macrophages (Fig. 70–5). The sexual state of *H. capsulatum* is designated *Ajellomyces capsulatus* and is classified as an ascomycete.

Epidemiology

The etiologic agent of histoplasmosis, *H. capsulatum* var. *capsulatum*, grows in soil with a high nitrogen content, especially in areas contaminated with the excreta of bats and birds (starlings and chickens, in particular). Birds are not infected, whereas natural infection does occur in bats. The fungi are isolated from soil samples taken from various bird and bat habitats (e.g., chicken coops, attics, barns, woodpiles, caves, roosting areas such as city parks and even schoolyards). Numerous

Saprobic phase
(25° C)

Parasitic phase
(37° C)

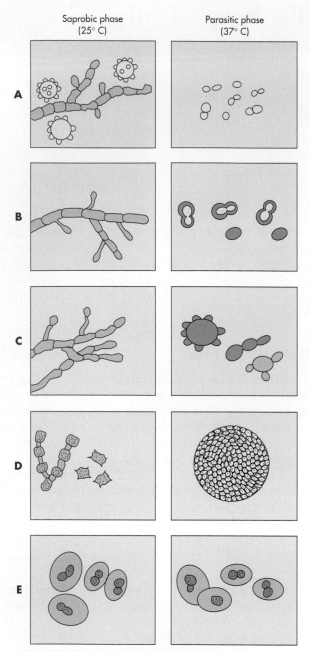

FIGURE 70–1. Saprobic and parasitic phases of systemic pathogenic fungi. *A, Histoplasma capsulatum. B, Blastomyces dermatitidis. C, Paracoccidioides brasiliensis* exhibits mold-to-yeast transition when infecting susceptible species. *D, Coccidioides immitis* exhibits mold-to-spherule transition when it infects susceptible species. *E, Cryptococcus neoformans* is an encapsulated yeast at 25°C, 37°C, and in infected tissues.

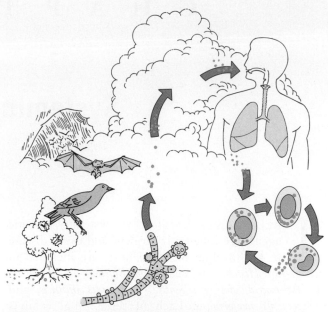

FIGURE 70–2. Natural history of the saprobic and parasitic cycles of *Histoplasma capsulatum.*

efforts to document the outbreaks, have accidentally acquired the disease while exploring suspected sites to obtain soil samples.

Histoplasmosis is widely distributed throughout the temperate, subtropical, and tropical zones of the world. Some areas within these zones are highly endemic, including the Ohio and Mississippi Valley regions of the United States, the southern fringes of the provinces of Ontario and Quebec in Canada, and scattered areas of Central and South America (see Fig. 70–3). Surveys of skin test reactivity to histoplasmin indicate that at

well-documented epidemics of respiratory histoplasmosis have occurred when environments harboring the fungi have been disturbed by activities such as exploring caves (spelunking), demolishing old buildings during urban renewal, cleaning chicken coops, and setting up campsites. Researchers and epidemiologists, in their

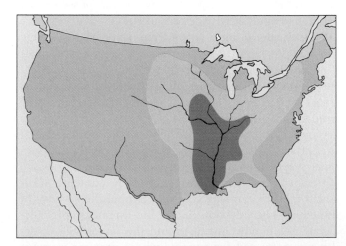

FIGURE 70–3. Endemic areas of histoplasmosis in North America. *Dark purple shading* indicates area of high endemism. *Light purple shading* indicates area of moderate endemism.

BOX 70–1. Summary of Histoplasmosis

Etiological Agent

Asexual phase: *Histoplasma capsulatum*.
Sexual phase: *Ajellomyces capsulatus*.

Mycology

Dimorphic; mycelia at 25°C; typical tuberculate macroconidia (8–14 μm in diameter); microconidia (2–4 μm
in diameter).
At 37°C and in tissue, this organism is a budding yeast
(2–3 × 3–4 μm in diameter).
Organism is found predominantly in histocytes.

Epidemiology and Ecology

Organism occurs throughout temperate, subtropical, and
tropical areas of the world. Endemic areas include the
Ohio and Mississippi River valleys and parts of Central
and South America.
The organism has been isolated from numerous soil samples, particularly those contaminated by bat, chicken,
and starling droppings. Bats are naturally infected, but
birds are not.
A unique clinical form occurs in Africa; it is caused by *H.
capsulatum* var. *duboisii*.

Clinical Disease

The clinical symptoms vary, depending on the degree of
individual exposure and immunologic state of the patient.
About 95% of all primary cases are not referable to
specific symptoms.
Acute pneumonia develops in 5% of cases.
Less than 1% of infections become progressive and require therapy. In this case, an underlying condition of
debilitation or immunosuppression usually makes these
people prone to life-threatening disease.

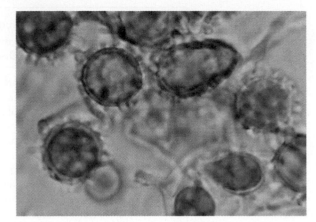

FIGURE 70–4. Tuberculate macroconidia and microconidia of *Histoplasma capsulatum*.

thereby containing the infection. Transient fungemia occurring before the development of immunity accounts for the distribution of calcified granulomas in the liver and spleen that are frequently seen at autopsy of patients from endemic areas. Viable organisms may persist in the host after resolution of uncomplicated histoplasmosis; they are the presumed source of disseminated disease in immunocompromised patients who do not have a history of recent exposure. The major clinical syndromes associated with *H. capsulatum* infection are summarized in Table 70–1.

An estimated 500,000 people in the United States are exposed to *H. capsulatum* each year; however, most people infected with *H. capsulatum* have a high degree of natural resistance to the organism. Few, if any, overt symptoms appear, and the disease resolves rapidly. Approximately 5% of infections result in symptomatic disease, usually as an acute, self-limited, influenza-like illness with various degrees of pulmonary involvement. Symptoms usually resolve without specific antifungal

least 80% of the long-term residents of the Ohio and Mississippi River valleys have been infected with *H. capsulatum*. Serial studies of individuals living in endemic areas show that skin test reactivity can be lost and reacquired, suggesting that the high incidence of reactivity in these areas results from reinfection.

Cases of histoplasmosis have also been reported in Europe and Asia. A variant form of histoplasmosis occurs in Africa; the etiologic agent of this disease has been designated *H. capsulatum* var. *duboisii*.

Clinical Syndromes

The lung is the usual portal of entry for infection. Conidia or hyphal fragments of *H. capsulatum* are inhaled, are phagocytosed by pulmonary macrophages, and then convert to yeasts, which are able to replicate in macrophages (see Fig. 70–5). In an immunocompetent host, macrophages acquire fungicidal activity,

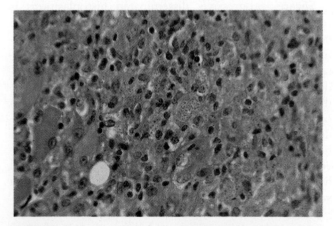

FIGURE 70–5. Yeast cells of *Histoplasma capsulatum* phagocytosed by mononuclear cells (Giemsa stain).

TABLE 70–1. Classification of Histoplasmosis

Type of Infection	Specific Disorder	Comments
Histoplasmosis in normal hosts	Asymptomatic or mild influenza-like illness	Occurrence with normal exposure
	Acute pulmonary histoplasmosis	Occurrence with heavy exposure
	Rare complications	Pericarditis, mediastinal fibrosis
Opportunistic infection	Disseminated histoplasmosis	Occurrence in people with immune defects
	Chronic pulmonary histoplasmosis	Occurrence in people with structural defects

therapy. An overly vigorous host immune response can occasionally result in complications such as mediastinal fibrosis, which is the development of hard fibrous tissue in the upper mediastinum that causes compression, distortion, or obliteration of the superior vena cava and sometimes constriction of the bronchi and large pulmonary vessels.

H. capsulatum can also cause progressive and potentially fatal disease when host defenses are impaired. In a small number of cases, the initial infection is not cleared and the disease progresses to disseminated histoplasmosis. This condition is characterized by continued intracellular replication of *H. capsulatum* yeasts within macrophages, presumably caused by a defect in cell-mediated immunity. Clinically, infection ranges from acute, life-threatening, disseminated histoplasmosis to chronic, mild, disseminated histoplasmosis, depending on the extent of parasitization of the mononuclear phagocytic system. Patients frequently complain of fever, night sweats, and weight loss. Mucosal lesions are also common and may be the primary clinical finding in an otherwise healthy-appearing individual.

Severe, progressive, disseminated histoplasmosis is reported with increasing frequency in adults who have hematologic malignancies and who are receiving immunosuppressive therapy (particularly chronic corticosteroid therapy) or who have acquired immunodeficiency syndrome (AIDS). In these settings, disseminated histoplasmosis is best described as an opportunistic infection. Infection with human immunodeficiency virus (HIV-1) may trigger reactivation of dormant *H. capsulatum*. Central nervous system involvement, an unusual complication of disseminated histoplasmosis, has also been reported in association with AIDS.

Chronic pulmonary histoplasmosis is most often encountered in patients with underlying chronic obstructive pulmonary disease. Because of structural defects in the lung, *H. capsulatum* can escape normal defense mechanisms and cause progressive, destructive lesions similar to tuberculosis.

In Africa, a distinct clinical form of histoplasmosis is seen. It involves primarily the bone and subcutaneous tissues.

Laboratory Diagnosis

The diagnosis of histoplasmosis is based on serologic findings, direct histopathologic examination of infected tissue, and culture of the etiologic agent. Diagnosis of disseminated histoplasmosis requires demonstration of the organism in extrapulmonary sites. This is best accomplished by a combination of culture and histopathologic examination of tissue.

The antigenic reagents used in the serologic tests for histoplasmosis are derived from two sources: the cell-free culture filtrate from the mycelial phase of growth (histoplasmin) and inactivated, whole yeast phase cells. Both reagents are used because neither type of antigen detects antibodies in all cases.

In general, delayed skin test reactivity to histoplasmin develops within 2 weeks after exposure. This test is of little diagnostic or prognostic value and may be misleading because in a significant percentage of the hypersensitive patients, serologic titers may become elevated as a result of skin testing with the reagent (anamnestic response). For this reason, the skin test should not be used in the diagnostic workup of a patient.

Two serologic tests are frequently used to diagnose histoplasmosis. The complement fixation test is the standard test, and the results are positive later in disease (6 weeks or longer after symptoms occur). Complement fixation tests, which measure antibodies directed against *H. capsulatum*, are performed using histoplasmin and intact formalin-treated yeast as the antigens. Serum complement fixation titers of at least 16 or a fourfold rise in titer suggests histoplasmosis;

however, false-positive reactions can occur because of cross-reactive antibodies associated with other fungal infections and tuberculosis. Complement fixation titers decline after infection in normal hosts. Fewer than 5% of individuals have a positive complement fixation reaction in areas where the rate of positive skin test results is high. A single serologic test does not allow a reliable diagnostic or prognostic interpretation and might cause a delay in instituting specific therapeutic measures. However, serologic tests of two or more serum specimens taken at suitable intervals during the acute and convalescent phases of infection yield information of great diagnostic and prognostic value.

The immunodiffusion test detects antibodies to the H and M antigens of *H. capsulatum* (Fig. 70–6) and is more specific but less sensitive than complement fixation. Serologic tests can aid in the diagnosis of histoplasmosis but do not distinguish disseminated disease from other forms of histoplasmosis. Furthermore, the results of these tests can be negative in 25% or more of patients who have disseminated histoplasmosis.

In contrast to traditional serologic tests, direct detection of *H. capsulatum* antigens in blood or urine may prove valuable for rapid diagnosis of disseminated disease. Intracellular yeast can often be seen by histopathologic examination of infected tissue, especially bone marrow, blood, and lung, using special stains, thus permitting rapid diagnosis. *H. capsulatum* can be cultured from bone marrow or blood in more than 75% of cases of disseminated histoplasmosis. Sputum cultures are useful in the diagnosis of chronic pulmonary histoplasmosis but are usually negative in cases of acute, self-limited disease. *H. capsulatum* usually takes 1 to 2 weeks to grow in culture. Preliminary identification of the isolate is based on morphologic features, including delicate septate hyphae with tuberculate macroconidia (see Fig. 70–4).

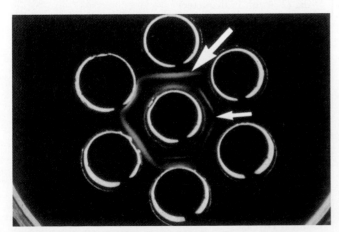

FIGURE 70–6. Immunodiffusion illustrating H *(short arrow)* and M *(long arrow)* precipitin bands that form when histoplasmin is tested against sera containing reactive antibodies.

In the past, confirmation was based on the ability to convert the culture morphology from the mycelial phase to the yeast phase, a process that can require weeks to months. Use of an exoantigen test now permits confirmation as soon as sufficient growth occurs. In the exoantigen test, antigens are extracted from the agar medium that supports fungal growth and are tested for their reaction against antihistoplasma antibody in an immunodiffusion test. Positive identification is made when precipitin lines of identity form with control histoplasmin antigens.

A rapid DNA probe test that has been developed uses nucleic acid hybridization for rapid identification of *H. capsulatum* grown from clinical material. The test is based on the ability of complementary nucleic acid strands specifically to align and associate to form stable, double-stranded complexes. A commercially available test uses a chemiluminescent-labeled, single-stranded DNA probe that is complementary to the ribosomal RNA isolated from the unidentified culture. The test result is read in a luminometer, which allows for the differentiation between hybridized and nonhybridized probes.

Treatment

Amphotericin B remains the mainstay of treatment for disseminated histoplasmosis and other severe forms of the disease. In patients with AIDS, however, relapses after the completion of therapy are a significant problem, and lifelong suppressive therapy must be considered.

Blastomycosis

Blastomycosis, also called Chicago disease, Gilchrist's disease, and North American blastomycosis, is caused by inhalation of conidia of *B. dermatitidis* (Fig. 70–7). Primary pulmonary infections are often inapparent and difficult to document, even radiologically. The forms of disease most often seen clinically are ulcerative lesions of the skin and lytic bone lesions, both of which represent systemic or disseminated disease (Box 70–2).

Morphology

B. dermatitidis is closely related biochemically and serologically to *H. capsulatum*. The sexual phase of *B. dermatitidis* has been discovered. It is classified as an ascomycete and designated *Ajellomyces dermatitidis*, the same genus as the sexual state of *H. capsulatum*.

Epidemiology

The geographic distribution of blastomycosis is limited to the North American continent and parts of Africa. Blastomycosis, like histoplasmosis, is endemic in the

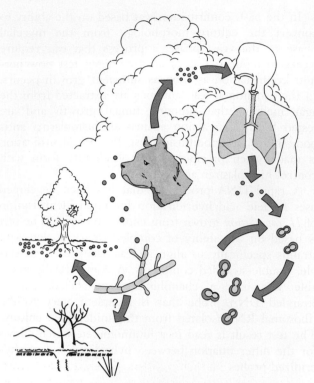

FIGURE 70–7. Natural history of the saprobic and parasitic cycle of *Blastomyces dermatitidis*.

Ohio and Mississippi Valley regions and to a lesser extent the Missouri and Arkansas River basins. Additional endemic sites have been found in Minnesota, Southern Manitoba, and Southwest Ontario, including the St. Lawrence River basin. Epidemics have occurred in Wisconsin, Minnesota, Illinois, and in the eastern states of Virginia and North Carolina. It has also been reported in a wide geographic area of Africa. In endemic areas, natural disease exists among dogs and horses and is an important veterinary problem. The veterinary profile is similar to the clinical and pathologic disease in human infections. Untreated, blastomycosis in animals may have a rapid and fatal course.

The natural reservoir for the agent of blastomycosis is unknown. Unlike *H. capsulatum*, *B. dermatitidis* is rarely cultured from soil in endemic areas. The organism is believed to be present in the soil but flourishes only in a narrow, yet undefined ecologic niche.

Clinical Syndromes

The natural history of *B. dermatitidis* infections is not as well documented as that of *H. capsulatum* infections because of the lack of reliable serologic tests and characteristic radiographic findings. Manifestations of symptomatic blastomycosis, an uncommon disease, often indicate systemic spread. Large numbers of asymptomatic infections presumably occur, analogous to histoplasmosis.

Inhalation of *B. dermatitidis* conidia produces a primary pulmonary infection in the host. As with *H. capsulatum*, *B. dermatitidis* conidia convert to yeast and are phagocytosed by macrophages, which may carry them to other organs. The initial infection can be symptomatic or asymptomatic. Chest radiographs may show nonspecific pulmonary infiltrates; however, unlike histoplasmosis, resolution of these lesions is not accompanied by calcifications. Primary pulmonary disease can have three outcomes: resolution without involvement of other organs, progressive pulmonary disease, or resolution of the pulmonary infection followed by systemic disease.

Laboratory Diagnosis

Serologic and immunologic findings for blastomycosis are unclear. Two antigenic preparations are used in tests to detect the immune response to infection by *B. dermatitidis*: cell-free culture filtrate of the mycelial phase (blastomycin) and inactivated whole yeast phase cells. The data obtained from skin testing and serologic studies are difficult to interpret because the antigenic preparations are poorly defined. The reagents tend to be highly cross-reactive with etiologic agents of other mycoses, particularly those of histoplasmosis and coccidioidomycosis.

An immunodiffusion test that appears to be specific

BOX 70–2. **Summary of Blastomycosis**

Etiological Agent

Asexual phase: *Blastomyces dermatitidis*.
Sexual phase: *Ajellomyces dermatitidis*.

Mycology

Dimorphic; mycelia at 25°C; typical pyriform microconidia (2–4 μm in diameter).
At 37°C and in tissue, this organism is a yeast (8–15 μm in diameter).
Buds produced singly are attached to the parent cell by a broad base.

Epidemiology and Ecology

Geographically, the organism is limited to the North American continent and parts of Africa. The area of endemism in the United States overlaps that for histoplasmosis.
Blastomycosis is an important veterinary problem, and dogs develop a disease similar to that in humans.
There are few reports of successful isolation of this organism from soil.

Clinical Disease

Primary infection in the lung is often inapparent, although epidemics of respiratory blastomycosis have been documented.

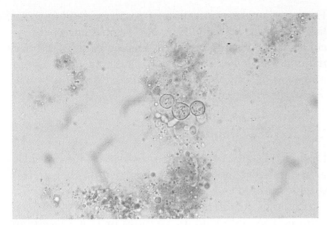

FIGURE 70–8. Broad-based budding yeast cells of *Blastomyces dermatitidis* seen in purulent material expressed from a microabscess.

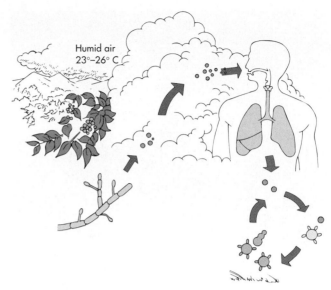

FIGURE 70–9. Natural history of the saprobic and parasitic cycle of *Paracoccidioides brasiliensis.*

for blastomycosis has been developed. It is based on a yeast phase culture filtrate, designated A antigen. Suitable control sera containing antibodies that react with A antigen must be included with patient sera in immunodiffusion studies.

Diagnosis of blastomycosis requires identification of the organism in infected tissue or isolation in culture. Microscopic examination reveals characteristic broad-based, budding yeast cells (Fig. 70–8) in purulent abscess fluid that has been treated with potassium hydroxide or in biopsy specimens of stained skin lesions. The organism grows readily in culture. It is identified by its conversion from the mycelial phase to the yeast phase or by the exoantigen test.

Treatment

Amphotericin B remains the mainstay of therapy for patients with systemic disease or serious pulmonary disease, particularly in immunocompromised patients. Uncomplicated pulmonary disease may respond to fluconazole.

Paracoccidioidomycosis

Paracoccidioidomycosis is a pulmonary disease resulting from inhalation of infectious conidia of *P. brasiliensis* (Fig. 70–9). Pulmonary infections are often asymptomatic. The most common form exhibits ulcerative lesions of the oral and nasal cavity. The disease is also called South American blastomycosis and Lutz-Splendore-Almeida disease (Box 70–3).

Morphology

P. brasiliensis is dimorphic, growing as a mold in the environment and as budding yeast in infected tissue. The yeast phase is characterized by multipolar budding

from a single cell (Fig. 70–10). The transition from mold to yeast can be induced in vitro by raising the temperature from 25°C to 37°C. Studies show that as little as 10^{10} M-17-β-estradiol significantly inhibits the transformation of mycelia to yeast at 37°C. Testoster-

---

BOX 70–3.   **Summary of Paracoccidioidomycosis**

Etiological Agent

Asexual phase: *Paracoccidioides brasiliensis.*
Sexual phase: Not known.

Mycology

Dimorphic; mycelia at 25°C; no typical pattern of sporulation.
At 37°C and in tissue, this organism is a yeast with several budding cells attached to the parent cell, some in a ship's wheel arrangement.
Yeasts are 2–30 μm in diameter.

Epidemiology and Ecology

This disease is geographically limited to Central and South America. The major focus of the disease is Brazil.
Females are as susceptible to infections as males, but the incidence of clinical disease is about 9 times higher in males.
The organism has been isolated from the soil on rare occasions.

Clinical Disease

Primary pulmonary disease is often inapparent.
Disseminated disease often causes ulcerative lesions of the buccal, nasal, and occasionally gastrointestinal mucosa.

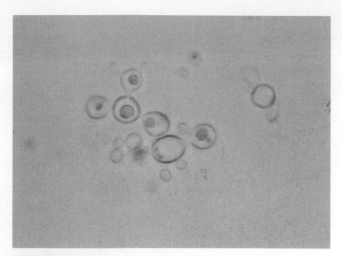

FIGURE 70–10. Multipolar budding characteristic of the yeast phase of *Paracoccidioides brasiliensis.*

one, corticosterone, and 17-α-estradiol have no inhibitory effect on the transition of the mycelia phase to the yeast phase at 37°C. The findings may have clinical significance (see the following discussion on epidemiology). A sexual state for *P. brasiliensis* has not been described.

Epidemiology

Paracoccidioidomycosis is geographically restricted to Central and South America, having a high incidence in Brazil, Venezuela, and Colombia. The endemic areas have been delineated by data taken from extensive skin test surveys and case reports. Like *B. dermatitidis, P. brasiliensis* cannot routinely be cultured from soil in endemic areas. Careful, retrospective epidemiologic studies and data from a report on the isolation of *P. brasiliensis* from soil samples suggest that the fungi reside in environments that have high humidity and average temperatures around 23°C.

Results of skin test surveys indicate an equal distribution of reactors between male and female patients. However, analysis of data from clinically significant disease indicates that the number of male patients affected is disproportionate to the number of female patients (9:1). This difference has been attributed to high-risk factors, underlying disease, malnourishment, and hormonal differences. Inhibition of the mycelia-to-yeast transition by β-estradiol may also account for the lower incidence of disseminated paracoccidioidomycosis in women.

Clinical Syndromes

The prominence of oral and nasal lesions led to the belief that infection resulted from local inoculation.

However, primary infection of paracoccidioidomycosis, like the other systemic mycoses, is now known to occur in the lungs as a result of inhaling conidia. Primary pulmonary paracoccidioidomycosis is frequently asymptomatic but can develop into progressive pulmonary disease or disseminated disease.

Laboratory Diagnosis

Diagnosis of paracoccidioidomycosis, as with histoplasmosis and coccidioidomycosis, is based on detection of specific antibodies, visualization of the organism in histopathologic material, and isolation of the organism in culture. Two antigenic preparations of *P. brasiliensis* are used for serologic diagnosis: a cell-free culture filtrate of the mycelial phase (paracoccidioidin) and an inactivated whole yeast phase preparation. These serologic reagents are not routinely available in the United States. Specific antibodies are measured by complement fixation and immunodiffusion.

The organism can be seen in potassium hydroxide preparations of infected material or in silver-stained histologic sections. The presence of numerous small, budding cells arranged around a large, mature cell (ship's wheel pattern) is diagnostic of *P. brasiliensis* (see Fig. 70–10). However, in the absence of buds, the yeast of *P. brasiliensis* may be confused with immature spherules of *C. immitis* or the nonbudding yeast of *B. dermatitidis* or *H. capsulatum.* Clinical material that is cultured on medium incubated at 25°C yields a slow-growing white mold after 10 to 14 days of incubation. Microscopic examination of the growth is usually not diagnostic because *P. brasiliensis* does not sporulate readily. Transfer of the culture to incubation at 37°C yields a yeastlike growth with characteristic multipolar budding cells.

Treatment

Successful treatment of paracoccidioidomycosis generally requires long-term therapy. Amphotericin B is effective against all forms of paracoccidioidomycosis, but because of toxicity and the difficulty of long-term administration, it is usually reserved for severe cases. Sulfa drugs have been used for decades to treat disease; however, treatment failures can occur despite therapy that lasts for years. Ketoconazole and the newer azole agents are very active in vitro against *P. brasiliensis* and appear to be clinically effective.

Coccidioidomycosis

Inhalation of the arthroconidia of *C. immitis* causes an acute, self-limited, and usually benign respiratory infection (Fig. 70–11). The condition may be asymptomatic, or it may vary in degree from the mildness of a

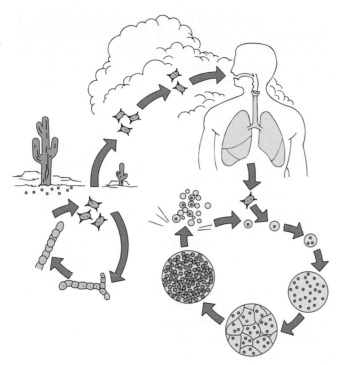

FIGURE 70–11. Natural history of the saprobic and parasitic cycle of *Coccidioides immitis*.

common cold to the severity of a disseminated life-threatening disease. Coccidioidomycosis has also been called Posada-Wernicke disease, San Joaquin Valley fever, and desert rheumatism (Box 70–4).

Morphology

C. immitis is a dimorphic fungus that grows as a filamentous mold in the environment. The mycelia fragment to produce cylindric arthroconidia (Fig. 70–12).

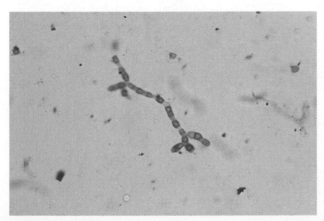

FIGURE 70–12. Hyphae and arthroconidia of *Coccidioides immitis*.

BOX 70–4. **Summary of Coccidioidomycosis**

Etiological Agent

Asexual phase: *Coccidioides immitis*.
Sexual phase: Not known.

Mycology

Dimorphic; mycelia at 25°C.
As the culture ages, the septate hyphae mature such that alternate cells develop into arthroconidia separated by vacuolated cells.
The arthroconidia separate readily and have a barrel-shaped appearance.
In tissue and at 37°C, the organism develops into large, spherical structures (10–60 μm in diameter) called *spherules* (sporangia) that are filled with endospores 2–5 μm in diameter.

Epidemiology and Ecology

This disease is geographically restricted to North, Central, and South America, where there are areas of high endemism. In North America, the disease is highly endemic in the San Joaquin Valley of California, the Southwestern part of the United States, and the northern states of Mexico.
Natural infection occurs in domestic and wild animals.
The organism has been repeatedly isolated from soil samples taken from an endemic area.

Clinical Disease

Approximately 60% of these infections are asymptomatic.
The most common symptoms of primary disease are cough, fever, and chest pain. Night sweats and joint pain are not unusual.
An epidemiologic history should be taken to determine whether the patient has been in an endemic area.

The tissue phase of *C. immitis* is the spherule (Fig. 70–13), a multinucleated structure that undergoes internal cleavage to produce uninucleate endospores that can then generate new spherules. A sexual state has not been observed for *C. immitis*.

Epidemiology

Coccidioidomycosis, which can be described as a disease of the New World, is geographically limited to the North, Central, and South American continents (Fig. 70–14). The areas of highest endemism have a semiarid climate and include the central San Joaquin Valley in California, Maricopa and Pima Counties in Arizona, and several western and southwestern counties in Texas. The disease is also endemic in the northern states of Mexico and parts of Venezuela, Paraguay, and Argentina. Cases of coccidioidomycosis have also been reported in Central America. The organism can be

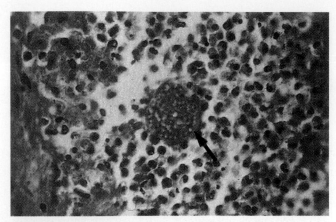

FIGURE 70–13. Spherule phase of *Coccidioides immitis* as seen in stained tissue section.

routinely isolated from soil in areas of high endemism. Although geographically restricted, the organism has on occasion spread extensively as a result of large dust storms.

Clinical Syndromes

The natural history of coccidioidomycosis has been well characterized because large groups of nonimmune individuals who have migrated to endemic areas could be studied (e.g., military personnel stationed in the San Joaquin Valley during World War II). Exposure to *C. immitis*, compared with *H. capsulatum*, causes a greater percentage of individuals to undergo a mild febrile to moderately severe respiratory disease. However, a high degree of innate immunity generally exists in the adult population. Approximately 40% of individuals develop a symptomatic pulmonary infection after exposure to the organism. These primary infections are usually self-limited, but in a small proportion of patients, *C. immitis* causes progressive pulmonary disease or disseminates to produce extrapulmonary disease that mainly involves the meninges, skin, or both.

Laboratory Diagnosis

Two sources of antigens, both of which are cell-free culture filtrates, are used in the preparation of serologic reagents: the mycelial phase of growth (coccidioidin) and the spherule phase (spherulin). Skin test reactivity to coccidioidin develops 2 to 4 weeks after symptoms. The tube precipitin and the complement fixation tests are the time-honored serologic procedures used to diagnose coccidioidomycosis. Precipitins appear early, between 2 and 4 weeks after symptoms, followed by the appearance of complement-fixing antibodies.

Other methods of detecting specific antibodies, such as latex particle agglutination and agar immunodiffusion, are now available. These tests largely replace the tube precipitin and complement fixation tests as routine screening methods because they are more sensitive in detecting specific antibodies of infected individuals, are commercially available, and are easily performed. In the immunodiffusion test, two lines of precipitation are significant: one line associated with the antigen that detects precipitin and agglutinating antibodies and another line associated with the complement-fixing antibodies. Once the presence of an infection has been established, complement fixation titers can yield important prognostic information. High, persistent, or rising titers indicate a high probability of disseminated disease. *C. immitis* spherules can be seen on infected tissue stained with hematoxylin and eosin. The organism can be cultured on conventional media; however, it must be handled with caution because *C. immitis* is a leading cause of laboratory-acquired infections. Although the mold phase of *C. immitis* is highly suggestive of the organism, arthroconidia are found in several saprobic fungi; therefore, definitive identification is based on conversion to spherules or a specific exoantigen test.

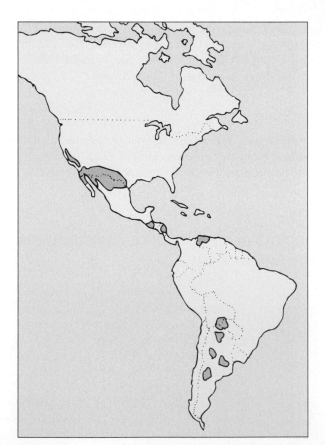

FIGURE 70–14. Geographic distribution of coccidioidomycosis in North, Central, and South America *(shaded).*

BOX 70–5. Summary of Cryptococcosis

Etiological Agent

Asexual phase: *Cryptococcus neoformans.*
Sexual phase: *Filobasidiella neoformans.*

Mycology

Monomorphic.
This organism is a yeast at 25°C and 37°C. The unique feature of the yeast is the acidic mucopolysaccharide capsule.

Epidemiology and Ecology

This disease is worldwide in distribution. This yeast has been repeatedly isolated from sites inhabited by pigeons, particularly from their roosts and droppings. Pigeons are not naturally infected.

Clinical Disease

Primary pulmonary cryptococcosis is usually inapparent but may be chronic, subacute, or acute.
The clinical entity most often seen is cryptococcal meningitis.
Osseous and cutaneous disease can be present without apparent neurologic involvement.

Treatment

Amphotericin B is the drug of choice for the treatment of serious coccidioidal infections. Meningeal infections are particularly difficult to treat, partly because of the poor penetration of amphotericin B into cerebrospinal fluid. Fluconazole is effective in suppressing infections, but relapses occur after ceasing therapy.

Cryptococcosis

Cryptococcosis, also called Busse-Buschke disease, torulosis, or European blastomycosis, is a chronic to acute infection caused by *C. neoformans* (Box 70–5). There are two varieties of *C. neoformans: C. neoformans* var. *neoforman* (serotypes A and D) and *C. neoformans* var. *gatti* (serotypes B and C). In contrast to the other systemic mycotic agents, dimorphism does not have a role in the pathogenesis of *C. neoformans* because the organism is an encapsulated yeast in culture at 25°C and 37°C and in tissues. Several putative virulence factors of *C. neoformans* have been identified. The capsular polysaccharide, for example, inhibits phagocytosis. Another virulence factor appears to be phenoloxidase, an enzyme that converts phenolic compounds to melanin. The lung is the primary site of infection; however, the organism has a high predilection for systemic spread to the brain and meninges (Fig. 70–15). *C. neoformans* is the leading cause of fungal meningitis and is an impor-

tant cause of morbidity and mortality in patients with AIDS and in transplant recipients. *C. neoformans* also produces systemic disease in patients who have no apparent underlying immunologic disorder.

Morphology

Unlike the other systemic mycotic agents, the asexual phase of *C. neoformans* is not dimorphic. The organism grows as a budding yeast in infected tissue and in culture at 25°C and 37°C. The most distinctive feature of *C. neoformans* is the presence of an acidic mucopolysaccharide capsule. This capsule is required for pathogenicity and is important diagnostically, in terms of both antigen detection and specific histologic staining. The sexual phase of *C. neoformans* has been discovered; it is *Filobasidiella neoformans* and is classified as a basidiomycete (see Chapter 7). There is speculation that the basidiospore may be the infectious propagule, but it has not been identified.

Epidemiology

C. neoformans serotypes A and D are recovered in large numbers from the excreta and debris of pigeons. Thus, the organism appears to survive well in a desiccated, alkaline, nitrogen-rich, and hypertonic environment. It has a close relationship with the habitats of pigeons, but the organism does not appear to infect the bird naturally. The natural reservoir of *C. neoformans* var.

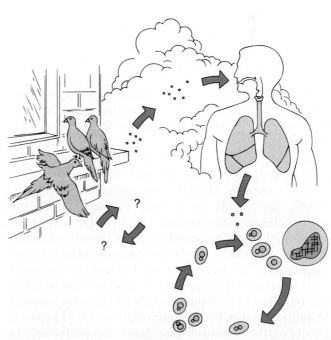

FIGURE 70–15. Natural history of the saprobic and parasitic cycle of *Cryptococcus neoformans.*

gatti (serotype B) was unknown until it was isolated from the tree sap of *Eucalyptus camaldulensis* (red gum). Cryptococcosis occurs throughout the world. The true prevalence of infection is unknown because of the lack of a reliable skin test or another serologic screening test, but subclinical infections are believed to be common. Symptomatic cryptococcal disease, mainly meningitis, is frequently encountered in individuals who are debilitated, immunosuppressed, or otherwise compromised. However, some patients who develop cryptococcal meningitis have no underlying immune or metabolic defects.

Clinical Syndromes

Primary pulmonary infections are frequently asymptomatic and may be detected as incidental findings on a routine chest radiographic examination. A solitary pulmonary nodule that can mimic a carcinoma is most commonly observed; the correct diagnosis is usually made when the mass is resected. *C. neoformans* can also produce a symptomatic pneumonia characterized by diffuse pulmonary infiltrates.

Cryptococcal meningitis, which is caused by hematogenous spread of yeast from the lungs to the meninges surrounding the brain, is the most frequently diagnosed form of cryptococcosis. Symptoms usually include the combinations of headache, mental status changes, and fever lasting several weeks. Cryptococcal disease of the central nervous system may occasionally take the form of an expanding intracerebral mass that causes focal neurologic deficits. Other common manifestations of disseminated cryptococcosis include skin lesions and osteolytic bone lesions.

Laboratory Diagnosis

Unlike the serologic procedures used to diagnose the other systemic mycoses, the serologic procedures used in the diagnosis of cryptococcosis are based on the detection of antigens, not antibodies. The latex agglutination test for the detection of cryptococcal polysaccharide antigens in cerebrospinal fluid and serum is routinely used in clinical laboratories; it is sensitive, specific, and simple to perform. The test involves the use of latex particles coated with a rabbit anticryptococcal antibody. The capsular polysaccharide present in a clinical specimen binds to the antibodies, thereby agglutinating the latex particles. Because the latex particles are coated with antibodies, false-positive reactions can be caused by rheumatoid factor (immunoglobulin M antibodies that bind immunoglobulin G). Therefore, an appropriate control test must be performed in which the clinical specimen is mixed with latex particles coated with nonimmune rabbit antibodies. In addi-

tion, the patient's serum can be treated with a protease to destroy any proteins that might cause nonspecific agglutination of the latex particles. Rare cross-reactions occur with sera from patients with disseminated infections caused by *Trichosporon beigelii*. To evaluate the clinical progress of a patient during therapy, serial samples of cerebrospinal fluid are examined for the presence of cryptococcal antigen. A favorable prognosis is indicated by a decrease in the titer of antigen.

A rapid diagnosis of cryptococcal meningitis can often be made by examination of an India ink preparation of cerebrospinal fluid. *C. neoformans* appears as a single cell or budding yeast surrounded by a clear halo because of the exclusion of the ink particles by the polysaccharide capsule (Fig. 70–16).

Although diagnosis may be rapid with the India ink preparation, test results are positive in only half of cryptococcal meningitis cases. Culture remains the definitive method for documenting infection. The organism grows well on standard, nonselective mycologic media but is inhibited by cycloheximide, an antibiotic used to suppress the growth of saprobes. Identification of *C. neoformans* is based on the presence of a capsule, the production of the enzyme urease, the assimilation pattern of carbon substrates, and other specific biochemical reactions.

Treatment

Whereas pulmonary cryptococcosis is frequently a self-limited infection or can be cured by surgical excision of a solitary nodule, disseminated cryptococcosis is almost always fatal if untreated. Cryptococcal meningitis remains the model for combination therapy with antifungal agents. Amphotericin B is active against *C. neoformans* but exhibits relatively poor penetration into cerebrospinal fluid. Although 5-fluorocytosine has good

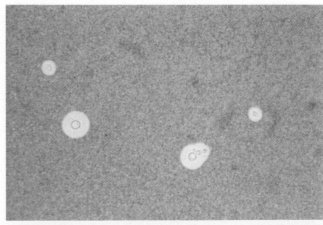

FIGURE 70–16. Encapsulated budding yeast cells of *Cryptococcus neoformans* highlighted with India ink.

cerebrospinal fluid penetration, the development of resistant cryptococci is a problem. Controlled clinical trials have shown that combination therapy with amphotericin B and 5-fluorocytosine for 6 weeks is as effective as amphotericin B alone for 10 weeks. Nonetheless, relapses after either treatment regimen remain a problem, particularly in patients with AIDS.

CASE STUDY AND QUESTIONS

■ About 7 to 10 days after exploring a bat cave in Missouri, three of five members of a spelunkers club who had gone on the expedition complained of influenza-like symptoms and made appointments to see their internist. Patient A was febrile and had a nonproductive cough but was otherwise fine. Patient B, who was HIV-positive, was febrile, had a very deep cough, and complained of night sweats, chest pains, and tender joints. Patient C could not see his internist immediately and waited a week for his appointment. When this patient was seen, he was asymptomatic and said that after taking a couple of aspirin with a lot of water and getting 3 days of rest, he felt "fit as a fiddle." The remaining two spelunkers said that they felt fine and did not experience any of the described symptoms. During the course of examination, all of the spelunkers remarked that bats had roosted in the cave and a great deal of dust was raised during their exploration.

1. What was the diagnosis, and what should have been done to confirm it?
2. What are the geographic distributions of and the endemic areas for (a) coccidioidomycosis, (b) histoplasmosis, (c) blastomycosis, (d) paracoccidioidomycosis, and (e) cryptococcosis?
3. What are the distinguishing morphologic features of the etiologic agents of the systemic mycoses (a) in nature and (b) in tissue?
4. What is interesting about the epidemiology of (a) paracoccidioidomycosis, (b) coccidioidomycosis, (c) histoplasmosis, (d) blastomycosis, and (e) cryptococcosis?
5. What concern should have been shown for the patient who was also HIV-positive?

BIBLIOGRAPHY

Hay RJ: Fungal infections. In Friedman IM et al: *Fitzpatrick's dermatology in general medicine*, ed 5, New York. 1999, McGraw-Hill.

Kwon-Chung KJ, Bennett JE: *Medical mycology*, Philadelphia, 1992, Lea & Febiger.

Sarosi GA, Davies SF, editors: *Fungal diseases of the lung*, Orlando, Fla, 1986, Grune & Stratton.

Szaniszlo PJ, editor: *Fungal dimorphism: with emphasis on fungi pathogenic for humans*, New York, 1985, Plenum.

CHAPTER 71

Opportunistic Mycoses

Humans are constantly exposed to viable fungal propagules. Most tolerate these exposures with no resulting sequelae, but some develop an allergic hypersensitivity (see Chapter 66). There are at least two reasons for this. First, healthy, immunologically competent people have a high degree of innate resistance to fungal colonization. Second, most fungi have low inherent virulence. Under conditions that lead to host debilitation, however, many people become susceptible to fungi. If the infection is not rapidly diagnosed and aggressively treated and if the underlying conditions causing host debilitation are not brought under control, the fungal infection may become life-threatening. These infections, once considered rare and exotic, have become more common and of great medical significance. This is because of acquired immunodeficiency syndrome (AIDS) and the increased use of radiation and cytotoxic drug therapy to treat organ transplant recipients or patients with malignancies. Because these fungi become pathogens by taking advantage of the host's debilitated condition, they are commonly called opportunistic fungi.

A growing list of exotic and rare fungi has been implicated in opportunistic infections, but most such infections are caused by various species of *Candida* (e.g., *Candida albicans*), *Aspergillus* (e.g., *Aspergillus fumigatus*), and various Zygomycetes (e.g., *Rhizopus arrhizus*). Although **opportunistic pathogens** is the term used to define these organisms, it is based on the clinical setting and has no taxonomic significance. Two of the most common opportunistic pathogens, *C. albicans* and *A. fumigatus*, have notably different biologic properties and host interactions. In addition, pathogenicity is not an all-or-nothing phenomenon. Individual species within both *Candida* and *Aspergillus* genera exhibit a range of pathogenicity.

Pneumocystis carinii is a noteworthy etiologic agent of opportunistic infections. It is a unicellular eukaryotic organism that causes a severe interstitial plasma cell pneumonia. This organism was once classified as a protozoan; however, ultrastructural studies providing immunologic and molecular genetic evidence indicate that it is closely related phylogenetically to fungi. This parasitic organism is unique, however, because it has features (in particular, its putative life cycle) that distinguish it from other fungi.

Numerous other fungi have been implicated as etiologic agents of opportunistic infections of humans. A cursory examination of the literature supports the contention that the list of exotic and rare species of fungi causing infectious problems is large and continues to grow. For further details, see the bibliography at the end of this chapter.

Candidiasis

Several species of *Candida* are implicated in candidiasis (Box 71–1). Candidiasis is a major disease problem of immunocompromised hosts. The clinical spectrum of manifestations ranges from superficial infections of the skin to systemic life-threatening infections. Under various conditions, *C. albicans*, *Candida tropicalis*, *Candida kefyr* (formerly *Candida pseudotropicalis*), *Candida glabrata* (formerly *Torulopsis glabrata*), and *Candida parapsilosis* are part of the normal flora of humans. They can be isolated from healthy mucosal surfaces of the oral cavity, vagina, gastrointestinal tract, and rectal area. As many as 80% of people may show colonization of these sites in the absence of disease.

In contrast, the organism is rarely isolated from the surface of normal human skin except sporadically from certain intertriginous areas (i.e., skin surfaces that appose each other) such as the groin. Under certain circumstances, these organisms gain hematogenous access from the oropharynx or gastrointestinal tract when the mucosal barrier is breached (e.g., inflammation of mucous membranes secondary to chemotherapy) or when intravenous catheters and syringes are contaminated. The organs most often involved include the lungs, spleen, kidneys, liver, heart, and brain. *Candida* organisms may produce endophthalmitis (inflammation involving the eyes), indicating hematogenous dissemination of *C. albicans* and the possibility of multiorgan involvement. Skin lesions may occur in 10% to 30% of

*Formerly called *Candida pseudotropicalis*.
†Formerly called *Torulopsis glabrata*.
AIDS = acquired immunodeficiency syndrome.

patients with disseminated infections. Early recognition of such lesions is important in diagnosis because antemortem blood cultures are negative in a high percentage of patients with autopsy-proven systemic candidiasis.

Morphology

With one exception, a striking morphologic feature of the yeasts in the genus *Candida* is that they multiply by forming blastospores, pseudohyphae, and septate hyphae (see Chapter 7). *C. glabrata*, a yeast implicated in urinary tract infections and systemic disease in debilitated people, is the exception, producing only yeast cells.

Clinical Syndromes

The spectrum of infections caused by organisms in the genus *Candida* includes localized diseases of the skin and nails; diseases that affect the mucosal surfaces of the mouth, vagina, esophagus, and bronchial tree; and diseases that disseminate and involve many organ systems. Candidal diseases involving the skin and nails frequently mimic dermatophyte infections. In all cases, the diagnosis must be supported by microscopically observing fungi in lesion specimens and must be confirmed by culture of the organism. Factors leading to a predisposition to the various candidal infections are summarized in Box 71–1.

Chronic mucocutaneous candidiasis (CMC) is a heterogenous group of clinical syndromes characterized by chronic treatment-resistant superficial *Candida* infections of the skin, nails, and oropharynx (see Immunity and Host Factors). Despite extensive cutaneous involvement, patients have virtually no propensity for disseminated visceral candidiasis. In many cases, narrow but specific abnormalities in T-cell–mediated immunity are found. In others, the defects are more general. Various underlying conditions, such as hypoparathyroidism, hypoadrenalism, hypothyroidism, and the presence of circulating autoimmune antibodies, have been associated with CMC. In adults, CMC is frequently associated with thymoma. When cutaneous candidiasis suggests the possibility of an immunologic or endocrine disorder, efforts must be made to uncover and to correct the underlying defect so that the fungal infection can be properly treated.

Disseminated candidiasis is usually spread through the blood stream and therefore involves many organs. Severe neutropenia is considered to be the most significant predisposing factor for life-threatening infections. The incidence of this form of candidiasis is steadily rising as more patients with serious hematologic malignancies are treated aggressively with potent immunosuppressive drugs and as more patients undergo bone marrow and organ transplantation (Fig. 71–1).

Whereas disseminated candidiasis continues to be a major problem in immunocompromised hosts, this is not the case in patients with AIDS, who develop serious infections of the oropharynx and upper gastrointestinal tract but rarely experience systemic disease. The development of oral candidiasis in previously healthy adults not receiving corticosteroid therapy or broad-spectrum antibiotic therapy should strongly alert the physician to consider infection with human immunodeficiency virus.

Immunity and Host Factors

Innate immunity to these organisms in healthy adults appears to be strong. The immune mechanisms responsible for protection against candidal infections include humoral and cell-mediated processes. Based on experiments with CMC indicating that a defect in cell-mediated immunity leads to extensive superficial candidiasis despite normal or exaggerated humoral defenses, cell-mediated processes are considered to be more important immune mechanisms.

Production of serum antibody to the principal wall

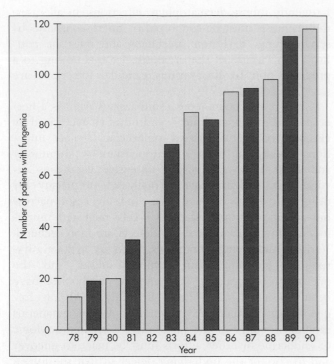

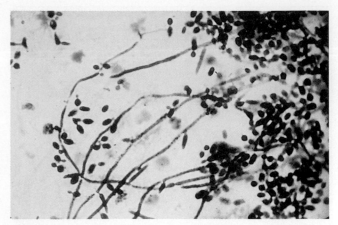

FIGURE 71–2. Sputum specimen illustrating budding yeast cells and pseudohyphae of *Candida* species.

FIGURE 71–1. Incidence of culture-proven candidal fungemia at Barnes Hospital (St. Louis) from 1978 to 1990.

glycoprotein antigens of the *Candida* species occurs in low titers in healthy people. The protective role of these antibodies, however, is controversial, and their presence may reflect only an immunologic response to colonization of the gastrointestinal tract early in life. For this reason, serodiagnosis of candidiasis is not routinely performed. In certain experimental studies, such as the passive transfer of serum, a slight degree of protection may be provided. In the clinical setting, however, it is clear that patients with primarily B-cell deficiency states are not at high risk for infection by *Candida* organisms. Evidence for the role of secretory immunoglobulin A in limiting mucosal infections is confusing. It is probable that various innate, non-immune host factors in conjunction with cell-mediated immunity and complement activation contribute more to host defense against *Candida* organisms than humoral immunity.

Laboratory Diagnosis

The *Candida* species most often responsible for these infections include *C. albicans*, *C. tropicalis*, *C. kefyr*, *C. glabrata*, *C. krusei*, and *C. parapsilosis*. In histopathologic sections and sputum, they may produce budding yeast cells, pseudohyphae, and septate hyphae (Fig. 71–2). On solid media, the organisms produce yeast and pseudohyphal cells, and the gross appearance of the colony is opaque, cream-colored, and pasty. The species of all yeasts cultured from blood, cerebrospinal fluid, and

surgical specimens should be identified. Laboratory standards should be set for identification of yeasts from sputum, urine, and other nonsterile sources, because yeasts may be part of the normal flora or transient colonizers. Several procedures are available for identification; most combine morphologic, physiologic, and biochemical tests. A rapid and reliable test to identify *C. albicans* is the germ tube test. Blastospores of *C. albicans* produce hyphal outgrowths (germ tubes) when they are suspended in serum and incubated at 37°C (Fig. 71–3).

For the test to be valid, the suspension must be examined within 2 to 3 hours after incubation because other species may form similar structures with longer incubation. A few isolates of *C. albicans* do not form germ tubes under these conditions. Therefore, other tests based on biochemical and physiologic properties of the organisms are performed, such as the ability to assimilate various sugars or produce morphologic struc-

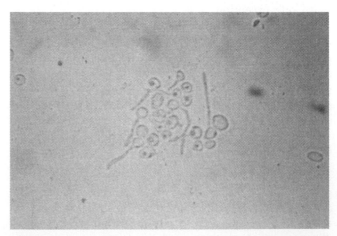

FIGURE 71–3. Development of germ tubes by *Candida albicans* yeast cells after incubation in serum for 2 hours at 37°C.

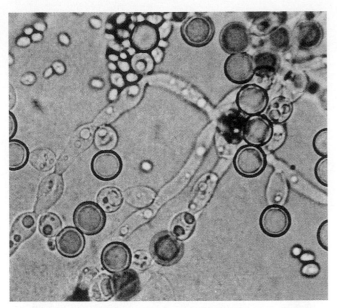

FIGURE 71-4. Formation of chlamydospores by *Candida albicans* when cultured on cornmeal agar at 25°C.

tures (e.g., chlamydospores) (Fig. 71-4) under certain growth conditions.

Treatment, Prevention, and Control

In immunologically competent patients, topical treatment is usually preferred for cutaneous and mucocutaneous disease, and except for disease of the nails, a good clinical response generally results when proper therapy is instituted. Therapy for systemic disease varies depending on the organ involvement and immune status of the patient. For systemic disease, amphotericin B alone or combined with 5-fluorocytosine may be indicated. Alternative therapy includes the use of the azole derivatives. Ketoconazole and fluconazole are preferred because they are active when given orally and less toxic than amphotericin B. The azole derivatives are fungistatic, however, and in many cases the disease recurs after therapy is discontinued. Fungal infections in immunosuppressed patients pose a problem because the underlying conditions leading to immunosuppression must be corrected to obtain maximal response from the antifungal treatment. Patients who are intubated or are connected to various support catheters must be monitored closely; lines must be changed frequently so that they do not become contaminated and serve as foci for fungal colonization. See Chapter 67 for further details about treatment, prevention, and control.

Aspergillosis

The spectrum of medical problems caused by various species of *Aspergillus* is broad (Table 71-1). Organisms belonging to this genus are extremely common in the environment. In contrast to most infections caused by *Candida* organisms, aspergillosis is acquired from exogenous sources. As a result, assessing the significance of culture reports may be difficult unless the organism is seen in histopathologic specimens.

Morphology

These organisms are identified in culture by their morphologic features, the pattern of conidiophore development, and the color of the formed conidia (Fig. 71-5). Species of *Aspergillus* are extremely common in the environment, and several have been implicated as etiologic agents. Of the approximately 900 described *Aspergillus* species, *A. fumigatus* and *A. flavus* have been most frequently associated with invasive disease.

Clinical Syndromes

Normal, healthy individuals are not susceptible to systemic aspergillosis. It is purely an opportunistic infection. As with candidiasis, the type of disease evoked depends on the local or general physiologic and immunologic state of the host. Factors that lead to host debilitation are also important in aspergillosis. In contrast to candidiasis, the etiologic agents implicated in aspergillosis are ubiquitous in the environment and are not part of the normal flora of humans, although transient colonization may occur. These agents are involved in many animal diseases, such as mycotic abortion of sheep and cattle and pulmonary infections of birds, and their metabolites serve as carcinogenic agents in animals that have ingested contaminated feed. Because of their diverse involvement in both human and animal disease, these agents pose a great economic problem.

Allergic aspergillosis may initially occur as a benign

TABLE 71-1. Diseases Associated with *Aspergillus* Species

Disease	Etiologic Agent
Mycotoxicoses	Ingestion of contaminated food products
Hypersensitivity pneumonitis	Allergic bronchopulmonary disease
Secondary colonization	Fungal colonization of preexisting cavity (e.g., pulmonary abscess) without invasion into contiguous tissues
Systemic disease	Invasive disease involving many organs

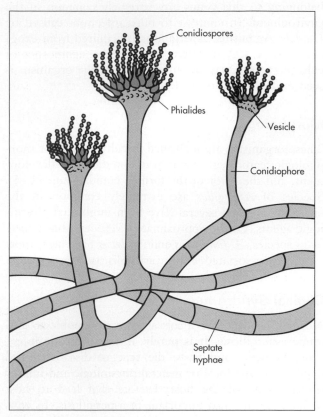

FIGURE 71–5. Asexual fruiting structure of *Aspergillus* species in culture.

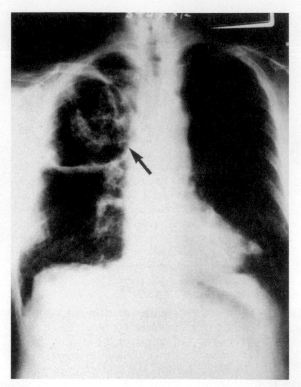

FIGURE 71–6. Chest film illustrating a cavity in the upper right lobe *(arrow)* with an organizing fungus ball.

process and then become severe as the patient grows older. Respiratory distress increases with age, leading to bronchiectasis (chronic dilatation of the air passages). Collapse of a segment of the lung eventually results in fibrosis (scarring).

In secondary colonization, a chronic clinical situation may exist with little distress, except occasional bouts of hemoptysis (coughing up of blood) and pathologic changes in the lungs that lead to the formation of a "fungus ball" (Fig. 71–6). Histopathologically, the fungus ball is a spherical mass of intertwined, branching, septate hyphal elements. These structures can also be visualized radiologically as space-occupying spherical structures that move within the cavity as a patient changes position.

Systemic aspergillosis is an extremely serious disorder that usually is rapidly fatal unless diagnosed early and treated aggressively. In immunosuppressed hosts, the organism spreads from its primary site to contiguous tissues without regard to tissue planes, and lesions frequently contain hyphae within blood vessels, causing infarcts and hemorrhage. As in disseminated candidiasis, the physiologic and immunologic conditions that contribute to the host's increased susceptibility to the infection must be reversed for proper management.

Laboratory Diagnosis

The diagnosis of invasive aspergillosis is considered when septate hyphae that branch at regular intervals and that tend to be oriented in the same direction are seen in clinical specimens (Fig. 71–7). Confirmation of invasive aspergillosis is sometimes difficult because cultures are not always performed or are often negative. Because these organisms exist everywhere in the environment, the clinical and histopathologic diagnosis of

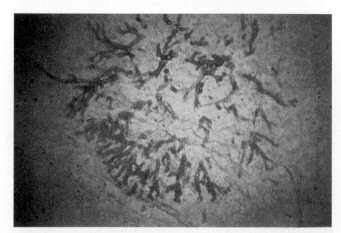

FIGURE 71–7. Dichotomous branching septate hyphae of *Aspergillus fumigatus* in tissue specimen.

invasive aspergillosis is strongly supported by repeated isolation of the organism in culture.

Zygomycosis

Fungi belonging to the Zygomycetes are abundant in the environment. The clinical entity zygomycosis, also termed mucormycosis or phycomycosis, encompasses a spectrum of infections similar to aspergillosis. As with candidiasis and aspergillosis, several underlying factors lead to the host's increased susceptibility to fungi belonging to the class Zygomycetes. Most notable are metabolic acidosis, diabetes mellitus, leukopenia, and other immunosuppressive disorders.

Morphology

Fungi causing the zygomycoses grow rapidly on all laboratory media not containing cycloheximide. *Rhizopus*, *Absidia*, and *Mucor* species have been implicated in zygomycosis. They form coenocytic hyphae (i.e., not separated by cross-walls) and reproduce asexually by producing sporangia, within which develop sporangiospores (Fig. 71–8). These organisms are ubiquitous in the environment and frequently are encountered as contaminants. The relevance of the isolate may be difficult to establish if coenocytic hyphal elements are not seen in the histopathologic section. Repeated isolation of the organism from consecutive specimens provides strong evidence that the organism may be relevant, even though coenocytic hyphal elements are not seen in histopathologic examination of tissue. A point to remember is that all fungi having coenocytic hyphae are classified as Zygomycetes, but not all Zygomycetes are coenocytic.

Clinical Syndromes

Various diseases are caused by organisms belonging to the class Zygomycetes order Mucorales. Rhinocerebral zygomycosis is the most common of the diseases. This infection originates in the paranasal sinuses and can involve the ocular orbit and palate with extension into the brain. It usually occurs as a terminal event in acidotic patients with metabolic disorders or uncontrolled diabetes mellitus. Other forms of zygomycosis afflicting immunosuppressed or otherwise debilitated patients involve the lungs, gastrointestinal tract, and subcutaneous tissues. In severely burned patients, these organisms colonize the damaged tissues and tend to become invasive. In disseminated disease, the organism shows a marked predilection for invading major blood vessels. The emboli (clots) that result cause ischemia (obstruction of blood vessels) and necrosis of adjacent tissues.

Laboratory Diagnosis

These organisms are filamentous, and their distinct morphology helps identify them in microscopic examination of pathologic material. The hyphal filaments are coenocytic and have a ribbon-like appearance in tissue specimens (Fig. 71–9). Cultures grown on medium not containing antibiotics are dense and appear hairy. Microscopic examination of this growth confirms the coenocytic nature of the hyphae, and sporulating species produce characteristic sporangia (asexual fruiting bodies) (see Fig. 71–8) that contain sporangiospores. The most frequently encountered agents of zygomycosis are *R. arrhizus* and *Absidia corymbifera*. Assessing reports on the number and variety of species that may cause disease is often difficult because culture frequently fails to isolate the organism. Therefore, the diagnosis is often based on histopathologic examination of tissue.

Pneumocystis carinii Pneumonia

Disease caused by *P. carinii* is associated with various clinical conditions of debilitation, particularly those associated with age, congenital and iatrogenically induced immunosuppression, and AIDS. It primarily afflicts premature and malnourished children in crowded insti-

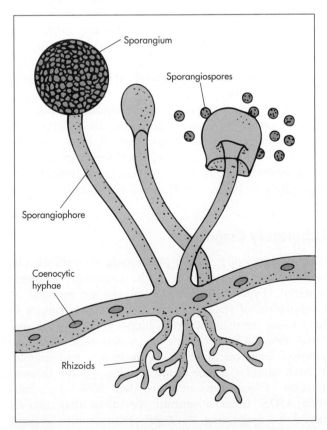

FIGURE 71–8. Asexual fruiting structure of *Rhizopus* species.

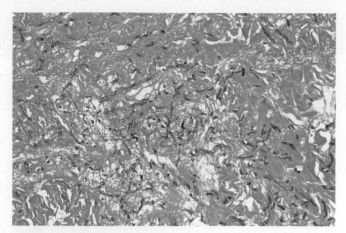

FIGURE 71–9. Histologic section from a case of zygomy-cosis. Ribbon-like, broad, nonseptate (coenocytic) hyphae (stained with Gomori methenamine silver) are illustrated.

tutions such as orphanages and hospitals. It is also encountered in adults in chronic disease wards and is a common opportunistic infection in patients with AIDS and other immune deficiencies. Many patients with AIDS develop pneumonia caused by *P. carinii*, which is a cosmopolitan organism in humans and other mammals. Although rodents are infected with this organism, they probably do not serve as a reservoir for its transmission to humans because comparison of surface antigens and nucleic acid sequences of various genes of rat and human isolates shows distinct differences between these. Transmission from host to host is apparently by droplet inhalation and close contact. This opportunistic organism is present in many persons whose disease is completely asymptomatic. Symptomatic disease develops when some imbalance or debilitating illness (e.g., AIDS) is present, suggesting reactivation of latent infection or a long-term carrier state.

Morphology and Taxonomic Status

Morphologic and molecular genetic evidence indicates that *P. carinii* is closely related phylogenetically to fungi. The cyst wall closely resembles that of fungi; there is excellent homology of the conserved domains of the 16S ribosomal RNA (rRNA) subunit with that of ascomycetes, the 5S rRNA with that of primitive zygomycetous fungi, and the protein synthesis elongation factor (EF-3) with that of *Saccharomyces cerevisiae*. The respiratory tract appears to be the portal of entry, because primary infection is in the lungs. Various stages of the organism's life cycle may be found in Giemsa- and methenamine-stained clinical specimens. The organism may appear in a trophic form (1.5 to 5.0 μm), as a uninucleated sporocyst (4.0 to 5.0 μm), or

as a mature spore case (5.0 μm) containing eight spherical or oval to fusiform spores (1.0 to 3.0 μm). After the mature spore case ruptures to release the intracystic bodies, the cyst wall remains and may be seen as empty oval or collapsed structures. *P. carinii* is atypical when it is compared with other fungi in terms of phenotypic features, the different morphologic forms found in infected tissue, and the refractoriness toward most antifungal antibiotics.

Clinical Syndromes

Evidence from serologic studies indicates that infection with *P. carinii* occurs at an early age and that the organism is common in the environment. Subclinical infections in healthy people are probably frequent, and the organism may remain dormant for a long time. Alveolar macrophages and CD4 T cells have an important role in host defense against *P. carinii*. Patients with AIDS are at high risk for developing disease when their CD4 T-cell count falls below 200 cells/μL^3. The onset of disease is insidious, but it can be suspected in patients who are malnourished or immunocompromised and who develop fever and pneumonitis that are not otherwise explainable.

Interstitial pneumonitis with plasma cell infiltrates is a hallmark of *P. carinii* infections. As the disease progresses, the patient experiences weakness, dyspnea, and tachypnea, leading to cyanosis. Radiologic study of the lungs shows infiltrations spreading from hilar areas, giving the lungs a so-called ground-glass appearance. In these cases, the arterial oxygen tension is low and carbon dioxide tension is normal or low. Death results from asphyxiation.

In the past few years, extrapulmonary infections with *P. carinii* have been described in patients with AIDS. Numerous sites of involvement have been observed, including the ear, eye, liver, and bone marrow. Most patients have received aerosolized pentamidine as a prophylactic to prevent *P. carinii* pneumonia.

Laboratory Diagnosis

The diagnosis of *P. carinii* pneumonia is established by morphologic identification of the organism in clinical material. Typical *P. carinii* organisms are revealed by examination of stained slides of impression smears of lung tissue obtained by brush biopsy (Fig. 71–10), material obtained by percutaneous transthoracic needle aspiration, aspirates of bronchial washings, and sputum. Bronchoalveolar lavage alone is adequate for demonstration of organisms in more than 90% of patients with AIDS. Induced sputum specimens may also be useful for diagnosing *P. carinii* pneumonia in patients with AIDS because of the tremendous number of organisms. The parasites can be stained by Gomori

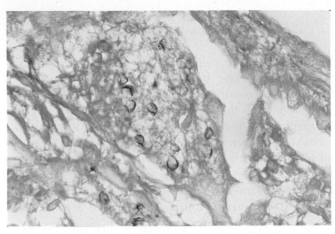

FIGURE 71–10. Gomori methenamine silver–stained section of lung biopsy specimen demonstrates groups of rounded, cup-shaped organisms, 4 to 5 μm in diameter within the intra-alveolar exudate. The staining of the cyst wall and intracystic bodies helps distinguish these organisms from yeast. The cuplike forms and indented shapes are characteristic of *Pneumocystis carinii*.

methenamine silver or the Giemsa method or with calcofluor or specific fluorescein-labeled antibodies. Radiology is of value in establishing the typical appearance of lungs infected with *P. carinii*. Serologic tests have been used for epidemiologic surveys but are not useful as a diagnostic procedure.

Treatment, Prevention, and Control

The treatment of choice includes trimethoprim-sulfamethoxazole or pentamidine isethionate; both may have toxic side effects. Supportive measures such as administration of oxygen and antibiotics may also be indicated. Treatment with amphotericin B or the azole derivatives is not clinically effective in patients with this infection.

Education about transmission of the organism, avoidance of close contact with infected patients, and elimination of possible contact with droplet transmission all are critical, as are prompt diagnosis and treatment. The organism and its transmission are difficult to control because of the extended carrier state and its presence as an opportunistic pathogen. Prophylaxis with trimethoprim-sulfamethoxazole or aerosolized pentamidine may be useful in people with AIDS.

Penicilliosis and Infections Caused by *Penicillium marnefeii*

Except for infections caused by *Penicillium marnefeii*, the role other species of *Penicillium* have in infections of the clinical entity penicilliosis is difficult to confirm because these organisms are ubiquitous in the environ-

ment and are frequently isolated in air samples and as contaminants in laboratory cultures. A historic event occurred in 1929 when Sir Alexander Fleming noticed that a species of *Penicillium* had contaminated his culture of *Staphylococcus aureus*, killing the bacteria in its immediate vicinity and leaving a clear halo around the mold. This serendipitous observation led to the discovery of penicillin.

Morphology

Fungi belonging to this genus are characterized by producing conidiophores at the tips of branching septate hyphae, which in turn may produce secondary structures termed metulae, from which flask-shaped structures called phialides bearing smooth- or rough-shaped conidia are produced in chains, giving the entire structure a brushlike appearance (Fig. 71–11). When mature cultures are disturbed by handling or by air currents, the chains of conidia fragment and contaminate the environment. When they lodge on surfaces such as agar media, they germinate and grow rapidly, producing white filamentous colonies that rapidly mature to produce a powdery bluish green surface growth.

Clinical Syndromes

Because these organisms are abundant in the environment, it is difficult to assess their significance when

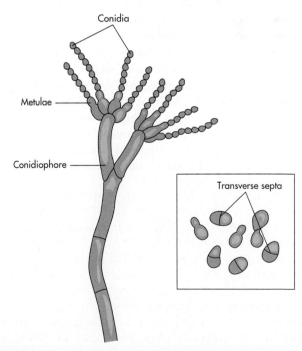

FIGURE 71–11. Conidiophore of *Penicillium marnefeii* illustrating conidiophore, metulae, and conidia growth at 25°C. *Inset* shows yeastlike cells containing transverse septa.

they are isolated from clinical specimens, the exception being *P. marnefeii*. Repeated isolation of the same species of *Penicillium* from clinical material may be significant, provided no other fungal organisms are isolated and branching septate hyphal elements are seen in microscopic examination of tissue taken from the patient. The medical literature cites several case reports that describe the isolation of *Penicillium* species from various clinical specimens taken from patients who are immunosuppressed or otherwise debilitated. However, the role of isolates as the primary etiologic agent has been questioned.

P. marnefeii is the only species of *Penicillium* that is a pathogen. It is primarily a pathogen of the Chinese bamboo rat, *Rhizomys sinisensis*, and has caused spontaneous infections of the human reticuloendothelial system involving the lymphatics, lungs, liver, spleen, and bone. The infection is endemic in Thailand, Vietnam, Indonesia, and neighboring areas of Southeast Asia but has also been diagnosed in some European countries as well as the United States of America. In most cases occurring outside the endemic area, patients have a strong history of having visited endemic sites. The infection has occurred in patients who have no underlying disease but is particularly devastating and severe in patients with AIDS. The organism is morphologically unique in that it is the only species of *Penicillium* that is dimorphic. In cultures at 25°C, it grows as a mold elaborating a pink to reddish pigment that diffuses into the medium. At 37°C on suitable media such as those containing sheep blood or wort agar, the organism transforms into a yeastlike organism that is characterized by globose, ovoid to elliptical cells that divide by producing a transverse septum. The primary site of infection is not known but presumed to be pulmonary. In progressive disease, yeastlike organisms are found in reticuloendothelial cells of various vital organs. Cutaneous lesions and subcutaneous abscesses have been reported. In vitro susceptibility studies indicate that clinical isolates of *P. marnefeii* are highly susceptible to the available antifungals, with itraconazole and ketoconazole being the primary drugs of choice, but in advanced disseminated disease, amphotericin B is recommended.

CASE STUDY AND QUESTIONS

■ A 42-year-old man with end-stage liver disease secondary to hepatitis B underwent liver transplantation. Immunosuppression was maintained with cyclosporine and prednisone therapy. Four months after the surgical procedure, the patient was admitted to the hospital because of persistent fever and hypotension. Examination of his skin revealed ecchymotic lesions over the abdominal surface. Biopsy specimens were taken for histologic examination and culture. Microscopic examination revealed granulomatous inflammation of the deep dermis, and dichotomously branching septate hyphae were seen on special stains. Cultures grew *A. flavus*.

1. What are some of the predisposing factors of opportunistic fungal infections?
2. Why are epidemics of fungal infections rare?
3. Which is more important in opportunistic fungal infections, humoral-mediated or cell-mediated immunity? Why?
4. Is contagion a problem (i.e., should a patient be placed on isolation)?
5. What is the current taxonomic status of *P. carinii* and why is it classified as such?

BIBLIOGRAPHY

Anker van den JN, Popele van NML, Sauer PJJ: Antifungal agents in neonatal candidiasis, *Antimicrob Agents Chemother* 39:1391–1397, 1995.

Dixon DM et al: Fungal infections: a growing threat, *Public Health Rep* 111:226–235, 1996.

Gradon JD, Timpone JG, Schnittman SM: Emergence of unusual opportunistic pathogens in AIDS: a review, *Clin Infect Dis* 15:134–157, 1992.

Hadley KW, Ng VL: Pneumocystis. In Murray PR et al, editors: *Manual of clinical microbiology*, ed 7, Washington, DC, 1999, American Society for Microbiology.

Laitge PF: *Aspergillus fumigatus* and aspergillosis, *Clin Microbiol Rev* 12:310–350, 1999.

Powderly WG: In Merigan TC Jr et al, editors: *Textbook of AIDS medicine*, ed 2, Baltimore, 1998, Williams & Wilkins.

Parasitology

C H A P T E R 7 2

Pathogenesis of Parasitic Disease

Given the wide diversity that exists among human parasites, it is not surprising that the pathogenesis of protozoan and helminthic disease is highly variable. Although the various human parasites exhibit a wide range of **direct** pathogenic mechanisms, in many instances the organisms themselves are not highly virulent or are unable to replicate within the host. Thus, the severity of illness caused by many parasites is related to the infecting dose and the number of organisms acquired over time. Unlike many bacterial and viral infections, parasitic infections are often chronic, lasting months to years. Repeated exposures result in an ever-increasing parasite burden. When infection with a particular organism is associated with a strong immune response, there is undoubtedly a considerable immunopathologic contribution to the disease manifestations attributed to the infection.

Important factors to consider when discussing parasite pathogenicity are listed in Box 72–1. Parasites are almost always exogenous to the human host and thus must enter the body through ingestion or direct penetration of anatomic barriers. Inoculum size and duration of exposure greatly influence the disease-causing potential of an organism. Likewise, the route of exposure is critical for most organisms. For example, pathogenic strains of *Entamoeba histolytica* are unlikely to cause disease on exposure to intact skin but may cause severe dysentery after oral ingestion. Many parasites have active, self-directed means of invading the human host. Once they have invaded, parasites attach to specific host cells or organs, avoid immune detection, replicate (most protozoa and some helminths), produce toxic substances that destroy tissue, and cause disease secondary to the host's own immunologic response (see Box 72–1). In addition, some parasites physically obstruct and damage organs and tissues because of their size alone. In this chapter, factors that are important for parasite pathogenicity are discussed and examples of organisms and disease processes related to each factor are provided.

Exposure and Entry

Although many infectious diseases are caused by **endogenous** organisms that are part of the normal flora of the human host, this is not the case with most diseases caused by protozoan and helminthic parasites. These organisms are virtually always acquired from an **exogenous** source, and, as such, they have evolved numerous ways to enter the body of the human host. The most common modes of entry are oral ingestion or direct penetration through the skin or other surfaces (Table 72–1). Transmission of parasitic diseases is frequently facilitated by contamination of the environment with human and animal wastes. This is most applicable to diseases transmitted by the fecal-oral route but also applies to helminthic infections such as hookworm disease and strongyloidiasis, which rely on larval penetration of the skin.

Many parasitic diseases are acquired via the bites of arthropod vectors. Transmission of disease in this manner is extraordinarily effective, as evidenced by the widespread distribution of diseases such as malaria, trypanosomiasis, and filariasis. Examples of parasites and their ports of entry are listed in Table 72–1. This compilation should not be considered exhaustive; rather, the list provides examples of some of the more common parasites and the means by which they enter the human body.

Additional factors that determine the outcome of the interaction between parasite and host are **route of exposure** and **inoculum size**. Most human parasites have a limited range of organs or tissues in which they can replicate or survive. For example, simple skin contact with most intestinal protozoa does not result in disease; rather, the organisms must be ingested for the disease process to be initiated. Likewise, a minimum number of organisms is required to establish infection. Although some parasitic diseases may be acquired by the ingestion or inoculation of only a few organisms, a sizable inoculum is usually required. Whereas an individual may acquire malaria by a single bite of an infected female mosquito, large inocula are usually necessary to produce diseases such as amebiasis in humans.

BOX 72–1. Factors Associated with Parasite Pathogenicity

Infective dose and exposure
Penetration of anatomic barriers
Attachment
Replication
Cell and tissue damage
Disruption, evasion, and inactivation of host defenses

TABLE 72–1. Parasite Ports of Entry

Route	Examples
Ingestion	*Giardia* species, *Entamoeba histolytica, Cryptosporidium* species, cestodes, nematodes
Direct penetration	
Arthropod bite	Malaria, *Babesia* species, filaria, *Leishmania* species, trypanosomes
Transplacental penetration	*Toxoplasma gondii*
Organism-directed penetration	Hookworm, *Strongyloides* species, schistosomes

Adherence and Replication

Most infections are initiated by the attachment of the organism to host tissues, followed by replication to establish colonization. The life cycle of a parasite is based on species and tissue tropisms, which determine the organs or tissues of the host in which a parasite can survive. The attachment of the parasite to host cells or tissue can be relatively nonspecific, can be mediated by mechanical or biting mouth parts, or can result from the interaction between structures on the parasite surface known as **adhesins** and specific glycoprotein or glycolipid receptors found on some cell types but not on others. Specific surface structures that facilitate parasite adhesion include surface glycoproteins such as glycophorin A and B, complement receptors, adsorbed components of the complement cascade, fibronectin, and N-acetylglucosamine conjugates. Examples of some of the adherence mechanisms identified in human parasites are listed in Table 72–2.

E. histolytica is a good model for the importance of adhesins in virulence. The pathogenesis of invasive am-

ebiasis requires adherence of amebae to the colonic mucous layer, parasite attachment to and lysis of colonic epithelium and acute inflammatory cells, and resistance of the amebic trophozoites to host humoral and cell-mediated immune defense mechanisms. Amebic adherence to colonic mucins, epithelial cells, and leukocytes is mediated by a surface lectin inhibitable by galactose (gal) or N-acetyl-D-galactosamine (GalNAc). Binding of the galactose-inhibitable adherence lectin to carbohydrates on the host cell surface is required for *E. histolytica* trophozoites to exert their cytolytic activity. The presence of the galactose-inhibitable adherence lectin is one feature that distinguishes pathogenic from nonpathogenic strains of *E. histolytica*.

Various attachment mechanisms have been associated with specific infections. For example, the Duffy

TABLE 72–2. Examples of Parasitic Adherence Mechanisms

Organism	Disease	Target	Mechanism of Attachment and Receptor
Plasmodium vivax	Malaria	Red blood cell	Merozoite (non–complement-mediated attachment), Duffy antigen
Plasmodium falciparum	Malaria	Red blood cell	Merozoite and glycophorin A and B
Babesia species	Babesiosis	Red blood cell	Complement-mediated C3b receptor
Giardia lamblia	Diarrhea	Duodenal and jejunal epithelium	Trypsin-activated *G. lamblia* lectin and mannose 6-phosphate *G. lamblia* adherence molecule–1 on disk
Entamoeba histolytica	Dysentery	Colonic epithelium	Lectin and N-acetylglucosamine conjugates
Trypanosoma cruzi	Chagas' disease	Fibroblast	Penetrin, fibronectin, and fibronectin receptor
Leishmania major	Leishmaniasis	Macrophage	Adsorbed C3bi and CR3
Leishmania mexicana	Leishmaniasis	Macrophage	Surface glycoprotein (gp63) and CR2
Necator americanus *Ancylostoma duodenale*	Hookworm	Intestinal epithelium	Mechanical and biting mouth parts

blood group antigen acts as an attachment site for *Plasmodium vivax*. Red blood cells of most West Africans, in contrast to those of Europeans, lack the Duffy antigen. Accordingly, malaria resulting from *P. vivax* is almost unknown in West Africa. The physical structures of parasites may interact with adhesion molecules to promote attachment to host cells. *Giardia lamblia* is a protozoan parasite that uses a ventral disk to attach to the intestinal epithelium by a clasping or suction-like mechanism. Two adhesins, trypsin-activated *G. lamblia* lectin (taglin) and *G. lamblia* adherence molecule-1 (GLAM-1), may also be important in attachment to enterocytes. It is believed that initial contact of the parasite with the intestinal surface is facilitated by taglin, which is distributed over the surface of the parasite, and that the disk-specific GLAM-1 is responsible for the avid attachment of the disk to the enterocyte surface.

After attaching to the specific cell or tissue type, the parasite may undergo replication as the next step in establishing infection. Most protozoan parasites replicate intracellularly or extracellularly in the human host, whereas replication is generally not observed among the helminths capable of establishing human infection.

Temperature may also play an important role in the ability of parasites to infect a host and cause disease. This is well illustrated by the *Leishmania* species. *Leishmania donovani* replicates well at 37°C and causes **visceral** leishmaniasis involving the bone marrow, liver, and spleen. In contrast, *Leishmania tropica* grows well at 25°C to 30°C but grows poorly at 37°C and causes an infection of the **skin** without involvement of deeper organs.

Cell and Tissue Damage

Although some microorganisms may cause disease by localized multiplication and elaboration of potent microbial toxins, most organisms initiate the disease process by invading normally sterile tissue with subsequent replication and destruction. Parasitic protozoa and helminths are generally not known to produce toxins with potencies comparable to those of classic bacterial toxins such as anthrax toxin and botulinum toxin; however, parasitic disease can be established by the elaboration of toxic products, mechanical tissue damage, and immunopathologic reactions (Table 72–3).

Numerous investigators have suggested that toxic products elaborated by parasitic protozoa are responsible for at least some aspects of pathology (see Table 72–3). Proteases and phospholipases may be secreted and are released on the destruction of the parasites. These enzymes can cause host cell destruction, inflammatory responses, and gross tissue pathology. For example, the intestinal parasite *E. histolytica* produces proteinases that can degrade epithelial basement membrane and cell-anchoring proteins, disrupting epithelial cell layers. Furthermore, the amoebae produce phospholipases and an ionophore-like protein that lyse the responding host neutrophils, resulting in the release of neutrophil constituents that are toxic to host tissues. The expression of certain proteinases increases relative to the virulence of the strain of *E. histolytica*.

In contrast to the protozoan parasites, many of the pathogenic consequences of helminthic infections are related to the size, movement, and longevity of the parasites. The host is exposed to long-term damage and immune stimulation as well as to the sheer physical consequences of being inhabited by large foreign bodies. The most obvious forms of **direct damage** from helminthic parasites are those resulting from **mechanical blockage** of internal organs or from the effects of pressure exerted by growing parasites. Large adult *Ascaris* organisms can physically block the intestine and the bile ducts. Likewise, blockage of lymph flow, leading to elephantiasis, is associated with the presence of adult *Wuchereria* organisms in the lymphatic system. Some neurologic manifestations of cysticercosis are due to the pressure exerted by the slowly

TABLE 72–3. Some Pathologic Mechanisms in Parasitic Diseases

Mechanism	Examples
Toxic Parasite Products	
Hydrolytic enzymes, proteinases, collagenase, elastase	Schistosomes (cercariae), *Strongyloides* species, hookworm, *Entamoeba histolytica*, African trypanosomes, *Plasmodium falciparum*
Amebic ionophore	*E. histolytica*
Endotoxins	African trypanosomes, *Plasmodium falciparum*
Indole catabolites	Trypanosomes
Mechanical Tissue Damage	
Blockage of internal organs	*Ascaris* species, tapeworms, schistosomes, filaria
Pressure atrophy	*Echinococcus* species, *Cysticercus* species
Migration through tissue	Helminthic larvae
Immunopathology	
Hypersensitivity	See Table 72–4
Autoimmunity	See Table 72–4
Protein-losing enteropathies	Hookworm, tapeworm, *Giardia* species, *Strongyloides* species
Metaplastic changes	*Opisthorchis* species (liver flukes), schistosomes

TABLE 72–4. Immunopathologic Reactions and Parasitic Diseases

Reaction	Mechanism	Result	Example
Type 1: anaphylactic	Antigen + Immunoglobulin E antibody attached to most cells: histamine release	Anaphylactic shock; bronchospasm; local inflammation	Helminth infection, African trypanosomiasis
Type 2: cytotoxic	Antibody + antigen on cell surface: complement activation or antibody-dependent cellular cytotoxicity	Lysis of cell-bearing microbial antigens	*Trypanosoma cruzi* infection
Type 3: immune complex	Antibody + extracellular antigen complex	Inflammation and tissue damage; complex deposition in glomeruli, joints, skin vessels, brain; glomerulonephritis, and vasculitis	Malaria, schistosomiasis, trypanosomiasis
Type 4: cell-mediated (delayed)	Sensitized T cell reaction with antigen, liberation of lymphokines, triggered cytotoxicity	Inflammation, mononuclear accumulation, macrophage activation; tissue damage	Leishmaniasis, schistosomiasis, trypanosomiasis

Modified from Mims C et al: *Mims' pathogenesis of infectious disease,* ed 4, London, 1995, Academic.

expanding larval cysts of *Taenia solium* on the central nervous system (CNS) and eyes. Migration of helminths (usually larval forms) through body tissues such as the skin, lungs, liver, intestines, eyes, and CNS can damage the tissues directly and initiate hypersensitivity reactions.

As with many infectious agents, the manifestations of parasitic disease are due not only to the mechanical or chemical tissue damage produced by the parasite, but also to the host responses to the presence of the parasite. Cellular hypersensitivity is observed in protozoan and helminthic disease (Table 72–4). During a parasitic infection, host cell products such as cytokines and lymphokines are released from activated cells. These mediators influence the action of other cells and may contribute directly to the pathogenesis of parasite infections. Immunopathologic reactions range from acute anaphylactic reactions to cell-mediated delayed hypersensitivity reactions (see Table 72–4). Because many parasites are long-lived, many inflammatory changes become irreversible, producing functional changes in tissues. Examples include hyperplasia of the bile ducts secondary to the presence of liver flukes and extensive fibrosis leading to genitourinary and hepatic dysfunction in chronic schistosomiasis. Migration of larval helminths through tissues such as the skin, lungs, liver, intestine, CNS, and eyes produces immune-mediated inflammatory changes in these structures. Finally, chronic inflammatory changes around parasites such as *Opisthorchis sinensis* and *Schistosoma haematobium* have been linked to induction of carcinomatous changes in the bile ducts and the bladder, respectively.

Disruption, Evasion, and Inactivation of Host Defenses

Although the processes of cell and tissue destruction are often sufficient to **initiate** clinical disease, the parasite must be able to evade the host's immune defense system for the disease process to be maintained. Like other organisms, parasites elicit humoral and cell-mediated immune responses; however, parasites are particularly adept at interfering with or avoiding these defense mechanisms (Table 72–5).

Organisms can shift antigenic expression, such as that observed with the African trypanosomes. Rapid variation of expression of antigens in the glycocalyces of these organisms occurs each time that the host exhibits a new humoral response. Similar changes have been observed with *Plasmodium, Babesia,* and *Giardia* species. Some organisms may produce antigens that mimic host antigens (mimicry) or acquire host molecules that conceal the antigenic site (masking), thus preventing immune recognition by the host.

Many protozoan parasites evade the immune response by assuming an intracellular location in the host. The organisms that reside in macrophages have developed a variety of mechanisms to avoid intracellular killing. These include prevention of phagolysosome fusion, resistance to killing after exposure to lysosomal enzymes, and escape of phagocytosed cells from the phagosome into the cytoplasm with subsequent replication of the organism (see Table 72–5).

Immunosuppression of the host is often observed during the course of parasitic infections. The immuno-

TABLE 72–5. Microbial Interference with or Avoidance of Immune Defenses

Type of Interference or Avoidance	Mechanism	Example
Antigenic variation	Variation of surface antigens within the host	African trypanosomes, *Plasmodium* species, *Babesia* species, *Giardia* species
Molecular mimicry	Microbial antigens mimicking host antigens, leading to poor antibody response	*Plasmodium* species, trypanosomes, schistosomes
Concealment of antigenic site (masking)	Acquisition of coating of host molecules	Hydatid cyst, filaria, schistosomes, trypanosomes
Intracellular location	Failure to display microbial antigen on host cell surface	*Plasmodium* species (RBC), trypanosomes, *Leishmania* species, *Toxoplasma* species
	Inhibition of phagolysosomal fusion	*Toxoplasma* species
	Escape from phagosome into cytoplasm with subsequent replication	*Leishmania* species, *Trypanosoma cruzi*
Immunosuppression	Suppression of parasite-specific B- and T-cell responses	Trypanosomes, *Plasmodium* species
	Degradation of immunoglobulins	Schistosomes

suppression may be parasite-specific or generalized, involving a response to various nonparasitic and parasitic antigens. Proposed mechanisms include antigen overload, antigenic competition, induction of suppressor cells, and production of lymphocyte-specific suppressor factors. Certain helminths, such as *Schistosoma mansoni*, may also produce proteinases that can degrade immunoglobulins.

QUESTIONS

1. What are the most common modes of entry of parasites into the human host?

2. Name two factors that determine the outcome of the interaction between parasite and host.

3. Give an example of an adhesin that is directly related to the virulence of a parasite.

4. Name three pathologic mechanisms believed to be important in parasitic diseases.

5. How can parasites resist immunologic clearance? Give at least one example of each mechanism.

6. Name the four types of immunopathologic reactions that occur in parasitic diseases and provide examples of each.

BIBLIOGRAPHY

Chen Q, Schlichtherle M, Wahlgren M: Molecular aspects of severe malaria, *Clin Microbiol Rev* 13:439–450, 2000.

Connor DH et al, editors: *Pathology of infectious disease*, vol 2, Stamford, Conn, 1997, Appleton and Lange.

Cunningham MW, Fujinami RS, editors: *Molecular mimicry, microbes, and autoimmunity*, Washington, DC, 2000, ASM Press.

Espinosa-Cantellano M, Martinez-Palomo A: Pathogenesis of intestinal amebiasis: from molecules to disease, *Clin Microbiol Rev* 13:318–331, 2000.

Hall LR, Pearlman E: Pathogenesis of onchocercal keratitis (river blindness), *Clin Microbiol Rev* 12:445–453, 1999.

Orihel TC, Ash LR, editors: *Parasites in human tissues*, Chicago, 1995, American Society for Clinical Pathology.

Sherman IW, editor: *Malaria: parasite biology, pathogenesis, and protection*, Washington DC, 1998, ASM Press.

Van Velthuysen M-LF, Florquin S: Glomerulopathy associated with parasitic infections, *Clin Microbiol Rev* 13:55–66, 2000.

CHAPTER 73

Antiparasitic Agents

The chemotherapeutic approach to the management of infectious diseases has clearly changed the face of medicine. Unfortunately, few of the anti-infective agents that have proved so successful against bacterial pathogens have been effective against parasites. In many instances, clinicians continue to rely on antiparasitic agents from the preantibiotic era. These and some newer agents remain limited in effectiveness and are relatively toxic. Many antiparasitic agents require prolonged or parenteral administration and may be effective only for certain disease states. Fortunately, during the 1990s, several new agents have appeared that constitute significant advances in the treatment of parasitic diseases. In each case, the previously available drugs were toxic and often ineffective.

In large part, treating parasitic diseases is difficult because parasites are eukaryotic organisms and thus are more similar to the human host than are the more successfully treated prokaryotic bacterial pathogens. Furthermore, the chronic and prolonged course of infection and the complex life cycles and multiple developmental stages of many parasites add to the difficulties of effective chemotherapeutic intervention. Additional complicating factors in developing countries, where the majority of parasitic diseases occurs, include (1) the presence of multiple infections and the high probability of reinfection, (2) the large number of persons immunocompromised by malnutrition and infection with the human immunodeficiency virus, and (3) the overwhelming influence of poverty and poor sanitation, which facilitate transmission of many parasitic infections. Although chemotherapeutic approaches may be used effectively to treat and prevent many parasitic infections, some agents have adverse effects or eventually meet with resistance (microbial and social). Most antiparasitic agents are too expensive for widespread use in developing countries. Thus, the global approach to the prevention and treatment of parasitic diseases must involve several strategies, including improved hygiene and sanitation, control of the disease vector, use of vaccinations if available (largely unavailable for parasitic diseases), and prophylactic and therapeutic administration of safe and effective chemotherapy. These strategies must now also include efforts to decrease transmission of infection by the human immunodeficiency virus.

Targets for Antiparasitic Drug Action

As mentioned previously, parasites are eukaryotic organisms and thus have more similarities than differences with the human host. Consequently, many antiparasitic agents act on pathways (nucleic acid synthesis, carbohydrate metabolism) or targets (neuromuscular function) shared by both the parasite and the host. For this reason, developing safe and effective antiparasitic drugs based on biochemical differences between the parasite and host has been difficult. Differential toxicity is commonly achieved by preferential uptake, metabolic alteration of the drug by the parasite, or differences in the susceptibility of functionally equivalent sites in the parasite and host. Fortunately, as our understanding of the basic biology and biochemistry of parasites and the mechanism of action of antimicrobial agents has improved, so has our recognition of potential parasite-specific targets for chemotherapeutic attack. Examples of the chemotherapeutic strategies that exploit the differences between parasite and host are provided in Table 73–1. These strategies are discussed in greater detail as we deal with the specific agents.

Drug Resistance

Resistance to antimicrobial agents is an important consideration in treating infections resulting from bacteria and fungal pathogens and certainly plays a role in the chemotherapy of parasitic diseases. Unfortunately, our understanding of the molecular and genetic basis for resistance to most antiparasitic agents is quite limited. Most of the information regarding the molecular mechanisms of drug resistance in parasites has come from studies in plasmodia. Resistance to chloroquine, a major antimalarial agent, is most likely due to the presence of an active chloroquine efflux mechanism similar

TABLE 73–1. Chemotherapeutic Strategies That Exploit Differences Between Parasite and Host

Unique Site of Attack	Drug	Organism
Drug-concentrating mechanism unique to parasite	Chloroquine	*Plasmodium* species
Folic acid pathway (parasite unable to use exogenous folate)	Pyrimethamine or trimethoprim-sulfamethoxazole	*Plasmodium* or *Toxoplasma* species
Inhibitor of trypanothion-dependent mechanism for reducing oxidized thiol groups	Arsenicals, difluoromethylornithine	Trypanosomes
Interference with neuromediators unique to parasites	Pyrantel pamoate, piperazine	*Ascaris* species
Inhibitors of GABA-mediated conduction in peripheral nervous system of parasites	Ivermectin	*Filaria*
Interaction with tubulin unique to parasites	Benzimidazoles	Many helminths
Inhibition of topoisomerase II	Pentamidine	Trypanosomes

GABA = γ-aminobutyric acid.

to that producing the rapid efflux of anticancer drugs observed in multidrug-resistant mammalian cancer cells. In addition, development of plasmodial resistance to antifolate compounds such as pyrimethamine is due to a series of mutations in the parasite's combined dihydrofolate reductase–thymidylate synthetase enzyme. Further insights into the mechanisms of action and resistance to antiparasitic agents are necessary to optimize the effectiveness of antiparasitic chemotherapy.

Antiparasitic Agents

Although the number of effective antiparasitic agents is small relative to the vast array of antibacterial agents, the list is expanding (Table 73–2). In many cases, certainly, the goal of antiparasitic therapy is similar to that of antibacterial therapy: to eradicate the organism rapidly and completely. Often, however, the agents and treatment regimens used for parasitic diseases are designed simply to decrease the parasite burden or to prevent the systemic complications of chronic infection, or both. Thus, the goals of antiparasitic therapy, particularly as applied in endemic areas, may be quite different from those usually considered for treatment of microbial infection in the United States or other developed countries. Given the significant toxicity of many of these agents, in every case, the need for treatment must be weighed against the toxicity of the drug. A decision to withhold therapy may often be correct, particularly when the drug can cause severe adverse effects.

Immunocompromised individuals pose a particular problem with respect to antiparasitic chemotherapy. On the one hand, prophylaxis, such as that administered for toxoplasmosis, may be effective in preventing infection. Once infection is established, however, radical cure may not be possible, and long-term suppressive therapy may be indicated. In some diseases, such as cryptosporidiosis and microsporidiosis, effective (curative) therapy is not available, and care must be taken to avoid unnecessary toxicity while providing supportive care for the patient.

The remainder of this chapter provides an overview of the major classes of antiprotozoal and antihelminthic agents. These and additional antiparasitic agents, their mechanisms of action, and their clinical indications are listed in Table 73–2. Treatment of specific infections is discussed in the chapters that deal with the parasites. The Bibliography lists several excellent reviews for more complete information and for discussions of the antiparasitic agents that are available.

Antiprotozoal Agents

Similar to antibacterial and antifungal agents, the antiprotozoal agents are generally targeted at relatively rapidly proliferating, young, growing cells. Most commonly, these agents target nucleic acid synthesis, protein synthesis, or specific metabolic pathways (e.g., folate metabolism) unique to the protozoan parasites.

Heavy Metals

The heavy metals used for the treatment of parasitic infections include arsenical (melarsoprol) and antimonial compounds (sodium stibogluconate, meglumine antimonate). These agents are believed to oxidize sulfhydryl groups of enzymes, which are essential catalysts in carbohydrate metabolism. Melarsoprol inhibits

TABLE 73–2. Mechanisms of Action and Clinical Indications for the Major Antiparasitic Agents

Drug Class	Mechanism of Action	Examples	Clinical Indication
Antiprotozoal Agents			
Heavy metals: arsenicals and antimonials	Inactivate sulfhydril groups	Melarsoprol Sodium stibogluconate Meglumine antimonate	Trypanosomiasis Leishmaniasis
Aminoquinoline analogues	Accumulate in parasitized cells; interfere with DNA replication; bind to ferriprotoporphyrin IX; raise intravesicular pH; interfere with hemoglobin digestion	Chloroquine Mefloquine Quinine Primaquine	Malaria prophylaxis and therapy Radical cure (exoerythrocytic-primaquine only)
Folic acid antagonists	Inhibit dihydropteroate synthetase and dihydrofolate reductase	Sulfonamides Pyrimethamine Trimethoprim	Toxoplasmosis Malaria Cyclosporiasis
Inhibitors of protein synthesis	Block peptide synthesis at level of ribosome	Clindamycin Spiramycin Paromomycin Tetracycline Doxycycline	Malaria Babesiosis Amebiasis Cryptosporidiosis
Diamidines	Bind DNA Interfere with uptake and function of polyamines	Pentamidine	Pneumocystosis Leishmaniasis Trypanosomiasis
Nitroimidazoles	Unclear; interact with DNA Inhibit metabolism of glucose and interfere with mitochondrial function	Metronidazole Benzimidazole Tinidazole	Amebiasis Giardiasis Trichomoniasis
Quinolones	Inhibit DNA gyrase	Ciprofloxacin	Malaria
Sesquiterpenes	React with heme, causing free-radical damage to parasite membranes	Artemisinin	Malaria
Ornithine analogue	Inhibits ornithine decarboxylase Interferes with polyamine metabolism	Difluoromethylornithine	African trypanosomiasis
Inhibitors of nucleic acid synthesis	Inhibit enzymes in purine salvage pathway	Allopurinol	Leishmaniasis
Acetanilide	Unknown	Diloxanide furoate	Intestinal amebiasis
Sulfated naphthylamine	Inhibits *sn*-glycerol phosphate oxidase and glycerol 3-phosphate dehydrogenase, causing decreased ATP synthesis	Suramin	African trypanosomiasis
Phenanthrenemethanols	Bind to ferriprotoporphyrin IX; affect mitochondria	Halofantrine	Malaria
Antihelminthic Agents			
Benzimidazoles	Inhibit fumarate reductase Inhibit glucose transport Disrupt microtubular function	Mebendazole Thiabendazole Albendazole	Broad-spectrum antihelminthics Nematodes Cestodes
Tetrahydropyrimidine	Blocks neuromuscular action Inhibits fumarate reductase	Pyrantel pamoate	Ascariasis Pinworm Hookworm
Piperazines	Are GABA agonists Cause neuromuscular paralysis Stimulate phagocytic cells	Piperazine Diethylcarbamazine	*Ascaris* and pinworm infections Filarial infections
Avermectins	Block neuromuscular action Are GABA antagonists Inhibit filarial reproduction	Ivermectin	Filarial infections

(continued)

Drug Class	Mechanism of Action	Examples	Clinical Indication
Pyrazinoisoquinoline	Is calcium agonist; causes tetanic muscular contractions; cause tegumental disruption; provides synergy with host defenses	Praziquantel	Broad-spectrum antihelminthics Cestodes Trematodes
Phenol	Uncouples oxidative phosphorylation	Niclosamide	Intestinal tapeworm
Quinolone	Alkylates DNA; inhibits DNA, RNA, and protein synthesis	Bithionol Oxamniquine	Paragonimiasis Schistosomiasis
Organophosphate	Is anticholinesterase; blocks neuromuscular action	Metrifonate	Schistosomiasis
Sulfated naphthylamidine	Inhibits glycerophosphate oxidase and dehydrogenase	Suramin	Onchocerciasis

ATP = adenosine triphosphate; GABA = γ-aminobutyric acid.

parasite pyruvate kinase, causing decreased concentrations of adenosine triphosphate (ATP), pyruvate, and phosphoenolpyruvate. Arsenicals also inhibit *sn*-glycerol 3-phosphate oxidase, which is needed for the regeneration of nicotinamide adenine dinucleotide in trypanosomes but is not found in mammalian cells. The antimonials, sodium stibogluconate and meglumine antimonate, inhibit the glycolytic enzyme phosphofructokinase and certain Krebs cycle enzymes in *Leishmania* organisms. In each instance, the inhibition of parasite metabolism is parasiticidal. Unfortunately, the heavy metal compounds are toxic to the host, as well as to the parasite. The toxicity is greatest on cells that are most metabolically active, such as neuronal, renal tubular, intestinal, and bone marrow stem cells. Their differential toxicity and therapeutic value are largely related to enhanced uptake by the parasite and its intense metabolic activity.

Melarsoprol is the drug of choice for trypanosomiasis involving the central nervous system. It can penetrate the blood-brain barrier and is effective in all stages of trypanosomiasis. The antimonial compounds are restricted to the management of leishmaniasis. Meglumine antimonate and sodium stibogluconate are the drugs of choice for leishmaniasis and are active against all forms of the disease. Prolonged therapy is usually required for disseminated leishmaniasis, and relapses are common.

Aminoquinoline Analogues

The aminoquinoline analogues include the 4-aminoquinolines (chloroquine), the 8-aminoquinolines (primaquine), and the 4-quinolinemethanols (mefloquine). Additional quinoline analogues include quinine, quinidine, quinacrine, and amodiaquine. These compounds all have antimalarial activity and accumulate preferentially in parasitized red blood cells. Several potential mechanisms of action have been proposed, including

(1) binding to DNA and interfering with DNA replication; (2) binding to ferriprotoporphyrin IX released from hemoglobin in infected erythrocytes, producing a toxic complex; and (3) raising the pH of the parasite's intracellular acid vesicles, thus interfering with its ability to degrade hemoglobin. Quinine, the 4-aminoquinolines, and 4-quinolinemethanols rapidly destroy the erythrocytic stage of malaria and thus may be used prophylactically to suppress clinical illness or therapeutically to terminate an acute attack. The 8-aminoquinolines (e.g., primaquine) accumulate in tissue cells and destroy the extraerythrocytic (hepatic) stages of malaria, resulting in a radical cure of the infection.

Chloroquine remains the drug of choice for the prophylaxis and treatment of susceptible malaria strains. Chloroquine is active against all four *Plasmodium* species (*Plasmodium falciparum*, *Plasmodium vivax*, *Plasmodium ovale*, *Plasmodium malariae*) and is well tolerated, inexpensive, and effective orally. Unfortunately, resistance of *P. falciparum* to chloroquine is widespread in Asia, Africa, and South America, which greatly limits the use of this agent. Likewise, resistance of *P. vivax* to chloroquine has been reported from Papua New Guinea, the Solomon Islands, Indonesia, and Brazil.

Quinine is used primarily to treat infection with chloroquine-resistant *P. falciparum*. Presumably, it is active against the chloroquine-resistant strains of *P. vivax*, as well. Quinine is used orally only to treat mild attacks and is used intravenously to treat acute attacks of multidrug-resistant *P. falciparum*. The drug is quite toxic and is not rapidly parasiticidal; thus, it is never used alone but is often used with a sulfonamide or tetracycline antibiotic with antimalarial activity.

Mefloquine is a 4-quinolinemethanol antimalarial agent used for the prophylaxis and treatment of falciparum malaria. It displays a high level of activity against most chloroquine-resistant parasites. Unfortunately, mefloquine-resistant strains of falciparum malaria have been reported from Southeast Asia.

Folic Acid Antagonists

As do other organisms, protozoan parasites require folic acid for the synthesis of nucleic acids and, ultimately, DNA. Protozoa are unable to absorb exogenous folate and thus are susceptible to drugs that inhibit folate synthesis. The folic acid antagonists that are useful in treating protozoan infections include the diaminopyrimidines (pyrimethamine and trimethoprim) and the sulfonamides. These compounds block separate steps in the folic acid pathway. The sulfonamides inhibit the conversion of aminobenzoic acid to dihydropteroic acid. The diaminopyrimidines inhibit dihydrofolate reductase, which effectively blocks the synthesis of tetrahydrofolate, a precursor necessary for the formation of purines, pyrimidines, and certain amino acids. These agents are effective at concentrations far less than those needed to inhibit the mammalian enzyme, so selectivity can be attained. When a diaminopyrimidine is used with a sulfonamide, a synergistic effect is achieved via the blockade of two steps in the same metabolic pathway, resulting in very effective inhibition of protozoan growth.

The diaminopyrimidine trimethoprim is used with sulfamethoxazole to treat toxoplasmosis. Another diaminopyrimidine, pyrimethamine, has a high affinity for sporozoan dihydrofolate reductase and has been very effective when combined with a sulfonamide in the treatment of malaria and toxoplasmosis. Resistance to antifolates is due to specific point mutations at the active site of the parasite's dihydrofolate reductase and has been largely confined to species of plasmodia.

Inhibitors of Protein Synthesis

Several antibiotics that inhibit protein synthesis in bacteria also exhibit antiparasitic activity in vitro and in vivo. These agents include clindamycin, spiramycin, tetracycline, and doxycycline.

Clindamycin and the tetracyclines are active against *Plasmodium* species, *Babesia* species, and amoebae. Doxycycline is used for the chemoprophylaxis of chloroquine-resistant *P. falciparum* malaria, and tetracycline may be used with quinine for the treatment of chloroquine-resistant *P. falciparum* infection. Clindamycin may be useful in the treatment of central nervous system toxoplasmosis. Spiramycin is recommended as an alternative to the antifolates in the treatment of toxoplasmosis. Although spiramycin appears active against *Cryptosporidium* species in vitro, it has not been shown to be effective clinically for human cryptosporidiosis. Recent studies suggest that paromomycin, an older aminoglycoside, may be at least partially effective in treating cryptosporidiosis. Paromomycin, which is not absorbed systemically, is also used as a secondary drug in amebiasis and in giardiasis.

Diamidines

Pentamidine, a diamidine, is a relatively toxic agent. Pentamidine is a polycation and may interact with DNA, or it may interfere with the uptake and function of polyamines.

Pentamidine is effective in treating the tissue forms of leishmania and the early (pre–central nervous system) forms of African trypanosomiasis. Pentamidine does not penetrate the central nervous system and is therefore not useful in the late stages of infection with *Trypanosoma brucei gambiense*. Recent information suggests that pentamidine may inhibit kinetoplast topoisomerase II activity and may act against trypanosomes in part by this mechanism.

Nitroimidazoles

The nitroimidazoles include the well-known antibacterial agent metronidazole as well as benzimidazole and tinidazole. The mechanism of action of these compounds is unclear. It has been suggested that they inhibit DNA and RNA synthesis and also inhibit the metabolism of glucose and interfere with mitochondrial function. Metronidazole binds to parasite guanine and cytosine residues, causing the loss of helical structure and breakage of DNA strands.

The nitroimidazoles have excellent penetration into body tissues and are therefore particularly effective for the treatment of disseminated amebiasis. Metronidazole is the drug of choice for trichomoniasis and is effective in the treatment of giardiasis. Tinidazole appears to be more effective and less mutagenic than metronidazole but is not widely available.

Other Antiprotozoal Agents

A number of additional agents used in therapy, their mechanism of action (if known), and clinical use are listed in Table 73–2.

Antihelminthic Agents

The strategy for the use of antihelminthic drugs is quite different from that for the use of drugs for treating most protozoal infections. Most antihelminthic drugs are targeted at nonproliferating adult organisms, whereas with protozoa, the targets are generally younger, more rapidly proliferating cells. The helminthic life cycle is frequently quite complex, and the adaptation to survival in the human host depends strongly on (1) neuromuscular coordination for feeding movements and for maintenance of a favorable location of the worm within the host; (2) carbohydrate metabolism as the major source of energy, with glucose the primary substrate; and (3) microtubular integrity, because egg laying and hatching, larval development, glucose transport, and enzyme activity and secretion are impaired when microtubules are modified. Most antihelminthic agents are targeted at one of these biochemical functions in the adult organism.

The mechanisms of action and clinical indications for common antihelminthic agents are listed in Table 73–2.

Benzimidazoles

The benzimidazoles are broad-spectrum antihelminthic agents and include mebendazole, thiabendazole, and albendazole. The basic structure of these agents consists of linked imidazole and benzene rings. Three mechanisms of action have been proposed for the benzimidazoles: (1) inhibition of fumarate reductase; (2) inhibition of glucose transport, resulting in glycogen depletion, cessation of ATP formation, and paralysis or death; and (3) disruption of microtubular function. Benzimidazoles block the assembly of tubulin dimers into tubulin polymers in a process mimicked by colchicine, a powerful antimitotic and embryotoxic drug. Because tubulin is important for parasite motility, drugs such as the benzimidazoles, which bind to parasite tubulin, are believed to act against nematode parasites by reducing or eliminating their motility.

The benzimidazoles have a wide spectrum of activity, including intestinal nematodes (*Ascaris*, *Trichuris*, *Necator*, and *Ancylostoma* species; *Enterobius vermicularis*), as well as a number of cestodes (*Taenia*, *Hymenolepis*, and *Echinococcus* species). Thiabendazole acts against larval and adult nematodes and is useful in the management of cutaneous larval migrans, trichinosis, and most intestinal nematode infections. Mebendazole is active against the intestinal nematodes and the cestodes listed previously. Albendazole has a spectrum similar to that of mebendazole and may have greater activity against *Echinococcus* species. In addition to its broad-spectrum antihelminthic activity, albendazole is active against *Giardia* species and appears promising in the treatment of intestinal microsporidiosis in patients with the acquired immunodeficiency syndrome.

Tetrahydropyrimidines

Pyrantel pamoate, a tetrahydropyrimidine, is a cholinergic agonist that has a powerful effect on nematode muscle cells by binding to cholinergic receptors, which results in cell depolarization and muscle contraction. This paralytic action on intestinal nematodes leads to expulsion of the worm from the host intestinal tract.

Pyrantel pamoate is not readily absorbed from the intestine and is active against *Ascaris*, pinworm, and hookworm. An analogue of pyrantel, oxantel, may be used with pyrantel to provide effective therapy for the three major soil-transmitted nematodes: *Ascaris*, hookworm, and *Trichuris*.

Piperazines

The piperazine antihelmintics include piperazine and diethylcarbamazine. Piperazine is believed to act by hyperpolarization of the muscle membrane, which produces a flaccid paralysis. The current hypothesis is that piperazine acts against nematodes as a low-potency γ-aminobutyric acid (GABA) agonist. Diethylcarbamazine may act by stimulating cholinergic receptors and depolarizing muscle cells, with subsequent paralysis of the worms. Additional evidence suggests, however, that it enhances the adherence of leukocytes to microfilariae and thus may act by altering the parasite surface membrane or by directly stimulating phagocytic cells.

The piperazines are active against *Ascaris* and pinworm (*E. vermicularis*). In addition, diethylcarbamazine is active against the filariae that produce river blindness (*Onchocerca volvulus*) and lymphatic filariasis (*Wuchereria bancrofti* and *Brugia malayi*). Unfortunately, destruction of the microfilariae in the tissues may increase the pathology because of the host inflammatory response to the parasite antigens released on exposure to diethylcarbamazine. Current information suggests that single-dose treatment with diethylcarbamazine may produce antiparasitic effects similar to those obtained with 14- to 21-day courses without the severe side effects observed with the multidose regimens.

Avermectins

Ivermectin, an avermectin, acts by interacting with the chloride channel on the helminth GABA receptor complex, thus inhibiting GABA-ergic synapses in the peripheral nervous system of nematode parasites. As a result, the parasites become paralyzed and may be eliminated by the host. The drug also inhibits the reproductive function of the adult female *O. volvulus* and alters the ability of the *O. volvulus* microfilariae to evade the host immune system.

Although ivermectin is used extensively to control gut-dwelling nematode infections in domestic and farm animals, its use in humans is limited primarily to treating ocular and lymphatic filariasis. Ivermectin is effective in the treatment of strongyloidiasis as well as several common intestinal parasitic nematodes including *Ascaris*, *Trichuris*, and *Enterobius* species. When used to treat filariasis, ivermectin has fewer side effects than has diethylcarbamazine, and a single dose can eliminate microfilariae for up to 6 months. Ivermectin has a dramatic effect on the tissue-dwelling microfilariae of *O. volvulus* and reduces the severity of the ocular pathology seen in onchocerciasis. Because of its ability to markedly reduce the number of microfilariae in the

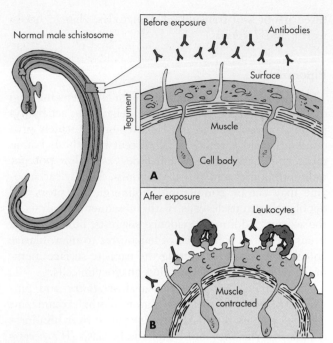

FIGURE 73–1. Before exposure to praziquantel, the schistosome is capable of avoiding the numerous antibodies directed toward surface and internally located antigens. *A,* Cross section of the dorsal surface of a normal male schistosome. Within 1 to 2 seconds after exposure to praziquantel, the muscles of the schistosome contract because of a drug-induced influx of calcium ions into the schistosome tegument. *B,* The change in permeability of the schistosome surface toward external ions initiates the appearance of small holes and balloon-like structures, making the parasite vulnerable to antibody-mediated adherence of host leukocytes that kill the helminth. (From Wingard LB Jr et al: *Human pharmacology: molecular to clinical,* St. Louis, 1991, Mosby.)

skin of persons with onchocerciasis, ivermectin has been effective in reducing the transmission of onchocerciasis in endemic areas.

Pyrazinoisoquinolines

Praziquantel, a pyrazinoisoquinoline, is an antihelminthic active against a broad spectrum of trematodes and cestodes. The drug is rapidly taken up by susceptible helminths in which it acts as a calcium agonist. The entry of calcium into various cells results in elevated intracellular calcium levels, tetanic muscular contraction, and destruction of the tegument. Praziquantel appears to act with the host immune system to produce a synergistic antihelminthic effect. The drug causes disruption of the parasite surface and tegument, allowing antibodies to attack parasite antigens not normally exposed on the surface (Fig. 73–1). Irreversible damage to the parasite probably occurs when complement

or host leukocytes are recruited to the sites where antibody is bound.

Praziquantel has extremely broad-spectrum activity against trematodes including *Fasciolopsis, Fasciola, Clonorchis, Opisthorchis, Paragonimus,* and *Schistosoma* species. It is also active against cestodes including *Echinococcus, Taenia,* and *Dipylidium* species. Praziquantel is the drug of choice for the treatment of schistosomiasis, clonorchiasis, opisthorchiasis, and neurocysticercosis. There is now reliable evidence that praziquantel reduces hepatosplenomegaly and portal hypertension in schistosomiasis. Effective activity has also been demonstrated against other common trematode and cestode infections.

Phenols

Niclosamide, a phenol, is a nonabsorbable antihelminthic with selective activity against intestinal tapeworms. The drug is absorbed by gut-dwelling cestodes but not by nematodes. It acts by uncoupling oxidative phosphorylation in mitochondria, resulting in a loss of helminth ATP that ultimately immobilizes the parasite so that it is expelled with the feces. Niclosamide is effective in the treatment of intestinal tapeworms in humans and animals.

Other Antihelminthic Agents

Additional antihelminthic agents, including oxamniquine, metrifonate, and suramin, are described in Table 73–2. These agents are generally considered secondary agents for the treatment of trematode (oxamniquine and metrifonate) and filarial (suramin) infections.

QUESTIONS

1. What are the obstacles to effective treatment and prophylaxis of parasitic diseases in developing countries?
2. What are the goals of antiparasitic therapy and how are they different from antibacterial therapy?
3. What is the importance of aminoquinoline analogues?
4. How does the strategy for the use of antihelminthic agents differ from that for the use of drugs for protozoal infections?

BIBLIOGRAPHY

Abiose A: Onchocercal eye disease and the impact of mectizan treatment, *Ann Trop Med Parasitol* 92:S11–S22, 1998.

Engers HD, Bergquist R, Modabber F: Progress on vaccines against parasites, *Dev Biol Stand* 87:73–84, 1996.

Faubert G: Immune response to *Giardia duodenalis, Clin Microbiol Rev* 13:35–54, 2000.

Geertz S, Gryseels B: Drug resistance in human helminths: current situation and lessons from livestock, *Clin Microbiol Rev* 13:207–222, 2000.

Gilbert DN, Moellering RC Jr, Sande MA, editors: *The Sanford guide to antimicrobial therapy*, ed 13, Hyde Park, Vt, 2000, Antimicrobial Therapy.

Khaw M, Panosian CB: Human antiprotozoal therapy: past, present, and future, *Clin Microbiol Rev* 8:427–439, 1995.

Liu LX, Weller PF: Antiparasitic drugs, *New Engl J Med* 334:1178–1184, 1996.

Petri WA, Singh V: Diagnosis and management of amebiasis, *Clin Infect Dis* 29:1117–11125, 1999.

Roose MH: The role of drugs in the control of parasitic nematode infections: must we do without? *Parasitology* 114:S137–S144, 1997.

Sangster NC: Anthelminthic resistance: past, present and future, *Int J Parasitol* 29:115–124, 1999.

Wahlgren M, Perlmann P, editors: *Malaria: molecular and clinical aspects*, the Netherlands, 1999, Harwood Academic.

Wingard LB Jr et al, editors: *Human pharmacology: molecular to clinical*, St. Louis, 1991, Mosby.

CHAPTER 74

Laboratory Diagnosis of Parasitic Diseases

The diagnosis of parasitic infections may be very difficult, particularly in the nonendemic setting. The clinical manifestations of parasitic diseases are seldom specific enough to raise the possibility of these processes in the mind of the clinician, and routine laboratory tests are seldom helpful. Although peripheral eosinophilia is widely recognized as a useful indicator of parasitic disease, this phenomenon is characteristic only of helminthic infection and, even in these cases, is frequently absent. Thus, the physician must maintain a heightened index of suspicion and must rely on detailed travel, food intake, transfusion, and socioeconomic history to raise the possibility of parasitic disease. The following conditions are required for proper diagnosis:

1. The physician must consider the possibility of parasitic infection.
2. Appropriate specimens must be obtained, and they must be transported to the laboratory in a timely fashion.
3. The laboratory must competently perform the appropriate procedures for the recovery and identification of the etiologic agent.
4. The laboratory test results must be effectively communicated to the physician.
5. The results must be correctly interpreted by the physician and applied to the care of the patient.

In addition, for most parasitic diseases, appropriate test selection and interpretation of results are based on an understanding of the life cycle of the parasite as well as the pathogenesis of the disease process in humans.

Numerous methods for diagnosing parasitic diseases have been described (Box 74–1). Some are useful in detecting a wide variety of parasites, and others are particularly useful for only one or a few parasites. Although the mainstay of diagnostic clinical microbiology is the isolation of the causative pathogen in culture, the diagnosis of parasitic diseases is accomplished almost entirely by morphologic (usually microscopic) demonstration of parasites in clinical material. Occasionally, demonstration of a specific antibody response (serodiagnosis) helps in establishing the diagnosis.

The detection of parasite antigens in serum, urine, or stool may provide a rapid and sensitive means of diagnosing infection with certain organisms. Likewise, newly developed nucleic acid probe–based assays may prove to be excellent means of detecting and identifying a number of parasites in biologic samples, such as blood, stool, urine, sputum, and tissue biopsy specimens, obtained from infected patients. In general, it is better for the laboratory to offer a limited number of competently performed procedures than to offer a wide variety of infrequently and poorly performed tests.

This chapter provides a general description of the principles of specimen collection and processing necessary for the diagnosis of most parasitic infections. Specific details of these and other procedures of general and limited usefulness may be found in several reference texts listed in the Bibliography.

Parasite Life Cycle as an Aid in Diagnosis

Parasites may have complex life cycles involving single or multiple hosts. Understanding the life cycles of parasitic organisms is a key to understanding important features of geographic distribution, transmission, and pathogenesis of many parasitic diseases. The life cycles of parasites often suggest useful clues for diagnosis as well.

For example, in the life cycle of filariae that infect humans, certain species, such as *Wuchereria bancrofti*, have a "nocturnal periodicity," in which greater numbers of microfilariae are found in the peripheral blood at night. Sampling the blood of such patients during daytime hours may fail to detect the microfilariae, whereas blood specimens collected between 10 PM and 4 AM may demonstrate many microfilariae. Likewise, intestinal nematodes such as *Ascaris lumbricoides* and hookworm, which reside in the lumen of the intestine, produce large numbers of eggs that can be detected easily in the stool of an infected patient. In contrast, another intestinal nematode, *Strongyloides stercoralis*, lays its eggs in the bowel wall rather than in the intestinal lumen. As a result, the eggs are rarely seen on stool examination; to make the diagnosis, the parasitologist must be alert for the presence of larvae. Finally, parasites may cause clinical symptoms at a time when diagnostic forms are not yet present in the usual site. For example, in certain intestinal nematode infections, the migration of larvae through the tissues may cause an intense symptomatology weeks before the characteristic eggs are present in the feces.

General Diagnostic Considerations

The importance of appropriate specimen collection, the number and timing of specimens, timely transport to the laboratory, and prompt examination by an experienced microscopist cannot be overemphasized. Because the majority of parasitologic examinations and identifications are based entirely on recognition of the characteristic morphology of the organisms, any condition that may obscure or distort the morphologic appearance of the parasite may result in an erroneous identification or missed diagnosis.

As noted previously and in Box 74-1, there may be alternatives to microscopy for the detection and identification of certain parasites. These tests (e.g., antigen detection, nucleic acid probes), although currently uncommon, may become more widely applied in the future. They offer the promise of more rapid, sensitive, and specific diagnostic testing for parasitic diseases. These diagnostic test options may expand the testing capabilities of many laboratories, allowing laboratories with limited proficiency in parasitology to offer diagnostic testing for certain parasitic diseases. A list of common and uncommon diagnostic procedures and specimens to be collected for selected parasitic infections is provided in Table 74-1.

Parasitic Infections of Intestinal or Urogenital Tract

Protozoa and helminths may colonize or infect the intestinal and urogenital tract of humans. Most commonly these parasites are amebae, flagellates, or nematodes (Table 74-2). However, infection with trematodes, cestodes, or ciliate, coccidian, or microsporidian parasites may also be encountered.

In intestinal and urogenital infections, a simple wet mount or stained smear is often inadequate. Repeated specimen collections and testing are often necessary to optimize the detection of organisms that are shed intermittently or in fluctuating numbers. Concentration of specimens by sedimentation or flotation techniques may be required to detect low numbers of ova (worms) or cysts (protozoa) in fecal specimens.

Occasionally, specimens other than stool or urine must be examined (see Table 74-1). Optimal detection of small bowel pathogens such as *Giardia lamblia* and *S. stercoralis* may require the aspiration of duodenal contents or even small bowel biopsy. Likewise, the detection of colonic parasites such as *Entamoeba histolytica* and *Schistosoma mansoni* may necessitate proctoscopic or sigmoidoscopic examination with aspiration or biopsy of mucosal lesions. Sampling of the perianal skin is a useful means of recovering the eggs of *Enterobius vermicularis* (pinworm) or *Taenia* species (tapeworm).

Fecal Specimen Collection

Patients, clinicians, and laboratory personnel must be properly instructed about collection and handling of specimens. All fecal specimens should be collected in a clean, wide-mouthed, waterproof container with a tight-fitting lid to ensure and maintain adequate moisture. Specimens must not be contaminated with water, soil, or urine, because water and soil may contain free-living organisms that can be mistaken for human parasites and urine can destroy motile trophozoites and may cause helminth eggs to hatch. Stool specimens should not contain barium, bismuth, mineral oil, antibiotics, antimalarials, or other chemical substances, because such substances compromise the detection of intestinal parasites. Specimen collection should be delayed for 5 to 10 days to allow barium to clear and for at least 2 weeks to allow intestinal parasites to recover from the toxic (but not curative) effects of antibiotics such as tetracycline.

TABLE 74–1. Body Sites, Specimen Collection, and Diagnostic Procedures for Selected Parasitic Infections

Infecting Organism	Specimen Options	Collection Methods	Diagnostic Procedure
Blood			
Plasmodium species, *Babesia* species, filaria	Whole blood, anticoagulated	Venipuncture	Microscopic examination (Giemsa stain) Thin film Thick film Blood concentration (filaria) Serology Antibody Antigen
Bone Marrow			
Leishmania species	Aspirate Serum	Sterile Venipuncture	Microscopic examination (Giemsa stain) Culture Serology (antibody)
Central Nervous System			
Acanthamoeba species, *Naegleria* species, trypanosomes *Angiostrongylus cantonensis*	Spinal fluid Serum	Sterile Venipuncture	Microscopic examination Wet mount Permanent stain Culture Serology (antibody)
Cutaneous Ulcers			
Leishmania species	Aspirate Biopsy Serum	Sterile plus smears Sterile, nonsterile to histology Venipuncture	Microscopic examination (Giemsa stain) Culture Serology (antibody)
Eye			
Acanthamoeba species	Corneal scrapings Corneal biopsy	Sterile saline, air-dried smear Sterile saline	Microscopic examination Wet mount Permanent stain Culture
Intestinal Tract			
Entamoeba histolytica	Fresh stool Preserved stool Sigmoidoscopy material Serum	Waxed container Formalin, PVA Fresh, PVA Schaudinn's smears Venipuncture	Microscopic examination Wet mount Permanent stains Serology Antigen (stool) Antibody (serum) Culture
Giardia species	Fresh stool Preserved stool Duodenal contents	Waxed container Formalin, PVA Entero-Test or aspirate	Microscopic examination Wet mount Permanent stains Antigen IFA EIA Culture
Cryptosporidium species	Fresh stool Preserved stool Biopsy	Waxed container Formalin, PVA Saline	Microscopic examination (acid-fast) Antigen IFA EIA
Microsporidia	Fresh stool Preserved stool Duodenal contents Biopsy	Waxed container Formalin, PVA Aspirate Saline	Microscopic examination Giemsa stain Gram stain Chromotrope stain
Pinworm	Anal impression smear	Cellophane tape	Macroscopic examination Microscopic examination (eggs)

(continued)

Infecting Organism	Specimen Options	Collection Methods	Diagnostic Procedure
Helminths	Fresh stool	Waxed container	Macroscopic examination (adults)
	Preserved stool	Formalin, PVA	Microscopic examination (larvae and eggs)
	Serum	Venipuncture	Serology (antibody)
			Culture (*Strongyloides* species)
Liver, Spleen			
E. histolytica, Leishmania species	Aspirates	Sterile, collected in four separate aliquots (liver)	Microscopic examination Wet mount
	Biopsy	Sterile; nonsterile to histology	Permanent stains
	Serum	Venipuncture	Serology
			Antigen
			Antibody
			Culture
Lung			
Rarely: amebae *(E. histolytica)*, trematodes *(Paragonimus westermani)*, larvae *(Strongyloides stercoralis)*, or cestode hooklets	Sputum	Induced, no preservative	Microscopic examination
	Lavage	No preservative	Giemsa stain
	Transbronchial aspirate	Air-dried smears	Gram stain
		Same as above	Hematoxylin and eosin
	Brush biopsy	Fresh squash preparation, nonsterile to histology	Antigen
	Open lung biopsy		IFA
			EIA
			Serum (antibody)
Muscle			
Trichinella spiralis	Biopsy	Nonsterile to histology	Microscopic examination (permanent stains)
Trypanosoma cruzi	Serum	Venipuncture	Serology
			Antibody
			Antigen
Skin			
Onchocerca volvulus, Leishmania species	Scrapings	Aseptic, smear, or vial	Microscopic examination
	Skin snip	No preservative	Wet mount
Cutaneous larval migrans	Biopsy	Nonsterile to histology	Permanent stains
	Serum	Venipuncture	Serology (antibody)
			Culture (*Leishmania* species)
Urogenital System			
Trichomonas vaginalis	Vaginal discharge	Saline swab, culture medium	Microscopic examination
	Urethral discharge		Wet mount
	Prostatic secretions	Same as above	Permanent stains
			Antigen (IFA)
			Culture *(T. vaginalis)*
			Serology (antibody)
			Nucleic acid probes *(T. vaginalis)*
Schistosoma haematobium	Urine	Single, unpreserved specimen	Microscopic examination
	Biopsy	Nonsterile to histology	

EIA = enzyme immunoassay; IFA = immunofluorescent assay; PVA = polyvinyl alcohol.

Purged specimens may be collected when organisms are not detected in normally passed fecal specimens; however, only certain purgatives (sodium sulfate and buffered sodium biphosphate [Fleet Phospho-Soda]) are satisfactory. One series of purged specimens may be examined in place of, or in addition to, a series of normally passed specimens.

Unpreserved formed fecal specimens should arrive in the laboratory within 2 hours after passage. If the stool is liquid and thus more likely to contain tropho-

zoites, it should reach the laboratory for examination within 30 minutes. Soft or loose stools should be examined within 1 hour of passage. All fresh fecal samples should be placed in preservatives such as 10% formalin, polyvinyl alcohol (PVA), Merthiolate-iodine-formalin (MIF), or sodium acetate–formalin (SAF) if examination is not possible within the recommended time limits. Fecal specimens may be stored at 4°C but should not be incubated or frozen.

The number of specimens required to demonstrate

TABLE 74–2. Most Commonly Identified Intestinal Parasites in U.S. Laboratories (1995)

Organism	Positive Specimens	Patients
Giardia lamblia	896	723
Cryptosporidium species	114	81
Dientamoeba fragilis	102	77
Ascaris lumbricoides	73	59
Entamoeba histolytica	66	52
Trichuris trichiura	58	44
Hookworm	53	45
Enterobius vermicularis	52	49
Strongyloides stercoralis	51	36
Hymenolepis nana	23	17
Isospora species	12	7
Microsporidia	8	6
Clonorchis or *Opisthorchis* species	5	4
Other helminths	24	22

Modified from Valenstein P et al: The use and abuse of routine stool microbiology: a College of American Pathologists Q-probes study of 601 institutions, *Arch Pathol Lab Med* 120:206–211, 1996.

intestinal parasites varies according to (1) the quality of the specimen submitted, (2) the accuracy of the examination performed, (3) the severity of the infection, and (4) the purpose for which the examination is made. If the physician is interested only in determining the presence or absence of helminths, one or two examinations may suffice, provided that concentration methods are used. For a routine parasitic examination, a total of three fecal specimens is recommended. The examination of three specimens with a combination of techniques ensures detection of more than 99% of infections. In a 1996 survey, examination of three specimens detected 99.8% of infected patients, and examination of four specimens detected an additional 0.1% (Table 74–3).

TABLE 74–3. Number of Specimens Required to Detect Intestinal Parasites

Number of Specimens per Patient	Percentage of Infected Patients Detected*
1	91.9
2	97.6
3	99.8
4	99.9

* n = 1159.

Modified from Valenstein P et al: The use and abuse of routine stool microbiology: a College of American Pathologists Q-probes study of 601 institutions, *Arch Pathol Lab Med* 120:206–211, 1996.

It is inappropriate for multiple specimens to be collected from the same patient on the same day. It is also not recommended for the three specimens to be submitted one each day for 3 consecutive days. The series of three specimens should be collected within a time no longer than 10 days. Many parasites do not appear in fecal specimens in consistent numbers on a daily basis; therefore, collection of specimens on alternate days tends to yield a higher percentage of positive findings.

It has become apparent that in the United States, submission of stool for parasitologic examination from patients with hospital-acquired diarrhea (onset more than 3 days after admission) is usually inappropriate. The reason is that the frequency of acquisition of protozoan or helminthic parasites in a hospital is vanishingly rare. A request for stool examination for ova and parasites in a hospitalized patient should be accompanied by a clear statement of clinical indications and only after the more common causes of hospital-acquired diarrhea (e.g., antibiotics) have been ruled out.

Techniques of Stool Examination

Specimens should be examined systematically by a competent microscopist for helminth eggs and larvae as well as intestinal protozoa. For optimal detection of these various infectious agents, a combination of several techniques of examination is required.

Macroscopic Examination

The fecal specimen should be examined for consistency and for the presence of blood, mucus, worms, and proglottids.

Direct Wet Mount

Fresh stools should be examined under the microscope with the use of the saline and iodine wet-mount technique to detect motile trophozoites or larvae (*Strongyloides* species). The saline and iodine wet mounts are also used to detect helminth eggs, protozoan cysts, and host cells such as leukocytes and red blood cells. This approach is also useful in examining material from sputum, urine, vaginal swabs, duodenal aspirates, sigmoidoscopy, abscesses, and tissue biopsy specimens.

Concentration

All fecal specimens should be placed in 10% formalin to preserve parasite morphology and should be concentrated by means of a procedure such as formalin–ethyl acetate (or formalin-ether) sedimentation or zinc sulfate flotation. These methods separate protozoan cysts and helminth eggs from the bulk of fecal material and thus enhance the ability to detect small numbers of organisms usually missed by the use of only a direct smear. After concentration, the material is stained with iodine and examined microscopically.

Permanently Stained Slides

The detection and correct identification of intestinal protozoa often depend on the examination of the permanently stained smear. These slides provide a permanent record of the protozoan organisms that are identified. The cytologic detail revealed by one of the permanent staining methods is essential for accurate identification, and most identifications should be considered tentative until confirmed by a permanently stained slide. The permanent stains commonly used are trichrome, iron hematoxylin, and Mallory's phosphotungstic acid–hematoxylin. Slides are made either by preparing smears of fresh fecal material and placing them in Schaudinn's fixative solution or by fixing a small amount of fecal material in PVA fixative.

Collection and Examination of Specimens Other Than Stool

Commonly, specimens other than fecal material must be collected and examined to diagnose infections by intestinal pathogens. Such specimens include perianal samples, sigmoidoscopic material, aspirates of duodenal contents and liver abscesses, and sputum, urine, and urogenital specimens.

Perianal Specimens

The collection of perianal specimens is frequently necessary to diagnose pinworm (*E. vermicularis*) and occasionally *Taenia* (tapeworm) infections. The methods include the preparation of a clear cellulose tape slide or an anal swab. The cellulose tape slide preparation is the method of choice for the detection of pinworm eggs. Specimens collected by either method should be obtained in the morning before the patient bathes or goes to the bathroom. The tape method requires that the adhesive surface of the tape be pressed firmly against the right and left perianal folds and then spread onto the surface of a microscope slide. Likewise, the anal swab should be rubbed gently over the perianal area and transported to the laboratory for microscopic examination. The slides or swabs should be kept at 4°C if transport to the laboratory is to be delayed.

Sigmoidoscopic Material

Material from sigmoidoscopy can be helpful in the diagnosis of *E. histolytica* infection that has not been detected by routine fecal examinations. The specimens consist of scraped or aspirated material from the muco-

sal surface. At least six areas should be sampled. After collection, the material should be placed in a tube containing 0.85% saline and should be kept warm during transport to the laboratory. The specimens should be examined immediately for motile trophozoites.

Duodenal Aspirates

Sampling and examination of duodenal contents is a means of recovering the following (1) *Strongyloides* larvae, (2) the eggs of *Clonorchis, Opisthorchis,* and *Fasciola* species, and (3) other small bowel parasites, such as *Giardia, Isospora,* and *Cryptosporidium* organisms. Specimens may be obtained with endoscopic intubation or with the use of the enteric capsule or string test (Entero-Test). Endoscopic biopsy of the small intestinal mucosa may reveal *Giardia* organisms, *Cryptosporidium* organisms, and microsporidia as well as *Strongyloides* larvae. Specimens should be collected in saline and transported directly to the laboratory for microscopic examination.

Liver Abscess Aspirate

Suppurative lesions of the liver and subphrenic spaces may be caused by *E. histolytica* (extraintestinal amebiasis). This disorder may occur in the absence of any history of symptomatic intestinal infection. The specimen should be collected from the liver abscess margin instead of the necrotic center. The first portion removed is usually yellowish white and seldom contains amebae. Later portions, which are reddish, are more likely to contain organisms. A minimum of two separate portions of exudative material should be removed. After aspiration, the collapse of the abscess and the subsequent inflowing of blood often release amebae from the tissue. Subsequent aspirations may have a greater chance of revealing organisms. The aspirated material should be transported immediately to the laboratory.

Sputum

Occasionally, intestinal parasites may be detected in sputum. These organisms include (1) the larvae of *Ascaris* species, *Strongyloides* species, and hookworm, (2) cestode hooklets, and (3) intestinal protozoa such as *E. histolytica* and *Cryptosporidium* species. The specimen should be deeply located sputum rather than primarily saliva, and it should be delivered immediately to the laboratory. Microscopic examination should include saline wet-mount and permanent stain preparations.

Urine

Examination of urine specimens may be useful in diagnosing infections caused by *Schistosoma haematobium* (occasionally other species as well) and *Trichomonas vaginalis*. Detection of eggs in urine can be accomplished either through direct detection or through concentration by the sedimentation centrifugation technique. Eggs may be trapped in mucus or pus and are more commonly present in the last few drops of the specimen rather than the first portion. The production of *Schistosoma* eggs fluctuates; therefore, multiple specimens should be collected and examined over several days. *T. vaginalis* may be found in the urinary sediment of male and female patients.

Urogenital Specimens

Urogenital specimens are collected if infection with *T. vaginalis* is suspected. Identification is based on wet-mount preparation examinations of vaginal and urethral discharges, prostatic secretions, or urine sediment. A specimen should be placed in a container with a small amount of 0.85% saline and sent immediately to the laboratory for examination. If no organisms are detected on direct wet mount, culture may be used.

Parasitic Infections of Blood or Tissue

Parasites localized within the blood or tissues of the host are more difficult to detect than intestinal and urogenital parasites. Microscopic examination of blood films is a direct and useful means of detecting malarial parasites, trypanosomes, and microfilariae. Unfortunately, the concentration of organisms often fluctuates; thus, the collection of multiple specimens over several days is required.

The preparation of both wet mounts (microfilariae and trypanosomes) and permanently stained thick and thin blood films is the mainstay of diagnosis. Examination of sputum may reveal helminth ova (lung flukes) or larvae (*Ascaris* and *Strongyloides* species) after appropriate concentration techniques. Biopsy of skin (onchocerciasis) or muscle (trichinosis) may be required for the diagnosis of certain nematode infections (see Table 74–1).

Blood Films

The clinical diagnosis of parasitic diseases such as malaria, leishmaniasis, trypanosomiasis, and filariasis largely rests on the collection of appropriately timed blood samples and the expert microscopic examination of properly prepared and stained thick and thin blood films. The optimal time for obtaining blood for parasitologic examination varies with the particular parasite suspected.

Because malaria is one of the few parasitic infections that can be life-threatening, blood collection and examination of blood films should be performed as soon as the diagnosis is suspected. Laboratories offering this service should be prepared to do so on a 24-hour basis, 7 days a week. Because the levels of parasitemia may be low or fluctuating, it is recommended that further specimens for blood films be obtained and examined at 6, 12, and 24 hours after the initial sample. Detection of trypanosomes in blood is occasionally possible during the early acute phase of the disease. *Trypanosoma cruzi* (Chagas' disease) may also be detected during subsequent febrile periods. After several months to a year, the trypomastigotes of African trypanosomiasis (*Trypanosoma brucei rhodesiense* and *Trypanosoma brucei gambiense*) are better demonstrated in spinal fluid than blood. Blood films for the detection of nocturnal microfilariae (*W. bancrofti* and *Brugia malayi*) should be prepared between 10 PM and 4 AM, whereas for the diurnal *Loa loa*, films are prepared around noon.

Two types of blood films are prepared for the diagnosis of blood parasite infections, thin films and thick films. Although wet-mount preparations of blood films can be examined for motile parasites (microfilariae and trypanosomes), most laboratories proceed directly to the preparation of thick and thin films for staining. In the thin film, the blood is spread over the slide in a thin (single-cell) layer, and the red blood cells remain intact after staining. In the thick film, the red cells are lysed before staining, and only the white blood cells, platelets, and parasites (if present) are visible. Thick films allow a larger amount of blood to be examined, increasing the possibility of detecting light infections. Unfortunately, greater distortion of the parasites makes species identification through the thick film particularly difficult. Proper use of this technique usually requires a great deal of expertise and experience.

Occasionally, other blood-concentration procedures may be used to detect light infections. Alternative concentration methods for detecting blood parasites include the use of microhematocrit centrifugation, the examination of buffy coat preparations, a triple centrifugation technique for the detection of low numbers of trypanosomes, and a membrane filtration technique for the detection of microfilariae.

Once prepared, blood films must be stained. The most dependable staining of blood parasites is obtained with Giemsa stain buffered to pH 7.0 to 7.2, although special stains may be occasionally used to identify species of microfilariae. Giemsa stain is particularly useful for the staining of protozoa (malaria and trypanosomes). The sheath of microfilariae, however, may not always stain with Giemsa stain; in this case, hematoxylin-based stains may be used.

Specimens Other Than Blood

On the basis of clinical presentation and epidemiologic considerations, tissue and body fluids other than blood may have to be examined. Smears and concentrates of cerebrospinal fluid are necessary to detect trophozoites of *Naegleria* species, trypanosomes, and larvae of *Angiostrongylus cantonensis* within the central nervous system. Cerebrospinal fluid must be promptly examined because the trophozoite forms of these parasites either are very labile (trypanosomes) or tend to round up and become nonmotile (*Naegleria* species). Examination of tissue impression smears of lymph nodes, liver biopsy material, spleen, or bone marrow stained with Giemsa stain is very useful for detecting intracellular parasites such as *Leishmania* and *Toxoplasma* species.

Biopsies of various tissues are excellent means of detecting localized or disseminated infections caused by protozoan and helminthic parasites. Saline mounts of superficial skin snips are very useful in detecting the microfilariae of *Onchocerca volvulus*. Examination of sputum (induced) is indicated when there is a question of pulmonary paragonimiasis (lung fluke) or abscess formation with *E. histolytica*. *Strongyloides* larvae may be detected in sputum from a patient with hyperinfection syndrome.

Alternatives to Microscopy

In most cases, the diagnosis of parasitic disease is made in the laboratory through microscopic detection and morphologic identification of the parasite in clinical specimens. Sometimes the parasite cannot be detected despite a careful search because of low levels or absence of organisms in readily available clinical material. In such cases, the clinician may need to rely on alternative methods based on the detection of parasite-derived material (antigens or nucleic acids) or on the host response to parasitic invasion (antibodies). Additional approaches used in selected infections include culture, animal inoculation, and xenodiagnosis.

Immunodiagnostics

Immunodiagnostic methods have long been used as aids in the diagnosis of parasitic diseases. Most of these serologic tests are based on the detection of specific antibody responses to the presence of the parasite. The analytical approaches include the use of classic procedures, such as agglutination, complement fixation, and gel diffusion methods as well as more modern techniques such as immunofluorescence assay (IFA), enzyme immunoassay (EIA), and Western blot analysis. Antibody detection is useful and is indicated in the diagnosis of many protozoan diseases (e.g., extraintestinal amebiasis, South American trypanosomiasis, leishmaniasis, transfusion-acquired malaria, toxoplasmosis) and helminthic diseases (e.g., clonorchiasis, cysticercosis, hydatidosis, lymphatic filariasis, schistosomiasis, trichinellosis, toxocariasis). There is a problem with the detection of antibody as a means of diagnosis. Because of the persistence of antibody for months to years after

the acute infection, demonstration of antibody can rarely differentiate between acute and chronic infections.

In contrast to antibody detection, the measurement of circulating parasite antigen in serum, urine, or feces may provide a more appropriate marker for the presence of active infection and may also indicate parasite load. Likewise, demonstrations of specific parasite antigen in lesion fluid, such as material from an amebic abscess or fluid from a hydatid cyst, may provide a definitive diagnosis of the infecting organism. Most common antigen-detection assays use an EIA format; however, immunofluorescence, radioimmunoassay, and immunoblot methods have also proved useful.

Several commercial assays for the detection of parasite antigens are now available in kits. These include EIA for the detection of *Giardia* and *Cryptosporidium* species in stool, EIA for the detection of *T. vaginalis* in urogenital specimens, and IFAs for the detection of *Giardia*, *Cryptosporidium*, and *Trichomonas* species. The reported sensitivity and specificity for most of these kits are quite good. The advantages of these approaches are labor savings and a potential increase in sensitivity. The disadvantages are the loss of parasitologic expertise and the fact that in each case, the available assay tests for only a single organism, whereas conventional microscopic examination provides the opportunity to recognize many different parasites.

Although antigen-detection assays have been described for many other parasites, they are not widely available. The availability of a broader panel of antigen-detection assays would make the use of an antigen screen a viable alternative to tedious microscopic examination.

Molecular Diagnostic Approaches

In addition to immunodiagnostic methods, the diagnosis of parasitic diseases has been enhanced considerably by the application of molecular diagnostic methods based on nucleic acid hybridization. This approach takes advantage of the fact that all organisms contain nucleic acid sequences that may be used in a hybridization assay to distinguish among strains, species, and genera. Thus, parasites may be simultaneously detected and identified in clinical material depending on the specificity of the nucleic acid probe used. Another advantage of nucleic acid–based detection systems is that their results are independent of the patients' immunologic status or previous infection history, thereby identifying active infection. Finally, the development of target amplification techniques, such as the polymerase chain reaction (PCR), provides exquisite sensitivity, allowing the detection of as little as one organism in a biologic sample (Table 74–4).

Nucleic acid probes can be used to detect parasites not only in clinical samples of blood, stool, or tissue

TABLE 74–4. Examples of Techniques for Detection of Parasitic Infections Based on Polymerase Chain Reaction (PCR) Analysis

Organism	Gene Target	Sensitivity (%)	Comment
Plasmodium vivax	Circumsporozoite gene	91–96	Dried blood–spotted filter paper samples are used.
Leishmania species	kDNA minicircle sequence	87–100	Results are compared with results of culture and microscopy of biopsy specimens.
Trypanosoma cruzi	kDNA minicircle sequence	100	Results are compared with results of serology and xenodiagnosis of blood samples.
Toxoplasma gondii	B1 repetitive gene P30 major surface antigen Recombinant DNA sequences	46–99	PCR of bronchoalveolar lavage, blood, cerebrospinal fluid, and amniotic fluid show great potential for diagnosis of toxoplasmosis.
Entamoeba histolytica	P145 tandem repeat sequence	96	Results are compared to microscopic diagnosis of stool samples. Test may distinguish pathogenic from nonpathogenic strains.

from infected patients but also in their natural vector. The application of DNA "fingerprinting" allows precise identification of the parasite or vector to the subspecies or strain level and has considerable value in epidemiologic studies. Assay formats using nucleic acid probes range from dot blot and Southern hybridization methods to in situ hybridization in tissue to PCR amplification coupled with solid- or solution-phase hybridization.

The use of nonisotopic DNA labeling techniques greatly expands the potential applicability of these assays worldwide. Diagnostic kits based on these methods are not widely available; however, several are under development and may be available for clinical use in the near future. A simple nucleic acid probe assay for *T. vaginalis* in urogenital specimens is now available commercially in kit form for use in clinics and physicians' offices.

Irrespective of the assay format, nucleic acid probes and amplification techniques are now being used on a research basis for the detection and identification of numerous species and strains, including *Plasmodium* species, *Leishmania* species, *T. cruzi*, *E. histolytica*, and *Toxoplasma gondii* (see Table 74–4). It must be understood that the application of nucleic acid hybridization methods to the diagnosis of parasitic diseases is still in its infancy. Before these techniques can be applied broadly to aid in clinical diagnosis, simple procedures must be developed for sample handling and preparation, and the techniques must undergo extensive clinical and field testing.

Culture

Although culture is the standard for the diagnosis of most infectious diseases, it is not commonly used in the parasitology laboratory. Certain protozoan parasites, such as *T. vaginalis*, *E. histolytica*, *Acanthamoeba* species, *Naegleria* species, *Leishmania* species, *T. cruzi*, and *Toxoplasma* species can be cultured with relative ease. However, culture of other parasites has not been successful or is too difficult or cumbersome to be of practical value in routine diagnostic efforts.

Animal Inoculation

Animal inoculation is a sensitive means of detecting infection caused by blood and tissue parasites, such as *T. b. gambiense*, *T. b. rhodesiense*, *T. cruzi*, *Leishmania* species, and *T. gondii*. Although useful, this approach is not practical for most diagnostic laboratories and is largely confined to research settings.

Xenodiagnosis

The technique of xenodiagnosis employs the use of laboratory-raised arthropod vectors to detect low levels of parasites in infected individuals. Classically, this approach was used to diagnose Chagas' disease, as follows:

1. An uninfected reduviid bug was allowed to feed on an individual suspected of having the disease.
2. The bug was dissected and examined microscopically for evidence of developmental stages of *T. cruzi*.

Although this technique may be used in endemic areas, it is obviously not practical for most diagnostic laboratories.

QUESTIONS

1. Why is it important to understand the life cycle of parasites in order to diagnose parasitic diseases?

2. What factors may confound the use of microscopy in the diagnosis of parasitic disease?

3. Describe the important considerations in collecting and submitting a fecal specimen for parasitologic examination.

4. Which parasites can be detected in blood?

5. What are the alternatives to microscopy for the diagnosis of parasitic infections?

BIBLIOGRAPHY

Connor DH et al, editors: *Pathology of infectious diseases*, vol II, Stamford, Conn, 1997, Appleton & Lange.

Garcia LS et al: *Slide preparation and staining of blood films for the laboratory diagnosis of parasitic diseases*, National Committee for Clinical Laboratory Standards document M15-T, Villanova, Pa, 1992.

Garcia LS, editor: *Diagnostic medical parasitology*, ed 4, Washington, DC, 2001, ASM Press.

Garcia LS, Schimizu RY, Bernard CN: Detection of *Giardia lamblia, Entamoeba histolytica/Entamoeba dispar*, and *Cryptosporidium parvum* antigens in human fecal specimens using the Triage Parasite Panel enzyme immunoassay, *J Clin Microbiol* 38:3337–3340, 2000.

Hague R et al: Diagnosis of amebic liver abscess and intestinal infection with the Tech Lab *Entamoeba histolytica* II antigen detection and antibody tests, *J Clin Microbiol* 38: 3235–3239, 2000.

Maddison SE: Serodiagnosis of parasitic diseases, *Clin Microbiol Rev* 4:457–469, 1991.

Marshall MM et al: Waterborne protozoan pathogens, *Clin Microbiol Rev* 10:67–85, 1997.

Valenstein P, Pfaller M, Yungbluth M: The use and abuse of routine stool microbiology: a College of American Pathologists Q-Probes study of 601 institutions, *Arch Pathol Lab Med* 120:206–211, 1996.

Weiss JB: DNA probes and PCR for diagnosis of parasitic infections, *Clin Microbiol Rev* 8:113–130, 1995.

C H A P T E R   7 5

Intestinal and Urogenital Protozoa

Protozoa may colonize and infect the oropharynx, duodenum and small bowel, colon, and urogenital tract of humans. The majority of these parasites belong to the amebae and flagellates; however, infection with ciliate, coccidian, or microsporidian parasites may also be encountered (see Table 74–2). These organisms are transmitted by the fecal-oral route. In the United States, transmission of intestinal protozoa is particularly problematic in daycare centers, where several outbreaks of diarrhea caused by *Giardia* or *Cryptosporidium* species have been documented. In other parts of the world, the spread of enteric protozoal infections may be controlled in part by improved sanitation and by chlorination and filtration of water supplies; however, these measures may be difficult or impossible to achieve in many developing countries.

Amebae

The amebae are primitive unicellular microorganisms. Their life cycle is relatively simple and divided into two stages, the actively motile feeding stage (trophozoite) and the quiescent, resistant, infective stage (cyst). Replication occurs through binary fission (splitting of the trophozoite) or through the development of numerous trophozoites within the mature multinucleated cyst. Motility is accomplished by extension of a pseudopod ("false foot") with extrusion of the cellular ectoplasm and then drawing up of the rest of the cell in a snail-like movement to meet this pseudopod. The amebic trophozoites remain actively motile as long as the environment is favorable. The cyst form develops when the environmental temperature or moisture level drops.

Most amebae found in humans are commensal organisms (*Entamoeba coli, Entamoeba hartmanni, Entamoeba dispar, Entamoeba gingivalis, Endolimax nana, Iodamoeba bütschlii*). However, *Entamoeba histolytica* is an important human pathogen. Other amebae, particularly *Entamoeba polecki*, can cause human disease but are rarely isolated. The pathogenicity of *Blastocystis hominis* is still controversial. Some free-living amebae (*Naegleria fowleri, Acanthamoeba* species) are present in soil and in warm freshwater ponds or swimming pools and can be opportunistic human pathogens, causing meningoencephalitis or keratitis.

Entamoeba histolytica

Physiology and Structure

Cyst and trophozoite forms of *E. histolytica* are detected in fecal specimens from infected patients (Fig. 75–1). Trophozoites can also be found in the crypts of the large intestine. In freshly passed stools, actively motile trophozoites can be seen, whereas in formed stools, the cysts are usually the only form recognized. For the diagnosis of amebiasis, distinguishing between the trophozoites and cysts of *E. histolytica* and those of commensal amebae is important.

Pathogenesis

After ingestion, the cysts pass through the stomach, where exposure to gastric acid stimulates the release of the pathogenic trophozoite in the duodenum. The trophozoites divide and produce extensive local necrosis in the large intestine. The basis for this tissue destruction is incompletely understood, although it is attributed to production of a cytotoxin. Attachment of *E. histolytica* trophozoites to host cells via a galactose-inhibitable adherence protein is required for cytolysis and tissue necrosis to occur. The lysis of colonic epithelial cells, human neutrophils, lymphocytes, and monocytes by trophozoites is associated with a lethal alteration of host cell membrane permeability, resulting in an irreversible increase in intracellular calcium levels. The release of toxic neutrophil constituents after the lysis of neutrophils may contribute to the tissue destruction. Flask-shaped ulcerations of the intestinal mucosa are present, with inflammation, hemorrhage, and secondary bacterial infection.

Invasion into the deeper mucosa with extension into the peritoneal cavity may occur. This can lead to secondary involvement of other organs, primarily the liver but also the lungs, brain, and heart. Extraintestinal am-

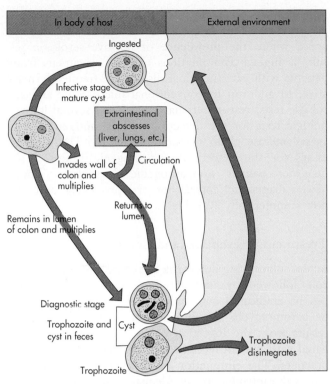

FIGURE 75–1. Life cycle of *Entamoeba histolytica.*

ebiasis is associated with trophozoites. Amebae are found only in environments that have a low oxygen pressure, because the protozoa are killed by ambient oxygen concentrations.

New procedures, such as lectin binding, zymodeme analysis, genomic DNA analysis, and staining with specific monoclonal antibodies, have been used as markers to identify invasive strains of *E. histolytica*. It is now recognized that the ameba morphologically identified as *E. histolytica* is actually two distinct species. The pathogenic species is *E. histolytica*, and the nonpathogenic species is *E. dispar*. The zymodeme profiles as well as the biochemical, molecular, and immunogic differences are stable and support the existence of two species.

Epidemiology

E. histolytica has a worldwide distribution. Although it is found in cold areas such as Alaska, Canada, and Eastern Europe, its incidence is highest in tropical and subtropical regions that have poor sanitation and contaminated water. The average prevalence of infection in these areas is 10% to 15%, with as many as 50% of the population infected in some areas. Many of the infected individuals are asymptomatic carriers, who represent a reservoir for the spread of *E. histolytica* to others. The prevalence of infection in the United States is 1% to 2%.

Patients infected with *E. histolytica* pass noninfectious trophozoites and the infectious cysts in their stools. The trophozoites cannot survive in the external environment or in transport through the stomach if ingested. Therefore, the main source of water and food contamination is the asymptomatic carrier who passes cysts. This is a particular problem in hospitals for the mentally ill, military and refugee camps, prisons, and crowded daycare centers. Flies and cockroaches can also serve as vectors for the transmission of *E. histolytica* cysts. Sewage containing cysts can contaminate water systems, wells, springs, and agricultural areas where human waste is used as fertilizer. Finally, cysts can be transmitted by oral-anal sexual practices, and amebiasis is prevalent in homosexual populations. Direct trophozoite transmission in sexual encounters can produce cutaneous amebiasis.

Clinical Syndromes

The outcome of infection may result in a carrier state, intestinal amebiasis, or extraintestinal amebiasis. If the strain of *E. histolytica* has a low virulence, if the inoculum is low, or if the patient's immune system is intact, the organisms may reproduce, and cysts may be passed in stool specimens with no clinical symptoms. Although infections with *E. histolytica* may be asymptomatic, most asymptomatic people are infected with the noninvasive *E. dispar*, as characterized by specific isoenzyme profiles (zymodemes), their susceptibility to complement-mediated lysis, and their failure to agglutinate in the presence of the lectin concanavalin A. Detection of carriers of *E. histolytica* in areas with a low endemicity is important for epidemiologic purposes.

Patients with intestinal amebiasis develop clinical symptoms related to the localized tissue destruction in the large intestine. Symptoms include abdominal pain, cramping, and colitis with diarrhea. More severe disease is characterized by the passing of numerous bloody stools in a day. Systemic signs of infection (fever, leukocytosis, rigors) are present in patients with extraintestinal amebiasis. The liver is primarily involved, because trophozoites in the blood are removed from the blood as it passes through this organ. Abscess formation is common. The right lobe is most commonly involved. Pain over the liver with hepatomegaly and elevation of the diaphragm is observed.

Laboratory Diagnosis

The identification of *E. histolytica* trophozoites (Fig. 75–2) and cysts in stools and trophozoites in tissue is diagnostic of amebic infection. Care must be taken to distinguish between these amebae and commensal amebae as well as between these amebae and polymorphonuclear leukocytes. Microscopic examination of stool

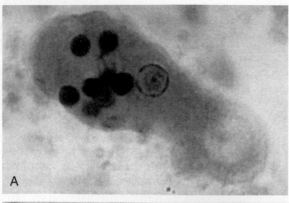

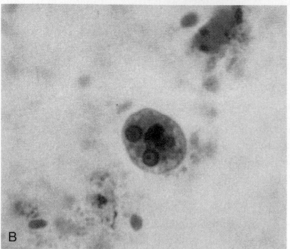

FIGURE 75–2. *Entamoeba histolytica* trophozoite *(A)* and cyst *(B).* Trophozoites are motile and vary in size from 12 to 60 μm (average, 15 to 30 μm). The single nucleus in the cell is round with a central dot (karyosome) and an even distribution of chromatin granules around the nuclear membrane. Ingested erythrocytes may be in the cytoplasm. The cysts are smaller (10 to 20 μm with an average size of 15 to 20 μm) and contain one to four nuclei (usually four). Round chromatoidal bars may be in the cytoplasm. *(A* from Lennette EH et al: *Manual of clinical microbiology,* ed 5, Washington, DC, 1991, American Society for Microbiology; *B* from Markell EK, Voge M, John DT: *Medical parasitology,* ed 7, Philadelphia, 1992, WB Saunders.)

specimens is inherently insensitive, because (1) the protozoa are not usually distributed homogeneously in the specimen and (2) the parasites are concentrated in the intestinal ulcers and at the margins of the abscess, not in the stool or the necrotic center of the abscess. For this reason, multiple stool specimens should be collected. Extraintestinal amebiasis is sometimes diagnosed through the use of scanning procedures for the liver and other organs. Specific serologic tests, together with microscopic examination of the abscess material, can confirm the diagnosis.

Virtually all patients with hepatic amebiasis and most patients (more than 80%) with intestinal disease have positive serologic findings at the time of clinical presentation. This fact may be less useful in endemic areas, where the prevalence of positive serologic results is higher. Examinations of stool specimens from patients with extraintestinal disease are frequently negative. In addition to conventional microscopic and serologic tests, researchers have developed several immunologic tests for the detection of fecal antigen as well as polymerase chain reaction (PCR) and DNA probe assays for the detection of pathogenic strains of *E. histolytica* (versus nonpathogenic *E. dispar*). These newer diagnostic approaches are promising and are now commercially available.

Treatment, Prevention, and Control

Acute, fulminating amebiasis is treated with metronidazole followed by iodoquinol. Asymptomatic carriage can be eradicated with iodoquinol, diloxanide furoate, or paromomycin. As already noted, human infection results from the ingestion of food or water contaminated with human feces or as a result of specific sexual practices. The elimination of the cycle of infection requires the introduction of adequate sanitation measures and education about the routes of transmission. The chlorination and filtration of water supplies may limit the spread of these and other enteric protozoal infections but are not possible to achieve in many developing countries. Physicians should alert travelers to developing countries of the risks associated with the consumption of water (including ice cubes), unpeeled fruits, and raw vegetables. Water should be boiled and fruits and vegetables thoroughly cleaned before consumption.

Other Intestinal Amebae

Other amebae that can parasitize the human gastrointestinal tract are *E. coli, E. hartmanni, E. polecki, E. nana, I. bütschlii* and *B. hominis. E. polecki,* which is primarily a parasite of pigs and monkeys, can cause human disease—a mild, transient diarrhea. The diagnosis of *E. polecki* infection is confirmed by the microscopic detection of cysts in stool specimens. Treatment is the same as for *E. histolytica* infections.

B. hominis, previously regarded as a nonpathogenic yeast, is now the center of considerable controversy concerning its taxonomic position and its pathogenicity. The organism is found in stool specimens from asymptomatic people as well as from people with persistent diarrhea. It has been suggested that the presence of large numbers of these parasites (five or more per oil-immersion microscopic field) in the absence of other intestinal pathogens indicates disease. Other investigators have concluded that "symptomatic blastocystosis" is attributable to an undetected pathogen or

TABLE 75–1. Morphologic Identification of *Entamoeba histolytica* and *Entamoeba coli*

	E. histolytica	E. coli
Size (diameter; μm)		
Trophozoite	12–50	20–30
Cyst	10–20	10–30
Pattern of peripheral nuclear chromatin	Fine, dispersed ring	Coarse, clumped
Karyosome	Central, sharp	Eccentric, coarse
Ingested erythrocytes	Present	Absent
Cyst structure		
No. of nuclei	1–4	1–8
Chromatoidal bars	Rounded ends	Splintered, frayed ends

functional bowel problems. The organism may be detected in wet mounts or trichrome-stained smears of fecal specimens. Treatment with iodoquinol or metronidazole has been successful in eradicating the organisms from the intestine and alleviating symptoms. However, the definitive role of *B. hominis* in disease remains to be demonstrated.

The nonpathogenic intestinal amebae are important, because they must be distinguished from *E. histolytica*, *E. polecki*, and *B. hominis*. This differentiation is particularly important for *E. coli*, which is frequently detected in stool specimens collected from patients exposed to contaminated food or water. Accurate identification of intestinal amebae requires careful microscopic examination of the cyst and trophozoite forms present in stained and unstained stool specimens (Table 75–1). Likewise, *E. dispar* may now be differentiated with specific immunologic reagents.

Flagellates

The flagellates of clinical significance include *Giardia lamblia (duodenalis)*, *Dientamoeba fragilis*, and *Trichomonas vaginalis*. Nonpathogenic commensal flagellates, such as *Chilomastix mesnili* (enteric) and *Trichomonas tenax* (oral), may also be observed. *Giardia* organisms, like *E. histolytica*, have cyst and trophozoite stages in their life cycles. In contrast, no cyst stage has been observed for *Trichomonas* or *Dientamoeba* species. Unlike the amebae, most flagellates move by the lashing of flagella that pull the organisms through fluid environments. Diseases produced by flagellates are primarily the result of mechanical irritation and inflammation. For example, *G. lamblia (duodenalis)* attaches to the intestinal villi with an adhesive disk, resulting in localized tissue damage. The tissue invasion with extensive tissue

destruction, as seen with *E. histolytica*, is rare with flagellates.

Giardia lamblia (duodenalis)

Physiology and Structure

Both cyst and trophozoite forms of *G. lamblia (duodenalis)* are detected in fecal specimens from infected patients (Fig. 75–3).

Pathogenesis

Infection with *G. lamblia (duodenalis)* is initiated by ingestion of cysts (Fig. 75–4). The minimum infective dose for humans is estimated to be 10 to 25 cysts. Gastric acid stimulates excystation, with the release of trophozoites in the duodenum and jejunum, where the organisms multiply by binary fission. The trophozoites can attach to the intestinal villi by means of a prominent ventral sucking disk. Although the tips of the villi may appear flattened and inflammation of the mucosa with hyperplasia of lymphoid follicles may be observed, frank tissue necrosis does not occur. In addition, metastatic spread of disease beyond the gastrointestinal tract is very rare.

Epidemiology

Giardia species have a worldwide distribution, and the flagellates have a sylvatic or "wilderness" distribution in many streams, lakes, and mountain resorts. This sylvatic distribution is maintained in reservoir animals such as beavers and muskrats. Giardiasis is acquired through the consumption of inadequately treated contaminated water, ingestion of contaminated uncooked vegetables or fruits, or person-to-person spread by the

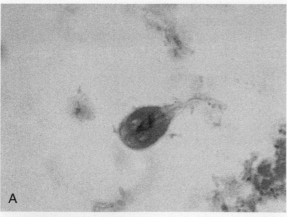

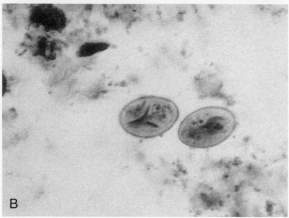

FIGURE 75–3. *Giardia lamblia (duodenalis)* trophozoite *(A)* and cyst *(B)*. Trophozoites are 9 to 12 μm long and 5 to 15 μm wide. Flagella are present, as are two nuclei with large central karysomes, a large ventral sucking disk for attachment of the flagellate to the intestinal villi, and two oblong parabasal bodies below the nuclei. The morphology gives the appearance that the trophozoites are "looking back" at the viewer. Cysts are smaller—8 to 12 μm long and 7 to 10 μm wide. Four nuclei and four parabasal bodies are present. (From Feingold SM, Baron EJ: *Bailey and Scott's diagnostic microbiology*, ed 7, St Louis, 1986, Mosby.)

fecal-oral or oral-anal route. The cyst stage is resistant to chlorine concentrations (1 to 2 parts per million) used in most water treatment facilities. Thus, adequate water treatment should include chemicals with filtration.

Risk factors associated with *Giardia* infections include poor sanitary conditions, travel to known endemic areas, consumption of inadequately treated water (e.g., from contaminated mountain streams), daycare centers, and oral-anal sexual practices. Infections may occur in outbreak and endemic forms within daycare centers and other institutional settings and among family members of infected children. Scrupulous attention to hand washing and treatment of all infected individuals are important in controlling the spread of infection in these settings.

Clinical Syndromes

Giardia infection can result in either asymptomatic carriage (observed in approximately 50% of infected individuals) or symptomatic disease ranging from mild diarrhea to a severe malabsorption syndrome. The incubation period before symptomatic disease develops ranges from 1 to 4 weeks (average, 10 days). The onset of disease is sudden and consists of foul-smelling, watery diarrhea; abdominal cramps; flatulence; and steatorrhea. Blood and pus are rarely present in stool specimens, a feature consistent with the absence of tissue destruction in this infection. Spontaneous recovery generally occurs after 10 to 14 days, although a more chronic disease with multiple relapses may develop. Chronic disease is particularly a problem for patients with immunoglobulin A deficiency or intestinal diverticula.

Laboratory Diagnosis

With the onset of diarrhea and abdominal discomfort, stool specimens should be examined for cysts and trophozoites (see Fig. 75–3). *Giardia* species may occur in "showers"; that is, many organisms may be present in the stool on a given day and few or none may be detected the next day. For this reason, the physician should never accept the results of a single negative stool specimen as evidence that the patient is free of intestinal parasites. One stool specimen per day for 3 days should be examined. If results of stool examina-

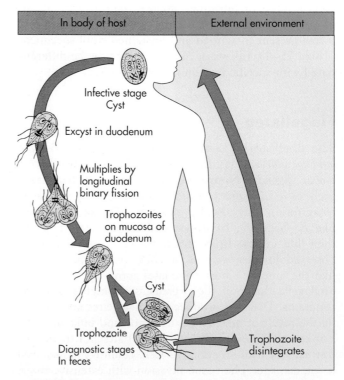

FIGURE 75–4. Life cycle of *Giardia lamblia (duodenalis)*.

tion remain persistently negative in a patient in whom giardiasis is highly suspected, additional specimens can be collected by duodenal aspiration, string test (Entero-Test), or biopsy of the upper small intestine.

In addition to conventional microscopy, several immunologic tests for the detection of fecal antigen are available commercially. They include countercurrent immunoelectrophoresis, enzyme immunoassay, and indirect immunofluorescent staining. Reported sensitivities range from 88% to 98%, and specificities from 87% to 100%.

Treatment, Prevention, and Control

It is important to eradicate *Giardia* species from asymptomatic carriers and diseased patients. The drug of choice is quinacrine, with metronidazole an acceptable alternative. The prevention and control of giardiasis involve the avoidance of contaminated water and food, especially by travelers and outdoor enthusiasts. People can protect themselves by boiling drinking water taken from streams and lakes or available in countries with a high incidence of endemic disease. Maintenance of properly functioning filtration systems in municipal water supplies is also required, because *Giardia* cysts are resistant to standard chlorination procedures. Public health efforts should be made to identify the reservoir of infection to prevent spread of disease. In addition, high-risk sexual behavior should be avoided.

Dientamoeba fragilis

Physiology and Structure

Dientamoeba fragilis was classified initially as an ameba; however, the internal structures of the trophozoite are typical of a flagellate. No cyst stage has been described.

Epidemiology

D. fragilis has a worldwide distribution. The transmission of the delicate trophozoite is not completely understood. Some observers believe the organism can be transported from person to person inside the protective shell of worm eggs such as those of *Enterobius vermicularis*, the pinworm. Transmission by the fecal-oral and oral-anal routes does occur.

Clinical Syndromes

Most infections with *D. fragilis* are asymptomatic, with colonization of the cecum and upper colon. However, some patients may develop symptomatic disease, consisting of abdominal discomfort, flatulence, intermittent diarrhea, anorexia, and weight loss. There is no evidence of tissue invasion with this flagellate, although irritation of the intestinal mucosa occurs.

Laboratory Diagnosis

Infection is confirmed by the microscopic examination of stool specimens in which typical trophozoites can be seen. The trophozoite is small (5 to 12 μm), with one or two nuclei. The central karyosome consists of four to six discrete granules. Excretion of the parasite may fluctuate markedly from day to day, and thus, collection of several stool samples may be necessary. Examination of a purged stool sample may also be useful.

Treatment, Prevention, and Control

The therapeutic agent of choice for *D. fragilis* infection is iodoquinol, with tetracycline and paromomycin acceptable alternatives. The reservoir for this flagellate and the organism's life cycle are unknown. Thus, specific recommendations for prevention and control are difficult. However, infections can be avoided by maintenance of adequate sanitary conditions. The eradication of infections with *Enterobius* organisms may also reduce the transmission of *Dientamoeba* infection.

Trichomonas vaginalis

Physiology and Structure

T. vaginalis is not an intestinal protozoan but, rather, the cause of urogenital infections. The flagellate's four flagella and short, undulating membrane are responsible for motility. *T. vaginalis* exists only as a trophozoite and is found in the urethras and vaginas of women and the urethras and prostate glands of men.

Epidemiology

This parasite has worldwide distribution, and sexual intercourse is the primary mode of transmission (Fig. 75–5). Occasionally, infections have been transmitted by fomites (toilet articles, clothing), although this transmission is limited by the lability of the trophozoite form. Infants may be infected by passage through the mother's infected birth canal. The prevalence of this flagellate in developed countries is reported to be 5% to 20% in women and 2% to 10% in men.

Clinical Syndromes

Most infected women are asymptomatic or have a scant, watery vaginal discharge. Vaginitis may occur with more extensive inflammation, along with erosion of the epithelial lining that is associated with itching, burning, and painful urination. Men are primarily asymptomatic carriers who serve as reservoirs for infections in women. However, men occasionally experience urethritis, prostatitis, and other urinary tract problems.

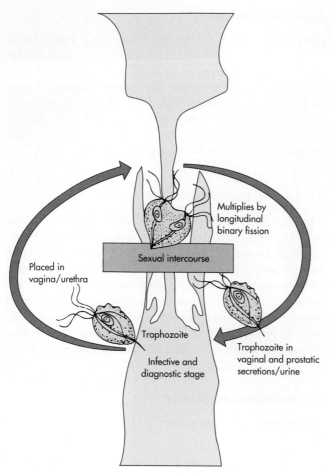

FIGURE 75–5. Life cycle of *Trichomonas vaginalis.*

Ciliates

The intestinal protozoan *Balantidium coli* is the only member of the ciliate group that is pathogenic for humans. Disease produced by *B. coli* is similar to amebiasis, because the organisms elaborate proteolytic and cytotoxic substances that mediate tissue invasion and intestinal ulceration.

Balantidium coli

Physiology and Structure

The life cycle of *B. coli* is simple, involving ingestion of infectious cysts, excystation, and invasion of trophozoites into the mucosal lining of the large intestine, cecum, and terminal ileum (Fig. 75–7). The trophozoite is covered with rows of hairlike cilia that aid in motility. Morphologically more complex than amebae, *B. coli* has a funnel-like primitive mouth called a cytostome, a large (macro) nucleus and a small (micro) nucleus involved in reproduction, food vacuoles, and two contractile vacuoles.

Epidemiology

B. coli is distributed worldwide. Swine and (less commonly) monkeys are the most important reservoirs. Infections are transmitted by the fecal-oral route; outbreaks are associated with contamination of water supplies with pig feces. Person-to-person spread, in-

Laboratory Diagnosis

Microscopic examination of vaginal or urethral discharge for characteristic trophozoites is the diagnostic method of choice (Fig. 75–6). Stained (Giemsa, Papanicolaou) or unstained smears can be examined. The diagnostic yield may be improved by culture of the organism (93% sensitivity) or use of monoclonal fluorescent antibody staining (86% sensitivity). A nucleic acid probe assay is also available commercially. Serologic tests may be useful in epidemiologic surveillance.

Treatment, Prevention, and Control

The drug of choice is metronidazole. Both male and female sex partners must be treated to avoid reinfection. Resistance to metronidazole has been reported and may require retreatment with higher doses. Good personal hygiene, avoidance of shared toilet articles and clothing, and safe sex practices are important preventive actions. Elimination of carriage in men is critical for the eradication of disease.

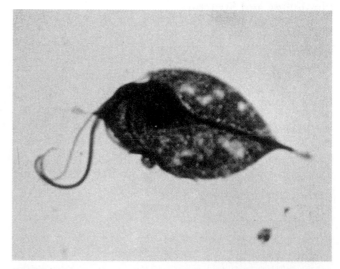

FIGURE 75–6. *Trichomonas vaginalis* trophozoite. The trophozoite is 7 to 23 μm long and 6 to 8 μm wide (average, 13 × 7 μm). The flagella and a short undulating membrane are present at one side, and an axostyle extends through the center of the parasite. (From Ash LR, Orihel TC: *Atlas of human parasitology*, ed 2, Chicago, 1984, American Society of Clinical Pathologists.)

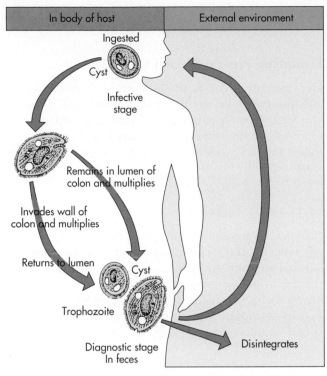

FIGURE 75–7. Life cycle of *Balantidium coli.*

cluding through food handlers, has been implicated in outbreaks. Risk factors associated with human disease include contact with swine and substandard hygienic conditions.

Clinical Syndromes

As with other protozoan parasites, asymptomatic carriage of *B. coli* can exist. Symptomatic disease is characterized by abdominal pain and tenderness, tenesmus, nausea, anorexia, and watery stools with blood and pus. Ulceration of the intestinal mucosa, as with amebiasis, can be seen; a secondary complication caused by bacterial invasion into the eroded intestinal mucosa can occur. Extraintestinal invasion of other organs is extremely rare in balantidiasis.

Laboratory Diagnosis

Microscopic examination of feces for trophozoites and cysts is performed. The trophozoite is very large, varying in length from 50 to 200 μm and in width from 40 to 70 μm. The surface is covered with cilia, and the prominent internal structure is a macronucleus. A micronucleus is also present. Two pulsating, contractile vacuoles are also seen in fresh preparations of the trophozoites. The cyst is smaller (40 to 60 μm in diameter), is surrounded by a clear refractile wall, and has a single nucleus in the cytoplasm. *B. coli* is a large organ-

ism compared with other intestinal protozoa and is readily detected in fresh, wet microscopic preparations.

Treatment, Prevention, and Control

The drug of choice is tetracycline; iodoquinol and metronidazole are alternative antimicrobials. Actions for prevention and control are similar to those for amebiasis. Appropriate personal hygiene, maintenance of sanitary conditions, and the careful monitoring of pig feces are all important preventive measures.

Coccidia

Coccidia constitute a very large group called Apicomplexa, some members of which are discussed in this section with the intestinal parasites and others with the blood and tissue parasites. All coccidia demonstrate typical characteristics, especially the existence of asexual (schizogony) and sexual (gametogony) reproduction. Most members of the group also share alternative hosts; for example, in malaria, mosquitoes harbor the sexual cycle and humans the asexual cycle. Coccidia discussed in this chapter are *Isospora*, *Sarcocystis*, *Cryptosporidium*, and *Cyclospora* species.

Isospora belli

Physiology and Structure

Isospora belli is a coccidian parasite of the intestinal epithelium. Both sexual and asexual reproduction can occur in the intestinal epithelium, resulting in tissue damage (Fig. 75–8). The end product of gametogenesis is the oocyst, which is the diagnostic stage present in fecal specimens.

Epidemiology

Isospora organisms are distributed worldwide but are infrequently detected in stool specimens. However, this parasite has been reported with increasing frequency in healthy and immunocompromised patients. The change is probably due to the greater awareness of disease caused by *Isospora* species in patients with the acquired immunodeficiency syndrome (AIDS). Infection with this organism follows ingestion of contaminated food or water or oral-anal sexual contact.

Clinical Syndromes

Infected individuals may be asymptomatic carriers or may experience mild to severe gastrointestinal disease. Disease most commonly mimics giardiasis, consisting of a malabsorption syndrome characterized by loose, foul-smelling stools. Chronic diarrhea with weight loss, anorexia, malaise, and fatigue can be seen, although it

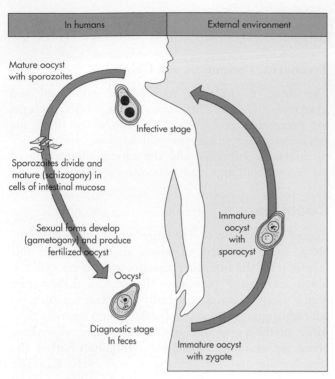

FIGURE 75–8. Life cycle of *Isospora* species.

In humans | External environment

Mature oocyst with sporozoites

Infective stage

Sporozoites divide and mature (schizogony) in cells of intestinal mucosa

Sexual forms develop (gametogony) and produce fertilized oocyst

Immature oocyst with sporocyst

Oocyst

Diagnostic stage In feces

Immature oocyst with zygote

is difficult to separate this manifestation from the patient's underlying disease.

Laboratory Diagnosis

Careful examination of concentrated stool sediment and special staining with iodine or a modified acid-fast procedure reveals the parasite (Fig. 75–9). Small-bowel

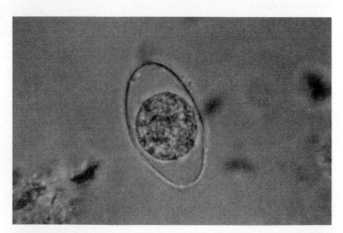

FIGURE 75–9. Immature oocyst of *Isospora* species. Oocysts are ovoid (approximately 25 μm long and 15 μm wide) with tapering ends. A developing sporocyst is seen within the cytoplasm. (From Lennette EH et al: *Manual of clinical microbiology*, ed 4, Washington, DC, 1985, American Society for Microbiology.)

biopsy has been used to establish the diagnosis when the results of tests on stool specimens are negative.

Treatment, Prevention, and Control

The drug of choice is trimethoprim-sulfamethoxazole, with the combination of pyrimethamine and sulfadiazine an acceptable alternative. Prevention and control are effected by maintaining personal hygiene and highly sanitary conditions and by avoiding oral-anal sexual contact.

Sarcocystis Species

Physician awareness of the genus *Sarcocystis* is important only for the recognition that its members can be detected in stool specimens. *Sarcocystis* species can be isolated from pigs and cattle and are identical in all aspects to *Isospora* species, with one exception: *Sarcocystis* oocysts rupture before passage in stool specimens, so only sporocysts are present.

Cryptosporidium parvum

Physiology and Structure

The life cycle of *Cryptosporidium parvum* is typical of coccidians, as is the intestinal disease, but this species differs in the intracellular location in the epithelial cells. In contrast to the deep intracellular invasion observed with *Isospora* species, *Cryptosporidium* organisms are found just within the brush border of the intestinal epithelium. The coccidia attach to the surfaces of the cells and replicate by a process that involves schizogony (Fig. 75–10).

Epidemiology

Cryptosporidium species are distributed worldwide. Infection is reported in a wide variety of animals, including mammals, reptiles, and fish. Waterborne transmission of cryptosporidiosis is now well-documented as an important route of infection. The massive outbreak of cryptosporidiosis in Milwaukee (approximately 300,000 individuals infected) was linked to contamination of the municipal water supply. Cryptosporidia are resistant to the usual water-purification procedures (chlorination and ozone), and it is believed that runoff of local waste water and surface water into municipal water supplies is an important source of contamination. Other common means of infection are zoonotic spread from animal reservoirs to humans and person-to-person spread by fecal-oral and oral-anal routes. Veterinary personnel, animal handlers, and homosexuals are at particularly high risk for infection. Many outbreaks have now been described in daycare centers, where fecal-oral transmission is common.

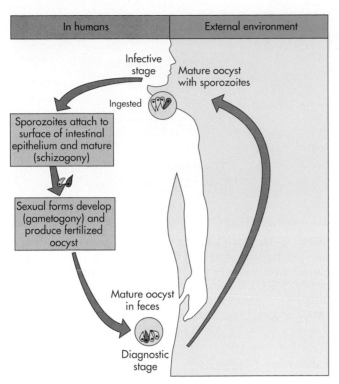

FIGURE 75-10. Life cycle of *Cryptosporidium* species.

Clinical Syndromes

As with other protozoan infections, exposure to *Cryptosporidium* organisms may result in asymptomatic carriage. Disease in previously healthy individuals is usually a mild, self-limited enterocolitis characterized by watery diarrhea without blood. Spontaneous remission after an average of 10 days is characteristic. In contrast, disease in immunocompromised patients (e.g., patients with AIDS), characterized by 50 or more stools per day and tremendous fluid loss, can be severe and can last for months to years. In some patients with AIDS, disseminated *Cryptosporidium* infections have been reported.

Laboratory Diagnosis

Cryptosporidium parvum may be detected in large numbers in unconcentrated stool specimens obtained from immunocompromised individuals with diarrhea. Oocysts may be concentrated with the modified zinc sulfate centrifugal flotation technique or by Sheather's sugar flotation procedure. Specimens may be stained with the modified acid-fast method (Fig. 75–11) or by an indirect immunofluorescence assay. An enzyme immunoassay for detecting fecal antigen is also commercially available. The number of oocysts shed in stool may fluctuate; therefore, a minimum of three specimens should be examined. Serologic procedures for diagnosing and monitoring infections are under investigation but are not yet widely available.

Treatment, Prevention, and Control

Unfortunately, no broadly effective therapy has been developed for managing *Cryptosporidium* infections in immunocompromised patients. No controlled studies have been published, and all therapeutic information is based on isolated reports and anecdotal information. Spiramycin may help control the diarrhea in some patients in the early stages of AIDS who have cryptosporidiosis but is ineffective in patients who have progressed to the later stages of AIDS. Spiramycin was no more effective than placebo in treating cryptosporidial diarrhea in infants. Reports concerning efficacy of azithromycin and paromomycin are promising, but these need confirmation. Therapy consists primarily of supportive measures to restore the tremendous fluid loss from the watery diarrhea.

Because of the widespread distribution of this organism in humans and other animals, preventing infection is difficult. The same methods of improved personal hygiene and sanitation used for other intestinal protozoa should be maintained for this disease. Contaminated water supplies should be treated with chlorination and filtration. In addition, avoidance of high-risk sexual activities is critical.

Cyclospora cayetanensis

Physiology and Structure

Cyclospora is a coccidian parasite that is taxonomically related to *Isospora* species, *Cryptosporidium parvum*, and *Toxoplasma gondii*. A single species infecting humans, *Cyclospora cayetanensis*, has been identified thus far.

Although the details of the life cycle have yet to be determined, *Cyclospora* organisms are similar to *Isospora*, in that oocysts are excreted unsporulated and require a period outside the host for maturation to occur. The pathogenic mechanisms by which *Cyclospora* species cause clinical illness are unknown; however, the organisms usually infect the upper small bowel and cause

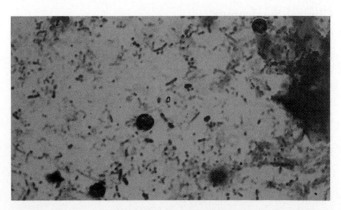

FIGURE 75-11. Acid-fast–stained *Cryptosporidium* oocysts (approximately 5 to 7 μm in diameter).

pronounced histopathologic changes. *C. cayetanensis* is found within vacuoles in the cytoplasm of jejunal epithelial cells, and its presence is associated with inflammatory changes, villous atrophy, and crypt hyperplasia.

The morphologic characteristics of *C. cayetanensis* are similar to those of *Isospora* species and *C. parvum*, with a few exceptions. The oocysts of *C. cayetanensis* are spherical and are 8 to 10 μm in diameter, as opposed to the smaller oocysts of *C. parvum* (4 to 6 μm) and the much larger elliptical oocysts of *Isospora* species (15 to 25 μm). The oocyst of *C. cayetanensis* contains two sporocysts, each of which contain two sporozoites; a sporozoite contains a membrane-bound nucleus and micronemes characteristic of the apicomplexans. In contrast, the *Cryptosporidium* oocyst contains four naked, or nonencysted, sporozoites, whereas the *Isospora* oocyst contains two sporocysts, each containing four sporozoites.

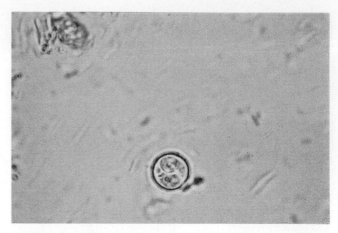

FIGURE 75-12. Sporulated oocyst of *Cyclospora cayetanensis*. The oocysts measure 8 to 10 μm in diameter and contain two sporocysts with two sporozoites. (Saline wet mount; ×900.) (Courtesy Mr. J Williams; from Peters W, Giles HM: *Color atlas of tropical medicine and parasitology*, ed 4, London, 1995, Mosby-Wolfe.)

Epidemiology

As with *Cryptosporidium*, *C. cayetanensis* is widely distributed throughout the world and infects a variety of reptiles, birds, and mammals. Although direct animal-to-human or person-to-person transmission has not been documented, there is now compelling evidence that *Cyclospora* infection is acquired through contaminated water. In areas of endemicity, such as Nepal, studies have documented an annual surge of cyclosporiasis that coincides with the rainy season. The prevalence of infection (symptomatic and asymptomatic) ranges from 2% to 18% in endemic areas and is estimated at 0.1% to 0.5% in developed countries. Outbreaks in the United States have occurred during the summer months, and although no source has been identified, transmission via contaminated water has been suggested. Like *Cryptosporidium*, *C. cayetanensis* is resistant to chlorination and is not readily detected by methods used currently to ensure the safety of supplies of drinking water.

Clinical Syndromes

The clinical manifestations of cyclosporiasis resemble those of cryptosporidiosis and include mild nausea, anorexia, abdominal cramping, and watery diarrhea. Fatigue, malaise, flatulence, and bloating have also been reported. In immunocompetent hosts, diarrhea is self-limited but may be prolonged and may last for weeks. Among immunocompromised people, specifically patients infected with the human immunodeficiency virus (HIV), clinical illness is typically prolonged and severe and is associated with a high rate of recurrence. Biliary tract infection with *Cyclospora* infection has been reported in two patients with AIDS.

Laboratory Diagnosis

The diagnosis of cyclosporiasis is based on the microscopic detection of oocysts in stool. Oocysts may be detected by light microscopic examination of unstained fecal material (wet mount), where they appear as nonrefractile, spherical to oval, slightly wrinkled bodies measuring 8 to 10 μm in diameter; they have an internal cluster of membrane-bound globules (Fig. 75–12). In fresh specimens, *Cyclospora* organisms fluoresce when examined with an ultraviolet fluorescence microscope fitted with a 365-nm excitation filter.

Cyclospora oocysts may be concentrated with the modified zinc sulfate centrifugal flotation technique or Sheather's sugar flotation procedure. Organisms are acid-fast and thus can be detected with the use of one of the many acid-fast staining techniques, including the modified Ziehl-Neelsen stain and the Kinyoun acid-fast stain (Fig. 75–13). A distinguishing feature of *C. cayetanensis* species is its variable appearance on acid-fast staining, which ranges from unstained to mottled pink to deep red.

The relative sensitivity, specificity, and predictive value of the various methods for diagnosing *Cyclospora* infection are not known. Currently, there are no immunodiagnostic techniques to aid in the diagnosis and monitoring of these infections. The rudimentary nature of the available diagnostic techniques and the incomplete understanding of the disease process may contribute to underrecognition of *Cyclospora* infection.

Treatment, Prevention, and Control

The effectiveness of trimethoprim-sulfamethoxazole has been demonstrated in anecdotal reports; in a large,

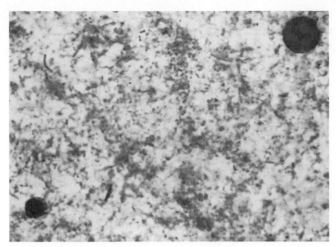

FIGURE 75–13. Oocysts of *Cryptosporidium parvum (lower left)* and *Cyclospora cayetanensis (upper right).* Both parasites strain red with Ziehl-Neelsen stain; however, *Cyclospora* organisms typically take up variable amounts of the stain, and oocysts are larger (8 to 10 μm compared with 4 to 6 μm). (Courtesy Mr. J. Williams: from Peters W, Giles HM: *Color atlas of tropical medicine and parasitology,* ed 4, London, 1995, Mosby-Wolfe.)

open-label study of patients infected with HIV; and in a placebo-controlled trial. In HIV-infected patients, it appears that the high rate of recurrence can be attenuated by long-term suppressive therapy with trimethoprim-sulfamethoxazole. Although numerous additional agents, including metronidazole, norfloxacin, quinacrine, nalidixic acid, tinidazole, and diloxanide furoate, have been used in various trials, the effectiveness of any one of these agents has not been proved.

Like *Cryptosporidium* infection, *Cyclospora* infection is difficult to prevent. Although *Cyclospora* organisms appear resistant to chlorination, the treatment of water supplies with chlorination and filtration remains a reasonable practice. In addition, the same methods used for other intestinal protozoa, such as improved personal hygiene and sanitation, should be used as preventive measures against this disease.

Microsporidia

Physiology and Structure

Microsporidia are obligate intracellular pathogens belonging to the phylum Microspora. They are considered primitive eukaryotic organisms because they lack mitochondria, peroxisomes, Golgi membranes, and other typically eukaryotic organelles. The parasites are characterized by the structure of their spores, which have a complex tubular extrusion mechanism used for injecting the infective material (sporoplasm) into cells. Microsporidia have been detected in human tissues and

implicated as participants in human disease. To date, six genera of microsporidia (*Encephalitozoon, Pleistophora, Nosema, Vittaforma, Trachipleistophora,* and *Enterocytozoon*) and unclassified *Microsporidium* species have been reported in humans.

Pathogenesis

Infection with microsporidia is initiated by the ingestion of spores. After ingestion, the spores pass into the duodenum, where the sporoplasm with its nuclear material is injected into an adjacent cell in the small intestine. Once inside a suitable host cell, the microsporidia multiply extensively either within a parasitophorous vacuole or free within the cytoplasm. The intracellular multiplication includes a phase of repeated divisions by binary fission (merogony) and a phase culminating in spore formation (sporogony). The parasites spread from cell to cell, causing cell death and local inflammation. Although some species are highly selective in the cell type that they invade, the microsporidia are collectively capable of infecting every organ of the body, and disseminated infections have been described in severely immunocompromised individuals. After sporogony, the mature spores containing the infective sporoplasm may be excreted into the environment, thus continuing the cycle.

Epidemiology

Microsporidia are distributed worldwide and have a wide host range among invertebrate and vertebrate animals. *Enterocytozoon bieneusi* and *Encephalitozoon* (previously known as *Septata*) *intestinalis* have gained increasing attention as causes of chronic diarrhea in patients with AIDS. Both *Encephalitozoon*-like and *Enterocytozoon*-like organisms have been reported in the tissues of patients with AIDS who have hepatitis and peritonitis. *Trachipleistophora* and *Nosema* are known to cause myositis in immunocompromised patients. *Nosema* species has caused localized keratitis as well as disseminated infection in a child with severe combined immunodeficiency. *Microsporidium* species and *Encephalitozoon hellem* have caused infection of the human cornea.

Although the reservoir for human infection is unknown, transmission is probably accomplished through ingestion of spores that have been shed in the urine and feces of infected animals or people. As with cryptosporidial infection, patients with AIDS and other cellular immune defects appear to be at greater risk for infection with microsporidia.

Clinical Syndromes

Clinical signs and symptoms of microsporidiosis are quite variable in the few human cases reported. Intesti-

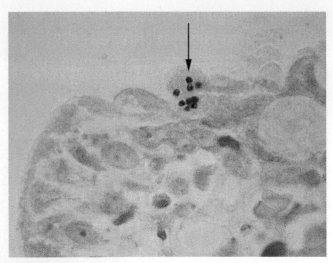

FIGURE 75–14. Gram-positive spores of microsporidia *(arrow)* in jejunal biopsy. (Brown-Brenn stain; ×1750). (From Weber R et al: Improved light-microscopical detection of microsporidia spores in stool and duodenal aspirates: The Enteric Opportunistic Infections Working Group, *N Engl J Med* 326:161–166, 1992.)

nal infection caused by *E. bieneusi* in patients with AIDS is marked by persistent and debilitating diarrhea similar to that seen in patients with cryptosporidiosis, cyclosporiasis, and isosporiasis. The clinical manifestation of infection with other species of Microspora depends on the organ system involved and ranges from localized ocular pain and loss of vision (*Microsporidium* and *Nosema* species) to neurologic disturbances and hepatitis (*Encephalitozoon cuniculi*) to a more generalized picture of dissemination with fever, vomiting, diarrhea, and malabsorption (*Nosema* species). In a report of disseminated infection with *Nosema connori*, the organism was observed to involve the muscles of the stomach, bowel, arteries, diaphragm, and heart and the parenchymal cells of the liver, lungs, and adrenal glands.

Laboratory Diagnosis

Diagnosis of microsporidia infection may be made through detection of the organisms in biopsy material and by light microscopy examination of cerebrospinal fluid and urine. Spores measuring between 1.0 and 2.0 μm may be visualized with Gram (gram-positive), acid-fast, periodic acid–Schiff, immunochemical, and Giemsa staining techniques (Fig. 75–14). A chromotrope-based staining technique for light microscopy detection of *E. bieneusi* and *E. (Septata) intestinalis* spores in stool and duodenal aspirates has been described (Fig. 75–15). Electron microscopy is considered the standard for diagnostic confirmation of microsporidiosis; however, its sensitivity is unknown. Additional diagnostic techniques, including polymerase chain reac-

tion, culture, and serologic testing, are under investigation. These techniques are not yet considered reliable enough for routine diagnosis.

Treatment, Prevention, and Control

There is no known effective treatment for microsporidian infections. Treatment with metronidazole has resulted in temporary improvement in patients with intestinal microsporidiosis. Likewise, some patients treated with sulfa drugs have survived. Preliminary reports with albendazole also appear promising. In vitro studies have demonstrated activity of trimethoprim-sulfisoxazole and of the antibiotic fumagillin against *E. cuniculi*, but these results have not been confirmed in vivo.

As with *Cryptosporidium* infections, preventing microsporidian infection is difficult. The same methods used for other intestinal protozoa, such as improved personal hygiene and sanitation, should be used as preventive measures against this disease.

CASE STUDY AND QUESTIONS

■ A 31-year-old female veterinarian complained of diarrhea that she had experienced for 2 weeks. The diarrhea was described as thin, watery, and nonbloody. The patient described 10 to 14 diarrheal stools per

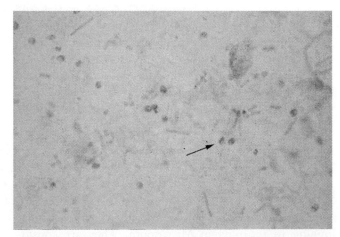

FIGURE 75–15. Smear of formalin-fixed stool specimen showing pinkish red–stained microsporidia spores, some with a distinct pinkish, beltlike stripe *(arrow)*. Bacteria are stained a faint green. (Chromotrope-based stain; ×1800.) (From Weber R et al: Improved light-microscopical detection of microsporidia spores in stool and duodenal aspirates: The Enteric Opportunistic Infections Working Group, *N Engl J Med* 326:161–166, 1992.)

day, the frequency of which was not influenced by a variety of over-the-counter antidiarrheal medications.

Physical examination revealed a well-developed, well-nourished woman who appeared somewhat fatigued and mildly dehydrated. Results of workup included a negative HIV serologic test, a normal flexible sigmoidoscope examination, and a negative stool culture for bacterial pathogens. A microscopic examination of the stool for white blood cells was negative, as was a test for *Clostridium difficile* toxin. A stool specimen was sent for ova and parasite examination and, after appropriate concentration measures, demonstrated acid-fast oocysts.

1. Which parasite was found in the patient's stool?

2. What was the likely source of this individual's infection?

3. If this individual were HIV-positive, what other intestinal pathogens would have been considered?

4. Other than conventional microscopy, what other methods could have been used to diagnose this infection?

5. Should this patient have received specific antimicrobial therapy? If so, what would have been prescribed? If not, why not?

BIBLIOGRAPHY

Clark DP: New insights into human cryptosporidiosis, *Clin Microbiol Rev* 12:554–563, 1999.

Connor DH et al, editors: *Pathology of infectious diseases*, vol II, Stamford, Conn, 1997, Appleton & Lange.

Espinosa-Cantellano M, Martinez-Palomo A: Pathogenesis of intestinal amebiasis: from molecules to disease, *Clin Microbiol Rev* 13:318–331, 2000.

Faubert G: Immune response to *Giardia duodenalis*, *Clin Microbiol Rev* 13:35–54, 2000.

Garcia LS, editor: *Diagnostic medical parasitology*, ed 4, Washington DC, 2001, ASM Press.

Gay JD et al: *Entamoeba polecki* infections in Southeast Asian refugees: multiple cases of a rarely reported parasite, *Mayo Clin Proc* 60:523–530, 1985.

Hayes EB et al: Large community outbreak of cryptosporidiosis due to contamination of a filtered public water supply, *N Engl J Med* 320:1372–1376, 1989.

Marshall MM et al: Waterborne protozoan pathogens, *Clin Microbiol Rev* 10:67–85, 1997.

May LP, Sidhu GS, Buchness MR: Diagnosis of *Acanthamoeba* infection by cutaneous manifestations in a man seropositive to HIV, *J Am Acad Dermatol* 26:352–355, 1992.

Peters W, Giles HM: *Color atlas of tropical medicine and parasitology*, ed 4, London, 1995, Mosby-Wolfe.

Schwartz DA et al: Pathology of microsporidiosis: emerging parasitic infections in patients with acquired immunodeficiency syndrome, *Arch Pathol Lab Med* 120:173–188, 1996.

Soave R: Cyclospora: an overview, *Clin Infect Dis* 23:429–437, 1996.

Weber R et al: Human microsporidial infections, *Clin Microbiol Rev* 7:426–461, 1994.

Weber R et al: Improved light-microscopical detection of microsporidia spores in stool and duodenal aspirate, *N Engl J Med* 326:161–166, 1992.

Wittner M, Weiss LM, editors: *The microsporidia and microsporidiosis*, Washington DC, 1999, ASM Press.

CHAPTER 76

Blood and Tissue Protozoa

The protozoa of blood and tissues are closely related to the intestinal protozoan parasites in practically all aspects except for their sites of infection (Box 76–1). The malaria parasites (*Plasmodium* species) infect both blood and tissues.

Plasmodium Species

Plasmodia are coccidian or sporozoan parasites of blood cells, and like other coccidia, they require two hosts, (1) the mosquito for the sexual reproductive stages, and (2) humans or other animals for the asexual reproductive stages.

The four species of plasmodia that infect humans are *Plasmodium vivax*, *Plasmodium ovale*, *Plasmodium malariae*, and *Plasmodium falciparum* (Table 76–1). These species have a common life cycle, as illustrated in Figure 76–1. Human infection is initiated by the bite of an *Anopheles* mosquito, which introduces infectious plasmodia sporozoites into the circulatory system via its saliva. The sporozoites are carried to the parenchymal cells of the liver, where asexual reproduction (schizogony) occurs. This phase of growth, termed the exoerythrocytic cycle, lasts 8 to 25 days, depending on the plasmodial species. Some species (e.g., *P. vivax*, *P. ovale*) can establish a dormant hepatic phase in which the sporozoites (called hypnozoites or sleeping forms) do not divide. The presence of these viable plasmodia can lead to the relapse of infections months to years after the initial clinical disease (relapsing malaria). The hepatocytes eventually rupture, liberating the plasmodia (termed merozoites at this stage), which in turn attach to specific receptors on the surface of erythrocytes and enter the cells, thus initiating the erythrocytic cycle.

Asexual replication progresses through a series of stages (ring, trophozoite, schizont) that culminates in the rupture of the erythrocyte, releasing up to 24 merozoites, which initiates another cycle of replication by infecting other erythrocytes. Some merozoites also develop within erythrocytes into male and female gametocytes. If a mosquito ingests mature male and female gametocytes during a blood meal, the sexual reproductive cycle of malaria can be initiated, with the eventual production of sporozoites infectious for humans. This sexual reproductive stage within the mosquito is necessary for the maintenance of malaria within a population.

Most malaria seen in the United States is acquired by visitors or residents of countries with endemic disease (imported malaria). However, the appropriate vector, *Anopheles* mosquito, is found in several sections of the United States, and domestic transmission of disease has been observed (introduced malaria). In addition to transmission by mosquitos, malaria can also be acquired through blood transfusions from an infected donor (transfusion malaria). This type of transmission can also occur among narcotic addicts who share needles and syringes ("mainline" malaria). Congenital acquisition, although rare, is also a possible mode of transmission (congenital malaria).

Plasmodium vivax

Physiology and Structure

P. vivax is selective, in that it invades only young, immature erythrocytes (Fig. 76–2). *P. vivax* infections have the following characteristics:

1. Infected red blood cells usually are enlarged and contain numerous pink granules or Schüffner's dots.
2. The trophozoite is ring-shaped but ameboid in appearance.
3. More mature trophozoites and erythrocytic schizonts containing up to 24 merozoites are present.
4. The gametocytes are round.

These characteristics are helpful in identification of the specific plasmodial species, which is important for the treatment of malaria.

Epidemiology

P. vivax is the most prevalent of the human plasmodia and has the widest geographic distribution, including the tropics, subtropics, and temperate regions.

BOX 76–1. Medically Important Blood and Tissue Protozoa

Plasmodium species
Babesia species
Toxoplasma species
Sarcocystis species
Acanthamoeba species
Balamuthia species
Naegleria species
Leishmania species
Trypanosoma species

Clinical Diseases

After an incubation period (usually 10 to 17 days), the patient experiences vague flu-like symptoms, such as headache, muscle pains, photophobia, anorexia, nausea, and vomiting.

As the infection progresses, increased numbers of rupturing erythrocytes liberate merozoites as well as toxic cellular debris and hemoglobin into the circulation. Together, these substances produce the typical pattern of chills, fever, and malarial rigors. These paroxysms usually reappear periodically (generally every 48 hours) as the cycle of infection, replication, and cell lysis progresses. The paroxysms may remain relatively mild or may progress to severe attacks, with hours of sweating, chills, shaking, persistently high temperatures (103°F to 106°F), and exhaustion.

P. vivax causes "benign tertian malaria." This term refers to the cycle of paroxysms every 48 hours (in untreated patients) and to the fact that most patients tolerate the attacks and can survive for years without treatment. If left untreated, however, chronic *P. vivax* infections can lead to brain, kidney, and liver damage as a result of the malarial pigment, cellular debris, and capillary plugging of these organs by masses of adherent erythrocytes.

Laboratory Diagnosis

Microscopic examination of thick and thin films of blood is the method of choice for confirming the clini-

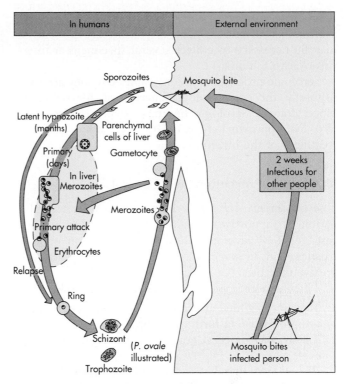

FIGURE 76–1. Life cycle of *Plasmodium* species.

cal diagnosis of malaria and identifying the specific species responsible for disease. The thick film is a concentration method that may be used to detect the presence of organisms. With training, thick films may also be used to diagnose the species. The thin film is most useful for establishing species identification. Specimens for blood films can be collected at any time over the course of the infection, but the best time is midway

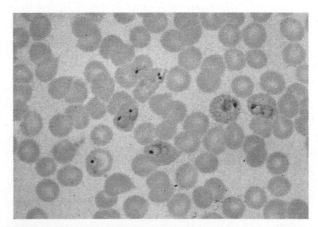

FIGURE 76–2. *Plasmodium vivax* ring forms and young trophozoites. Note the multiple stages of the parasite seen in the peripheral blood smear, the enlarged parasitized erythrocytes, and the presence of Schüffner's dots with the trophozoite form. These are characteristic of *P. vivax* infections.

TABLE 76–1. Human Malarial Parasites

Parasite	Disease
Plasmodium vivax	Benign tertian malaria
Plasmodium ovale	Benign tertian or ovale malaria
Plasmodium malariae	Quartan or malarial malaria
Plasmodium falciparum	Malignant tertian malaria

between paroxysms of chills and fever, when the greatest number of intracellular organisms are present. It may be necessary to collect several specimens at intervals of 4 to 6 hours.

Serologic procedures are available, but they are used primarily for epidemiologic surveys or for screening blood donors. Serologic findings usually remain positive for approximately a year, even after complete treatment of the infection.

Treatment, Prevention, and Control

The treatment of *P. vivax* infection involves a combination of supportive measures and chemotherapy. Bed rest, relief of fever and headache, regulation of fluid balance, and, in some cases, blood transfusion are supportive therapies.

The chemotherapeutic regimens are as follows:

1. *Suppressive*: aimed at avoiding infection and clinical symptoms (i.e., a form of prophylaxis).
2. *Therapeutic*: aimed at eradicating the erythrocytic cycle.
3. *Radical cure*: aimed at eradicating the exoerythrocytic cycle in the liver.
4. *Gametocidal*: aimed at destroying erythrocytic gametocytes to prevent their transmission by mosquito.

Chloroquine is the drug of choice for the suppression and therapeutic treatment of *P. vivax*, followed by primaquine for radical cure and elimination of gametocytes. Reports now suggest the emergence of chloroquine-resistant forms of *P. vivax* in Indonesia, the Solomon Islands, New Guinea, and Brazil. Patients infected with chloroquine-resistant *P. vivax* may be treated with other agents, including mefloquine, quinine, pyrimethamine-sulfadoxine (Fansidar), and doxycycline. Primaquine is especially effective in preventing a relapse with the latent forms of *P. vivax* in the liver. Because antimalarial drugs are potentially toxic, it is imperative that physicians carefully review the recommended therapeutic regimens.

Chemoprophylaxis and prompt eradication of infections are critical in breaking the mosquito-human transmission cycle. Control of mosquito breeding as well as protection of individuals by screening, netting, protective clothing, and insect repellents are also essential. Immigrants from and travelers to endemic areas must be carefully screened, through the use of blood films or serologic tests, to detect possible infection. The development of vaccines to protect persons living in or traveling to endemic areas is under investigation.

Plasmodium ovale

Physiology and Structure

P. ovale is similar to *P. vivax* in many respects, including its selectivity for young, pliable erythrocytes. As a

consequence, the host cell becomes enlarged and distorted, usually in an oval form. Schüffner's dots appear as pale pink granules, and the cell border is commonly fimbriated or ragged. The schizont of *P. ovale*, when mature, contains about half the number of merozoites seen in *P. vivax*.

Epidemiology

P. ovale is distributed primarily in tropical Africa, where it is often more prevalent than *P. vivax*. It is also found in Asia and South America.

Clinical Diseases

The clinical picture of tertian attacks for *P. ovale* (benign tertian or ovale malaria) infection is similar to that for *P. vivax*. Untreated infections last only about a year instead of the several years for *P. vivax*. Both the relapse and recrudescence phases are similar to those for *P. vivax*.

Laboratory Diagnosis

As with *P. vivax*, thick and thin blood films are examined for the typical oval host cell with Schüffner's dots and a ragged cell wall. Serologic tests reveal cross-reaction with *P. vivax* and other plasmodia.

Treatment, Prevention, and Control

The treatment regimen, including the use of primaquine to prevent relapse from latent liver forms, is similar to that used for *P. vivax* infections. Preventing *P. ovale* infection involves the same measures as those for *P. vivax* and other plasmodia.

Plasmodium malariae

Physiology and Structure

In contrast with *P. vivax* and *P. ovale*, *P. malariae* can infect only mature erythrocytes with relatively rigid cell membranes. As a result, the parasite's growth must conform to the size and shape of the red blood cell. This requirement produces no red cell enlargement or distortion, as seen in *P. vivax* and *P. ovale*, but it does result in distinctive shapes of the parasite seen in the host cell: "band and bar forms" as well as very compact, dark-staining forms. The schizont of *P. malariae* shows no red cell enlargement or distortion and is usually composed of eight merozoites appearing in a rosette. Occasionally, reddish granules called Ziemann's dots appear in the host cell.

Unlike hypnozoites for *P. vivax* and *P. ovale*, hypnozoites for *P. malariae* are not found in the liver, and relapse does not occur. Recrudescence does occur, however, and attacks may develop after apparent abatement of symptoms.

Epidemiology

P. malariae infection occurs primarily in the same subtropical and temperate regions as infections with the other plasmodia but is less prevalent.

Clinical Diseases

The incubation period for *P. malariae* is the longest of the plasmodia, usually 18 to 40 days but possibly several months to years. The early symptoms are flu-like, with fever patterns of 72 hours (quartan or malarial) in periodicity. Attacks are moderate to severe and last several hours. Untreated infections may last as long as 20 years.

Laboratory Diagnosis

Observing the characteristic bar and band forms and the rosette schizont in thick and thin films of blood establishes the diagnosis of *P. malariae* infection. As noted, serologic tests cross-react with other plasmodia.

Treatment, Prevention, and Control

Treatment is similar to that for *P. vivax* and *P. ovale* infections and must be undertaken to prevent recrudescent infections. Treatment to prevent relapse caused by latent liver forms is not required, because these forms do not develop with *P. malariae*. Preventive and controlling mechanisms are as discussed for *P. vivax* and *P. ovale*.

Plasmodium falciparum

Physiology and Structure

P. falciparum demonstrates no selectivity in host erythrocytes and invades any red blood cell at any stage in its existence. Also, multiple sporozoites can infect a single erythrocyte. Thus, three or even four small rings may be seen in an infected cell. *P. falciparum* is often seen in the host cell at the very edge or periphery of the cell membrane, appearing almost as if it were "stuck" on the outside of the cell. This appliqué or accolé position is distinctive for the species.

Growing trophozoite stages and schizonts of *P. falciparum* are rarely seen in blood films, because their forms are sequestered in the liver and spleen. Only in very heavy infections are they found in the peripheral circulation. Thus, peripheral blood smears from patients with *P. falciparum* malaria characteristically contain only young ring forms and occasionally gametocytes. The typical crescentic gametocytes are diagnostic for the species. Infected red blood cells do not enlarge

and become distorted like they do with *P. vivax* and *P. ovale*. Occasionally, reddish granules known as Maurer's dots are observed in *P. falciparum*.

P. falciparum, like *P. malariae*, does not produce hypnozoites in the liver. Relapses from the liver are not known to occur.

Epidemiology

P. falciparum occurs almost exclusively in tropical and subtropical regions.

Clinical Diseases

Of all the plasmodia, *P. falciparum* has the shortest incubation period, which ranges from 7 to 10 days rather than extending for months to years. After the early flu-like symptoms, *P. falciparum* rapidly produces daily (quotidian) chills and fever as well as severe nausea, vomiting, and diarrhea. The periodicity of the attacks then becomes tertian (36 to 48 hours), and fulminating disease develops. The term malignant tertian malaria is appropriate for this infection. Because the symptoms of this type of malaria are similar to those of intestinal infections, the nausea, vomiting, and diarrhea have led to the observation that malaria is "the malignant mimic."

Although any malaria infection may be fatal, *P. falciparum* disease is the most likely to result in death if left untreated. The greater numbers of erythrocytes infected and destroyed result in toxic cellular debris, adherence of red blood cells to vascular endothelium and to adjacent red blood cells, and formation of capillary plugging by masses of red blood cells, platelets, leukocytes, and malarial pigment.

Involvement of the brain (cerebral malaria) is most often seen in *P. falciparum* infection. Capillary plugging from an accumulation of malarial pigment and masses of cells can result in coma and death.

Kidney damage is also associated with *P. falciparum* malaria, resulting in an illness called blackwater fever. Intravascular hemolysis with rapid destruction of red blood cells produces a marked hemoglobinuria and can result in acute renal failure, tubular necrosis, nephrotic syndrome, and death. Liver involvement is characterized by abdominal pain, vomiting of bile, severe diarrhea, and rapid dehydration.

Laboratory Diagnosis

Thick and thin blood films are searched for the characteristic rings of *P. falciparum*, which frequently occur in multiples within a single cell as well as in the accolé position (Fig. 76-3). Also diagnostic are the distinctive crescentic gametocytes (Fig. 76-4).

Laboratory personnel must perform a thorough search of the blood films, because mixed infections can

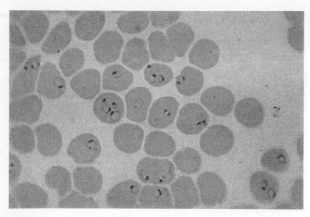

FIGURE 76–3. Ring forms of *Plasmodium falciparum*. Note the multiple ring forms within the individual erythrocytes, a feature characteristic of this organism.

occur with any combination of the four species but most often the combination is *P. falciparum* and *P. vivax*. The detection and proper reporting of a mixed infection directly affect the treatment chosen, as discussed in the next section.

Treatment, Prevention, and Control

The treatment of malaria is based on the history regarding travel to endemic areas, prompt clinical review and differential diagnosis, accurate and rapid laboratory work, and correct use of antimalarial drugs.

Because chloroquine-resistant strains of *P. falciparum* are present in many parts of the world, physicians must review all current protocols for the proper treatment of *P. falciparum* infections, noting particularly where chloroquine resistance is known to occur. If the patient's history indicates that the origin is not from a chloroquine-resistant area, the drug of choice is either chlo-

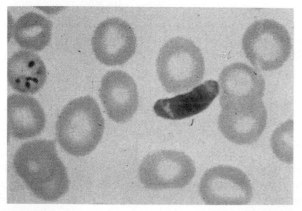

FIGURE 76–4. Mature gametocyte of *Plasmodium falciparum*. The presence of this sausage-shaped form is diagnostic of *P. falciparum* malaria.

roquine or parenteral quinine. Patients infected with chloroquine-resistant *P. falciparum* (or *P. vivax*) may be treated with other agents, including mefloquine, quinine, quinidine, pyrimethamine-sulfadoxine, and doxycycline. Because quinine and pyrimethamine-sulfadoxine are potentially toxic, they are used more often for treatment than for prophylaxis. Amodiaquine, an analogue of chloroquine, is effective against chloroquine-resistant *P. falciparum*; however, toxicity limits its use. Newer agents with promising activity against multiple-drug–resistant strains of *P. falciparum* include halofantrine, a phenanthrenemethanol, and artemisinin, a sesquiterpene derivative of qinghaosu. They are not yet available in the United States.

When there is uncertainty whether the *P. falciparum* is chloroquine resistant, it is advisable to assume that the strain is resistant and to treat the patient accordingly. If the laboratory reports a mixed infection involving *P. falciparum* and *P. vivax*, the treatment must eradicate not only *P. falciparum* from the erythrocytes but also the liver stages of *P. vivax* to avoid relapses. Failure on the part of the laboratory to detect and report such a mixed infection can result in inappropriate treatment and unnecessary delay in accomplishing a complete cure.

P. falciparum infection can be prevented and controlled exactly like *P. vivax* infection and the other human malarias. Chloroquine resistance complicates the management of these diseases but can be overcome by the physician's awareness of appropriate regimens.

Babesia Species

Members of the genus *Babesia* are intracellular sporozoan parasites that morphologically resemble plasmodia. Babesiosis is a zoonosis infecting a variety of animals, such as deer, cattle, and rodents; humans are accidental hosts. Infection is transmitted by ixodid ticks. *Babesia microti* is the usual cause of babesiosis in the United States.

Physiology and Structure

Human infection follows contact with an infected tick (Fig. 76–5). The infectious pyriform bodies are introduced into the blood stream and infect erythrocytes. The intraerythrocytic trophozoites multiply by binary fission, forming tetrads, and then lyse the erythrocytes, releasing the merozoites. The merozoites can reinfect other cells to maintain the infection. Infected cells can also be ingested by feeding ticks, in which additional replication can take place. Infection in the tick population can also be maintained by transovarian transmission. The infected cells in humans resemble the ring forms of *P. falciparum*, but malarial pigment or other stages of growth characteristically seen with plasmodial

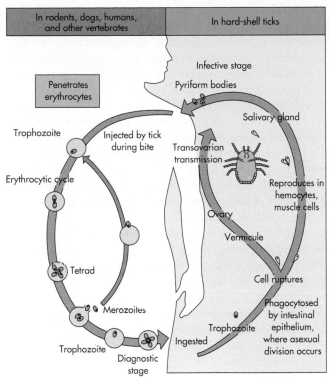

FIGURE 76–5. Life cycle of *Babesia* species.

infections are not observed on careful examination of blood smears.

Epidemiology

More than 70 different species of *Babesia* are found in Africa, Asia, Europe, and North America, with *B. microti* responsible for disease along the northeastern seaboard of the United States (e.g., Nantucket Island, Martha's Vineyard, Shelter Island). *Ixodes dammini* is the tick vector responsible for transmitting babesiosis in this area, and the natural reservoir hosts are field mice, voles, and other small rodents. Serologic studies in endemic areas have demonstrated a high incidence of previous exposure to *Babesia*. Presumably, most infections are asymptomatic or mild. *Babesia divergens*, which has been reported more frequently from Europe, causes severe, often fatal infections in people who have undergone splenectomies. Although most infections follow tick bites, transfusion-related infections have been demonstrated.

Clinical Diseases

After an incubation period of 1 to 4 weeks, symptomatic patients experience general malaise, fever without periodicity, headache, chills, sweating, fatigue, and weakness. As the infection progresses with greater de-

struction of erythrocytes, hemolytic anemia develops, and the patient may experience renal failure. Hepatomegaly and splenomegaly can occur in advanced disease. Low-grade parasitemia may persist for weeks. Splenectomy or functional asplenia, immunosuppression, and advanced age increase a person's susceptibility to infections as well as to more severe disease.

Laboratory Diagnosis

Examination of blood smears is the diagnostic method of choice. Laboratory personnel must be experienced in differentiating *Babesia* and *Plasmodium* species. Infected patients may have negative smears because of the low-grade parasitemia. These infections can be diagnosed through inoculation of samples of blood into hamsters, which are highly susceptible to infection. Serologic tests are also available for diagnostic use.

Treatment, Prevention, and Control

The drug of choice is clindamycin combined with quinine. Other antiprotozoal regimens, including chloroquine and pentamidine, have been used with variable results. However, most patients with mild disease recover without specific therapy. Exchange blood transfusion has also been successful in patients who have undergone splenectomy and have severe infections caused by *B. microti* or *B. divergens*.

The use of protective clothing and insect repellents can minimize tick exposure in endemic areas, a measure critical for the prevention of disease. Ticks must feed on humans for several hours before the organisms are transmitted, so prompt removal of ticks can be protective.

Toxoplasma gondii

Toxoplasma gondii is a typical coccidian parasite related to *Plasmodium*, *Isospora*, and other members of the phylum Apicomplexa. *T. gondii* is an intracellular parasite, and it is found in a wide variety of animals, including birds and humans. Only one species exists, and there appears to be little strain-to-strain variation. The essential reservoir host of *T. gondii* is the common house cat and other felines.

Physiology and Structure

Organisms develop in the intestinal cells of the cat as well as during an extraintestinal cycle with passage to the tissues via the blood stream (Fig. 76–6). The organisms from the intestinal cycle are passed in cat feces and mature into infective cysts within 3 to 4 days in the external environment. These oocysts are similar to those of *Isospora belli*, the human intestinal protozoan

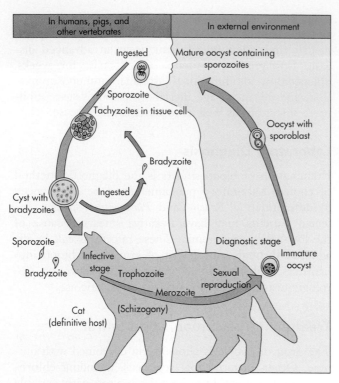

FIGURE 76-6. Life cycle of *Toxoplasma gondii*.

parasite; they can be ingested by mice and other animals (including humans) and can produce acute and chronic infection of various tissues, including brain. Infection in cats is established when the animals eat the tissues of infected rodents.

Some infective forms, or trophozoites, from the oocyst develop as slender, crescentic types called tachyzoites. These rapidly multiplying forms are responsible for the initial infection and the tissue damage. Slow-growing, shorter forms called bradyzoites also develop and form cysts in chronic infections.

Epidemiology

Human infection with *T. gondii* is ubiquitous; however, it is increasingly apparent that certain immunocompromised people, such as patients with the acquired immunodeficiency syndrome (AIDS), are more likely to have severe manifestations. The wide variety of animals that harbor the organism—carnivores and herbivores as well as birds—accounts for the widespread transmission.

Humans become infected from the following two sources: (1) ingestion of improperly cooked meat from animals that serve as intermediate hosts and (2) ingestion of infective oocysts from contaminated cat feces. Serologic studies show an increased prevalence in human populations in which the consumption of uncooked meat or meat juices is popular. It is noteworthy

that serologic tests of human and rodent populations are negative in the few geographic areas where cats have not existed. Outbreaks of toxoplasmosis in the United States are usually traced to poorly cooked meat (e.g., hamburgers) as well as contact with cat feces.

Transplacental infection can occur in pregnancy either from infection acquired from meat and meat juices or from contact with cat feces. Transfusion infection via contaminated blood can occur but is not common. Transplacental infection from an infected mother has a devastating effect on the fetus.

Although the rate of seroconversion is similar for individuals within a geographic location, the rate of severe infection is dramatically affected by the immune status of the individual. Patients with defects in cell-mediated immunity, especially those who are infected with the human immunodeficiency virus (HIV) or who have undergone organ transplantation or immunosuppressive therapy, are most likely to have disseminated or central nervous system (CNS) disease. Illness in this setting is generally believed to be caused by reactivation of previously latent infection rather than new exposure to the organism.

Clinical Diseases

Most *T. gondii* infections are benign and asymptomatic, with symptoms occurring as the parasite moves in the blood to tissues, where it becomes an intracellular parasite. When symptomatic disease occurs, the infection is characterized by cell destruction, reproduction of more organisms, and eventual cyst formation. Many tissues may be affected; however, the organism has a particular predilection for cells of the lung, heart, lymphoid organs, and CNS, including the eye.

Symptoms of acute disease include chills, fever, headaches, myalgia, lymphadenitis, and fatigue; the symptoms occasionally resemble those of infectious mononucleosis. In chronic disease, the signs and symptoms comprise lymphadenitis, occasionally a rash, evidence of hepatitis, encephalomyelitis, and myocarditis. In some of the cases, chorioretinitis appears and may lead to blindness.

Congenital infection with *T. gondii* also occurs in infants born to mothers infected during pregnancy. If infection occurs in the first trimester, the result is spontaneous abortion, stillbirth, or severe disease. Manifestations in the infant infected after the first trimester include epilepsy, encephalitis, microcephaly, intracranial calcifications, hydrocephalus, psychomotor or mental retardation, chorioretinitis, blindness, anemia, jaundice, rash, pneumonia, diarrhea, and hypothermia. Infants may be asymptomatic at birth, only to experience disease months to years later. Most often these children develop chorioretinitis with or without blindness or other neurologic problems, including retardation, seizures, microcephaly, and hearing loss.

In immunocompromised older patients, a different spectrum of disease is seen. Reactivation of latent toxoplasmosis is a special problem for such people. The presenting symptoms of *Toxoplasma* infection in immunocompromised patients are usually neurologic, most frequently consistent with diffuse encephalopathy, meningoencephalitis, or cerebral mass lesions. Reactivation of cerebral toxoplasmosis has emerged as a major cause of encephalitis in patients with AIDS. The disease is usually multifocal, with more than one mass lesion appearing in the brain at the same time. Symptoms, which are related to the location of the lesions, include hemiparesis, seizures, visual impairment, confusion, and lethargy. Other reported sites of infection are the eye, lung, and testes. Although disease is seen predominantly in patients with AIDS, it may also occur with similar manifestations in other immunocompromised patients, in particular those undergoing solid organ transplantation.

Laboratory Diagnosis

Serologic testing is required for the diagnosis of acute active *Toxoplasma* infection; the diagnosis is established by the finding of rising antibody titers documented in serially collected blood specimens. Because contact with the organism is common, attention to rising titers is essential to distinguish acute, active infection from previous asymptomatic or chronic infection. Currently, the enzyme-linked immunosorbent assay (ELISA) for detecting immunoglobulin M antibodies appears to be the most reliable procedure because of its simplicity and rapidity in documenting acute infections. The test is not generally satisfactory in patients with AIDS who have latent or reactivated infections, because they do not produce an immunoglobulin M response or rising immunoglobulin G titer.

Demonstration of these organisms as trophozoites and cysts in tissue and body fluids is the definitive method of diagnosis (Fig. 76–7). Biopsy specimens from lymph nodes, brain, myocardium, or other suspected tissue as well as body fluids, including cerebrospinal fluid, amniotic fluid, and bronchoalveolar lavage fluid, can be directly examined for the organisms. Newer monoclonal antibody–based fluorescent stains may facilitate direct detection of *T. gondii* in tissue. Culture methods for *T. gondii* are largely experimental and are not usually available in clinical laboratories. The two available methods involve inoculation of potentially infected material into either mouse peritoneum or tissue culture. Advances in developing detection methods based on polymerase chain reaction (PCR) are promising and may provide rapid and sensitive approaches for detecting the organism in blood,

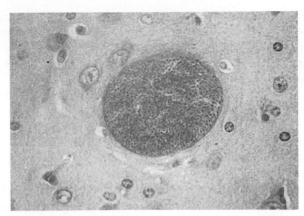

FIGURE 76–7. Cyst of *Toxoplasma gondii* in mouse brain. Hundreds of organisms may be present in the cyst, which may become active and may initiate disease with decreased host immunity (e.g., immunosuppression in transplant recipients and patients with AIDS).

cerebrospinal fluid, amniotic fluid, and other clinical specimens.

Treatment, Prevention, and Control

The therapy for toxoplasmosis depends on the nature of the infectious process and the immunocompetence of the host. Most mononucleosis-like infections in normal hosts resolve spontaneously and do not require specific therapy. In contrast, disseminated or CNS infection in immunocompromised people must be treated. Before the association of *T. gondii* with HIV infection, immunocompromised patients with toxoplasmosis were treated for 4 to 6 weeks. In the setting of HIV infection, discontinuing therapy after 4 to 6 weeks is associated with a relapse rate of 25%. Such patients are currently treated with an initial high-dose regimen of pyrimethamine plus sulfadiazine followed by lower doses of both drugs given for an indefinite period.

Although this drug combination is the regimen of choice, toxicity (rash and bone marrow suppression) may necessitate changes to alternative agents. Clindamycin plus pyrimethamine is the best-studied alternative. Atovaquone and azithromycin (each alone or with pyrimethamine) also have some activity, although their efficacy and safety in comparison with clindamycin plus pyrimethamine must be assessed. Trimethoprim-sulfamethoxazole is not an acceptable alternative to pyrimethamine plus sulfadiazine for treatment of disseminated or CNS toxoplasmosis. The use of corticosteroids is indicated as part of therapy for cerebral edema and ocular infections that involve or threaten the macula.

Infections in the first trimester of pregnancy are difficult to manage because of the teratogenicity of pyrimethamine in laboratory animals. Both clindamycin and spiramycin have been substituted with apparent success. Spiramycin does not appear to be effective for the treatment of toxoplasmosis in immunocompromised patients.

As more immunocompromised patients at risk for disseminated infection are identified, greater emphasis is being placed on preventive measures and specific prophylaxis. Serologic screening of patients before organ transplantation and early in the course of HIV infection has become routine. Individuals with positive serologic results are at much higher risk for the development of disease and are now being considered for prophylaxis. Trimethoprim-sulfamethoxazole, which is also used as prophylaxis to prevent *Pneumocystis carinii* infections, also appears to be effective in preventing infections with *T. gondii*. Additional preventive measures for pregnant women and immunocompromised hosts should include avoiding (1) consumption and handling of raw or undercooked meat and (2) exposure to cat feces.

Sarcocystis lindemanni

Sarcocystis lindemanni is a typical coccidian closely related to the intestinal forms *Sarcocystis suihominis*, *Sarcocystis bovihominis*, and *I. belli* and the blood and tissue parasite *T. gondii*. *S. lindemanni* occurs worldwide in various animals, especially sheep, cattle, and pigs. Humans are accidentally infected only as the result of eating meat from these animals. Most infections are asymptomatic, but occasionally, an infection may cause myositis, swelling of muscle, dyspnea, and eosinophilia. Infection of the myocardium has been observed but is extremely rare. There is no specific treatment for the muscle infection.

Free-Living Amebae

Naegleria species, *Acanthamoeba* species, *Balamuthia* species, and other free-living amebae are found in soil and in contaminated lakes, streams, and other water environments. Most human infections with these amebae are acquired during the warm summer months by people exposed to them while swimming in contaminated water. Inhalation of cysts present in dust may account for some infections, whereas ocular infections with *Acanthamoeba* species are associated with the contamination of contact lenses with nonsterile cleaning solutions.

Clinical Diseases

Naegleria, *Acanthamoeba*, and *Balamuthia* organisms are opportunistic pathogens. Although colonization of the nasal passages is usually asymptomatic, these amebae can invade the nasal mucosa and extend into the brain.

Acute primary amebic meningoencephalitis is most commonly caused by *Naegleria fowleri*. Destruction of brain tissue is characterized by a fulminant, rapidly fatal meningoencephalitis. Symptoms include intense frontal headache, sore throat, fever, blocked nose with altered senses of taste and smell, stiff neck, and Kernig's sign. The cerebrospinal fluid is purulent and may contain many erythrocytes and motile amebae. Clinically, the course of the disease is rapid, with death usually occurring within 4 or 5 days. Postmortem findings show *Naegleria* trophozoites present in the brain but no evidence of cysts. Although all cases of this disease were fatal before 1970, survival has now been reported in a few cases in which the disease was rapidly diagnosed and treated.

In contrast to *Naegleria*, *Acanthamoeba* and *Balamuthia* organisms produce granulomatous amebic encephalitis and single or multiple brain abscesses, primarily in immunocompromised individuals. The course of the disease is longer, with an incubation period of at least 10 days. The resulting disease is a chronic granulomatous encephalitis with edema of the brain tissue.

Eye and skin infection by *Acanthamoeba* organisms may also occur. Keratitis is usually associated with eye trauma that occurred before contact with contaminated soil, dust, or water. The use of improperly cleaned contact lenses is also associated with this disease. Invasion by *Acanthamoeba* species produces corneal ulceration and severe ocular pain. Cases of apparent disseminated cutaneous and subcutaneous infection with *Acanthamoeba* and *Balamuthia* organisms have been described in patients with AIDS. These infections include multiple soft tissue nodules that on biopsy are found to contain amebae. CNS or deep tissue involvement may also be present with this form of infection.

Laboratory Diagnosis

For the diagnosis of *Naegleria*, *Acanthamoeba*, and *Balamuthia* infections, specimens of nasal discharge and cerebrospinal fluid and, in the case of eye infections, corneal scrapings should be collected. The specimens should be examined with the use of a saline wet preparation and iodine-stained smears. *Naegleria* and *Acanthamoeba* species are difficult to differentiate except by experienced microscopists. However, the observation of an ameba in a normally sterile tissue is diagnostic (Fig. 76–8). In *Naegleria* infection, only the ameboid trophozoites are found within the tissue, whereas with *Acanthamoeba* and *Balamuthia* infection, both trophozoites and cysts are found in tissues. The clinical specimens can be cultured on agar plates seeded with live gram-negative enteric bacilli. Amebae present in the specimens use the bacteria as a nutritional source and

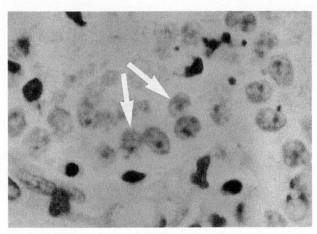

FIGURE 76–8. Numerous *Naegleria* trophozoites *(arrows)* in a section of spinal cord from a patient with amebic meningoencephalitis. (From Rothrock JF, Buchsbaum HW: *JAMA* 243:2329–2330, 1980.)

TABLE 76–2. Leishmaniasis in Humans	
Parasite	**Disease**
Leishmania donovani	Visceral leishmaniasis (kala-azar, dumdum fever)
Leishmania tropica	Cutaneous leishmaniasis (Oriental sore, Delhi boli)
Leishmania braziliensis	Mucocutaneous leishmaniasis (American leishmaniasis, espundia, chiclero ulcer)

can be detected within 1 or 2 days by the presence of the trails that form on the agar surface as the amebae move. *Balamuthia* do not grow on agar plates used for *Naegleria* and *Acanthamoeba* but have been recovered in tissue culture using mammalian cell lines.

Treatment, Prevention, and Control

Treatment of free-living amebic infections is largely ineffective. Amebic meningoencephalitis due to either *Naegleria*, *Acanthamoeba*, or *Balamuthia* is unresponsive to antibacterial and antiamebic drugs. The treatment of choice for *Naegleria* infections is amphotericin B combined with miconazole and rifampin. *Acanthamoeba* and *Balamuthia* appear resistant to ketoconazole, miconazole, itraconazole, sulfadiazine, flucytosine, pentamidine, and polymyxin B. Amebic keratitis and cutaneous infections may respond to topical miconazole, chlorhexidine gluconate, or propamidine isethionate. Treatment of amebic keratitis may require repeated corneal transplantation or, rarely, enucleation of the eye.

The wide distribution of these organisms in fresh and brackish waters makes the prevention and control of infection difficult. It has been suggested that known sources of infection be declared "off limits" to bathing, diving, and water sports, although this ruling is generally difficult to enforce. Swimming pools with cracks in the walls, allowing soil seepage, should be repaired to avoid creation of a source of infection.

Leishmania

The hemoflagellates are flagellated, insect-transmitted protozoa that infect blood and tissues. Three species of *Leishmania*, a protozoan hemoflagellate, produce hu-

man disease: *Leishmania donovani*, *Leishmania tropica*, and *Leishmania braziliensis* (Table 76–2). The diseases are distinguished by the ability of the organism to infect deep tissues (visceral leishmaniasis) or replicate only in cooler superficial tissues (cutaneous or mucocutaneous leishmaniasis). The reservoir hosts and geographic distribution differ for the three species, but transmission by sandflies (belonging to the genera *Phlebotomus* or *Lutzomyia*) is common to all leishmanial species.

Leishmania donovani

Physiology and Structure

The life cycles of all leishmanial parasites differ in epidemiology, tissues affected, and clinical manifestations (Fig. 76–9). The promastigote stage (long, slender form with a free flagellum) is present in the saliva of infected sandflies. Human infection is initiated by the bite of an infected sandfly, which injects the promastigotes into the skin, where they lose their flagella, enter the amastigote stage, and invade reticuloendothelial cells. Reproduction occurs in the amastigote stage, and as cells rupture, destruction of specific tissues (e.g., cutaneous tissues, visceral organs such as the liver and spleen) develops. The amastigote stage (Fig. 76–10) is diagnostic for leishmaniasis, and is the infectious stage for sandflies. Ingested amastigotes transform in the sandfly into the promastigote stage, which multiplies by binary fission in the fly midgut. After development, this stage migrates to the fly proboscis, where new human infection can be introduced during feeding.

Epidemiology

L. donovani infection of the classic kala-azar or dumdum fever type occurs in many parts of Asia, Africa, and Southeast Asia. Except for some rodents in Africa, there are few reservoir hosts. The vector is the *Phlebotomus* sandfly. Variants of *L. donovani* are also recognized. *L. donovani infantum* is present in countries

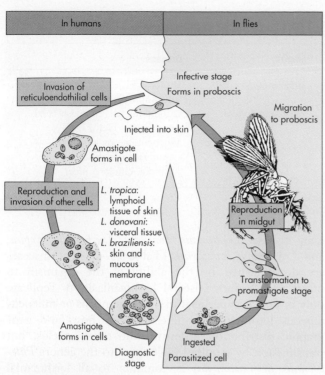

FIGURE 76–9. Life cycle of *Leishmania* species.

along the Mediterranean basin (European, Near Eastern, and African) and is found in parts of China and the former Soviet Union. Reservoir hosts of this organism include dogs, foxes, jackals, and porcupines. The vector is also the *Phlebotomus* sandfly. *L. donovani chagasi* is found in South America, Central America, especially Mexico, and the West Indies. Reservoir hosts

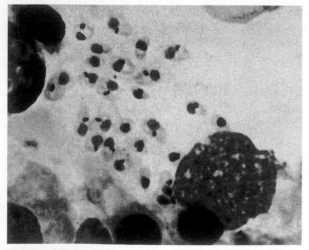

FIGURE 76–10. Giemsa-stained amastigotes (Leishman-Donovan bodies) of *Leishmania donovani* present in bone marrow. A small, dark-staining kinetoplast can be seen next to the spherical nucleus in some parasites. (From Ash LR, Orihel TC: *Atlas of human parasitology,* ed 2, Chicago, 1984, American Society of Clinical Pathologists.)

are dogs, foxes, and cats, and the vector is the *Lutzomyia* sandfly.

Clinical Diseases

The incubation period for visceral leishmaniasis may be several weeks to a year, with a gradual onset of fever, diarrhea, and anemia. Chills and sweating that may resemble malaria symptoms are common early in the infection. As organisms proliferate and invade cells of the liver and spleen, marked enlargement of these organs, weight loss, and emaciation occur. Kidney damage may also occur as cells of the glomeruli are invaded. With persistence of the disease, deeply pigmented, granulomatous areas of skin, referred to as post–kala-azar dermal leishmaniasis, occur. If untreated, visceral leishmaniasis develops into a fulminating, debilitating, and lethal disease in a few weeks or may persist as a chronic debilitating disease, leading to death in 1 or 2 years.

Laboratory Diagnosis

The amastigote stage can be demonstrated by tissue biopsy, bone marrow aspiration or lymph node aspiration, and thorough examination of properly stained smears. Culture of blood, bone marrow, and other tissues often demonstrates the promastigote stage of the organisms. Serologic testing is also available.

Treatment, Prevention, and Control

Visceral leishmaniasis is treated with pentavalent antimonial compounds. The drug of choice is stibogluconate. Therapy is not uniformly successful, and relapse rates of 2% to 8% are seen. Alternative approaches include the addition of allopurinol and the use of pentamidine or amphotericin B. Prompt treatment of human infections and control of reservoir hosts, along with insect control, help eliminate transmission of disease. Protection from sandflies by screening and insect repellents is also essential.

Leishmania tropica

Physiology and Structure

The life cycle of *L. tropica* is illustrated in Figure 76–9.

Epidemiology

Cutaneous leishmaniasis produced by *L. tropica* is present in many parts of Asia, Africa, Mediterranean Europe, and the southern region of the former Soviet Union. In these regions, the reservoir hosts are dogs, foxes, and rodents, and the vector is the *Phlebotomus* sandfly. Two related species are also recognized.

Leishmania aethiopica is endemic in Ethiopia, Kenya, and Yemen; dogs and rodents are reservoir hosts, and the vector is the *Phlebotomus* sandfly. *Leishmania mexicana* occurs in South and Central America, especially in the Amazon basin, with sloths, rodents, monkeys, and raccoons as reservoir hosts. The vector is the *Lutzomyia* sandfly.

Clinical Diseases

The incubation period after a sandfly bite may be as short as 2 weeks or as long as 2 months. The first sign, a red papule, appears at the site of the fly's bite. This lesion becomes irritated, with intense itching, and begins to enlarge and ulcerate. Gradually, the ulcer becomes hard and crusted and exudes a thin, serous material. At this stage, secondary bacterial infection may complicate the disease. The lesion may heal without treatment in a matter of months but usually leaves a disfiguring scar. A disseminated nodular type of cutaneous leishmaniasis has been reported from Ethiopia, probably caused by an allergy to *L. aethiopica* antigens. A viscerotropic form of *L. tropica* has been described in people returning from the Persian Gulf.

Laboratory Diagnosis

Demonstration of the amastigotes in properly stained smears from touch preparations of ulcer biopsy specimens and cultures of ulcer tissue determines the diagnosis. Serologic tests are also available. DNA probes have also been developed for the direct examination of cutaneous lesions. There are no commercially available products for these tests, and careful studies to determine the accuracy of testing procedures have not yet been performed.

Treatment, Prevention, and Control

The drug of choice is stibogluconate, with an alternative treatment of applying heat directly to the lesion. Protection from sandfly bites through the use of screening, protective clothing, and repellents is essential. Prompt treatment and eradication of the ulcers to prevent transmission, along with control of sandflies and reservoir hosts, reduce the incidence of human infection.

Leishmania braziliensis

Physiology and Structure

The life cycle of *L. braziliensis* is illustrated in Figure 76–9.

Epidemiology

Mucocutaneous leishmaniasis produced by *L. braziliensis* is seen from the Yucatan peninsula into Central and South America, especially in rain forests where workers are exposed to sandfly bites while harvesting the chicle sap for chewing gum (thus the name chiclero ulcer). There are many jungle reservoir hosts, and domesticated dogs serve as reservoirs as well. The vector is the *Lutzomyia* sandfly. The variant *Leishmania braziliensis panamensis* is similar in all respects to *L. braziliensis*, except for its more common occurrence in Panama and slight difference in growth in cultures. Reservoir hosts and the vector are similar to those for *L. braziliensis*.

Clinical Diseases

The incubation period and appearance of ulcers for *L. braziliensis* are similar to those for *L. tropica*, requiring a few weeks to months for the papule to appear. The essential difference in clinical disease is the involvement and destruction of mucous membranes and related tissue structures. These signs are often combined with edema and secondary bacterial infection to produce severe and disfiguring facial mutilation.

Laboratory Diagnosis

The diagnostic tests are similar for all *Leishmania* infections. Organisms are demonstrated in ulcers or cultured tissue. Serologic testing is also performed.

Treatment, Prevention, and Control

The drug of choice is stibogluconate; an alternative is amphotericin B. As with all the other *Leishmania* complexes, screening, protective clothing, insect repellents, and prompt treatment are needed to prevent transmission and control disease. The protection of forest and construction workers in endemic areas is most difficult, and disease in those places may be effectively controlled only by vaccination. Work to develop a vaccine is under way.

Trypanosomes

Trypanosoma, another hemoflagellate, causes two distinctly different forms of disease (Table 76–3). One is called African trypanosomiasis, or sleeping sickness, and is produced by *Trypanosoma brucei gambiense* and *Trypanosoma brucei rhodesiense*. It is transmitted by tsetse flies. The second infection, called American trypanosomiasis, or Chagas' disease, is produced by *Trypanosoma cruzi*. It is transmitted by true bugs (triatomids and reduviids, also called kissing bugs).

TABLE 76-3. *Trypanosoma* Species Responsible for Human Diseases

Parasite	Vector	Disease
Trypanosoma brucei gambiense and *Trypanosoma rhodesiense*	Tsetse fly	African trypanosomiasis (sleeping sickness)
Trypanosoma cruzi	Reduviids	American trypanosomiasis (Chagas' disease)

Trypanosoma brucei gambiense

Physiology and Structure

The life cycle of the African forms of trypanosomiasis is illustrated in Figure 76–11. The infective stage of the organism is the trypomastigote, which is present in the salivary glands of transmitting tsetse flies. The organism in this stage has a free flagellum and an undulating membrane running the full length of the body. The trypomastigotes enter the wound created by the fly bite and find their way into blood and lymph, eventually invading the CNS. Reproduction of the trypomastigotes in blood, lymph, and spinal fluid is by binary or longitudinal fission. These trypomastigotes in

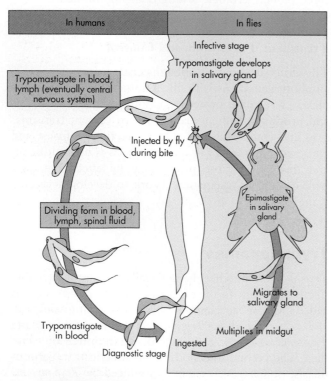

FIGURE 76-11. Life cycle of *Trypanosoma brucei*.

blood are then infective for biting tsetse flies, in the midgut of which further reproduction occurs. The organisms then migrate to the salivary glands, where an epimastigote form (with a free flagellum but only a partial undulating membrane) continues reproduction to the infective trypomastigote stage. Tsetse flies become infective 4 to 6 weeks after feeding on blood from a diseased patient.

Epidemiology

T. b. gambiense is limited to tropical West and Central Africa, correlating with the range of the tsetse fly vector. The tsetse flies transmitting *T. b. gambiense* prefer shaded stream banks for reproduction and proximity to human dwellings. People who work in such areas are at greatest risk of infection. An animal reservoir has not been proved, although several species of animals have been infected experimentally.

Clinical Diseases

The incubation period of Gambian sleeping sickness varies from a few days to weeks. *T. b. gambiense* produces chronic disease that often ends fatally, with CNS involvement after several years' duration. One of the earliest signs of disease is an occasional ulcer at the site of the fly bite. As reproduction of organisms continues, the lymph nodes are invaded, and fever, myalgia, arthralgia, and lymph node enlargement result. Swelling of the posterior cervical lymph nodes is characteristic of Gambian disease and is called Winterbottom's sign. Patients in this acute phase often exhibit hyperactivity.

Chronic disease progresses to CNS involvement with lethargy, tremors, meningoencephalitis, mental retardation, and general deterioration. In the final stages of chronic disease, convulsions, hemiplegia, and incontinence occur. The patient becomes difficult to arouse or obtain a response from, eventually progressing to a comatose state. Death is the result of CNS damage and other infections, such as malaria and pneumonia.

Laboratory Diagnosis

Organisms can be demonstrated in thick and thin blood films, in concentrated anticoagulated blood preparations, and in aspirations from lymph nodes and concentrated spinal fluid (Fig. 76–12). Methods for concentrating parasites in blood may be helpful. Approaches include centrifugation of heparinized samples and anion-exchange chromatography. Levels of parasitemia vary widely, and several attempts to visualize the organism over a number of days may be necessary. Preparations should be fixed and stained immediately to avoid disintegration of the trypomastigotes.

Serologic tests are also useful diagnostic techniques.

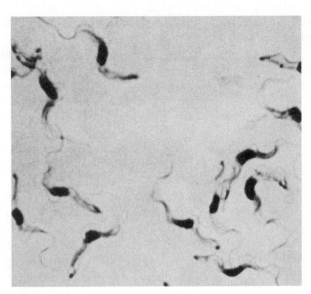

FIGURE 76-12. Trypomastigote stage of *Trypanosoma brucei gambiense* in a blood smear. (From Ash LR, Orihel TC: *Atlas of human parasitology*, ed 2, Chicago, 1984, American Society of Clinical Pathologists.)

Immunofluorescence, ELISA, precipitin, and agglutination methods have been used. Most reagents are not available commercially.

Treatment, Prevention, and Control

For the acute stages of the disease, the drug of choice is suramin, with pentamidine as an alternative. In chronic disease with CNS involvement, the drug of choice is melarsoprol; alternatives include tryparsamide combined with suramin. Difluoromethylornithine has also been introduced and holds promise for the treatment of all stages of disease.

The most essential elements for prevention are (1) control of breeding sites of the tsetse flies by clearing brush, (2) use of insecticides, and (3) treatment of human cases to reduce transmission to flies. People going into known endemic areas should wear protective clothing and use screening, bed netting, and insect repellents.

Trypanosoma brucei rhodesiense

Physiology and Structure

The life cycle of *T. b. rhodesiense* is similar to that of *T. b. gambiense* (see Fig. 76-11), with both trypomastigote and epimastigote stages and transmission by tsetse flies.

Epidemiology

The organism is found primarily in East Africa, especially the cattle-raising countries, where tsetse flies breed in the brush rather than along stream banks. *T. b. rhodesiense* also differs from *T. b. gambiense* in that domestic animal hosts (cattle and sheep) and wild game animals act as reservoir hosts. This transmission and vector cycle makes the organism more difficult to control than *T. b. gambiense*.

Clinical Diseases

The incubation period for *T. b. rhodesiense* is shorter than that for *T. b. gambiense*. Acute disease (fever, rigors, and myalgia) occurs more rapidly and progresses to a fulminating, rapidly fatal illness. Infected people are usually dead within 9 to 12 months if their disease is untreated.

This more virulent organism also develops in greater numbers in the blood. Lymphadenopathy is uncommon, and early in the infection, CNS invasion occurs, resulting in lethargy, anorexia, and mental disturbance. The chronic stages described for *T. b. gambiense* are not often seen, because in addition to rapid CNS disease, the organism produces kidney damage and myocarditis, leading to death.

Laboratory Diagnosis

Examination of blood and spinal fluid is carried out as for *T. b. gambiense*. Serologic tests are available; however, the marked variability of the surface antigens of trypanosomes limits the diagnostic usefulness of this approach.

Treatment, Prevention, and Control

The same treatment protocol applies as for *T. b. gambiense*, with early treatment for the more rapid neurologic manifestations. Similar prevention and control measures are needed, such as control of tsetse flies and the use of protective clothing, screens, netting, and insect repellent. In addition, early treatment is essential to control transmission, detect infection, and determine treatment in domestic animals. Control of infection in game animals is difficult, but infection can be reduced if measures to control the tsetse fly population, specifically, eradication of brush and grassland breeding sites, are applied.

Trypanosoma cruzi

Physiology and Structure

The life cycle of *T. cruzi* (Fig. 76-13) differs from that of *T. brucei* in that it includes the development of an additional form called an amastigote (Fig. 76-14). The amastigote is an intracellular form with no flagellum and no undulating membrane. It is smaller than the trypomastigote, oval in shape, and is found in tissues.

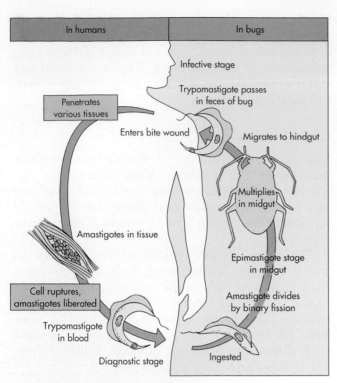

FIGURE 76–13. Life cycle of *Trypanosoma cruzi.*

The infective trypomastigote, which is present in the feces of a reduviid bug (kissing bug), enters the wound created by the biting, feeding bug. The bugs have been called kissing bugs because they frequently bite people around the mouth and in other facial sites. They are notorious for biting, feeding on blood and tissue juices, and then defecating into the wound. The organisms in the feces of the bug enter the wound; penetration is

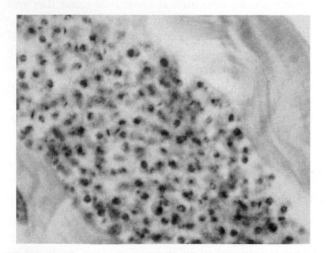

FIGURE 76–14. Amastigote stage of *Trypanosoma cruzi* in skeletal muscle. (From Ash LR, Orihel TC: *Atlas of human parasitology,* ed 2, Chicago, 1984, American Society of Clinical Pathologists.)

usually aided when the patient rubs or scratches the irritated site.

The trypomastigotes then migrate to other tissues (e.g., cardiac muscle, liver, brain), lose the flagellum and undulating membrane, and become the smaller, oval, intracellular amastigote form. These intracellular amastigotes multiply by binary fission and eventually destroy the host cells. Then they are liberated to enter new host tissue as intracellular amastigotes or to become trypomastigotes infective for feeding reduviid bugs.

Ingested trypomastigotes develop into epimastigotes in the midgut of the insect and reproduce by longitudinal binary fission. The organisms migrate to the hindgut of the bug, develop into metacyclic trypomastigotes, and then leave the bug in the feces after biting, feeding, and defecating, initiating a new human infection.

Epidemiology

T. cruzi occurs widely in both reduviid bugs and a broad spectrum of reservoir animals in North, Central, and South America. Human disease is found most often among children in South and Central America, where there is a direct correlation between infected wild animal reservoir hosts and the presence of infected bugs whose nests are found in human homes. Cases are rare in the United States, because the bugs prefer nesting in animal burrows and homes are not as open to nesting as those in South and Central America.

Clinical Diseases

Chagas' disease may be asymptomatic, acute, or chronic. One of the earliest signs is development at the site of the bug bite of an erythematous and indurated area called a chagoma. This is often followed by a rash and edema around the eyes and face. The disease is most severe in children younger than 5 years and frequently is seen as an acute process with CNS involvement. Acute infection is also characterized by fever, chills, malaise, myalgia, and fatigue. Parasites may be present in the blood during the acute phase; however, they are sparse in patients older than 1 year. Death may ensue a few weeks after an acute attack, the patient may recover, or the patient may enter the chronic phase as organisms proliferate and invade the heart, liver, spleen, brain, and lymph nodes.

Chronic Chagas' disease is characterized by hepatosplenomegaly, myocarditis, and enlargement of the esophagus and colon as a result of the destruction of nerve cells (e.g., Auerbach's plexus) and other tissues that control the growth of these organs.

Megacardia and electrocardiographic changes are

commonly seen in chronic disease. Involvement of the CNS may produce granulomas in the brain with cyst formation and a meningoencephalitis. Death from chronic Chagas' disease results from tissue destruction in the many areas invaded by the organisms, and sudden death results from complete heart block and brain damage.

Laboratory Diagnosis

T. cruzi can be demonstrated in thick and thin blood films or concentrated anticoagulated blood early in the acute stage. As the infection progresses, the organisms leave the blood stream and become difficult to find. Biopsy of lymph nodes, liver, spleen, or bone marrow may demonstrate the organisms in the amastigote stage. Culture of blood or inoculation into laboratory animals may be useful when the parasitemia is low. Serologic tests are also available. In endemic areas, xenodiagnosis is widely used. Gene amplification techniques, such as polymerase chain reaction, have been used to detect the organism in the blood stream. These approaches are not widely available and have not been adapted for use in the field.

Treatment, Prevention, and Control

Treatment of Chagas' disease is limited by the lack of reliable agents. The drug of choice is nifurtimox. Although it has some activity against the acute phase of disease, it has little activity against tissue amastigotes and also has a number of side effects. Alternative agents include allopurinol and benzimidazole. Education regarding the disease, its insect transmission, and the wild animal reservoirs is critical. Bug control, eradication of nests, and construction of homes to prevent nesting of bugs are also necessary. The use of dichlorodiphenyltrichloroethane (DDT) in bug-infested homes has demonstrated a drop in the transmission of malaria and Chagas' disease. Screening of blood by serologic means or exclusion of blood donors from endemic areas prevents some infections that would otherwise be associated with transfusion therapy.

Development of a vaccine is possible, because *T. cruzi* does not have the wide antigenic variation observed with the African trypanosomes.

CASE STUDY AND QUESTIONS

■ A 44-year-old woman who has received a heart transplant complains to her primary physician about headache, nausea, and vomiting approximately 1 year after transplantation. She has no skin lesions. A computed tomographic scan of the head demonstrates ring-enhancing lesions. A biopsy of the lesions is performed. All cultures (bacterial, fungal, viral) are negative. Special stains of the tissue reveal multiple cystlike structures of varying size.

1. What is the differential diagnosis of infectious agents in this patient? What is the most likely etiologic agent?
2. What other tests could have been performed to confirm the diagnosis?
3. What aspects of the medical history might suggest a risk for infection with this agent?
4. What are the therapeutic options and the likelihood that therapy will be successful?

BIBLIOGRAPHY

Boland PB, Neafie RC, Marty AM: Malaria: a re-emerging disease. In Nelson AM, Horsburgh CR Jr, editors: *Pathology of emerging infections*, Washington DC, 1998, American Society of Microbiology.

Connor DH et al, editors: *Pathology of infectious disease*, vol II, Stamford, Conn, 1997, Appleton & Lange.

Evans TG: Leishmaniasis, *Infect Dis Clin North Am* 7:527–546, 1993.

Garavelli PL, Corti E: Chloroquine resistance in *Plasmodium vivax*: the first case in Brazil, *Trans R Soc Trop Med Hyg* 86:128, 1992.

Garcia LS, editor: *Diagnostic medical parasitology*, ed 4, Washington DC, 2001, American Society of Microbiology.

Homer MJ et al: Babesiosis, *Clin Microbiol Rev* 13:451–469, 2000.

Strickland GT, editor: *Hunter's tropical medicine and emerging infectious diseases*, ed 8, Philadelphia, 2000, WB Saunders.

Wahlgren M, Perlman P, editors: *Malaria: molecular and clinical aspects*, The Netherlands, 1999, Harwood Academic.

CHAPTER 77

Nematodes

The most commonly recognized helminths in the United States are primarily intestinal nematodes, although in other countries nematode infections of blood and tissues can cause devastating disease. The nematodes are the most easily recognized form of intestinal parasite because of their large size and cylindrical, unsegmented bodies; hence, the common name roundworms. These parasites live primarily as adult worms in the intestinal tract, and nematode infections are most commonly confirmed by detecting the characteristic eggs in feces. The identification of eggs should be approached in a systematic manner, with the size and shape of the egg, the thickness of the shell, and the presence or absence of specialized structures, such as polar plugs, knobs, spines, and opercula, taken into account. The presence and characteristics of larvae within the eggs may also be useful. The most common nematodes of medical importance are listed in Table 77–1.

The filariae are long, slender roundworms that are parasites of blood, lymph, subcutaneous, and connective tissues. All of these nematodes are transmitted by mosquitoes or biting flies. Most produce larval worms called microfilariae that are demonstrated in blood specimens or in subcutaneous tissues and skin snips.

Enterobius vermicularis

Physiology and Structure

E. vermicularis, the pinworm, is a small, white worm that is familiar to parents, who find them in the perianal folds or vagina of an infected child. Infection is initiated by ingestion of embryonated eggs (Fig. 77–1). Larvae hatch in the small intestine and migrate to the large intestine, where they mature into adults in 2 to 6 weeks. Fertilization of the female by the male produces the characteristic asymmetrical eggs. These eggs are laid in the perianal folds by the migrating female. As many as 20,000 eggs are deposited on the perianal skin. The eggs rapidly mature and are infectious within hours.

Epidemiology

E. vermicularis occurs worldwide but is most common in the temperate regions, where person-to-person spread is greatest in crowded conditions, such as in daycare centers, schools, and mental institutions. An estimated 500 million cases of pinworm infection are reported worldwide, and it is the most common helminthic infection in North America.

Infection occurs when the eggs are ingested and the larval worm is free to develop in the intestinal mucosa. These eggs may be transmitted from hand to mouth by children scratching the perianal folds in response to the irritation caused by the migrating, egg-laying female worms, or the eggs may find their way to clothing and play objects in daycare centers. They can also survive long periods in the dust that accumulates over doors, on windowsills, and under beds in the rooms of infected people. Egg-laden dust can be inhaled and swallowed to produce infestation. In addition, autoinfection ("retrofection") can occur, wherein eggs hatch in the perianal folds and the larval worms migrate into the rectum and large intestine. Infected individuals who handle food can also be a source of infection.

No animal reservoir for *Enterobius* is known. Physicians should be aware of the related epidemiology of *Dientamoeba fragilis*; this organism correlates well with the presence of *E. vermicularis*, in that *D. fragilis* is transported in the pinworm eggshell.

Clinical Diseases

Many children and adults show no symptoms and serve only as carriers. Patients who are allergic to the secretions of the migrating worms experience severe pruritus, loss of sleep, and fatigue. The pruritus may cause repeated scratching of the irritated area and may lead to secondary bacterial infection. Worms that migrate into the vagina may produce genitourinary problems and granulomas.

Worms attached to the bowel wall may produce inflammation and granuloma formation around the eggs. Although the adult worms may occasionally in-

TABLE 77–1. Nematodes of Medical Importance

Parasite	Common Name	Disease
Enterobius vermicularis	Pinworm	Enterobiasis
Ascaris lumbricoides	Roundworm	Ascariasis
Toxocara canis	Dog ascaris	Visceral larva migrans
Toxocara cati	Cat ascaris	Visceral larva migrans
Trichuris trichiura	Whipworm	Trichuriasis
Ancylostoma duodenale	Old World hookworm	Hookworm infection
Necator americanus	New World hookworm	Hookworm infection
Ancylostoma braziliense	Dog or cat hookworm	Cutaneous larva migrans
Strongyloides stercoralis	Threadworm	Strongyloidiasis
Trichinella spiralis	—	Trichinosis
Wuchereria bancrofti	Bancroft's filariasis	Filariasis
Brugia malayi	Malayan filariasis	Filariasis
Loa loa	African eye worm	Loiasis
Mansonella species	Mansonelliasis	Filariasis
Onchocerca volvulus	River blindness	Onchocerciasis
Dirofilaria immitis	Dog heartworm	Filariasis
Dracunculus medinensis	Guinea worm	Dracunculosis

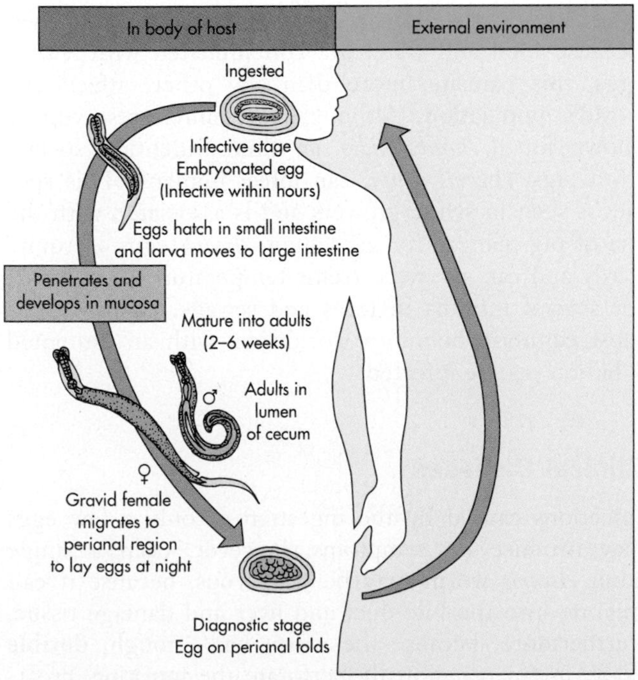

vade the appendix, there remains no proven relationship between pinworm invasion and appendicitis. Penetration through the bowel wall into the peritoneal cavity, liver, and lungs has been infrequently recorded.

Laboratory Diagnosis

The diagnosis of enterobiasis is usually suggested by the clinical manifestations and confirmed by detection of the characteristic eggs on the anal mucosa. Occasionally, the adult worms are seen by laboratory personnel in stool specimens, but the method of choice for diagnosis involves use of an anal swab with a sticky surface that picks up the eggs (Fig. 77–2) for microscopic examination. Sampling can be done with clear tape or commercially available swabs. The sample should be collected when the child arises and before bathing or defecation, so that eggs laid by migrating worms during the night can be picked up. Parents can collect the specimen and deliver it to the physician for immediate microscopic examination. Three swabbings, one per day for 3 consecutive days, may be required to detect the diagnostic eggs. The eggs are rarely seen in fecal specimens. Systemic signs of infection such as eosinophilia are rare.

Treatment, Prevention, and Control

The drug of choice is pyrantel pamoate; as an alternative drug, mebendazole is used. To avoid reintroduc-

FIGURE 77–1. Life cycle of *Enterobius vermicularis*.

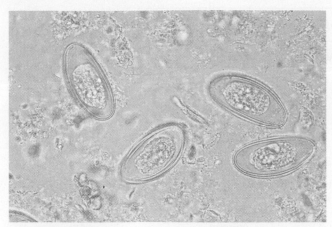

FIGURE 77–2. *Enterobius vermicularis* egg. The thin-walled eggs are 50 to 60 × 20 to 30 μm, ovoid, and flattened on one side (not because children sit on them, but this is an easy way to correlate the egg morphology with the epidemiology of the disease).

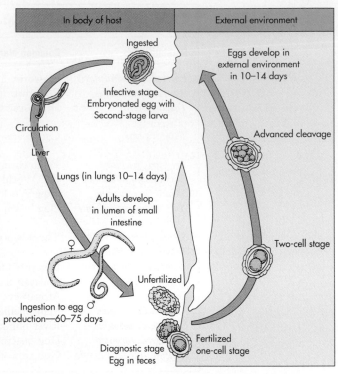

FIGURE 77–3. Life cycle of *Ascaris lumbricoides.*

tion of the organism and reinfection in the family environment, it is customary to treat the entire family simultaneously. Although cure rates are high, reinfection is common. A second course of treatment after 2 weeks may be useful in preventing reinfection.

Good personal hygiene, clipping of fingernails, thorough washing of bed clothes, and prompt treatment of infected individuals all contribute to control. When housecleaning is done in the home of an infected family, dusting under beds, on window sills, and over doors should be done with a damp mop to avoid inhalation of infectious eggs.

Ascaris lumbricoides

Physiology and Structure

Ascaris lumbricoides are large (20 to 35 cm long), pink worms that have a more complex life cycle than *E. vermicularis* (Fig. 77–3) but are otherwise typical of an intestinal roundworm.

The ingested infective egg releases a larval worm that penetrates the duodenal wall, enters the blood stream, is carried to the liver and heart, and then enters the pulmonary circulation. The larvae break free in the alveoli of the lungs, where they grow and molt. In about 3 weeks, the larvae pass from the respiratory system to be coughed up, swallowed, and returned to the small intestine.

As the male and female worms mature in the small intestine (primarily jejunum), fertilization of the female by the male initiates production of eggs, which may number 200,000 per day for as long as a year. Female worms can also produce unfertilized eggs in the absence of males. Eggs are found in the feces 60 to 75

days after the initial infection. Fertilized eggs become infectious after approximately 2 weeks in the soil.

Epidemiology

A. lumbricoides is prevalent in areas where sanitation is poor and where human feces are used as fertilizer. Because food and water are contaminated with *Ascaris* eggs, this parasite, more than any other, affects the world's population. Although no animal reservoir is known for *A. lumbricoides*, an almost identical species from pigs, *Ascaris suum*, can infect humans. This species is seen in swine growers and is associated with the use of pig manure for gardening. *Ascaris* eggs are quite hardy and can survive extreme temperatures and persist for several months in feces and sewage. *Ascaris* is the most common helminth worldwide, with an estimated 1 billion people infected.

Clinical Diseases

Infections caused by the ingestion of only a few eggs may produce no symptoms; however, even a single adult *Ascaris* worm may be dangerous, because it can migrate into the bile duct and liver and damage tissue. Furthermore, because the worm has a tough, flexible body, it can occasionally perforate the intestine, creating peritonitis with secondary bacterial infection. The adult worms do not attach to the intestinal mucosa but depend on constant motion to maintain their position within the bowel lumen.

After infection with many larvae, migration of worms to the lungs can produce pneumonitis resembling an asthmatic attack. Pulmonary involvement is related to the degree of hypersensitivity induced by previous infections and the intensity of the current exposure and may be accompanied by eosinophilia and oxygen desaturation. Also, a tangled bolus of mature worms in the intestine can result in bowel obstruction or perforation as well as occlusion of the appendix. As mentioned previously, migration into the bile duct, gallbladder, and liver can produce severe tissue damage. This migration can occur in response to fever, drugs other than those used to treat ascariasis, and some anesthetics. Patients with many larvae may also experience abdominal tenderness, fever, distention, and vomiting.

Laboratory Diagnosis

Examination of the sediment of concentrated stool reveals the knobby-coated, bile-stained, fertilized and unfertilized eggs. Eggs are oval, 55 to 75 μm long, and 50 μm wide. The thick-walled outer shell can be partially removed (decorticated egg). Occasionally, adult worms pass with the feces, an occurrence that can be quite dramatic because of their large size (20 to 35 cm long). Radiologists may also visualize the worms in the intestine, and cholangiograms often disclose their presence in the biliary tract of the liver. The pulmonary phase of the disease may be diagnosed from the finding of larvae and eosinophils in sputum.

Treatment, Prevention, and Control

Treatment of symptomatic infection is highly effective. The drug of choice is mebendazole; pyrantel pamoate and piperazine are alternatives. Patients with mixed parasitic infections (*A. lumbricoides* and other helminths, *Giardia lamblia*, and *Entamoeba histolytica*) in the stool should be treated for ascariasis first to avoid provoking worm migration and possible intestinal perforation. Education, improved sanitation, and avoidance of human feces as fertilizer are critical. A program of mass treatment in highly endemic areas has been suggested, but such a program may not be economically feasible. Furthermore, eggs can persist in contaminated soil for 3 years or more. Certainly, improved personal hygiene among people who handle food is an important aspect of control.

Toxocara canis and *Toxocara cati*
Physiology and Structure

Toxocara canis and *Toxocara cati* are ascarid worms, naturally parasitic in the intestines of dogs and cats, that accidentally infect humans, producing a disease called **visceral larva migrans** or *toxocariasis*. When ingested by humans, the eggs of these worms can hatch into larval forms that cannot follow the normal developmental cycle seen in the natural dog or cat host. They can penetrate the human gut, reach the blood stream, and then migrate as larvae to various human tissues. They do not develop beyond the migrating larval form.

Epidemiology

Whenever infected dogs and cats are present, the eggs are a threat to humans. This is especially true for children, who are exposed more readily to contaminated soil and who tend to put objects in their mouths.

Clinical Diseases

The clinical manifestations of toxocariasis in humans are related to the migration of the larvae through tissues. The larvae may invade any tissue of the body, where they can induce bleeding, the formation of eosinophilic granulomas, and necrosis. Patients may be asymptomatic and have only eosinophilia, but they can also have serious disease directly related to the number and location of the lesions caused by the migrating larvae as well as the extent to which the host is sensitized to the larval antigens. The organs most commonly involved are the lungs, heart, kidneys, liver, skeletal muscles, eyes, and central nervous system. Signs and symptoms include cough, wheezing, fever, rash, anorexia, seizures, fatigue, and abdominal discomfort. On examination, patients may have hepatosplenomegaly and nodular pruritic skin lesions. Death may result from respiratory failure, cardiac arrhythmia, or brain damage. Ocular disease can also occur with the movement of larvae through the eye and may be mistaken for malignant retinoblastoma. Prompt diagnosis is required to avoid unnecessary enucleation.

Laboratory Diagnosis

The diagnosis of visceral larva migrans is based on clinical findings, the presence of eosinophilia, known exposure to dogs or cats, and serologic confirmation. Enzyme-linked immunosorbent assay (ELISA) is readily available and appears to offer the best serologic marker for disease. The examination of feces from infected patients is not useful, because egg-laying adult worms are not present. However, examination of fecal material from infected pets often supports the diagnosis. Tissue examination for larvae may provide a definitive diagnosis but may have negative results because of sampling error.

Treatment, Prevention, and Control

Treatment is primarily symptomatic, because antiparasitic agents are not of proven benefit. The drug of choice is diethylcarbamazine or thiabendazole. Mebendazole is an acceptable alternative. Corticosteroid therapy may be life-saving if the patient has serious pulmonary, myocardial, or central nervous system involvement, because a major component of the infection is an inflammatory response to the organism. This zoonosis can be greatly reduced if pet owners conscientiously eradicate worms from their animals and clean up pet fecal material from yards and school playgrounds. Children's play areas and sandboxes should be carefully monitored.

Trichuris trichiura

Physiology and Structure

Commonly called **whipworm** because it resembles the handle and lash of a whip, *Trichuris trichiura* has a simple life cycle (Fig. 77–4). Ingested eggs hatch into a larval worm in the small intestine and then migrate to the cecum, where they penetrate the mucosa and mature into adults. Some 3 months after the initial infection, the fertilized female worm starts laying eggs, possibly producing 3000 to 10,000 per day. Female worms can live for as long as 8 years. Eggs passed into the soil mature and become infectious in 3 weeks. *T.*

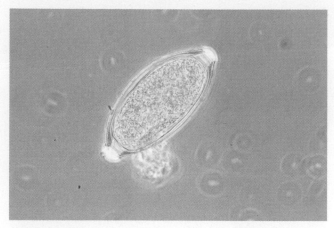

FIGURE 77–5. *Trichuris trichiura* egg. The eggs are barrel-shaped, measuring 50 × 24 μm, with a thick wall and two prominent plugs at the ends. Internally, an unsegmented ovum is present.

trichiura eggs are distinctive, with dark bile staining, a barrel shape, and the presence of polar plugs in the eggshell (Fig. 77–5).

Epidemiology

Like *A. lumbricoides*, *T. trichiura* has worldwide distribution, and its prevalence is directly correlated with poor sanitation and the use of human feces as fertilizer. No animal reservoir is recognized.

Clinical Diseases

The clinical manifestations of trichuriasis are generally related to the intensity of the worm burden. Most infections are with small numbers of *Trichuris* organisms and are usually asymptomatic. Secondary bacterial infection may occur, however, because the heads of the worms penetrate deep into the intestinal mucosa. Infections with many larvae may produce abdominal pain and distention, bloody diarrhea, weakness, and weight loss. Appendicitis may occur as worms fill the lumen of the organ, and prolapse of the rectum is seen in children as a result of the irritation and straining during defecation. Anemia and eosinophilia are also seen in severe infections.

Laboratory Diagnosis

Stool examination reveals the characteristic bile-stained eggs with polar plugs. Light infestations may be difficult to detect because of the paucity of eggs in the stool specimens.

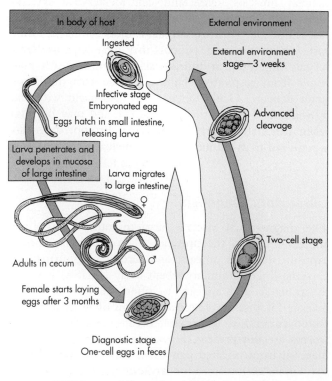

FIGURE 77–4. Life cycle of *Trichuris trichiura*.

Treatment, Prevention, and Control

The drug of choice is mebendazole. As with *A. lumbricoides*, prevention of *T. trichiura* depends on education, good personal hygiene, adequate sanitation, and avoidance of the use of human feces as fertilizer.

Hookworms

Ancylostoma duodenale and *Necator americanus*

Physiology and Structure

The two human hookworms are *Ancylostoma duodenale* (Old World hookworm) and *Necator americanus* (New World hookworm). Differing only in geographic distribution, structure of mouthparts, and relative size, these two species are discussed together as agents of hookworm infection. The human phase of the hookworm life cycle is initiated when a **filariform** (infective form) larva penetrates intact skin (Fig. 77–6). The larva then (1) enters the circulation, (2) is carried to the lungs, (3) like that of *A. lumbricoides*, is coughed up and swallowed, and (4) develops to adulthood in the small intestine. The adult *N. americanus* has a hooklike head, which accounts for the name commonly used.

Adult worms lay as many as 10,000 to 20,000 eggs per day, which are released into feces. Egg laying is initiated 4 to 8 weeks after the initial exposure and can persist for as long as 5 years. On contact with soil, the **rhabditiform** (noninfective) larvae are released from the eggs and within 2 weeks develop into filariform larvae. The filariform larvae can then penetrate exposed skin (e.g., bare feet) and initiate a new cycle of human infection.

Both species have mouthparts designed for sucking blood from injured intestinal tissue. *A. duodenale* has chitinous teeth, and *N. americanus* has shearing chitinous plates.

Epidemiology

Transmission of hookworm infection requires the deposition of egg-containing feces on shady, well-drained soil and is favored by warm, humid (tropical) conditions. Hookworm infections are reported worldwide in places where direct contact with contaminated soil can lead to human disease, but they occur primarily in warm subtropical and tropical regions and in southern parts of the United States. It is estimated that more than 900 million individuals worldwide are infected with hookworms, including 700,000 in the United States.

Clinical Diseases

Skin-penetrating larvae may produce an allergic reaction and rash at sites of entry, and larvae migrating in the lungs can cause pneumonitis. Adult worms produce the gastrointestinal symptoms nausea, vomiting, and diarrhea. As blood is lost from feeding worms, a microcytic hypochromic anemia develops. Daily blood loss is estimated at 0.15 to 0.25 mL for each adult *A. duodenale* and 0.03 mL for each adult *N. americanus*. In severe chronic infections, emaciation and mental and physical retardation, related to anemia from blood loss and nutritional deficiencies, may occur. Also, intestinal sites may be secondarily infected by bacteria when the worms migrate along the intestinal mucosa.

Laboratory Diagnosis

Stool examination reveals the characteristic non–bile-stained segmented eggs shown in Figure 77–7. Larvae are not found in stool specimens unless the specimens are left at ambient temperature for a day or more. The eggs of *A. duodenale* and *N. americanus* cannot be distinguished. The larvae must be examined to identify these hookworms specifically, although the distinction is clinically unnecessary.

Treatment, Prevention, and Control

The drug of choice is mebendazole; pyrantel pamoate is an alternative. In addition to eradication of the worms to stop blood loss, iron therapy is indicated to raise hemoglobin levels to normal. Blood transfusion may be necessary in severe cases of anemia. Education, improved sanitation, and controlled disposal of human

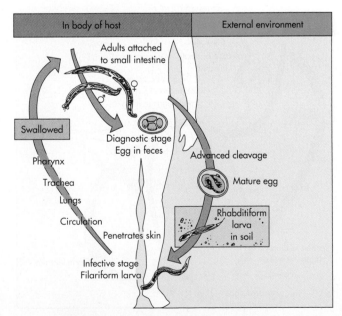

FIGURE 77–6. Life cycle of human hookworms.

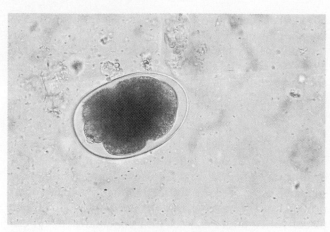

FIGURE 77-7. Human hookworm egg. The eggs are 60 to 75 μm long and 35 to 40 μm wide, are thin-shelled, and enclose a developing larva.

feces are critical preventive measures. Wearing shoes in endemic areas helps reduce the prevalence of infection.

Ancylostoma braziliense

Physiology and Structure

A. braziliense, a species of hookworm, is naturally parasitic in the intestines of dogs and cats and accidentally infects humans. It produces a disease properly called **cutaneous larva migrans** but also called *ground itch* and *creeping eruption*. The filariform larvae of this hookworm penetrate intact skin but can develop no further in humans. The larvae remain trapped in the skin of the "wrong" host for weeks or months, wandering through subcutaneous tissue and creating serpentine tunnels.

Epidemiology

Similar to the situation with *Ascaris* worms, the threat of infection with *A. braziliense* is greatest among children coming into contact with soil or sandboxes contaminated with animal feces containing hookworm eggs. Infections are prevalent throughout the year on beaches in subtropical and tropical regions; in the summer, infection is reported as far north as the Canadian-U.S. border.

Clinical Diseases

The migrating larvae may provoke a severe erythematous and vesicular reaction. Pruritus and scratching of the irritated skin may lead to secondary bacterial infection. About half of patients develop transient pulmonary infiltrates with peripheral eosinophilia (Löffler's syndrome), presumably as a result of pulmonary migration of the larvae.

Laboratory Diagnosis

Occasionally, larvae are recovered in skin biopsy specimens or after freezing of the skin, but most diagnoses are based on the clinical appearance of the tunnels and a history of contact with dog and cat feces. The larvae are rarely found in sputum.

Treatment, Prevention, and Control

The drug of choice is thiabendazole. Antihistamines may be helpful in controlling pruritus. Risk for this zoonosis, as with animal *Ascaris* infection, can be reduced by educating pet owners to treat their animals for worm infections and to pick up pet feces from yards, beaches, and sandboxes. In endemic areas, shoes or sandals should be worn to prevent infection.

Strongyloides stercoralis

Physiology and Structure

Although *Strongyloides stercoralis* resembles hookworm in morphology and epidemiology, the life cycle of these worms (Fig. 77–8) differs in the following three aspects:

1. Eggs hatch into larvae in the intestine and before they are passed in feces.
2. Larvae can mature into filariforms in the intestine and cause autoinfection.

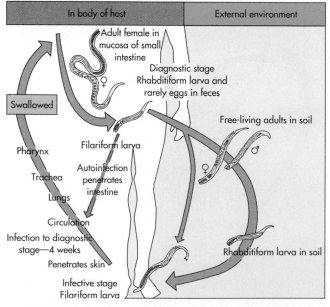

FIGURE 77-8. Life cycle of *Strongyloides stercoralis*.

3. A free-living, nonparasitic cycle can be established outside the human host.

In direct development, like the hookworm, a skin-penetrating *S. stercoralis* larva enters the circulation and follows the pulmonary course. It is coughed up and swallowed, and adults develop in the small intestine. Adult females burrow into the mucosa of the duodenum and reproduce parthenogenetically. Each female produces about a dozen eggs each day, which hatch within the mucosa and release rhabditiform larvae into the lumen of the bowel. The rhabditiform larvae are distinguished from the larvae of hookworms by their short buccal capsule and large genital primordium. The rhabditiform larvae are passed in the stool and may either continue the direct cycle by developing into infective filariform larvae or develop into free-living adult worms and initiate the indirect cycle.

In indirect development, the larvae in soil develop into free-living adults that produce eggs and larvae. Several generations of this nonparasitic existence may occur before new larvae become skin-penetrating parasites.

Finally, in **autoinfection**, rhabditiform larvae in the intestine do not pass with feces but become filariform larvae. These larvae penetrate the intestinal or perianal skin and follow the course through the circulation and pulmonary structures, are coughed up, and then are swallowed. At this point, they become adults, producing more larvae in the intestine. This cycle can persist for years and can lead to hyperinfection and massive or disseminated, often fatal infection.

Epidemiology

Similar to hookworms in its requirements for warm temperatures and moisture, *S. stercoralis* demonstrates low prevalence but a somewhat broader geographic distribution, including parts of the northern United States and Canada. Sexual transmission also occurs. Animal reservoirs, such as domestic pets, are recognized.

Clinical Diseases

Individuals with strongyloidiasis frequently are afflicted with pneumonitis from migrating larvae similar to that seen in ascariasis and hookworm infection. The intestinal infection is usually asymptomatic. However, heavy worm loads may involve the biliary and pancreatic ducts, the entire small bowel, and the colon, causing inflammation and ulceration leading to epigastric pain and tenderness, vomiting, diarrhea (occasionally bloody), and malabsorption. Symptoms mimicking peptic ulcer disease coupled with peripheral eosinophilia should strongly suggest the diagnosis of strongyloidiasis.

Autoinfection may lead to chronic strongyloidiasis that can last for years even in nonendemic areas. Although many of these chronic infections may be asymptomatic, as many as two thirds of patients have recurring episodic symptoms referable to the involved skin, lungs, and intestinal tract. People with chronic strongyloidiasis are at risk for development of severe, life-threatening **hyperinfection syndrome** if the host-parasite balance is disturbed by any drug or illness that compromises the host's immune status. Hyperinfection syndrome is seen most commonly in people who are immunocompromised by malignancies (especially hematologic malignancies), corticosteroid therapy, or both. Hyperinfection syndrome has also been observed in patients who have undergone solid organ transplantation and in malnourished people.

Loss of cellular immune function may be associated with the conversion of rhabditiform larvae to filariform larvae, followed by dissemination of the larvae via the circulation to virtually any organ. Most commonly, extraintestinal infection involves the lung and includes bronchospasm, diffuse infiltrates, and occasionally cavitation. Widespread dissemination that involves the abdominal lymph nodes, liver, spleen, kidneys, pancreas, thyroid, heart, brain, and meninges is common.

Intestinal symptoms of hyperinfection syndrome consist of diarrhea, malabsorption, and electrolyte abnormalities. Notably, hyperinfection syndrome is associated with a mortality rate of approximately 86%. Bacterial sepsis, meningitis, peritonitis, and endocarditis secondary to larval spread from the intestine are common and often fatal complications of hyperinfection syndrome.

Laboratory Diagnosis

The diagnosis of strongyloidiasis may be difficult because of the intermittent passage of low numbers of first-stage larvae in stool. Examination of concentrated stool sediment reveals the larval worms (Fig. 77–9), but in contrast with hookworm infections, eggs are generally not seen in stool specimens from patients with *S. stercoralis* infections. Collecting samples from three stools, one per day for 3 days, as for *G. lamblia*, is recommended, because *S. stercoralis* larvae may occur in "showers," with many present one day and few or none the next.

Several authorities favor the Baermann method of concentrating living *S. stercoralis* larvae from fecal specimens. This method uses a funnel with a stopcock and a gauze insert. The funnel is filled with lukewarm water to a level just covering the gauze, and a specimen of stool is placed on the gauze, partially in contact with the water. The larvae in the stool migrate through the gauze into the water and then sediment into the neck of the funnel, where they may be detected by low-power microscopy.

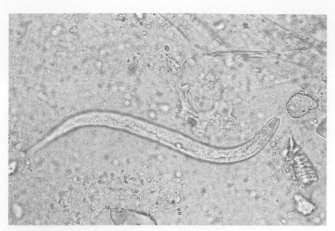

FIGURE 77–9. *Strongyloides stercoralis* larvae. The larvae are 180 to 380 μm long and 14 to 24 μm wide. They can be differentiated from hookworm larvae on the basis of (1) the length of the buccal cavity and esophagus and (2) the structure of the genital primordium.

When absent from stool, larvae may be detected in duodenal aspirates or in sputum in the case of massive infection. Finally, culture of the larvae from stool using charcoal cultures or an agar plate method may be used, although these procedures are not routine in most laboratories. Serologic tests are generally not available.

Treatment, Prevention, and Control

All infected patients should be treated to prevent autoinfection and potential dissemination of the parasite (hyperinfection). The drug of choice is thiabendazole, with mebendazole as an alternative. Patients in endemic areas who are preparing to undergo immunosuppressive therapy should undergo at least three stool examinations to rule out *S. stercoralis* infection and thus avoid the risks of autoinfection. Strict infection-control measures should be enforced when clinicians care for patients with hyperinfection syndrome, because stool, saliva, vomitus, and body fluids may contain infectious filariform larvae. As with hookworm, control of *Strongyloides* species requires education, proper sanitation, and prompt treatment of existing infections.

Trichinella spiralis

Physiology and Structure

Trichinella spiralis is the etiologic agent of trichinosis. The adult form of this organism lives in the duodenal and jejunal mucosa of flesh-eating mammals worldwide. The infectious larval form is present in the striated muscles of carnivorous and omnivorous mammals. Among domestic animals, swine are most commonly affected. Figure 77–10 illustrates the simple, direct life

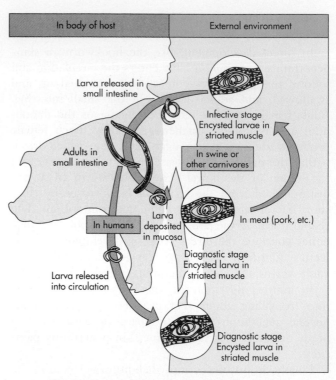

FIGURE 77–10. Life cycle of *Trichinella spiralis*.

cycle, which terminates in the musculature of humans, where the larvae eventually die and calcify.

The infection begins when meat that contains encysted larvae is digested. The larvae leave the meat in the small intestine and within 2 days develop into adult worms. A single fertilized female produces more than 1500 larvae in 1 to 3 months. These larvae move from the intestinal mucosa into the blood stream and are carried in the circulation to various muscle sites

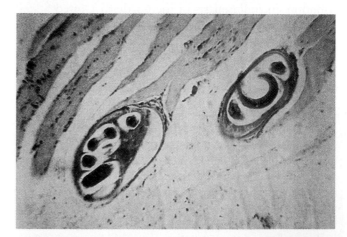

FIGURE 77–11. Encysted larva of *Trichinella spiralis* in a muscle biopsy specimen. (From Finegold SM, Baron EJ, editors: *Bailey and Scott's diagnostic microbiology*, ed 7, St Louis, 1986, Mosby.)

throughout the body, where they coil in striated muscle fibers and become encysted (Fig. 77–11). The muscles invaded most commonly are (1) the extraocular muscles of the eye, (2) the tongue, (3) the deltoid, pectoral, and intercostal muscles, (4) the diaphragm, and (5) the gastrocnemius muscle. The encysted larvae remain viable for many years and are infectious if ingested by a new animal host.

Epidemiology

Trichinosis occurs worldwide in humans, and its greatest prevalence is associated with the consumption of pork products. In addition to pigs, many carnivorous and omnivorous animals harbor the organism and are potential sources of human infection. Notably, polar bears and walruses in the Arctic account for outbreaks in human populations, especially with a strain of *T. spiralis* that is more resistant to freezing than the *T. spiralis* strains found in the continental United States and other temperate regions. It is estimated that more than 1.5 million Americans carry live *Trichinella* cysts in their musculature and that 150,000 to 300,000 acquire new infection annually.

Clinical Diseases

Trichinosis is one of the few tissue parasitic diseases still seen in the United States. As with other parasitic infections, most patients have minimal or no symptoms. The clinical presentation depends largely on the tissue burden of organisms and the location of the migrating larvae. Patients in whom no more than 10 larvae are deposited per gram of tissue are usually asymptomatic; those with at least 100 larvae per gram of tissue generally have significant disease; and those with 1000 to 5000 larvae per gram of tissue have a very serious course that occasionally ends in death.

In mild infections with few migrating larvae, patients may experience only a flu-like syndrome with slight fever and mild diarrhea. More extensive larval migration leads to persistent fever, gastrointestinal distress, marked eosinophilia, muscle pain, and periorbital edema. "Splinter" hemorrhages beneath the nails, a common finding, are probably caused by vasculitis resulting from toxic secretions of the migrating larvae. In heavy infections, severe neurologic symptoms, including psychosis, meningoencephalitis, and cerebrovascular accident, may occur.

Patients who survive the migration, muscle destruction, and encystment of larvae in moderate infections experience a decline in clinical symptoms in 5 or 6 weeks. Lethal trichinosis results when myocarditis, encephalitis, and pneumonitis combine; the patient dies 4 to 6 weeks after infection. Respiratory arrest often follows heavy invasion and muscle destruction in the diaphragm.

Laboratory Diagnosis

The diagnosis is usually established with clinical observations, especially when an outbreak can be traced to consumption of improperly cooked pork or bear meat. The laboratory may confirm the diagnosis if the encysted larvae are detected in the implicated meat or in a muscle biopsy specimen from the patient. Marked eosinophilia is characteristically present in patients with trichinosis. Serologic procedures are also available for confirmation of the diagnosis. Significant antibody titers are usually absent before the third week of illness but then may persist for years.

Treatment, Prevention, and Control

Treatment of trichinosis is primarily symptomatic, because there are no good antiparasitic agents for tissue larvae. Treatment of the adult worms in the intestine with mebendazole may halt the production of new larvae. Steroids, along with thiabendazole or mebendazole, are recommended for severe symptoms. Education regarding disease transmission from pork and bear meat is essential, especially the recommendation that pork and bear meat be cooked until the interior is gray. Microwave cooking and smoking or drying meat do not kill all larvae.

Laws regulating the feeding of garbage to pigs help control transmission of trichinosis, as may measures taken to control the foraging of bears in garbage pits and public parks. Freezing pork, as conducted in federally inspected meat packing plants, has reduced transmission. Quick freezing of pork at −40°C effectively destroys the organisms, as does low-temperature storage at −15°C for 20 days or more.

Wuchereria bancrofti and *Brugia malayi*

Physiology and Structure

Because of their many similarities, *Wuchereria bancrofti* and *Brugia malayi* are discussed together. Human infection is initiated by the introduction of infective larvae, which is present in the saliva of a biting mosquito, into a bite wound (Fig. 77–12). Various species of *Anopheles*, *Aedes*, and *Culex* mosquitoes are vectors of both Bancroft's filariasis and Malayan filariasis.

The larvae migrate from the location of the bite to the lymphatic system, primarily in the arms, legs, or groin, where they grow to adulthood. From 3 to 12 months after the initial infection, the adult male worm fertilizes the female, which in turn produces the

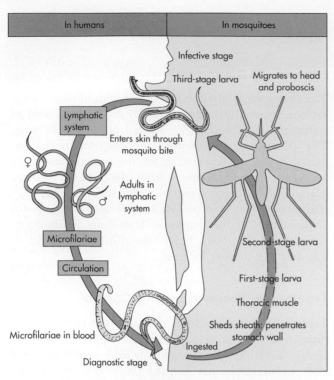

| In humans | In mosquitoes |

FIGURE 77–12. Life cycle of *Wuchereria bancrofti*.

sheathed larval microfilariae that find their way into the circulation. The presence of microfilariae in blood is diagnostic for human disease and is infective for feeding mosquitoes. In the mosquito, the larvae move through the stomach and thoracic muscles in developmental stages and finally migrate to the proboscis. There, they become infective third-stage larvae and are transmitted by the feeding mosquito. The adult form in humans can persist for as long as 10 years.

Epidemiology

W. bancrofti occurs in tropical and subtropical areas and is endemic in central Africa, along the Mediterranean coast, and in many parts of Asia, including China, Korea, Japan, and the Philippines. It is also present in Haiti, Trinidad, Surinam, Panama, Costa Rica, and Brazil. No animal reservoir has been identified. *B. malayi* is found primarily in Malaysia, India, Thailand, Vietnam, and parts of China, Korea, Japan, and many Pacific islands. Animal reservoirs such as cats and monkeys are recognized.

Clinical Diseases

In some patients there is no sign of disease, even though blood specimens may show the presence of many microfilariae. Other patients experience early acute symptoms, such as fever, lymphangitis and

lymphadenitis with chills, and recurrent febrile attacks. The acute presentation is thought to result from the inflammatory response to the presence of molting adolescent worms and dead or dying adults within the lymphatic vessels.

As the infection progresses, the lymph nodes enlarge, possibly involving many parts of the body, including the extremities, the scrotum, and the testes, with occasional abscess formation. This process results from the physical obstruction of lymph in the vessels caused by the presence of adult worms and host reactivity in the lymphatic system. The process may be complicated by recurrent bacterial infections, which contribute to the tissue damage. The thickening and hypertrophy of tissues infected with the worms may lead to the enlargement of tissues, especially the extremities, progressing to **filarial elephantiasis.** Filariasis of this type is thus a chronic, debilitating, and disfiguring disease requiring prompt diagnosis and treatment. Occasionally, ascites and pleural effusions secondary to rupture of the enlarged lymphatic vessels into the peritoneal or pleural cavity may be observed.

Laboratory Diagnosis

Eosinophilia is usually present during acute inflammatory episodes; however, demonstration of microfilariae in the blood is required for definitive diagnosis. As with malaria, microfilariae can be demonstrated in Giemsa-stained blood films in infection with *W. bancrofti* or *B. malayi* (Fig. 77–13). Concentrations of anticoagulated blood specimens and urine specimens are also valuable procedures. Buffy coat films concentrate the white blood cells and are useful for the detection of microfilariae.

The presence of small numbers of microfilariae in blood can be detected by a membrane-filtration tech-

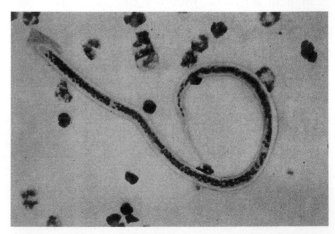

FIGURE 77–13. *Wuchereria bancrofti* microfilaria in blood smear.

nique, in which anticoagulated blood is mixed with saline and forced through a 5-mm membrane filter. After several washes with saline or distilled water, the filter either is examined microscopically for living microfilariae or is dried, fixed, and stained as for a thin blood film.

W. bancrofti and *B. malayi* have a periodicity in the production of microfilariae called **nocturnal periodicity.** There are greater numbers of microfilariae in blood at night. It is recommended that blood specimens be collected between 10 PM and 4 AM for detection of infection.

W. bancrofti, as well as *B. malayi* and *Loa loa*, demonstrate a sheath on their microfilariae. This feature can be the first step in identifying the specific types of filariasis. Further identification is based on study of head and tail structures (Fig. 77–14). Clinically, an exact species identification is not critical, because treatment for all infections with the filariae except *Onchocerca volvulus* is identical.

Serologic testing is also available through reference laboratories so that a diagnosis can be reached. Detection of circulating filarial antigens is promising but is not widely available as a diagnostic test.

Treatment, Prevention, and Control

Treatment is of little benefit in most cases of chronic lymphatic filariasis. The drug of choice for treatment of *W. bancrofti* and *B. malayi* infections is diethylcarbamazine. Ivermectin appears promising, although controlled studies have not yet been performed. Supportive and surgical therapy for lymphatic obstruction may

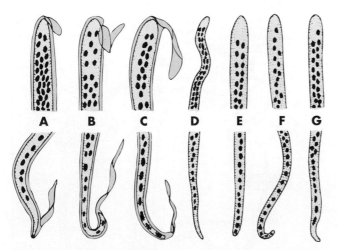

FIGURE 77–14. Differentiation of microfilariae. Identification of microfilariae is based on the presence of a sheath covering the larvae as well as the distribution of nuclei in the tail region. *A, Wuchereria bancrofti. B, Brugia malayi. C, Loa loa. D, Onchocerca volvulus. E, Mansonella perstans. F, Mansonella streptocerca. G, Mansonella ozzardi.*

be of some cosmetic help. Education regarding filarial infections, mosquito control, use of protective clothing and insect repellents, and treatment of infections to prevent further transmission is essential. Control of *B. malayi* infections is more difficult because of the presence of disease in animal reservoirs.

Loa loa

Physiology and Structure

The life cycle of *L. loa* is similar to that illustrated in Figure 77–12, except that the vector is a biting fly called *Chrysops*, the mango fly. The production of microfilariae begins approximately 6 months after infection and can persist for 17 years or more. Adult worms can migrate through subcutaneous tissues, through muscle, and in front of the eyeball.

Epidemiology

L. loa is confined to the equatorial rain forests of Africa and is endemic in tropical West Africa, the Congo basin, and parts of Nigeria. Monkeys in these areas serve as reservoir hosts in the life cycle, with mango flies as vectors.

Clinical Diseases

Symptoms usually do not appear until a year or so after the fly bite, because the worms are slow in reaching adulthood. One of the first signs of infection is the so-called fugitive or **Calabar swellings.** These swellings are transient and usually appear on the extremities, produced as the worms migrate through subcutaneous tissues, creating large, nodular areas that are painful and pruritic. Because eosinophilia (50% to 70%) is observed, Calabar swellings are believed to result from allergic reactions to the worms or their metabolic products.

Adult *L. loa* worms can also migrate under the conjunctiva, producing irritation, painful congestion, edema of the eyelids, and impaired vision. The presence of a worm in the eye can obviously cause anxiety in the patient. The infection may be long-lived and, in some cases, asymptomatic.

Laboratory Diagnosis

The clinical observation of Calabar swellings or migration of worms in the eye, combined with eosinophilia, should alert the physician to consider infection with *L. loa*. The microfilariae can be found in the blood. In contrast to the other filariae, *L. loa* is primarily present during the daytime. Serologic testing can also be useful for confirming the diagnosis but is not readily available.

Treatment, Prevention, and Control

Diethylcarbamazine is effective against adults and microfilariae; however, destruction of the parasites may induce severe allergic reactions that require treatment with corticosteroids. The role of ivermectin remains undefined for this infection. Surgical removal of a worm that is migrating across the eye or bridge of the nose can be accomplished by immobilizing the worm with instillation of a few drops of 10% cocaine.

Education about the infection and its vector, especially for people entering the known endemic areas, is essential. Protection from fly bites by means of screening, appropriate clothing, and insect repellents, along with treatment of cases, is also critical in reducing the incidence of infection. However, the presence of disease in animal reservoirs (e.g., monkeys) limits the feasibility of controlling this disease.

Mansonella Species

Filarial infections by *Mansonella* species are less important than those by parasites previously discussed. Physicians should be aware of the names, however because they may encounter patients with *Mansonella* infections. Infections caused by these organisms are generally asymptomatic but may cause dermatitis, lymphadenitis, hydrocele, and, rarely, lymphatic obstruction resulting in elephantiasis.

All of the *Mansonella* species produce nonsheathed microfilariae in blood and subcutaneous tissues, and all are transmitted by biting midges (*Culicoides* species) or black flies (*Simulium* species). As with previous filarial infections, infections by all *Mansonella* species are treatable with diethylcarbamazine. Species identification, if desired, can be accomplished with examination of blood smears and observation of the structure of the microfilariae. Serologic tests are also available.

Prevention and control require measures that involve insect repellents, screening, and other precautions as for all insect-transmitted diseases.

Mansonella perstans

Mansonella perstans occurs primarily in parts of tropical Africa and Central and South America. It may produce allergic skin reactions, edema, and Calabar swellings like those of *L. loa* infection. Reservoir hosts are chimpanzees and gorillas.

Mansonella ozzardi

Mansonella ozzardi is found primarily in Central and South America and the West Indies. It may produce swelling of the lymph nodes and occasional hydrocele. There are no known reservoir hosts.

Mansonella streptocerca

Mansonella streptocerca occurs primarily in Africa, especially in the Congo basin. It may produce edema in the skin and, rarely, a form of elephantiasis. Monkeys serve as reservoir hosts.

Onchocerca volvulus
Physiology and Structure

Infection by *Onchocerca volvulus* occurs after the introduction of larvae through the skin during the biting and feeding of the *Simulium* or black fly vector (Fig. 77–15). The larval worms migrate from the skin to subcutaneous tissue and develop into adult male and female worms. The adults become encased in fibrous subcutaneous nodules, within which they may remain viable for as long as 15 years. The female worm, after fertilization by the male, begins producing as many as 2000 nonsheathed microfilariae each day. The microfilariae exit the capsule and migrate to the skin, the eyes, and other body tissues. These nonsheathed microfilar-

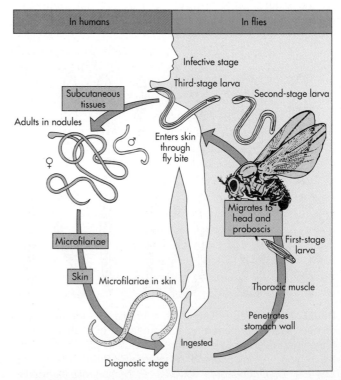

FIGURE 77–15. Life cycle of *Onchocerca volvulus*.

iae appearing in skin tissue are infective for feeding black flies.

Epidemiology

O. volvulus is endemic in many parts of Africa, especially in the Congo basin and the Volta River basin. In the western hemisphere, it occurs in many Central and South American countries. Onchocerciasis affects more than 50 million people worldwide and causes blindness in approximately 5% of infected people.

Several species of the black fly genus *Simulium* serve as vectors, but none so appropriately named as the principal vector, *Simulium damnosum* ("the damned black fly"). These black flies, or buffalo gnats, breed in fast-flowing streams; control or eradication by insecticides is almost impossible, because the chemicals are rapidly washed away from the eggs and larvae.

There is a greater prevalence of infection in men than women in endemic areas because of their work in or near the streams where the black flies breed. Studies in endemic areas in Africa have shown that 50% of men are totally blind before they reach 50 years of age. This fact accounts for the common term **river blindness** applied to the disease onchocerciasis. The fear of blindness has created an additional problem in many parts of Africa, because whole villages leave the areas near streams and farmland that could produce food. The migrating populations then find themselves in areas where they face starvation.

Clinical Diseases

Clinical onchocerciasis is characterized by infection involving the skin, subcutaneous tissue, lymph nodes, and eyes. The clinical manifestations of the infection are due to the acute and chronic inflammatory reaction to antigens released by the microfilariae as they migrate through the tissues. The incubation period from infectious larvae to adult worms is several months to a year. The initial signs of disease are fever, eosinophilia, and urticaria. As the worms mature, copulate, and produce microfilariae, subcutaneous nodules begin to appear on any part of the body. These nodules are most dangerous when they are present on the head and neck, because the microfilariae may migrate to the eyes and cause serious tissue damage, leading to blindness. The mechanisms for development of eye disease are thought to be a combination of both direct invasion by the microfilaria and antigen-antibody complex deposition within the ocular tissues. Patients progress from conjunctivitis with photophobia to punctate and sclerosing keratitis. Internal eye disease with anterior uveitis, chorioretinitis, and optic neuritis may also occur.

Within the skin, the inflammatory process results in loss of elasticity and areas of depigmentation, thickening, and atrophy. A number of skin conditions, including pruritus, hyperkeratosis, and myxedematous thickening, are related to the presence of this parasite. A form of elephantiasis called hanging groin also occurs when the nodules are located near the genitalia.

Laboratory Diagnosis

The diagnosis of onchocerciasis is made from the demonstration of microfilariae in skin snip preparations from the infrascapular or gluteal region. A sample is obtained by raising the skin with a needle and shaving the epidermal layer with a razor. The specimen is incubated in saline for several hours and is then inspected with a dissecting microscope for the presence of nonsheathed microfilariae. In patients with ocular disease, the organism may also be seen in the anterior chamber with the aid of a slit lamp. Serologic and culture methods are not helpful, although efforts to develop serologic detection methods are ongoing.

Treatment, Prevention, and Control

Surgical removal of the encapsulated nodule is often performed to eliminate the adult worms and stop production of microfilariae. In addition, treatment with ivermectin is recommended. A single oral dose of ivermectin (150 μg/kg) greatly reduces the number of microfilariae in the skin and eyes, thus diminishing the likelihood of development of a disabling onchocerciasis. In endemic areas, the dose of ivermectin can be repeated every 6 to 12 months to maintain suppression of dermal and ocular microfilariae. Suppression of dermal microfilariae reduces the transmission of this vector-borne disease, and thus, mass chemotherapy may prove to be a successful strategy for the prevention of onchocerciasis.

Education regarding the disease and its transmission is essential. Protection from black fly bites through the use of protective clothing, screening, and insect repellents, as well as prompt diagnosis and treatment of infections to prevent further transmission, is critical.

Although control of black fly breeding is difficult because insecticides wash away in the streams, some form of biologic control of this vector may reduce fly reproduction and disease transmission.

Dirofilaria immitis

Several mosquito-transmitted filariae infect dogs, cats, raccoons, and bobcats in nature and occasionally are found in humans. *Dirofilaria immitis*, the dog heartworm, is notorious for forming a lethal worm bolus in the dog's heart. This nematode may also infect humans, producing a subcutaneous nodule called a **coin** lesion in the lung. Only very rarely have these worms been found in human hearts.

The coin lesion in the lung presents a problem for the radiologist and the surgeon, because it resembles a malignancy requiring surgical removal. Unfortunately, no laboratory test can provide an accurate diagnosis of dirofilariasis. Peripheral eosinophilia is rare, and the radiographic features are insufficient to allow the clinician to distinguish pulmonary dirofilariasis from bronchogenic carcinoma. Serologic tests are not sufficiently sensitive or specific to preclude the surgical intervention. A definitive diagnosis is made when a thoracotomy specimen is examined microscopically, revealing the typical cross-sections of the parasite.

Transmission of the filarial infections can be reduced by mosquito control and the prophylactic use of the drug ivermectin in dogs.

Dracunculus medinensis

The name *Dracunculus medinensis* means "little dragon of Medina." This is a very ancient worm infection thought by some scholars to be the "fiery serpent" noted by Moses with the Israelites at the Red Sea.

Physiology and Structure

D. medinensis is not a filarial worm but a tissue-invading nematode of medical importance in many parts of the world. The worms have a very simple life cycle, depending on fresh water and a microcrustacean (copepod) of the genus *Cyclops* (Fig. 77–16). When *Cyclops* species harboring larval *D. medinensis* are ingested in drinking water, the infection is initiated with liberation of the larvae in the stomach. These larvae penetrate the wall of the digestive tract and migrate to the retroperitoneal space, where they mature. These larvae are not microfilariae and do not appear in the blood or other tissues. Male and female worms mate in the retroperitoneum, and the fertilized female then migrates to the subcutaneous tissues, usually in the extremities. When the fertilized female worm becomes gravid, a vesicle is formed in the host tissue, which ulcerates. When the ulcer is completely formed, the worm protrudes a loop of uterus through the ulcer. On contact with water, the larval worms are released. The larvae are then ingested by the *Cyclops* species in fresh water, where they are then infective for humans or animals drinking the water containing the *Cyclops* species.

Epidemiology

D. medinensis occurs in many parts of Asia and equatorial Africa, infecting an estimated 10 million people. Reservoir hosts include dogs and many fur-bearing ani-

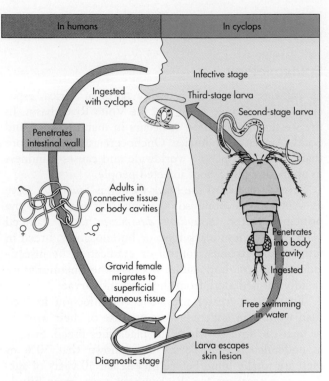

FIGURE 77–16. Life cycle of *Dracunculus medinensis*.

mals that come into contact with drinking water containing infective *Cyclops* species.

Human infections usually result from ingestion of water from so-called step wells, where people stand or bathe in the water, at which time the gravid female worm discharges larvae from lesions on the arms, legs, feet, and ankles to infect *Cyclops* species in the water. Ponds and standing water are occasionally the source of infection when humans use them for drinking water.

Clinical Diseases

Symptoms of infection usually do not appear until the gravid female creates the vesicle and the ulcer in the skin for the liberation of larval worms. This step occurs usually 1 year after initial exposure. Symptoms at the site of the ulcer consist of erythema and pain as well as an allergic reaction to the worm. There is also the possibility of abscess formation and secondary bacterial infection, leading to further tissue destruction and inflammatory reaction with intense pain and sloughing of skin.

If the worm is broken in attempts to remove it, there may be toxic reactions, and if the worm dies and calcifies, there may be nodule formation and some allergic reaction. Once the gravid female worm has discharged all the larvae, it may retreat into deeper tissue, where it is gradually absorbed, or it may simply be expelled from the site.

Laboratory Diagnosis

Diagnosis is established by observing the typical ulcer and by flooding the ulcer with water to recover the larval worms when they are discharged. Occasionally, radiographic examination reveals worms in various parts of the body.

Treatment, Prevention, and Control

The ancient method of slowly wrapping the worm on a twig is still used in many endemic areas (Fig. 77–17). Surgical removal is also a practical and reliable procedure for the patient. The drug of choice for treatment is niridazole; alternative drugs are metronidazole and thiabendazole. These drugs have an anti-inflammatory effect and either eliminate the worm or make surgical removal easier.

Education regarding the life cycle of the worm and avoidance of water contaminated with *Cyclops* species are critical. Protection of drinking water by prohibition of bathing and washing of clothing in wells is essential. Persons who live in or travel to endemic areas should boil water before drinking it. The treatment of water with chemicals and the use of fish that consume *Cyclops* species as food also help control transmission. Prompt diagnosis and treatment of cases also limit further transmission. These preventive measures have been incorporated into an ongoing global effort to eliminate dracunculiasis.

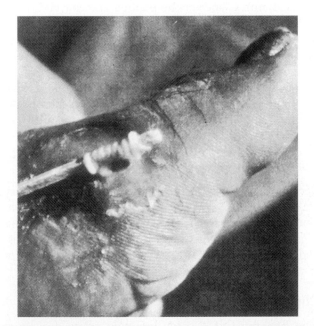

FIGURE 77–17. Removal of a *Dracunculus medinensis* adult from an exposed ulcer by winding of the worm slowly around a stick. (From Binford CH, Conner DH: *Pathology of tropical and extraordinary diseases,* Washington DC, 1976, Armed Forces Institute of Pathology.)

CASE STUDY AND QUESTIONS

■ A 10-year-old boy was brought in to the hospital by his father for evaluation of crampy abdominal pain, nausea, and mild diarrhea that had persisted for approximately 2 weeks. On the day before evaluation, the boy reported to his parents that he passed a large worm into the toilet during a bowel movement. He flushed the worm before the parents could see it. Physical examination was completely unremarkable. The boy had no fever, cough, or rash and did not complain of anal pruritus. His travel history was also unremarkable. Examination of a stool specimen revealed the diagnosis.

1. Which intestinal parasites of humans are nematodes?
2. Which nematode was likely in this case? What organisms may be found in stool?
3. What was the most likely means of acquisition of this parasite?
4. Was this patient at risk of autoinfection?
5. Describe the life cycle of this parasite.
6. Can this parasite cause extraintestinal symptoms? What other organs may be invaded, and what might stimulate extraintestinal invasion?

BIBLIOGRAPHY

Garcia LS, editor: *Diagnostic medical parasitology,* ed 4, Washington DC, 2001, American Society for Microbiology.

Hall LR, Pearlman E: Pathogenesis of onchocercal keratitis (river blindness), *Clin Microbiol Rev* 12:445–453, 1999.

Liu LX, Weller PF: Antiparasitic drugs, *N Engl J Med* 334: 1178–1184, 1996.

Markell EK, John DT, Krotoski WA, editors: *Markell and Voge's medical parasitology,* ed 8, Philadelphia, 1999, WB Saunders.

Orihel TC, Ash LR, editors: *Parasites in human tissues,* Chicago, 1995, American Society of Clinical Pathologists.

Orihel TC, Eberhard ML: Zoonotic filariasis, *Clin Microbiol Rev* 11:366–381, 1998.

Strickland GT, editor: *Hunter's tropical medicine and emerging infectious diseases,* Philadelphia, 2000, WB Saunders.

C H A P T E R 7 8

Trematodes

The trematodes (flukes) are members of the Platyhelminthes phylum and are flat, fleshy, leaf-shaped worms. In general, they are equipped with two muscular suckers: an oral type, which is the beginning of an incomplete digestive system, and a ventral sucker, which is simply an organ of attachment. The digestive system consists of lateral tubes that do not join to form an excretory opening. Most flukes are hermaphroditic, with both male and female reproductive organs in a single body. Schistosomes are the only exception; they have cylindrical bodies (like the nematodes), and separate male and female worms exist.

All flukes require intermediate hosts for the completion of their life cycles, and without exception the first intermediate hosts are mollusks (snails and clams). In these hosts, an asexual reproductive cycle is a type of germ cell propagation. Some flukes require various second intermediate hosts before reaching the final host and developing into adult worms. This variation is discussed in the sections on the individual species.

Fluke eggs are equipped with a "lid" at the top of the shell. Called an operculum, the lid opens to allow the larval worm to find its appropriate snail host. The schistosomes do not have an operculum; rather, the eggshell splits to liberate the larva. The medically significant trematodes are summarized in Table 78–1.

Fasciolopsis buski

A number of intestinal flukes are recognized, including *F. buski*, *Heterophyes heterophyes*, *Metagonimus yokogawai*, *Echinostoma ilocanum*, and *Gastrodiscoides hominis*. *F. buski* is the largest, most prevalent, and most important intestinal fluke. The other flukes are similar to *F. buski* in many respects (epidemiology, clinical syndromes, treatment) and are not discussed further. It is important only that physicians recognize the relationship among these different flukes.

Physiology and Structure

This large intestinal fluke has a typical life cycle (Fig. 78–1). Humans ingest the encysted larval stage (metacercaria) when they peel the husks from aquatic vegetation (e.g., water chestnuts) with their teeth. The metacercariae are scraped from the husk and swallowed, and they develop into immature flukes in the duodenum. The fluke attaches to the mucosa of the small intestine with two muscular suckers, develops into an adult form, and undergoes self-fertilization. Egg production is initiated 3 months after the initial infection with the metacercariae. The operculated eggs pass in feces to water, where the operculum at the top of the eggshell pops open, liberating a free-swimming larval stage (miracidium). Glands at the pointed anterior end of the miracidium produce lytic substances that allow penetration of the soft tissues of snails. In the snail tissue, the miracidium develops through a series of stages by asexual germ cell propagation. The final stage (cercaria) in the snail is a free-swimming form that, after release from the snail, encysts on the aquatic vegetation, becoming the metacercariae, or infective stage.

Epidemiology

Because it depends on the distribution of its appropriate snail host, *F. buski* is found only in China, Vietnam, Thailand, parts of Indonesia, Malaysia, and India. Pigs, dogs, and rabbits serve as reservoir hosts in these endemic areas.

Clinical Diseases

The symptoms of *F. buski* infection relate directly to the worm burden in the small intestine. Attachment of the flukes in the small intestine can produce inflammation, ulceration, and hemorrhage. Severe infections produce abdominal discomfort similar to that of a duodenal ulcer, as well as diarrhea. Stools may be profuse, a malabsorption syndrome similar to giardiasis is common, and intestinal obstruction can occur. Affected

TABLE 78–1. Medically Significant Trematodes

Trematode	Common Name	Intermediate Host	Biologic Vector	Reservoir Host
Fasciolopsis buski	Giant intestinal fluke	Snail	Water plants (e.g., water chestnuts)	Pigs, dogs, rabbits, humans
Fasciola hepatica	Sheep liver fluke	Snail	Water plants (e.g., watercress)	Sheep, cattle, humans
Opisthorchis (Clonorchis) sinensis	Chinese liver fluke	Snail, freshwater fish	Uncooked fish	Dogs, cats, humans
Paragonimus westermani	Lung fluke	Snail, freshwater crabs, crayfish	Uncooked crabs, crayfish	Pigs, monkeys, humans
Schistosoma species	Blood fluke	Snail	None	Primates, rodents, domestic pets, livestock, humans

persons also show marked eosinophilia. Although death can occur, it is rare.

Laboratory Diagnosis

Stool examination reveals the large, golden, bile-stained eggs with an operculum on the top (Fig. 78–2). The measurements and appearance of *F. buski* eggs are similar to that of the liver fluke, *Fasciola hepatica*, and differentiation of the eggs of these species usually is not possible. Large (approximately 1.5 × 3.0 cm) adult flukes can rarely be found in feces or specimens collected at surgery.

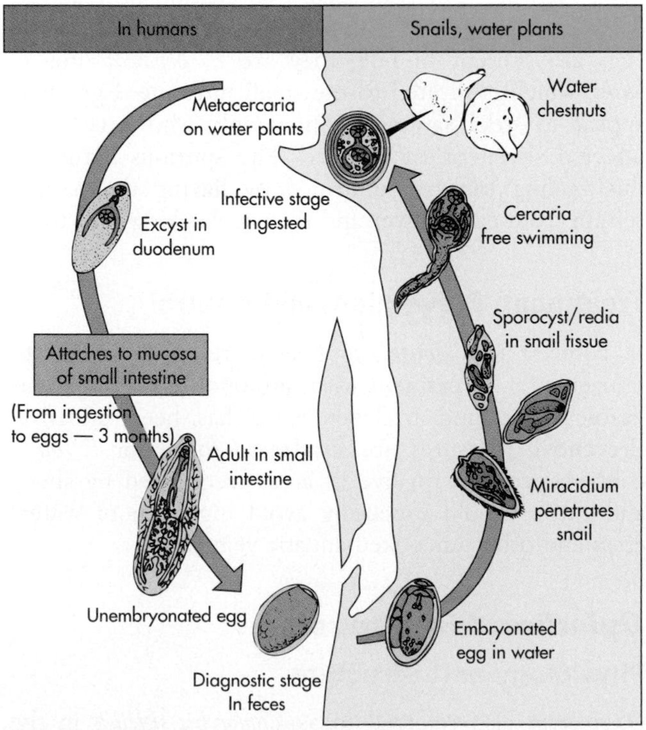

Treatment, Prevention, and Control

The drug of choice is praziquantel, and the alternative is niclosamide. Education about the safe consumption of infective aquatic vegetation (particularly water chestnuts), proper sanitation, and control of human feces reduces the incidence of disease. In addition, the snail population may be eliminated with molluscacides. When infection occurs, treatment should be initiated promptly to minimize its spread. Control of the reservoir hosts also reduces transmission of the worm.

FIGURE 78–1. Life cycle of *Fasciolopsis buski* (giant intestinal fluke).

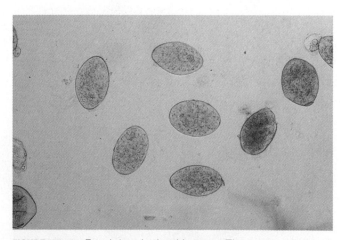

FIGURE 78–2. *Fasciolopsis buski* eggs. The eggs are oval, large (75 to 100 × 130 to 150 μm) and surrounded by a thin shell. Although an operculum is present, it is rarely seen.

Fasciola hepatica

A number of liver flukes are recognized, including *F. hepatica*, *Opisthorchis sinensis*, *O. felineus*, and *Dicrocoelium dendriticum*. Only *F. hepatica* and *O. sinensis* are discussed in this chapter, although the eggs of other flukes are occasionally detected in the feces of patients in other geographic areas.

Physiology and Structure

Commonly called the sheep liver fluke, *F. hepatica* is a parasite of herbivores (particularly sheep and cattle) and humans. Its life cycle (Fig. 78–3) is similar to that of *F. buski*, with human infection resulting from ingestion of watercress that harbors the encysted metacercariae. The larval flukes then migrate through the duodenal wall and across the peritoneal cavity, penetrate the liver capsule, pass through the liver parenchyma, and enter the bile ducts to become adult worms. Approximately 3 to 4 months after the initial infection, the adult flukes start producing operculated eggs that are identical to those of *F. buski*, as seen in stool specimens.

Epidemiology

Infections have been reported worldwide in sheep-raising areas, with the appropriate snail as an intermediate host. These areas include the former Soviet Union, Japan, Egypt, and many Latin American countries. Outbreaks are directly related to human consumption of contaminated watercress in areas where infected herbivores are present. Human infection is rare in the United States, but several well-documented cases have been reported in travelers from endemic areas.

Clinical Diseases

Migration of the larval worm through the liver produces irritation of this tissue, tenderness, and hepatomegaly. Pain in the right upper quadrant, chills, and fever with marked eosinophilia are commonly observed. As the worms take up residence in the bile ducts, their mechanical irritation and toxic secretions produce hepatitis, hyperplasia of the epithelium, and biliary obstruction. Some worms penetrate eroded areas in the ducts and invade the liver to produce necrotic foci referred to as *liver rot*. In severe infections, secondary bacterial infection can occur, and portal cirrhosis is common.

Laboratory Diagnosis

Stool examination reveals operculated eggs indistinguishable from the eggs of *F. buski*. Exact identification is a therapeutic problem because treatment is not the same for both infections. Whereas *F. buski* responds favorably to praziquantel, *F. hepatica* does not. When exact identification is desired, examination of a sample of the patient's bile differentiates the species; if the eggs are present in bile, they are *F. hepatica*, not *F. buski*, which is limited to the small intestine. Eggs may appear in stool samples from people who have eaten infected sheep or cattle liver. The spurious nature of this finding can be confirmed by having the patient refrain from eating liver and then rechecking the stool.

Treatment, Prevention, and Control

In contrast to *F. buski*, *F. hepatica* responds poorly to praziquantel. Treatment with bithionol or the benzimidazole compound triclabendazole has been effective. Preventive measures are similar to those for *F. buski* control; people who live in areas frequented by sheep and cattle should especially avoid ingestion of watercress and other uncooked aquatic vegetation.

Opisthorchis sinensis
Physiology and Structure

O. sinensis, also referred to as *Clonorchis sinensis* in the older literature, is commonly called the Chinese liver fluke. Figure 78–4 illustrates its life cycle, which involves two intermediate hosts. This trematode differs

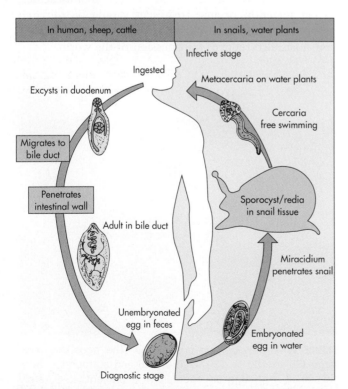

FIGURE 78–3. Life cycle of *Fasciola hepatica* (sheep liver fluke).

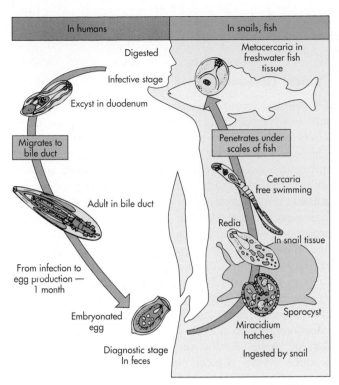

FIGURE 78–4. Life cycle of *Opisthorchis sinensis* (Chinese liver fluke).

from other fluke cycles because the eggs are eaten by the snail and reproduction then begins in the soft tissues of the snail. *O. sinensis* also requires a second intermediate host, freshwater fish, in which the cercariae encyst and develop into infective metacercariae. When uncooked freshwater fish harboring metacercariae are eaten, flukes develop first in the duodenum and then migrate to the bile ducts, where they become adults. The adult fluke undergoes self-fertilization and begins producing eggs. *O. sinensis* may survive in the biliary tract for as long as 50 years, producing approximately 2000 eggs per day. These eggs pass with feces and are once again eaten by snails, reinitiating the cycle.

Epidemiology

O. sinensis is found in China, Japan, Korea, and Vietnam, where it is estimated to infect approximately 19 million people. It is one of the most frequent infections among Asian refugees, and it can be traced to the consumption of raw, pickled, smoked, or dried freshwater fish that harbor the viable metacercariae. Dogs, cats, and fish-eating mammals can also serve as reservoir hosts.

Clinical Diseases

Infection in humans is usually mild and asymptomatic. Severe infection with many flukes in the bile ducts produces fever, diarrhea, epigastric pain, hepatomegaly, anorexia, and occasionally jaundice. Biliary obstruction may occur, and chronic infection can result in adenocarcinoma of the bile ducts. Invasion of the gallbladder may produce cholecystitis, cholelithiasis, and impaired liver function, as well as liver abscesses.

Laboratory Diagnosis

The diagnosis is made by recovering the distinctive eggs from stool. The eggs measure 27 to 35 × 12 to 19 μm and are characterized by a distinct operculum with prominent shoulders and a tiny knob at the posterior (abopercular) pole (Fig. 78–5). In mild infections, repeated examinations of stool or duodenal aspirates may be necessary. Persons with acute symptomatic infection usually have eosinophilia and an elevation of serum alkaline phosphatase levels. Radiographic imaging procedures may detect abnormalities of the biliary tract.

Treatment, Prevention, and Control

The drug of choice is praziquantel. Infection is prevented by not eating uncooked fish and by implementing proper sanitation policies, including disposal of human, dog, and cat feces in adequately protected sites so that they cannot contaminate water supplies with the intermediate snail and fish hosts.

Paragonimus westermani

Physiology and Structure

P. westermani, commonly called the lung fluke, is one of several species of *Paragonimus* that infect humans and many other animals. Figure 78–6 shows a familiar

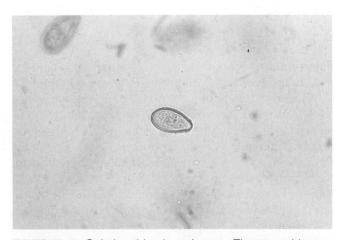

FIGURE 78–5. *Opisthorchis sinensis* egg. These ovoid eggs are small (22 to 30 μm long and 12 to 19 μm wide) and have a yellowish brown, thick shell with a prominent operculum at one end and a small knob at the other.

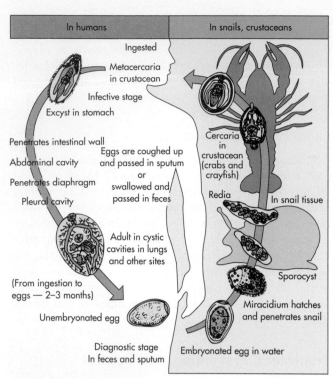

FIGURE 78–6. Life cycle of *Paragonimus westermani* (Oriental lung fluke).

fluke life cycle from egg to snail to infective metacercaria. The infective stage occurs in a second intermediate host: the muscles and gills of freshwater crabs and crayfish. In humans who ingest infected meat, the larval worm hatches in the stomach and follows an extensive migration through the intestinal wall to the abdominal cavity, then through the diaphragm, and finally to the pleural cavity. Adult worms reside in the lungs and produce eggs that are liberated from ruptured bronchioles and appear in sputum or, when swallowed, in feces.

Epidemiology

Paragonimiasis occurs in many countries in Asia, Africa, India, and Latin America. It can be encountered in refugees from Southeast Asia. Its prevalence is directly related to the consumption of uncooked freshwater crabs and crayfish. It is estimated that approximately 3 million people are infected with this lung fluke. As many as 1% of all Indochinese immigrants to the United States are infected with *P. westermani*. A wide variety of shore-feeding animals (e.g., wild boars, pigs, and monkeys) serve as reservoir hosts, and some human infections result from ingestion of meat containing migrating larval worms from these reservoir hosts. Human infections endemic to the United States are usually caused by a related species, *Paragonimus*

kellicotti, which is found in crabs and crayfish in eastern and midwestern waters.

Clinical Diseases

The clinical manifestations of paragonimiasis may result from larvae migrating through tissues or from adults established in the lungs or other ectopic sites. The onset of disease coincides with larval migration and is associated with fever, chills, and marked eosinophilia. The adult flukes in the lungs first produce an inflammatory reaction that results in fever, cough, and increased sputum. As the destruction of lung tissue progresses, cavitation occurs around the worms, sputum becomes blood-tinged and dark with eggs (so-called rusty sputum), and patients experience severe chest pain. The resulting cavity may become secondarily infected with bacteria. Dyspnea, chronic bronchitis, bronchiectasis, and pleural effusion may ensue. Chronic infections lead to fibrosis in the lung tissue. The location of larvae, adults, and eggs in ectopic sites may produce severe clinical symptoms depending on the site involved. Migration of larval worms may result in invasion of the spinal cord and brain, producing severe neurologic disease (visual problems, motor weakness, and convulsive seizures), referred to as *cerebral paragonimiasis*. Migration and infection may also occur in subcutaneous sites, the abdominal cavity, and the liver.

Laboratory Diagnosis

Examination of sputum and feces reveals golden brown operculated eggs (Fig. 78–7). Pleural effusions, when present, should be examined for eggs. Chest radiographs often show infiltrates, nodular cysts, and pleural

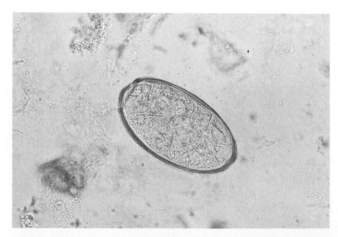

FIGURE 78–7. *Paragonimus westermani* egg. These large ovoid eggs (80 to 120 μm long and 45 to 70 μm wide) have a thick, yellowish brown shell and a distinct operculum.

effusion. Marked eosinophilia is common. Serologic procedures are available through reference laboratories and can be helpful, particularly in cases with extrapulmonary (e.g., central nervous system) involvement.

Treatment, Prevention, and Control

The drug of choice is praziquantel; bithionol is an alternative. Education about the consumption of uncooked freshwater crabs and crayfish, as well as the flesh of animals found in endemic areas, is critical. Pickling and wine soaking of crabs and crayfish do not kill the infective metacercarial stage. Proper sanitation and control of the disposal of human feces are essential.

Schistosomes

Schistosomiasis is a major parasitic infection of tropical areas, with some 200 million infections worldwide. The three schistosomes most frequently associated with human disease are *Schistosoma mansoni*, *Schistosoma japonicum*, and *Schistosoma haematobium*. They collectively produce the disease schistosomiasis, also known as bilharziasis or snail fever. As discussed earlier, the schistosomes differ from other flukes: They are male and female rather than hermaphroditic, and their eggs do not have an operculum. They also are obligate intravascular parasites and are not found in cavities, ducts, and other tissues. The infective forms are skin-penetrating cercariae liberated from snails, and these differ from other flukes in that they are not eaten on vegetation, in fish, or in crustaceans.

Figure 78–8 illustrates the life cycle of the different schistosomes. Infection is initiated by ciliated, free-swimming cercariae in fresh water that penetrate intact skin, enter the circulation, and develop in the intrahepatic portal circulation (*S. mansoni* and *S. japonicum*) or in the vesical, prostatic, rectal, and uterine plexuses and veins (*S. haematobium*). The female has a long, slender, cylindrical body, whereas the shorter male, which appears cylindrical, is actually flat. The cylindrical appearance derives from folding the sides of the body to produce a groove, the gynecophoral canal, in which the female resides for fertilization. Both sexes have oral and ventral suckers and an incomplete digestive system, which is typical of a fluke.

As the worms develop in the portal circulation, they elaborate a remarkable defense against host resistance. They coat themselves with substances that the host recognizes as itself; consequently, little host response is directed against their presence in blood vessels. This protective mechanism accounts for chronic infections that may last 20 to 30 years or longer.

After developing in the portal vein, the male and female adult worms pair up and migrate to their final

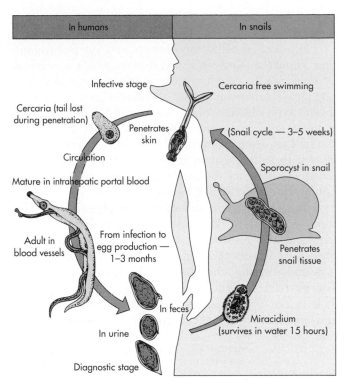

FIGURE 78–8. Life cycle of schistosomes.

locations, where fertilization and egg production begin *S. mansoni* and *S. japonicum* are found in mesenteric veins and produce intestinal schistosomiasis; *S. haematobium* resides in veins around the urinary bladder and causes vesicular schistosomiasis. On reaching the submucosal venules of their respective locations, the worms initiate oviposition, which may continue at the rate of 300 to 3000 eggs daily for 4 to 35 years. Although the host inflammatory response to the adult worms is minimal, the eggs elicit an intense inflammatory reaction with mononuclear and polymorphonuclear cellular infiltrates and the formation of microabscesses. In addition, the larvae inside the eggs produce enzymes that aid in tissue destruction and allow the eggs to pass through the mucosa and into the lumen of the bowel and bladder, where they are passed to the external environment in the feces and urine, respectively.

The eggs hatch quickly on reaching fresh water to release motile miracidia. The miracidia then invade the appropriate snail host, where they develop into thousands of infectious cercariae. The free-swimming cercariae are released into the water, where they are immediately infectious for humans and other mammals.

The infection is similar in all three species of human schistosomes in that disease results primarily from the host's immune response to the eggs. The very earliest signs and symptoms are due to penetration of the cercariae through the skin. Immediate and delayed hypersensitivity to parasite antigens result in an intensely pruritic papular skin rash.

The onset of oviposition results in a symptom complex known as Katayama's syndrome, which is marked by fever, chills, cough, urticaria, arthralgias, lymphadenopathy, splenomegaly, and abdominal pain. This syndrome typically develops 1 to 2 months after primary exposure and may persist for 3 months or more. It is thought to result from massive release of parasite antigens with subsequent immune complex formation. Associated laboratory findings include leukocytosis, eosinophilia, and polyclonal gammopathy.

The more chronic and significant phase of schistosomiasis is due to the presence of eggs in various tissues and the resulting formation of granulomas and fibrosis. The retained eggs induce extensive inflammation and scarring, the clinical significance of which is directly related to the location and number of eggs.

Because of differences in some aspects of disease and epidemiology, these worms are discussed as separate species.

Schistosoma mansoni

Physiology and Structure

S. mansoni usually resides in the small branches of the inferior mesenteric vein near the lower colon. The species of *Schistosoma* can be differentiated by their characteristic egg morphology (Figs. 78–9 through 78–11). The eggs of *S. mansoni* are oval, possess a sharp lateral spine, and measure 115 to 175 × 45 to 70 μm (see Fig. 78–9).

Epidemiology

The geographic distribution of the various species of *Schistosoma* depends on the availability of a suitable

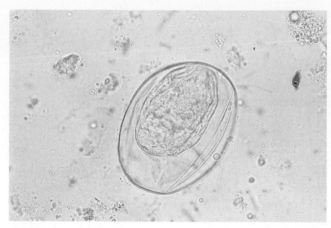

FIGURE 78–10. *Schistosoma japonicum* egg. These eggs are smaller than those of *Schistosoma mansoni* (70 to 100 μm long and 55 to 65 μm wide) and have a spine that is inconspicuous.

snail host. *S. mansoni* is the most widespread of the schistosomes and is endemic in Africa, Saudi Arabia, and Madagascar. It has also become well established in the Western Hemisphere, particularly in Brazil, Surinam, Venezuela, parts of the West Indies, and Puerto Rico. Cases originating in these areas occur in the United States. In all of these areas there are also reservoir hosts, specifically primates, marsupials, and rodents. Schistosomiasis may be considered a disease of economic progress; the development of massive land irrigation projects in desert and tropical areas has resulted in dispersion of infected humans and snails to previously uninvolved areas.

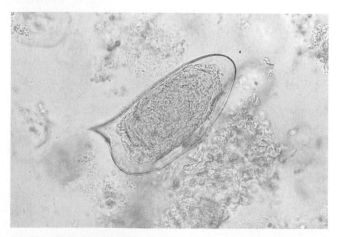

FIGURE 78–9. *Schistosoma mansoni* egg. These eggs are 115 to 175 μm long and 45 to 70 μm wide, contain a miracidium, and are enclosed in a thin shell with a prominent lateral spine.

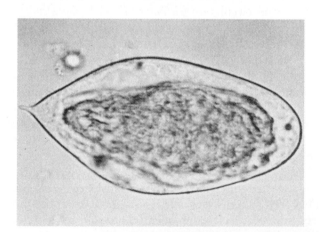

FIGURE 78–11. *Schistosoma haematobium* egg. These eggs are similar in size to those of *Schistosoma mansoni* but can be differentiated by the presence of a terminal spine. (From Ash LR, Orihel TC: *Atlas of human parasitology*, ed 2, Chicago, 1984, American Society of Clinical Pathologists.)

Clinical Diseases

As noted before, cercarial penetration of the intact skin may be seen as dermatitis with allergic reactions, pruritus, and edema. Migrating worms in the lungs may produce cough; as they reach the liver, hepatitis may appear.

Infections with *S. mansoni* may produce hepatic and intestinal abnormalities. As the flukes take up residence in the mesenteric vessels and egg laying begins, fever, malaise, abdominal pain, and tenderness of the liver may ensue. Deposition of eggs in the bowel mucosa results in inflammation and thickening of the bowel wall with associated abdominal pain, diarrhea, and blood in the stool. Eggs may be carried by the portal vein to the liver, where inflammation can lead to periportal fibrosis and eventually to portal hypertension and its associated manifestations.

Chronic infection with *S. mansoni* produces dramatic hepatosplenomegaly with large accumulations of ascitic fluid in the peritoneal cavity. On gross examination, the liver is studded with white granulomas (pseudotubercles). Although *S. mansoni* eggs are primarily deposited in the intestine, eggs may appear in the spinal cord, lungs, and other sites. A similar fibrotic process occurs at each site. Severe neurologic problems may follow when eggs are deposited in the spinal cord and brain. In fatal schistosomiasis caused by *S. mansoni*, fibrous tissue, reacting to the eggs in the liver, surrounds the portal vein in a thick, grossly visible layer ("clay pipestem fibrosis").

Laboratory Diagnosis

The diagnosis of schistosomiasis is usually established by demonstration of characteristic eggs in feces. Stool examination reveals the large golden eggs with a sharp lateral spine (see Fig. 78–9). Concentration techniques may be necessary in light infections. Using rectal biopsy, the clinician can see the egg tracks laid by the worms in rectal vessels. Measurement of egg output in stool is useful in estimating the severity of infection and in monitoring the response to therapy. Serologic tests are also available but are largely of epidemiologic interest only. The development of newer tests using stage-specific antigens may allow the distinction of active from inactive disease, and these tests thus may have greater clinical application.

Treatment, Prevention, and Control

The drug of choice is praziquantel, and the alternative is oxamniquine. Antihelminthic therapy may terminate oviposition but does not affect lesions caused by eggs already deposited in tissues. Schistosomal dermatitis and Katayama's syndrome may be treated with administration of antihistamines and corticosteroids. Educa-

tion regarding the life cycles of these worms and control of snails using molluscacides are essential. Improved sanitation and control of human fecal deposits are critical. Mass treatment may one day be practical, and the development of a vaccine may be forthcoming.

Schistosoma japonicum

Physiology and Structure

S. japonicum resides in branches of the superior mesenteric vein around the small intestine and in the inferior mesenteric vessels. *S. japonicum* eggs (see Fig. 78–10) are smaller than those of *S. mansoni*, are almost spherical, and possess a tiny spine. These eggs are produced in greater numbers than those of *S. mansoni* and *S. haematobium*. Because of the size, shape, and numbers of these eggs, they are carried to more sites in the body (liver, lungs, brain), and infection with a few *S. japonicum* adults can be more severe than infections involving similar numbers of *S. mansoni* or *S. haematobium*.

Epidemiology

This Oriental blood fluke is found only in China, Japan, and the Philippines and on the island of Sulawesi, Indonesia. Epidemiologic problems correlate directly with a broad range of reservoir hosts, many of which are domestic (cats, dogs, cattle, horses, and pigs).

Clinical Diseases

The initial stages of infection with *S. japonicum* are similar to those of *S. mansoni*, with dermatitis, allergic reactions, fever, and malaise, followed by abdominal discomfort and diarrhea. Katayama's syndrome associated with the onset of oviposition is observed more commonly with *S. japonicum* than with *S. mansoni* infection. In chronic *S. japonicum* infection, hepatosplenic disease, portal hypertension, bleeding esophageal varices, and accumulation of ascitic fluid are common. Granulomas that appear as pseudotubercles in and on the liver are common, along with the clay pipestem fibrosis as described for *S. mansoni*.

S. japonicum frequently involves cerebral structures when eggs reach the brain and granulomas develop around them. The neurologic manifestations include lethargy, speech impairment, visual defects, and seizures.

Laboratory Diagnosis

Stool examination demonstrates the small golden eggs with tiny spines; rectal biopsy usually is similarly revealing. Serologic tests are available.

Treatment, Prevention, and Control

The drug of choice is praziquantel. Prevention and control may be achieved by measures similar to those for *S. mansoni*, especially education of populations in endemic areas about proper water purification, sanitation, and control of human fecal deposits. Control of *S. japonicum* must also involve the broad range of reservoir hosts and must consider the fact that people work in rice paddies and on irrigation projects where infected snails are present. Mass treatment may offer help, and a vaccine may be developed someday.

Schistosoma haematobium

Physiology and Structure

After development in the liver, these blood flukes migrate to the vesical, prostatic, and uterine plexuses of the venous circulation; they occasionally migrate to the portal blood stream and only rarely to other venules.

Large eggs with a sharp terminal spine (see Fig. 78–11) are deposited in the wall of the bladder and occasionally in the uterine and prostatic tissues. Those deposited in the bladder wall can break free and are found in urine.

Epidemiology

S. haematobium occurs throughout the Nile Valley and in many other parts of Africa, including islands off the eastern coast. It also appears in Asia Minor, Cyprus, southern Portugal, and India. Reservoir hosts include monkeys, baboons, and chimpanzees.

Clinical Diseases

Early stages of infection with *S. haematobium* are similar to those of infections involving *S. mansoni* and *S. japonicum*, with dermatitis, allergic reactions, fever, and malaise. Unlike the other two schistosomes, *S. haematobium* produces hematuria, dysuria, and urinary frequency as early symptoms. Associated with hematuria, bacteriuria is frequently a chronic condition. Egg deposition in the walls of the bladder may eventually result in scarring with loss of bladder capacity and the development of obstructive uropathy.

Patients with *S. haematobium* infections involving many flukes frequently demonstrate squamous cell carcinoma of the bladder. It is commonly stated that the leading cause of cancer of the bladder in Egypt and other parts of Africa is *S. haematobium*. The granulomas and pseudotubercles seen in the bladder may also be present in the lungs. Fibrosis of the pulmonary bed caused by egg deposition leads to dyspnea, cough, and hemoptysis.

Laboratory Diagnosis

Examination of urine specimens reveals the large, terminally spined eggs. Bladder biopsy is occasionally helpful in establishing the diagnosis. *S. haematobium* eggs may appear in stool if worms have migrated to mesenteric vessels. Serologic tests are also available.

Treatment, Prevention, and Control

The drug of choice is praziquantel. At present, education, possible mass treatment, and development of a vaccine are the best approaches to the control of *S. haematobium* disease. The basic problems of irrigation projects (e.g., dam building), migratory human populations, and numerous reservoir hosts make prevention and control extremely difficult.

Cercarial Dermatitis

Several nonhuman schistosomes have cercariae that penetrate human skin, producing a severe dermatitis ("swimmer's itch"), but these schistosomes cannot develop into adult worms. The natural hosts are birds and other shore-feeding animals from freshwater lakes throughout the world and from a few marine beaches. The intense pruritus and urticaria from this skin penetration may lead to secondary bacterial infection due to scratching the sites of infection.

Treatment consists of oral trimeprazine and topical applications of palliative agents. When indicated, sedatives may be given. Control is difficult because of bird migration and the transfer of live snails from lake to lake. Molluscacides such as copper sulfate have produced some reduction in the snail populations. Immediate drying of the skin when people leave such waters offers some protection.

CASE STUDY AND QUESTIONS

■ A 45-year-old Egyptian man was referred for evaluation of hematuria and urinary frequency of 2 months' duration. This man had lived in the Middle East for most of his life but for the past year lived in the United States. He denied previous renal or urologic problems. Results of his physical examination were unremarkable. A midstream urine specimen was grossly bloody.

1. What was the differential diagnosis of hematuria in this patient?

2. What was the etiologic agent of this patient's urologic process?

3. What exposures might put an individual at risk for this infection?

4. What are the major complications of this infection?

5. How is this disease treated?

BIBLIOGRAPHY

Ash LR, Orihel TC: Intestinal helminths. In Murray PR et al, editors: *Manual of clinical microbiology*, ed 7, Washington, DC, 1999, American Society for Microbiology.

Connor DH et al, editors: *Pathology of infectious diseases*, vol 2, Stamford, Conn, 1997, Appleton & Lange.

Garcia LS, editor: *Diagnostic medical parasitology*, ed 4, Washington, DC, 2001, American Society for Microbiology.

Markell EK, John DT, Krotoski WA, editors: *Markell and Voges' medical parasitology*, ed 8, Philadelphia, 1999, WB Saunders.

Strickland GT, editor: *Hunter's tropical medicine and emerging infectious diseases*, Philadelphia, 2000, WB Saunders.

CHAPTER 79

Cestodes

The bodies of cestodes, tapeworms, are flat and ribbon-like, and the heads are equipped with organs of attachment. The head, or scolex, of the worm usually has four muscular, cup-shaped suckers and a crown of hooklets. An exception is *Diphyllobothrium latum*, the fish tapeworm, whose scolex is equipped with a pair of long, lateral muscular grooves and lacks hooklets.

The individual segments of tapeworms are called proglottids, and the chain of proglottids is called a strobila.

All tapeworms are hermaphroditic, with male and female reproductive organs present in each mature proglottid. The eggs of most tapeworms are nonoperculated and contain a six-hooked hexacanth embryo; the one exception, *D. latum*, has an unembryonated, operculated egg similar to a fluke egg. Tapeworms have no digestive system, and food is absorbed from the host intestine through the soft body wall of the worm. Most tapeworms found in the human intestine have complex life cycles involving intermediate hosts, and in some instances (cysticercosis, echinococcosis, sparganosis) humans serve as a form of intermediate host that harbors larval stages. The presence of extraintestinal larvae is at times more serious than that of adult worms in the intestine. The most common cestodes of medical importance are listed in Table 79–1.

Taenia solium

Physiology and Structure

After a person ingests pork muscle containing a larval worm called a cysticercus ("bladder worm"), attachment of the scolex with its four muscular suckers and crown of hooklets initiates infection in the small intestine (Fig. 79–1). The worm then produces proglottids until a strobila of proglottids, which may be several meters in length, is developed. The sexually mature proglottids contain eggs, and as these proglottids leave the host in feces, they can contaminate water and vegetation ingested by swine. In swine, the eggs become a six-hooked larval form called an oncosphere that penetrates the pig's intestinal wall, migrates in the circulation to the tissues, and becomes a cysticercus to complete the cycle.

Epidemiology

T. solium infection is directly correlated with eating insufficiently cooked pork and is prevalent in Africa, India, Southeast Asia, China, Mexico, Latin American countries, and Slavic countries. It is infrequently encountered in the United States.

Clinical Diseases

Adult *T. solium* in the intestine seldom causes appreciable symptoms. The intestine may be irritated at sites of attachment, and abdominal discomfort, chronic indigestion, and diarrhea may occur. Most patients become aware of the infection only when they see proglottids or a strobila of proglottids in their feces.

Laboratory Diagnosis

Stool examination may reveal proglottids and eggs, and treatment may produce the entire worm for identification. The eggs are spherical, 30 to 40 μm in diameter, and possess a thick, radially striated shell containing a six-hooked hexacanth embryo (Fig. 79–2). The eggs are identical to those of *Taenia saginata* (beef tapeworm); thus, eggs alone are not sufficient for species identification. Critical examination of the proglottids reveals their internal structure, which is important for differentiating *T. solium* and *T. saginata*. Gravid proglottids of *T. solium* are smaller than those of *T. saginata* and contain only 7 to 13 lateral uterine branches versus 15 to 30 for the beef tapeworm.

Treatment, Prevention, and Control

The drug of choice is niclosamide; praziquantel, paromomycin, or quinacrine is an effective alternative. Prevention of pork tapeworm infections requires that pork

TABLE 79–1. Medically Important Cestodes

Cestode	Common Name	Reservoir for Larvae	Reservoir for Adults
Taenia solium	Pork tapeworm	Hogs	Humans
	Cysticercosis	Humans	—
Taenia saginata	Beef tapeworm	Cattle	Humans
Diphyllobothrium latum	Fish tapeworm	Freshwater crustaceans and fish	Humans, dogs, cats, bears
Echinococcus granulosus	Unilocular hydatid cyst	Herbivores, humans	Canines
Echinococcus multilocularis	Alveolar hydatid cyst	Herbivores, humans	Foxes, wolves, dogs, cats
Hymenolepis nana	Dwarf tapeworm	Rodents, humans	Rodents, humans
Hymenolepis diminuta	Dwarf tapeworm	Insects	Rodents, humans
Dipylidium caninum	Pumpkinseed tapeworm	Fleas	Dogs, cats

be either cooked until the interior of the meat is gray or frozen at −20°C for at least 12 hours. Sanitation is critical; every effort must be made to keep human feces containing *T. solium* eggs out of water and vegetation ingested by pigs.

Cysticercosis

Physiology and Structure of the Causative Organism

Cysticercosis is human infection with the larval stage of *T. solium*, the cysticerci, which normally infect pigs (Fig. 79–3). Human ingestion of water or vegetation contaminated with *T. solium* eggs from human feces initiates the infection. Autoinfection may occur when eggs from a person infected with the adult worm are transferred from the perianal area to the mouth on contaminated fingers. Once ingested, the eggs hatch in the stomach of the intermediate host, releasing the hexacanth embryo or oncosphere. The oncosphere penetrates the intestinal wall and migrates in the circulation to the tissues, where it develops into a cysticercus over 3 to 4 months. The cysticerci may develop in muscle, connective tissue, brain, lungs, and eyes and remain viable for as long as 5 years.

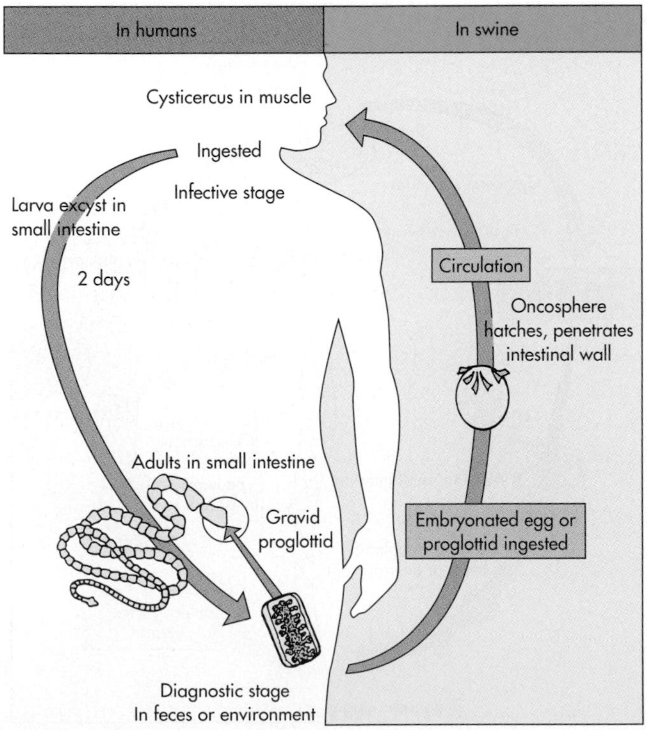

Epidemiology

Cysticercosis is found in the areas where *T. solium* is prevalent and is directly correlated with human fecal contamination. In addition to fecal-oral transmission,

FIGURE 79–1. Life cycle of *Taenia solium* (pork tapeworm).

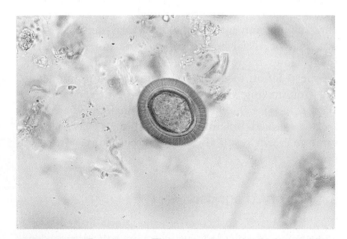

FIGURE 79–2. *Taenia* egg. The eggs are spherical, are 30 to 40 μm in diameter, and contain three pairs of hooklets internally. The eggs of the different *Taenia* species cannot be differentiated.

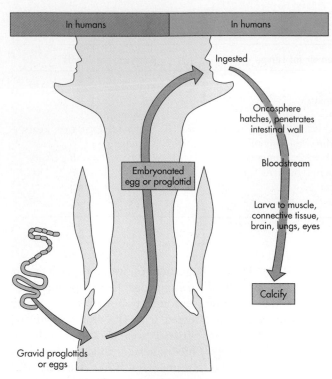

FIGURE 79–3. Development of human cysticercosis.

autoinfection may occur when a proglottid containing eggs is regurgitated from the small intestine into the stomach, allowing the eggs to hatch and release the infectious oncosphere.

Clinical Diseases

A few cysticerci in nonvital areas (e.g., subcutaneous tissues) may not provoke symptoms, but serious disease may follow as the cysticerci lodge in vital areas such as the brain and eyes. In the brain, they may produce hydrocephalus, meningitis, cranial nerve damage, seizures, hyperactive reflexes, and visual defects. In the eye, loss of visual acuity may occur, and if the larvae lodge along the optic tract, visual field defects result. Tissue reaction to viable larvae may be only moderate, thus minimizing symptoms. Death of the larvae, however, results in release of antigenic material that stimulates a marked inflammatory reaction; exacerbation of symptoms can result in fever, muscle pains, and eosinophilia.

Laboratory Diagnosis

The presence of cysticerci is usually established by the appearance of calcified cysticerci in soft tissue roentgenograms, surgical removal of subcutaneous nodules, and visualization of cysts in the eye. Central nervous system lesions may be detected by computed tomogra-

phy, radioisotope scanning, or ultrasonography. Serologic studies may be useful; false-positive results may occur in people with other helminthic infections.

Treatment, Prevention, and Control

The drug of choice for treating cysticercosis is praziquantel. Albendazole has also been used successfully in the treatment of parenchymal neurocysticercosis. Concomitant steroid administration may be necessary to minimize the inflammatory response to dying larvae. Surgical removal of cerebral and ocular cysts may be necessary. Critical to the prevention and control of human infection are treatment of human cases harboring adult *T. solium* (to reduce egg transmission) and controlled disposal of human feces. These measures also reduce the likelihood of infection in pigs.

Taenia saginata

Physiology and Structure

The life cycle of *T. saginata*, the beef tapeworm, is similar to that of *T. solium* (Fig. 79–4), with infection resulting after cysticerci are ingested in insufficiently cooked beef. After excystment, the larvae develop into adults in the small intestine and initiate egg production in maturing proglottids. The adult worm may parasitize the jejunum and small intestine of humans for as

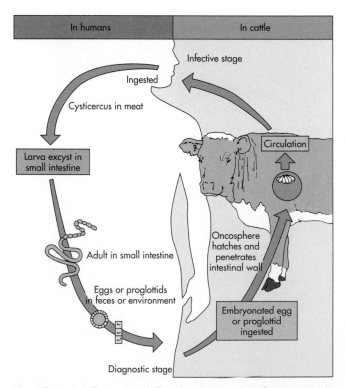

FIGURE 79–4. Life cycle of *Taenia saginata* (beef tapeworm).

long as 25 years, attaining a length of 10 m. In contrast to *T. solium* infections, cysticercosis produced by *T. saginata* does not occur in humans. The adult *T. saginata* worm also differs from *T. solium* because it lacks a crown of hooklets on the scolex and has a different proglottid uterine branch structure. These facts are important in differentiating between the two tapeworms but do not affect therapy.

Epidemiology

T. saginata occurs worldwide and is one of the most frequent causes of cestode infections in the United States. Humans and cattle perpetuate the life cycle: Human feces contaminate water and vegetation with eggs, which are then ingested by cattle. The cysticerci in cattle produce adult tapeworms in humans when rare or insufficiently cooked beef is eaten.

Clinical Diseases

The syndrome that results from *T. saginata* infection is similar to the intestinal infection with *T. solium*. Patients are generally asymptomatic or may complain of vague abdominal pains, chronic indigestion, and hunger pains. Proglottids may pass out of the anus directly.

Laboratory Diagnosis

The diagnosis of *T. saginata* infection is similar to that of *T. solium*, with recovery of proglottids and eggs or recovery of an entire worm whose scolex lacks hooklets. Study of the uterine branches in the proglottids differentiates *T. saginata* from *T. solium*.

Treatment, Prevention, and Control

Treatment is identical to that for the intestinal phase of *T. solium*. A single dose of niclosamide is highly effective in eliminating the adult worm. Education about cooking beef and controlling disposal of human feces is a critical measure.

Diphyllobothrium latum

Physiology and Structure

One of the largest tapeworms (20 to 30 feet long), *D. latum* (fish tapeworm) has a complex life cycle involving two intermediate hosts: freshwater crustaceans and freshwater fish (Fig. 79–5). The ribbon-like larval worm in the flesh of freshwater fish is called a sparganum. Ingestion of this sparganum in raw or insufficiently cooked fish initiates infection. The scolex of *D. latum* is shaped like a lance and has long, lateral

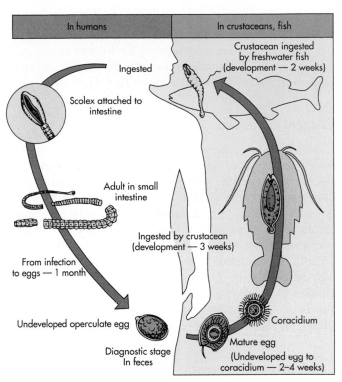

FIGURE 79–5. Life cycle of *Diphyllobothrium latum* (fish tapeworm).

grooves (bothria), which serve as organs of attachment. The proglottids of *D. latum* are broad, have a central uterine structure resembling a rosette, and produce eggs with an operculum, like fluke eggs, and a knob on the shell at the bottom of the egg. The adult worms may produce eggs for months or years. More than 1 million eggs per day are released into the fecal stream. On reaching fresh water, the unembryonated, operculate eggs require a period of 2 to 4 weeks to develop a ciliated, free-swimming larval form called a coracidium. The fully developed coracidium leaves the egg via the operculum and is ingested by tiny crustaceans called copepods (e.g., *Cyclops* and *Diaptomus* species); the coracidium then develops into a procercoid larval form. The crustacean harboring the larval stage is then eaten by a fish, and the infectious plerocercoid or sparganum larvae develop in the musculature of the fish. If the fish is in turn eaten by another fish, the sparganum simply migrates into the muscles of the second fish. Humans are infected when they eat raw or undercooked fish containing the larval forms.

Epidemiology

D. latum infection occurs worldwide, most prevalently in cool lake regions where raw or pickled fish is popular. Insufficient cooking over campfires and tasting and seasoning gefilte fish account for many infections. A reservoir of infected wild animals, such as bears, minks, walruses, and members of the canine and feline families that eat fish, are also sources for human infections. The practice of dumping raw sewage into freshwater lakes contributes to propagation of this tapeworm.

Clinical Diseases

Clinically, as is the case with most adult tapeworm infections, most *D. latum* infections are asymptomatic. People occasionally complain of epigastric pain, abdominal cramping, nausea, vomiting, and weight loss. As many as 40% of *D. latum* carriers may have low serum levels of vitamin B_{12}, presumably because of the competition between the host and the worm for dietary vitamin B_{12}. A small percentage (0.1% to 2%) of people infected with *D. latum* develop clinical signs of vitamin B_{12} deficiency, including megaloblastic anemia and neurologic manifestations such as numbness, paresthesia, and loss of vibration sense.

Laboratory Diagnosis

Stool examination reveals the bile-stained, operculated egg with its knob at the bottom of the shell (Fig. 79–6). Typical proglottids with the rosette uterine structure may also be found in stool specimens. Con-

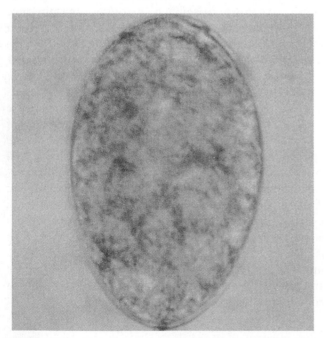

FIGURE 79–6. *Diphyllobothrium latum* egg. Unlike other tapeworm eggs, *D. latum* eggs are operculated. They are 45 × 70 μm in size. (From Lennette EH, Balows A, Hausler WJ, Shadomy HJ: *Manual of clinical microbiology*, ed 4, Washington, DC, 1985, American Society for Microbiology.)

centration techniques are usually not necessary because the worms produce large numbers of ova.

Treatment, Prevention, and Control

The drug of choice is niclosamide; praziquantel and paromomycin are acceptable alternatives. Vitamin B_{12} supplementation may be necessary in people with evidence of clinical vitamin B_{12} deficiency. The prevalence of this infection is reduced by avoiding ingestion of insufficiently cooked fish; controlling the disposal of human feces, especially by proper treatment of sewage before disposal in lakes; and promptly treating infections.

Sparganosis

Physiology and Structure of the Causative Organisms

The larval forms of several tapeworms closely related to *D. latum* (most often *Spirometra* species) can produce human disease in subcutaneous sites and in the eyes. In these cases, humans act as the end-stage host for the larval stage, or sparganum. Infections are acquired primarily by drinking pond or ditch water that contains crustaceans (copepods) that carry a larval tapeworm. This larval form penetrates the intestinal wall and migrates to various sites in the body, where it develops into a sparganum. Infections may also occur if tadpoles, frogs, and snakes are ingested raw or if the flesh of these animals is applied to wounds as a poultice. The larval worm leaves the relatively cold flesh of the dead animal and migrates into the warm human flesh.

Epidemiology

Cases have been reported from various parts of the world, including the United States, but the infection is most prevalent in Asia. Regardless of location, drinking contaminated water and eating raw tadpole, frog, and snake flesh lead to infection.

Clinical Diseases

In subcutaneous sites, sparganosis can produce painful inflammatory tissue reactions and nodules. In the eye, the tissue reaction is intensely painful, and periorbital edema is common. Corneal ulcers may develop with ocular involvement. Ocular disease is frequently associated with the use of frog or snake flesh as a poultice over a wound near the eye.

Laboratory Diagnosis

Sections of tissue removed surgically show characteristic tapeworm features, including highly convoluted parenchyma and dark-staining calcareous corpuscles.

Treatment, Prevention, and Control

Surgical removal is the customary approach. The drug praziquantel may be used; however, no clinical data support its efficacy. Education about possible contamination of drinking water with crustaceans that harbor larval worms is essential, and contamination most likely occurs in pond and ditch water. Ingestion of raw frog and snake flesh or their use as poultices over wounds also should be avoided.

Echinococcus granulosus

Physiology and Structure

Infection with *E. granulosus* is another example of accidental human infection, with humans serving as dead-end intermediate hosts in a life cycle that occurs naturally in other animals. *E. granulosus* adult tapeworms are found in nature in the intestines of canines (dog, fox, wolf, coyote, jackal, dingo); the larval cyst stage is present in the viscera of herbivores (sheep, cattle, swine, deer, moose, elk) (Fig. 79–7). The worm consists of a *Taenia*-like scolex with four sucking disks and a double row of hooklets as well as strobila containing three proglottids: one immature, one mature, and one gravid. Adult tapeworms in the canine intestine produce infective eggs that pass in feces. The eggs are identical in appearance to those of the *Taenia* species. When these eggs are ingested by humans, a six-hooked larval stage called an oncosphere hatches. The oncosphere penetrates the human intestinal wall and enters the circulation to be carried to various tissue sites, primarily the liver and lungs but also the central nervous system and bone. This same cycle occurs in the viscera of herbivores. When the herbivore is killed by a canine predator or viscera is fed to canines, the ingestion of cysts produces adult tapeworms in the canine intestine to complete the cycle and initiate new egg production. Adult tapeworms do not develop in the intestines of herbivores or humans.

In humans, the larvae form a unilocular hydatid cyst, which is a slow-growing, tumor-like, space-occupying structure enclosed by a laminated germinative membrane. This membrane produces structures on its wall called brood capsules, where tapeworm heads (protoscolices) develop. Daughter cysts may develop in the original mother cyst and produce brood capsules and protoscolices. The cysts and daughter cysts accumulate fluid as they grow. This fluid is potentially

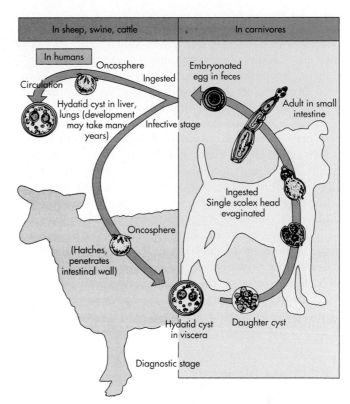

FIGURE 79–7. Life cycle of *Echinococcus granulosus*.

toxic; if it is spilled into body cavities, anaphylactic shock and death can result. Spillage and the escape of protoscolices can lead to the development of cysts in other sites because the protoscolices have the germinative potential to form new cysts. The brood capsules and daughter cysts eventually disintegrate within the mother cyst, liberating the accumulated protoscolices. These become known as hydatid sand. This type of *Echinococcus* cyst is called a unilocular cyst to differentiate it from related cysts that grow differently. The unilocular cyst is generally about 5 cm in diameter, but some as large as 20 cm, containing almost 2 L of cyst fluid, have been reported. The cyst may die and become calcified over long periods.

Epidemiology

Human infection with *E. granulosus* unilocular cyst is directly correlated with raising sheep in many countries in Europe, South America, Africa, Asia, Australia, and New Zealand. It occurs in Canada and in the United States, with cases reported from Alaska, Utah, New Mexico, Arizona, California, and the lower Mississippi Valley. Human infection follows ingestion of contaminated water or vegetation as well as hand-to-mouth transmission of canine feces carrying the infective eggs.

Clinical Diseases

Because the unilocular cyst grows slowly, 5 to 20 years may pass before any symptoms appear. In many instances, it appears that the cyst is as old as its host. The pressure of the expanding cyst in an organ is usually the first sign of infection. In most cases, the cysts are located in the liver or lung. In the liver, the cyst may exert pressure on both bile ducts and blood vessels and create pain and biliary rupture. In the lungs, cysts may produce cough, dyspnea, and chest pains. Rupture of the cysts may occur in 20% of cases, producing fever, urticaria, and occasionally anaphylactic shock and death, which are caused by the release of antigenic cyst contents. Cyst rupture may also lead to dissemination of infection resulting from the release of thousands of protoscolices. In bone, the cyst is responsible for erosion of the marrow cavity and the bone itself. In the brain, severe damage may occur as a result of the cyst's tumor-like growth into brain tissue.

Laboratory Diagnosis

The diagnosis of hydatid disease is difficult and depends primarily on clinical, radiographic, and serologic findings. Radiologic examination, scanning procedures, tomography, and ultrasonographic techniques all are valuable and may provide the first evidence of the cyst's presence. Aspiration of cyst contents may demonstrate the presence of the protoscolices (hydatid sand); however, it is contraindicated because of the risk of anaphylaxis and dissemination of the infection. Serologic testing may be useful, but results are negative in 10% to 40% of infections.

Treatment, Prevention, and Control

Surgical resection of the cyst is the treatment of choice. In some instances, the cyst is first aspirated to remove the fluid and hydatid sand, and then it is instilled with formalin to kill and detoxify remaining fluid; finally, it is rolled into a marsupial pouch and sewn shut. If the condition is inoperable because of the cyst's location, medical therapy with high-dose albendazole, mebendazole, or praziquantel may be considered. The most important factor in preventing and controlling echinococcosis is education about the transmission of infection and the role of canines in the life cycle. Proper personal hygiene and the washing of hands and cooking utensils in environments inhabited by dogs are critical. Dogs should not be allowed in the vicinity of animal slaughter and should never be fed the viscera of slain animals. In some areas, killing stray dogs has reduced the incidence of infection.

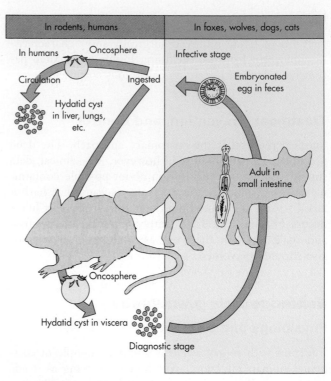

FIGURE 79–8. Life cycle of *Echinococcus multilocularis*.

Echinococcus multilocularis

Physiology and Structure

Like infection with *E. granulosus*, human infection with *E. multilocularis* is accidental (Fig. 79–8). Adult *E. multilocularis* tapeworms are primarily found in foxes and wolves, although farm dogs and cats harbor them in some rural environments. The intermediate hosts that harbor the cyst stage are rodents (mice, voles, shrews, and lemmings). Humans become infected with the cyst stage as a result of contact with fox, dog, or cat feces contaminated with eggs. Trappers and workers who handle fur pelts may become infected by inhaling fecal dust that carries eggs.

Infective eggs hatch in and penetrate the intestinal tract to become oncospheres. These forms enter the circulation and take up residence primarily in the liver and lungs but also possibly in the brain.

The alveolar hydatid cyst develops as an alveolar or honeycombed structure that is not covered by a unilocular-limiting mother cyst–laminated membrane. The cyst grows via exogenous budding, eventually resembling a carcinoma. In humans, individual cysts are said to be sterile and rarely produce protoscolices (hydatid sand).

Epidemiology

E. multilocularis is found primarily in northern areas such as Canada, the former Soviet Union, northern

Japan, Central Europe, and Alaska, Montana, North and South Dakota, Minnesota, and Iowa in the United States. There is evidence that the life cycle may be extending to other Midwestern states, where foxes and mice transmit the organism to dogs and cats and eventually to humans.

Clinical Diseases

E. multilocularis, because of its slow growth, may be present in human tissues for many years before symptoms appear. In the liver, cysts eventually mimic a carcinoma, with liver enlargement and obstruction of biliary and portal pathways. The growth often metastasizes to the lungs and brain. Malnutrition, ascites, and portal hypertension produced by *E. multilocularis* create the appearance of hepatic cirrhosis. Among all of the worm infections of humans, *E. multilocularis* is one of the most lethal. If infection is left untreated, the mortality rate is approximately 70% of infected people.

Laboratory Diagnosis

Unlike *E. granulosus*, the tissue form of *E. multilocularis* presents no protoscolices, and the material so resembles a neoplasm that even pathologists mistake it for carcinoma. Radiologic procedures and scanning techniques are helpful, and serologic methods are available.

Treatment, Prevention, and Control

Surgical removal of the cyst is indicated, especially if an entire hepatic area can be resected. The same surgical approach applies to lesions in the lung in which a lobe can be resected. Mebendazole and albendazole, as used for the treatment of *E. granulosus* infection, have produced clinical cures. As with *E. granulosus* infection, education, proper personal hygiene, and deworming of farm dogs and cats are critical. It is extremely important to treat animals that have contact with children.

Hymenolepis nana

Physiology and Structure

H. nana, the dwarf tapeworm, is only 2 to 4 cm in length, unlike *Taenia* organisms, which measure several meters. The life cycle is also simple and does not require an intermediate host (Fig. 79–9), although mice and beetles may be infected and enter the cycle.

Infection begins when the embryonated eggs are ingested and develop in the intestinal villi into a larval cysticercoid stage. This cysticercoid larva attaches its four muscular suckers and crown of hooklets to the small intestine, and the adult worm produces a strobila of egg-laden proglottids. Eggs passing in the feces are

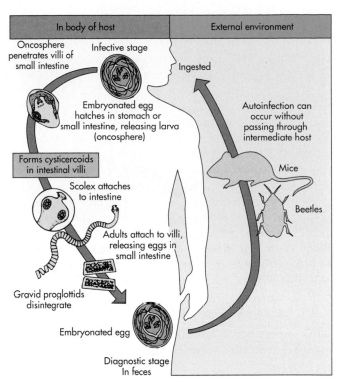

FIGURE 79–9. Life cycle of *Hymenolepis nana* (dwarf tapeworm).

then immediately and directly infective, initiating another cycle. Infection may also be acquired by ingesting infected insect intermediate hosts.

H. nana also can cause autoinfection, with a subsequent increased worm burden. Eggs are able to hatch in the intestine, develop into cysticercoid larvae, and then grow into adult worms without leaving the host. This can lead to hyperinfection with very heavy worm burdens and severe clinical symptoms.

Epidemiology

H. nana occurs worldwide in humans and is also a common parasite of mice. The most common tapeworm infection in North America, it occasionally develops its cysticercoid stage in beetles; humans and mice may ingest these beetles in contaminated grain and flour. Children are especially at risk of infection, and because of the simple life cycle of the parasite, families with children in daycare centers experience problems in controlling transmission of this organism.

Clinical Diseases

With only a few worms in the intestine, affected persons experience no symptoms. In heavy infections, especially if autoinfection and hyperinfection occur, pa-

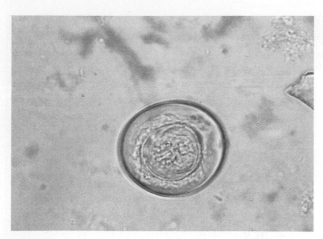

FIGURE 79–10. *Hymenolepis nana* egg. The eggs are 30 to 45 μm in diameter and have a thin shell containing a six-hooked embryo.

tients experience diarrhea, abdominal pain, headache, anorexia, and other vague complaints.

Laboratory Diagnosis

Stool examination reveals the characteristic *H. nana* egg with its six-hooked embryo and polar filaments (Fig. 79–10).

Treatment, Prevention, and Control

The drug of choice is praziquantel; an alternative is niclosamide. Treatment of cases, improved sanitation, and proper personal hygiene, especially in the family and institutional environments, are essential for controlling the transmission of *H. nana*.

Hymenolepis diminuta
Physiology and Structure

H. diminuta, closely related to *H. nana*, is primarily a tapeworm of rats and mice, but it is also found in humans. It differs from *H. nana* in length, measuring 20 to 60 cm. The scolex lacks hooklets, and the egg is larger, is bile-stained, and has no polar filaments. The life cycle of *H. diminuta* is more complex than that of *H. nana*, and it requires larval insects ("mealworms") to reach the infective cysticercoid stage.

Epidemiology

Infections have been found all over the world, including in the United States. Larval beetles and other larval insects become infected when they feed on rat feces that carry *H. diminuta* eggs. Humans are infected by

ingesting the larval insects (mealworms) in contaminated grain products (e.g., flour, cereals).

Clinical Diseases

Mild infections produce no symptoms, but heavier worm burdens produce nausea, abdominal discomfort, anorexia, and diarrhea.

Laboratory Diagnosis

Stool examination demonstrates the characteristic bile-stained egg that lacks polar filaments.

Treatment, Prevention, and Control

The drug of choice is niclosamide, with praziquantel an alternative. Rodent control in areas where grain products are produced or stored is essential. Thorough inspection of uncooked grain products to detect mealworms is also important.

Dipylidium caninum
Physiology and Structure

D. caninum, a small tapeworm averaging about 15 cm in length, is primarily a parasite of dogs and cats, but it can infect humans, especially children whose mouths are licked by infected pets. The life cycle involves the development of larval worms in dog and cat fleas. These fleas, when crushed by the teeth of the infected pet, are carried on the tongue to the child's mouth when the child kisses the pet or the pet licks the child. Swallowing the infected flea leads to intestinal infection.

Because of the size and shape of the mature and terminal proglottids, *D. caninum* is often called the pumpkinseed tapeworm. The eggs are distinctive because they occur in packets covered with a tough, clear membrane. A packet may contain as many as 25 eggs, and a single egg free of the packet is seldom seen.

Epidemiology

D. caninum occurs worldwide, especially in children. Its distribution and transmission are directly correlated with dogs and cats infected with fleas.

Clinical Diseases

Light infections are asymptomatic; heavier worm burdens produce abdominal discomfort, anal pruritus, and diarrhea. Anal pruritus results from active migration of the motile proglottid.

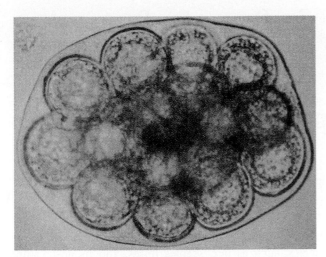

FIGURE 79–11. *Dipylidium caninum* eggs. Free eggs are rarely seen. Instead, egg packets that contain 8 to 15 six-hooked oncospheres enclosed in a thin membrane are most commonly found in fecal specimens. (From Lennette EH, Balows A, Hausler WJ, Shadomy HJ: *Manual of clinical microbiology*, ed 4, Washington, DC, 1985, American Society for Microbiology.)

Laboratory Diagnosis

Stool examination reveals the colorless egg packets (Fig. 79–11), and proglottids may be in feces brought to physicians by patients.

Treatment, Prevention, and Control

The drug of choice is niclosamide; praziquantel and paromomycin are alternatives. Dogs and cats should be dewormed and should not be allowed to lick the mouths of children. Pets should be treated to eradicate fleas.

CASE STUDY AND QUESTIONS

■ A 30-year-old Hispanic man entered the emergency department after a focal neurologic seizure. The patient had recently emigrated from Mexico and was in his usual state of good health before the seizure. Neu-rologic examination revealed no focal findings. A computed tomographic scan of his head revealed numerous small cystic lesions in both cerebral hemispheres. Punctate calcification was noted in several of the lesions. A lumbar puncture revealed a glucose level of 65 mg/dL (normal) and a protein level of 38 mg/dL (normal) in cerebrospinal fluid. The white blood cell count was 20/mm^3 (abnormal), with a differential of 5% neutrophils, 90% lymphocytes, and 5% monocytes. A purified protein derivative skin test was negative with positive controls. The result of a serologic test for human immunodeficiency virus was negative.

1. What was the differential diagnosis of this patient's neurologic process?

2. Which parasite or parasites may have caused this condition?

3. What diagnostic tests were available for this infection?

4. What were the therapeutic options for this patient?

5. How do people become infected with this parasite?

6. What tissue sites (besides the central nervous system) may be involved? How would these additional foci of infection be documented?

BIBLIOGRAPHY

Ash LR, Orihel TC: Intestinal helminths. In Murray PR et al, editors: *Manual of clinical microbiology*, ed 7, Washington, DC, 1999, American Society for Microbiology.

Botero D et al: Taeniasis and cysticercosis, *Infect Dis Clin North Am* 7:683–697, 1993.

Garcia LS, editor: *Diagnostic medical parasitology*, ed 4, Washington, DC, 2001, American Society for Microbiology.

Gottstein B: Molecular and immunologic diagnosis of echinococcosis, *Clin Microbiol Rev* 5:248–261, 1992.

Kammerer WS, Schantz PM: Echinococcal disease, *Infect Dis Clin North Am* 7:605–618, 1993.

Liu LX, Weller PF: Drug therapy: antiparasitic drugs, *N Engl J Med* 334:1178–1184, 1996.

Markell EK, John DT, Krotoski WA, editors: *Markell and Voges medical parasitology*, ed 8, Philadelphia, 1999, WB Saunders.

Strickland GT, editor: *Hunters tropical medicine and emerging infectious diseases*, Philadelphia, 2000, WB Saunders.

CHAPTER 80

Arthropods

The Arthropoda is the largest of the animal phyla, with more than 1 million species. The phylum Arthropoda comprises invertebrate animals with a segmented body, several pairs of jointed appendages, bilateral symmetry, and a rigid, chitinous exoskeleton that is molted periodically as the animal grows. Arthropods characteristically develop from egg to adult by a process known as metamorphosis. As they mature, the organisms pass through several distinct morphologic stages including egg, larvae or nymph, pupa (certain insects), and adult. Five classes of arthropods are of medical importance on the basis of the number or the severity of the illnesses they cause: the Chilopoda, Pentastomida, Crustacea, Arachnida, and Insecta (Table 80–1).

The arthropods or their larvae may affect human health in many ways. Most arthropods function indirectly in human disease; they transmit disease but do not produce it. Arthropods may transmit disease mechanically, as when flies carry enteric bacterial pathogens from feces to human food. Of outstanding importance is the ability of many arthropods to act as biologic vectors and intermediate hosts in the transmission and developmental cycle of viruses, bacteria, protozoa, and metazoa (Table 80–2). Certain arthropods

may inflict direct injury by their bites or stings. Other species, such as lice, scabies mites, and tissue-invading maggots, may act as true parasites. Still other species may function as both parasites and vectors of disease.

It is not the purpose of this chapter to consider medical entomology in detail. Rather, the purpose is to provide a brief overview of several of the more important aspects of arthropods and their relationship to human disease. More detailed information on arthropods of medical importance and the therapy and control of arthropod infestations may be found in the references listed in the bibliography.

Chilopoda
Centipedes

Physiology and Structure. The centipedes are elongated, multisegmented (15 to more than 181 segments), many-legged, tracheate arthropods. They possess a distinct head and trunk. The body is dorsoventrally flattened, and each trunk segment bears a single pair of legs. Maxillipeds or poison claws are situated on the first segment and are used for capturing prey. The centipedes are sometimes classified with the millipedes; however, millipedes lack the poison claws of centipedes and have two pairs of legs per segment.

Epidemiology. Most centipedes are predacious insectivores and are commonly found in dark, damp environments such as the areas beneath logs, among rubbish, and inside old buildings. Humans are almost invariably bitten as a result of accidental exposure to the organism during outdoor activities.

Clinical Diseases. Centipede bites may be extremely painful and may cause swelling at the site of the bite. Reports of the effects of centipede bites on humans are conflicting. One species, *Scolopendra gigantea*, which is found in Central and South America and the Galapagos Islands, reportedly has caused several deaths. With

TABLE 80–1. Medically Important Classes of Arthropods

Phylum	Class	Organisms
Arthrodpoda	Chilopoda	Centipedes
	Pentastomida	Tongue worms
	Crustacea	Copepods
		Decapods (crabs, crayfish)
	Arachnida	Spiders, scorpions, mites, ticks
	Insecta	Flies, mosquitoes, lice, fleas, bugs, stinging insects

TABLE 80–2. Select Human Illnesses Transmitted by Arthropods

Primary Vector or Intermediate Host	Disease	Etiologic Agent
Arachnida		
Mite: *Leptotrombidium*	Scrub typhus (tsutsugamushi disease)	*Rickettsia tsutsugamushi*
Mite: *Liponyssoides sanguineus*	Rickettsial pox	*Rickettsia akari*
Tick: *Dermacentor*	Tularemia	*Francisella tularensis*
Tick: *Dermacentor* and other ixodid ticks	Rocky Mountain spotted fever	*Rickettsia rickettsii*
Tick: *Dermacentor, Boophilus*	Q fever	*Coxiella burnetii*
Tick: *Dermacentor*	Colorado tick fever	Orbivirus
Tick: *Ornithodoros*	Relapsing fever	*Borrelia*
Tick: *Ixodes*	Babesiosis	*Babesia microti*
Tick: *Ixodes*	Lyme disease	*Borrelia burgdorferi*
Tick: *Dermacentor variabilis, Amblyomma americanum*	Ehrlichiosis	*Ehrlichia risticii*
Crustacea		
Copepod: *Cyclops*	Diphyllobothriasis	*Diphyllobothrium latum*
Copepod: *Cyclops*	Dracunculiasis	*Dracunculus medinensis*
Crabs, crayfish: various freshwater species	Paragonimiasis	*Paragonimus westermani*
Insecta		
Lice: *Pediculus humanus*	Epidemic typhus	*Rickettsia prowazekii*
Lice: *P. humanus*	Trench fever	*Bartonella quintana*
Lice: *P. humanus*	Louse-borne relapsing fever	*Borrelia recurrentis*
Flea: *Xenopsylla cheopis,* various other rodent fleas	Plague	*Yersinia pestis*
Flea: *X. cheopis*	Murine typhus	*Rickettsia typhi*
Flea: various species	Dipylidiasis	*Dipylidium caninum*
Bug: *Triatoma, Panstrongylus*	Chagas' disease	*Trypanosoma cruzi*
Beetles: flour beetle	Hymenolepiasis	*Hymenolepis nana*
Fly, gnat: *Glossina* (tsetse flies)	African trypanosomiasis	*Trypanosoma brucei rhodesiense* and *T. b. gambiense*
Fly, gnat: *Simulium*	Onchocerciasis	*Onchocerca volvulus*
Fly, gnat: *Chrysops*	Tularemia	*Francisella tularensis*
Fly, gnat: *Phlebotomus, Lutzomyia* (sandfly)	Leishmaniasis	*Leishmania* species
Fly, gnat: *Phlebotomus*	Bartonellosis	*Bartonella bacilliformis*
Mosquito: *Anopheles*	Malaria	*Plasmodium*
Mosquito: *Aedes aegypti*	Yellow fever	Flavivirus
Mosquito: *Aedes*	Dengue fever	Flavivirus
Mosquito: *Culiseta melanura, Coquillettidia perturbans, Aedes vexans*	Eastern equine encephalitis	Alphavirus
Mosquito: *Aedes triseriatus*	La Crosse encephalitis	Bunyavirus
Mosquito: *Culex*	St. Louis encephalitis	Flavivirus
Mosquito: *Culex*	Venezuelan equine encephalitis	Alphavirus
Mosquito: *Culex tarsalis*	Western equine encephalitis	Alphavirus
Mosquito: various species	Bancroftian filariasis	*Wuchereria bancrofti*
Mosquito: various species	Malayan filariasis	*Brugia*
Mosquito: various species	Dirofilariasis	*Dirofilaria immitis*

the exception of *Scolopendra* and related tropical genera, the bite of most centipedes is harmless to humans.

Treatment, Prevention, and Control. Treatment of a centipede bite includes local measures such application of compresses of sodium bicarbonate or solutions of Epsom salts. Control consists of removing rubbish near dwellings.

Pentastomida

Tongue Worms

The pentastomids, or tongue worms, are bloodsucking endoparasites of reptiles, birds, and mammals. Their taxonomic status is uncertain. Some scientists include pentastomids among the arthropods because their larvae superficially resemble those of mites. Others consider them annelids, and still others place them in an entirely separate phylum. For purposes of this discussion, they are considered with the arthropods.

Physiology and Structure. Tongue worms are degenerate, wormlike arthropods that live primarily in the nasal and respiratory passages of reptiles, birds, and mammals. Adult pentastomids are white, cylindrical, or flattened parasites that possess two distinct body regions: an anterior head, or cephalothorax, and an abdomen. The adults are elongated and may attain a length of 1 to 10 cm. The head has a mouth and two pairs of hooks. Although the abdomen may appear annulated, it is not segmented (Fig. 80–1). The pentastomids possess digestive and reproductive organs; however, they lack circulatory and respiratory systems.

The adult pentastomids are found in the lungs of reptiles and the nasal passages of mammals. Many vertebrates, including humans, may serve as intermediate hosts. The embryonated eggs are discharged in the feces or respiratory secretions of the infected definitive host and contaminate vegetation or water, which is in turn ingested by one of several possible intermediate hosts (fish, rodents, goats, sheep, or humans). The eggs hatch in the intestine, and the primary larvae penetrate the intestinal wall and attach to the peritoneum. The larvae mature in the peritoneum and develop into infective larvae, encyst in viscera, or die and become calcified. In tissue sections, encysted larvae can be identified by acidophilic glands, a chitinous cuticle, and

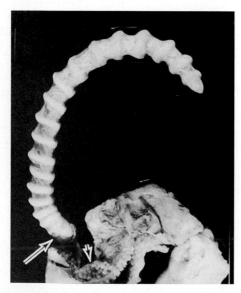

FIGURE 80–1. Adult female pentastome *(Armillifer armillatus)* attached to the respiratory surface of the lung *(short arrow)* of a rock python. Note the short cephalothorax *(long arrow)* and a long, annulated abdomen. (From Binford CH, Connor DH: *Pathology of tropical and extraordinary diseases,* vol 2, Washington, DC, 1976, Armed Forces Institute of Pathology.)

prominent hooks, which are present in the anterior end of the organism. Subcuticular glands and striated muscle fibers may also be observed beneath the cuticle.

Humans may also become infected by ingesting the inadequately cooked flesh of infected reptiles or other definitive hosts or by eating the infected flesh of intermediate hosts (e.g., goats, sheep) containing infective larvae. In the latter instance, the infective larvae migrate from the stomach to the nasopharyngeal tissues, where they develop into adult pentastomids and produce the symptoms of the halzoun syndrome (see the later section on clinical syndromes). In this case, the human host is considered a temporary definitive host.

Epidemiology. Most tongue worm infections are reported in Europe, Africa, and South and Central America. The infection is common in Malaysia, where autopsy studies reveal pentastomiasis in up to 45% of people. As previously described, the infection is acquired by ingesting raw vegetables or water contaminated with pentastome eggs or by consuming raw or undercooked flesh of infected animals.

Clinical Diseases. In most cases, infection is asymptomatic and is discovered accidentally during roentgenographic examination (calcified larvae), at surgery, or at autopsy. Pneumonitis, pneumothorax, peritonitis, meningitis, nephritis, and obstructive jaundice all have been ascribed to pentastomid infections; however, definitive proof of a causal relationship between disease and the presence of the parasite is frequently lacking. Localized infection of the eye has been reported, presumably secondary to direct inoculation.

Halzoun syndrome, caused by the attachment of adult pentastomes to the nasopharyngeal tissues, is characterized by pharyngeal discomfort, paroxysmal coughing, sneezing, dysphagia, and vomiting. Asphyxiation has been rarely reported.

Laboratory Diagnosis. The diagnosis is made by identifying a pentastomid in a biopsy specimen obtained at surgery or at autopsy. Calcified larvae may occasionally be observed on radiographs of the abdomen or chest, providing a presumptive diagnosis. No serologic tests are useful.

Treatment, Prevention, and Control. Treatment is not usually warranted. In symptomatic patients, surgical removal of free or encysted parasites should be attempted. Preventive measures include thorough cooking of meat and vegetables and avoidance of contaminated water.

Crustacea

The crustaceans are primarily gill-breathing arthropods of fresh and salt water. Those of medical importance are found in fresh water and serve as intermediate hosts of various worms (see Table 80–2).

The copepods, or water fleas, are represented by the genera *Cyclops* and *Diaptomus*. The larger crustaceans, called decapods, include crabs and crayfish. These crustaceans also serve as the second intermediate hosts of the lung fluke *Paragonimus westermani* (see Table 80–2).

Copepods

Physiology and Structure. Copepods are small, simple aquatic organisms. They lack a carapace, have one pair of maxillae, and have five pairs of biramous swimming legs. Free and parasitic forms exist. The genera *Diaptomus* and *Cyclops* are medically important.

Copepods are an intermediate host in the life cycle of several human parasites, including *Dracunculus medinensis* (dracunculiasis), *Diphyllobothrium latum* (diphyllobothriasis), *Gnathostoma spinigerum* (gnathostomiasis), and *Spirometra* species (sparganosis). Copepods have been associated with a single case of a perirectal abscess but generally are not considered a primary cause of human infection.

Epidemiology. Copepods have a worldwide distribution and serve as intermediate hosts for helminthic diseases in the United States and Canada as well as in Europe and the tropics. Human infection with these helminthic parasites results from ingesting water contaminated with copepods or from eating the raw or insufficiently cooked flesh of infected fish. Pseudo-outbreaks of copepods in human stool specimens submitted for ova and parasite examination have been reported from New York. As many as 40% of concentrated stool samples submitted for ova and parasite examination were found to contain copepods, presumably as a result of contamination of a hospital water supply. The single reported case of apparent human infection with copepods occurred in this hospital.

Clinical Diseases. The clinical signs and symptoms associated with helminthic infections in which copepods serve as intermediate hosts are described in Chapters 77, 78, and 79. The single case of apparent human infection with copepods occurred in a 22-year-old man with Crohn's disease and a perirectal abscess. Drainage of the abscess revealed purulent material that on microscopic examination contained numerous copepods surrounded by leukocytes. It was hypothesized that the copepods were introduced into preexisting perirectal lesions during sitz baths, which were prepared with unfiltered tap water and may have contained copepods. Although the copepods contained within the abscess material were viable and may have been successfully feeding on body tissue, it was believed that the copepods were unlikely to have been the primary cause of the abscess.

Laboratory Diagnosis. The laboratory diagnosis of helminthic infections in which copepods serve as intermediate hosts are described in Chapters 77, 78, and 79. In general, infection is demonstrated by microscopic examination of clinical material.

Treatment, Prevention, and Control. Specific treatment of copepod-associated helminthic infection is described in Chapters 77, 78, and 79. Prevention of these infections requires attention to standard public health measures such as chlorination and filtration of water and thorough cooking of all fish. Infected people must not be allowed to bathe in water used for drinking, and suspected water should be avoided.

Decapods

The decapods include the prawns, shrimps, lobsters, crayfish, and crabs. The cephalothorax of these animals is always covered by a carapace. They have three anterior pairs of thoracic appendages that are modified into biramous maxillipeds and five posterior pairs that are developed into uniramous legs. Crabs and crayfish are medically important as the second intermediate hosts of the lung fluke *P. westermani*. The parasitic, epidemiologic, and clinical aspects of infection with *P. westermani* are described in Chapter 78. Thorough cooking of crabs and crayfish is the most effective means of preventing infection with *P. westermani*.

Arachnida

Spiders

Spiders have a number of characteristic features that permit easy identification. Specifically, they possess eight legs, no antennae, a body divided into two regions (cephalothorax and abdomen), and an unsegmented abdomen with spinnerets posteriorly. All true spiders produce venom and kill their prey by biting; however, few have fangs (chelicerae) powerful enough to pierce human skin or venom potent enough to produce more than a transitory local skin irritation. Venomous spiders may be classified as those that cause systemic arachnidism and those that cause necrotic arachnidism. This classification is based on the type of tissue damage produced.

Systemic arachnidism is primarily caused by tarantulas and black widow spiders. Tarantulas (family Theraphosidae) are large, hairy spiders of the tropics and subtropics. The tarantulas are of little importance because they are not very aggressive and avoid human habitations. Their bite causes intense pain and a phase of agitation, followed by stupor and somnolence. The black widow spider, *Latrodectus mactans*, is widespread through the southern and western United States. Related species of *Latrodectus* are found throughout temperate and tropical regions of all continents, but none is primarily domestic; thus, their contact with humans is limited.

Necrotic arachnidism is produced by spiders that belong to the genus *Loxosceles*. The bites of these spiders may produce severe tissue reaction. *Loxosceles reclusa*, the brown recluse spider, is a medically important spider of this genus.

Black Widow Spiders

Physiology and Structure. The female black widow spider *(L. mactans)* is easily recognized by the presence of a globose, shiny, black abdomen bearing the characteristic orange or reddish hourglass marking on the ventral surface (Fig. 80–2). Females vary from 5 to 13.5 mm in body length, but the males are much smaller.

The venom of the black widow spider is a potent peripheral neurotoxin, which is delivered by a pair of jawlike structures, or chelicerae. Only the female *Latrodectus* spider is dangerous to humans; the small, feeble male delivers an ineffective bite.

Epidemiology. These spiders frequent woodpiles and brushpiles, old wooden buildings, cellars, hollow logs, and privies. Given these locations, the bite is often located on the genitalia, buttocks, or extremities. Black widow spiders are common in the southern United States but are found throughout the temperate and tropical regions of both the New and Old World.

Clinical Diseases. As is true with most cases of envenomation, the clinical profile depends on factors such as the amount of the venom injected, the location of the bite, and the age, weight, and sensitivity of the patient. Shortly after the bite, the victim feels a sharp pain but shows little or no immediate swelling. This is followed

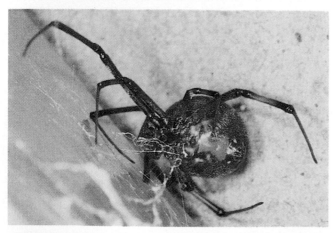

FIGURE 80–2. Female black widow spider *(Latrodectus mactans)*. (From Peters W: *A colour atlas of arthropods in clinical medicine*, London, 1992, Wolfe.)

by local redness, swelling, and burning. Systemic signs and symptoms generally occur within an hour of the bite and include muscle cramps, chest pains, nausea, vomiting, diaphoresis, intestinal spasms, and visual difficulties. Abdominal tetanic cramps producing a board-like abdomen are highly characteristic and may mimic an acute surgical abdomen. The acute symptoms usually subside within 48 hours; however, in severe cases, paralysis and coma may precede cardiac or respiratory failure. Mortality from the bite of the black widow spider is estimated at 4% to 5%.

Treatment, Prevention, and Control. Healthy adults usually recover, but small children or weakened people suffer considerably from these bites and may die without treatment. Muscle spasms may be severe and may require intravenous administration of calcium gluconate or other muscle relaxant agents. A specific antivenin is available and remains the treatment of choice. It is valuable if given shortly after the bite. Because it is prepared from the serum of hyperimmunized horses, patients must be tested for sensitivity to horse serum before administration. Hospitalization is advisable for the care of people with known or suspected black widow spider bites.

Good housekeeping can be the simplest and most effective control for spiders in homes. This includes dusting webs and carefully removing debris from around homes and adjacent sheds. Children should be discouraged from playing on woodpiles and in woodsheds.

Brown Recluse Spiders

Physiology and Structure. Spiders producing necrotic arachnidism belong to the genus *Loxosceles*. These spiders are yellow to brown and are of medium size (5 to 10 mm long) with relatively long legs (Fig. 80–3). They commonly display two distinguishing characteristics: a dark fiddle- or violin-shaped marking on the dorsal side of the cephalothorax and six eyes arranged in three pairs forming a semicircle. The venom injected by the female or male spider is a necrotoxin that may also have hemolytic properties and that causes necrotic lesions with deep tissue damage.

Epidemiology. Four species of the genus *Loxosceles* are found in the Americas. *L. reclusa* is found in the south and central United States, *Loxosceles arizonica* in the western states, and *Loxosceles laeta* in South America. *L. reclusa* is found outdoors in woodpiles and debris in warmer climates and in basements or storage areas in cooler regions. *L. laeta* is found in closets and corners of rooms. Humans are bitten only when the spider is threatened or disturbed.

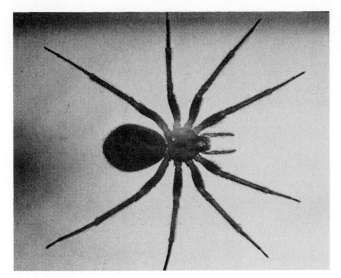

FIGURE 80–3. Female brown recluse spider *(Loxosceles laeta)*. (Courtesy Professor H Schenone; from Peters W: *A colour atlas of arthropods in clinical medicine*, London, 1992, Wolfe.)

Clinical Diseases. The bite of *Loxosceles* species initially tends to be painless; however, several hours later, itching, swelling, and soreness may develop in the area of the bite. A vesicle or bleb may frequently form at the site. General systemic symptoms are unusual but when present may include chills, headache, and nausea. Within 3 to 4 days, the bleb sloughs and may be followed by ulceration and radiating necrosis, which does not heal but continues to spread for weeks or months.

Intravascular coagulation and hemolysis may occur and be accompanied by hemoglobinuria and cardiac and renal failure. This hemolytic syndrome may be life-threatening and occurs more commonly after the bite of *L. laeta*. In South America, this syndrome is known as visceral loxoscelism.

Diagnosis. Identifying a species of spider on the basis of the appearance of the lesion alone is not possible; however, a working diagnosis is commonly based on the appearance of bleb formation around puncture marks and the nature of the developing lesion. The spider may be identified easily by the characteristic features previously described. An enzyme-linked immunosorbent assay has been developed to confirm the diagnosis of brown recluse spider bite but is not widely available.

Treatment, Prevention, and Control. The treatment of brown recluse spider bites is variable and based on the severity of the necrotic reaction. Most bites in the United States are inconsequential and require no specific therapy. Cleansing the bite wound and providing tetanus prophylaxis and antibiotics to prevent second-ary infection may be all that is indicated. Healing is generally uncomplicated, and débridement or excision should not be performed for 3 to 6 weeks to allow natural healing to commence. Excision and skin grafting may be necessary for bites that have not healed in 6 to 8 weeks. Systemic therapy with corticosteroids may be useful in treating the hemolytic syndrome but is of little proven value in preventing or treating cutaneous necrosis. Although not available in the United States, an antivenin is used in South America for the treatment of visceral loxoscelism.

Preventive measures are similar to those recommended for black widow spiders. *Loxosceles* (and other) spiders may be controlled in dwellings by applying insecticide compounds.

Scorpions

Physiology and Structure. The typical scorpion is elongated with conspicuous, pincer-like claws, or pedipalps, at the anterior end of the body; four pairs of walking legs; and a distinctly regimented abdomen that tapers to a curved, hollow, needle-like stinger (Fig. 80–4). When the scorpion is disturbed, it uses its stinger for defense. Both male and female scorpions can sting. Venom is injected through the stinger from two venom glands in the abdomen. Most scorpions are unable to penetrate human skin or inject enough venom to cause real damage; however, a few species are capable of inflicting painful wounds that may cause death.

Epidemiology. Scorpions considered dangerous may be found in the southwestern United States, Mexico, and Venezuela. This includes several species of the genus *Centruroides*, which accounts for as many as 1000 deaths annually. Also important are several species of *Tityus*, found in Trinidad, Argentina, Brazil, Guyana,

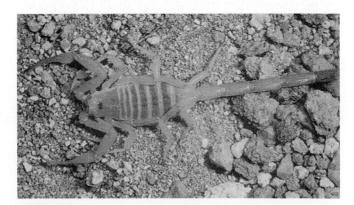

FIGURE 80–4. Scorpion (*Centruroides* species). (Courtesy Dr JC Cokendolpher; from Peters W: *A colour atlas of arthropods in clinical medicine*, London, 1992, Wolfe.)

and Venezuela. Children younger than 5 years are most likely to be fatally stung by scorpions.

Scorpions are nocturnal, and during the day, they remain concealed under logs and rocks and in other dark, moist places. They invade human habitations at night, where they may hide in shoes, towels, clothing, and closets.

Clinical Diseases. The effect of a scorpion sting on its victim is highly variable and depends on factors such as the species and age of the scorpion, the kind and amount of venom injected, and the age, size, and sensitivity of the person who was stung. Although the sting of many scorpions is relatively nontoxic and produces only local symptoms, other stings may be serious. Scorpions produce two types of venom: a neurotoxin and hemorrhagic or hemolytic toxin. The hemolytic toxin is responsible for local reactions at the site of the sting, including radiating, burning pain; swelling; discoloration; and necrosis. The neurotoxin produces minimal local reaction but rather severe systemic effects, including chills, diaphoresis, excessive salivation, difficulty speaking and swallowing, muscle spasm, tachycardia, and generalized seizures. In severe cases, death may result from pulmonary edema and respiratory paralysis.

Diagnosis. Local or systemic signs and symptoms coupled with physical evidence of a single point of skin penetration are usually sufficient to establish the diagnosis. The patient may have observed the scorpion or brought it in for identification. Although scorpions are relatively easy to identify, it is important to realize that other nonpoisonous arachnids strongly resemble scorpions. An entomologist or parasitologist should be consulted if there is a taxonomic question.

Treatment, Prevention, and Control. The management of scorpion stings varies. In the absence of systemic symptoms, palliative treatment may be all that is necessary. Pain may be relieved by analgesics or local injection of lidocaine, however, opiates appear to increase toxicity. Local cryotherapy may reduce swelling and retard the systemic absorption of the toxin. Hot packs produce vasodilatation and may accelerate toxin distribution systemically and are therefore contraindicated. Antivenin is available and is effective if administered soon after the sting. Very young children with systemic symptoms should be treated as medical emergencies. Systemic symptoms and shock should be treated supportively.

Preventive measures include the use of chemical pesticides to reduce scorpion populations. Removal of debris around dwellings can reduce hiding and breeding places.

Mites

Mites are small, eight-legged arthropods characterized by a saclike body and no antennae. A large number of mite species are free-living or are normally associated with other vertebrates (e.g., birds, rodents) and may cause dermatitis in humans on rare occasions. The number of mites that are considered true human parasites or that present real medical problems is small and includes the human itch mite (*Sarcoptes scabiei*), the human follicle mite (*Demodex folliculorum*), and the chigger mite. Mites affect humans in three ways: by causing dermatitis, by serving as vectors of infectious diseases, and by acting as a source of allergens.

Itch Mites

Physiology and Structure. The itch mite (*S. scabiei*) causes an infectious skin disease variably known as scabies, mange, or the itch. The adult mites average 300 to 400 μm in length and have an oval, saclike body in which the first and second pairs of legs are widely separated from the third and fourth pairs (Fig. 80–5). The body has dorsal transverse parallel ridges, spines, and hairs. The ova measure 100 to 150 μm.

Adult mites enter the skin, creating serpiginous burrows in the upper layers of the epidermis. The female mite lays her eggs in the skin burrows, and the larval and nymph stages that develop also burrow in the skin. The female mites live and deposit eggs and feces in epidermal burrows for up to 2 months. Characteristically, the preferred sites of infestation are the interdigital and popliteal folds, the wrist and inguinal regions, and the inframammary folds. The presence of the mites and their secretions causes intense itching of the involved areas. The mite is an obligate parasite and can perpetuate itself in a single host indefinitely.

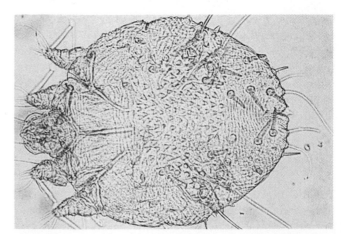

FIGURE 80–5. Scabies mite (*Sarcoptes* species). (From Peters W: *A colour atlas of arthropods in clinical medicine*, London, 1992, Wolfe.)

Epidemiology. Scabies is cosmopolitan in distribution, with an estimated global prevalence of about 300 million cases. The mite is an obligate parasite of domestic animals and humans; however, it may survive for hours to days away from the host, thus facilitating its spread. Transmission is accomplished by direct contact or by contact with contaminated objects such as clothing. Sexual transmission has been well documented. Spread of the infection to other areas of the body is accomplished by scratching and manual transfer of the mite by the affected person. Scabies may occur in epidemic fashion among people in crowded conditions such as daycare centers, nursing homes, military camps, and prisons.

Clinical Diseases. The outstanding clinical diagnostic symptom is intense itching, usually in the interdigital folds and sides of the fingers, buttocks, external genitalia, wrists, and elbows. The uncomplicated lesions appear as short, slightly raised cutaneous burrows. At the end of the burrow frequently is a vesicle containing the female mite. The intense pruritus usually leads to excoriation of the skin secondary to scratching, which in turn produces crusts and secondary bacterial infection. Patients experience their first symptoms within weeks to months after exposure; however, the incubation period may be as little as 1 to 4 days in persons sensitized by prior exposure. Host hypersensitivity (delayed or type IV) probably has an important role in determining the variable clinical manifestations of scabies.

Some immunodeficient people may develop a variant of scabies, so-called Norwegian scabies, characterized by generalized dermatitis with extensive scaling and crusting and the presence of thousands of mites in the epidermis. This disease is highly contagious and suggests that host immunity also plays a part in suppressing *S. scabiei*.

Diagnosis. The clinical diagnosis of scabies is based on the characteristic lesions and their distribution. The definitive diagnosis of scabies depends on demonstration of the mite in skin scrapings. Because the adult mite is most frequently found in the terminal portions of a fresh burrow, it is best to make scrapings in these areas. The scrapings are placed on a clean microscope slide, cleared by the addition of one or two drops of a 20% solution of potassium hydroxide, covered with a coverslip, and examined under a low-power microscope. With experience, the mite and ova may be recognized. Skin biopsy may also reveal the mites and ova in tissue sections.

Treatment, Prevention, and Control. The standard and very effective treatment for scabies is 1% γ-benzene hexachloride (lindane) in a lotion base. One or two applications (head to toe) at weekly intervals is effective against scabies. Lindane is absorbed through the skin, and repeated applications may be toxic. For this reason, it is not advisable to use it in treating infants, small children, or pregnant or lactating women.

A 5% permethrin cream (Elimite) has replaced lindane lotions as the treatment of choice for scabies. Clinical trials have shown permethrin to be more effective and less toxic than lindane. Other preparations used to treat scabies include crotamiton, sulfur (6%) preparations, benzyl benzoate, and tetraethylthiuram monosulfide. The last two preparations are not available in the United States.

Primary prevention of scabies is best achieved with correct hygiene habits, personal cleanliness, and routine washing of clothing and bed linens. Secondary prevention includes identification and treatment of infected people and possibly their household and sexual contacts. In an epidemic situation, simultaneous treatment of all affected people and their contacts may be necessary. This is followed by thorough cleansing of the environment (e.g., boiling clothing and linens) and ongoing surveillance to prevent recurrence.

Human Follicle Mites

Physiology and Structure. The human follicle mites include two species of the genus *Demodex*, *D. folliculorum* and *D. brevis*. These mites are minute (0.1 to 0.4 mm) organisms with a wormlike body, four pairs of stubby legs, and an annulate abdomen. *D. folliculorum* parasitizes the hair follicles of the face of most adult humans, whereas *D. brevis* is found in the sebaceous glands of the head and trunk.

Epidemiology. Organisms of the *Demodex* genus are obligate parasites of the human integument and are cosmopolitan in their distribution. Infestations are uncommon in young children and increase at the time of puberty. It is estimated that 50% to 100% of adults are infested with these mites.

Clinical Diseases. The role of *Demodex* species in human disease is uncertain. They have been associated with acne, blackheads, blepharitis, abnormalities of the scalp, and truncal rashes. More recently, extensive papular folliculitis resulting from *Demodex* infestation has been described in people with acquired immunodeficiency. Factors such as poor personal hygiene, increased sebum production, mite hypersensitivity, and immunosuppression may increase host susceptibility and enhance the clinical presentation of *Demodex* infestation. Most people infested with these mites remain asymptomatic.

Diagnosis. Mites may be demonstrated microscopically in material expressed from an infested follicle. They may be seen as incidental findings in histologic sections of facial skin.

Treatment. Effective treatment consists of a single application of 1% γ-benzene hexachloride.

Chigger Mites

Physiology and Structure. Chiggers are the larvae of mites of the family Trombiculidae. The adult trombiculid mites infest grass and bushes, and their larvae (i.e., chiggers) attack humans and other vertebrates, producing severe dermatitis. The larvae have three pairs of legs and are covered with characteristic branched, feather-like hairs.

The larvae appear as minute, barely visible reddish dots attached to the skin, where they use their hooked mouth parts to ingest tissue fluids. Chiggers typically attach to the skin areas where clothing is tight or restricted, such as the wrists, ankles, armpits, groin, and waistline. After feeding, the engorged larvae fall to the ground, where they molt and undergo development into nymphs and adults.

Epidemiology. Chiggers that are important in North America include the larvae of *Eutrombicula alfreddugèsi* and *Eutrombicula splendens.* In Europe, the important species is the harvest mite, *Trombicula autumnalis.* Chiggers are a particular problem for outdoor enthusiasts such as campers and picnickers. In Europe and the Americas, they are associated with intensely pruritic lesions; however, in Asia, Australia, and the western Pacific rim, they serve as vectors of the rickettsial disease scrub typhus or tsutsugamushi fever *(Rickettsia tsutsugamushi)* (see Table 80–2).

Clinical Diseases. Saliva injected into the skin at the time of mite attachment produces intense pruritus and dermatitis. The skin lesions appear as small erythematous marks that progress to papules and may persist for weeks. Mite larvae may be visible in the center of the reddened, swollen area. The irritation may be so severe that it causes fever and disrupts sleep. Secondary bacterial infection of the excoriated lesions may occur.

Treatment, Prevention, and Control. Treatment for dermatitis caused by chiggers is largely symptomatic and consists of antipruritics, antihistamines, and steroids. The use of insect repellents such as *N,N*9-diethyl-m-toluamide (DEET) may be of some help in prevention for persons going into chigger-infested areas.

Ticks

Physiology and Structure. Ticks are bloodsucking ectoparasites of a number of vertebrates, including humans.

Ticks are opportunistic rather than host-specific and tend to suck blood from a number of large and small animals. Ticks have a four-stage life cycle that includes the egg, larva, nymph, and adult. Although the larva, nymph, and adult all are bloodsuckers, it is the adult tick that usually bites humans.

Ticks comprise two large families, the Ixodidae, or hard ticks, and the Argasidae, or soft ticks. Soft ticks have a leathery body that lacks a hard dorsal scutum, and the mouthparts are located ventrally and are not visible from above (Fig. 80–6). Hard ticks have a hard dorsal plate or scutum, and the mouthparts are clearly visible from above (Fig. 80–7). Both hard and soft ticks serve as ectoparasites of humans. Soft ticks differ from hard ticks primarily in their feeding behavior. Soft ticks complete engorgement in a matter of minutes or at most a few hours; hard ticks feed slowly, taking 7 to 9 days to become engorged.

Epidemiology. Ticks are found in wooded and rural areas worldwide. In North America, the important species of hard ticks include *Dermacentor variabilis* (the American dog tick), *Dermacentor andersoni* (the Rocky Mountain wood tick), *Amblyomma americanum* (the Lone Star tick), *Rhipicephalus sanguineus* (the brown dog tick), and *Ixodes dammini* (the deer tick). These ticks are found variably throughout the United States and are important vectors of several infectious diseases, including Rocky Mountain spotted fever *(Dermacentor* species), tularemia *(Dermacentor* species), Q fever *(Dermacentor* species), Lyme disease *(Ixodes* species), babesiosis *(Ixodes* species), and ehrlichiosis *(D. variabilis* and *A. americanum)* (see Table 80–2). Soft ticks of the genus *Ornithodoros* transmit relapsing fever spirochetes

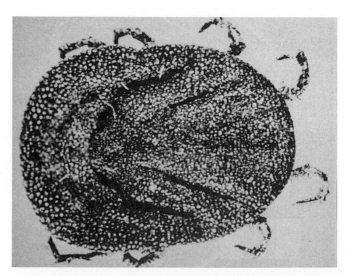

FIGURE 80–6. Soft tick (*Ornithodoros* species). (From Strickland GT: *Hunter's tropical medicine*, ed 7, Philadelphia, 1991, WB Saunders.)

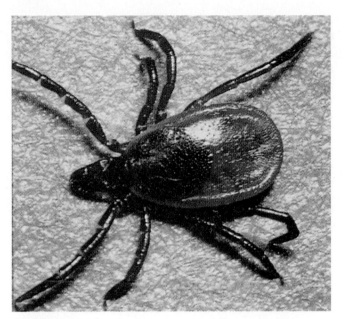

FIGURE 80–7. Hard tick *(Ixodes dammini).* (Courtesy Professor A Spielman; from Peters W: *A colour atlas of arthropods in clinical medicine,* London, 1992, Wolfe.)

(*Borrelia* species) in limited areas in the West (see Table 80–2). In general, people at risk for tick exposure are involved in outdoor activities in wooded areas. Tick exposure may also occur during stays in rural cabins inhabited by small rodents, which commonly serve as hosts for ticks and other ectoparasites.

Clinical Diseases. Tick bites are generally of minor consequence and are limited to small erythematous papules. More serious consequences of tick bite include the development of a type of paralysis resulting from substances released by ticks during feeding, as well as transmission of a number of rickettsial, bacterial, viral, spirochetal, and protozoan diseases of humans and other animals.

Ticks may attach at any point on the body but typically favor the scalp hairline, ears, axillae, and groin. The initial bite is usually painless, and the presence of the tick may not be detected for several hours after contact. After the tick has dropped off or has been removed manually, the area may become reddened, painful, and pruritic. The wound may become secondarily infected and necrotic, particularly if the mouthparts remain attached after manual removal.

Three species of tick, *D. andersoni,* *D. variabilis,* and *A. americanum,* all have been reported to cause tick paralysis. This is characterized by an ascending flaccid paralysis, fever, and general intoxication, which may lead to respiratory compromise and death. The paralysis is due to toxic substances released in the saliva of the tick and may be reversed by tick removal. Tick paralysis is observed more commonly in young chil-

dren and when tick attachment is in opposition to the central nervous system (e.g., scalp, head, neck).

Ticks are also involved in the transmission of infections such as Lyme disease, Rocky Mountain spotted fever, ehrlichiosis, Colorado tick fever, relapsing fever, tularemia, Q fever, and babesiosis (see Table 80–2). The reader is referred to the appropriate sections of this book for discussion of the clinical and microbiologic aspects of these infections.

Diagnosis. The diagnosis of tick bites and tick-borne diseases usually rests on finding a tick or eliciting a history of exposure to tick-infested areas. Identification of an organism as an adult tick is usually straightforward and based on the observations of an organism that is dorsoventrally flattened and possesses four pairs of legs and no visible segmentation (see Figs. 80–6 and 80–7). An entomologist or parasitologist should be consulted if further identification is desired. The diagnosis of specific tick-borne infectious diseases is covered in the respective sections of this book.

Treatment, Prevention, and Control. Early removal of attached ticks is of primary importance and may be accomplished by steady traction on the tick body, grasped with forceps as close to the skin as possible. Care should be taken to avoid twisting or crushing the tick, which may leave the mouthparts attached to the skin or inject potentially infectious material into the wound. Steady traction is superior to noxious stimuli or occlusive techniques for removing ticks. After removal, the wound should be cleansed and observed for secondary infection. Because ticks may harbor highly infectious agents, the clinician should use appropriate infection-control precautions (e.g., use of gloves, hand washing, proper disposal of ticks and contaminated material) during tick removal.

Preventive measures used in tick-infested areas include wearing protective clothing that fits snugly about the ankles, wrists, waist, and neck so that ticks cannot gain access to the skin. Insect repellents such as DEET are generally effective. People and pets should be inspected for ticks after visits to tick-infested areas.

Insecta

The insects, or hexapods, constitute the largest and most important of all the classes of arthropods, accounting for approximately 70% of all known species of animals. Insects include animals such as mosquitoes, flies, fleas, lice, roaches, bees, wasps, beetles, and moths, to name just a few. The insect body is divided into three parts—head, thorax, and abdomen—and is equipped with one pair of antennae, three pairs of appendages, and one or two pairs of wings or no wings at all. The medical significance of any insect is related to its way of life, particularly its mouthparts and feeding habits. Insects may serve as vectors for a number of bacterial, viral, protozoan, and metazoan pathogens. Certain insects may serve merely as mechanical vectors for the transmission of pathogens, whereas in other insects the pathogens undergo multiplication or cyclic development within the insect host. The methods by which the insects transmit pathogens vary and are discussed here. Insects can also be pathogens themselves by causing mechanical injury through bites, chemical injury through the injection of toxins, and allergic reactions to materials transmitted by bites or stings. There are more than 30 orders of insects, but only those of major medical importance are discussed in this section.

Bloodsucking Diptera

Diptera is the large order of flying insects. All dipterans have a single pair of functional membranous wings and various modifications of the mouthparts, which have been adapted for piercing the skin and sucking blood or tissue juices. Their most important feature is their role as mechanical or biologic vectors of a number of infectious diseases, including leishmaniasis, trypanosomiasis, malaria, filariasis, onchocerciasis, tularemia, bartonellosis, and the viral encephalitides (see Table 80–2). The bloodsucking flies include mosquitoes, sandflies, and black flies, all of which are capable of transmitting diseases to humans. Other dipterans such as horseflies and stable flies are capable of inflicting painful bites but are not known to transmit human pathogens. Although the common housefly does not bite, it certainly is capable of mechanical transmission of a number of viral, bacterial, and protozoan infections to human hosts. The infectious diseases transmitted by bloodsucking flies are well covered in other chapters of this book. The following section deals only with injury resulting from the bite of these insects and the effects of salivary substances introduced into the human skin and tissues.

Mosquitoes

Physiology and Structure. Adult mosquitoes are small and have delicate legs, one pair of wings, long antennae, and greatly elongated mouthparts adapted for piercing and sucking. The two major families of mosquitoes (Culicidae), the Anophelinae and the Culicinae, share a number of similarities in their life cycles and development. They lay eggs on or near water, are good fliers, and feed on nectar and sugars. The females of most species also feed on blood, which they require for each clutch of 100 to 200 eggs. Females may take a blood meal every 2 to 4 days. In the act of feeding, the female mosquito injects saliva, which produces me-

chanical damage to the host and may transmit disease and produce immediate and delayed immune reactions.

Epidemiology. Within the family Anophelinae, the genus *Anopheles* contains the species responsible for the transmission of human malaria. In the tropics, these mosquitoes breed continually in relation to rainfall. These species vary in their capacity for the transmission of malaria, and within each geographic area the number of species that serves as malaria vectors is small. *Anopheles gambiae* is an important vector of malaria in sub-Saharan Africa.

Mosquitoes of the genus *Aedes*, the largest genus of the subfamily Culicinae, are found in all habitats ranging from the tropics to the Arctic. *Aedes* may develop overwhelming populations in marsh or tundra and pasture or floodwater and may have a severe impact on wildlife, livestock, and humans. *Aedes aegypti*, the yellow fever mosquito, usually breeds in man-made containers (flower pots, gutters, cans) and is the primary vector of yellow fever and dengue in urban environments throughout the world.

Clinical Diseases. Mechanical damage induced by the feeding mosquito is usually minor but may be accompanied by mild pain and irritation. The bite is usually followed within a few minutes by a small, flat wheal surrounded by a red flare. The delayed reaction consists of itching, swelling, and reddening of the wound region. Secondary infection may follow as a result of scratching.

Treatment, Prevention, and Control. Medical attention is usually not sought for a bite unless secondary infection occurs. Local anesthetics or antihistamines may be useful in treating reactions to mosquito bites.

Preventive measures in mosquito-infested areas include the use of window screens, netting, and protective clothing. Insect repellents such as DEET are generally effective. Mosquito-control measures that involve the use of insecticides have been effective in some areas.

Gnats and Biting Midges

Physiology and Structure. Ceratopogonids represent an assortment of tiny flies with names such as gnats, midges, and punkies. Most of the flies that attack humans belong to the genus *Culicoides;* they are minute (0.5 to 4 mm long) and slender enough to pass through the fine mesh of ordinary window screens. The females suck blood and typically feed at dusk, when they may attack in large numbers.

Epidemiology. Biting midges may be important pests in beach and resort areas near salt marshes. Those of the genus *Culicoides* are the main vectors of filariasis in Africa and the New World tropics.

Clinical Diseases. The mouthparts of biting midges are lancet-like and produce a painful bite. Bites may produce local lesions lasting hours or days.

Treatment, Prevention, and Control. Local treatment is palliative with lotions, anesthetics, and antiseptic measures. The treatment of breeding sites with pesticides and repellents may be useful against some of the common species of these pests.

Sandflies

Physiology and Structure. Sandflies, or moth flies, belong to a single subfamily of the Psychodidae, the Phlebotominae. They are small (1 to 3 mm), delicate, hairy, weakly flying insects that suck the blood of humans, dogs, and rodents. They transmit a number of infections, including leishmaniasis (see Table 80–2). Female flies become infected when they feed on infected people.

Epidemiology. Phlebotomine larvae develop in non-aquatic habitats such as moist soil, stone walls, and rubbish heaps. In many areas, sandflies cause problems as pests. They also serve as vectors of infectious diseases such as leishmaniasis in the Mediterranean, the Middle East, Asia, India, and Latin America.

Clinical Diseases. The bite may be painful and pruritic around the local lesion. Sensitized people may have allergic reactions. Sandfly fever is characterized by severe frontal headaches, malaise, retro-orbital pain, anorexia, and nausea.

Treatment, Prevention, and Control. Sandflies are sensitive to insecticides, which should be applied to breeding sites and window screens. Various insect repellents may also be useful.

Black Flies

Physiology and Structure. Members of the family Simuliidae are commonly called black flies or buffalo gnats. They are 1 to 5 mm long, are hump-backed, and have mouthparts consisting of six "blades" that are capable of tearing skin (Fig. 80–8). Black flies are bloodsucking insects and breed in fast-flowing streams and rivers. They are of major importance as vectors of onchocerciasis (see Table 80–2).

Epidemiology. Black flies are common in Africa and South America, where they serve as vectors of onchocerciasis. In North America they are common around the lake regions of Canada and the northern United

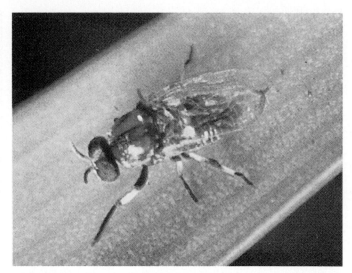

FIGURE 80–8. Black fly (*Simulium* species), the vector of onchocerciasis. (Courtesy Dr S Meredith; from Peters W: *A colour atlas of arthropods in clinical medicine*, London, 1992, Wolfe.)

States. They are pests to hunters and fisherman in these areas. In large numbers they may cause significant blood loss and pose a major threat to wild and domestic animals.

Clinical Diseases. Various responses have been observed in humans after the bite of black flies. The bite of the female can tear the skin surface and induce bleeding that continues for some time after the fly has departed. A distinct hemorrhagic spot usually develops at the site of the bite. Multiple bites may result in considerable blood loss. The bite is painful and is accompanied by local inflammation, itching, and swelling.

The local reaction may also be accompanied by a systemic response that varies according to the number of bites and the sensitivity of the person. This syndrome is known as black fly fever and is marked by headache, fever, and adenitis. It usually subsides within 48 hours and is considered a hypersensitivity reaction to the salivary secretions of the fly.

In addition to local and systemic responses to black fly bites, a hemorrhagic syndrome has been described after bites of black flies in certain areas of Brazil. This syndrome resembles thrombocytopenic purpura and is characterized by local and disseminated cutaneous hemorrhages associated with mucosal bleeding. It is thought that this hemorrhagic syndrome may be produced by a hypersensitivity phenomenon or response to a toxin following numerous black fly bites.

Diagnosis. The black fly bite is marked characteristically by a point of dried blood and subcutaneous hemorrhage at the wound site. In people with the hemorrhagic syndrome, platelet counts are reduced; prolonged bleeding time and poor clot retraction are noted in about half of patients.

Treatment, Prevention, and Control. Treatment includes the usual palliative measures (e.g., anesthetics, antihistamines, lotions) to relieve local pruritus and swelling. Patients with the hemorrhagic syndrome have shown marked improvement in response to corticosteroid therapy.

Preventive measures include protective clothing. In general, insect repellents are ineffective against black flies. Some control is achieved by pouring insecticides into rivers and streams.

Horseflies and Deer Flies

The family Tabanidae consists of species that attack mainly animals, including horseflies, deer flies, gadflies, and mango flies. They are large, ranging in length from 7 to 30 mm. The males feed on plant juices, the females on blood. In the act of biting, the female fly leaves a deep wound drawing blood, which the fly laps up. The fly may serve as a mechanical vector of infectious diseases when the fly's mouthparts become contaminated on one host and transfer organisms to the next. These flies are not considered important vectors of infectious disease in humans.

Muscoid Flies

Physiology and Structure. The muscoid flies include the important insects, the housefly, *Musca domestica;* the stable fly, *Stomoxys calcitrans;* and the tsetse flies of the genus *Glossina.* The stable fly, often mistaken for the housefly, is a true bloodsucker capable of serving as a short-term mechanical vector of a number of bacterial, viral, and protozoal infections. The tsetse fly (Fig. 80–9) is also a biting fly and serves as the biologic vector and intermediate host for the agents of African trypanosomiasis, *Trypanosoma brucei rhodesiense* and *Trypanosoma brucei gambiense.* The common housefly represents a host of genera that are nonpiercing or contaminating flies. Because of their living and feeding habits, they mechanically transmit diverse agents to humans.

Epidemiology. The tsetse fly is found in the eastern and central regions of Africa, where it is of major medical and veterinary importance as the intermediate host and biologic vector of a number of trypanosomes that infect humans and animals. The housefly and stable fly are cosmopolitan in distribution and serve as indicators of poor sanitation. The housefly, *M. domestica,* lays eggs on any matter that will serve as food for developing fly larvae, or maggots (feces, garbage, decaying plant matter). Stable flies commonly lay eggs in

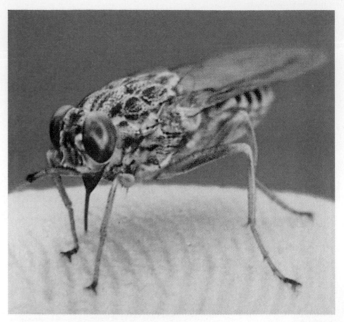

FIGURE 80–9. Tsetse fly, the vector of African trypanosomiasis. (Courtesy Wellcome Foundation, Ltd, Berkhamsted; from Peters W: *A colour atlas of arthropods in clinical medicine,* London, 1992, Wolfe.)

moist, decaying vegetable matter such as grass clippings or compost heaps found in suburban communities.

Prevention and Control. Control of tsetse fly populations has been problematic because of their widespread distribution in primarily rural and undeveloped areas. Insect repellents and insecticides may be effective against adult flies. Improved sanitation is important in controlling houseflies. Plant refuse should be protected from rain or destroyed.

Myiasis-Causing Flies

Myiasis is the term applied to the disease produced by maggots that live parasitically in human tissues. Clinically, myiasis may be classified according to the body part involved (e.g., nasal, intestinal, or urinary myiasis). The number of myiasis-producing flies and the diversity in lifestyle requirements are enormous. Only the host relations and sites of predilection of some of the more important species are covered in this section.

Specific myiasis refers to myiasis caused by flies that require a host for larval development. One important example is the human botfly, *Dermatobia hominis,* which is found in the humid regions of Mexico and Central and South America. The adult botfly attaches her eggs to the abdomen of bloodsucking flies or mosquitoes, which in turn distribute the eggs while obtaining a blood meal from an animal or human. The larvae enter the skin through the wound created by the biting insect. The larvae develop over 40 to 50 days, during which time a painful lesion known as a warble appears. When the larvae reach maturity, they leave the host to pupate. The resulting lesion may take weeks to months to heal and may become secondarily infected. If the larva dies before leaving the skin, an abscess forms.

Semispecific myiasis is caused by flies that normally lay their eggs on decaying animal or plant matter but develops in a host if entry is facilitated by the presence of wounds or sores. Representatives of this group include the greenbottle fly, *Phaenicia*; bluebottle flies, *Cochliomyia*; and blackbottle flies, *Phormia*. These flies are worldwide in distribution, and their presence is encouraged by poor sanitation. They occasionally lay their eggs on the open sores or wounds of animals and humans. Another group that causes myiasis in humans is the flesh flies, or sarcophagids. These flies have a worldwide distribution and normally breed in decomposing matter. They may deposit their larvae on foods that, if ingested, may serve as a source of infection.

Flies that produce **accidental myiasis** have no requirement for development in a host. Accidental infection may occur when eggs are deposited on oral or genitourinary openings and the resulting larvae gain entry into the intestinal or genitourinary tract. Flies that may produce accidental myiasis include *M. domestica*, the common housefly.

Sucking Lice

Physiology and Structure. Although several species of lice *(Anoplura)* infest humans as blood-feeding parasites, only the body louse is important in medicine as the vector of the rickettsia of typhus and trench fevers and the vector of the spirochetes of relapsing fever (see Table 80–2). The body louse, *Pediculus humanus*, and the head louse, *Pediculus humanus capitis*, are elongated, wingless, flattened insects with three pairs of legs and mouthpieces adapted for piercing flesh and sucking blood (Fig. 80–10). The pubic or crab louse, *Phthirus pubis*, has a short, crablike abdomen with clawed second and third legs (Fig. 80–11).

Epidemiology. Epidemics of head lice are reported frequently in the United States, particularly among school children. The head lice inhabit the hairs of the head and are transmitted by physical contact or sharing of hairbrushes or hats. Crab lice survive on blood meals around the hairs of the pubic and perianal areas of the body. They are transmitted frequently from one person to another by sexual contact and contaminated toilet seats or clothing. Body lice are usually found on clothing. Unlike head or crab lice, they move to the body for feeding and return to the clothing after obtaining a blood meal. All of the lice inject salivary fluids into the

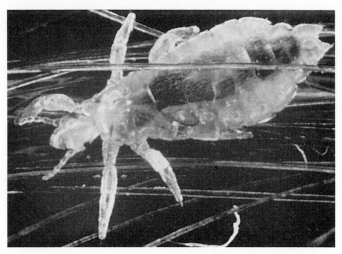

FIGURE 80–10. Body louse *(Pediculus humanus).* (Courtesy Oxford Scientific Films, Ltd [Dr RJ Warren]; from Peters W: *A colour atlas of arthropods in clinical medicine,* London, 1992, Wolfe.)

body during the ingestion of blood, causing various degrees of sensitization in the human host.

Clinical Diseases. Intense itching is the usual characteristic of infestation by lice (pediculosis). Patients may have pruritic red papules around the ears, face, neck,

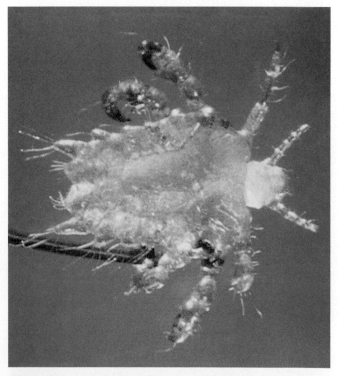

FIGURE 80–11. Crab louse *(Phthirus pubis).* (Courtesy Dr RV Southcott; from Peters W: *A colour atlas of arthropods in clinical medicine,* London, 1992, Wolfe.)

or shoulders. Secondary infection and regional adenopathy may be present.

Diagnosis. The diagnosis is made by demonstration of the lice or eggs from a patient complaining of pruritus. The patient frequently has noticed the insects, and the diagnosis may be made over the telephone. The eggs, or nits, are round white objects that may be found attached to the hair shafts (head and crab lice) or on clothing (body lice).

Treatment, Prevention, and Control. γ-Benzene hexachloride (lindane) lotion applied to the entire body and left on for 24 hours is an effective treatment for lice. Shaving the hair of affected areas is a desirable adjunct. Adult lice in clothing must be destroyed by the application of lindane or DDT powder or by boiling. Lice may survive in the environment for up to 2 weeks; thus, items such as brushes, combs, and bedding must be treated with a pediculicide or by boiling.

The best strategy for primary prevention is education and practice of appropriate hygiene habits. Secondary prevention may be practiced by a policy of routine surveillance (e.g., scalp inspections) in schools, daycare centers, military camps, and other institutions. Repellents may be necessary for people who run a high risk of exposure in crowded conditions.

Fleas

Physiology and Structure. Fleas *(Siphonaptera)* are small, wingless insects with laterally compressed bodies and long legs adapted for jumping (Fig. 80–12). Their mouthparts are adapted for sucking or "siphoning" blood from the host.

Epidemiology. Fleas are cosmopolitan in distribution. Most species are adapted to a particular host; however, they can readily feed on humans, particularly when deprived of their preferred host. Fleas are important as vectors of plague and murine typhus and as intermediate hosts for dog *(Dipylidium caninum)* and rodent *(Hymenolepis* species) tapeworms that occasionally infect humans.

In contrast to most fleas, which do not invade the human integument, the chigoe flea, *Tunga penetrans*, may cause considerable damage by actively invading the skin. The female chigoe flea burrows into the skin, often under the toenails or between the toes, where she sucks blood and lays her eggs. The chigoe flea is found in tropical and subtropical regions of America as well as in Africa and the Far East. It is not known to transmit human pathogens.

Clinical Diseases. As with the bites of other bloodsucking arthropods, flea bites result in pruritic, erythematous lesions of varying severity, which depends on the intensity of the infestation and the sensitivity of the bitten person. The irritation caused by the flea's saliva may produce physical findings that vary from small red welts to a diffuse red rash. Secondary infection may be a complication.

Cutaneous invasion by the chigoe flea produces an erythematous papule that is painful and pruritic. Infested tissue can become severely inflamed and ulcerated. Secondary infection is common. In severe cases, the infestation may be complicated by tetanus or by gas gangrene, requiring amputation.

Diagnosis. The diagnosis of flea infestation is inferred in a patient who has annoying bites and is also a pet (dog or cat) owner. Examination of the patient and pet usually reveals the characteristic insect. Diagnosis of tungiasis is made by detecting the dark portion of the chigoe flea's abdomen as it protrudes from the skin surface in the center of an inflamed lesion.

Treatment, Prevention, and Control. Palliative treatment with antipruritics and antihistamines is indicated for most flea bites. Surgical removal of the chigoe flea is indicated.

Commercially available insecticides may control fleas at the source. Topically applied repellents can protect people against flea bites. Flea collars or powders on pets are also effective preventive measures.

Bugs

Physiology and Structure. Bugs are two specific bloodsucking insects: the bedbug and the triatomid bug

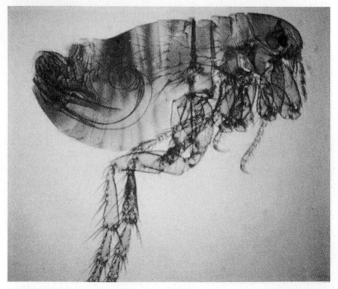

FIGURE 80–12. Flea. (From Peters W: *A colour atlas of arthropods in clinical medicine,* London, 1992, Wolfe.)

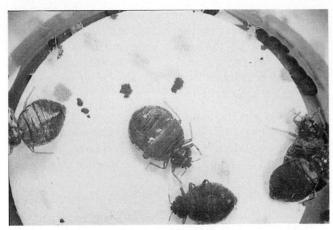

FIGURE 80–13. Bedbug *(Cimex lectularius)*. (From Peters W: *A colour atlas of arthropods in clinical medicine*, London, 1992, Wolfe.)

(Figs. 80–13 and 80–14). Both bugs are characterized by a long proboscis that is folded ventrally under the body when not in use. The bedbug *(Cimex lectularius)* is a reddish brown insect approximately 4 to 5 mm long. It has short wing pads but cannot fly. The triatomid, or "kissing" bug, has yellow or orange markings on the body and an elongated head. Triatomid bugs have wings and are aerial.

Epidemiology. Both bedbugs and triatomid bugs are nocturnal and feed indiscriminately on most mammals. Bedbugs are cosmopolitan in distribution, whereas triatomid bugs are limited to the Americas. Bedbugs hide during the day in cracks and crevices of wooden furniture, under loose wallpaper, in the tufts of mattresses, and in box springs. Triatomid bugs live in the cracks and crevices of walls and in thatched roofs. Bedbugs do

not have a role in the transmission of human disease; however, triatomid bugs are important vectors of Chagas' disease (see Table 80–2 and Chapter 76).

Clinical Diseases. The bites of bedbugs and triatomid bugs produce lesions that range from small red marks to hemorrhagic bullae. Bedbugs tend to bite in linear fashion on the trunk and arms, whereas triatomid bugs bite with higher frequency on the face. The classic periorbital edema secondary to a triatomid bite is known as Romaña's sign. The intensity of reaction to a bite depends on the degree of sensitization of the patient. In addition to causing local lesions, bedbugs may be associated with nervous disorders and sleeplessness in children and adults.

Diagnosis. The pattern and location of bites suggest bedbugs or triatomid bugs. The detection of tiny spots of blood on bedding or the dead insects themselves is frequently the first sign of bedbug infestation.

Treatment, Prevention, and Control. Topical palliatives are appropriate for the relief of pruritus. Antihistamines may be indicated if dermatitis is severe. Control consists of proper hygiene and environmental applications of insecticides.

Stinging Insects

Physiology and Structure. The order Hymenoptera comprises the bees, wasps, hornets, and ants. The modified ovipositor of the female, the apparatus for egg laying, serves as a stinging organ and is used for defense or to capture prey for food. Members of Hymenoptera are known for their complex social systems, castes, and elaborate hive or nest structures.

Epidemiology. Of the hymenopterans, the bees, or Apidae, live in complex social organizations such as hives or in less structured underground nests. Only honeybees and bumblebees are of concern to humans because of their ability to sting. The Vespidae include wasps, hornets, and yellow jackets; all are aggressive insects and a major cause of stings in humans. In the act of stinging, the aroused insects inserts the sheath to open the wound. The thrust of the stylets and injection of venom immediately follow.

One group of ants of concern in the United States is the fire ant, *Solenopsis invicta*. Fire ants are particularly common in the southeastern states. They are well camouflaged in large, hard-crusted mounds and attack when disturbed. They bite their victim with strong mandibles and then sting repeatedly.

Clinical Diseases. An estimated 50 to 100 people die each year in the United States of reactions to stings of

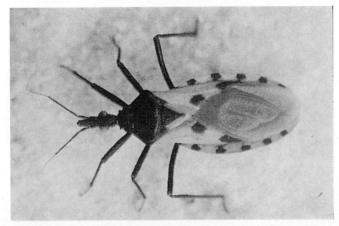

FIGURE 80–14. Triatomid bug. (Courtesy Dr D Minter; from Peters W: *A colour atlas of arthropods in clinical medicine*, London, 1992, Wolfe.)

the hymenopterans. Severe toxic reactions such as fever and muscle cramps can be caused by as few as 10 stings. Allergic reactions are the most serious consequence, but others include pain, edema, pruritus, and a heat sensation at the site of the sting. Anaphylactic shock due to bee stings has resulted in death in some instances.

Treatment, Prevention, and Control. No satisfactory treatment has been discovered for stings. If left in the wound, the sting apparatus should be removed immediately. Injection of epinephrine is sometimes necessary to counteract anaphylaxis. (Emergency kits are available by prescription for sensitive people.) For the relief of local discomfort, calamine lotion or a topical corticosteroid cream for more severe local lesions is helpful.

Although no repellents are effective against these insects, their nests can be destroyed with any of several commercially available insecticidal compounds. General avoidance of areas inhabited by hymenopterans is advised for sensitive people.

CASE STUDY AND QUESTIONS

■ A 4-year-old child was brought in by her mother with a complaint of itchy hands. The child stayed at a daycare center during the day while her mother worked. The girl had intense itching and a rash on her hands and arms for about 2 weeks. The itching became more severe and interfered with the child's sleep. On physical examination, the child appeared well-nourished and cared for. The skin on her hands, wrists, and forearms appeared red and excoriated. Raised, serpiginous tracks were noted on the sides of her fingers, on the ventral aspects of her wrists, and in the popliteal folds. Several of the tracks were inflamed and were beginning to form pustules. The mother stated that several other children at the daycare center were experiencing a similar problem.

1. What was the likely diagnosis?
2. How could this diagnosis have been confirmed?
3. How could this child have been treated, and what advice could have been given to the mother about prevention?
4. Did this child require antibiotic therapy? If so, why?
5. What should have been done about the other children at the daycare center?

BIBLIOGRAPHY

Binford CH, Connor DH: *Pathology of tropical and extraordinary diseases*, vol 3, Washington, DC, 1976, Armed Forces Institute of Pathology.

Fritsche TR: Arthropods of medical importance. In Murray PR et al, editors: *Manual of clinical microbiology*, ed 7, Washington, DC, 1999, American Society for Microbiology.

Markell EK, John DT, Krotoski WA: *Markell and Voges medical parasitology*, ed 8, Philadelphia, 1999, WB Saunders.

Najarian HH: *Textbook of medical parasitology*, Baltimore, 1967, Williams & Wilkins.

Peters W: *A colour atlas of arthropods in clinical medicine*, London, 1992, Wolfe.

Strickland GT: *Hunter's tropical medicine and emerging infectious diseases*, ed 8, Philadelphia, 2000, WB Saunders.

Van Horn KG et al: Copepods associated with a perirectal abscess and copepod pseudo-outbreaks in stools for ova and parasite examinations, *Diagn Microbiol Infect Dis* 15: 561–565, 1992.

Index

Note: Page numbers followed by the letter f refer to figures;
those followed by the letter t refer to tables; and those followed by the letter b indicate boxes.